Cancer Chemotherapy, Immunotherapy and Biotherapy

SIXTH EDITION

Principles and Practice

Cancer Chemotherapy, Immunotherapy and Biotherapy

SIXTH EDITION

Principles and Practice

Bruce A. Chabner, MD
Clinical Director, Emeritus
Massachusetts General Hospital Cancer
 Center
Professor of Medicine
Harvard Medical School
Boston, Massachusetts

Dan L. Longo, MD
Senior Physician
Division of Hematology
Brigham and Women's Hospital
Professor of Medicine
Harvard Medical School
Deputy Editor
New England Journal of Medicine
Boston, Massachusetts

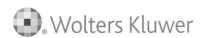

Philadelphia • Baltimore • New York • London
Buenos Aires • Hong Kong • Sydney • Tokyo

Acquisitions Editor: Ryan Shaw
Editorial Coordinator: Tim Rinehart
Marketing Manager: Rachel Mante Leung
Production Project Manager: David Saltzberg
Design Coordinator: Elaine Kasmer
Art Director: Jennifer Clements
Manufacturing Coordinator: Beth Welsh
Prepress Vendor: SPi Global

Sixth Edition

Copyright © 2019 Wolters Kluwer

9 8 7 6 5 4 3 2 1

Printed in China

Library of Congress Cataloging-in-Publication Data
Names: Chabner, Bruce, editor. | Longo, Dan L. (Dan Louis), 1949- editor.
Title: Cancer chemotherapy, immunotherapy, and biotherapy : principles and practice / [edited by] Bruce A. Chabner, Dan L. Longo.
Other titles: Cancer chemotherapy and biotherapy
Description: Sixth edition. | Philadelphia : Wolters Kluwer, [2019] | Preceded by Cancer chemotherapy and biotherapy : principles and practice / editors, Bruce A. Chabner, Dan L. Longo. 5th ed. 2011.
Identifiers: LCCN 2018022251 | ISBN 9781496375148
Subjects: | MESH: Neoplasms—drug therapy | Antineoplastic Agents—therapeutic use | Biological Products—therapeutic use | Neoplasms—therapy
Classification: LCC RC271.C5 | NLM QZ 267 | DDC 616.99/4061—dc23 LC record available at https://lccn.loc.gov/2018022251

LWW.com

Carmen J. Allegra, MD
Professor of Medicine
Chief of Hematology-Oncology
University of Florida School of Medicine
Gainesville, Florida

Lauren Amable, MD
Staff Scientist
Division of Intramural Research
National Institute on Minority Health and Health Disparities
Bethesda, Maryland

Tracy T. Batchelor, MD
Count Giovanni Auletta Armenise Professor of Neurology
Harvard Medical School
Massachusetts General Hospital
Boston, Massachusetts

Susan E. Bates, MD
Professor of Medicine
Department of Medicine, Division of Hematology/Oncology
Columbia University Irving Medical Center
New York, New York

Gideon Blumenthal, MD
Acting Deputy Director
Office of Hematology Oncology Products
U.S. Food and Drug Administration
Silver Spring, Maryland

Andrew M. Brunner, MD
Instructor in Medicine
Harvard Medical School
Massachusetts General Hospital
Boston, Massachusetts

Bruce A. Chabner, MD
Director of Clinical Research
Massachusetts General Hospital Cancer Center
Professor of Medicine
Harvard Medical School
Boston, Massachusetts

Cindy H. Chau, PharmD, PhD
Scientist
Genitourinary Malignancies Branch
Center for Cancer Research
National Cancer Institute
National Institutes of Health
Bethesda, Maryland

Jerry M. Collins, PhD
Associate Director
Developmental Therapeutics Program
National Cancer Institute
Bethesda, Maryland

Katherine D. Cummins, MD, FRACP, FRCPA
Post-doctoral Research Fellow
Center for Cellular Immunotherapies
The University of Pennsylvania
Philadelphia, Pennsylvania

Ibiayi Dagogo-Jack, MD
Center for Thoracic Cancers
Massachusetts General Hospital
Instructor in Medicine
Harvard Medical School
Boston, Massachusetts

Robert B. Diasio, MD
Director
Mayo Clinic Cancer Center
Professor of Molecular Pharmacology and Experimental
    Therapeutics and Oncology
Rochester, Minnesota

Jean Grem, MD
Professor, Internal Medicine
Division of Oncology and Hematology
University of Nebraska Medical Center
Omaha, Nebraska

William D. Figg, PharmD, MBA
Senior Investigator
Clinical Pharmacology Program and Molecular Pharmacology
    Section
Center for Cancer Research
National Cancer Institute
National Institutes of Health
Bethesda, Maryland

Keith T. Flaherty, MD
Director, Termeer Center for Targeted Therapy
Director, Clinical Research; Professor of Medicine
Department of Medicine
Massachusetts General Hospital Cancer Center
Harvard Medical School
Boston, Massachusetts

Justin F. Gainor, MD
Center for Thoracic Cancers
Massachusetts General Hospital
Assistant Professor of Medicine
Harvard Medical School
Boston, Massachusetts

Stanton L. Gerson, MD
Director, Case Comprehensive Cancer Center
Case Western Reserve University School of Medicine
National Center for Regenerative Medicine, CWRU, UH, CC
President, Association of American Cancer Institutes
Cleveland, Ohio

William J. Gradishar, MD, FASCO, FACP
Professor of Medicine
Northwestern University-Feinberg School of Medicine
Lurie Cancer Center
Chicago, Illinois

Kenneth R. Hande, MD
Professor Medicine
Vanderbilt University School of Medicine
Vanderbilt-Ingram Cancer Center
Nashville, Tennessee

Gabriela Hobbs, MD
Clinical Director, Leukemia Service
Instructor of Medicine
Department of Medicine
Massachusetts General Hospital
Harvard Medical School
Boston, Massachusetts

Harper G. Hubbeling, MD
Medical Student
Harvard Medical School
Boston, Massachusetts

Douglas B. Johnson, MD, MSCI
Assistant Professor of Medicine
Department of Medicine
Vanderbilt University Medical Center
Nashville, Tennessee

Carl H. June, MD
Richard W. Vague Professor in Immunotherapy
Department of Pathology and Laboratory Medicine
Director Center for Cellular Immunotherapies
Director, Parker Institute for Cancer Immunotherapy
Perelman School of Medicine
University of Pennsylvania
Philadelphia, Pennsylvania

James A. Kennedy, MD, PhD
Clinical Fellow
Leukemia/MPN Program
Division of Medical Oncology and Hematology
Princess Margaret Cancer Centre
Toronto, Ontario, Canada

E. Bridget Kim, PharmD, BCPS, BCOP
Clinical Pharmacist
Ambulatory Oncology
Massachusetts General Hospital
Boston, Massachusetts

Henry B. Koon, MD
Associate Professor
Department of Medicine
Case Western Reserve School of Medicine
Cleveland, Ohio

Nicole M. Kuderer, MD
Chief Medical Officer
Advanced Cancer Research Group, LLC
Kirkland, Washington

Jacob Laubach, MD, MPP
Senior Physician
Department of Medical Oncology
Dana Farber Cancer Institute
Boston, Massachusetts

Richard J. Lee, MD, PhD
Assistant Professor of Medicine
Harvard Medical School
Massachusetts General Hospital
Boston, Massachusetts

Jessica J. Lin, MD
Clinical Fellow in Medicine
Dana-Farber/Partners
Boston, Massachusetts

Samantha O. Luk, PharmD, BCOP
Clinical Oncology/Hematology Pharmacist
Department of Pharmacy
Massachusetts General Hospital
Boston, Massachusetts

K. Ina Ly, MD
Fellow in Neuro-Oncology
Department of Neurology, Pappas Center for Neuro-Oncology
Massachusetts General Hospital
Boston, Massachusetts

Gary H. Lyman, MD, MPH, FRCP(Edin), FASCO
Professor Medicine
Duke University School of Medicine
Durham, North Carolina

David F. McDermott, MD
Director, Biologic Therapy and Cutaneous Oncology Programs
Beth Israel Deaconess Medical Center
Leader, Kidney Cancer Program
Dana-Farber/Harvard Cancer Center
Professor of Medicine
Harvard Medical School
Boston, Massachusetts

Constantine S. Mitsiades, MD, PhD
Assistant Professor of Medicine
Harvard Medical School
Dana Farber Cancer Institute
Boston, Massachusetts

Beverly Moy, MD, MPH
Associate Professor
Department of Medicine
Massachusetts General Hospital
Boston, Massachusetts

Maciej M. Mrugala, MD, PhD, MPH
Associate Professor, Director Comprehensive Multidisciplinary
    Neuro-Oncology Program
Department of Neurology, Neurosurgery and Medical
    Oncology
Mayo Clinic
Phoenix, Arizona

Christopher S. Nabel, MD
Fellow in Hematology-Oncology
Dana Farber Partners Cancer Care
Boston, Massachusetts

Rudolph M. Navari, MD, PhD, FACP
Professor of Medicine
Division of Hematology Oncology
University of Alabama at Birmingham School of Medicine
Senior Scientist, Experimental Therapeutics Program
University of Alabama at Birmingham Comprehensive Cancer
    Center
Birmingham, Alabama

Steven M. Offer, PhD
Assistant Professor of Pharmacology
Mayo Clinic College of Medicine
Rochester, Minnesota

Adam C. Palmer, PhD
Research Fellow
Program in Therapeutic Science
Harvard Medical School
Boston, Massachusetts

Yves Pommier, MD, PhD
Chief, Developmental Therapeutics Branch and Laboratory
    of Molecular Pharmacology
Center for Cancer Research
National Cancer Institute
National Institutes of Health
Bethesda, Maryland

Noopur Raje, MD
Director, Center for Multiple Myeloma
Department of Hematology/Oncology
Massachusetts General Hospital Cancer Center
Boston, Massachusetts

Ramya Ramaswami, MBBS, MRCP(UK), MPH
Assistant Research Physician
HIV/AIDS Malignancy Branch
Center for Cancer Research
National Cancer Institute
National Institutes of Health
Bethesda, Maryland

Eddie Reed, MD[†]
Professor
Mitchell Cancer Institute
University of South Alabama
Clinical Director
Mitchell Cancer Institute
University of South Alabama Hospitals
Mobile, Alabama

Rachel P. G. Rosovsky, MD, MPH
Assistant Professor of Medicine
Harvard Medical School
Department of Hematology/Oncology
Massachusetts General Hospital
Boston, Massachusetts

Antonia Rotolo, MD
Clinical Research Fellow
Department of Medicine
Imperial College London, Hammersmith Hospital
London, United Kingdom

Marco Ruella, MD
Assistant Professor of Medicine
Hematology and Oncology Division
Department of Medicine and Center for Cellular
    Immunotherapies
University of Pennsylvania
Philadelphia, Pennsylvania

David P. Ryan, MD
Professor of Medicine
Harvard Medical School
Chief of Hematology-Oncology
Massachusetts General Hospital
Boston, Massachusetts

Ami N. Shah, MD
Assistant Professor of Medicine
Division of Hematology and Oncology
Department of Medicine
Robert H. Lurie Comprehensive Cancer Center
Northwestern University Feinberg School of Medicine
Chicago, Illinois

Geoffrey I. Shapiro, MD, PhD
Director, Early Drug Development Center
Department of Medical Oncology
Dana-Farber Cancer Institute
Professor of Medicine
Harvard Medical School
Boston, Massachusetts

[†]Deceased.

Alice T. Shaw, MD, PhD
Director, Center for Thoracic Cancers
Massachusetts General Hospital
Professor of Medicine
Harvard Medical School
Boston, Massachusetts

Laura Spring, MD
Instructor
Department of Medicine
Massachusetts General Hospital
Boston, Massachusetts

Jeffrey G. Supko, PhD
Associate Professor of Medicine
Harvard Medical School
Massachusetts General Hospital
Boston, Massachusetts

Ira Surolia, MD, MPH
Instructor in Medicine
Division of Hematology–Oncology
Department of Medicine
Columbia University Vagelos College of Physicians and Surgeons
New York, New York

Anish Thomas, MBBS, MD
Investigator, NIH Lasker Clinical Research Scholar
Developmental Therapeutics Branch
Center for Cancer Research
National Cancer Institute
National Institutes of Health
Bethesda, Maryland

Lachelle D. Weeks, MD, PhD
Clinical Fellow in Hematology and Oncology
Dana Farber Cancer Institute
Harvard Medical School
Boston, Massachusetts

David C. Yao, MD, PhD
Medical Oncology Fellow
Department of Hematology/Oncology
University Hospitals Cleveland Medical Center
Cleveland, Ohio

Andrew J. Yee, MD
Instructor of Medicine
Harvard Medical School
Center for Multiple Myeloma
Massachusetts General Hospital Cancer Center
Boston, Massachusetts

All substances are poisonous; there is none that is not a poison. The right dose differentiates a poison from a remedy.

—Paracelsus (1538 AD)

For physicians who care for patients with cancer daily, Paracelsus was clairvoyant. Cancer therapy has developed its set of expectations: seriously toxic measures, often without positive results, but undertaken in the hope of averting a potentially fatal outcome. Stem cell transplantation probably represents the epitome of this state of affairs, but, with the exception of hormonal therapies, most cancer treatments fulfilled this forbidding description. However, remarkable progress in the past few years has significantly broadened the therapeutic landscape and improved the outlook for patients with advanced disease. We particularly take notice of the development of new and less toxic targeted therapies, the use of predictive molecular tests for response to treatment, the potential for long-term benefit for patients with advanced disease who are candidates for immune therapies, and continued progress in supportive and palliative care.

Research in both the public and private sectors has added new tools, both drugs and biological compounds, and new biomarkers and diagnostic tests. There is a growing appreciation that not all tumors with the same histological appearance share a common genetic origin. Genomic testing is allowing physicians to select the right treatment for patients with lung, melanoma, thyroid, breast, and many other tumors, contributing to improved survival in patients with the most common forms of malignancy.

Advances that affect patient survival are clear. Adjuvant therapy reduces recurrence rates in node-positive colon cancer and breast cancer by 40%, and the quality of adjuvant therapy is improving with combinations of drugs and biologicals in the earliest stages of disease. The adjuvant use of immunotherapies is now a reality in melanoma and in lung cancer, and neoadjuvant applications are also burgeoning. While this is clear progress, it remains disappointing that in many instances patients are treated with therapies that produce toxic effects but no antitumor effects. Gene arrays that convey useful prognostic information have become common tools for assessing the need for adjuvant therapy in breast cancer, but at present, we lack biomarkers to guide chemotherapy. A further challenge is the need to identify patients with node-negative breast, colon, lung, bladder, and other cancers who have residual disease after primary surgery. Will circulating tumor DNA or circulating tumor cell assays allow us to identify these high risk patients?

Agents with improved design based on studies of drug resistance to first-line agents are demonstrating better activity in many clinical settings. Third-generation drugs, such as osimertinib and alectinib, that evade resistance mechanisms are improving the treatment of epidermal growth factor receptor (EGFR) or ALK-mutant lung cancers. The principle of expecting improvements in established therapies applies to common agents such as 5-fluorouracil, where alternative fluoropyrimidines (TAS 102, S-1) have achieved success.

The field of antiangiogenic drugs has shown promise for enhancing therapy for solid tumors. Improved small molecules, such as cabozantinib, have yielded significantly better results in clear cell carcinoma of the kidney as compared to earlier antiangiogenic drugs. Significant benefit has accrued from advances in hormonal therapy with receptor degrading molecules and inhibitors of adrenal steroid biosynthesis.

Novel targets of drug action have led to surprising results with novel agents, including the CDK4/6 inhibitors in breast cancer and the PARP inhibitors in breast and ovarian cancer, and the IDH1 and 2 inhibitors in acute leukemia. Discovery of the mechanism of action of the IMiD class of compounds should open new fields of drug development targeting the ubiquitin ligases and associated proteins.

Most impressive has been the rapid evolution of immunotherapies in the past 5 years, as checkpoint antibodies and CAR-T cell therapies enter clinical practice. Much work needs to be done to make these expensive and at times dangerous therapies less toxic and more selective. The challenge of understanding their mechanism of action, developing suitable biomarkers to guide patient selection, and averting serious toxicity remains an unsolved problem, but their benefits cannot be ignored.

This brief but impressive list of advances in the past 5 years indicates not only the quickening pace of new cancer treatments, but the changing nature of the enterprise. The emphasis now is on developing agents that block key targets in tumor growth, with limited effects on normal tissues. Integration of these new therapies with traditional chemotherapy and with other targeted drugs will require well-planned, biomarker-driven trials. The task ahead of us is daunting. With each new agent acting by a distinct mechanism, the number of potential combinations of agents increases factorially.

In planning the new edition of this book, we have sought to provide the wisdom of experts. The facts contained herein can form a framework from which clinical decisions can be made. However, the facts are not a substitute for excellent clinical judgment. While adherence to protocols is critical, the practice of oncology cannot appropriately be reduced to recipes and algorithms that are universally applicable to every patient. Each physician must develop a sense of what the agents can and cannot do and apply that knowledge to the individual patient, who becomes the host for these foreign molecules. We hope the information in this book can be a useful guide in the development of clinical skills that subsequent experience will embellish and refine.

ACKNOWLEDGMENTS

The sixth edition of *Cancer Chemotherapy, Immunotherapy, and Biotherapy: Principles and Practice* was a labor of love. The last five editions were published by Lippincott Williams & Wilkins, which was acquired by Wolters Kluwer. We were guided by Tim Rinehart, Editorial Coordinator at Wolters Kluwer, who was helpful at every turn. The distinguished roster of contributors wrote remarkably up-to-date chapters and were patient with the iterative process of making requested revisions in a timely fashion. Their motivation to educate the reader about the rapidly changing cancer treatment landscape drove the project to fruition. And lastly, our colleagues have been the inspiration for this book, as they show us how to employ these agents in increasingly effective ways.

The editors are also grateful for having been able to watch and contribute to the development of the field of cancer treatment from its earliest days of exploration of single alkylating agent activity, radical surgery, and localized radiation therapy to the amazing expansion in the number of available tools. Radical surgery, the first curative intervention, is largely being replaced by more limited operations often performed robotically. Technology has continuously improved the capacity to deliver radiation to various tumors with increasing focus and specificity. The improvements in surgery and radiation therapy have led to a closer interdigitation of these treatments with chemotherapy and biological therapies in earlier phases of disease, making a knowledge of pharmacology of even greater importance to multidisciplinary care. The burgeoning of effective drug classes aiming at an increasing number of targets has steadily improved response rates and survival and, somewhat paradoxically, has complicated the process of developmental therapeutics given that we are still quite naive about how to combine agents that interfere with distinct (or even overlapping) targets to achieve optimal anticancer effects at acceptable levels of toxicity. The field of immunotherapy is also beginning to deliver on its enormous promise after years of modest results. We experienced the disappointment when the much-hyped interferon was introduced to enormous fanfare but produced only modest successes in a few rare tumor types and settings at a cost of often intolerable toxicity. However, persistence and accumulating new knowledge is paying off as immune interventions are now achieving long-term disease control in advanced solid tumors that were formerly universally fatal. Antibodies, naked and armed with drugs and radionuclides, cytokines, and adoptive cellular therapies are now essential tools for physicians treating patients with cancer. And the advances are not only helping cancer patients. Therapies such as rituximab and technologies such as bone marrow transplantation, initially developed for cancer, are improving the lives of patients with nonmalignant autoimmune or inherited diseases.

We have moved from the initial successes of single agent (choriocarcinoma) and combination chemotherapy (lymphoma, adjuvant therapy) and are now seeing the emerging successes of myriad novel rational interventions. It is extremely gratifying to have witnessed the change from the revolutionary findings of first our mentors, then our colleagues, and now our mentees. We dedicate this book to all of them in the hope that something between these covers stimulates a thought that leads to something new.

CONTENTS

Section I

Basic Principles of Cancer Treatment

Clinical Strategies for Cancer Treatment: The Role of Drugs

Bruce A. Chabner and Adam C. Palmer

Cancer treatment requires the cooperative efforts of multiple medical specialties. Although surgeons are often the first specialists to treat the cancer patient, the radiation oncologist and medical oncologist have become increasingly important in the initial management of cancer patients, and responsibility for care of patients with metastatic cancer is usually in their hands. The array of alternatives for the treatment of cancer is constantly expanding. As new drugs and new biologics demonstrate effectiveness in advanced disease, and with the evolution of strategies for integrated multimodality treatment, the development of an initial plan of treatment requires the combined input of specialists from pertinent disciplines. The plan must be based on a thorough understanding of the potential benefit and likely acute and delayed toxicities of each component of the treatment regimen, as well as their possible positive and negative interactions.

As a general rule, the medical oncologist is urged to use standard regimens as described in the *Physician Data Query (PDQ)* system of the National Cancer Institute (NCI) (https://www.cancer.gov/publications/pdq). *PDQ* contains information on state-of-the-art treatments for each pathologic type of cancer, as well as a listing of experimental protocols for each disease. A separate list of recommended therapies for different stages and presentations of cancer is offered by the expert panels of the National Cancer Center Network (https://www.nccn.org/professionals/physician_gls/f_guidelines.asp). An important alternative to "standard" therapy is the clinical trial, which should be considered for every eligible patient. Such trials are listed in cancer center and cooperative group websites, and on" Clinical Trials.gov". Trials offer new and potentially more effective treatments for specific subsets of cancer. While response rates have historically been less than 5% in phase I trials of chemotherapy drugs, much higher response and disease control rates have been achieved in genomically selected subsets of lung and other cancers in trials of molecularly targeted drugs, leading to drug approval even after phase I.[1] With either choice, standard therapy or a clinical trial, the medical oncologist and the patient must understand the potential benefits and risks of new and established drugs or combinations of drugs, often integrated with surgery and irradiation. Steps in the decision-making process are discussed to provide the reader with an understanding of strategies for drug treatment of cancer.

Determinants of Treatment Planning

The first and primary determinant of treatment is the histologic diagnosis. Malignant neoplasms occur in many different pathologic forms, each with a characteristic natural history, pattern of progression, and responsiveness to treatment. Thus, the *histologic diagnosis*, usually made by biopsy or excision of a primary tumor, is of critical importance as a first step in treatment planning. The clinical oncologist must be alert to the possibility of atypical presentations of treatable and even curable tumors, such as germ cell tumors of the testis, lymphomas, and breast cancer, and must ask for special immunohistologic or molecular tests to rule in or rule out a potentially curable tumor type.

In a growing number of cases—for example, lung carcinoma or the non-Hodgkin's lymphomas—accurate pathological and molecular *subtyping* of tumors is important because the subtypes of these diseases have different natural histories and responses to treatment. Genomic analysis may be necessary for further delineation and more effective therapy of subsets of the lung, colon, melanoma, gastric, and esophageal cancer but may be complicated by the intratumoral heterogeneity of molecular subclones.[2] Mutant forms of the epidermal growth factor receptor (EGFR), ALK, and ROS-1 identify unique subgroup of patients with non–small cell lung cancer highly responsive to targeted drugs, while the absence of *KRAS* mutation in colorectal cancers implies a reasonable chance of response to the anti-EGFR receptor antibodies, cetuximab, and panitumumab.[3] In breast cancer, the status of estrogen or progesterone receptors and amplification of the *HER-2* oncogene guide the decision to use hormonal therapy or adjuvant chemotherapy, with an anti-Her2 antibody, and influence the selection of specific drugs or regimens. Predictors for response and benefit for checkpoint inhibitors include microsatellite instability in colorectal cancer and other microsatellite unstable tumors,[4] and the status of beta-2-microglubulin expression, and PDL-1 expression in non–small cell lung cancer.[5] These and other molecular and immunohistochemical tests are indispensable in making appropriate therapeutic decisions. Molecular profiling of tumors will contribute more significantly in the future, as targeted molecules gain a greater foothold in cancer treatment.

Staging

Following the precise workup of pathological samples, the next step in treatment planning is to determine the clinical extent of disease and specifically to determine whether the tumor is curable by local treatment or requires systemic treatment. This *staging* process requires radiological studies and biopsies of suspicious lesions. The treatment of Hodgkin's lymphomas, while primarily based upon combination chemotherapy, will require radiation therapy if a large mediastinal mass is present and does not regress completely on PET scanning. Patients with disease confined to a single lymph node site or area (stage I) are curable with a limited number of cycles of reduced intensity chemotherapy, while more advanced stages (II to IV) must be treated with aggressive chemotherapy regimens. Further, in planning treatment for apparently localized breast cancer, the choice of modalities for definitive therapy may vary depending on the size of the primary tumor, the presence of cancer at the margins of resection or the involvement of lymph nodes. Similarly, the need for adjuvant chemotherapy for breast and colorectal cancers and adenocarcinoma of the lung will depend on, among other factors, whether regional lymph nodes are involved with tumor.

For metastatic cancer, the number and locations of metastases may require multiple interventions such as resection of a solitary lung or brain lesion or radiation therapy to a site of potentially dangerous vertebral or hip metastasis, in addition to systemic chemotherapy. Thus, accurate determination of the location and extent of disease is critical to the planning of initial therapy.

Individualizing Treatment Choice

An additional factor, the patient's probable tolerance for the side effects of the various possible treatments, must also be considered. Not all cancer patients are suitable candidates for intensive treatment. Severely debilitated patients and those with underlying comorbid problems—for example, heart disease, renal or hepatic dysfunction, advanced diabetes, neurological impairment, or chronic obstructive pulmonary disease—might well suffer severely disabling or fatal complications from the side effects of a potentially curative regimen. Common drugs such as cisplatin, doxorubicin, and methotrexate can have devastating side effects if used in the wrong patient. The physician may have to reduce doses in cases of organ dysfunction or choose a less toxic, palliative regimen. The ultimate decision to use drugs must be based on a comprehensive understanding of the disease and the patient in question, the *clinical* pharmacology of drugs, and the potential benefits and risks of alternatives, such as radiation therapy, or surgery.

Pharmacogenomic differences are increasingly identified as influencing response and toxicity of cancer drugs. Polymorphisms of genes responsible for inactivating irinotecan (UGT1A1), 6-mercaptopurine (thiopurine methyltransferase, TMPT), and 5-fluorouracil (5-FU; dihydropyrimidine dehydrogenase, DPD) may be responsible for delayed drug clearance, leading to unexpected toxicity (see Chapters 5 and 8). Tests for the inherited gene variants are available through genomics companies or specialized laboratories in cancer centers (Table 1.1).

The design of multidrug treatment regimens is based on a number of considerations. These include (a) responsiveness of the pathologic and molecular type of tumor to specific drugs, (b) the biochemical mechanisms of cytotoxicity of each drug, (c) drug cross-resistance patterns, and (d) potential drug interactions affecting pharmacokinetics, toxicity, or response. The molecular actions and pharmacokinetic features of individual drugs are considered in detail in succeeding chapters, but a brief review of the impact of these factors on trial design at this juncture provides a framework for understanding regimen design.

Finally, in the context of information about tumor histology, stage, and molecular features, and with information about the patient's age and baseline health, the oncologist must decide whether a realistic opportunity exists for cure. A decision to treat with curative intent demands a high degree of adherence to drug dosage and schedule, as specified in the standard or experimental regimen, and a willingness to accept treatment-related toxicity. When cure is not a realistic expectation, treatment decisions are based on an expectation for

TABLE **1.1**	*Pharmacogenomic tests for cancer chemotherapy*		
Genetic Test	**Disease**	**Clinical Impact**	**Commercial Laboratory (Examples)[a]**
Thiopurine methyltransferase[b]	Childhood ALL	Identifies patients at high risk of 6-MP toxicity	ARUP Laboratories (Salt Lake City) (https://www.aruplab.com/oncology/tests) Promethius Laboratories (San Diego); Mayo Clinic (http://mayoresearch.mayo.edu/center-for-individualized-medicine/drug-gene-testing.asp)
UDP glucuronyltransferase 1A1[b]	Colorectal cancer	Identifies patients at high risk of irinotecan toxicity	ARUP Laboratories (https://www.aruplab.com/oncology/tests)
Dihydropyrimidine dehydrogenase[b]	Any 5-FU containing regimen	Identifies patients at high risk for 5-FU toxicity	ARUP Laboratories (Salt Lake City) (https://www.aruplab.com/oncology/tests)

[a]Many cancer centers and hospitals offer an array of diagnostic molecular tests.
[b]Test of host DNA for polymorphism.

prolonging life or improving the quality of life through relief of pain or disability. In patients receiving purely palliative treatment, dosage adjustments or treatment delays help to minimize the impact of myelosuppression or mucositis but at the cost of antitumor efficacy.

The Various Roles of Drug Therapies in Cancer Treatment

Following the diagnostic workup and initial surgical biopsy or excision of tumor, multiple treatment options are available to the team of physicians who treat cancer (Table 1.2).

Among these options, drugs (including chemotherapy, targeted agents, and immunotherapies) may be used with or without irradiation, depending on the tumor presentation, sites of disease, and specific kind of cancer. Although initially developed for treatment of patients with metastatic cancers, drugs are now routinely used before or after the primary surgical excision of tumor. Cytotoxic drugs cure some disseminated cancers and are effective in decreasing tumor

volume, alleviating symptoms, and prolonging life in many forms of metastatic cancer, even those that are not curable. *Adjuvant* therapy regimens are used in patients who have had primary tumors resected and who, although possibly cured by surgery, are at significant risk of recurrence. Adjuvant therapy decreases tumor recurrence rates and prolongs survival in patients with breast cancer, colorectal cancer, non–small cell lung cancer, osteosarcoma, and other tumors. *Neoadjuvant* drug therapy effectively reduces the bulk of locally extensive tumors *prior to* initial surgical resection, allowing less destructive and more effective resection. Neoadjuvant therapy with drugs or hormonal agents is often used with or without irradiation in patients with locally advanced breast cancer; head and neck, bladder, esophageal, prostate, and non–small cell lung cancer; osteosarcoma; and soft tissue sarcomas. This approach potentially preserves the breast and reduces the extent of surgery for the bladder, anus, head and neck, and other sites of cancers. In the treatment of osteogenic sarcoma, the clinical response of the tumor mass to chemotherapy, prior to resection, can serve as an indication of tumor sensitivity to the drugs used and therefore a signal to continue chemotherapy after surgery.

TABLE

1.2   *Options for treating cancer*

Modality	Example Disease	Example Treatment
1. Surgery		
Removal of primary tumor	Breast cancer	Lumpectomy or mastectomy
Reduction of tumor volume	Ovarian cancer	Debulking of intra-abdominal disease
Resection of solitary metastasis	Soft tissue sarcoma with isolated lung metastasis	Resection of lung lesion
Biopsy of metastasis	Non–small cell lung cancer	Provide tissue for molecular analysis
2. Radiation therapy		
Curative therapy for local disease	Hodgkin disease, stage 1	Regional lymph node irradiation
Local control of primary tumor, cure unlikely	Locally advanced cervical cancer	Pelvic irradiation
Combined irradiation and chemotherapy for local control and potential cure	Locally advanced head and neck cancer	Irradiation to tumor and regional lymph nodes, with concurrent cisplatin
Postsurgical treatment to prevent local disease recurrence	Breast cancer with lymph node involvement	Irradiation to chest wall and axillary lymph nodes
Palliative treatment of metastatic lesion to prevent serious complication	Breast cancer	Irradiation to brain, spinal cord, or hip lesion
3. Chemotherapy		
Curative treatment of systemic disease	Hodgkin disease	ABVD chemotherapy
Adjuvant chemotherapy	Breast cancer, hormone and HER-2 receptor negative, stage I–II	Adriamycin, cyclophosphamide, taxane
Palliative treatment of metastatic cancer	Colon cancer, stage IV	FOLFOX chemotherapy
Regional chemotherapy	Meningeal leukemia	Intrathecal methotrexate
4. Targeted molecular therapy		
Treatment of metastatic disease	Non–small cell lung cancer	Erlotinib for EGFR-mutated lung cancer, stage IV
Adjuvant therapy, with chemotherapy	Breast cancer, stage I-II, HER-2 positive	Trastuzumab with paclitaxel
5. Immunotherapy		
Palliative treatment of metastatic disease	Melanoma, stage IV	Anti-PD1 antibody
Adjuvant therapy	Melanoma, stage III	Anti-PD1 antibody

Kinetic Basis of Drug Therapy

The objective of cancer treatment is to reduce the tumor cell population to zero. Chemotherapy experiments with rapidly growing transplanted leukemias in mice established the validity of the *fractional cell kill hypothesis*, as developed by Skipper et al.,[6] which states that a given drug concentration applied for a defined time period will kill a constant fraction of the tumor population, independent of the absolute number of cells. Regrowth of tumor occurs during the drug-free interval between cycles of treatment. Thus, each treatment cycle kills a specific fraction of the remaining cells. Assuming that drug-resistant cells do not outgrow, the results of treatment are a function of (a) the dose of drug administered, (b) the fraction of tumor cells killed with each treatment, and (c) the number and frequency of repetitions of treatment. Based on these cytokinetic considerations, most chemotherapy regimens from the 1950s to 1990s consisted of cycles of intensive therapy repeated as frequently as allowed by the tolerance of dose-limiting tissues, such as bone marrow or gastrointestinal tract. The object of these cycles was to reduce the absolute number of remaining tumor cells to 0 (or <1) through the multiplicative effect of successive fractional cell kills (e.g., given

99% cell kill per cycle, a tumor burden of 10^{11} cells will be reduced to <1 cell with six cycles of treatment: $[10^{11} \text{ cells}] \times [0.01]^6 < 1$).

Regimens of intensive, cyclic chemotherapy, based on the fractional cell kill hypothesis, were successfully implemented to cure human leukemia and lymphoma. These regimens combined multiple active drugs selected for nonoverlapping toxicities, in order to maximize the tolerable combined dose, and therefore the extent of cell kill per cycle. This approach was less successful in treating the more slowly growing and clonally diverse solid tumors in humans. It is now realized that a number of confounding factors alter the fundamental assumption of a constant fractional cell kill per treatment cycle (see Fig. 1.1, The Cell Cycle).

The assumptions that a uniform cell growth rate and uniform drug sensitivity characterized all cells in a given tumor were incorrect. Many solid tumors (such as lung and colon cancers) become clinically apparent at a stage of decelerating growth, when tumor vascularity is not uniform and not adequate to provide oxygen and nutrients to the bulk of the tumor, leading to nonuniformity of growth rate. These large tumors contain a significant fraction of slowly dividing or noncycling cells (termed "G_0 cells") (Fig. 1.1).

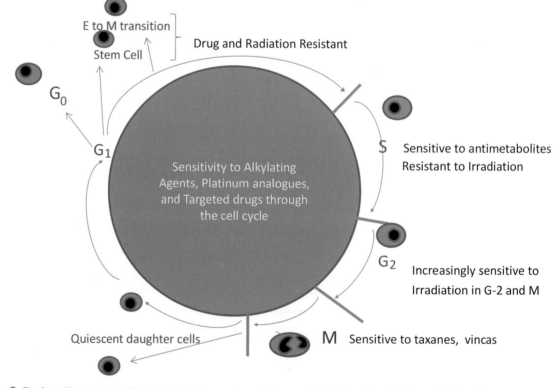

The Cell Cycle: Specific Periods of Drug and Radiation Sensitivity

FIGURE **1.1** The figure illustrates the different phases of the growth cycle of tumor cells. G_1 is the phase of cell growth prior to the DNA replication (S). Cells are most vulnerable to antimetabolites damage during S-phase. Cells enter an interphase (G_2) prior to actual cell division in M, or mitotic, phase. A small subpopulations of nondividing, or slowly dividing cells, may be generated during mitosis (quiescent cells and stem cell like G-0 cells). These cells are less vulnerable to cancer treatment and may re-enter active proliferation, depending on oxygenation, perfusion, or other growth stimuli. The relative sensitivity of common treatment modalities for each of these phases of the cell cycle is indicated. Oncogene regulation, p53 status and responses to DNA damage may also influence drug and radiation sensitivity of normal and malignant cells. (From Comaills V, Kabeche L, Morris R, et al. Genomic instability is induced by persistent proliferation of cells undergoing epithelial-to-mesenchymal transition. *Cell Rep.* 2016;17:2632-2647.)

Since most antineoplastic agents, particularly the antimetabolites and antitumor antibiotics, are most effective against rapidly dividing cells, cell killing will not be uniform throughout the tumor. Some drugs selectively kill cells during specific phases of the cell cycle (S-phase, for cytosine arabinoside, and mitosis, for the vincas and taxanes) and depend on there being a rapid rate of cell division. Others are most active during other brief phases in the cell cycle, as for example, radiation therapy in G-2, the interphase between DNA synthesis and mitosis or the taxanes and vinca alkaloids during mitosis (M phase). The initial kinetic features of cells in a large, poorly vascularized, and slowly growing tumor are unfavorable for treatment with cell-cycle phase-specific drugs.[7] To address this heterogeneity, alkylators and adduct-forming platinum derivatives, which attack DNA in all phases of the cell cycle, are used in combination with antimetabolites such as 5-FU and pemetrexed and antimitotic drugs such as the taxanes. An initial reduction in cell numbers produced by surgery, radiotherapy, or non–cell-cycle-specific drugs may improve blood flow (and drug delivery) and thereby push the slowly dividing cells into a state of more rapid cell division, where they become increasingly susceptible to therapy with cell-cycle-specific agents. Fractional cell kill may actually increase with sequential courses of treatment, as in the treatment of bulky tumors, such as testicular cancers and lymphomas, that are cured by chemotherapy.

Assumptions that a tumor population is biologically uniform are inaccurate.[8] The clonal evolution and molecular diversity of any given population of tumor cells, all derived from a common founder cell, have now been amply demonstrated in human tumors. That diversity encompasses not only the emergence of unique *driver mutations* in subsets of tumor, but a diversity of *mutations that confer drug resistance* may be found in subpopulations in a single site of tumor, and in multiple different metastatic sites. When a diverse population of tumor cells is subjected to the selective pressure of drug treatment, drug-sensitive tumor cells are destroyed, but subpopulations of resistant cells survive and proliferate. With some notable exceptions (treatment of chronic myelogenous leukemia [CML] with imatinib, gestational choriocarcinoma treated with methotrexate, cyclophosphamide treatment for African Burkitt's lymphoma, and cladribine treatment for hairy cell leukemia), single-agent therapy rarely produces long-term remission or cure of advanced malignancies. The diversity of resistance mechanisms and secondary driver mutations has been demonstrated in solid tumors and leukemias following treatment with molecularly targeted agents.[9]

An additional flaw in the kinetic theory, and a reason for failure of cyclic combination chemotherapy, is the existence of stem cell populations within the tumor; these nondividing cells possess a multidrug-resistant and radiation-resistant phenotype and may lie dormant for years.[10] They possess the capacity of unlimited self-renewal when awakened by unknown stimuli. The origin of these stem cells is uncertain. The process of cell division, while assigning equal complements of DNA to each daughter, consistently generates a small population of nondividing or quiescent cells, impervious to treatment, but capable of resuming cell-cycle progression.[11] Thus, the failure of therapy may result from the persistence of quiescent and relatively drug-resistant cells after eradication of the more drug-sensitive and actively dividing bulk of tumor.

Selection of Therapy Based on Molecular Profiling: Precision Medicine

Clinical trials have set the standard for treatment of most types of cancer, but for most metastatic cancers, only a fraction of patients respond to chemotherapy, and those responses are temporary and incomplete. To avoid the needless toxicity of ineffective treatment, especially in diseases with only modest rates of response, it would be desirable to predict sensitivity for the specific tumor and patient at hand. Various systems have been established to predict response to chemotherapy and some even commercialized for testing tumor cells in vitro, but only fragmentary evidence, and no prospective controlled trial data, exists to justify their routine use. However, with the advent of routine genomic profiling of many histological categories of human cancer, treatments are increasingly based on the idea of matching the drug to the tumor genomics in an approach often called Precision Medicine.

The strategy of patient selection based on molecular biomarkers has proven to be a powerful tool in the development of molecularly targeted drugs. These agents are designed to block the biochemical function of driver mutations, to which certain tumors are addicted; inhibiting these drivers lead to cell death. The first successful use of biomarkers to select patients was employed for hormonal therapy in breast cancer treatment (estrogen and progesterone receptor). With the discovery of specific molecular changes (mutations, translocations, amplifications) that drive human cancers, drug development changed course in the late 1990s. The first of many targeted therapies was directed against the bcr-abl tyrosine kinase that underlies CML. Imatinib, an inhibitor of the kinase, introduced in 2001, proved to have striking activity in the chronic phase of CML and has limited toxicity for normal bone marrow cells.[12] Because imatinib also inhibits the c-kit tyrosine kinase, it is effective against gastrointestinal stromal tumors (GIST). Most patients with GIST express a mutated and activated form of the *c-kit* receptor. Pretreatment sequencing of the *C-KIT* gene provides important prognostic information and allows appropriate selection of patients for treatment with imatinib (exon 11 mutations), sunitinib (exon 9 mutations), or other experimental drugs.[13]

The strategy was successful applied to the use of drugs that block the HER-2-amplified kinase in breast cancer, C-KIT in GIST, the tyrosine kinases that drive melanoma, non–small cell lung cancer, and thyroid cancer, and other molecular subsets of cancer (see relevant chapters). Selection of patients for specific targeted therapies, based on molecular biomarkers, has dramatically improved response rates in early drug trials, leading to approvals for marketing after phase II or even after phase I for 10 to 20 new targeted agents yearly in the time period from 2010 to 2017, in contrast to the 1 to 4 new agents approved each year for cancer in the chemotherapy era.

The list of molecularly targeted agents, discussed in various chapters of this book, is constantly growing. Effective agents target the oncoproteins produced by the *EML4-ALK* mutation in non–small cell lung cancer, the *RET* mutation in medullary thyroid cancer, and the polyadenosyl ribose phosphatase (PARP) DNA repair function in breast and ovarian cancer.[14] Monoclonal antibodies (trastuzumab and cetuximab) are proving most effective when used in combination with cytotoxic agents. These results give hope that in the future, cancer treatment will be much more grounded in individualized treatment selection based on tumor genomics.

With rapid approval of new targeted agents, oncologists must undertake genomic profiling for both common and rare tumors and must be able to interpret molecular findings in these reports in their choice of drugs. Genomic profiling is not only useful in choosing the initial therapy. Repeat tumor biopsies at the time of tumor progression or monitoring of circulating tumor DNA in plasma are undertaken for characterization of drug resistance and for choosing the next therapy, as drugs specific for certain resistance mutations (osimertinib for T790M in EGFR-mutated lung cancer, and ponatinib for the highly drug-resistant mutation [T315I] in CML) come into practice. A cogent example of clonal evolution during therapy was provided by studies of prostate cancer, which usually presents as a modestly mutated primary tumor. In contrast, multiple different mutations are found after androgen deprivation therapy in castration-resistant disease, in which a diversity of mechanisms are found, often in a single patient: PTEN loss or activation of AKT (promoting tumor survival), androgen receptor mutations, and receptor splice mutations or amplification, all leading to antiandrogen resistance.[15] Each of these changes would call for a different choice of next therapy (Chapter 28).

It is important to realize the limitations of precision medicine. The drugs are costly, have idiosyncratic and unpredictable toxicities, often inhibit off-target kinases, and as single agents do not address the genomic complexity of many drug-resistant cancers and do not account for the "tissue context" (e.g., BRAF inhibitors in melanoma versus colon cancer) that may determine response versus resistance.[16] Nonetheless, genomic profiling and patient selection are clearly a step forward toward rational cancer therapy.

Pharmacokinetic Determinants of Response

Although the outcome of cancer treatment depends in large part on the inherent sensitivity of the tumor being treated, the chances for success can be compromised by the oncologist's failure to consider important pharmacokinetic factors such as drug absorption, metabolism, elimination, and drug interactions in designing experimental regimens and in clinical practice.

The pharmacokinetics of a given schedule of administration are subject to significant interindividual variability in drug concentration over time (see Chapter 5). The origin of this variability is multifactorial. Pharmacogenetic variants (polymorphisms in expression of drug-metabolizing enzymes and receptors) determine the rate of elimination and thus the toxicity of some drugs, including irinotecan (glucuronyl transferase UGT 1A1), 6-mercaptopurine (thiopurine methyltransferase), and 5-FU (dihydropyrimidine dehydrogenase). In addition, variability in hepatic microsomal isoenzyme activity, serum albumin levels that affect protein binding of drug, and age-related changes in renal tubular function all contribute to variability of drug clearance and drug toxicity in elderly patients. As a result, in a patient population with apparently normal renal and hepatic function, measurement of drug levels in plasma will reveal at least a three- to fourfold variability around the mean drug concentration at any given time point and an equal interindividual variability in drug exposure, expressed as the area under the drug concentration in plasma (times) time curve (AUC) for a given dose of drug.

Pharmacokinetic factors are important not only in general protocol design but also in determining specific modifications of dosage in individual patients. Dosage may be increased or decreased empirically, based on observed patterns of toxicity (neutrophil count following cytotoxic drug, acneform rash after EGFR inhibitor therapy). Drug levels are routinely measured in only a few settings, as for example, to identify patients at high risk of toxicity in high-dose methotrexate and to adjust dosage to achieve optimal blood levels in children receiving methotrexate for acute lymphocytic leukemia (ALL) (see Chapter 7). Response rates improve and episodes of extreme toxicity are unusual when 5-FU drug levels are monitored and doses adjusted to reach prespecified pharmacokinetic end points.[17] However, monitoring of 5-FU drug levels is not accepted as a routine practice.

Most drugs are cleared through hepatic metabolism or renal excretion. Renal or hepatic dysfunction may delay drug elimination and result in overwhelming toxicity (see Chapter 4). To avoid such toxicity, doses of certain agents must be modified based on estimates of renal or hepatic function, as will be discussed in the individual drug chapters.

Rationale for Combination Therapy

Although the first effective drugs for treating cancer were brought to clinical trial in the late 1940s, initial therapeutic results were disappointing. As single agents, methotrexate and nitrogen mustard caused impressive regressions of ALL and adult lymphomas, respectively, but responses were of short duration, and relapse was invariably associated with resistance to further treatment by the same agent. Both historically with cytotoxic chemotherapy, and presently with targeted therapies, with rare exceptions resistance to a given single agent emerges eventually if not quickly, even for the most responsive tumors. In patients with Hodgkin's disease, for example, the complete response rate to alkylating agents or procarbazine does not exceed 20%, and virtually all patients relapse within weeks or months. Studies of imatinib resistance in CML have verified the long-standing hypothesis that untreated tumors harbor spontaneously resistant cells, which are selected and emerge clinically following drug exposure. Additionally, anticancer drugs and radiation therapy increase the rate of mutation to resistance in experimental studies, as does hypoxia.[18] Experiments with human solid tumors suggest that a subset of tumor cells, probably harboring either genetic or epigenetic features that promote survival, may persist after treatment and may spontaneously give rise to drug-resistant clones.[10]

The first motivation proposed for combination therapy was to address the heterogeneity of drug response found within a single tumor (which we call intratumor heterogeneity) and the selection for drug-resistant cells during treatment; application of combination therapy to the cancer problem was inspired by the success of multidrug regimens to cure tuberculosis infections. The use of multiple agents, each with cytotoxic activity in the disease under consideration but with different mechanisms of action, allows independent cell killing by each agent and discourages the outgrowth of malignant clones resistant to any single agent. If the frequency of resistance to one drug is low, and a second drug (or third drug and so on) lacks cross-resistance to the first agent, then the frequency of simultaneous resistance in any single cell to all agents shrinks rapidly with an increasing number of active drugs that lack cross-resistance. The success of this approach was demonstrated by cyclic combination chemotherapy ("total therapy") for ALL of childhood in the early 1960s,[19] which marked a turning point in the effective treatment of neoplastic disease.

The heterogeneity of response to chemotherapeutic agents found among a cohort of patients with tumors of a given histological type (intertumor heterogeneity) is a second motivation for combination therapy, the need for which became evident early in the history of combination therapy.[20,21] The chances of establishing remission for a population of patients harboring genetically diverse tumors, all of the same histological type, meant that increasing the number of agents, each with a different mechanism of action, was required to produce maximal numbers of responses. The benefit achieved can be represented as the sum of independent drug action, in which the remission rate depends on the probabilities that either drug alone induces remission (see Figs. 1.2 and 1.3). Put simply, two chances for remission are superior to one, although this depends on the drugs not sharing cross-resistance. The first cures for ALL demonstrated that combination therapy is an effective approach in addressing both inter- and intratumor heterogeneity, because more patients respond and also their responses are categorically superior. In childhood ALL combining two or three chemotherapies increased the rate of remission (as in Fig. 1.2), combining four or five chemotherapies produced cures in a minority of patients, and combinations of up to eight different drugs made cures commonplace (Fig. 1.4).[20] Variability in drug response across patient populations is a near-ubiquitous feature of cancer treatment, and for this reason, managing intertumor heterogeneity remains a challenge and an important rationale for combination therapy.

The question arises as to whether the benefits of combination therapy reflect actual drug synergy: a greater effect than would be expected from the sum of the independent actions of the drugs rather than simply additive benefit. While synergy may apply in specific regimens, many successful combinations achieve an observed result that equals the expected effect of *independent drug action*; as shown in Figure 1.3, improvements in the average survival of a patient population can be explained without imposing the idea that drug combinations are synergistic in each individual patient.[23] But it is also possible for multiple active drugs to deliver enhanced control of individual tumors. Here the notion of *independent* drug action applies in a different way: if two cancer killing drugs are not cross-resistant, then cells have statistically independent chances of being killed by either drug. Statistically, independent drug action means that the log-kills achieved by each drug in a combination will simply add up: for example, if each of two drugs can alone kill 90% of cancer cells (1 log-kill per drug), their independent combined effect is to kill 99% of cancer cells (2 log-kills). Note that when measuring the fractional killing of cancer cells, *drug independence* therefore has the same meaning as *drug additivity* (this is not generally true in other domains of pharmacology). Synergistic interaction between the effects of multiple drugs can further enhance response to treatment, but it is not necessary to invoke synergy to achieve a clinically beneficial combination therapy.

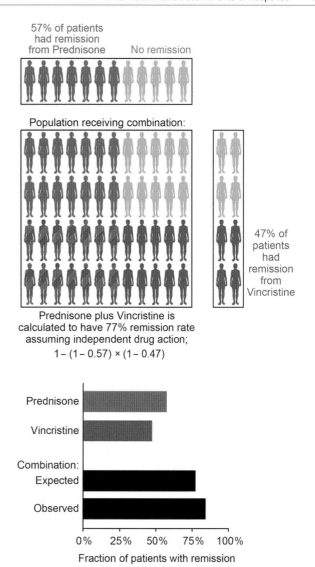

FIGURE **1.2** The benefit of independent drug combinations. In childhood acute lymphocytic leukemia, early trials of single-drug treatments showed that prednisone induces remission in 57% of patients, and vincristine induces remission in 47% of patients. Frei III et al. surmised that if the drugs act independently, then the combination of both drugs should have a remission rate of 77% [1 – (1 – 0.57) × (1 – 0.47)]; this proved similar to the observed rate of 84%. Independent drug action, calculated in this manner, accurately described the superior remission rates of a number of different combination regimens. (From Frei E III. The effectiveness of combinations of antileukemic agents in inducing and maintaining remission in children with acute leukemia. *Blood.* 1965;26:641-656; Palmer AC, Sorger PK. Combination cancer therapy can confer benefit via patient-to-patient variability without drug additivity or synergy. *Cell.* 2017;171:1678-1691.e13.)

As discussed, patterns of cross-resistance must be taken into consideration in formulating drug combinations. Cross-resistance between drugs affects the capacity of drug combinations to manage both intratumor and intertumor heterogeneity. Resistance to many agents may result from unique and specific mutations or amplifications, for example, as may occur in the genes coding for enzymes or receptors inhibited by antimetabolites (such as dihydrofolate reductase or thymidylate synthase) or the mutant tyrosine kinases blocked by molecularly targeted drugs (BCR-ABL, EGFR, EML4-ALK).[24]

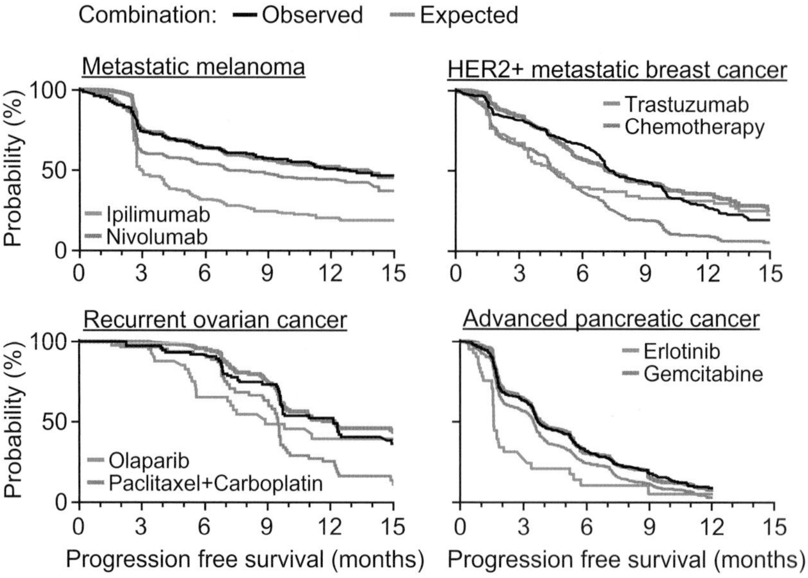

Combination: —Observed   —Expected

Metastatic melanoma

HER2+ metastatic breast cancer
— Trastuzumab
— Chemotherapy

— Ipilimumab
— Nivolumab

Recurrent ovarian cancer

Advanced pancreatic cancer
— Erlotinib
— Gemcitabine

— Olaparib
— Paclitaxel+Carboplatin

Progression free survival (months)   Progression free survival (months)

FIGURE **1.3** Longer progression-free survival from inde-pendent drug combinations. When two or more active drugs are combined, which each individually confer some probability of durable progression-free survival, then their combination may be expected to further increase the probability of progression-free survival, provided that the drugs are not cross-resistant. This demonstrates that drug combinations do not need to act syner-gistically to meaningfully improve patient survival, although if synergy occurs it can further improve benefit. (From Palmer AC, Sorger PK. Combination cancer therapy can confer benefit via patient-to-patient variability without drug additivity or synergy. *Cell.* 2017;171:1678-1691.e13.)

Drug resistance mutations affecting cell survival pathways, such as the bcl-2 or PI-3 Kinase cascades, or multidrug resistance trans-porters may lead to broad cross-resistance (see Table 1.3).

The most thoroughly studied and undoubtedly one of the more important mechanisms of multidrug resistance is increased expres-sion of the *MDR-1* gene[25] and its gene product, the P-glycoprotein (*pgp*). This gene codes for *pgp*, which promotes the efflux of vinca alkaloids, anthracyclines, taxanes, actinomycin D, epipodophyl-lotoxins, other natural products, and even small molecules that target tyrosine kinases. This protein occurs constitutively in many

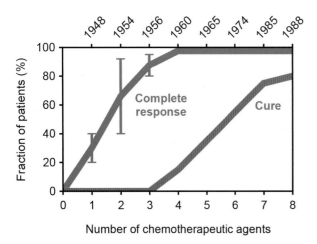

FIGURE **1.4** Combination chemotherapy is essential to curing childhood acute lymphoblastic leukemia. Early combinations of small numbers of chemo-therapeutic agents produced a higher rate of complete remission, and subsequent development of combinations of larger numbers of agents produced cures with increasing frequency. Chemotherapeutics were introduced in the sequence: metho-trexate, 6-mercaptopurine, prednisone, vincristine, intrathecal methotrexate, adri-amycin, asparaginase, ara-C. (From Frei E III. Studies of sequential and combination antimetabolite therapy in acute leukemia: 6-mercaptopurine and methotrexate. *Blood.* 1961;18:431-454; Frei E III. The effectiveness of combinations of antileuke-mic agents in inducing and maintaining remission in children with acute leukemia. *Blood.* 1965;26:641-656; Eder JP, et al. Principles of dose, schedule and combina-tion chemotherapy. In: Hong WK, Holland JR, Frei E III, eds. *Cancer Medicine.* 8th ed. People's Medical Publishing House; 2016.)

normal tissues, including most stem cells, and mature epithelial cells of the kidney, colon, and adrenal gland and has been identified in tumors derived from these tissues. It is prominently expressed in many tumors recurring after chemotherapy, including lympho-mas, myeloid leukemias, multiple myeloma, and other cancers. *Pgp*-mediated resistance, and the associated decrease in intracellu-lar drug levels, can be reversed experimentally by calcium-channel blockers, various steroid hormones, and cyclosporine analogues. Results of clinical trials investigating the use of agents to reverse multidrug resistance have been confounded by pharmacokinetic interactions, increased toxicity, and inconclusive therapeutic results.

A second class of efflux transporters, the multidrug-resistance proteins (MRPs), may also confer complex patterns of cross-resis-tance. In experimental tumors, these efflux pumps promote drug efflux and confer resistance to anthracyclines, etoposide, taxanes, and vinca alkaloids, as well as many of the targeted small molecules. Members of the MRP family may also mediate efflux of methotrex-ate, 6-mercaptopurine, and camptothecin derivatives.[25] The MRP family of genes is widely expressed in epithelial tumors, and their potential for mediating multiagent resistance deserves further study.

Finally, classic alkylating agents (cyclophosphamide, melpha-lan hydrochloride, nitrogen mustard) may share cross-resistance related to enhanced DNA repair or by increased intracellular nucleophilic thiols, such as glutathione. Increased expression of nucleotide excision repair (NER) components correlates with a poor outcome in ovarian cancer (ERCC1) and in bladder cancer (ERCC2) treated with platinum-based regimens.[26] Not all alkylat-ing agents share cross-resistance. As mentioned earlier, resistance to the nitrosourea, procarbazine, dacarbazine, and other methylat-ing alkylators is mediated by increased levels of a different enzyme, methyl guanine methyl transferase, which removes the adduct from purine bases in DNA (Chapter 12).

DNA repair defects may have either synergistic interactions or may confer resistance to therapy. Increased expression of NER components mediates resistance to bischloroethyl alkyl-ators. Alternatively, defective mismatch repair (MMR) is associ-ated with a high number of genomic mutations and *increases the response rate to* checkpoint inhibitors in colon cancer treatment.

Mechanism of Resistance	Drug	Alteration
Decreased drug uptake	Methotrexate sodium	Decreased expression of the folate transporter
Decreased drug activation	Cytosine arabinoside, fludarabine, cladribine	Decreased deoxycytidine kinase
	Methotrexate	Decreased folylpolyglutamyl synthetase
Increased drug target	Methotrexate	Amplified DHFR
	5-Fluorouracil	Amplified TS
Absent or mutated drug target	Etoposide	Altered topo II
	Doxorubicin	
Enhanced DNA repair	Alkylating agents, platinum analogs	Increased nucleotide excision repair
	Nitrosoureas, procarbazine, temozolomide	Increased O^{6M}-alkyl-guanine alkyl transferase
Defective recognition of DNA adducts	Cisplatin, 6-mercaptopurine	Mismatch repair defect
Increased drug efflux	Doxorubicin, etoposide, vinca alkaloids, paclitaxel, topotecan	Increased MDR expression or MDR gene amplification
Defective checkpoint function and apoptosis	Most anticancer drugs	*p53* mutations, bcl2 activation or overexpression
Molecularly Targeted Drugs		
Mutation of target	Most tyrosine kinase inhibitors: for example, EGFR inhibitors	T790M in EGFR
	Imatinib, nilotinib, dasatinib	T315 I in BCR- ABL
Activation of an alternative pathway	EGFR inhibitors	c-MET amplification
	BRAF inhibitors	RAS family mutation
	PIK3CA kinase Inhibitor	Activation of AKT, loss of PTEN
Hormonal Therapies		
Mutation of target	Androgen receptor	Mutation prevents binding of antagonist
	Estrogen receptor	
Amplification of target	Androgen receptor	Increased target prevents shut down of pathway
	Estrogen receptor	
Splice variants	Androgen receptor	Ligand-independent signaling maintains pathway
	Estrogen receptor	
Activation of cell survival pathway	PTEN loss, PI3Kinase mutation	PI3Kinase pathway activation promotes cell survival

DHFR, dihydrofolate reductase; MDR, multidrug resistance; topo II, topoisomerase II; TS, thymidylate synthase; EGFR, epidermal growth factor receptor.

Alternatively, an MMR complex recognizes areas of altered DNA duplex pairing and activates apoptosis and is required for sensitivity to methylating drugs and platinating agents. A single mutation in one component of this system, such as *MSH6*, *confers resistance* to platinating drugs and methylating agents, as well as 6-mercaptopurine.[27]

Multiple different mechanisms of resistance can be detected in tumor cells in a single patient. Inherited polymorphisms may contribute to resistance. Hormonal therapies are affected by mutations that alter splice splicing of the androgen or estrogen receptor, leading to constitutive receptor activation in the absence of ligand; hormonal therapy resistance can also result from receptor amplification or mutation, all of which can be detected in circulating tumor cells or circulating tumor DNA in single patients who display resistance to therapy[26,28] (see Chapters 27 and 28).

The introduction of monoclonal antibodies for cancer treatment has led to the successful use of trastuzumab with taxanes for breast cancer, rituximab with various chemotherapies for lymphoid tumors, bevacizumab with 5-flurouracil and oxaliplatin for colon cancer, and cetuximab (erbitux) with irinotecan for colon cancer (Chapter 29). This success is attributed to several mechanisms: (a) the ability of bevacizumab to normalize blood flow and improve cytotoxic drug delivery to otherwise poorly perfused tumors; (b) the proapoptotic effects of receptor inhibitors such as trastuzumab and cetuximab, which block the antiapoptotic signaling from mutated, overexpressed, or amplified tyrosine kinases; and (c) invocation of immune mechanisms (cell mediated or complement mediated) of cell death by antibodies (Chapter 29). Unfortunately, targeted small molecules have exhibited less synergy than have antibodies in combination with chemotherapy. Small molecular weight inhibitors of EGFR and VEGFR have not enhanced the efficacy of chemotherapy in the lung and breast cancer. The reasons for the greater effectiveness of monoclonal antibodies in combination therapy may relate to their additional ability to mobilize the immune response, such as complement-mediated cytotoxicity or T cell–mediated effects. Trials of checkpoint inhibitor antibodies with chemotherapy are showing promising results for lung cancer and Hodgkin's disease,[29] in spite of the immunosuppressive effects of chemotherapy.

A further step in rational therapy will be the use of multiple targeted agents in rational combinations to block parallel pathways that account for resistance to single agents. Laboratory experiments with human tumor cells in culture suggest that synergistic combinations of targeted drugs can be identified for many lung cancer patients, but limited evidence has been presented for this strategy in improving patient outcomes.[30] To date, the most successful example is the combination of a BRAF inhibitor with a MEK inhibitor for melanoma (see Chapter 22). However, effective implementation of a strategy for combination therapies will depend on accurate genomic profiling of tumor prior to therapy and early introduction of a second agent when genomic evidence of resistance is detected in the bloodstream. Circulating tumor DNA may reveal the necessary information without invasive biopsy.[9] This issue of combining multiple targeted agents is more fully discussed in Chapters 21 and 22.

Schedule Development in Combination Therapy: Kinetic and Toxicity Considerations

The detailed scheduling of drugs in multidrug regimens is based on both practical and theoretical considerations. Intermittent cycles of treatment permit periods of recovery for host bone marrow, gastrointestinal tract, and immune function, with the expectation that recovery of the tumor cell population would be slower than that of the injured normal tissues. A commonly used strategy in designing chemotherapy regimens is to incorporate myelotoxic agents on day 1 of each cycle, while delivering nonmyelosuppressive agents, such as bleomycin, vincristine, prednisone, or high-dose methotrexate with leucovorin rescue, during the period of bone marrow suppression (e.g., on day 8 of a 21-day cycle) to provide continuous inhibition of tumor growth while allowing maximum time for marrow recovery. Effective interdigitation of immunotherapy with cytotoxic or targeted therapies, or with radiation therapy, is still in development. It is unclear whether the suppressive therapies are optimally effective if used prior to, with, or after checkpoint inhibitors. Drugs or radiation have the potential of suppressing the systemic immune response to immunotherapies, and destroying T-cells that are infiltrating a tumor. On the other hand, cytotoxic treatment that releases tumor antigens might enhance immune recognition. Further studies are needed to determine if chemotherapy, targeted drugs, or radiotherapy can be used either concurrently or sequentially with checkpoint therapy without compromising the latter although early studies with combined checkpoint anti-PD1 and chemotherapy show positive results in lung cancer.[31]

Although most of the common anticancer drugs are administered as bolus infusions, continuous infusions provide longer exposure to chemotherapy above the threshold for cytotoxicity and may improve or change the toxicity profile for normal tissues. The R-EPOCH (rituximab, etoposide, prednisone, vincristine, cyclophosphamide, doxorubicin) regimen, in which chemotherapy drugs are given as a 96-hour infusion, has produced impressive rates of response and long-term disease free survival in greater than 90% of AIDS-associated Burkitt's lymphoma and in other high-grade lymphomas. Infusional regimens cause less nausea, vomiting, bone marrow suppression, and cardiotoxicity as compared to bolus regimens (R-CHOP).[32] Extended infusion regimens have improved therapeutic ratios, decreasing bone marrow toxicity and increasing response rates for 5-FU when given as a multiday infusions rather than in a bolus dose.[33] The continuous infusion of a cell-cycle-phase–specific agent such as cytosine arabinoside or 5-FU allows a greater fraction of the tumor cell population to be exposed to drug during the sensitive S-phase of the cell cycle, as compared to the more limited exposure after intermittent bolus therapy. The same prolongation of exposure can be achieved by designing prodrugs that are slowly metabolized to the active parent, as accomplished by capecitabine, an orally administered fluoropyrimidine, or by changing the formulation of the drug, as with liposomal encapsulation of doxorubicin and cytosine arabinoside.[34]

Additional Considerations in Combination Chemotherapy: Taking Advantage of Mutations in DNA Repair and Apoptosis

Mutations in DNA repair pathways predispose to malignancy. These repair processes and the common lesions that impair their function in cancer are shown in Table 1.4.

Drug discovery efforts are aimed at taking advantage of these alterations in repair or apoptosis. For example, double-strand breaks in DNA are repaired through homologous recombination, a process that requires BRCA1 and BRCA2. Alkylating agents, anthracyclines, and platinum analogues cause double-strand DNA breaks and show strong activity against BRCA1- or BRCA2-mutant tumors.[35] BRCA1- and BRCA2-mutant breast cancer and prostate cancer lack the capacity to repair double-strand breaks and therefore depend on the PARP enzyme complex to repair single-stranded breaks. If not repaired, these single-strand breaks become double-strand lesions that lead to apoptosis. An inhibitor of PARP-mediated repair of single-strand breaks has significant activity against BRCA1/2-mutant breast and ovarian cancers[14] and BRCA2-deficient prostate cancer.[36] Since many chemotherapeutic agents produce double-strand breaks (alkylating agents, platinating drugs), combining PARP inhibitors with chemotherapy is a logical approach but has been impaired by bone marrow suppression of combinations of olaparib and cisplatin.

Apoptosis is an active, energy-requiring, and protein synthesis–dependent process whereby cells, in response to specific signals, undergo an orderly, programmed series of intracellular events that lead to death. This process is a necessary component of normal development in all multicellular organisms and is required to control the cell population of many normal proliferating or renewable tissues such as the lymphatic and hematopoietic systems. Suppression of apoptosis, as for example, through loss or mutation of p53, is a common feature of neoplastic transformation.[37] It may be the direct result of mutation or overexpression of antiapoptotic genes such as BCL-2 as in lymphomas, or indirectly, through activation of growth factor pathways such as the PI-3 kinase and epidermal growth factor

TABLE

1.4   *DNA repair processes and role in drug sensitivity or resistance (see applicable chapter for reference)*

Repair Process	DNA Lesion Repaired	Example of Drug Sensitivity or Resistance
Polyadenosyl ribose polymerase (PARP)	Signals need for excision and repair of damaged DNA Base	Olaparib inhibits PARP, causes regression of BRCA1- or BRCA2-deficient tumor
Nucleotide excision repair	Excision of alkylated or platinated DNA	Overexpression of ERCC2 in bladder cancer leads to resistance to cisplatin
Homologous recombination	Repair of cross-linked DNA	BRCA1- or BRCA2-deficient tumors are sensitive to cisplatin and olaparib
Methylguanine methyltransferase	Removes alkylated bases	Presence in brain tumors leads to resistance to procarbazine or temozolomide
Mismatch repair	Recognizes alkylated DNA lesions, inducing apoptosis	Loss of mismatch repair component leads to temozolomide resistance

(EGF) pathways in epithelial cancers or through amplification of *HER-2* in breast cancer. Translocation and overexpression of BCL-2 are a hallmark of follicular B-cell lymphomas, but the same gene is commonly overexpressed in epithelial tumors. Activation of other protective factors such as NF-κB and the PI-3 kinase pathway in response to DNA damage suppresses cytotoxicity of chemotherapy drugs and radiation. Lowe et al.[37] elegantly demonstrated that the presence of wild-type *p53* conferred tumor sensitivity to doxorubicin, 5-FU, and etoposide, as well as x-irradiation, while the same cells lacking a functional p53 gene were drug and irradiation resistant. This and other studies link the loss of cell-cycle control to resistance to chemotherapeutic agents and explain the high rate of inherent drug resistance of many p53-mutated solid tumors. Furthermore, these results suggest potential targets for effectively bypassing the elaborate defense machinery available to the cancer cell. Drugs are currently in development that activate apoptosis (TRAIL receptor agonists, MDM inhibitors) or attack antiapoptotic proteins, such as the BH3 domain proteins. Venetoclax, a drug that inhibits the antiapoptotic bcl-2, has been approved for drug-resistant chronic lymphocytic leukemia.[38]

Dose-Intensification Strategies

Dose intensification has received increasing emphasis in recent years as a strategy for overcoming resistance to chemotherapy. The intensity of conventional treatment, that is, the dose per time unit, correlates with decreased recurrence rates in adjuvant therapy of breast cancer.[39] By decreasing the interval between treatments, a "dose-dense" regimen, improves relapse-free survival. Drug-responsive tumors have a steep dose-response curve, thus indicating the importance of delivering maximum tolerated doses as rapidly as possible. The following dosing principles derived from the treatment of Hodgkin's disease are broadly applicable to other curable cancers: (a) Do not modify planned doses or schedules of chemotherapy in anticipation of toxicity that has not yet happened, nor for short-term, non–life-threatening toxicity, such as emesis or mild neuropathy. (b) Because significant individual variation may exist in the pharmacokinetics of drugs or in the sensitivity of the bone marrow (and other normal organs) to drug-related toxicity,

the granulocyte count should be used as an in vivo biologic assay of the individual dosage limits of myelotoxic agents. Dose escalation is built into many chemotherapy protocols to achieve a target nadir of $1,000/mm^3$.

While readily tolerable ("standard") doses of combination chemotherapy drugs are sufficient for patients with sensitive tumors, greater dose intensity may be necessary for the subset of patients with drug-resistant tumors. The challenge is to identify reliable predictive tumor markers (such as, potentially, bcl-2 overexpression in large cell lymphoma or mutations in p53 or K-RAS genes) or pharmacokinetic parameters that identify patients who will benefit from more intensive therapy. In the absence of such markers, the only alternative is to treat every potentially curable patient with maximally tolerated doses, as established by the published or experimental protocol. An alternative strategy for dose intensification is to shorten the interval between courses, as has been done in dose-dense breast cancer chemotherapy.[39]

Recombinant hematopoietic growth factors can mitigate the bone marrow toxicity of chemotherapy. Granulocyte colony-stimulating factor is effective in decreasing the duration of granulocyte nadir after myelotoxic chemotherapy. However, erythropoietin preparations decrease survival in some settings and should only be used to correct chemotherapy induced anemia with Hg < 10 g/mm³ in symptomatic patients (see Chapter 34).

High-Dose Chemotherapy

Marrow-ablative dosages of chemotherapy represent the ultimate extrapolation of the dose intensity concept. In practice, it is possible to rescue the host with either autologous bone marrow or peripheral blood stem cells or with stem cells or marrow from an allogeneic but histocompatible donor. During the past 45 years, marrow-ablative chemotherapy with stem cell rescue has become standard as salvage therapy for patients relapsing after primary treatment for leukemias, Hodgkin's and non-Hodgkin's lymphomas, multiple myeloma, other hematologic malignancies, and testicular cancers. Marrow from a human leukocyte antigen (HLA)-compatible donor has the advantage of being free of malignant cells and contains T lymphocytes that generate a strong, and potentially curative, graft versus tumor response. The drugs and doses used in these programs would otherwise cause fatal myelosuppression as their primary dose-limiting toxicity, but with marrow transplantation, extramedullary toxicities become limiting. Alkylators such as busulfan, ifosfamide, and cyclophosphamide are prominent in most ablative regimens because characteristically their extramyeloid toxicity becomes dose limiting only at multiples of their standard dosage. *High-dose regimens exaggerate the extramyeloid toxicities of each drug and introduce new sites of organ damage.* Virtually every organ in the body, including the heart, lungs, liver, gastrointestinal epithelium, and the nervous system, may suffer significant acute and/or chronic toxicity during or after high-dose chemotherapy, and the specific patterns of such toxicity and their reversibility are discussed in relevant chapters.

Randomized trials comparing high-dose regimens with best conventional therapy generally have not proven the value of dose escalation in patients with metastatic solid tumors, with the possible exception of relapsed testicular cancer.[40] High-dose regimens with allogeneic bone marrow transplant are curative in approximately 40% to 50% of patients with acute myeloid leukemia, whereas autologous bone marrow or peripheral blood stem cell transplant regimens are equally effective in drug-responsive Hodgkin Disease in first or second relapse and in intermediate-grade and high-grade non-Hodgkin lymphoma in first relapse. One should remember that both the acute and the late toxicities of high-dose chemotherapy in both autologous and allogeneic bone marrow transplant regimens are formidable and may decrease long-term survival due to later development of myelodysplasia, acute myeloid leukemia, and cardiovascular disease.[41] Acute and chronic graft versus host disease, opportunistic infection, acute gastrointestinal and pulmonary toxicity, and venoocclusive disease of the liver result from drug damage to bone marrow, epithelial tissue, and vascular endothelium, respectively, contribute to mortality of high-dose alkylator regimens.

Drug Interactions in Combination Chemotherapy: Pharmacokinetic Interactions and Overlapping Toxicity

Specific drug interactions, both favorable and unfavorable, must be considered in developing combination regimens. These interactions may take the form of pharmacokinetic, cytokinetic, or biochemical effects of one drug that influences the pharmacokinetic or pharmacodynamic properties of a second component of a combination. Patterns of overlapping toxicity are a primary concern. Drugs that cause renal toxicity, such as cisplatin, must be used cautiously in combination with other agents (such as methotrexate, pemetrexed, the purine analogues, or bleomycin) that depend on renal elimination as a primary mechanism of excretion. It is particularly important to monitor renal function in regimens that incorporate cisplatin with pemetrexed or etoposide, as dose adjustment of the second agent may be necessary to avoid toxicity. Paclitaxel delays the clearance of doxorubicin and increases the risk of cardiotoxicity.[42]

Overlapping toxicities are a primary impediment to some combinations. Trastuzumab and doxorubicin cause incremental cardiac toxicity. Induction of microsomal metabolism by phenytoin or phenobarbital accelerates the clearance of irinotecan, paclitaxel, vincristine, and imatinib. Most "targeted" drugs are cleared by microsomal metabolism and may be ineffective when used with an inducer (see Chapter 21), omeprazole, rifampin, statins, ritonavir,

or adrenal steroids. The opposite effect, a diminished clearance of the cancer drugs, results from their combined use with cytochrome inhibitors, such as ketoconazole. The potential for important interactions between cancer drugs and other medications must always be kept in mind during the routine care of cancer patients, who are often receiving concurrent antibiotics and other agents.

Biochemical interactions between cancer drugs also may be important considerations in determining the choice of agents and their sequence of administration. Both synergistic and antagonistic interactions have been described. A cancer drug may be modulated by a second agent that has no antitumor activity in its own right, but that enhances the intracellular activation or target binding of the primary agent or inhibits the repair of lesions produced by the primary drug. An example of this synergy is the use of leucovorin (5-formyl tetrahydrofolate), which itself has no cytotoxic effect but which, when converted to the active cofactor N-5,10-methylene-tetrahydrofolic acid, enhances the binding of 5-FU to its target, thymidylate synthase, forming a ternary complex with enzyme and 5-dFUMP (see Chapter 8).

Combined Chemotherapy and Radiotherapy

A further innovation in the use of antineoplastic drugs is to combine drugs with irradiation to take advantage of the well-documented synergy between irradiation and cisplatin, 5-fluorouracil, paclitaxel, or cetuximab. Gemcitabine, a most potent sensitizer to irradiation, must be used at fractional doses with irradiation. The mechanism of synergy for each drug is discussed in detail in specific chapters.

The design of integrated chemotherapy-radiotherapy combinations presents special problems because of the synergistic therapeutic, and toxic, effects of the two therapies on both normal and malignant tissue. The normal tissue of greatest concern is the bone marrow, although intestinal epithelium, heart, lungs, brain and any other organ in the path of the beam may be affected. Radiation given to the pelvic or midline abdominal areas produces a decline in blood counts, and a decrease in bone marrow reserve. This can severely compromise the ability to deliver myelotoxic chemotherapy, even months or years after the radiation. Conformal irradiation narrows the irradiation field and preserves a greater portion of the marrow-bearing tissue. For some toxicities, the sequence of administration of drugs and irradiation may be crucial. For example, mediastinal irradiation after combination chemotherapy for massive mediastinal Hodgkin's disease has proven to be practicable and effective. Because the initial chemotherapy results in significant shrinkage of the mediastinal tumor, smaller radiation portals can be used to encompass the residual tumor with proportionately less radiation damage to lungs and heart. Concurrent irradiation and chemotherapy is superior to radiotherapy alone in adjuvant therapy for head and neck cancer (with cisplatin and 5-FU),[43] anal cancer (with mitomycin or 5-FU),[44] cervical cancer (with cisplatin),[45] and rectal cancer (with 5-FU).[46] Thus, although it is important to consider the cumulative toxicities of chemotherapy and radiation on bone marrow and other vulnerable tissues in the radiation field, the therapeutic benefits of simultaneous irradiation and chemotherapy often outweigh the disadvantages.

Many chemotherapeutic agents greatly potentiate the effects of irradiation and may lead to unacceptable toxicity for organs usually resistant to radiation damage. Doxorubicin sensitizes both normal and malignant cells to radiation damage, possibly because both doxorubicin and x-rays produce free-radical damage to tissues. Doxorubicin adjuvant chemotherapy given in conjunction with irradiation to the left chest wall increases the risk of intense skin reactions and cardiac toxicity in patients with left breast cancer.[47] Extreme care must be taken in treatment planning to the dose of irradiation to the heart. Bleomycin and gemcitabine strongly enhance the toxicity of irradiation.

Chemotherapy and irradiation are both carcinogenic. In patients treated with both modalities and cured of Hodgkin disease, the risk for secondary solid tumors in the irradiation field, including breast cancers and sarcomas, increases to approximately 15% at 15 years and 20% at 25 years.[48] The most important chemotherapy-related second malignancy is leukemia due to DNA alkylating or methylating agents. Among the most potently leukemogenic agents are the mustard-type alkylators, nitrosoureas, and procarbazine. A qualitatively different type of secondary non-lymphocytic leukemia is associated with topoisomerase II inhibitors, including etoposide, and doxorubicin (see Chapter 14).[49] Characteristically, acute myelogenous leukemia associated with topoisomerase II inhibitor therapy (anthracyclines or etoposide) has a shorter latency period (1 to 4 years) than does alkylator-induced myelodysplasia and leukemia (3 to 7 years after treatment). Leukemias arising after topoisomerase inhibitor treatment are often associated with reciprocal translocations involving the *MLL* gene at chromosome band 11q23.

Conclusion

The physician must use her/his intimate knowledge of drug efficacy and toxicity to achieve maximum benefit. The foregoing discussion emphasizes that tumor biology, drug mechanisms, drug disposition, and drug interactions, as well as acute and late side effects, are critical considerations in the design and application of effective cancer chemotherapy. Most recently, research is moving the chemotherapy field very rapidly in the direction of personalizing therapy; the hope is that understanding the biology of each tumor at the molecular level at every step in the treatment continuum will add highly relevant information and improve the specificity of treatment, but it will bring additional complexity to the challenge of selecting appropriate therapy for individual patients. The following chapters present information on individual drugs and, if mastered, will enhance the success of our efforts to treat cancer.

References

1. Chabner BA. Breakthrough drugs and turtle soup. *Oncologist*. 2015;20: 845-846.
2. Gerlinger M, Rowan AJ, Horswell S, et al. Intratumor heterogeneity and branched evolution revealed by multiregion sequencing. *N Engl J Med*. 2012; 366:883-892.
3. Rankin A, Klempner SJ, Erlich R, et al. Broad Detection of alterations predicted to confer lack of benefit from EGFR antibodies or sensitivity to targeted therapy in advanced colorectal cancer. *Oncologist*. 2016;21: 1306-1314.
4. Lee V, Murphy A, Le DT, Diaz LA Jr. Mismatch repair deficiency and response to immune checkpoint blockade. *Oncologist*. 2016;21: 1200-1211.
5. Ayvar BV, Arora S, O'Kennedy R. Coming-of-age of antibodies in cancer therapeutics. *Trends Pharmacol Sci*. 2016;12:1009-1028.
6. Skipper HE, Schabel FM Jr, Mellett LB, et al. Implications of biochemical, cytokinetic, pharmacologic, and toxicologic relationships in the design of optimal therapeutic schedules. *Cancer Chemother Rep*. 1970;54:431-450.
7. Rahbari NN, Kedrin D, Incio J, et. al. Anti-VEGF therapy induces ECM remodeling and mechanical barriers to therapy in colorectal cancer liver metastases. *Sci Transl. Med* 2016;360. DOI: 10.1126/scitranslmed. aaf5219.
8. Russo M, Siravegna G, Blaszkowsky LS, et al. Tumor heterogeneity and lesion-specific response to targeted therapy in colorectal cancer. *Cancer Discov*. 2016;6:147-153.
9. Corcoran RB, Chabner BA. Application of cell-free DNA analysis to cancer treatment. *New Engl J Med* 2018: in press.
10. Hata AN, Niederst MJ, Archibald HL, et al. Tumor cells can follow distinct evolutionary paths to become resistant to epidermal growth factor receptor inhibition. *Nat Med*. 2016;22:262-269.
11. Comaills V, Kabeche L, Morris R, et al. Genomic instability is induced by persistent proliferation of cells undergoing epithelial-to-mesenchymal transition. *Cell Rep*. 2016;17:2632-2647.
12. Druker BJ, Talpaz M, Resta DJ. Efficacy and safety of a specific inhibitor of the BCR-ABL tyrosine kinase in chronic myeloid leukemia. *N Engl J Med*. 2001;344:1031-1037.
13. Demetri G. Tales of personalized cancer treatment. *Semin Nephrol*. 2016;36:462-467.
14. Swisher EM, Lin KK, Oza AM, et al. Rucaparib in relapsed, platinum-sensitive high-grade ovarian carcinoma (ARIEL2Part1): an international, mulit-centre, open-label phase 2 trial. *Lancet Oncol*. 2017;18:75-87.
15. Miyamoto DT, Zhao Y, Wittner BS, et al. RNA-Seq of single prostate CTCs implicates noncanonical Wnt signaling in antiandrogen resistance. *Science*. 2015;349:1351-1356.
16. Ahronian LG, Sennott EM, Van Allen EM, et al. Clinical acquired resistance to RAF inhibitor combinations in B-RAF mutant colorectal cancer through MAPK pathway alterations. *Cancer Discov*. 2015;5:358-367.
17. Haragwwoin A, Kaldate RR, Hamilton SA, et al. Modeling 5-FU AUC-dose relationship to develop a PK dosing algorithm. *J Clin Oncol*. 2011;29(suppl):547.
18. Saito S, Lin YC, Tsai MH, et al. Emerging roles of hypoxia-inducible factors and reactive oxygen species in cancer and pluripotent stem cells. *Kaohsiung J Med Sci*. 2015;31:279-286.
19. Pinkel D. Five year follow-up of "total therapy" of childhood lymphocytic leukemia. *JAMA*. 1971;216:648-652.
20. Frei E III. Studies of sequential and combination antimetabolite therapy in acute leukemia: 6-mercaptopurine and methotrexate. *Blood*. 1961;18: 431-454.
21. Frei E III. The effectiveness of combinations of antileukemic agents in inducing and maintaining remission in children with acute leukemia. *Blood*. 1965;26:641-656.
22. Eder JP, et al. Principles of dose, schedule and combination chemotherapy. In: Hong WK, Holland JR, Frei E III, eds. *Cancer Medicine*. 8th ed. Beijing: People's Medical Publishing House; 2016.
23. Palmer AC, Sorger PK. Combination cancer therapy can confer benefit via patient-to-patient variability without drug additivity or synergy. *Cell*. 2017;171:1678-1691.e13.
24. Druker BJ. Circumventing resistance to kinase-inhibitor therapy. *N Engl J Med*. 2006;354:2594-2596.
25. Li W, Zhang H, Assaraf YG, et al. Overcoming ABC transporter-mediated multidrug resistance: molecular mechanisms and novel therapeutic drug strategies. *Drug Resist Updat*. 2016;27:14-29.
26. Van Ellen EM, Mouw KW, Kin P, et al. Somatic ERCC2 mutations correlate with cisplatin sensitivity in muscle-invasive urothelial carcinoma. *Cancer Discov*. 2014;4:1140-1153.
27. Cahill DP, Codd PJ, Batchelor TT, et al. MSH6 inactivation and emergent temozolomide resistance in human glioblastomas. *Clin Neurosurg*. 2008;55:165-171.
28. Hearn JWD, AbuAli G, Reichard CA, et al. HSD3B1 and resistance to androgen-deprivation therapy in prostate cancer: a retrospective, multico-hort study. *Lancet Oncol*. 2016;17(10):1435-1444.

29. Ansell SM, Lesokhin AM, Borrello I, et al. PD-1 blockade with nivolumab in relapsed or refractory Hodgkin's lymphoma. *N Engl J Med.* 2015;372:311-319.

30. Crystal AS, Shaw AT, Sequist LV, et al. Patient-derived models of acquired resistance can identify effective drug combinations for cancer. *Science.* 2014;346:1480-1486.

31. Schartsman G, Ferrarotto R, Massarelli E. Checkpoint inhibitors in lung cancer: latest developments and clinical potential. *Ther Adv Med Oncol.* 2016;8:460-473.

32. Wilson WH, Dunleavy K, Pittaluga S, et al. Phase II study of dose-adjusted EPOCH and Rituximab in untreated diffuse large B-Cell lymphoma with analysis of Germinal Center and Post-Germinal Center biomarkers. *J Clin Oncol.* 2008;26:2717-2724.

33. De Gramont A, Bosset JF, Milan C, et al. Randomized trial comparing monthly low-dose leucovorin and fluorouracil bolus with bimonthly high-dose leucovorin and fluorouracil bolus plus continuous infusion for advanced colorectal cancer: a French intergroup study. *J Clin Oncol.* 1997;15:808-815.

34. Lancet JE, Cortes JE, Hogge DE, et al. Phase 2 trial of CPX-351, a fixed 5:1 molar ratio of cytarabine/daunarubicin vs. cytarabine/daunorubicin in older adults with untreated AML. *Blood.* 2014;123:3239-3246.

35. Taniguchi T, Tischkowitz M, Ameziane N, et al. Disruption of the Fanconi anemia-BRCA pathway in cisplatin-sensitive ovarian tumors. *Nat Med.* 2003;9:568-574.

36. Mateo J, Carreira S, Sandhu S, et al. DNA-repair defects and olaparib in metastatic prostate cancer. *N Engl J Med.* 2015;373:1697-1708.

37. Lowe SW, Ruley HE, Jacks T, et al. *p53*-dependent apoptosis modulates the cytotoxicity of anticancer agents. *Cell.* 1993;74:957-967.

38. Roberts AW, Davids MS, Pagel JM, et al. Targeting BCL2 with venetoclax in relapsed chronic lymphocytic leukemia. *N Engl J Med.* 2016;374:311-322.

39. Citron M. Dose-dense chemotherapy: principles, clinical results and future perspectives. *Breast Care (Basel).* 2008;3:251-255.

40. Lewin J, Dickinson M, Voskoboynik M, et al. High-dose chemotherapy with autologous stem cell transplantation in relapsed or refractory germ cell tumours: outcome and prognostic variables in a case series of 17 patients. *Intern Med J.* 2014;44:771-778.

41. Chow EJ, Cushing-Haugen KL, Cheng GS, et al. Morbidity and mortality differences between hematopoietic cell transplantation survivors and other cancer survivors. *J Clin Oncol.* 2017;35(3):306-313.

42. Holmes FA, Rowinsky EK. Pharmacokinetic profiles of doxorubicin in combination with taxanes. *Semin Oncol.* 2001;28(suppl 12):8-14.

43. Cohen EEW, Harar DJ, List MA, et al. High survival and organ function rates after primary chemoradiotherapy for intermediate-stager squamous cell carcinoma of the head and neck in a multicenter phase II trial. *J Clin Oncol.* 2006;24:3436-3444.

44. Ajani JA, et al. Fluorouracil, mitomycin and radiotherapy vs fluorouracil, cisplatin, and radiotherapy for carcinoma of the anal canal: a randomized controlled trial. *JAMA.* 2008;299:1914-1921.

45. Rose PG, Bundy BN, Watkins EB, et al. Concurrent cisplatin-based chemoradiation improves progression-free and overall survival in advanced cervical cancer: results of a randomized Gynecologic Oncology Group study. *N Engl J Med.* 1999;340:1144-1153.

46. Fisher B, Wolmark N, Rockette H, et al. Postoperative adjuvant chemotherapy or radiation therapy for rectal cancer: results from NSABP protocol R-01. *J Natl Cancer Inst.* 1988;80:21-29.

47. Shapiro CL, Hardenbergh P, Gelman R, et al. Cardiac effects in adjuvant doxorubicin and radiation therapy in breast cancer patients. *J Clin Oncol.* 1998;16:3493-3501.

48. Grantzau T, Overgaard J. Risk of second non-invasive cancer among patients treated with and without postoperative radiotherapy for primary breast cancer: a systematic review and meta-analysis of population-based studies including 522,739 patients. *Radiother Oncol.* 2016;121(3):402-413.

49. Winters AC, Bernt KM. MLL-rearranged leukemias—an update on science and clinical approaches. *Front Pediatr.* 2017;5:4.

Target Identification and Drug Discovery

Bruce A. Chabner

This chapter provides an overview of the discovery and preclinical development of small molecules for anticancer treatment. The Reader is referred to Chapters 29 to 32 for in depth discussion of immunotherapies, and for other specialized chapters dealing with hormonal agents and biological molecules.

A Brief History of Cancer Drug Discovery

The history of cancer drug discovery begins with the initial experiments of Goodman and Gilman during and after the second World War[1,2]; they showed that alkylating mustards produced antitumor effects in murine test systems, leading to the first trials of nitrogen mustard against a patient with Hodgkin's disease. Their work and the subsequent establishment of the initial cancer drug development program at the National Cancer Institute (NCI) in 1956 led to the successful identification of other chemotherapeutic drugs in industry and at the NCI, and the incorporation of multiple drugs into curative regimens for leukemia, lymphomas, and testicular cancer.[2] These agents, identified in empirical screening systems that used murine leukemias, were primarily antiproliferative, targeting steps in DNA synthesis or physically interacting with and damaging DNA. They were nonselective in the sense that they were toxic to all proliferating cells, including bone marrow and intestinal epithelium, and for poorly understood reasons, had a positive therapeutic index: the injury to normal tissues was reversible, while some tumors were completely eradicated. For these early drug discovery efforts, screening libraries were composed of random chemicals, nucleotide analogues, electrophilic alkylating type analogues, and randomly collected fermentation or plant-derived products. The yield in new drugs rarely exceeded 1 to 2 new active chemical entities approved for human use in any given year. Prior to 1990, screening systems for new drugs consisted primarily of tumor cell lines, first of murine origin (L1210, P388 leukemias) and later, in 1984, a panel of 60 human tumor cell lines.[3] There was no specific molecular target in this strategy, although the cell line panel was developed with the intention, not realized, of finding tumor-specific drugs. In subsequent years, the 60 cell line panel has been extensively characterized with regard to genomics, mechanisms of DNA repair, and drug resistance[4,5] and has become a widely used tool for evaluation of compounds in development against cancer. The screening systems used by NCI yielded a number of very active and ultimately useful products, including taxanes[6] and platinum analogues.[7] The empirical screens proved particularly adept at identifying basic classes of cytotoxic compounds, including antimetabolites, antimitotic drugs, topoisomerase inhibitors, and a variety of unusual natural products, such as taxanes and podophyllotoxins.

A Transition to Targeting "Driver" Mutations

A revolution of cancer drug discovery occurred in the years from 1990 forward, as the result of burgeoning biological understanding of cancer as a disease driven by oncogenic mutations that could be targeted for cancer-specific drug development. The biological basis for the concept of "driver mutations" arose from discoveries in the NCI's viral oncology program. Harold Varmus and Michael Bishop's discovery of the SRC viral oncogene, and its counterpart c-SRC in animal tissues, won a Nobel Prize in 1989 and set in motion a search for similar genes in human tumors.[8] These oncogenic drivers have since been revealed in many different subsets of human tumors through genomic analysis[9] and through reference to a comprehensive genome wide sequencing of thousands of human tumors, such as now available in the NCI's The Cancer Genome Atlas. Through the application of statistical algorithms, highly suspect and recurrent mutations associated with specific subsets of human cancer are earmarked for studies that establish their role as oncogenes.[10] In assessing the probability that a given recurrent mutations is fact a "driver" in a given subset of human cancer, Getz's analysis[10] takes into account the underlying frequency of mutations in that group of tumors, as well as the biological function of the gene in question.

Once a suspected driver mutation is found recurrently in human tumor specimens, a process for *validation* of the target is necessary before embarking on an expensive and multiyear drug discovery effort. The target should be present in a defined subset of human cancer, such as the epidermal growth factor receptor (EGFR) mutant subset of lung cancer.[11] The target should be essential to the growth and survival of the tumor cells, as is established by studies of cell lines in which the oncogene activity can be knocked down by siRNAs or by CRISPR technology. These studies require access to human tumor cell lines or to human tumor xenografts, and have been able to define multiple individual subset of common tumors, such as non–small cell lung cancer, each amenable to effective treatment with specifically designed targeted drugs (Fig. 2.1).

RNA interference is an essential tool for target discovery and validation. It was first recognized after seeking to define mechanisms for regulating gene expression in model invertebrate systems. Briefly (Fig. 2.2), siRNAs are double-stranded

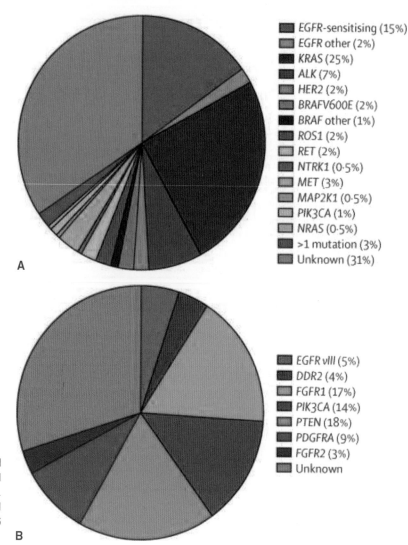

EGFR-sensitising (15%)
EGFR other (2%)
KRAS (25%)
ALK (7%)
HER2 (2%)
BRAFV600E (2%)
BRAF other (1%)
ROS1 (2%)
RET (2%)
NTRK1 (0·5%)
MET (3%)
MAP2K1 (0·5%)
PIK3CA (1%)
NRAS (0·5%)
>1 mutation (3%)
Unknown (31%)

A

EGFR vIII (5%)
DDR2 (4%)
FGFR1 (17%)
PIK3CA (14%)
PTEN (18%)
PDGFRA (9%)
FGFR2 (3%)
Unknown

B

Figure 2.1 Subsets of non–small cell lung cancer, as defined by molecular drivers. Adenocarcinomas **(A)** and squamous cell carcinomas **(B)**. (Reprinted from Hirsch FR, Suda K, Wiens J, et al. New and emerging targeted treatments in advanced non-small-cell lung cancer. *Lancet.* 2016;388(10048):1012-1024. Copyright © 2016 Elsevier. With permission.)

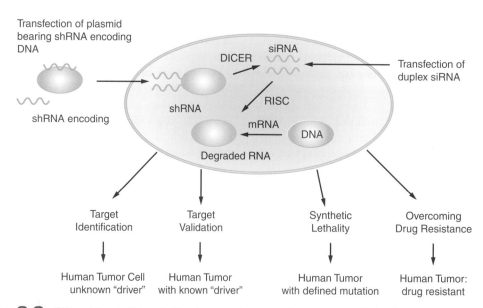

Figure 2.2 siRNA and its potential applications for cancer drug target discover, target validation, "synthetic lethal" targets, and elucidation of drug and radiation sensitivity/resistance. siRNA binds to its target messenger RNA, and the complex is degraded, preventing synthesis of the oncoprotein.

"short interfering RNA" (siRNA), one strand of which has homology to a target sequence in the mRNA of a gene of interest. It forms a complex with the target cellular RNA leading to the target's degradation through formation of an RNA-induced silencing complex (RISC). The loss of mRNAs bearing the target sequence changes the tumor cell phenotype, and when directed against a "driver" mutations, may lead to an abrupt cessation of proliferation and cell death. siRNAs may be introduced directly into cells, or may be cleaved intracellularly from "short hairpin RNAs" (shRNAs) that are introduced into cells via plasmids or into embryos by lentivirus. RNA interference technology has utility in virtually all aspects of cancer drug discovery[12,13] including target identification and validation, synthetic lethal screening, identification of tumor suppressor genes,[13] and exploration of drug sensitization or resistance mechanisms. CRISPR screens offer the advantage of identifying genes essential for proliferation of tumor subsets, such as *RAS*-driven tumors, and searching for partner genes that become essential to survival only when the oncogene of interest is expressed or the suppressor gene of interest is lost (synthetic lethal screening, see below).[14] This type of screen becomes particularly valuable when the driver gene is "undruggable" or the function of the suppressor gene cannot be replaced. The "essential" partner can then be targeted as an alternative.

Establishing a Screen: Assay Development

The era of oncogene discovery has generated a multitude of new targets for drug discovery. As the field of cancer biology expanded, small biotechnology companies have seized the opportunity to rationalize cancer drug development. The biotechnology industry has grown remarkably in the past two decades. There are currently over 2,000 companies engaged in the cancer therapeutics area at the present time. Figure 2.3 illustrates the generic flow of drug discovery from target identification and validation, devising a screening assay and choosing an appropriate library of chemicals for lead identification and lead optimization and finally refinement of the lead compound as a drug. Assays for high throughput screening in general employ the protein product of cancer driver genes, and will make it possible to survey vast libraries of synthetic compounds in the search for a lead compound.

To screen for inhibitors or activators of a given molecular target, the activity of the target protein or pathway must be linked to a readily detectable readout.[15] Commonly used types of screening assays employ an immobilized target protein that captures compounds capable of moderately high affinity binding. The bound small chemical can then be identified by its molecular or fluorescent tag

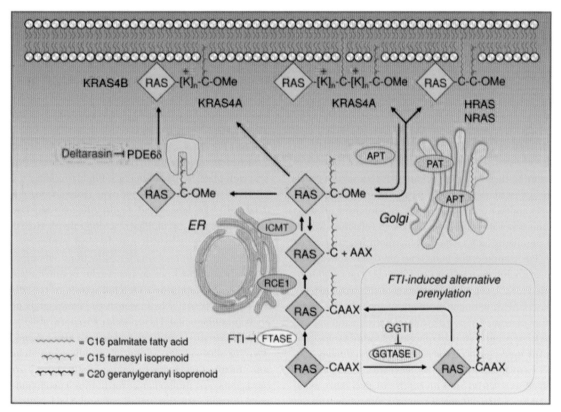

FIGURE 2.3 Mechanisms of RAS protein modification and insertion in the cell membrane, presenting multiple opportunities for inhibition at steps to modify the terminal CAAX domain of RAS: add lipid (farnesyl or geranyl), add a methyl group to the terminal cysteine, cleave the terminal three amino acids, and direct membrane insertion through phosphodiesterase 6-gamma (PDE6-gamma). The enzymatic steps include FTASE (farnesyltransferase), RCE1 (endocarboxypeptidase 1), ICMT (isoprenylcysteine carboxymethyl transferase), GGTase I (geranylgeranyltransferase), PAT (protein acyltransferase), and APT1/2 (acyl protein thioesterase). Recycling of acyl groups by the action of ATP1/2 is essential to the preservation of the intracellular pool of lipid. Each RAS isoform is subject to different modification. (Reprinted from Cox AD, Der CJ, Philips MR. Targeting RAS membrane association: back to the future for anti-RAS drug Discovery? *Clin Cancer Res.* 2015;21(8):1819-1827. Copyright © 2015 American Association for Cancer Research. With permission from AACR.)

and further evaluated in cell-free or cell-based assays to confirm target engagement. Other assays may be employed, such as enzyme inhibition or *in vitro* binding with detection of the enzyme reaction or protein binding as reported by fluorescence polarization, fluorescent resonance energy transfer, scintillation proximity, and luminescent proximity (ALPHA Screen). The target protein may be labeled with a fluorescent amino acid, such as 19-fluoro-tryptophan, and affinity of binding can be quantified by shifts in fluorescence spectra.[16] Assays may also measure changes in light absorbance (UV/vis), in the activity of luciferase, or in the expression of green fluorescent or other related proteins. In general, the throughput of samples is highest when the binding of candidate molecules is easily imaged without separation from the unbound fraction.

In the past, cell-based assays for inhibitors of proliferation were frequently employed as the initial screen[3] and had the advantage of identifying compounds that crossed cell membranes and retained their activity intracellularly. However, these cell-based screens lacked specificity for a target or pathway, excluded compounds that might have become useful leads that could be refined into active drugs, and in general were limited in their capacity to handle thousands of library candidates. *However, once a lead compound has been detected in a cell-free assay, further evaluation and refinement of structure will require cell lines chosen for the expression of the target of interest.*

Innovations in screening have become important in expanding the scope of drug discovery. Zon et al.[17] have employed zebrafish, which generate hundreds of offspring after each mating. These fish preserve the same signaling pathways that have undergone mutations in human cancers. Mutant targets in the fish can generate tumors such as B-RAF–driven melanoma, allowing in vivo screening in fish tanks and in microplate wells containing tiny fish with visible melanotic tumors.[18]

Quality Control and Standardization of Assay

A major restriction to the development of new HTS assays has been the acquisition and standardization of reagents, particularly for innovative targets and assays. In some cases, recombinant proteins are required, and innovative biochemical assays reflecting activities of protein modifiers such as the histone methyltransferase or demethylases.[19] For example, the basic screening assay for histone methyltransferase inhibitors employed by Epizyme required purification of histone H3K27 peptide fragments as a substrate and the methyltransferase EZH2, with enhancement of the relatively slow catalytic reaction *in vitro*. Even with substantial miniaturization, many molecularly targeted screens require much more target protein (and/or many more cells) than is needed for basic research on the target. It is essential that sufficient reagents are available for the entire screening effort to avoid batch-to-batch variation. Also, many of the newer highly sensitive technologies, although affordable on a small scale, become prohibitively expensive when screening large libraries. The availability and cost of reagents can be pivotal factors in deciding whether to screen a selected target.

An ideal assay plate design includes untreated, negative control well and wells with compound or a condition known to affect the target (positive controls). These provide clear definition of the maximum and minimum signal on an individual plate and, therefore, the window in which compound activity can be measured. However,

when studying a newly identified and incompletely characterized target, a specific inhibitor (or activator) may not be known. For some targets, a more generic method of inhibition can be used in the absence of a specific inhibitor (e.g., ethylenediaminetetraacetic acid [EDTA] inhibits most metal-dependent enzymes). The reproducibility among the control wells within a plate and the reproducibility of the control wells among the plates within a set are indicative of the quality of the screen. Once a new screening assay has been designed and standardized, it is important to characterize its performance by completing pilot-scale screens. For example, application of a consistent set of "training compounds" of different structural types can provide a quantitative measure of the reproducibility of the assay, sometimes even leading to the identification of intriguing lead.[20] In establishing a cell-free biochemical screening system, it is necessary to define the kinetics of interaction with natural substrates, cofactor requirements, pH optima, and a detection system for the reaction product.

Screening Libraries

When an assay for target binding and/or inhibition has been established and validated, the next step is to choose an initial library of candidate compounds in the search for "hits." Compound libraries employed in target-directed assays are enriched for potentially active structures for a given target; thus, ATP analogs, S-adenosyl-L-methionine analogs,[19] and analogs of substrates for acetyl transferases (Chapter 16) become the fertile soil for lead discovery. Many libraries are available commercially, while others are provided by the NCI (see below). Using such enriched libraries, researchers have elevated the hit rate to 0.1% to 1% of compounds that enter the screening process, with even higher hit rates for chemical fragments.[21]

Over the years, collections of pure compounds and natural product extracts coalesced into libraries, arrayed into 96-well plates or 384-well plates suitable for HTS. Popular commercial libraries are available from ChemBridge Corp. (San Diego, CA), Maybridge (Cornwall, England), and Sigma-Aldrich (St. Louis, MO; and notably the Library of Pharmacologically Active Compounds or LOPAC), many of which may be cost prohibitive for academic researchers. Additional smaller collections of compounds are commercially available from an assortment of other suppliers. The NCI Open Source Repository (OSR) of approximately 250,000 samples is the publicly available subset of the compounds obtained by the NCI Developmental Therapeutics Program (DTP) over the past 50 years for use in anticancer drug screening (http://dtp.nci.nih.gov). Smaller subsets of the DTP collection, including diversity sets of natural product extracts and collections of approved oncology agents, are also available; for both nonprofit and small business entities (subject to limitations of available substance and costs of shipping).

Natural Products in Cancer Drug Screening

A crucial issue in any screening project for new anticancer drugs is the acquisition of compound libraries. Whether the initial screen is a target-directed biochemical screen or an empirical antiproliferation screen, the greater the structural diversity in the set of molecules examined, the more likely a novel inhibitor will be identified. Historically, natural products, defined here as extracts from plants, microbial, and animal sources, have provided an excellent source of chemically unique bioactive molecules with novel mechanisms of action.

The advantages and disadvantages of natural product extracts as sources for cancer drug discovery have been extensively reviewed.[22,23] There are over 52,000 unique molecules in the most complete dataset of natural products, many built on approximately 6,500 unique scaffolds that found only in subsets of natural sources.[22] While having quite diverse structure found only in subgroups of marine organisms, fungi, bacteria, and other sources, the useful cancer active natural products often fall into one of several categories: antimetabolites derived as fermentation products, topoisomerase inhibitors (anthracyclines and etoposide), antimitotics (vinca alkaloids and taxanes), and alkylating entities (mitomycin). Other cancer drugs derived from natural products, but not members of these classes, include DNA minor groove binders (calicheamicin) and inhibitors of histone deacetylase (romidepsin), RNA polymerase 2 (trabectedin),[24] various kinases, phosphodiesterases,[25] and other targets. The significant disadvantages of natural products are the need to purify the active component from the extract or from a fermentation broth, to resolve the structure of the active principle, to define its mechanism of action, to recollect starting material from the parent source, and ultimately, if the product is of high interest, to synthesize analogues of the often complex structure. The considerable challenge of derivatizing the product to adjust drug-like properties adds to the complexity of natural product work. At the present time, efforts to derive bioactive natural products have plateaued at about 1,600 novel structures per year, and about 200 "low similarity" compounds per year, few of which make it into clinical trials.[22] Most drug discovery efforts are employing chemical libraries rather than natural products.

Synthetic Chemical Libraries

Advances in combinatorial chemistry have greatly magnified the number of compounds available for screening. The method of synthesizing multiple derivative compound as a result of a single reaction began approximately 35 years ago with the synthesis by Geysen et al.[26] of multiple peptides on polyethylene rods. These early endeavors, confined to the synthesis of small peptide libraries, were of limited value to cancer drug discovery because peptides tend not to enter cells and generally are not suitable drug candidates. Subsequent advances in the field included development of more efficient ways to track the compounds, use of a greater number of scaffolds on which to construct libraries, and use of a wider variety of reagents and amenable reaction conditions. Now, combinatorial chemistry provides an efficient method of exploring chemical space in a focused manner and, when applicable, an excellent means of rapidly defining structure activity relationships around active compounds. "Fragment libraries" are a further refinement; small molecular weight chemical fragments can be screened in silico, and hits can be confirmed through an *in vitro* binding assay.

These results may suggest helpful modifications that increase drug potency or modify other pharmacological properties of the parent molecule.[27]

Alternative to Small Molecule Libraries for Drug Discovery

While the traditional approach to drug discover utilizes synthetic small molecules against protein targets, there is growing interest in radically different compounds and targets. RNA interference, produced by small, complimentary RNA molecules that bind and degrade oncogene specific RNAs, has proven effective in early clinical trials against lipid disorders,[28] porphyria, and neurological disease, and has potential uses against cancer.[29] This technology is currently limited by the slow uptake of these molecules in most tumors, the tendency of synthetic RNAs to localize in the liver, and their spectrum of unusual toxicity (thrombocytopenia).

A second novel approach employs highly potent cytotoxins bound to monoclonal antibodies that are directed against cancer membrane antigens.[30,31] Many cytotoxins prove too toxic to normal tissues when administered systemically as conventional drugs. Among the most prominent failures have been the antimitotic maytansine and a number of highly potent, but toxic DNA minor groove binding candidates. Attaching these molecules to monoclonal antibodies directs the toxin to cancer cells, where they are bound to a surface antigen, internalized in a lysosome, and cleaved to release the active drug intracellularly. Critical to the technology of ADC's has been the development of stable linker systems, which release the drug in the lysosome either through hydrolysis of a disulfide bond or through the action of a lysosomal protease. Improvements, such as inserting a succinimide linker, which is cleaved in the lysosome, have stabilized the bond between the "warhead" and antibody and have increased the effectiveness and decreased toxicity of these compounds, more than 60 of which are currently in clinical trial (see Chapter 29). FDA has approved brentuximab (an auristatin-armed antibody to CD30) for Hodgkin's disease[32] and myelotarg[33] (a calicheamicin-armed anti-CD33) for acute myeloid leukemia. The advantages of ADCs are their ability to deliver the toxin specifically to the tumor, avoiding systemic toxicity, with limited leakage of the toxin into normal tissues.

"Undruggable" Targets

Some targets remain elusive despite concerted attempts to identify and develop active drugs; among these "undruggable" targets, perhaps the most important are some of the most commonly mutated oncogenes in human cancer: the RAS oncogenes, c-MYC, P53, and oncogenic transcription factors activated in human sarcomas. Early attempts to target the RAS group of oncogenes through inhibition of its lipid modification (farnesyltransferase inhibition) failed in clinical trials[34] due to the presence of unforeseen alternative pathways for lipid attachment and membrane insertion of RAS protein. Progress in understanding the structure and function of the RAS molecules, their modification by lipid, their membrane insertion, and their interaction with effector molecules has led to new opportunities for RAS drug discovery (Fig. 2.3).[35–37] Innovative electrophilic compounds that attack the G12C mutant of KRAS that drives 20% of non–small cell lung cancer have evoked great interest, but effective drug-like derivatives have not yet reached the clinic. Others are attempting to block RAS function through inhibition of its interaction with effector proteins[37] that block GTP recycling, promote membrane insertion by phosphodiesterase[34] (Fig. 2.3), and transmit signals downstream through the RAL, PI3K, and MAPK pathways,[37] but RAS remains an elusive target.[38]

Mutations that altered transcription factor interaction with regulatory sequences in DNA are a frequent finding in human sarcomas, but attempt to block these pathways for anticancer drug development have not yet been successful. The large surfaces of molecular interaction between proteins or between protein and DNA provide few high affinity pockets for drug attack. Bromodomain inhibitors represent one of the few promising classes of new inhibitors, and have displayed initial activity in clinical trials against NUT midline carcinomas and multiple myeloma[39,40] (see below).

Among the many new targets for drug development, the processes involved in repair of DNA have attracted increasing interest. Environmental insults such as ionizing irradiation and toxic chemicals, as well as chemotherapy and radiation therapy create single-strand DNA adducts and breaks that are converted to double-strand breaks (DSBs) when encountered by replication forks. These DSBs present challenges to the cellular repair process. The first challenge is to repair the DSBs by homologous recombination (HR). Cancers often contain mutations or loss of expression of key repair genes, such as BRCA1 and 2, PALB2, Chk2, and ATM, which participate in recognition and repair of double-strand DNA breaks by the multistep process of homologous recombination. Additionally, if unprotected, stalled replication forks (SRFs) at the site of DSBs are susceptible to nuclease digestion, leading to cell death. Key to the protection of SRFs is ATR, a kinase for which inhibitors have been developed.[41] These ATR inhibitors, as expected, sensitize cells to chemotherapy, irradiation, and are "synthetically lethal" against cancers with underlying mutations in repair components, including ATM, ARIDIA complex, and ALT telomerase function.[41] Mutations in BRCA1 and 2, and PALB2 underlie inherited breast cancer and ovarian cancer, and are components of the DSB repair pathway, and, when defective, lead to vulnerability to inhibitors of ATR, PARP, or chemotherapy-induced DSBs. This vulnerability is a clear example of "synthetic lethality."[42,43] PARP inhibitors are now approved for treatment of ovarian cancers in patients with mutations in BRCA 1 or 2, and approvals will likely be expanded to the same mutations in breast cancers and other tumors.[44] Active programs in ATR kinase inhibition have progressed to early clinical trials.

The concept of "synthetic lethality"[45] is based on findings from yeast genetics, in which two genes are "synthetic lethal" to survival if mutation of both genes results in cell death even though mutation of either alone is compatible with cell viability. In the presence of an initial mutation, cells become dependent for their survival on the function of a second gene. In drug discovery, this concept is applied to identifying second targets that are synthetic lethal to cancer cells containing a mutation such as BRCA 1, but leaving normal cells with intact DNA repair pathways unaffected. Synthetic lethal screening, employing libraries of siRNA, allows the identification of second genes, which is vital to the survival of cells bearing oncogenic mutations.

Targeting Drug Resistance in Drug Development

Early in the clinical development of targeted drugs, such as imatinib for chronic myelogenous leukemia, it was recognized that following exposure to an effective anticancer drug-resistant cancer cells emerge[46] creating new and increasingly complex targets for drug discovery. Resistance to cancer drugs may take many forms, including amplification of the target gene, activation of an alternative pathway, reversion to a stem cell phenotype, or mutation of the drug target. These mutations often prevent drug binding within the catalytic site of the enzyme, but permit continued activity with normal substrates. The mutated drug binding site can be analyzed through crystallography and compounds with improved fit can be designed (see Chapter 24). Second- and third-generation drugs for CML such as nilotinib and dasatinib accommodate many of these drug-resistant mutations, but are uniformly ineffective against the T315I mutation. Ponatinib is the lone compounds active against T315 I, although its use is compromised by its tendency to cause vascular occlusions.[47] Other second- and third-generation compounds have improved activity against drug-resistant mutations found in *EGFRm* non–small cell lung cancer (NSCLC)[48] and *EML4-ALKm* NSCLC.[49] For example, alectinib overcomes multiple drug-resistant *EML4-ALK* mutations and has the added significant advantage of improved penetration into the central nervous system, preventing metastases at that site (Chapter 21). It is superior to the first-line agent, crizotinib in time to progression on therapy, and has become the first-line agent of choice.[50] However, it, too, is the subject of drug resistance mutations and activation of secondary oncogenic pathways: some of the alectinib-resistant mutations are sensitive to lorlatinib, a "fourth-generation" EML4-ALK antagonist. Resistance to lorlatinib is mediated by the dual mutations, L1198F and C1156Y, which individually remain sensitive to the drug, but together, confer resistance. Interestingly, these combinations of mutations restore sensitivity to crizotinib (see Chapter 21).[51] With virtually every successful targeted drug, a second- or third-generation drug with improved pharmacological and mutation-specific features has come into practice.

Qualifying a Lead Compound for Further Development

Once the screening process has revealed promising lead compounds, it is necessary to confirm target engagement and antitumor activity in intact cells containing the target of interest. The process for culling hits is multifold and usually begins by confirming compound identity and activity and demonstrating a dose-response relationship in a cell-based assay. Ideally, the proposed mechanism of action of compounds identified in *in vitro* assays is corroborated in cell-based assays, which demonstrate the ability to inhibit the target and a lack of toxicity for cells not expressing the target. A broad collection of well-annotated human tumor cells is required. Often, confirmed active compounds are filtered through one or more algorithms designed to recognize drug-like molecules and purge compounds known to be toxic, chemically reactive, unstable in solution, and/or nonselective. Filtering software packages are available from several companies, including Leadscope, Inc. (Columbus, OH),

Accelrys, Inc. (Burlington, MA), Bioreason, Inc. (Santa Fe, NM), and Golden Helix, Inc. (Bozeman, MT). Eventually, the most active, most unique compounds are selected as the basis for lead optimization and development.

Refinement of Hits

"Hits" are compounds that bind to target proteins or inhibit enzymatic activity in micromolar concentrations, and they become the subject for modification, enhancement of potency, and refinement of drug-like properties. These hits are then typically used for optimization through studies of crystallographic imaging of inhibitor binding to its target protein. Likewise, in silico modeling can help identify appropriate structures to improve the hit rate from otherwise random screening.

It is exceptionally unusual for an initial screening effort to yield compounds suitable for clinical study. Most require further chemical refinement to increase potency and specificity, and to incorporate favorable "drug-like" properties. The path for refinement of a lead compounds is now heavily dependent upon obtaining crystallographic structures of the different confirmations of protein-substrate and protein-inhibitor binding. It requires an analysis of hydrogen or van der Waals bonding between drug candidate and target pocket, and aspects of the binding inhibitor or binding pocket that interfere with stability of binding. Chemical modification of the inhibitor may engage sites neighboring the inhibitor binding pocket, or induce favorable changes in the conformation of the target protein.

The importance of understanding the multiple configurations of the target protein is illustrated by Gray's work on receptor tyrosine kinases.[51] Gray has described four potential classes of RTK inhibitors: type I is highly specific for the deep binding cavity of ATP as it requires a perfect fit within a rigid binding site. Type II inhibitors, such as imatinib, attack the enzyme in its inactive or relaxed state by engaging an adjacent binding pocket (the Mg^{++} binding site in the DFG "out" conformation), thereby preventing activation of the enzyme in a less specific manner. Type II inhibitors have been the favored approach for kinase inhibition. Multiple interactions of inhibitors and enzyme in the inactive conformations may markedly strengthen binding, including engagement of the phosphate-binding loop, or P-loop, while also improving selectivity. Type III inhibitors, such as the MEK inhibitor trametinib, bind to sites outside the catalytic pocket but exert allosteric effects on ATP binding. Type IV inhibitors block interaction with accessory proteins. Based on the above approach, increasingly potent and specific RTK inhibitors have emerged from the laboratory of Gray[52] and others.[53] For example, recent interest has focused on ATP analogues that contain electrophilic substituents that bind covalently to cysteines in the catalytic pocket of the kinases[37] culminating in the synthesis of ibrutinib and other analogues[53] for targeting *BTK*-driven lymphoid tumors, osimertinib for T790M *EGFR*,[49] and G12M-mutated K-RAS.[37] Like many other kinase targets, BTK, achieving specificity is a challenge. Eleven kinases, including BTK, share a highly homologous sequence that includes the key cysteine in its catalytic pocket; one candidate covalent inhibitor, CHMFL-BTK-11, a potent anti-inflammatory compound, achieved greater specificity, and greater than 10-fold potency versus the only other kinase inhibited, through its interaction with the adjacent hinge region outside the catalytic domain of BTK.[53]

Successive efforts to "build" higher-affinity derivatives can utilize both in silico modeling and structural studies in solution by nuclear magnetic resonance (NMR) or by crystallography to enhance interaction with targets. These studies may be done with modified fragments of the drug scaffold, and when improved binding is confirmed, these fragments may then be incorporated into the parent drug.[27] Second-generation leads are built by combining fragments into molecules to yield high-affinity binders.

Where there is already a richness of information about a target, crystallographic selection strategies can be defined that can improve lead structures. This is exemplified by the refinement of active inhibitor of CSF1R kinase.[54] In the latter case, a nanomolar inhibitor, PLX3397, was modified based upon structural information, to allow a juxtamembrane portion of the receptor to stabilize the inhibitor and enzyme complex in an inactive confirmation (Fig. 2.4).

Recent progress on the difficult problem of inhibiting protein-protein interactions is exemplified by the work of Bradner and colleagues[55] who have led efforts to block the bromodomain proteins that interact with *N*-acetyl lysine side chains of histones and transcriptions factors. BET (bromodomain and extraterminal) proteins have become an important target for blocking male fertility (the BrdT protein), or regulating the c-MYC oncogene (BRD4).[54] Their lead compound, JQ1, a pan BET inhibitor, caused memory defects in mice, leading to an instructive search for more specific BrdT inhibitors. Six million compounds were screened in silico against the protein structure of BrdT, yielding 24,000 "hits"; non–drug-like structures were eliminated, leaving 22 commercially available compounds that satisfied "Lipinski and Weber" rules for solubility, charge, and ease of modification. Of the nine most highly bound to BrdT in a fluorescence assay, six contained a dihydropyridopyrimidine structure that proven most selective in fluorescent binding assays with BrdT and Brd4. A 6-amino-1-ethyluracil derivative of the basic scaffold proved to be the tightest binder (Fig. 2.5), as confirmed by crystallography. Cell line testing against a myeloma cell line further suggested the advantage of a lactam derivative of the 6-amino-1-ethyl form of the drug.

In practical terms, modifications of structure typically improve the potency of binding of the "hit" by 100- to 1,000-fold, creating IC_{50}'s in the low nanomolar range, increasing the candidate's specificity for the target, and, as a final step introducing favorable drug properties such as a suitable bioavailability (at least 50%), plasma half-life (ideally 4 to 12 hours), and lack of susceptibility to the multidrug-resistant exporters. Examples of such refinement are found in the development of potent, highly specific, and clinically effective second- and third-generation inhibitors of receptor tyrosine kinases noted above. Some newer targets for which potent clinical inhibitors have been discovered include NTRK[56]; epigenetic modifiers such as vorinostat[57] and histone methyl transferases[19]; isocitrate dehydrogenase[58]; and many other oncogenic drivers. Specificity of inhibitors for specific oncogenic proteins has been a recurrent challenge, as many of the drugs in current clinical practice have multiple sites of action, leading both to additional antitumor uses, but also to toxicities (see Table 2.1). Since there is high homology of the ATP binding sites of subset of receptor tyrosine kinases (Fig. 2.6), toxicities to

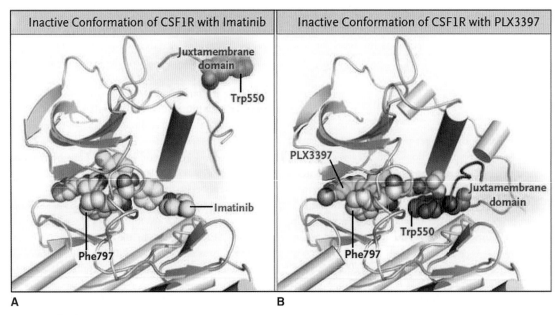

FIGURE 2.4 Molecular modeling of CSF1R inhibitor engagement of the catalytic pocket. CSF1R receptor inhibitors imatinib and PLX3397 enter the catalytic domain of the receptor when it is in an inactive confirmation. However, while imatinib binding **(A)** prevents the further conformational binding of a juxtamembrane (JM domain) into the pocket, the more potent inhibitor, PLX33977, **(B)** allows space for the Trp550 amino acid of the JM domain to enter the catalytic site and fix the receptor in the closed position. The drug proved highly effective in patients with tenosynovial giant cell tumors, which contain an activating mutation in CSF1R. (From Chabner B, Richon V. Structural Approaches to Cancer Drug Development. *N Engl J Med.* 2015;373(5):402-403. Copyright © 2015 Massachusetts Medical Society. Reprinted with permission from Massachusetts Medical Society.)

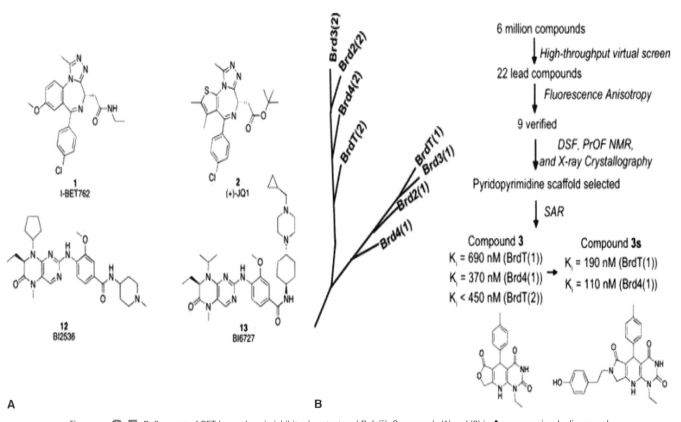

FIGURE 2.5 Refinement of BET bromodomain inhibitor (see text and Ref. [55]). Compounds (1) and (2) in **A** were previously discovered inhibitors built on a triazoloazepine scaffold, but (2) exhibited neurotoxicity in early clinical trials. Alternative scaffolds were known, compounds (12) and (13), and others were sought. The sequence of screening shown in the figure yielded compound (3) in the right hand panel of **B**, incorporating the 6-amino-1-ethyl dihydropyrimidine lead fragment, and inhibiting multiple members of the BET domain tree (shown in **B**). Further studies in myeloma cells led to a lactam derivative of (3s) with submicromolar antitumor potency. (Reprinted with permission from Ayoub A, Hawk LM, Herzig RJ, et al. BET bromodomain inhibitors with one-step synthesis discovered from virtual screen. *J Med Chem.* 2017;60(12):4805-4817. Copyright © 2017 American Chemical Society.)

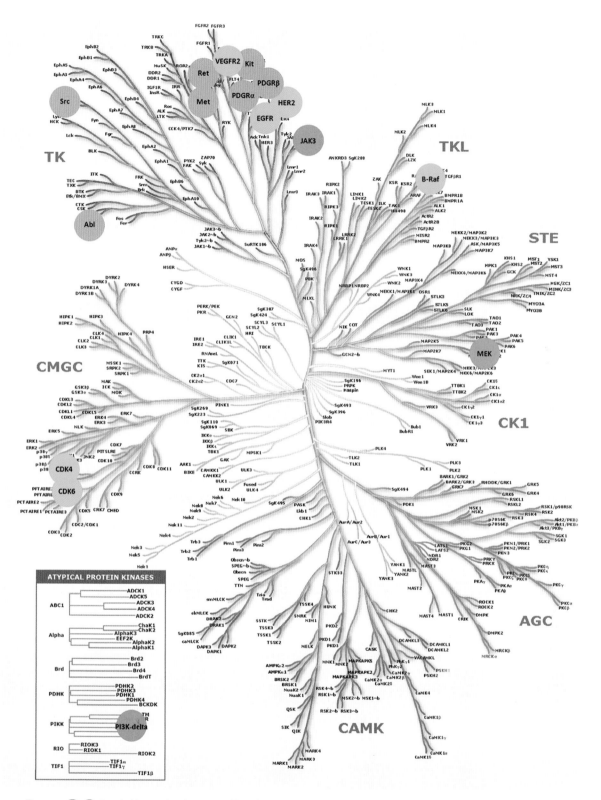

FIGURE 2.6 Protein kinase relatedness trees. There is extensive crossover of inhibitors that may target kinases from multiple families, although tightest binding usually occurs within a related subset of a given family. Examples of kinases targeted by drugs approved or in advances stages of development are highlighted by colored circles. The generic process of high-throughput, molecular-targeted screening (HTS) requires initial identification and validation of a target, and characterization of its specificity for inhibiting the kinases closely related to its primary target kinase, followed by development and characterization of an assay suitable for HTS. This assay is then used to screen chemical collections or "libraries" to identify active samples that are the focus of additional testing to establish potency, selectivity, and other features important for further development. Screening is typically conducted in a "campaign" mode, with primary screening data from a particular library undergoing evaluation after the whole library has been tested. (From Li YH, Wang PP, Li XX, et al. The human kinome targeted by FDA approved multi-target drugs and combination products: a comparative study from the drug-target interaction network perspective. *PLoS One.* 2016;11(11): e0165737, under a Creative Commons Attribution License.)

skin and GI epithelium are common side effects for compounds of this class. However, it has been possible to synthesize drugs highly specific for a single, specific target unique to cancer cells, as for example osimertinib,[48] a highly active and specific inhibitor of the T790M mutant *EGFR* gene. It is 100-fold more potent against the mutant enzyme as compared to the wild-type EGFR.

Cell-Based and *In Vivo* Testing of Candidate Molecules

The above examples illustrate the critical cooperation between a team of experts in chemistry, structural biology, in silico modeling, and biochemistry to improve leads directed to a particular target and activity in a "target-dependent" tumor model in cells and ultimately *in vivo*. This refinement of a lead is an iterative process, requiring an active interplay between team members.

While cell-based testing served historically as an empirical source of lead compounds,[3] it now serves as a confirmatory hurdle following identification of a lead from a high throughput screen. A key criticism of the NCI 60 cell-based screen is that although it was an early example of how cell-based screening can be useful in tying the action of a compound to the presence of particular targets or detoxifying mechanisms, it was not sufficiently representative of the diversity of human malignancy. Six lung cancer cell lines do not come close to matching the full spectrum of mutants within NSCLC. Much broader cell panels are now routinely used to search for subsets of cells susceptible to a given inhibitor. In this manner, it was found that crizotinib, a known inhibitor of c-met and the EML4-alk kinase, had potent activity against a lung cancer cell line containing a *ROS1* activating mutation. This cell line was one of 70 lung cancers represented in a broad panel of 1,000 human tumor lines at the Massachusetts General Hospital Laboratories.[59] This discovery led to the clinical testing and approval of crizotinib in the rare *ROS1* mutant NSCLC.

In Vivo Efficacy Testing

At the completion of the *in vitro* screening process, including confirmation of hits, definition of lead structures, and their structural optimization (ideally using information derived from binding of the lead to its intended target molecule), a limited set of promising compounds should be available for preliminary pharmacology studies in animal models, using immune-compromised mice bearing human tumor xenografts, or genetically engineered mouse models containing the target of interest. Data relating antitumor activity to pharmacodynamic and pharmacokinetic properties can be invaluable in planning the earliest clinical testing. Pharmacokinetic data are essential for guiding preclinical development of promising lead compounds and choosing schedule and starting dose. Lack of target inhibition in preclinical experiments or failure to achieve adequate drug levels would be an early indication to modify the candidate molecule or reassess the overall strategy. Conversely, clear evidence of target inhibition in mouse models at drug levels associated with *in vitro* preclinical activity argues strongly for accelerated clinical development, and may provide useful information in the transition to clinical evaluation, where blood levels of drug are crucial indicators of therapeutic potential. Studies of drug metabolism in mice can suggest further modifications in structure to prevent rapid metabolic inactivation or induction of drug-metabolizing enzymes such as CYP3A4/5. It is critical for a promising candidate for clinical development to demonstrate antitumor activity in *in vivo* animal models. Despite the best efforts to optimize a candidate molecule, many fail because of poor absorption from the gut, rapid degradation in a drug's first pass through the liver, poor tissue uptake or distribution, and unexpected toxic reactions. Often pharmaceutical firms will identify multiple candidates for *in vivo* testing because of the unpredictability of results of any single compound in animals.

While early strategies employed mice bearing syngeneic tumors, the shift to targeted drug development has led to a reliance on well-characterized human tumor cell lines, organoids,[60] xenografts, and GEMM models for confirmation of candidate drug activity and initial explorations of pharmacological properties. Organoids that maintain the histology and three-dimensional structure of human tumors in a culture environment have attracted interest as possible vehicles for drug testing; they are relatively easy to derive from common human tumors such as breast, ovary, and gastrointestinal tract tumors. Whether they will more accurately mirror drug response *in vivo* is still under investigation. These tumor models are selected for testing based on the presence of the desired drug target, usually an activated, amplified, or otherwise mutated oncogenic driver. In essence, the tumors contain the biomarker that will eventually guide the selection of patients for initial clinical trials. Thus, a validated assay, often called a companion diagnostic for the biomarker that discloses the presence of the "target," is required prior to drug approval. The assay may be a genomic assay, an immunohistochemical assay, or an in situ hybridization procedure for detecting the genetic lesion or the presence of its product.

Patient-derived tumor xenografts (PDXs) grown in immunocompromised (SCID, nu/nu, NIH-III, SCID/bg, NOD.SCID) mice are now widely available.[61] Tumors have been successfully generated following tumor cell inoculation into various anatomic sites: the peritoneal cavity, the subcutaneous tissues, the vascular network via cardiac or tail vein puncture, under the renal capsule, and intracerebrally. The information forthcoming from xenograft trials is summarized in Table 2.1. For most drugs intended for treatment of extracerebral tumors, subcutaneous flank locations are preferred, as tumor growth and response to drug treatment can be easily monitored, either visually or by fluorescent labeling. Tumor cell lines, explants, and organoids can now be developed with variable efficiency from human tumors or even circulating tumor cells in the peripheral blood. In general, these tumors are essential tools for drug development, and for studies of tumor genomic heterogeneity and mechanisms of drugs resistance. They are not yet practical vehicles for selecting treatment for individual patients.

Transgenic animals expressing targets of interest have been used for *in vivo* assessment of drug action. Intrinsic limitations to their use include variability in penetrance and an unpredictable latency in tumor development. However, the impact of chemotherapeutic agents on tumor development and growth may be assessed following treatment at various times. A drawback to their use in drug development is the fact that they represent an "artificial" mouse tumor developed against a genetic background that may not reflect the variety of features of human tumor containing the same oncogene. A *KRAS*

<table>
<tr><td>

TABLE

2.1 *Parameters for assessing drug efficacy in subcutaneous xenograft models*

</td></tr>
</table>

Efficacy against a subset of human tumors bearing the intended selective biomarker
- Tumor weight (treated/control)
- Median days to tumor reaching specified weight or doubling volumes
- Growth delay at a specified tumor weight or doubling volume
- Net log cell kill
- Number of complete and partial tumor regressions
- Dose-response relationship
- Pharmacodynamic biomarkers

Toxicity
- Dose-toxicity relationship
- Organ-specific toxicity
- Treatment-related weight loss

Pharmacokinetics
- Bioavailability
- Plasma levels over time
- Metabolism and route of clearance

GEMMS model of lung cancer may not be representative of human *KRAS*-driven lung cancer, let alone *KRAS*-driven pancreatic, or colon cancer.

While transgenic mice may be of research interest, their use as a routine subject is further limited by the time required for tumor development, the lack of synchrony in tumor development among litter mates, and the need for multiple animals to obtain statistically meaningful results.

Improving Drug-Like Properties

As a compound approaches development for clinical trials, the molecule may have to be modified to yield acceptable bioavailability, distribution, metabolism, and excretion. Historically, considerable effort in drug discovery programs has been spent refining drug leads that subsequently fail in the development process because of inability to correct toxicity issues or poor pharmacokinetic properties.

The development of predictive, inexpensive, *in vitro* assays and computer models to quantify pharmacologic properties is helping to alleviate this lead development bottleneck and substantially enhancing the multidisciplinary character of drug discovery. For example, assays such as those developed by Exelixis, Inc. (San Francisco, CA) use parameters including partition coefficients, P-glycoprotein efflux, P-450 induction and metabolism, and protein binding to predict the pharmacokinetics of novel compounds. These assays have been refined with the use of *in vivo* data from animals and humans. Commercially available software packages rely entirely on "well-trained" computer algorithms to predict compound absorption (e.g., GastroPlus [Simulations Plus, Inc., Lancaster, CA]), subcompartment penetration, plasma protein binding, and metabolism (MetabolExpert [CompuDrug International Inc., Sedona, AZ], META [Multicase, Beachwood, OH], and Meteor LHASA,

Department of Chemistry, Leeds, UK). These and other similar model systems permit analysis of the pharmacologic properties of a larger number of compounds early in the development process, and hopefully reduce the rates of compound failure later in development.

Conclusion

The process of cancer drug discovery has dramatically changed over the past 50 years. At first, based on empirical screening in murine tumors, it has progressed to a highly targeted approach employing all the tools of structural analysis, computer-based decision making, and highly sophisticated chemistry to develop potent and specific inhibitors. The importance of selectivity is still under debate. Most clinically effective kinase inhibitors such as imatinib and cabozantinib inhibit multiple kinases. Although, the traditional teaching is that high specificity is most desirable in terms of limiting toxicity, in the case of cabozantinib, a highly effective drug for renal cell cancers and hepatocellular cancer, it is not clear to what degree its multiple sites of action (VEGFR2, C-MET, AXL, MNK) contribute to its antitumor activity.[62] Despite these improvements in specificity and biological focus, it remains a risky and unpredictable adventure, surely worthwhile and deserving of reward for those that succeed in reaching the goal line of drug approval. Whether drugs will ultimately defeat cancer will depend on an improved understanding of cancer biology, tumor heterogeneity, and drug resistance.

References

1. Gilman A. The initial clinical trial of nitrogen mustard. *Am J Surg.* 1963;105:574-578.
2. Chabner BA, Roberts TG Jr. Chemotherapy and the war on cancer. *Nat Rev Cancer.* 2005;5:65-72.
3. Chabner BA. NCI-60 cell line screening: a radical departure in its time. *J Natl Cancer Inst.* 2016;108:pii: doi: 10.1093/jnci/djv388.
4. Abaan OD, Polley EC, Davis SR, et al. The exomes of the NCI-60 panel: a genomic resource for cancer biology and systems pharmacology. *Cancer Res.* 2013;73: 4372-4382.
5. Reinhold WC, Varma S, Sunshine M, et al. The NCI-60 methylome and its integration into CellMiner. *Cancer Res.* 2017;77:601-612.
6. Wall ME, Wani MC. Camptothecin and taxol: from discovery to clinic. *J Ethnopharmacol.* 1996;51:239-253.
7. Rosenberg B. Anticancer activity of cis-dichlorodiammineplatinum(II) and some relevant chemistry. *Cancer Treat Rep.* 1979;63(9-10):1433-1438.
8. Varmus HE. Nobel lecture. Retroviruses and oncogenes. *Biosci Rep.* 1990;10:413-430.
9. Ross JS, Ali SM, Block J, et al. ALK fusions in a wide variety of tumor types respond to anti-ALK targeted therapy. *Oncologist.* 2017;22:1444-1450. doi: 10.1634/the oncologist.2016-0488.
10. Ramos AH, Lichtenstein L, Gupta M, et al. Oncotator: cancer variant annotation tool. *Hum Mutat.* 2015;36:E2423-E2429. doi: 10.1002/humu.22771.
11. Lynch TJ, Bell DW, Sordella R, et al. Activating mutations in the epidermal growth factor receptor underlying responsiveness of non-small-cell lung cancer to gefitinib. *N Engl J Med.* 2004;350:2129-2139.
12. Schramek D, Sendoel, A, Segal JP, et al. Direct in vivo RNAi screen unveils myosin IIa as a tumor suppressor of squamous cell carcinoma. *Science.* 2014;343:309-317.
13. Iorns E, Lord CJ, Turner N, et al. Utilizing RNA interference to enhance drug discovery. *Nat Rev Drug Discov.* 2007;6:556-568.
14. Wang T, Yu H, Hughes NW, et al. Gene Essentiality profiling reveals gene networks and synthetic lethal interactions with oncogenic RAS. *Cell.* 2017;168:890-903.

15. Coussens NP, Braisted JC, Peryea T, Sittampalam GS, Simeonov A, Hall MD. Small-molecule screens: a gateway to cancer therapeutic agents with case studies of food and drug administration-approved drugs. *Pharmacol Rev.* 2017;69:479-496.

16. Zhang G-J, Safran M, Weil W, et al. Bioluminescent imaging of Cdk2 inhibition in vivo. *Nat Med.* 2004;10:643-648.

17. Wiley DS, Redfield SE, Zon LI. Chemical screening in zebrafish for novel biological and therapeutic discovery. *Methods Cell Biol.* 2017;138:651-679.

18. Kaufman CK, Mosimann C, Fan ZP, et al. A zebrafish melanoma model reveals emergence of neural crest identity during melanoma initiation. *Science.* 2016;351:aad2197. doi: 10.1126/science.aad2197.

19. Ribich S, Harvey D, Copeland RA. Drug discovery and chemical biology of cancer epigenetics. *Cell Chem Biol.* 2017;24:1120-1147.

20. Shoemaker RH, Scudiero DA, Melillo G, et al. Application of high-throughput, molecular targeted screening to anticancer drug discovery. *Curr Top Med Chem.* 2002;2:229-246.

21. Hajduk PJ, Huth JR, Fesik SW. Druggability indices for protein targets derived from NMR-based screening data. *J Med Chem.* 2005;48:2518-2525.

22. Pye CR, Berlin MJ, Lokey RS, et al. Retrospective analysis of natural products provides insights for future discovery trends. *Proc Natl Acad Sci U S A.* 2017;114:5601-5606.

23. Cragg GM, Grothaus PG, Neuman DJ. Impact of natural products on developing new anticancer agents. *Chem Rev.* 2009;109:3012-3043.

24. Cai X, Gray PJ, von Hoff DD. DNA minor groove binders: back in the groove. *Cancer Treat Rev.* 2009;35:437-460.

25. Zimmerman G, Papke B, Ismail S, et al. Small molecule inhibition of the KRAS-PDE delta interaction impairs oncogenic signaling. *Nature.* 2013;497:638-642.

26. Geysen HM, Meloen RH, Barteling SJ. Use of peptide synthesis to probe viral antigens for epitopes to resolution of a single amino acid. *Proc Natl Acad Sci U S A.* 1984;81:3998-4002.

27. Marchand JR, Dalle Vedove A, Lolli G, Caflisch A. Discovery of inhibitors of four bromodomains by fragment-anchored ligand docking. *J Chem Inf Model.* 2017;57:2584-2597.

28. Fitzgerald K, Kallend D, Simon A. A highly durable RNAi therapeutic inhibitor of PCSK9. *N Engl J Med.* 2017;376:41-51. doi: 10.1056/NEJMoa1609243.

29. Malek-Adamian E, Guenther DC, Matsuda S, et al. 4′-C-methoxy-2′-deoxy-2′fluoro modified ribonucleotides improve metabolic stability and elicit efficient RNAi -mediated gene silencing. *J Am Chem Soc.* 2017;139:14542-14555.

30. Beck A, Goetsch L, Dumontet C, Corvaia N. Strategies and challenges for the next generation of antibody-drug conjugates. *Nat Rev Drug Discov.* 2017;16:315-337.

31. Nagayama A, Ellisen LW, Chabner B, Bardia A. Antibody-drug conjugates for the treatment of solid tumors: clinical experience and latest developments. *Target Oncol.* 2017;12:719-739. doi: 10.1007/s11523-01700535-0.

32. Eichenauer DA, Plutschow A, Kreissi S. Incorporation of brentuximab vedotin into first-line treatment of advanced classical Hodgkin's lymphoma: final analysis of a phase 2 randomised trial by the German Hodgkin Study Group. *Lancet Oncol.* 2017;18:1680-1687. doi: 101016/S1470-2045(17)30696-4.

33. Goodwin CD, Gale RP, Walter RB. Gemtuzumab ozogamicin in acute myeloid leukemia. *Leukemia.* 2017;31:1865-1868.

34. Cox AD, Der CJ, Philips MR. Targeting RAS membrane association: back to the future for anti-RAS drug Discovery? *Clin Cancer Res.* 2015;21(8):1819-1827.

35. Ostrem JML, Shokat KM. Direct small-molecule inhibitors of KRAS: from structural insights to mechanism-based designs. *Nat Rev Drug Discov.* 2016;15:771-784.

36. Singh H, Longo DL, Chabner BA. Improving prospects for targeting RAS. *J Clin Oncol.* 2015;33:3650-3659.

37. Keeton AB, Salter EA, Piazza GA. The RAS-effector interaction as a drug target. *Cancer Res.* 2017;77:221-226.

38. Westover KD, Janne PA, Gray NS. Progress on Covalent inhibition of KRAS(G12C). *Cancer Discov.* 2016;6:233-234.

39. Braun T, Gardin C. Investigational BET bromodomain protein inhibitors in early stage clinical trials for acute myelogenous leukemia (AML). *Expert Opin Investig Drugs.* 2017;26(7):803-811.

40. Urick AK, Hawk LML, Cassel MK, et al. Dual screening of BPTF and Brd4 using protein-observed fluorine NMR uncovers new bromodomain probe molecules. *ACS Chem Biol.* 2015;10:2246-2256.

41. Flynn Rl, Jeitany M, Wakimoto H, et. al. Alternative lengthening of telomerase renders cancer cells hypersensitive to ATR inhibitors. *Science.* 2015;347:273-277.

42. Flynn RL, Cox KE, Jeitany M, et al. Alternative lengthening of telomeres renders cancer cell hypersensitive to ATR inhibitors. *Science.* 2015;347(6219):273-277.

43. Lord CJ, Ashworth A. PARP inhibitors: synthetic lethality in the clinic. *Science.* 2017;355:1152-1158.

44. Balasubramaniam S, Kim GS, McKee AE, Pazdur R. Regulatory considerations on endpoint in ovarian cancer drug development. *Cancer.* 2017;123:2604-2608.

45. Kaelin WG Jr. The concept of synthetic lethality in the context of anticancer screening. *Nat Rev Cancer.* 2005;5:689-698.

46. Izar B, Rotow J, Jainor J et al. Pharmacokinetics, clinical indications and resistance mechanisms in molecular targeted therapies in cancer. *Pharmacol Rev.* 2013;65:1351-1395.

47. Massaro F, Molica M, Breccia M. Ponatinib: a review of efficacy and safety. *Curr Cancer Drug Targets.* 2017. doi: 10.2174/1568009617666171002142659.

48. Soria JC, Ohe Y, Vansteenkiste J, et al. Osimertinib in untreated EGFR-mutated advanced non-small cell lung cancer. *N Engl J Med.* 2018;378:113-125. doi: 10.1056/NEJMMos1713137.

49. Yvers A. Osimertinib (AZD9291)—a science-driven, collaborative approach to rapid drug design and development. *Ann Oncol.* 2016;27:1165-1170.

50. Peters S, Camidge DR, Shaw AT, et al. Alectinib versus crizotinib in untreated ALK-positive non-small cell lung cancer. *N Engl J Med.* 2017;377:829-838.

51. Shaw AT, Friboulet L, Leshchiner I, et al. Resensitization to crizotinib by the lorlatinib ALK resistance mutation L1198F. *N Engl J Med.* 2016;374:54-61.

52. Muller S, Chaikuad C, Fray NA, Knapp S. The ins and outs of selective kinase inhibitor development. *Nat Chem Biol.* 2015;11:818-822.

53. Xing L, Huang A. Bruton's TK inhibitors: structural insights and evolution of clinical candidates. *Future Med Chem.* 2014;6:675-695.

54. Tap WD, Wainberg ZA, Anthony SP, et al. Structure-guided blockade of CSF 1R Kinase in tenosynovial giant-cell tumor. *N Engl J Med.* 2015;373:428-437.

55. Ayoub A, Hawk LM, Herzig Rj, et al. BET bromodomain inhibitors with one-step synthesis discovered from virtual screen. *J Med Chem.* 2017;60:4805-4817.

56. Khotskkaya YB, Holla VR, Farago AF, et al. Targeting TRK family proteins in cancer. *Pharmacol Ther.* 2017;173:58-66.

57. Richon VM, Zhou X, Rifkind RA, Marks PA. Histone deacetylase inhibitors: development of suberoylanilide hydroxamic acid (SAHA) for the treatment of cancers. *Blood Cells Mol Dis.* 2001;1:260-264.

58. Dang L, Su SM. Isocitrate dehydrogenase mutation and (R)-2-hydroxyglutarate: from basic discovery to therapeutics development. *Annu Rev Biochem.* 2017;86:305-331.

59. Ember SW, Lambert QT, Berndt N, et al. Potent Dual BET bromodomain-kinase inhibitors as value-added multitargeted chemical probes and cancer therapeutics. *Mol Cancer Ther.* 2017;16:1054-1067.

60. Weeber R, Ooft SN, Dijkstra KK, Voest EE. Tumor organoids as a pre-clinical cancer model for drug discovery. *Cell Chem Biol.* 2017;24:1092-1100.

61. Clohessy JG, Pandolfi PP. Mouse hospital and co-clinical trial project—from bench to bedside. *Nat Rev Clin Oncol.* 2015;12:491-498.

62. Tannir NM, Schwab G, Grunwald V. Cabozantinib: an active novel multikinase inhibitor in renal cell carcinoma. *Curr Oncol Rep.* 2017;19:14.

Clinical Drug Development and Approval

Gideon M. Blumenthal

In the past decade, improved understanding of the underlying molecular and immunologic foundations of cancer has led to an unprecedented pace of oncology drug development. While there has been progress in the prevention and treatment of cancer,[1] the global burden of cancer in the United States and around the world remains vast and is likely to increase as the population ages and deaths due to infectious disease decrease. Oncology drug development has attracted overwhelming interest from the international pharmaceutical and biotechnology sectors and now accounts for about 40% of the global clinical pipeline with two to three times the active compounds in development compared with any other therapeutic area. In addition, the number of active compounds in development has reportedly quadrupled since 1996 and nearly doubled since 2008. For the U.S. Food and Drug Administration (FDA) Office of Hematology Oncology Products (OHOP), the pace of approval of oncology drugs has also quickened, as reflected in the average number of approvals of New Molecular Entity (NME) New Drug Applications (NDA) or Biologics License Applications (BLA), which increased from 4.5 per year from 1993 to 1996 to 9 per year from 2013 to 2016 (Fig. 3.1). This chapter will briefly review the drug approval process for cancer drugs, highlighting the changes that have taken place in response to the scientific evolution of the cancer research field and the need for a more flexible and responsive regulatory process.

Investigational New Drug

An investigational new drug (IND) is an exemption under the Interstate Commerce Act that allows for the interstate shipment of nonapproved drugs, also known as investigational drugs. There are certain legal requirements applicable to IND sponsors and clinical investigators when conducting a clinical investigation under an IND. These include informed consent requirements and Institutional Review Board (IRB) requirements.

A drug is defined as an article that is intended for use in the diagnosis, cure, mitigation, treatment, or prevention of disease *and* is an article (other than food) intended to affect the structure or any function of the body. Biological products (e.g., therapeutic cellular products, monoclonal antibodies, therapeutic cytokines) subject to licensure under section 351 of the Public Health Service Act may also be considered drugs within the scope of the Food, Drug, and Cosmetic Act. An IND is required in the United States to administer an unapproved drug to humans. If an investigator intends to conduct a clinical trial using commercial supplies of a lawfully marketed drug product, an IND may be exempt if certain conditions are met.

FDA Review of INDs

The FDA's major objectives during the review of an IND are to assure the safety and rights of subjects and to assure that the quality of a scientific investigation (particularly in phase 2 and 3 trials) is adequate to permit an evaluation of safety and efficacy. Within 30 days of receipt of a new IND, FDA will either allow the IND to proceed or will place the IND on hold. An IND must contain information pertaining to a drug's chemistry, manufacturing, and controls (CMC) and the drug's pharmacology and toxicology. A clinical protocol must also be submitted. In most cases, the IND must contain an Investigator's Brochure.

When an IND is received, quality staff (e.g., chemists, biologists, or microbiologists) will review data to assure the proper identification, quality, purity, and strength (or potency) of the product. Toxicology reviewers assess animal studies and other toxicology data. The clinical reviewer assesses the adequacy of protocols and risks to patients, as supported by animal or human data. A statistician may evaluate the appropriateness of the statistical analysis plan. A clinical pharmacologist evaluates the characterization of the investigational drug's pharmacokinetic profile in the target patient population and in special populations (e.g., in patients with hepatic or renal impairment).

Opportunities to Obtain Feedback from the FDA During the IND Process

Given the complexity of oncology drug development, the FDA recommends obtaining feedback during the drug development process in the form of meetings.[2] For example, a milestone meeting is an opportunity for sponsors to meet with the FDA to discuss the development program. Examples of meetings include pre-IND meetings, end-of-phase 1 or end-of-phase 2 meetings, and pre-New Drug Application or pre-Biologics License Application meetings.

New Drug Application and Biologics License Application

For a drug to be marketed in the United States, it must demonstrate efficacy and an acceptable safety profile in adequate and well-controlled clinical trials, with acceptable benefit–risk. The sponsor will submit the results of the clinical trials in clinical study reports, the primary and derived data sets, the summary of clinical

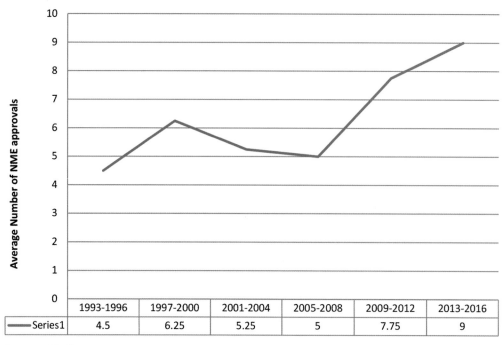

FIGURE **3.1** Average number of Office of Hematology Oncology Approvals of New Drug Applications and Biologics License Applications that are New Molecular Entities in 4-year intervals 1993 to 2016.

effectiveness, summary of clinical safety, an integrated summary of effectiveness, an integrated summary of safety, and draft product labeling in a NDA or BLA submission. The FDA will convene a multidisciplinary review team to review the application, including experts in clinical, pharmacology-toxicology, clinical pharmacology, biostatistics, chemistry manufacturing, product labeling, and drug safety. In addition to the multidisciplinary review, the FDA will often dispatch inspectors to the manufacturing sites and the clinical trial sites. Depending on the type of application, the review may be a standard review (typically a 10- to 12-month review clock) or a priority review (typically a 6- to 8-month review clock). Should advice on an NDA or BLA be necessary, FDA will convene the Oncologic Drugs Advisory Committee (ODAC).

Changes in the FDA Oncology Review Office

With the improved scientific understanding of the molecular and immunologic underpinnings of cancer, better drug discovery and drug development tools, and the urgency to make effective treatments available to patients with cancer, the FDA Oncology office has evolved. Contrary to public assertions, the median time for review of new cancer medicines in the United States outpaces the rest of the world, including Europe, with a median time of 6 to 7 months for FDA cancer drug review, versus 12 months for cancer drug review in the European Medicines Agency (EMA).[3,4] The evolving science has also led to instances, which have defied the typical estimated decade of drug development, from first-in-human (FIH) IND filing to FDA approval, with examples of drugs such as ceritinib and osimertinib taking 3 years or less to go from FIH to approval.[5,6] This chapter will review recent approvals in targeted therapy and immunotherapy, as well as regulatory initiatives to expedite the development of safe and effective anticancer agents.

Targeted Therapies

The landmark approvals of trastuzumab in 1998 for HER2-positive metastatic breast cancer and imatinib in 2003 for chronic myeloid leukemia paved the way for precision oncology or finding the right drug for the right patient at the right time. Since then, the FDA has considered an increasing number of impressively active drugs in molecularly defined subsets of otherwise poorly responsive tumor types and has developed an increasingly rapid and sophisticated approach to reviewing and approving these agents. For example, for patients with metastatic non–small cell lung cancer (mNSCLC), three epidermal growth factor receptor (EGFR) tyrosine kinase inhibitors (erlotinib, afatinib, and gefitinib) have been approved for treatment-naïve patients whose tumors harbor mutations in exon 19 or exon 21 in *EGFR*, and one (osimertinib) was approved for patients who develop the *EGFR* exon 20 T790M resistance mutation.[7–9] These actions required that clinicians have access to assays that reliably detect the specific mutations for which the drugs are active; thus, the FDA approved three tissue-based and one blood-based ctDNA companion diagnostic tests to detect EGFR mutations in NSCLC. Similar approvals, with companion diagnostics, occurred for patients with *ALK*-rearranged mNSCLC (crizotinib and ceritinib in the treatment-naive setting, and ceritinib, alectinib, and brigatinib for *ALK*-positive patients who have progressed on crizotinib)[10–12] and crizotinib for ROS1-rearranged mNSCLC, based on an expansion cohort of 50 patients in a phase 1 study.[13] For patients with BRAF V600E mutation–positive mNSCLC, the FDA approved the combination of dabrafenib and trametinib, based on sequential cohorts in a nonrandomized clinical trial.[14]

Identifying the right patient for these trials and for routine use of these drugs has required readily available and rapid molecular analysis of tumors. The development of next-generation sequencing

(NGS) platforms has addressed this challenge. These NGS platforms have replaced the earlier development paradigm of testing for single-gene/single-drug companion diagnostic model to a single multiplex platform that is able to detect mutations in hundreds of genes and thousands of variants in a single assay.[15] In June 2017, FDA approved the first NGS OncoPanel, the ThermoFisher Oncomine test to detect EGFR mutations, ROS1 translocations, and BRAF V600 mutations in patients with advanced NSCLC.

Targeted therapies now offer new treatment options for a broad range of solid and hematologic malignancies. Table 3.1 summarizes recent approvals of targeted therapy in oncology. Included in this table are the approvals of olaparib and rucaparib for patients with

TABLE

3.1   *Selected recent oncology targeted and immunotherapy approvals*

Therapy	Putative Target	Indication	First Approval/Most Recent Indication
Afatinib	EGFR L858R or del19	mNSCLC	2013/2016
Alectinib	ALK rearrangement	mNSCLC	2015
Atezolizumab	PD-L1	Urothelial, mNSCLC	2016
Avelumab	PD-L1	Merkel cell, urothelial	2017
Blinatumomab	CD19/CD3	Philadelphia-negative ALL	2014
Brentuximab vedotin	CD30	Hodgkin lymphoma, ALCL	2011/2015
Brigatinib	ALK rearrangement	mNSCLC	2017
Carfilzomib	Proteasome	Multiple myeloma	2012/2016
Ceritinib	ALK rearrangement	mNSCLC	2014
Cobimetinib	BRAF V600/Mek	Metastatic melanoma	2015
Crizotinib	ALK/ROS-1	mNSCLC	2011/2016
Dabrafenib	BRAF V600	Metastatic melanoma, mNSCLC	2013/2015
Daratumumab	CD38	Multiple myeloma	2015/2016
Dinutuximab	GD2	Pediatric neuroblastoma	2015
Durvalumab	PD-L1	Urothelial	2017
Elotuzumab	SLAMF7	Multiple myeloma	2015
Erlotinib	EGFR L858R or del19	mNSCLC	2004/2016
Gefitinib	EGFR L858R or del19	mNSCLC	2015
Ibrutinib	BTK	Mantle cell lymphoma, CLL, WM	2013/2016
Idelalisib	PI3K delta	CLL, B-cell NHL	2014
Ipilimumab	CTLA4	Melanoma	2011/2015
Ixazomib	Proteasome	Multiple myeloma	2015
Midostaurin	FLT3	AML	2017
Neratinib	HER2/neu	HER2+ extended adjuvant breast	2017
Nivolumab	PD-1	Melanoma, NSCLC, RCC, HL, HNSCC, urothelial	2014/2017
Obinutuzumab	CD20	Follicular lymphoma, CLL	2013/2016
Ofatumumab	CD20	CLL	2009/2016
Olaparib	BRCA/PARP	Ovarian	2014
Olaratumab	PDGFR-α	Soft tissue sarcoma	2016
Osimertinib	EGFR T790M	mNSCLC	2015
Palbociclib	CDK 4 and 6	Breast	2015/2016
Pembrolizumab	PD-1	NSCLC, melanoma, HNSCC, HL, urothelial, MSI-high	2014/2017
Pertuzumab	HER2/neu	Breast	2012/2013
Sonidegib	Hedgehog pathway	Basal cell	2015
Ribociclib	CDK 4 and 6	Breast cancer	2017
Rucaparib	BRCA/PARP	ovarian	2016
Trametinib	BRAF V600/Mek	Metastatic melanoma, mNSCLC	2013/2015
Vemurafenib	BRAF V600	Melanoma	2011
Venetoclax	BCL-2/17p deletion	CLL	2016

ALL, acute lymphoblastic leukemia; ALCL, anaplastic large cell lymphoma; CLL, chronic lymphocytic leukemia; HNSCC, head and neck squamous cell carcinoma; HL, Hodgkin lymphoma; mNSCLC, metastatic non–small cell lung cancer; NHL, non-Hodgkin lymphoma; WM, Waldenström's macroglobulinemia; MSI, microsatellite instability.

TABLE

3.2 *FDA-approved oncology drugs with companion diagnostics*

Therapy	Biomarker and Disease	Device Trade Name(s)
Afatinib; gefitinib	EGFR mutations in mNSCLC	Therascreen EGFR RGQ PCR Kit
Erlotinib; osimertinib	EGFR mutations in mNSCLC	Cobas EGFR Mutation Test V2 (for both tissue and plasma)
Pembrolizumab	PD-L1 expression mNSCLC	PD-L1 IHC 22C3 pharmDx
Crizotinib	ALK rearrangement in mNSCLC	Vysis ALK Break Apart FISH Probe Kit, VENTANA ALK (D5F3) CDx Assay
Trametinib; dabrafenib	BRAF mutations in melanoma	THxID BRAF Kit
Dabrafenib; trametinib, crizotinib; gefitinib	BRAF mutations, ROS1 rearrangements, EGFR mutations in mNSCLC	Oncomine Dx Target Test (NGS)
Vemurafenib; cobimetinib	BRAF mutations in melanoma	Cobas 4800 BRAF V600 Mutation Test
Trastuzumab	HER2 expression in breast cancer	INFORM HER-2/NEU, PATHVYSION HER-2 DNA Probe Kit, PATHWAY ANTI-HER-2/NEU (4B5) Rabbit Monoclonal Primary Antibody, INSITE HER-2/NEU KIT, SPOT-LIGHT HER2 CISH Kit, Bond Oracle Her2 IHC System, HER2 CISH PharmDx Kit, INFORM HER2 DUAL ISH DNA Probe Cocktail
Trastuzumab	HER2 expression in breast and gastric cancer	HER2 FISH PharmaDx Kit, HERCEPTEST
Olaparib	BRCA variants in ovarian cancer	BRCAnalysis CDx
Rucaparib	BRCA variants in ovarian cancer	FoundationFocus CDx BRCA Assay—NGS
Cetuximab; panitumumab	EGFR expression in colorectal cancer	DAKO EGFR PharmDx Kit
Cetuximab; panitumumab	KRAS mutations in colorectal cancer	Therascreen KRAS RGQ PCR Kit, Cobas KRAS Mutation Test
Panitumumab	RAS (KRAS, NRAS) mutations in colorectal cancer	Praxis Extended RAS Panel (NGS)
Imatinib	c-kit expression in GIST	DAKO c-kit pharmDx
Imatinib	KIT D816V aggressive systemic mastocytosis	KIT D816V Mutation Detection by PCR
Imatinib	PDGFRB gene rearrangement MDS/MPD	PDGFRB FISH
Venetoclax	17 p deletion in CLL	Vysis CLL FISH Probe Kit
Midostaurin	FLT3 Mutation in AML	LeukoStrat CDx FLT3 Mutation Assay

advanced refractory ovarian cancer, along with companion diagnostic test to detect deleterious germline mutations in the *BRCA* gene.[16,17] In addition, for melanoma patients with *BRAF* V600 mutations, the FDA approved two combinations of BRAF and MEK inhibitors (dabrafenib and trametinib; vemurafenib and cobimetinib), along with two companion diagnostics to detect these mutations.[18,19] Table 3.2 summarizes FDA-approved companion diagnostics in oncology.

Immunotherapies

The entry of targeted therapies into cancer treatment in the past two decades has been accompanied by an equally important development of immunotherapies in the past 10 years. Beginning with the 2011 FDA approval of ipilimumab, an anti-CTLA4 monoclonal antibody for treatment of advanced metastatic melanoma, the development of immune checkpoint inhibitors, predominantly targeting PD-1 and PD-L1, has moved at an unprecedented pace.[20] As of July 2017, FDA had approved two anti-PD-1—nivolumab and pembrolizumab—and three PDL-1 inhibitors, avelumab and atezolizumab,

for indications including melanoma, NSCLC, renal cell carcinoma, urothelial carcinoma, Hodgkin's lymphoma, squamous cell carcinoma of the head and neck, and Merkel cell carcinoma. A unique approval of a PD-1 inhibitor for tumors of any histological type harboring a mismatch repair defect (MSI-high) represented a major conceptual advance in the FDA approach. The number of new indications in various tumor types is rapidly expanding.[21–25] The FDA also approved one companion diagnostic test and two complementary diagnostic tests to detect PD-L1 expression on the tumor and/or immune cells in the tumor microenvironment.

As new immune checkpoint therapies enter late phases of clinical testing, novel combinatorial approaches that address resistance are being investigated. Furthermore, there is great interest in the development of new multiplex biomarkers assessing DNA, RNA, and protein aberrations, both within the tumor and the tumor microenvironment, to predict which patients will respond or are resistant to immune checkpoint inhibitors.[26] These predictive assess will allow the much needed refinement of the choice of drug and patient for immunotherapy.

Despite the progress and robust development of new immunotherapies and targeted therapies in certain advanced cancers, additional intermediate end points will be needed to detect signals of early activity, to prioritize combinations, and to interpret exploratory study results. Response and progression by conventional RECIST criteria may not fully reflect the clinical benefit of the immune checkpoint inhibitors. For example, in the "all-comer" second-line mNSCLC studies of anti–PD-1/PD-L1 therapy versus docetaxel, the ORR was relatively modest (roughly 15% to 20%), there were no improvements in PFS, and yet the overall survival (OS) was demonstrably superior, leading to drug approvals. Clinical trials of patients with other cancer types, including advanced head and neck cancer and urothelial cancer, have yielded similar results (modest ORR, no PFS improvement, OS improvements). These results require a reassessment of traditional reliance on radiographic responses to determine clinical benefit.

In addition, perhaps due to the delayed effect of certain immunotherapies in some patients, the rare unconventional radiographic patterns (such as immune cell infiltration of a tumor-mimicking disease progression) and the heterogeneity of patient populations studied, the Kaplan-Meier (K-M) curves that compare PFS or OS of patients treated with immunotherapy as compared to those treated with chemotherapy show nonproportionality and delayed separation.[27] While most patients do not appear to benefit from anti–PD-1 or anti–PD-L1 antibodies, a subset of patients derive long-term benefit. This may be analogous to anti–CTLA-4 therapy in metastatic melanoma, where long-term follow-up of patients demonstrated a "tail of the survival curve" indicating that a subset of patients are long-term survivors.[28]

Biomarker Development

In Vitro Diagnostic Devices

Devices, including in vitro diagnostic devices, can be classified based on the regulation necessary to provide reasonable assurance of its safety and effectiveness.[29] There are three classifications: class I, class II, and class III. The higher the classification, the more regulation the device is subjected to. The classification determines the type of premarket submission, namely, premarket approval application (PMA) submission, evaluation of automatic class III devices (de novo submissions), and premarket notification [510(k)] submissions.[30]

Companion Diagnostics

For the foregoing discussion, it is clear that biomarkers for patient selection and for predicting long-term benefit are exceedingly useful in expediting approval and understanding the limitations of new therapies. Once data have been collected in clinical trials, at the time of the NDA or BLA submission, the Center for Drug Evaluation and Research (CDER) performs the NDA or BLA review of clinical results, while the Center for Devices and Radiological Health (CDRH) reviews the companion diagnostic devices accompanying the submissions. The CDRH analysis determines whether the proposed biomarker test is validated as a laboratory assay, and whether it produces clinically useful and accurate results, and thus meets the standard for marketing authorization for the intended use.[31] In general, when FDA determines that a device (assay) is essential for the safe and effective use of a therapeutic product, the new drug product or new indication would not be approved absent the approval or clearance of the companion diagnostic. However, in some circumstances, FDA may decide to approve a therapeutic product if the companion diagnostic is not approved or cleared contemporaneously. For example, FDA did not approve a companion diagnostic for crizotinib for the ROS1 indication or for pembrolizumab for the histology-agnostic MSI-high solid tumor indication. In these cases, the compelling clinical benefit of these drugs in rare patient populations with fatal cancers outweighed the risks and uncertainties associated with a lack of companion diagnostic. Instead, the approval relied upon the local diagnostics performed in cancer centers and reached agreement with the drug sponsors on a plan to the develop companion diagnostics as a postmarketing commitment.

Complementary Diagnostics

During the device and drug review, the FDA may determine that the test is helpful but not essential for the safe and effective use of the drug. In these cases, where the test identifies a biomarker-defined subset of patients that responds differently to a drug and aids in the benefit–risk assessment for patients, the FDA may approve a complementary diagnostic and provide a description of the biomarker subset in product labeling. To date, there have been several "complementary diagnostic" determinations related to immunotherapies.[32,33]

Clinical Considerations: End Points

The appropriate primary efficacy end point(s) for a clinical trial will depend on the trial design and disease context, including specific disease site, organ of interest, and intent of therapy. Efficacy end points in cancer trials include radiographic end points, such as progression-free survival or objective response rate and duration of response, molecular end points such as major molecular response, and clinical outcomes such as OS or measures of symptoms or function.

Overall Survival End Point

Demonstration of an improvement in OS is the gold standard end point in oncology and has been commonly for oncology drug approval. Over the past 20 years, as cancer therapies have improved and as new strategies have allowed the very early identification of effective therapies in selected subsets of patients, FDA oncology and hematology reviews have evolved from the traditional requirement of two randomized, controlled trials demonstrating an improvement in OS for approval of a new therapy.[34] It is not always practical or feasible to demonstrate OS in diseases where patients can live for years following treatment, such as multiple myeloma or chronic lymphocytic leukemia, because trials required would delay the development and clinical use of effective therapies that address unmet needs. In addition, it may be unreasonable or even impossible to demonstrate improved OS with newer breakthrough therapies that target specific tumor mutations found in a very limited number of patients, making randomized studies impractical. In addition, equipoise may be lost, and a randomized trial against obviously inferior therapy may be unethical, when emerging data show that a new drug demonstrates overwhelming benefit, with acceptable safety, compared to other available drugs. FDA discussion with its ODAC and with patient advocacy groups has indicated a need for flexibility. Alternative end points such as objective response rate of sufficient duration and prolonged progression-free survival can be clinically relevant and meaningful and may be acceptable for drug approval in these circumstances. Other end points, employing pharmacokinetic assays, radiological assessment, and even pathological evaluations, have proved useful in the drug approval process.

Radiographic End Points (Overall Response Rate, Duration of Response, Progression-Free Survival)

For approvals based on ORR, the FDA has accepted single-arm, historically controlled trials, because (with rare exceptions) tumors do not shrink in the absence of therapy.[35] For approval, the response rate and duration should be of sufficient magnitude to either be considered as a surrogate *reasonably likely* to predict benefit (for accelerated approval) or to be considered as a clinical benefit in and of itself for regular approval.[36] PFS as a study end point generally requires smaller sample sizes and shorter follow-up compared to OS. Furthermore, PFS will not be influenced by subsequent therapies, which could potentially confound assessments of effects on OS. Nevertheless, PFS can be subject to unintentional ascertainment bias by investigators with knowledge of the treatment administered; therefore, blinded independent assessments of radiographs are often required by the FDA to mitigate the effects of such bias. Furthermore, attention to trial conduct is important in a study with a PFS end point, because missing data can complicate the analysis of PFS. To overcome these uncertainties, PFS improvements of large magnitude may provide reasonable assurance of clinical benefit if the overall benefit–risk is favorable.

Biomarker End Points

With the evolution of targeted therapies for cancer, biomarkers of tumor response may be valuable end points in the review of a new agent for approval. In CML, major molecular response is a validated surrogate and has been used for accelerated and regular approval in nonrandomized trials. Pharmacokinetic biomarkers may be sufficient in some circumstances. For example, the FDA approved glucarpidase, a folate-cleaving enzyme, for inactivation of toxic plasma methotrexate concentrations in patients with delayed methotrexate clearance due to impaired renal function. This approval was based on the demonstration of rapid and sustained clearance of otherwise toxic plasma methotrexate concentrations. Similarly, the FDA approved asparaginase *Erwinia chrysanthemi* for acute lymphoblastic leukemia in patients with hypersensitivity to *Escherichia coli*–derived asparaginase based on the proportion of patients who achieved a serum trough asparaginase level greater than or equal to 0.1 IU/mL, a level which correlates with effective antitumor activity.

Pathologic End Points

In 2013, the FDA granted accelerated approval to pertuzumab in combination with trastuzumab and docetaxel as neoadjuvant treatment of patients with HER2-positive, locally advanced, inflammatory, or early-stage breast cancer (either >2 cm in diameter or node positive) as part of a complete treatment regimen for early breast cancer based on demonstration of an improvement in pathological

complete response rate (pCR) and previous data in the metastatic setting demonstrating that pertuzumab improves OS of patients with HER2-postive breast cancer. In 2014, FDA finalized a guidance on pCR in neoadjuvant treatment of high-risk early-stage breast cancer as a potential end point to support accelerated approval.[37]

Expedited Programs

Demand for more rapid approval of drugs for patients with serious or life-threatening diseases and the improved ability to select the right patients for therapy have led to expedited development programs.[38] These new programs are particularly important in accelerating development and review of new drugs intended to address an unmet medical need in the treatment of a serious or life-threatening condition. Often, these patients have few or no other treatment options. Applicants must demonstrate how the product addresses an unmet medical need, such as providing greater benefit to patients than an available therapy, if one exists. The four FDA expedited programs are:

1. **Fast-Track Designation:** A therapy may be designated as fast-track product if intended for the treatment of a serious or life-threatening disease or condition and demonstrates the potential to address an unmet medical need. Preclinical or clinical evidence may be used for determining this designation. Under fast-track designation, applicants may meet frequently with the review team prior to filing an IND, as well as for meetings at the end-of-phase 1 and end-of-phase 2 to discuss study design and other issues that could address safety and efficacy as required to support approval. In addition, fast-track designation qualifies an applicant for a rolling BLA or NDA review.

2. **Breakthrough Therapy Designation (BTD):** The FDA Safety and Innovation Act (FDASIA) of 2012 established BTD with the understanding that given the rapidly evolving knowledge of the molecular basis of cancer and the discovery of new targets for drug development, FDA and industry need tools for those therapies that have transformative potential in providing benefit to patients.[39] BTD is available for drugs intended to treat a serious condition *and* where preliminary clinical evidence *indicates* that the drug may demonstrate substantial improvement on a clinically significant end point over available therapies.[40] This designation provides for an all-hands-on-deck commitment of FDA senior managers and experienced review staff. The designation allows the applicant to meet multiple times with the FDA on issues, such as manufacturing that arise within a compressed timeline. BTD does not guarantee future approval and may be rescinded if criteria are no longer met. As of July 2017, FDA approved drugs for 35 unique cancer indications that were granted BTD. The FDA has also approved many additional (supplemental) indications for already-approved BTD drugs.

3. **Accelerated Approval:** FDA published the final rule for the accelerated approval regulations in 1992. Accelerated approval is based on a surrogate end point reasonably likely to predict clinical benefit. This pathway may result in smaller and faster trials, as opposed to standard pathways for regular approval, which requires demonstration of an improvement in survival, or in quality of life, or an established surrogate. In addition, the

drug must treat a serious condition and provide a meaningful advantage over available therapies. Applicants must agree to complete postmarketing trials to confirm clinical benefit. If confirmatory trials fail, the FDA may take action to withdraw approval for the indication. Since its enactment, 92 oncology indications have received accelerated approval. Five of these indications have been withdrawn from the market; two of these (gefitinib and gemtuzumab ozogamicin) were subsequently approved for marketing after the correct patient population was identified (in the case of EGFR mutations in NSCLC for gefitinib) or the dose was optimized (gemtuzumab ozogamicin).

4. **Priority Review:** This designation provides a shorter time period for review of the application: within 8 months of receipt, compared with 12 months under standard review (this includes a 60-day filing period, after which the PDUFA clock begins). Priority review may be granted to a drug that treats a serious condition and, if approved, would provide a significant improvement in safety or effectiveness.

Seamless Oncology Drug Development

Increasingly in the clinical development of cancer drugs, the historical definitions for "phases" of clinical investigations (e.g., as described in 21 CFR 312.21) are devoid of meaning, as sponsors conduct the entire development program within a single clinical trial (which have exceeded 1,500 patients). For example, the keynote 001 trial began as a FIH dose escalation trial for pembrolizumab; following multiple protocol amendments and expansion cohorts ultimately led to accelerated approvals in advanced melanoma and PD-L1 high refractory NSCLC.[41,42] Such developmental approaches can be efficient and facilitate early access to investigational drugs; however, some are concerned that these protocols do not provide adequate oversight for drug-related toxicity. To ensure that "seamless" development plans are efficient and scientifically driven, these protocols should have statistical plans that provide justification for the sample size for each discrete phase, stage, or cohort.[43] Furthermore, an informed consent document appropriate for FIH use may require multiple modifications as the trial progresses and its objectives change or focus. Such trials require active, frequent, and clear communication between the sponsor, the investigational sites, and the agency.

The FDA has stated that these trial designs may be appropriate for certain drugs that appear highly active (i.e., drugs granted BTD). Nevertheless, trials should be carefully designed to ensure they are efficient and subject to external oversight of safety and more frequent real-time communication among sponsors, investigators, IRBs, regulators, and patients.

Biomarker-Directed Drug Development and "Master Protocols"

Master protocols offer another opportunity to increase the efficiency of drug development and bring promising new treatments to patients faster. A master protocol may include an evaluation of multiple drugs or may evaluate patients with multiple diseases,

with or without a common control arm. Furthermore, a master protocol may be amended to add or drop new treatment arms or substudies.[44] A common master protocol design allows for a patient's tumor to be tested for the presence of various biomarkers in order to assign the patient to treatment with drugs specifically targeted to treat that patient's particular tumor. Efficiency may be increased when such protocols use adaptive designs that, based on prespecified criteria, substitute a new investigational drug if one is not active or proceed to a randomized component (e.g., an adaptive trial) designed to formally evaluate the safety and effectiveness of the drug if promising activity is seen in a biomarker-positive population.

The design and conduct of master protocols can be challenging and require involvement from multiple stakeholders, including industry, patients, academia, and government (e.g., the NCI and the FDA). From a regulatory perspective, participation of both drug (or biologic) reviewers and device reviewers (CDRH) may be necessary. Several master protocols have been successfully launched and are awaiting results.

FDA Oncology Center of Excellence

Authorized by the 21st Century Cures Act and as part of the National Cancer Moonshot program, the FDA announced the planned formation of the Oncology Center of Excellence (OCE) on June 29, 2016. The OCE's role is to leverage the combined skills of the Agency's regulatory scientists and reviewers with expertise in drugs, biologics, and devices, to support an integrated approach to addressing cancer. One model for this approach is the academic cancer centers, which increasingly are structured in a multidisciplinary fashion to improve collaboration.[45] The OCE facilitates communication among the FDA's medical product centers, including the CDER, the Center for Biologics Evaluation Research (CBER), and the CDRH. The FDA formally announced the OCE's establishment on January 19, 2017.[46] On August 30, 2017, FDA approved tisagenlecleucel for the treatment of patients up to 25 years of age with B-cell precursor acute lymphoblastic leukemia that is refractory or in second or later relapse. This was the first CAR T-cell therapy approved by the FDA and the clinical review of this BLA was coordinated by the OCE.[47]

References

1. Garcia MC, Bastian B, Rossen LM, et al. Potentially preventable deaths among the five leading causes of death United States, 2010 and 2015. *MMWR Morb Mortal Wkly Rep.* 2016;65:1245-1255. doi: http://dx.doi.org/10.15585/mmwr.mm6545a1; doi:10.15585/mmwr.mm6545a1#_self

2. U.S. Food and Drug Administration. *Guidance for Industry: Formal Meetings between FDA and Sponsors or Applicants.* Silver Spring, MD: US Food and Drug Administration. Available at https://www.fda.gov/downloads/Drugs/.../Guidances/ucm153222.pdf, Accessed August 30, 2017.

3. Roberts SA, Allen JD, Sigal EV. Despite criticism of the FDA review process, new cancer drugs reach patients sooner in the United States than in Europe. *Health Aff.* 2011;30(7):1375-1381.

4. Downing NS, Zhang AD, Ross JS. Regulatory review of new therapeutic agents—FDA versus EMA, 2011–2015. *N Engl J Med.* 2017;376:1386-1387.

5. Chabner BA. Approval after phase 1: ceritinib runs the three-minute mile. *Oncologist.* 2014;19(6):577-578.

6. Yver A. Osimertinib (AZD9291)—a science-driven, collaborative approach to rapid drug design and development. *Ann Oncol.* 2016;6(1):1165-1170.

7. Khozin S, Blumenthal GM, Jiang X, et al. U.S. Food and Drug Administration approval summary: Erlotinib for the first-line treatment of metastatic non-small cell lung cancer with epidermal growth factor receptor exon 19 deletions or exon 21 (L858R) substitution mutations. *Oncologist.* 2014;19(7):774-779.

8. Kazandjian D, Blumenthal GM, Yuan W, et al. FDA approval of Gefitinib for the treatment of patients with metastatic EGFR mutation-positive non-small cell lung cancer. *Clin Cancer Res.* 2016;22(6):1307-1312.

9. Khozin S, Weinstock C, Blumenthal GM, et al. Osimertinib for the treatment of metastatic epidermal growth factor T790M positive non-small cell lung cancer. *Clin Cancer Res.* 2017;23(9):2131-2135.

10. Kazandjian D, Blumenthal GM, Chen HY, et al. FDA Approval Summary: Crizotinib for the treatment of metastatic non-small cell lung cancer with anaplastic kinase rearrangements. *Oncologist.* 2014;19(10):e5-e11.

11. Khozin S, Blumenthal GM, Zhang L, et al. FDA approval: ceritinib for the treatment of metastatic anaplastic lymphoma kinase-positive non-small cell lung cancer. *Clin Cancer Res.* 2015;21(11):2436-2439.

12. Larkins E, Blumenthal GM, Chen H, et al. FDA approval: alectinib for the treatment of metastatic, ALK-positive non-small cell lung cancer following crizotinib. *Clin Cancer Res.* 2016;22(21):5171-5176.

13. Kazandjian D, Blumenthal GM, Luo L, et al. Benefit-risk summary of crizotinib for the treatment of patients with ROS1 alteration-positive, metastatic non-small cell lung cancer. *Oncologist.* 2016;21(8):974-980.

14. Planchard D, Besse B, Groen HJM, et al. Dabrafenib plus trametinib in patients with previously treated BFAF(V600E)-mutant metastatic non-small cell lung cancer: an open-label, multicentre phase 2 trial. *Lancet Oncol.* 2016;17(7):984-993.

15. Blumenthal GM, Mansfield E, Pazdur R. Next-generation sequencing in oncology in the era of precision medicine. *JAMA Oncol.* 2016;2(1):13-14.

16. Balasubramaniam S, Beaver JA, Horton S, et al. FDA Approval Summary: Rucaparib for the treatment of patients with deleterious BRCA mutation-associated advanced ovarian cancer. *Clin Cancer Res.* 2017;23(23):7165-7170.

17. Kim G, Ison G, McKee AE, et al. FDA Approval Summary: Olaparib monotherapy in patients with deleterious germline BRCA-mutated advanced ovarian cancer treated with three or more lines of chemotherapy. *Clin Cancer Res.* 2015;21(19):4257-4261.

18. Robert C, Karaszewska B, Schachter J, et al. Improved overall survival in melanoma with combined dabrafenib and trametinib. *N Engl J Med.* 2015;372:30-39.

19. Larkin J, Ascierto PA, Dreno B, et al. Combined vemurafenib and cobimetinib in BRAF-mutated melanoma. *N Engl J Med.* 2014;371:1867-1876.

20. Hoos A. Development of immune-oncology drugs—from CTLA4 to PD1 to the next generations. *Nat Rev Drug Discov.* 2016;15(4):235-247.

21. Brawley L. With 20 agents, 803 trials, and 166,736 patient slots, is pharma investing too heavily in PD-1 drug development? *The Cancer Letter.* 2016;42(37).

22. Rosenberg JE, et al. Atezolizumab in patients with locally advanced and metastatic urothelial carcinoma who have progressed following treatment with platinum-based chemotherapy: a single-arm, multicenter, phase 2 trial. *Lancet.* 2016;387:1909-1920.

23. Ferris RL, et al. Nivolumab for recurrent squamous-cell carcinoma of the head and neck. *N Engl J Med.* 2016;375:1856-1867.

24. Kazandjian D, Khozin S, Blumenthal G, et al. Benefit-risk summary of nivolumab for patients with metastatic squamous cell lung cancer after platinum-based chemotherapy: a report from the U.S. Food and Drug Administration. *JAMA Oncol.* 2016;2(1):118–122.

25. Sul J, Blumenthal GM, Jiang X, et al. FDA Approval Summary: Pembrolizumab for the treatment of patients with metastatic non-small cell lung cancer whose tumors express programmed death ligand-1. *Oncologist.* 2016;21(5):643-650.

26. Melero I, Berman DM, Aznar MA, et al. Evolving synergistic combinations of targeted immunotherapies to combat cancer. *Nat Rev Cancer.* 2015;15:457-472.

27. Hellman DM, Kris MG, Rudin CM. Medians and milestones in describing the path to cancer cures: telling 'tails'. *JAMA Oncol.* 2016;2(2):167-168.

28. Maio M, Grob JJ, Aamdal S, et al. Five-year survival rates for treatment-naïve patients with advanced melanoma who received ipilimumab plus dacarbazine in a phase III trial. *J Clin Oncol.* 2015;33(10):1191-1196.

29. Tezak Z, Kondratovich MV, Mansfield E. US FDA and personalized medicine: in vitro diagnostic regulatory perspective. *Personalized Med.* 2010;7:517-530.

30. U.S. Food and Drug Administration. *FDA Overview of IVD Regulation.* Silver Spring, MD: US Food and Drug Administration Available at https://www.fda.gov/MedicalDevices/DeviceRegulationandGuidance/IVDRegulatoryAssistance/ucm123682.htm. Accessed August 30, 2017.

31. U.S. Food and Drug Administration. *In Vitro Companion Diagnostic Devices Guidance for Industry and FDA Staff.* Silver Spring, MD: US Food and Drug Administration. Available at https://www.fda.gov/downloads/medicaldevices/deviceregulationandguidance/guidancedocuments/ucm262327.pdf. Accessed August 30, 2017.

32. U.S. Food and Drug Administration. *FDA PD-L1 IHC 28-8 pharmDx Summary of Safety and Effectiveness Data.* Silver Spring, MD: US Food and Drug Administration. Available at https://www.accessdata.fda.gov/cdrh_docs/pdf15/P150027b.pdf. Accessed August 30, 2017.

33. U.S. Food and Drug Administration. *FDA VENTANA PD-L1 (SP142) Assay Summary of Safety and Effectiveness Data.* Silver Spring, MD: US Food and Drug Administration. Available at https://www.accessdata.fda.gov/cdrh_docs/pdf16/P160002B.pdf. Accessed August 30, 2017.

34. Blumenthal GM, Kluetz PG, Schneider J, et al. Oncology drug approvals: evaluating endpoints and evidence in an era of breakthrough therapies. *Oncologist.* 2017;22:762-767.

35. Blumenthal GM, Pazdur R. Response rate as an approval end point in oncology: back to the future. *JAMA Oncol.* 2016;2(6):780-781.

36. Simon R, Blumenthal GM, Rothenberg ML, et al. The role of nonrandomized trials in the evaluation of oncology drugs. *Clin Pharmacol Ther.* 2015;97(5):502-507.

37. U.S. Food and Drug Administration. *Guidance for Industry: Pathological Complete Response in Neoadjuvant Treatment of High-Risk Early-Stage Breast Cancer: Use as an Endpoint to Support Accelerated Approval.* Silver Spring, MD: US Food and Drug Administration. Available at https://www.fda.gov/downloads/drugs/guidances/ucm305501.pdf. Accessed August 30, 2017.

38. U.S. Food and Drug Administration. *Guidance for Industry: Expedited Programs for Serious Conditions—Drugs and Biologics.* Silver Spring, MD: US Food and Drug Administration. Available at https://www.fda.gov/downloads/drugs/guidancecomplianceregulatoryinformation/guidances/ucm358301.pdf. Accessed August 30, 2017.

39. Chabner BA. Breakthrough drugs and turtle soup. *Oncologist.* 2015;20(8):845-846.

40. Sherman RE, Li J, Shapley S, et al. Expediting drug development—the FDA's new "breakthrough therapy" designation. *N Engl J Med.* 2013;369:1877-1880.

41. Garon EB, Rizvi NA, Hui R, et al. Pembrolizumab for the treatment of non-small-cell lung cancer. *N Engl J Med.* 2015;372(21):2018-2028.

42. Caroline C, Ribas A, Wolchok JD, et al. Anti-programmed-death-receptor-1 treatment with pembrolizumab in ipilimumab-refractory advanced melanoma: a randomized dose-comparison cohort of a phase 1 trial. *Lancet.* 2014;9948:20-26.

43. Prowell TM, Theoret MR, Pazdur R. Seamless oncology—drug development. *N Engl J Med.* 2016;374(21):2001-2003.

44. Woodcock J, LaVange LM. Master protocols to study multiple therapies, multiple diseases, or both. *N Engl J Med.* 2017;377(1):62-70.

45. Pazdur R. Leveraging the power of collaboration at FDA's New Oncology Center of Excellence. June 29, 2016. Available at https://blogs.fda.gov/fdavoice/index.php/2016/06/leveraging-the-power-of-collaboration-fdas-new-oncology-center-of-excellence/

46. *Statement from FDA Commissioner Robert Califf, M.D., announcing FDA Oncology Center of Excellence launch.* January 19, 2017. Available at http://www.fda.gov/NewsEvents/Newsroom/PressAnnouncements/ucm537564.htm

47. *Statement from FDA Commissioner Scott Gottlieb, M.D., announcing FDA approval brings first gene therapy to the United States.* August 30, 2017. Available at https://www.fda.gov/NewsEvents/Newsroom/PressAnnouncements/ucm574058.htm

Principles of Pharmacokinetics

Jeffrey G. Supko and Jerry M. Collins

It is generally accepted that the biologic effects of a drug are related to the time course of the concentration of the administered compound or an active metabolite in the bloodstream. The realization of this association has evolved through advances in the discipline of pharmacokinetics. This discipline is defined as the study of rate processes involved in the absorption of drug from the administration site into the bloodstream, its subsequent distribution to extravascular regions throughout the body, and its eventual elimination from the body. From a broader perspective, pharmacokinetics may be thought of as the effect that the body has on a drug, whereas the pharmacologic effects that a drug has on the body are the realm of pharmacodynamics (PDs).

In anticancer chemotherapy, the general goal of killing tumor cells or inhibiting their proliferation and metastasis is clearly defined. However, in most cases, we are severely limited by an inability to deliver drugs in a manner that separates antitumor effects from normal tissue toxicity. Much remains to be learned about the exploitable differences between normal and tumor tissues. Thus, although pharmacokinetics is a tool that can be used to evaluate the feasibility of a drug delivery strategy based on intended PD effects, it does not replace knowledge of exploitable differences between host and tumor.

Studies to characterize the pharmacokinetic behavior of a drug have become integral to the preclinical and clinical development of new anticancer agents. One group[1] has even suggested that "it is now inconceivable to perform clinical research in cancer chemotherapy without obtaining adequate pharmacokinetic data." The objectives for undertaking a pharmacokinetic study in the context of a phase I or II clinical trial in cancer patients include (a) initial characterizing of the pharmacokinetic behavior of new chemotherapeutic agents in humans, (b) assessing whether or not an administration schedule provides a potentially effective pattern of systemic exposure to drug, (c) determining the magnitude of intrapatient and interpatient variability in pharmacokinetic parameters, (d) assessing the influence of patient characteristics on drug disposition, (e) establishing predictive correlations between biologic effects and pharmacokinetic parameters, and (f) determining whether combining drugs results in pharmacokinetic interactions. In addition, pharmacokinetic drug level monitoring has been used to improve therapy through dose individualization, to evaluate patient compliance during chronic therapy, and to assess whether alterations in drug disposition or metabolism are associated with the development of toxicity or the lack of effect.

The fundamental obstacle to greater success in the application of pharmacokinetics and clinical drug level monitoring to anticancer

therapy is our limited knowledge of PD. A complete understanding of the actions of a drug necessarily requires discerning the nature of the association between its pharmacokinetic behavior and PD effects. Relationships between pharmacokinetics and the severity of toxicity have been established for many anticancer drugs. However, pharmacokinetic associations accounting for the therapeutic effects of a chemotherapeutic agent are more difficult to establish because of the multiplicity of factors involving the host and tumor that influence response, as noted above, as well as the time lapse from initiating treatment to the first indications of a therapeutic response. In succeeding chapters, these relationships are discussed for individual agents. Nevertheless, elucidating the pharmacokinetic behavior of an anticancer drug may benefit efforts to determine the dose, route of administration, and schedule that maximize the therapeutic potential while minimizing serious toxic effects.

The intention of this chapter is to provide readers with a fundamental understanding of clinical pharmacokinetics and its practical application to the development and use of anticancer chemotherapy. Numerous texts with widely varying levels of complexity and focus are available for those interested in a more comprehensive discourse of the subject, ranging from easily understood introductions to the discipline[2] to more advanced texts with a mathematical approach.[3]

Acquisition and Analysis of Pharmacokinetic Data

Sample Collection and Drug Concentration Measurement

Pharmacokinetic studies involve collecting serial specimens of blood and other biologic fluids, such as urine, at predetermined time intervals from subjects following administration of the drug. Plasma is the blood component in which drugs are most commonly measured during pharmacokinetic studies, although determinations are also made in serum and, less frequently, in whole blood. The concentration of drug present in the study samples is measured using an appropriate bioanalytical method. Technical advances in separation and detection methods, especially the maturation of high-performance liquid chromatography coupled to mass spectrometry into a technique suitable for routine use, have provided a greatly improved basis for drug concentration measurement during the past decade. Review articles surveying the current techniques used for assaying drugs in biologic fluids regularly appear in the literature.[4]

Many anticancer drugs are difficult to measure because of inherent instability, either spontaneously degrading in solution or being degraded by enzymes in blood or tissues. It is therefore important to recognize that the quality of data derived from any pharmacokinetic study ultimately depends on the reliability of the assay used to measure the drug as well as the manner by which samples were processed and stored prior to analysis. The majority of bioanalytical methods used for pharmacokinetic studies measure the total concentration of drug, that is, free drug plus that which is reversibly associated with plasma proteins. However, the reversible binding of a drug to plasma proteins, such as albumin and α_1-acid glycoprotein, needs to be considered in the interpretation of total drug concentrations.[5] Only the free or unbound drug is pharmacologically active. Protein binding is usually assessed experimentally by ultrafiltration or equilibrium dialysis.

The Plasma Concentration-Time Profile

Except for cases in which a drug is given by bolus intravenous injection, the plasma concentration-time ($C \times T$) profile of any drug exhibits an initial region of increasing concentration, the achievement of a peak or maximum concentration (C_{max}), followed by a continual decline in concentration (Fig. 4.1A). The concentration of drug in plasma increases as long as the rate of input into systemic circulation exceeds the rate of loss due to distribution into other extracellular fluids, intracellular spaces, and tissues throughout the body and elimination from the body. The C_{max} is achieved when the rate of drug input is equivalent to the rate of loss from plasma, a time point that occurs at the instant that an intravenous injection or short infusion is terminated. During a continuous intravenous infusion, plasma levels of the drug increase at a progressively decreasing rate and eventually become constant, indicative of achieving steady-state conditions, if the infusion is continued for a sufficiently long time (Fig. 4.1C).

Figure 4.1 shows the same $C \times T$ data plotted on graphs with semilog axes (panel A) and rectangular coordinate axes (panel B). Presenting pharmacokinetic drug $C \times T$ profiles on semilog graphs provides a better visual depiction of the entire data set than a coordinate plot because plasma levels of a drug frequently differ by several orders of magnitude during the course of the observation period. Furthermore, the concentration of many drugs in systemic circulation decays in an apparent first-order manner, exemplified by a terminal region in the plasma profile in which the logarithm of the drug concentration is a linear function of time. Thus, a semilog plot provides some immediate inferences regarding the nature of the pharmacokinetic behavior of a drug.

The pattern of decay in the plasma concentration of a drug that exhibits first-order kinetics comprises one or more exponential phases. In the case of a plasma profile with drug concentrations that decline in a single log-linear phase, the entire body appears to be kinetically homogenous. In this case, the equilibrium of the drug between plasma and other fluids or tissues into which it distributes is very rapidly achieved, before the first blood specimen has been acquired. Polyexponential behavior results from distinguishable differences in the reversible transfer of drug from plasma to various

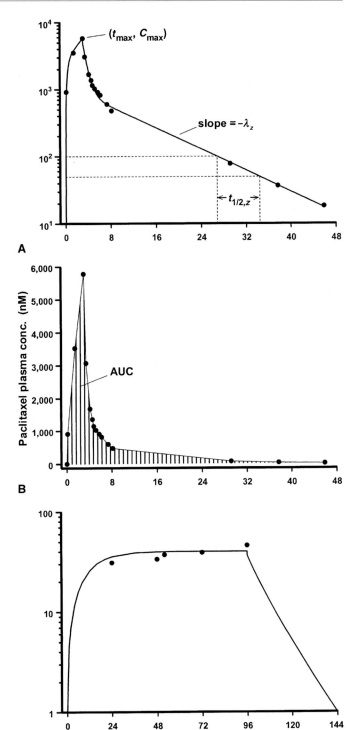

FIGURE 4.1 **A.** Plasma C × T profile for a 175 mg/m² dose of paclitaxel administered as a 3-hour continuous intravenous infusion shown on a graph with log-linear axes. Pharmacokinetic variables that can be estimated by visual inspection are indicated: maximum drug concentration (C_{max}), the time at which the peak concentration (t_{max}) occurs, and the biological half-life ($t_{1/2,z}$). **B.** Presentation of the same data shown in the upper panel on rectangular coordinate axes. The shaded area corresponds to the area under the curve (AUC). **C.** Time course of paclitaxel in plasma when given as a 96-hour continuous intravenous infusion at a rate of 25 mg/m²/d. The steady-state plasma concentration of the drug is approximately 40 nM.

regions or compartments of the body. Thus, for example, the presence of two exponential decay phases implies that the body behaves as if it is composed of two kinetically distinct compartments: the first comprising plasma and tissues with which equilibrium is rapidly established and the second "deeper" compartment comprising all other regions of the body into which drug distributes more slowly.

For some purposes, a mathematical equation or model is necessary to interpret pharmacokinetic data, but often questions may be answered without a formal model construction. Recently, there has been a growing trend toward analyzing pharmacokinetic data by empirical approaches that consider only the concentration of drug in the sampled fluid and require few assumptions about model structure. In these techniques, which include model-independent analysis[6] and noncompartmental analysis,[7] the various exponential decay phases are usually referred to simply as the initial, intermediate, and terminal disposition phases. Regardless of the particular method of analysis employed, the ultimate objective is the same, which is to estimate values of descriptive pharmacokinetic parameters from the C × T data.

Physiologic Pharmacokinetic Models

For pharmacologists interested in developing an understanding of drug disposition in individual tissue compartments, models that incorporate physiologic compartments are of considerable interest. These models require measurements of actual physiologic parameters, such as volumes and blood flow rates, as well as drug concentrations in various compartments, and therefore are based primarily on data from experimental animals. Entry into specific areas such as the central nervous system may be of critical importance in the use of drugs, and physiologic models can allow comparisons of C × T profiles for various schedules and routes of administration. Physiologic models have been constructed for many anticancer drugs. Models have been published for the most important drugs in clinical practice, among which are methotrexate (MTX),[8] 5-fluorouracil (5-FU),[9] cisplatin,[10] and doxorubicin.[11]

In the most general form, physiologic pharmacokinetic models are overly complex and require too large a database for routine clinical use. However, they provide a basis for understanding a drug's kinetic behavior that can be incorporated into simpler models, either physiologic or hybrid, assimilating both empiric observations and physiologic information. Physiologic modeling goes beyond the usual goals of empiric pharmacokinetic modeling to allow for incorporation of data obtained in other species or in vitro. The compartments comprising a physiologic pharmacokinetic model have an anatomic basis, and the transfer processes in the model have a physiologic or pharmacologic identity. Each organ is modeled separately; then, the model connections are provided by blood flow. The structure for the physiologic model for cytarabine is presented in Figure 4.2.[12]

Pharmacokinetic Parameters

Area Under the Curve

Noncompartmental analysis is considerably simpler than any equation-defining method of pharmacokinetic data analysis. All calculations and data manipulations can be performed by most spreadsheet software programs. The observed plasma C × T data are numerically integrated, most commonly by the trapezoidal method. In its

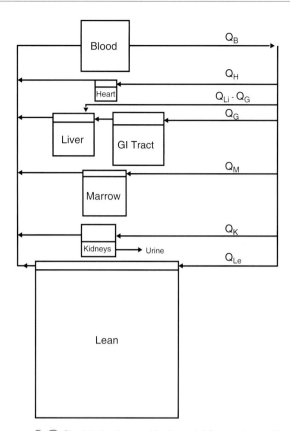

FIGURE 4.2 Physiologic pharmacokinetic model for cytosine arabinoside. GI, gastrointestinal. (Reprinted from Dedrick RL, Forrester DD, Cannon JN, et al. Pharmacokinetics of 1-β-D-arabinofuranosylcytosine (ARA-C) deamination in several species. *Biochem Pharmacol.* 1973;22(19):2405-2417. Copyright © 1973 Elsevier. With permission.)

simplest application, each successive set of data points, beginning with time zero, is used to define a trapezoid, the area of which is readily calculated. The cumulative sum of the areas of all such trapezoids affords an estimation of the area under the C × T curve to the last sample with a measurable drug concentration ($[C_t]$ $AUC_{0\rightarrow t}$). The slope of the terminal log-linear phase of the C × T profile ($-\lambda_z$) is then determined by linear regression using log-transformed concentration values (see Fig. 4.1A). The area under the curve from time zero to infinity (AUC) can then be calculated as

$$AUC = AUC_{0\rightarrow t} + C_t / \lambda_z$$

Although the AUC is not a pharmacokinetic parameter per se, because its magnitude depends on the administered dose of drug, it represents an important quantitative measure of total systemic drug exposure, as illustrated in Figure 4.1B. In addition, knowledge of the AUC is required to calculate values of pharmacokinetic parameters, as described in the following section.

Total Body Clearance

The total body clearance (CL) of a drug is formally defined as the volume of plasma from which drug is completely removed per unit time. It is readily calculated as

$$CL = D_{iv} / AUC$$

where D_{iv} is the dose of the drug given by intravenous injection or infusion. CL reflects the combined contribution of all processes by which drug is removed from the body, as represented by the equation

$$CL = CL_R + CL_{NR}$$

where CL_R and CL_{NR} designate renal and nonrenal clearance, respectively.[13] Renal clearance is usually the only route of drug elimination that can be directly and quantitatively determined in patients by noninvasive procedures. All other mechanisms of drug elimination that cannot be readily estimated, including biliary excretion of unchanged drug, metabolism, nonenzymatic irreversible reactions with endogenous molecules, and spontaneous chemical degradation, are grouped together as CL_{NR}. CL has units of volume per time (e.g., milliliters per minute, liter per hour) and is frequently normalized to the body weight or body surface area (BSA) of subjects (e.g., milliliters per minute per kilogram, liter per hour per square meter) under the presumption of minimizing interpatient variability in the magnitude of the parameter. However, the underlying presumption of a relationship between unnormalized clearance values and BSA does not exist for a significant number of anticancer drugs.[14] The CL values are often compared with glomerular filtration rate and hepatic blood flow, average values of which are approximately 125 mL/min (4.6 L/h/m²) and 1,500 mL/min (56 L/h/m²), respectively, in normal adults.[15,16] Although often informative, these comparisons can be extremely misleading unless the extent of plasma protein binding has been taken into account because only the free fraction of drug that is not bound to plasma proteins is usually subject to organ-mediated excretion or metabolism.

Apparent Volume of Distribution

The total body apparent volume of distribution, V_z, is strictly a proportionality constant relating the total amount of drug in the body to plasma concentration. It may be calculated by the equation

$$V_z = CL/\lambda_z$$

and has units of volume, typically expressed in terms of milliliters or liters normalized to body weight or BSA (e.g., milliliters per kilogram, liters per square meter). V_z is designated as an apparent volume because it is a hypothetical value that is not directly related to any real physiologic space. Nevertheless, it is an informative parameter, providing an indication of the relative extent of drug distribution from plasma. Specifically, for a given amount of drug in the body, the fraction present in plasma decreases as its distribution into peripheral tissues increases, leading to greater values of V_z.[17] Therefore, the effective lower limit of V_z is the plasma volume, which is approximately 4.5% of body weight (i.e., 45 mL/kg, 1.7 L/m²) for a normal adult. There really is no upper limit, as V_z can assume extremely large values in cases where the half-life of the terminal disposition phase is long relative to that of the preceding disposition phase, and drug levels decrease by several orders of magnitude before the terminal phase is achieved. For example, some anticancer agents, such as the anthracyclines, have V_z values exceeding 1,000 L/m² (27 times body weight).

Biologic Half-Life

The biologic half-life of a drug ($t_{1/2,z}$) is the time required for its plasma concentration to decrease by 50% any time during the terminal log-linear phase in the C × T profile (see Fig. 4.1A). It is only applicable to drugs that exhibit apparent first-order pharmacokinetics (see later discussion). As indicated by the relationship,

$$t_{1/2,z} = 0.693 \cdot V_z /CL$$

$t_{1/2,z}$ reflects both the ability of the body to eliminate the drug as well as the extent to which the drug distributes throughout the body. Nevertheless, there is a recurrent tendency in the anticancer drug literature to place undue emphasis on the value of $t_{1/2,z}$ as an indicator of drug elimination. The $t_{1/2,z}$ has an important practical application in that steady-state conditions during administration of a drug by continuous intravenous infusion or a multiple dosing regimen are achieved when the duration of treatment exceeds four times the value of $t_{1/2,z}$.

Linear and Nonlinear Pharmacokinetics

The majority of clinically used anticancer agents exhibit linear or first-order pharmacokinetics, whereby plasma concentrations of the drug decline in an exponential manner following intravenous administration. A distinguishing and defining characteristic of linear pharmacokinetics is that the plasma concentration of drug at a given time after dosing is directly proportional to the administered dose. Thus, the AUC increases proportionally with the dose and values of the pharmacokinetic parameters (i.e., CL, V_z) are independent of the dose. When a drug is predominantly eliminated by a potentially saturable process, such as hepatic metabolism or active tubular secretion, departures from linear pharmacokinetic behavior may become evident if sufficiently high doses can be administered to patients. As illustrated in Figure 4.3, classic nonlinear pharmacokinetics is indicated by a change in the appearance of the plasma profile from exponential character at lower doses to the appearance of a distinct downward curvature in the semilog plot of the plasma profile at higher doses.[18] In addition, the apparent CL exhibits a progressive decrease in magnitude as the dose is escalated. A clear

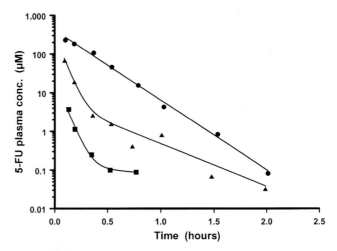

FIGURE 4.3 Plasma profiles of 5-flourouracil determined at doses of 25 mg/m² (■), 125 mg/m² (▲), and 375 mg/m² (●) illustrating the effect of classic nonlinear pharmacokinetics. Values of the apparent total body clearance decreased progressively from 142 L/h/m² for the 25 mg/m² dose to 47 L/h/m² at 125 mg/m² and 30 L/h/m² at 375 mg/m². There would be no significant difference between the clearance determined at different doses if the pharmacokinetic behavior of the drug was linear.

example of this phenomenon was reported recently for high-dose cytarabine given by continuous intravenous infusions in which small changes in the infusion rate produced disproportionately large increases in the steady-state drug concentration in plasma.[19]

Drug Elimination

Renal and Hepatic Excretion

Establishing the major pathways of drug elimination in patients is also an important objective of clinical pharmacokinetic studies. Disease states that compromise the function of a major drug-eliminating organ, such as the kidneys or liver, can enhance a patient's sensitivity to the toxic effects of the drug as a result of increased drug exposure. For this reason, patients with significant organ impairment are usually excluded from initial phase I studies to avoid possibly confounding sources of toxicity.

Renal excretion is a quantitatively significant route of elimination for many relatively small compounds, with molecular weights less than about 300, that are also highly to moderately hydrophilic,[20] if they are not substantially metabolized. Larger compounds and those with a more lipophilic character tend to be predominantly eliminated by biliary excretion, either directly or after metabolism. Determining CL_R involves measuring the amount of unchanged drug present in the urine (A_e) collected during one or more defined time intervals (Δt) following intravenous drug administration. It may be calculated by either of the following equations

$$CL_R = A_e / AUC_{0 \to t}$$

$$CL_R \approx (\Delta A_e / \Delta D_t) / C_{mid}$$

depending on whether urine has been continuously collected and pooled from the beginning of dose administration throughout the time that plasma specimens were obtained or during one or more discrete time intervals after dosing. In the second equation, C_{mid} is the plasma concentration of drug at the midpoint of the urine collection interval. The amount of unchanged drug in feces cannot be taken as a direct indication of biliary excretion because of the potential for drug metabolism by the gastrointestinal microflora.[21]

In cases in which renal or biliary excretion is a significant pathway of drug elimination, a predictive correlation may exist between clinical indicators of renal or hepatic function, such as serum creatinine and bilirubin levels, respectively, and CL. Establishing these relationships serves as the basis for defining guidelines pertaining to the minimal organ function required for patient eligibility in phase II studies and devising an empirical algorithm for dosage adjustment, including those documented in Table 4.1[22] (see also "Organ Dysfunction and its Effect on Drug Clearance").

Drug Metabolism

Metabolism represents a quantitatively important route of elimination for most anticancer agents. Xenobiotic biotransformation reactions may be broadly categorized into two classes, designated phase I and phase II. The principal phase I reactions are oxidation, reduction, and hydrolysis. Phase II reactions involve the conjugation or coupling of endogenous molecules, including glucuronide, sulfate,

TABLE **4.1**	*Predominant elimination mechanisms and dose adjustment recommendations for anticancer drugs*	
Major Route of Elimination	**Anticancer Agent**	**Dose Adjustment for Organ Dysfunction**[a]
Renal excretion	Bleomycin	b
	Carboplatin, cisplatin	b
	Etoposide	b
	Fludarabine	b
	Hydroxyurea	b
	Methotrexate	b
	Pentostatin	b
	Topotecan	b
Hepatic metabolism CYP450	Busulfan	c
	Chlorambucil	No
	Cyclophosphamide[b]	No
	Ifosfamide[b]	No
	Imatinib	b,c
	Irinotecan	No
	Paclitaxel	c
	Thiotepa	No
	Vinca alkaloids	c
Conjugation	Etoposide SN-38	c
Ubiquitous enzymes	Cytarabine	No
	Gemcitabine	No
	6-Mercaptopurine	d
Nonenzymatic hydrolysis	BCNU[b]	No
	Mechlorethamine	No
	Melphalan	No
Biliary excretion	Doxorubicin	No
	Irinotecan	No
	Vinca alkaloids	c

[a]b, decrease dose in proportion to the reduction in creatinine clearance below 60 mL/min; c, serum bilirubin: 1.5 to 3.0 mg/100 mL, 50% dose reduction; >3.0 mg/100 mL, 75% dose reduction; d, patients with *S*-methyltransferase deficiency; e, insufficient data to determine if dose reduction is necessary in hepatic dysfunction.
[b]Enzymatic or spontaneous chemical reactions required for drug activation.

amino acid, methyl, and glutathione moieties to the parent drug or a precursory phase I metabolite. Hepatic oxidation mediated by the cytochrome P450 (CYP450), a large family of heme-containing isozymes, undoubtedly plays the greatest overall role in drug metabolism among the phase I reactions.[23] The CYP450 enzymes are most abundantly expressed in the liver, but they are also present in the kidney, lung, and gastrointestinal epithelium. The predominant enzyme in this family, CYP3A4, catalyzes the oxidation of a multitude of structurally diverse compounds.[24–26] These include imatinib, gefitinib (and most other synthetic inhibitors of tyrosine kinases), docetaxel, etoposide, ifosfamide, vincristine, and paclitaxel. In addition to hepatic metabolism, some important phase I reactions are mediated by ubiquitous enzymes found in virtually all tissues of the body, such as dihydropyrimidine dehydrogenase, which catalyzes the reduction of 5-FU, and cytidine deaminase, which inactivates cytarabine.[27,28] Glucuronide conjugation catalyzed by uridine diphosphate glucuronosyltransferases (UGT) is the most commonly encountered phase II reaction. In contrast to phase I metabolism, which may yield a biologically active product, glucuronidation almost exclusively represents a detoxification mechanism that inactivates a compound and facilitates its excretion through enhanced hydrophilicity and recognition by biliary canalicular efflux proteins.[29] Glucuronidation is a clinically important route of elimination for 7-ethyl-10-hydroxycamptothecin (SN-38), the active metabolite of irinotecan, as the extent of its glucuronidation has been associated with the risk of severe diarrhea for the weekly treatment schedule of irinotecan.[30]

Chemical Degradation

Chemical degradation can be a significant elimination mechanism for drugs that are susceptible to hydrolysis or conjugation with sulfhydryls, such as many of the alkylating agents. Nonenzymatic reactions between drugs and endogenous molecules can also contribute prominently to elimination. For example, platinum-alkylating agents form covalent adducts with serum albumin and with small molecular weight sulfhydryls such as glutathione.[31]

Factors Contributing to Pharmacokinetic Variability

Obtaining an indication of interpatient variability in the values of pharmacokinetic parameters and related variables is an important objective of phase I trials. This information has considerable practical utility with regard to clinical drug development. These findings provide the basis for assessing the ability to reliably predict the C_{max} and AUC of a drug following the administration of any given dose to patients who have not been previously studied. The recommended dose of cytotoxic anticancer drugs is typically close to the maximum tolerated dose, and dose-limiting toxicities are often related in some manner to the levels of drug achieved in plasma. Thus, the margin of safety of these agents very much depends on the consistency of their pharmacokinetic behavior between patients. Conversely, the existence of a high degree of interpatient pharmacokinetic variability can result in unpredictable episodes of toxicity at the maximum tolerated dose, which may make it difficult to establish a potentially effective and safe dose. Although rarely employed in these circumstances, drug level monitoring to establish the optimal dosing regimen in individual patients may be warranted.

Patient Characteristics

Clinically significant associations between CL and patient characteristics including age, gender, weight, BSA, race or ethnicity, diet, and global region have been identified for many anticancer drugs. For example, it has been shown that the CL of 5-FU in females is significantly lower than in males and that formation of the glucuronide metabolite of SN-38 by UGT is subject to pharmacogenetic variations related to both race and gender.[32,33] The apparent oral clearance of alisertib, an investigational Aurora A kinase inhibitor, was found to be 40% lower in patients residing in East Asian countries as compared to patients from Western countries, resulting in 70% greater systemic

exposure to the drug at steady state when given by the same dose and schedule.[34] These factors are now being examined extensively during the global clinical development of new anticancer drugs.

Currently, more than half of all cancers occur in patients over 65. However, relatively few elderly patients are entered into early-stage clinical trials because of referral patterns, physiological limitations such as renal or hepatic function, or investigator bias. As a consequence, the pharmacokinetic behavior of most anticancer drugs has not been adequately characterized in elderly patients.[35] Older cancer patients display considerable heterogeneity in their handling of drugs as a result of age-related changes in body composition, including decreased muscle mass, increasing adipose tissue, and decreased renal function. Aging is accompanied by a 25% to 35% decrease in liver volume and a 35% to 40% decrease in hepatic blood flow.[36,37] Thus, the CL of drugs with a high hepatic extraction ratio, which is limited by liver blood flow, may be decreased in the elderly.[38,39] Age-associated decreases in the function of some drug-metabolizing enzymes have been identified, but their clinical significance remains uncertain.[40,41]

At the other end of the age spectrum, experience has shown that safe and effective doses of anticancer agents for children very often cannot be determined by scaling down from adult doses, using body weight or BSA.[42] Age-related changes are profoundly responsible for drug elimination and can have a profound effect on pharmacokinetics.[43] Thus, the rational use (alone or in combination) of drug eliminated by hepatic metabolism in adults requires the thorough characterization of pharmacokinetics and metabolism in children.

Organ Dysfunction and Its Effect on Drug Clearance

Physiologic conditions that affect hepatic or renal function, including blood flow to the liver or kidneys, can have a dramatic effect on the pharmacokinetic behavior of a drug in individual patients.[44] Powis[45] reviewed the effects of both renal and hepatic dysfunction for anticancer drugs. The estimation of creatinine clearance from serum creatinine concentration is a conveniently measured indicator of renal function. Hepatic function is more difficult to quantify. Serum transaminase and bilirubin concentrations provide indirect but somewhat useful information on hepatic function. Empirical guidelines for dose reduction in patients with underlying renal or hepatic dysfunction are devised by establishing relationships between these biochemical parameters and CL. In general, these adjustments would be expected to be less precise than adjustments based on drug level measurements. Occasionally, there is a close relationship between a renal function indicator and plasma pharmacokinetics. Egorin et al.[46] have elegantly applied such correlations for dose adjustments of carboplatin (Fig. 4.4) and other agents.[47] In fact, individualizing the dose of carboplatin to target a specific AUC value based on estimated creatinine clearance in patients has become a routine clinical practice.[48] Table 4.1 summarizes the recommended dose modifications for the standard anticancer drugs.

Drug Interactions

Essentially, all treatment protocols include combinations of drugs, encompassing two or more anticancer drugs, as well as various other drugs related to general symptomatic and supportive therapy of the patient. Many adjuvant medications that are routinely used in the management of cancer patients can potentially affect the pharmacokinetics of chemotherapeutic agents by either inhibiting or enhancing metabolic elimination (Table 4.2). Because cytotoxic

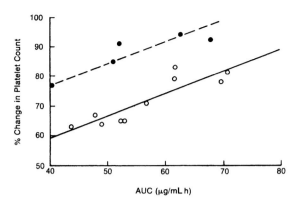

FIGURE **4.4** Relationship between thrombocytopenia and plasma levels of carboplatin. AUC, area under the concentration × time curve. Open circles (○) represent values in drug naive patients, while solid circles (●) represent values in heavily pretreated patients. (Data from Egorin MJ, Van Echo DA, Olman EA, et al. Prospective validation of a pharmacologically based dosing scheme for the cis-diamminedichloroplatinum(II) analog diamminecyclobutanedicarboxylatoplatinum. *Cancer Res* 1985;46:6502-6506.)

anticancer drugs are usually administered at their maximum tolerated doses, there is a substantially greater risk for pharmacokinetic interactions resulting in clinically significant toxicity than exists with drugs for most other indications. Accordingly, whenever possible, physicians should avoid administration of an anticancer agent together with another drug that modulates (induces or inhibits) the activity of an enzyme required for elimination of the first agent. Another important consideration is the highly variable pharmacokinetics of drugs predominantly eliminated by hepatic metabolism.[49] It is becoming increasingly apparent that genetic polymorphisms and mutations affecting key drug-metabolizing enzymes, including the cytochrome P450 enzymes, may account for aberrant pharmacokinetics in some patients or an otherwise high degree of interpatient variability (see Chapter 6).[50]

The serious adverse reactions caused by administration of ketoconazole to patients taking terfenadine,[51] which had been widely used and

considered to be a relatively safe antihistamine, provide a cautionary note for potential interactions with anticancer drugs because of their much narrower therapeutic index. Another common drug, cimetidine, is reported to inhibit the metabolism of cyclophosphamide[52] and hexamethylmelamine.[53] On the other hand, anticancer drugs interfere with the absorption of noncancer drugs, such as digoxin.[54] Balis[55] has reviewed the literature of drug interactions related to anticancer drugs. When evaluating drug-drug interactions, recent findings with paclitaxel illustrate the difficulties generated by interspecies differences in metabolic pathways.[56] Thus, animal studies may yield inaccurate predictions of drug interactions and metabolic pathways in humans.

Chemotherapeutic agents that are metabolized by the hepatic CYP450 system, especially members of the CYP3A subfamily, are particularly prone to pharmacokinetic interactions from the multitude of drugs and compounds of dietary origin that are inhibitors or inducers of CYP450.[57] A particularly serious example is the use of the dietary supplement, St. John's wort. This product induces drug-metabolizing enzymes and produces lack of drug efficacy.[58] Repeated daily administration of glucocorticoids, commonly used as antiemetics, can induce the expression of hepatic CYP450 and thereby enhance the CL of anticancer drugs that are CYP3A4 substrates.[59] In addition to hepatic drug-metabolizing enzymes, there are examples of pharmacokinetic interactions resulting from effects directed on other enzyme systems, excretory pathways, and even drug absorption. Salicylates can reduce the renal tubular secretion of MTX.[60,61] Morphine and its derivatives can alter the rate and extent of absorption of orally administered cytotoxic drugs by reducing gastrointestinal motility.[62] As discussed in a subsequent chapter, antiseizure drugs (dilation and phenobarbital) often used in brain tumor patients enhance the clearance of many anticancer agents, including most targeted agents, by inducing CYP450 enzymes.

Dose Individualization

The existence of a high degree of interpatient pharmacokinetic variability can result in unpredictable episodes of toxicity and make it difficult to establish a potentially effective and safe dose for the

TABLE

4.2 *Clinically significant pharmacokinetic drug interactions involving anticancer agents (for details of interactions, see relevant chapters)*

Chemotherapeutic Agent	Interacting Drug	Effect on Clearance of Anticancer Agent	Probable Mechanism
Cyclophosphamide	Phenobarbital	↑	CYP450 enzyme induction
Doxorubicin	Cyclosporin A	↓	Inhibits biliary excretion
Etoposide	Phenytoin	↑	CYP450 enzyme induction
Irinotecan		↑	
Paclitaxel		↑	
6-Mercaptopurine	Allopurinol	↓	Inhibits xanthine oxidase
	Methotrexate	↓	
Methotrexate	Aspirin	↓	Inhibits tubular secretion
	Probenecid	↓	
Paclitaxel	Verapamil	↓	Inhibits CYP450 metabolism or biliary excretion
Targeted small molecules	CYP inducers and inhibitors	↑↓	Altered CYP metabolism
Vinblastine	Erythromycin	↓	Inhibits CYP450 metabolism

population. For the individual, clinical monitoring and pharmacokinetics offer the possibility of tailoring drug delivery to the particular patient's needs. The standard doses derived from group studies do not allow for interindividual variability. However, doses may be adjusted on the basis of direct measurements of drug concentration in the individual patient, indicators of renal or hepatic dysfunction, or interactions of the anticancer drug with concomitant medications. Under these circumstances, it may also be beneficial to individualize doses of the drug based on plasma levels of the compound afforded by a test dose or a biochemical parameter that is predictive of CL.[63]

Tyrosine kinase inhibitors, including imatinib, erlotinib, sunitinib, and pazopanib, are a class of targeted anticancer agents for which good relationships between trough plasma concentrations of the drug and therapeutic efficacy have been established. Treatment with the approved dosing regimen for these drugs, which are administered orally once or twice daily on a continuous basis, failed to achieve their target steady-state trough plasma concentration at frequencies as high as 73% in patients receiving outpatient therapy.[64] It may be possible to improve the efficacy for these agents by dose adjustment based upon therapeutic drug monitoring in individual patients.[65,66] Improved response to anticancer treatment resulting from therapeutic drug monitoring and dose adjustment has been demonstrated in a number of clinical trials. Dose individualization significantly improved the outcome and minimized toxicity for children with B lineage acute lymphocytic leukemia (ALL) treated with MTX.[67] Adjusting the dose of *Escherichia coli* L-asparaginase every 3 weeks based upon measurement of trough serum asparaginase activity significantly improved 5-year event-free survival in children with ALL as compared to patients who received the same standard dose of the enzyme throughout the 30-week course of therapy.[68]

Dosing Regimens

For the average patient, or the general population, pharmacokinetics can help answer the fundamental questions in delivery of drugs: (a) What route of administration? (b) How much to give (dose)? (c) How often to administer (schedule)? These questions are answered using empiric observation (what works best in an experimental or clinical setting) as well as biochemical, cell kinetic, and pharmacokinetic considerations.

Routes of Drug Administration

The choice of drug administration *route* is based primarily on the ability to formulate an acceptable dose preparation for intravenous, oral, intramuscular, intrathecal, or subcutaneous use and pharmacokinetic assessment of the pattern of systemic drug exposure that they provide. Although current trends point toward the preferential development of orally administered drugs, cytotoxic anticancer drugs are still most commonly given by the intravenous route as this provides complete control over the actual dosage delivered to the systemic circulation and the rate at which it is presented. This results in maximum safety because the variability in systemic drug exposure between and within patients achieved with direct intravenous administration is typically much lower than that resulting from oral administration. Furthermore, for agents given by continuous intravenous infusion, drug delivery can be readily terminated, if necessary, because of the occurrence of an acute adverse reaction during administration.

All routes of administration other than intravenous, including oral, subcutaneous, intramuscular, intraperitoneal, and intrathecal delivery, involve an absorption process whereby dissolved drug molecules are transferred from the site of administration into the vasculature. Accordingly, drug given by an extravascular route is conceptualized as being outside the body until gaining access to the systemic circulation. Oral dosage forms are available for an ever-increasing number of anticancer drugs including hydroxyurea, MTX, etoposide, idarubicin, fludarabine, and many of the receptor tyrosine kinase inhibitors. The development of oral dosage forms is preferable for new anticancer agents that require chronic administration for optimal benefit, such as cytostatic drugs and many molecularly targeted drugs.

The bioavailability of a drug given by any extravascular route is defined as the rate and extent of absorption into systemic circulation. The absolute systemic availability (*F*) of a drug is ascertained by determining the AUC in the same patient following intravenous and extravascular administration of the agent, with an adequate time interval period between the two treatments. For the same dose given intravenously and extravascularly,

$$F = (AUC_{ev} / AUC_{iv}) \cdot (D_{iv} / D_{ev})$$

where *D* is the dose. In studies where an agent is administered exclusively by the oral route, CL and *F* are indeterminable, as explicitly indicated by the relationship

$$D_{ev} / AUC_{ev} = CL / F$$

Many factors influence oral bioavailability, including release of the drug from the dosage form, dissolution of drug within the gastrointestinal tract, drug stability under conditions encountered in the gastrointestinal tract, transport of dissolved drug across the intestinal epithelium into the vasculature, and the extent of first-pass hepatic metabolism. Mercaptopurine is an example of a drug with very low and erratic bioavailability,[69] whereas imatinib is a drug with consistently high bioavailability.[70]

Absorption through the lipid bilayer cell membrane of the intestinal mucosa is determined by molecular size, lipid solubility, and the presence of transport systems. As cancer chemotherapy shifts increasingly toward oral drug delivery, the importance of many general carrier systems, such as the "ABC" transporters, is becoming more widely appreciated alongside such specialized carriers as the folate transport mechanisms for antifolates. The physiologic state of the intestinal tract may be affected adversely by disease or by previous drug therapy. Vomiting induced by chemotherapeutic drugs such as cisplatin may lead to loss of a major portion of an oral dose. In addition to intestinal absorption, presystemic metabolism and biliary excretion may prevent orally administered drugs from reaching the systemic circulation in an active form. Presystemic metabolism, also known as the "first-pass effect," is a unique concern for the oral route because a drug is exposed to metabolism both in the gastrointestinal mucosa and in the liver, which it enters through the portal vein before returning to the heart.[71]

A tumor may grow in a region of the body, such as the central nervous system, that is not penetrated readily by systemically administered drugs. Accordingly, several unusual routes of administration have been implemented to maximize delivery of drugs to the site of the tumor and to reduce the deleterious effects associated with ordinary systemic administration. At least two of these routes have become accepted therapeutic practice: intrathecal delivery for meningeal leukemia[72] and intravesical delivery for transitional-stage bladder carcinoma. As discussed in detail in Chapter 6, intrathecal administration has been used primarily to obtain adequate drug levels in the cerebrospinal fluid to eradicate cancer cells that are otherwise protected from effective therapy. Intra-arterial drug administration, especially hepatic arterial delivery of 5-fluorodeoxyuridine (see Chapter 8), is another route that has been actively investigated but has not emerged as standard therapy.

Peritoneal dialysis continues to be evaluated as a delivery vehicle for anticancer drugs when disease is localized to the abdomen.[73] The pharmacokinetic rationale suggests that tumor tissue may be exposed to high local concentrations, whereas systemic levels are no greater than normally encountered with intravenous therapy. In an analogous fashion to intrathecal delivery, only cells in close contact with the peritoneal fluid will benefit from this mode of drug delivery. The intraperitoneal route has been the subject of many pilot studies and formal phase I and phase II trials by our group and others. Some promising pharmacologic results have been obtained and more definitive therapeutic trials are in progress. Three randomized phase III trials totaling approximately 3,000 patients with ovarian cancer have shown an advantage for intraperitoneal delivery compared with intravenous delivery for both time to disease recurrence/progression[74,75] and survival.[74,76] Pharmacokinetic analysis can help to evaluate the potential usefulness of these approaches. Of course, the pharmacokinetic advantage of achieving greater drug exposure is not always associated with improved responses.

Dose

Dose is usually determined by an empiric phase I trial using a fixed treatment schedule, with stepwise evaluation of toxicity at progressively higher doses. In certain circumstances, dose also may be determined by setting pharmacologic objectives, such as a target drug concentration in a specific body compartment such as plasma, cerebrospinal fluid, or ascites. This type of regimen planning requires pharmacokinetic design and verification by drug level monitoring and has been used in only a few clinical oncologic settings, such as intrathecal chemotherapy with MTX and intraperitoneal therapy with MTX and 5-FU. Additional information on the relationship of drug concentration to tumor cell kill, as provided by in vitro assays, may provide a basis for more precise pharmacokinetic adjustment of dosage.

Pharmacologically guided dose escalation was developed as an alternative to the predetermined escalation procedures such as the modified Fibonacci method for phase I trials.[77] After the first group of patients has been treated with the starting dose in a phase I clinical trial, the rate of dose escalation is determined by the plasma levels of drug relative to target plasma levels measured in mice at the maximum tolerated dose. With this approach, investigators can estimate the difference between the target concentration and plasma levels produced by the current dose level. Such information provides the opportunity to intervene at an early stage in the phase I trial. Cautious escalation may be indicated if it is determined that plasma levels of the drug are close to the target. If the current plasma levels are substantially below the targeted value, then a more rapid escalation of the dose could generate considerable savings in time and clinical resources, and fewer patients will be exposed to

doses that have little potential of being therapeutically effective. Although this procedure is conceptually attractive and found support in Europe and Japan, as well as the United States,[78-80] it has not been widely used, primarily because of logistical difficulties in its implementation.

Individualizing the dose of anticancer drugs by normalization to BSA has been a long-standing and generally accepted practice in clinical oncology.[81] This practice is ultimately based upon the presumed existence of a relationship between the CL of a drug and BSA. The intended objective is to minimize the variability in systemic drug exposure between patients and thereby enhance safety and efficacy. However, as previously mentioned, it has become appreciated that CL is not well correlated with BSA for numerous chemotherapeutic agents, particularly compounds that are predominantly eliminated by the liver.[14] Treating patients with the same absolute amount of a drug without adjustment for body weight or BSA, known as fixed dosing, is becoming increasingly common for new anticancer drugs that are administered orally. Fixed dosing has also been advocated as being appropriate for monoclonal antibody chemotherapeutic agents.[82] Establishing an alternative generally applicable method to better individualize the dose of anticancer drugs, such as low mass as measured by cross-sectional computed tomography imaging, to more accurately dose patients and minimize the occurrence of severe adverse effects remains a topic of considerable interest.[83]

Administration Schedule

The frequency of administration evaluated in the initial phase I trial of an anticancer agent is typically derived from the schedule that produces an optimal therapeutic effect against an appropriate preclinical tumor model. However, it has been repeatedly demonstrated that impressive preclinical antitumor activity is not a reliable predictor of clinical efficacy. A reasonable argument can be advanced to support the hypothesis that a candidate drug has little likelihood of being therapeutically effective unless a clinically tolerable dosing regimen provides a pattern of systemic exposure to the drug that is at least comparable with that required for activity against appropriate in vivo or in vitro preclinical models. Accordingly, when considered together with toxicologic and physiologic response factors, pharmacokinetic data acquired during phase I studies can facilitate efforts to optimize dosing regimens. Alternatively, withdrawing an agent from continued clinical development may be an option that warrants serious consideration in situations in which the plasma concentrations achieved in patients treated at the maximum tolerated dose are considerably lower than target levels, given the availability of limited clinical resources and ethical considerations of entering patients into a phase II trial of a compound that has little prospect of being therapeutically effective.

The *schedule* of drug administration depends highly on pharmacokinetic considerations and requires a choice of the duration of administration (e.g., bolus intravenous injection versus prolonged intravenous infusion), frequency of repeated dosing, and the sequencing of multiple drugs or drugs and other treatment modalities such as radiation. Bolus intravenous injection provides maximal peak drug levels in plasma but a rapid decline thereafter as the drug is eliminated from the plasma compartment by metabolism or excretion. This very convenient dosing method is appropriate for drugs that are not cell cycle–phase dependent and therefore do not have to be present during a specific phase of the cell cycle. Examples are the alkylating agents, such as chloroethyl nitrosoureas, nitrogen mustards, and procarbazine, as well as other drugs that chemically interact with DNA.

Administration by prolonged intravenous infusion (i.e., 6 to 120 hours) is advantageous for agents that act preferentially in discrete phases of the cell cycle, such as S-phase–specific drugs (e.g., cytarabine, MTX, camptothecins), particularly if the drug is rapidly cleared from systemic circulation. Prolonged infusions have the additional advantage of providing a specific and constant plasma concentration of the drug, a desirable feature if information regarding the chemosensitivity of the tumor is available, as determined experimentally by various in vitro tests. Intermediate-length infusions (i.e., 1 to 4 hours) may provide a means to overcome the acute toxicities that are produced by exposing host organs to high peak drug levels. Particularly for acutely neurotoxic or cardiotoxic compounds, rapid intravenous infusions may present unacceptable dangers, but intermediate-length infusions may reduce peak drug levels adequately while retaining some of the convenience of bolus dosing.

It may be desirable to achieve the steady-state concentration rapidly for a drug given as a continuous intravenous infusion, in which case a *loading dose* may be given by bolus injection at the same time that the infusion is started. This is now standard practice for the administration of 5-FU (see Chapter 6). The bolus dose is usually selected to achieve an initial concentration near the steady-state target value. In this way, the time lag to achieve the plateau in the $C \times T$ profile, which may be considerable for some drugs, is eliminated. As an alternative to administering a drug by continuous intravenous infusion, it may be possible to maintain reasonably constant plasma levels using a repeated bolus injection dosing regimen. There is an approach to steady-state conditions in which the peak and trough plasma concentrations increase successively during repeated doses before becoming constant. As with the continuous intravenous infusion, steady state can be reached immediately with the proper choice of loading dose. The most common such schedule targets the peak concentration as twice the trough concentration. This design requires dosing once each half-life. An initial dose of twice the successive (maintenance) doses abolishes the time lag. As the dosing frequency increases, the ratio of peak-to-trough concentrations approaches 1, and the $C \times T$ curve appears more like that of a constant infusion. These same scheduling considerations also apply to the timing of oral drug delivery.

Relationships with Pharmacological Effects

The toxicities of anticancer drugs are often better correlated with a pharmacokinetic variable than the administered dose. Relationships between the severity of toxicity and the AUC are most commonly encountered. However, other variables such as the C_{max} and duration of time that the drug concentration in plasma exceeds a particular threshold level are also predictive of toxicity. For example, the time interval that plasma levels of paclitaxel remain above 50 nM is better correlated with neutropenia, the principal dose-limiting toxicity, than either C_{max} or AUC.[84] The nature of these relationships can often be described by a sigmoidal E_{max} model, but they may appear linear unless patients have been evaluated across a sufficiently broad range of doses.[85]

As previously indicated, therapeutic response ultimately depends on the delivery of drug from the bloodstream to the tumor in such a way that malignant cells are exposed to biologically effective concentrations of the active form of the agent for an adequate duration of time. The rate processes associated with drug distribution and elimination depend on the physicochemical properties of the drug and numerous physiologic factors. As is the case with any specific organ or tissue, the time course of the concentration of a drug within a solid tumor cannot be defined from experimental data restricted to measurements made in plasma, serum, or whole blood. Although there is undoubtedly some temporal relationship between drug concentrations in plasma and the tumor, elucidating the intratumoral concentration-time profile requires the measurement of drug levels within the tumor itself, which presents considerable practical and technical challenges. Determining the drug concentration in a single biopsy specimen is typically not very informative. Microdialysis has been shown to be a very informative technique for characterizing the intratumoral pharmacokinetics of drugs in brain tumors, although its application presents some considerable technical challenges.[86] Efforts to determine whether adequate concentrations of the active form of a drug are achieved in cancer cells should be considered an important objective of early-phase clinical trials to evaluate new anticancer drugs in hematologic malignancies. The availability of this information will better facilitate the rational selection of drugs warranting further clinical evaluation.

Conclusions

There are numerous reasons for acquiring pharmacokinetic data during various stages in the clinical development of anticancer drugs. The therapeutic indices of many drugs used in the treatment of cancer are inherently narrow because they are used at doses close to the upper limit of tolerability. Furthermore, cancer patients frequently exhibit increased sensitivity to many medications due to compromised organ function or diminished overall tolerance due to their underlying disease state, augmenting the potential for an undesirable pharmacokinetic interaction with the host of concurrent medications used in the clinical management of cancer patients. The chances for an adverse event resulting from inappropriate dosing of a chemotherapeutic agent to a cancer patient are, therefore, considerably greater than experienced with most other patient groups. Since the dose-limiting toxicities of a chemotherapeutic agent are very often related to some measure of systemic exposure to the drug, the margin of safety of a potentially effective dose is dependent upon the consistency of its pharmacokinetic behavior among patients.

Pharmacokinetics can also serve a useful role in the process of drug development by assisting the overall integration of data between preclinical testing and early clinical trials.[87] Initial human studies rely heavily on toxicologic and pharmacologic data obtained in mice and dogs, and pharmacokinetics provides a convenient approach to comparative analysis.

The ultimate goal of pharmacokinetics is to assist in the optimization of therapy. Although progress has been made in pharmacokinetic areas, the limiting step for optimization of therapy is inadequate knowledge of the relationship between drug $C \times T$

profiles and drug effects. Pharmacokinetics can serve as a useful tool to help elucidate PD relationships by determining which profiles are feasible and by helping design administration strategies. Also, because overall drug effect results from both kinetic and dynamic variables, studies can be designed to adjust doses individually so that kinetic differences between patients can be minimized and attention can be focused solely on drug dynamics.

Our ability to find useful relationships between drug exposure and clinical outcomes is greatest for drugs that offer substantial benefits for patients. The success of imatinib in patients with chronic myeloid leukemia (CML) and gastrointestinal stromal tumors (GISTs) has provided immediate tangible benefits for these individuals. This success has also provided a major boost to the field of drug development. In the domain of pharmacokinetics, oral delivery of imatinib and other drugs presents substantial challenges in areas such as patient adherence to dosing regimens, erratic drug absorption, and drug-drug interactions. The rationale for efforts to emphasize improvement in these areas must be driven by solid indications of concentration-response relationships.

The demonstration of associations between plasma concentrations of imatinib and both complete cytogenetic response and major molecular response in CML supplies the impetus for further exploration.[88] Similarly, the report of associations in GIST between plasma concentrations of imatinib and both overall objective benefit and time to tumor progression provides additional incentive.[89] Although observational studies are not as powerful as prospective interventional studies, these strong signals have been replicated by other groups. Thus, research into the possibility of improving therapy via pharmacokinetic monitoring of plasma concentrations should be a high priority for continuing to optimize the use of imatinib in CML and GIST.

References

1. Donelli MG, D'Incalci M, Garattini S. Pharmacokinetic studies of anticancer drugs in tumor-bearing animals. *Cancer Treat Rep.* 1984;68:381-400.
2. Notari RE. *Biopharmaceutics and Clinical Pharmacokinetics.* New York, NY: Marcel Dekker; 1987.
3. Gilbaldi M, Perrier D, eds. *Pharmacokinetics.* 2nd ed. New York, NY: Marcel Dekker; 1982.
4. Timmerman PM, de Vries R, Ingelse BA. Tailoring bioanalysis for PK studies supporting drug discovery. *Curr Top Med Chem.* 2001;1:443-462.
5. Wright JD, Boudinot FD, Ujhelyi MR. Measurement and analysis of unbound drug concentrations. *Clin Pharmacokinet.* 1996;30:445-462.
6. Dunne A. An iterative curve stripping technique for pharmacokinetic parameter estimation. *J Pharm Pharmacol.* 1986;38:97-101.
7. Gillespie WR. Noncompartmental versus compartmental modelling in clinical pharmacokinetics. *Clin Pharmacokinet.* 1991;20:253-262.
8. Dedrick RL, Myers CE, Bungay PM, et al. Pharmacokinetic rationale for peritoneal drug administration in the treatment of ovarian cancer. *Cancer Treat Rep.* 1978;62:1-11.
9. Speyer JL, Sugarbaker PH, Collins JM, et al. Portal levels and hepatic clearance of 5-fluorouracil after intraperitoneal administration in humans. *Cancer Res.* 1981;41:1916-1922.
10. Farris FF, King FG, Dedrick RL, et al. Physiologic model for the pharmacokinetics of cis-dichlorodiammineplatinum(II) (DDP) in the tumored rat. *J Pharmacokinet Biopharm.* 1985;13:13-39.
11. Chan KK, Cohen JL, Gross JF, et al. Prediction of adriamycin disposition in cancer patients using a physiologic, pharmacokinetic model. *Cancer Treat Rep.* 1978;62:1161-1171.
12. Dedrick RL, Forrester DD, Cannon JN, et al. Pharmacokinetics of 1-β-D-arabinofuranosylcytosine (ARA-C) deamination in several species. *Biochem Pharmacol.* 1973;22:2405-2417.
13. Rowland M, Benet LZ, Graham GG. Clearance concepts in pharmacokinetics. *J Pharmacokinet Biopharm.* 1973;1:123-136.
14. Sawyer M, Ratain M. Body surface area as a determinant of pharmacokinetics and drug dosing. *Invest New Drugs.* 2001;19:171-177.
15. Carlisle KM, Halliwell M, Read AE, et al. Estimation of total hepatic blood flow by duplex ultrasound. *Gut.* 1992;33:92-97.
16. Cockcroft DW, Gault MH. Prediction of creatinine clearance from serum creatinine. *Nephron.* 1976;16:31-41.
17. Gibaldi M, McNamara PJ. Apparent volumes of distribution and drug binding to plasma proteins and tissues. *Eur J Clin Pharmacol.* 1978;13:373-380.
18. Collins JM, Dedrick RL, King FG, et al. Nonlinear pharmacokinetic models for 5-fluorouracil in man: intravenous and intraperitoneal routes. *Clin Pharmacol Ther.* 1980;28:235-246.
19. Donehower RC, Karp JE, Burke PJ. Pharmacology and toxicity of high-dose cytarabine by 72-hour continuous infusion. *Cancer Treat Rep.* 1986;70:1059-1065.
20. Besseghir K, Roch-Ramel F. Renal excretion of drugs and other xenobiotics. *Ren Physiol.* 1987;10:221-241.
21. Ilett KF, Tee LB, Reeves PT, et al. Metabolism of drugs and other xenobiotics in the gut lumen and wall. *Pharmacol Ther.* 1990;46:67-93.
22. Balis FM, Holcenberg JS, Bleyer WA. Clinical pharmacokinetics of commonly used anticancer drugs. *Clin Pharmacokinet.* 1983;8:202-232.
23. Glue P, Clement RP. Cytochrome P450 enzymes and drug metabolism—basic concepts and methods of assessment. *Cell Mol Neurobiol.* 1999;19:309-323.
24. von Moltke LL, Greenblatt DJ, Schmider J, et al. Metabolism of drugs by cytochrome P450 3A isoforms. Implications for drug interactions in psychopharmacology. *Clin Pharmacokinet.* 1985;29:33-43.
25. Gillum JG, Israel DS, Polk RE. Pharmacokinetic drug interactions with antimicrobial agents. *Clin Pharmacokinet.* 1993;25:450-482.
26. Kivisto KT, Kroemer HK, Eichelbaum M. The role of human cytochrome P450 enzymes in the metabolism of anticancer agents: implications for drug interactions. *Br J Clin Pharmacol.* 1995;40:523-530.
27. Chabot GG, Bouchard J, Momparler RL. Kinetics of deamination of 5-aza-2′-deoxycytidine and cytosine arabinoside by human liver cytidine deaminase and its inhibition by 3-deazauridine, thymidine or uracil arabinoside. *Biochem Pharmacol.* 1983;32:1327-1328.
28. Milano G, McLeod HL. Can dihydropyrimidine dehydrogenase impact 5-fluorouracil-based treatment? *Eur J Cancer.* 2000;36:37-42.
29. Clarke DJ, Burchell B. The uridine diphosphate glucuronosyltransferase multigene family: function and regulation. In: Kauffman FC, ed. *Handbook of Experimental Pharmacology, Conjugation-Deconjugation Reactions in Drug Metabolism and Toxicity.* Berlin: Springer-Verlag; 1994:3-43.
30. Ratain MJ. Insights into the pharmacokinetics and pharmacodynamics of irinotecan. *Clin Cancer Res.* 2000;6:3393-3394.
31. Ivanov AI, Christodoulou J, Parkinson JA, et al. Cisplatin binding sites on human albumin. *J Biol Chem.* 1998;273:14721-14730.
32. Milano G, Etienne MC, Cassuto-Viguier E, et al. Influence of sex and age on fluorouracil clearance. *J Clin Oncol.* 1992;10:1171-1175.
33. Innocenti F, Iyer L, Ratain MJ. Pharmacogenetics of anticancer agents: lessons from amonafide and irinotecan. *Drug Metab Dispos.* 2001;29:596-600.
34. Zhou X, Mould DR, Takubo T, et al. Global population pharmacokinetics of the investigational Aurora A kinase inhibitor alisertib in cancer patients: Rationale for lower dosage in Asia. *Br J Clin Pharmacol.* 2018;84(1):35-51. doi: 10.1111/bcp.13430.
35. Lichtman SM, Skirvin JA. Pharmacology of antineoplastic agents in older cancer patients. *Oncology.* 2000;14:1743-1752.
36. Geokas M, Haverback B. The aging gastrointestinal tract. *Am J Surg.* 1969;117:881-892.
37. Bender A. The effect of increasing age on the distribution of peripheral blood flow in man. *J Am Geriatr Soc.* 1965;13:192-198.
38. Bach B, Hansen J, Kampmann J, et al. Disposition of antipyrine and phenytoin correlated with age and liver volume in men. *Clin Pharmacokinet.* 1981;6:389-396.
39. Durnas C, Loi C, Cusack BJ. Hepatic drug metabolism and aging. *Clin Pharmacokinet.* 1990;19:359-389.

40. Baker SD, Grochow LB. Pharmacology of cancer chemotherapy in the older person. *Clin Geriatr Med.* 1997;13:169-183.

41. Kinirons MT, O'Mahony MS. Drug metabolism and ageing. *Br J Clin Pharmacol.* 2004;57:540-544.

42. Anderson GD. Children versus adults: pharmacokinetic and adverse-effect differences. *Epilepsia.* 2002;43(suppl 3):53-59.

43. Hammerlein A, Derendorf H, Lowenthal DT. Pharmacokinetic and pharmacodynamic changes in the elderly. Clinical implications. *Clin Pharmacokinet* 1998;35:49-64.

44. Barre J, Houin G, Brunner F, et al. Disease-induced modifications of drug pharmacokinetics. *Int J Clin Pharmacol Res.* 1983;3:215-226.

45. Powis G. Effect of human renal and hepatic disease on the pharmacokinetics of anticancer drugs. *Cancer Treat Rev.* 1982;9:85-124.

46. Egorin MJ, Van Echo DA, Olman EA, et al. Prospective validation of a pharmacologically based dosing scheme for the cis-diamminedichloroplatinum(II) analogue diamminecyclobutanedicarboxylatoplatinum. *Cancer Res.* 1985;45:6502-6506.

47. Egorin MJ, Sigman LM, Van Echo DA, et al. Phase I clinical and pharmacokinetic study of hexamethylene bisacetamide (NSC95580) administered as a five-day continuous infusion. *Cancer Res.* 1987;47:617-623.

48. van den Bongard HJ, Mathot RA, Beijnen JH, et al. Pharmacokinetically guided administration of chemotherapeutic agents. *Clin Pharmacokinet.* 2000;39:345-367.

49. Shimada T, Yamazaki H, Mimura M, et al. Interindividual variations in human liver cytochrome P-450 enzymes involved in the oxidation of drugs, carcinogens and toxic chemicals: studies with liver microsomes of 30 Japanese and 30 Caucasians. *J Pharmacol Exp Ther.* 1994;270:414-423.

50. Watters JW, McLeod HL. Cancer pharmacogenomics: current and future applications. *Biochim Biophys Acta.* 2003;1603:99-111.

51. Peck CC, Temple R, Collins JM. Understanding consequences of concurrent therapies. *JAMA.* 1993;269:1550-1552.

52. Dorr RT, Soble MJ, Alberts DS. Interaction of cimetidine but not ranitidine with cyclophosphamide in mice. *Cancer Res.* 1986;46:1795-1799.

53. Hande K, Combs G, Swingle R, et al. Effect of cimetidine and ranitidine on the metabolism and toxicity of hexamethylmelamine. *Cancer Treat Rep.* 1986;70:1443-1445.

54. Bjornsson TD, Huang AT, Roth P, et al. Effects of high-dose cancer chemotherapy on the absorption of digoxin in two different formulations. *Clin Pharmacol Ther.* 1986;39:25-28.

55. Balis FM. Pharmacokinetic drug interactions of commonly used anticancer drugs. *Clin Pharmacokinet.* 1986;11:223-235.

56. Jamis-Dow CA, Klecker RW, Katki AG, et al. Metabolism of taxol by human and rat liver in vitro: a screen for drug interactions and interspecies differences. *Cancer Chemother Pharmacol.* 1995;36:107-114.

57. van Meerten E, Verweij J, Schellens JH. Antineoplastic agents. Drug interactions of clinical significance. *Drug Saf.* 1995;12:168-182.

58. Markowitz JS, Donovan JL, DeVane CL, et al. Effect of St John's wort on drug metabolism by induction of cytochrome P450 3A4 enzyme. *JAMA.* 2003;290:1500-1504.

59. McCune JS, Hawke RL, LeCluyse EL, et al. In vivo and in vitro induction of human cytochrome P4503A4 by dexamethasone. *Clin Pharmacol Ther.* 2000;68:356-366.

60. Bannwarth B, Pehourcq F, Schaeverbeke T, et al. Clinical pharmacokinetics of low-dose pulse methotrexate in rheumatoid arthritis. *Clin Pharmacokinet.* 1996;30:194-210.

61. Evans WE, Christensen ML. Drug interactions with methotrexate. *J Rheumatol.* 1985;12(suppl 12):15-20.

62. Wood M. Pharmacokinetic drug interaction in anaesthetic practice. *Clin Pharmacokinet.* 1991;21:285-307.

63. Kerr IG, Jolivet J, Collins JM, et al. Test dose for predicting high-dose methotrexate infusions. *Clin Pharmacol Ther.* 1983;33:44-51.

64. Lankheet NAG, Knapen LM, Schellens JHK, et al. Plasma concentrations of tyrosine kinase inhibitors imatinib, erlotinib, and sunitinib in routine clinical outpatient cancer care. *Ther Drug Monit.* 2014;36:326-334.

65. Teng JFT, Mabasa VH, Ensom MHH, et al. The role of therapeutic drug monitoring of imatinib in patients with chronic myeloid leukemia and metastatic or unresectable gastrointestinal stromal tumors. *Ther Drug Monit.* 2012;34:85-97.

66. Lankheet NAG, Desar IME, Mulder SF, et al. Optimizing the dose in cancer patients treated with imatinib, sunitinib, and pazopanib. *Br J Clin Pharmacol.* 2017;83:2195-2204.

67. Evans WE, Relling MV, Rodman JH, et al. Conventional compared with individualized chemotherapy for childhood acute lymphoblastic leukemia. *N Engl J Med.* 1998;338:499-505.

68. Vrooman LM, Stevenson KE, Supko JG, et al. Postinduction dexamethasone and individualized dosing of *Escherichia coli* L-asparaginase each improve outcome of children and adolescents with newly diagnosed acute lymphoblastic leukemia: Results from a randomized study—Dana-Farber Cancer Institute ALL Consortium Protocol 00-01. *J Clin Oncol.* 2013;31:1202-1210.

69. Zimm S, Collins JM, Riccardi R, et al. Variable bioavailability of oral mercaptopurine: is maintenance chemotherapy in acute lymphoblastic leukemia being optimally delivered? *N Engl J Med.* 1983;308:1005-1009.

70. Peng B, Dutreix C, Mehring G, et al. Absolute bioavailability of imatinib (Glivec) orally versus intravenous infusion. *J Clin Pharmacol.* 2004;44:158-162.

71. Rubin GM, Tozer TN. Theoretical considerations in the calculation of bioavailability of drugs exhibiting Michaelis-Menten elimination kinetics. *J Pharmacokinet Biopharm.* 1984;12:437-450.

72. Blasberg R, Patlak CS, Fenstermacher JD. Intrathecal chemotherapy: brain tissue profiles after ventriculocisternal perfusion. *J Pharmacol Exp Ther.* 1975;195:73-83.

73. Myers CE, Collins JM. Pharmacology of intraperitoneal chemotherapy. *Cancer Invest.* 1983;1:395-407.

74. Markman M, Bundy BN, Alberts DS, et al. Phase III trial of standard-dose intravenous cisplatin plus paclitaxel versus moderately high-dose carboplatin followed by intravenous paclitaxel and intraperitoneal cisplatin in small-volume stage III ovarian carcinoma: an intergroup study of the Gynecologic Oncology Group, Southwestern Oncology Group, and Eastern Cooperative Oncology Group. *J Clin Oncol.* 2001;19:921-923.

75. Alberts DS, Markman M, Armstrong D, et al. Intraperitoneal therapy for stage III ovarian cancer: a therapy whose time has come! *J Clin Oncol.* 2002;20:3944-3946.

76. Alberts DS, Liu PY, Hannigan EV, et al. Intraperitoneal cisplatin plus intravenous cyclophosphamide versus intravenous cisplatin plus intravenous cyclophosphamide for stage III ovarian cancer. *N Engl J Med.* 1996;335:1950-1955.

77. Collins JM, Zaharko DS, Dedrick RL, et al. Potential roles for preclinical pharmacology in phase I trials. *Cancer Treat Rep.* 1986;70:73-80.

78. EORTC Pharmacokinetics and Metabolism Group. Pharmacokinetically guided dose escalation in phase I clinical trials. *Eur J Cancer Clin Oncol.* 1987;23:1083-1087.

79. Fuse E, Kobayashi S, Inaba M, et al. Application of pharmacokinetically guided dose escalation with respect to cell cycle phase specificity. *J Natl Cancer Inst.* 1994;86:989-996.

80. Collins JM, Grieshaber CK, Chabner BA. Pharmacologically guided phase I trials based upon preclinical development. *J Natl Cancer Inst.* 1990;82:1321-1326.

81. Gurney H. Dose calculation of anticancer drugs: a review of the current practice and introduction of an alternative. *J Clin Oncol.* 1996;14:2590-2611.

82. Hendrikx J, Haanen J, Voest EE, et al. Fixed dosing of monoclonal antibodies in oncology. *Oncologist.* 2017;22:1212-1221.

83. Hopkins JJ, Sawyer MB. A review of body composition and pharmacokinetics in oncology. *Expert Rev Clin Pharmacol.* 2017;10:947-956.

84. Gianni L, Kearns CM, Giani A, et al. Nonlinear pharmacokinetics and metabolism of paclitaxel and its pharmacokinetic/pharmacodynamic relationships in humans. *J Clin Oncol.* 1995;13:180-190.

85. Holford NH. Clinical pharmacokinetics and pharmacodynamics of warfarin. Understanding the dose-effect relationship. *Clin Pharmacokinet.* 1986;11:483-504.

86. Blakeley JO, Olson J, Grossman SA, et al. Effect of blood brain permeability in recurrent high grade gliomas on the intratumoral pharmacokinetics of methotrexate: a microdialysis study. *J Neurooncol.* 2009;91:51-58.

87. Collins JM. Pharmacology and drug development. *J Natl Cancer Inst.* 1988;80:790-792.

88. Larson RA, Druker BJ, Guilhot F, et al. Imatinib pharmacokinetics and its correlation with response and safety in chronic-phase chronic myeloid leukemia: a subanalysis of the IRIS study. *Blood.* 2008;111:4022-4028.

89. Demetri GD, Wang Y, Wehrle E, et al. Imatinib plasma levels are correlated with clinical benefit in patients with unresectable/metastatic gastrointestinal stromal tumors. *J Clin Oncol.* 2009;27:3141-3147.

Pharmacogenomics and the Role of Genomics in Cancer Therapeutics

Steven M. Offer and Robert B. Diasio

Introduction

Cancer patients often demonstrate variability in both responses and side effects to anticancer treatments. While some of this variability can be attributed to differences in age, sex, organ function, and underlying medical conditions, it has become increasingly evident that genetic variants are key to pharmacologic variability. In some cases, genetics have been shown to be the fundamental predictors of both the efficacy and the risk of severe side effects associated with specific therapies.

Pharmacogenetics is generally defined as the study of how inherited genetic differences in a single gene influence the therapeutic effect of and/or risk of toxicity to a single drug. Pharmacogenomics represents a broader field that studies how differences in all genes (i.e., the genome) influence drug responses.[1] Although the terms pharmacogenetics and pharmacogenomics are often used interchangeably, the latter term more appropriately captures the breadth of current studies that aim to identify genetic variants (both protein-coding variants and variants located in noncoding regions of the genome), as well as epigenetic factors, that influence drug efficacy and/or toxicity at a genome-wide scale. Therefore, pharmacogenomics will be used throughout this chapter. Within the field of pharmacogenomics, studies often focus on variants that affect either the pharmacokinetics (i.e., factors that affect drug bioavailability, including factors that are involved in determining drug absorption, distribution, metabolism, or elimination), or pharmacodynamics (i.e., factors that affect the biochemical and physiological effects of a drug). Cancer pharmacogenomics have an extra layer of complexity over noncancer pharmacogenomics in that both inherited germ-line variants and somatically acquired tumor variants need to be considered.

There is perhaps no area of modern pharmacology where genomics has had a larger role in influencing how drugs are used clinically than in the discipline of cancer therapeutics. For decades, oncologists have been aware that certain drugs, such as 6-mercaptopurine (6-MP), were associated with severe toxicity in a subset of patients.[2] Importantly, the severity of these toxicities was far outside the range of toxic side effects observed in the majority of patients receiving the same dose and schedule of the drug. This, together with family and population studies, led to an early appreciation of pharmacogenomics, even before the human gene structure had been fully elucidated.[3] As the structure of the human genome became more defined, it became increasingly possible to

pinpoint changes in specific genome regions that associate with these toxicities.[4] Awareness of the various cancer pharmacogenomic syndromes has provided an appreciation for the causes of accentuated responses. In most cases, these responses represent increased host toxicity; interestingly, in some instances, the genes that are responsible for these responses provide insight into factors that also determine tumor response.[5]

Impact of Genetic Variants on Cancer Therapy

Human genetic variability is a determinant of anticancer efficacy and safety. This variability, which is the basis of pharmacogenomics, encompasses an array of different types of DNA sequence modifications as well as differences in gene expression and regulation. The majority of this chapter focuses on the most common form of variation in genetic sequence, the single nucleotide polymorphism (SNP). While it has become increasingly acceptable to refer to any small genetic variant as an "SNP," the remainder of this chapter will use the broader term "variant," which more correctly accounts for genetic change of more than one nucleotide as well as deletion/insertion variations. Variants can be divided into classes based on the known or predicted effect on protein function and/or expression. For example, nonsynonymous variants result in a change to the encoded amino acid sequence and are generally found in the open reading frame of a gene. There are a number of different types of nonsynonymous variants, including missense, nonsense, insertion/deletion, and splice-site variations. Missense variants are single base changes that cause a codon to encode a different amino acid. Nonsense variants are also single base changes. However, instead of encoding a different amino acid, nonsense variants introduce a premature stop codon into the reading frame. Insertion and deletion variants (commonly known collectively as indels) can add or delete the entire codons from the reading frame or alter all downstream codons by introducing a frameshift. Splice-site variants typically occur at splice donor or acceptor sites and can lead to the exclusion of an entire exon of coding sequence or, in some instances, inclusion of additional intron sequence as part or all of an exon. Due to the biology of mRNA splicing, splice-site variants can be located in either exons or introns. Synonymous variants are located in the open reading frame, but they do not alter the amino acid sequence of the translated protein. This is possible due to degeneracy in the genetic code, where multiple three-base codons can encode the same amino acid. While synonymous variants do not alter the amino acid sequence, they can affect the transcription, splicing, transport, stability, and/or translation of mRNA, all of which can also result in phenotype changes.[6–8] Genome rearrangements of varying sizes, as well as other variants in regulatory, intronic, and noncoding regions, can also contribute to the complex and multi-factorial phenotypes of drug efficacy and safety.

Coinciding with the initial publications of the human genome,[9,10] the International SNP Map Working Group reported the first complete map of human genome sequence variation in early 2001.[11] They described a map of 1.42 million SNPs that were variably distributed across the genome.[11] Since that initial report, it has become increasingly evident that the human genome is far more varied than previously believed. The Database for Short Genetic Variations (dbSNP[12]) is a centralized catalog of short variations in humans. Currently, build 150 of dbSNP contains records of nearly 350 million human SNPs, over half of which have been mapped to a known gene.[12]

Impact of Allele Frequencies

There is a long-standing debate in biomedical genetics pertaining to the likelihood of variants of differing frequencies contributing to a given disease or condition. At opposite ends of the spectrum are the "common disease, common variant" hypothesis, which argues that variants that are relatively common (but low penetrance) alleles can elicit disease, and the "common disease, rare variant" hypothesis, which argues that multiple high-penetrance rare alleles are the major contributors to genetic disorders.[13] While common variants may impact a greater percentage of the population and, therefore, be attractive from a clinical diagnostic perspective, it is increasingly recognized that rare variants are more likely to be responsible for variations in phenotypes that are clinically relevant.[14–16] In support of these findings, a sequence-based strategy to evaluate all exon region variants in the *SLCO1B1* gene for association with altered methotrexate clearance in acute lymphoblastic leukemia (ALL) revealed that rare nonsynonymous variants with minor allele frequencies less than 1% displayed greater effect sizes than common nonsynonymous variants.[17] A study of whole-genome sequence data also concluded that rare variants are significantly more likely to alter function than common variants.[18] A correlation was noted between the rarity of a variant and the likelihood that the variant exerted a functional impact.[18] This correlation was observed for allele frequencies lower than 8% to 10%, with all alleles at higher frequencies showing similar risk for affecting function.[18] These findings suggest that even though pharmacogenomic syndromes typically do not manifest outside of the context of drug treatment, they likely remain subject to purifying selection.

It is well recognized that variants are unequally distributed between various racial, ethnic, and geographical groups. This distribution can have profound effects on implementing and interpreting pharmacogenomic tests, particularly when only genotype-level data, and not sequence-level data, are available. In the context of risk variants to 5-fluorouracil (5-FU) toxicity, several well-recognized risk variants for increased toxicity risk in the *DPYD* gene have been shown to be primarily carried by individuals of European descent, whereas additional deleterious variants are carried on other racial/regional haplotypes.[19–21] Therefore, pharmacogenomic tests based solely on risk variants identified in populations that are largely of European ancestry likely have limited ability to identify individuals at increased risk of severe 5-FU toxicity in individuals with non-European ancestry.[19–21]

Differences Between Host/Patient and Tumor Genomes

Chemotherapeutic drug response is a complex phenotype that is affected by interactions between networks of different genes and also by interactions between the patient and tumor genomes. The distinction between patient and tumor genomes is important because most anticancer agents do not solely affect tumor tissues. Therefore, genetic variants in pharmacokinetic pathways may differentially impact drug efficacy and host or tumor toxicity through regulation of drug bioavailability, retention, and detoxification; these effects depend on where the variant is carried—the host genome, the tumor genome, or both. The concept of using anticancer drugs to specifically target cancer cells is not new and can be traced back to the roots of cancer pharmacology. However, the use of specialized drugs that exploit specific genetic changes within a tumor has shown great potential; as a result, the field of "targeted therapeutics" has experienced incredible growth and development in the past few decades (Table 5.1). Most of this chapter is directed toward the role of patient germ-line genome pharmacogenomics in cancer. A primer on pharmacogenomic approaches using tumor

TABLE 5.1	*General classes of targeted therapeutics*

Angiogenesis inhibitors
These inhibitors block the growth of new vessels within tumors (angiogenesis), which limits the ability of a tumor to grow beyond certain size by limiting access to blood/oxygen.

Apoptosis inducers
This class of molecule bypasses the mechanisms by which cancer cells evade controlled cell death (apoptosis) to induce cell death.

Cancer vaccines
Cancer vaccines (sometimes called biological therapies) stimulate the patient's ability to prevent cancer from forming or to treat an existing cancer.

Gene expression modulators
These compounds affect the pathways through which cancer-related genes are regulated.

Hormone therapies
These drugs slow or stop the growth of cancers that have become reliant upon certain hormones for growth and survival.

Immunotherapies
This approach triggers the patient's own immune system to destroy cancer cells.

Monoclonal antibodies
Toxic molecules are bound to antibodies that recognize features that are specific to tumor cells.

Signal transduction inhibitors
These compounds block the function of molecules that direct how a cancer cell responds to signals from its environment.

genome information is presented toward the end of this chapter to provide an overview of the current status of the rapidly evolving field of targeted cancer therapeutics.

Approaches for Assessing Genotypes in Pharmacogenomic Studies

There are two major approaches to conducting genetic association studies: the candidate gene approach and the genome-wide association study (GWAS) approach. Note that the term "GWAS" can be singular (as in study) or plural (as in studies). As the names imply, candidate gene studies and GWAS differ mainly in the breadth of targets being evaluated. Both approaches have advantages and limitations relative to the other, and despite much discussion and debate, both will likely form the basis of pharmacogenomic studies for the foreseeable future. Within each approach, correlations between variants and disease/condition can be assessed using groups of related individuals (i.e., family studies) or unrelated individuals (i.e., population studies), which are discussed in greater detail later in this chapter.

Candidate Gene Approaches

In the candidate gene approach, variants are assessed within a single gene or within a group of prespecified genes. The gene or genes are typically chosen based on *a priori* knowledge related to gene function within a pharmacological condition[22]; therefore, candidate gene studies are often hypothesis-based. The roots of candidate gene approaches in pharmacogenomics can be traced back to three key discoveries in the 1950s.[23] First, deficiency of glucose-6-phosphate dehydrogenase was found to correlate with hemolysis in primaquine-treated patients.[24] Second, acetylcholinesterase deficiency was shown to have a genetic component that was associated with prolonged paralysis following succinylcholine anesthesia.[25,26] Third, the rate of isoniazid acetylation was shown to influence the development of peripheral neuropathy.[27] Since these initial gene-drug relationships were reported, candidate gene approaches have identified numerous additional pharmacogenomic pairings that will be discussed in greater detail later in this chapter.

GWAS Approaches

Whereas candidate gene approaches rely upon knowledge of potential pathways that are relevant to drug effects, GWAS attempt to identify genomic associations using a more global approach. As such, GWAS approaches epitomize the "genomics" aspect of pharmacogenomics and are increasingly being used to identify variants that affect drug response.[28] Evolving technologies such as microarrays and, more recently, high-throughput sequencing have fueled the growth of GWAS as cost-effective means to perform association studies that are unbiased by pre-existing mechanistic knowledge.

GWAS have historically utilized linkage disequilibrium (LD) as a method to assess the variability throughout the entire genome without needing to actually genotype all potential variant nucleotides. LD is defined by nonrandom segregation of alleles in a population, which results in higher rates of cotransmission of variants in LD than would be expected if the alleles were independent.[29] LD between two variants can be measured in a given population and the correlation expressed in terms of D' and r^2. Generally, D' provides an indication of how likely two variants are to be coinherited; r^2 provides an indication of how suitable the two SNPs are as proxies for each other by considering allele frequencies. Using this information, researchers can identify proxy SNPs that are not genotyped on a microarray, but their genotype can be inferred using information for one or more other variants.[30] Array manufacturers have taken advantage of this principle and designed microarrays that contain numerous "tag" SNPs that can be used to ascertain the genotype of other variants. Therefore, an array that directly genotypes 1 million SNPs can actually yield genotype information for a far greater number of SNPs. A consequence of this principle is that microarrays typically genotype only common variants (i.e., often defined in the context of GWAS as variants with allele frequencies ≥1%) and ignore the contributions of rare variants. This phenomenon can be traced back to the premise of GWAS, which generally posited that common variants were likely responsible for the risk of most complex genetic disorders.

As the costs of high-throughput sequencing have dropped, GWAS are increasingly being conducted using sequence-based approaches. The scope of the target regions used for high-throughput sequencing can blur the lines somewhat between candidate gene and GWAS approaches because sequence capture can be performed on highly targeted regions of the genome (e.g., cancer-specific panels of genes), the entire exome (i.e., exon-coding region of the genome), or the entire genome. Whereas SNP-based GWAS approaches (e.g., microarrays) rely on LD to increase coverage of the genome (and therefore primarily investigate common variants), sequence-based approaches can yield genotypes for rare variants that do not have a tag SNP present on the array, provided that the variant is located in the sequenced region. As such, sequence-based GWAS are not limited to only testing common variants; they are also able to potentially determine if one or more rare variants contribute to pharmacogenomic conditions. This paradigm shift in GWAS is significant because the substantial number of GWAS published for a wide variety of disorders has identified few common associated variants, and those variants explain only a small fraction of genetic risk for a disorder even when considered in aggregate tests.[31]

Because GWAS methods involve the study of thousands (potentially millions) of SNPs, multiple testing must be considered when interpreting results. Multiple testing is the principle that the outcome for one variable, in this case a genetic variant, can affect the outcome for a second variable. Generally speaking, as the number of variants being tested increases, the likelihood of detecting a false-positive result and incorrectly rejecting the null hypothesis (i.e., type I error) also increases. Various methods have been devised and implemented to address multiple testing in GWAS.[32] One of the more straightforward, but statistically conservative, of these methods is a Bonferroni correction, in which the threshold for significance (i.e., the p-value threshold that is needed to be reached for a result to be considered significant) is reduced by dividing by the number of statistical tests being performed (i.e., the number of SNPs tested). For instance, if the nominal threshold for a single marker association test is $p = 5 \times 10^{-2}$, the nominal Bonferroni threshold for each variant in a GWAS evaluating one million SNPs would be 5×10^{-8}. This approximation is used as the significance threshold for most GWAS because it is remarkably close to empirical estimates for genome-wide significance.[30,33]

Pharmacogenomic Research Strategies

Many of the well-known cancer pharmacogenomic syndromes described below were first characterized by phenotype alone, without the benefit of knowledge of the underlying gene(s) that might be involved. With an improved understanding of the biochemistry that underlies the altered phenotypic effect (e.g., variability in drug metabolism or transport), the search for specific genes responsible for the observed phenotypes has begun. Three major approaches have been generally utilized to identify clinical pharmacogenomic correlates: case/"N-of-1" studies, family studies, and association studies.

Case Reports and N-of-1 Studies

Case reports represent the most basic form of clinical research and are largely considered anecdotal. Nevertheless, case reports do serve important roles in pharmacogenomics by helping to generate plausible hypotheses regarding disease mechanisms through the in-depth evaluation of a limited number of clinical cases (in many instances, a single case). This type of publication generally reports on novel and/or remarkable cases. Within the field of pharmacogenomics, case reports can be used to document extreme responders to therapy at both ends of the spectrum to better guide future studies. As case studies move toward presenting individualized approaches to medicine, they have increasingly been considered as "n-of-1" or single-subject trials in the pharmacology spectrum and, in many instances, have yielded highly relevant information on the applications of personalized medicine.[34]

Family Studies

The use of pedigree data predates pharmacogenomics strategies; it has long been recognized that diseases, as well as responses to certain pharmacological compounds, often cluster in related individuals. The earliest pharmacogenomic studies were often an attempt to understand the pattern of inheritance for specific pharmacological traits without overt capacity at the time to identify the underlying genetic cause. While these early studies could not identify risk for toxicities to specific therapies without the toxicity first manifesting in related individuals (which undoubtedly contributed to high rates of both false-positive and false-negative associations), the practice of using pedigree information to inform clinical care remains an integral part of current practice, particularly in the absence of other data.

It can often be difficult to trace inheritance patterns for most pharmacological conditions because of the lack of an observable outward phenotype until after a drug has been administered. In the case of cytotoxic agents used for cancer treatment, pedigree information is generally not available unless multiple individuals in a family happen to have been treated using similar pharmacological regimens. Due to the potentially dangerous side effects, administering small test doses of many potentially toxic compounds is not considered an ethical course of action. However, in some instances, biological surrogate compounds, which are metabolized using the same pathways as specific drugs, can be used to assess inheritance patterns. For example, caffeine has been utilized as a surrogate for identifying and characterizing *N*-acetyltransferase (NAT) deficiency.[35] NAT is a phase II conjugating liver enzyme that catalyzes the N- and O-acetylation of heterocyclic amines. Individuals with NAT deficiency often experience toxicity to isoniazid, sulfonamide, procainamide, and hydralazine. NAT-deficient individuals are at high risk for developing peripheral neuropathy, idiopathic lupus erythematosus, and other drug-induced toxicities.[27,36] Caffeine can be administered as a relatively inert proxy compound to identify individuals in a family that are NAT-deficient without unnecessarily exposing people to the pharmacological compounds. Likewise, inert analogous test compounds may be used to test family members in the context of chemotherapy.[37]

As an alternative to measuring the in vivo metabolism of an analogous test compound, the activity of enzymes can be measured ex vivo. The ex vivo measurement of enzyme function often allows researchers to expand upon case reports to establish an inheritance pattern, particularly when rare variants are studied. For instance, the dihydropyrimidine dehydrogenase (DPD) enzyme (discussed in greater detail later in this chapter) rapidly inactivates approximately 85% of the chemotherapeutic 5-FU within minutes of administration.[38] This function primarily occurs in the liver; however, peripheral blood mononuclear cells (PBMCs) also express measurable levels of DPD. By measuring ex vivo DPD activity in PBMC lysates, researchers determined that causal variants for DPD deficiency exhibit codominant inheritance patterns.[39] Importantly, these variants were all later confirmed to be strongly associated with an increased risk of severe toxicity to 5-FU–containing treatments in large-scale clinical studies as discussed below.

Association Studies

Association studies aim to determine if the presence of a specific genotype correlates with a given outcome. In pharmacogenomics, outcome can be adverse response to a drug (e.g., toxicity) or pharmacological response to a drug (e.g., indicators of drug effectiveness). Association studies evaluate risk using two or more groups of unrelated individuals. As with pedigree studies, association studies can also utilize nonpharmacological test compounds and/or ex vivo measurements to determine the distribution of metabolic activity in the population. In pharmacogenomic association studies, patients are divided by genotype, and differences between endpoint frequency, timing, or other quantifiable variables are studied. Endpoints for efficacy can include overall survival, disease-free survival, progression-free survival, and adverse toxicity at or above a threshold (e.g., grade 3 or higher). The nature of the scientific question being asked often dictates the specific endpoint(s) to be studied. In many cases, multiple endpoints can be evaluated simultaneously.

When interpreting association studies, it is important to consider the contribution of other factors that may be exerting an effect on the endpoint, not just the genotype. For instance, older patients are often at greater risk for developing adverse toxicities to chemotherapy, regardless of genotype. Generalized differences in drug responses have also been observed between men and women for a multitude of therapeutic compounds. While many association studies strive to standardize treatment regimens, clinical practice often necessitates the administration of other drugs for potentially unrelated conditions. These covariates may exert some effect on the risk of experiencing an endpoint event that is likely independent of the genotype being studied. Therefore, statistical models need to be carefully designed to account for covariates in order to maintain adequate study power to address the primary hypothesis(es). Additionally, endpoints are not limited to binary variables. Commonly studied survival endpoints are nearly continuous variables that require specialized statistical tests to interpret (e.g., Kaplan-Meier statistics). When planning an association study, it is important to have *a priori* knowledge regarding the effect size that is expected for a given variant on an outcome. This helps to ensure that a study is adequately powered to accurately interpret results and to test the study's hypothesis.

Meta-analyses represent another class of association study that many consider to be the gold standard in clinical decision-making. Meta-analyses attempt to combine the results of multiple studies into a single statistical test. In meta-analyses, the power to interpret an association is not necessarily tied linearly to the overall population size. The power of evaluating multiple smaller studies can be greater than that of one large study. Careful consideration must also go into the design, analysis, and reporting of meta-analyses. Not all association studies are conducted using the same conditions, treatments, and assessments of endpoints. Therefore, statistical corrections are often applied to individual data sets in order to group analyses of results.

Guidelines for Tailoring Treatment Based on Genome Data

Several groups have begun to compile pharmacogenomic data with the goal of providing guidance for the appropriate implementation of genomic data into the clinical decision-making process (Table 5.2). The Pharmacogenomics Knowledge Base (PharmGKB) is a National Institutes of Health (NIH)-funded pharmacogenomics knowledge resource that contains clinical information including dosing guidelines and drug labels, as well as potentially clinically actionable gene-drug associations and genotype-phenotype correlations.[40] PharmGKB currently contains information on 631 drugs and 128 different pharmacokinetics/pharmacodynamics pathways.[1] Ninety-eight pharmacogenomic dosing guidelines and 488 drug labels are also reported on PharmGKB.[1] The dosing guidelines presented on PharmGKB are published by the Clinical Pharmacogenetics Implementation Consortium (CPIC), the Royal Dutch Association for the Advancement of Pharmacy—Pharmacogenomics Working Group (DPWG)—the Canadian Pharmacogenomics Network for Drug Safety (CPNDS), and other professional societies.

The three aforementioned professional societies are responsible for the vast majority of the curated clinical pharmacogenomics guidance that is available. CPIC is an international consortium of individual volunteers and a small, dedicated staff who are interested in facilitating the use of pharmacogenomic tests to improve patient care. The goal of CPIC is to reduce the barriers associated with translating genetic test results into actionable prescribing decisions by creating, curating, and freely disseminating peer-reviewed, evidence-based, updatable, and detailed gene/variant-drug clinical practice guidelines.[41–44] CPIC guidelines do not provide instruction on whether or not a specific pharmacogenomic test should be ordered; rather, they discuss how to interpret pharmacogenomic information and translate that information into clinical practice. The goals of DPWG are largely similar to those of CPIC

TABLE 5.2	*Resources for interpreting pharmacogenomic information*

Pharmacogenomics Knowledge Base (PharmGKB) https://www.pharmgkb.org/

PharmGKB is a knowledge repository that contains dosing guidelines and drug labels for potentially actionable gene-drug associations and genotype-phenotype relationships. PharmGKB curates information from many sources, including additional resources listed in this table.

Clinical Pharmacogenetics Implementation Consortium (CPIC) https://cpicpgx.org

CPIC is an international collaboration that is interested in overcoming barriers to the clinical implementation of pharmacogenomic test results by translating genetic information into actionable prescribing decisions. This is accomplished by CPIC by creating, curating, and making freely available, peer-reviewed, evidence-based, and detailed gene-drug clinical practice guidelines.

Dutch Pharmacogenetics Working Group (DPWG) https://www.pharmgkb.org/page/dpwg

DPWG's goals are to develop pharmacogenomics-based therapeutic recommendations and to assist with the integration of recommendations into computerized systems. Guidelines authored by DPWG are currently presented as individual research publications; however, the group is in the process of establishing a centralized and publically available repository for authored guidelines.

Canadian Pharmacogenomics Network for Drug Safety (CPNDS) http://cpnds.ubc.ca

The goals of CPNDS are directed toward reducing adverse drug responses in children through the development of predictive pharmacogenomic tests.

U.S. Food and Drug Administration (U.S. FDA) https://www.fda.gov

The U.S. FDA is a direct resource for approved drug labeling information.

in that they aim to develop pharmacogenetics-based therapeutic recommendations.[45,46] DPWG is also interested in assisting with the integration of recommendations into computerized systems for prescribing and automated medication surveillance.[45,46] As the name suggests, the scientists that comprise DPWG are all affiliated with research and/or medical centers in the Netherlands. CPNDS is a multicenter Canadian active surveillance and pharmacogenomic consortium that seeks to uncover the genetic and mechanistic basis of drug response phenotypes and to develop clinical pharmacogenomic implementation tools to improve the safety and efficacy of medications used in children and adults.[47] CPNDS is largely focused on adverse drug responses in pediatric care. The major sites for CPNDS activities are distributed throughout Canada; however, they also leverage a number of international collaborations.[47] In addition to the above-listed resources, information pertaining to pharmacogenomic biomarkers and implications for drug labeling can be obtained from the U.S. Food and Drug Administration (FDA).[48]

Actionable Gene Variants in Anticancer Drug Response

Several pharmacological syndromes are associated with specific genomic variants that can have profound effects not only on the efficacy of a drug but also on the toxicity profile and severity of toxicity associated with that compound. The levels of evidence linking specific variants to pharmacological conditions can vary. For instance, in the case of *DPYD*, there is reproducible and strong evidence that certain variants (e.g., *DPYD* *2A) can profoundly impact a patient's risk of severe and potentially lethal toxicity to 5-FU. The evidence correlating additional genes/variants with drug toxicity and/or response can vary greatly in strength.

5-Fluorouracil

The antimetabolite drug 5-FU was first synthesized nearly 60 years ago and is still widely used in cancer therapy. 5-FU is an analog of the naturally occurring pyrimidine uracil, which is taken up into cells and metabolized by the same enzymes that act on uracil.[38,39,49] Following uptake into cells, anabolism occurs via sequential steps to form the active 5-FU metabolites.[38,50,51] The biological activity of 5-FU is largely mediated through the anabolism product 5-fluoro-2′-deoxyuridine monophosphate (5-FdUMP). 5-FdUMP irreversibly inhibits the thymidylate synthase (TS) enzyme, which blocks the formation of thymidylate that is needed for DNA synthesis and repair.[52,53] Additional nucleotide products of 5-FU anabolism also contribute to the mode of action for 5-FU through integration of the fluorinated products into RNA and DNA. The activation of 5-FU via anabolism is detailed in Chapter 8 of this textbook. Catabolism, which occurs primarily in the liver, effectively limits the amount of circulating 5-FU that is available for anabolism by catalyzing the rapid and largely irreversible catabolic inactivation of approximately 85% of 5-FU (see Fig. 5.1).[38,54] DPD is the initial and rate-limiting enzyme of uracil and 5-FU catabolism. As such, DPD function has emerged as a key determinant of 5-FU toxicity risk.

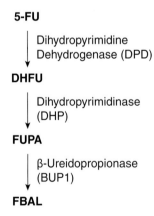

FIGURE　5.1 Approximately 85% of administered 5-fluorouracil (5-FU) is inactivated in the liver by the enzymes of the uracil catabolism pathway. The initial and rate-limiting enzyme of this pathway, dihydropyrimidine dehydrogenase (DPD), coverts 5-FU to 5,6-dihydro-5-fluorouracil (DHFU). Subsequently, DHFU is converted to α-fluoro-β-ureidopropionic acid (FUPA) by dihydropyrimidinase (DHP) enzymes. In the final step, β-ureidopropionase (BUP1) catalyzes the conversion of FUPA to fluoro-β-alanine (FBAL), which can subsequently undergo further modifications by both enzymatic and nonenzymatic processes. 5-FU and the downstream catabolites are all cleared from the circulation by the renal system.

A number of oral prodrugs of 5-FU have been developed. In the United States, capecitabine is the only one that is currently approved for clinical use. Capecitabine is activated to 5-FU by the action of three enzymes and exhibits a more sustained release of 5-FU into the circulation than intravenous bolus administration of 5-FU.[55,56] 5-FU and capecitabine are both used to treat two of the most common malignancies, colorectal and breast cancer, in approximately 2 million patients annually in the United States.

Dihydropyrimidine Dehydrogenase

Dihydropyrimidine dehydrogenase (DPD, encoded by the *DPYD* gene) is the enzyme that catalyzes the first step of the uracil catabolic pathway (Fig. 5.1) and is critically involved in the degradation of approximately 85% of administered 5-FU.[38] The inactivation of 5-FU via DPD occurs in an essentially unidirectional manner. Any inhibition of DPD by biochemical, pharmacologic, or genetic means can have profound effects on the circulating levels of 5-FU and increase the amount of 5-FU available for activation by the anabolic pathway. Therefore, factors that reduce DPD function increase toxicity in a similar manner as an overdose of 5-FU. While DPD is mainly expressed in the liver, measurable levels are also found in PBMCs, which can be sampled in a relatively noninvasive manner. DPD activity levels show a high degree of interindividual variability. Initial studies indicated that PBMC DPD activity levels were normally distributed in the general population; however, DPD activity varied between individuals by as much as 20-fold.[57] DPD activity inversely correlates with the half-life of 5-FU, and individuals with low DPD activity have extended half-lives for 5-FU in circulation.[38] Additionally, markedly reduced or even absent DPD activity has been observed in outliers from the observed normal distribution.[39]

Genetic variants in *DPYD* can cause complete or partial loss of DPD function and thus are thought to be responsible for much of the patient-to-patient variability in 5-FU toxicity and therapeutic efficacy.[20,39,58–60] *DPYD* is a relatively large gene that spans approximately 950 kb on chromosome 1p21.3.[61] The major isoform of *DPYD* (isoform 1, NM_000110) is composed of 4,451 nucleotides in 23 coding exons.[61–63] Familial studies have indicated that DPD deficiency is inherited in an autosomal codominant fashion and that DPD deficiency can be due to multiple mutations within the *DPYD* gene.[39,64] More than 100,000 inherited genetic variants have been reported in the genomic region encoding *DPYD*.[65] These include almost 700 nonsynonymous variants in the coding region that encompass 521 missense, 21 nonsense, 38 frameshift, and 107 splice variants, among other classes. The most widely studied variant that is associated with severe 5-FU toxicity is a splice junction variant known as *DPYD* *2A (also known as rs3918290, *DPYD*:IVS14 + 1G>A, c.1905+1G>A).[66–68] This variant causes the obligate expression of a truncated *DPYD* mRNA lacking sequence for exon 14, which results in a nonfunctional protein.[58,69–71] Other variants that have been shown to be associated with toxicity include rs55886062 (*DPYD* *13, c.1679A>C, p.I560S),[64] rs67376798 (c.2846T>A, p.D949V),[68,72] and rs75017182 (c.1129–5923C>G, a genetic tag for the *DPYD* haplotype HapB3).[73–76] Of these variants, rs3918290 and rs55886062 have the most deleterious impact on DPD activity,[71] whereas rs67376798 and rs75017182 result in moderately reduced DPD activity.[19,76] It should be noted that most clinical pharmacogenomic studies of 5-FU toxicity have largely studied Caucasian/European populations. Recently, an additional variant (rs115232898, c. 557A>G, p.Y186C) has been associated with reduced DPD function[20,77] and 5-FU toxicity[77–79] in African Americans.

The sensitivity of a genetic test for toxicity risk is dependent on the number of variants investigated. By combining the four well-established decreased/no function *DPYD* variants (rs3918290, rs67376798, rs55886062, and rs75017182), it is estimated that approximately 20% to 30% of early-onset 5-FU toxicities can be explained.[80] However, comprehensive data are not yet available to estimate the combined power of these four variants at predicting toxicity across all cycles of therapy. Regardless, any test that includes only a subset of those *DPYD* variants (e.g., only rs3918290) would have reduced sensitivity. Finally, given the existence of many additional deleterious *DPYD* variants,[19,21] the accuracy of genetic tests can potentially be improved by using sequence-based approaches instead of targeted genotyping approaches.

Recent preclinical studies have provided significant details regarding the contribution of rare genetic variants in *DPYD* to 5-FU toxicity risk.[19,21,71,77,81,82] These analyses have confirmed the level by which DPD function is reduced by commonly studied variants and have also identified the phenotypic effects of rare *DPYD* variants using in vitro and cellular systems. Importantly, many of the deleterious variants identified in these studies are enriched in or unique to non-European populations, which have been largely unrepresented in previous clinical studies.[19,21,77,82] It is estimated that the rare *DPYD* variants identified as deleterious in the above studies are present at similar and often higher cumulative frequencies in non-European populations as the well-studied toxicity-associated variants rs3918290, rs55886062, and rs67376798 (combined allele frequency).[82]

CPIC has established specific recommendations for using 5-FU in individuals who carry specific *DPYD* genotypes.[83,84] Current CPIC guidelines for *DPYD* recommend calculating a "DPD activity score" based on known/tested genetic variants. This score is tied to the number of variants identified, the known impact of the variants on function, and whether or not it is known if multiple variants are carried in *cis* on the same chromosome copy or in *trans* on opposite sister chromosome copies. The resulting score is used to calculate the starting dose of 5-FU, and it is suggested that subsequent doses be adjusted based on tolerance for therapy and therapeutic dose monitoring, if available. The strongest evidence for these recommendations has come from large clinical studies and meta-analyses. A recent large, well-controlled, clinical study established that 88% of heterozygous carriers of rs3918290/*2A develop a severe grade ≥3 toxicity to 5-FU.[68] The risk of severe toxicity remains extremely high in carriers of the partially deleterious variant rs67376798, with 82% of heterozygous carriers experiencing grade ≥3 toxicity.[68] Estimates for toxicity risk vary between studies, depending on the overall frequency of toxicity for a given treatment regimen.[68,73,80,85,86] It is also notable that patients without a detected deleterious *DPYD* variant may still experience severe toxicity due to additional genetic, environmental, or other factors.

Thymidylate Synthase

Over the past few decades, there has been considerable attention directed to thymidylate synthase (TS, encoded by the *TYMS* gene), one of the most important steps in 5-FU anabolism, as a source of variability for pharmacogenomic response. The 5-FU metabolite 5-FdUMP forms a stable complex with TS, inhibiting deoxythymidine monophosphate (dTMP) synthesis.[87] Variability in response to 5-FU has been suggested for some *TYMS* variants.[88,89] Additionally, high expression of TS has been linked to therapeutic resistance to 5-FU[5,90]; however, TS protein levels did not correlate with survival in a study of 391 stage III colon cancer patients treated with 5-FU–based regimens.[91] Overall, there are inadequate data at this time to include TS/*TYMS* expression or *TYMS* variations in the clinical decision-making process. A summary of additional relevant findings is presented below.

To date, several polymorphisms in the *TYMS* gene have been identified.[92] These include 74 missense, 1 nonsense, 1 frameshift, and 9 splice variants. The most commonly studied *TYMS* variant is a variable number tandem repeat of 28 base pairs located in the gene's enhancer region. This variant is denoted as TSER (for TS enhancer region) and typically contains 2 (TSER*2) to 9 (TSER*9) copies of the tandem repeat.[93] The TSER*2 and TSER*3 (i.e., 3 repeats) alleles are observed most frequently in Caucasian populations, and larger repeat expansions (e.g., TSER*4 through TSER*9) are detected more frequently in African populations.[94] The homozygous TSER*3 genotype is approximately twice as frequent in Asian populations (67%) as in Caucasian populations (38%). Using restriction fragment length polymorphism analysis, the allele frequency of TSER*3 in different ethnic populations was determined to be 56%, 47%, 28%, and 37% for non-Hispanic Whites, Hispanic Whites, African Americans, and Singapore Chinese, respectively.[95] The role of most of these alleles in TS expression is currently unknown; however, patients homozygous for the TSER*3 genotype have increased intratumor *TYMS* expression and elevated TS protein levels compared with patients with the homozygous TSER*2 genotype.[96,97]

The efficacy of 5-FU is reduced in patients with overexpressed TS due to an increased number of tandem repeats in the enhancer region.[98–103] Patients with metastatic colorectal cancer treated with 5-FU who are homozygous for TSER*3 have increased TS levels and reduced median survival (12 months) compared to patients homozygous for TSER*2 (16-month median survival).[104] *TYMS* expression has been shown to be increased greater than threefold in homozygous TSER*3 carriers compared to homozygous TSER*2 carriers.[96] 5-FU response has also been suggested to be correlated with TSER status. One study showed response rates of 50% in patients homozygous for TSER*2 and 9% in patients homozygous for TSER*3.[96] In a second study, colorectal cancer patients that were homozygous for TSER*3 were less likely to display improvements in tumor staging following 5-FU–based neoadjuvant therapy compared to TSER*2 homozygous or TSER*2/*3 heterozygous patients.[97] The TSER*3 allele has also been associated with reduced incidence of grade 3 or 4 toxicity.[105] A meta-analysis conducted in 2012 suggested that TSER*2 might be associated with clinical benefit and increased 5-FU toxicity; however, the authors noted publication bias in the data used for the analysis.[106] As a result, the contribution of TSER status to 5-FU response and toxicity remains unclear.[106] A recent study has suggested that another variant located in the enolase superfamily member 1 (*ENOSF1*) gene, which is adjacent to *TYMS*, is in LD with TSER variants and might contribute to 5-FU toxicity instead of *TYMS*.[107] At this time, 5-FU dose adjustments based on TSER status are not recommended by CPIC.[83]

Data for additional *TYMS* variants are generally lacking with regard to toxicity, efficacy, and/or tumor resistance. For instance, a single nucleotide variation within the second repeat of the TSER*3 allele (G→C, 3RG, and 3RC alleles) has been identified.[95] This variant has been suggested to reduce TS expression by abolishing a USF1 transcription factor binding site.[95] A 6–base pair deletion in the 3′ UTR of *TYMS* (located at nucleotide 1,496 of the mRNA, 447 nucleotides downstream of the stop codon) has also been reported.[108,109] This variant is in LD with TSER variants and has been shown to affect *TYMS* transcript levels, potentially by reducing mRNA stability.[108] An additional nonsense variant has been detected in a patient with longer-than-average survival, accompanied by grade 4 neutropenia, following 5-FU–based therapy for metastatic colorectal cancer.[110] Overall, there is general consensus that the evidence linking *TYMS* variants with response and/or toxicity to 5-FU is inadequate at present to be considered in the clinical decision-making process.

Methylenetetrahydrofolate Reductase

5,10-Methylenetetrahydrofolate (MTHF) is needed to form the ternary complex of 5-FdUMP and TS. It is this complex that essentially blocks the function of TS to convert deoxyuridine monophosphate (dUMP) to thymidylate. Methylenetetrahydrofolate reductase (MTHFR, encoded by the *MTHFR* gene) catalyzes the conversion of MTHF to 5-methyltetrahydrofolate, which itself does not complex with TS. A change in the availability of MTHF (due to MTHFR deficiency) would, therefore, be expected to augment the efficacy of 5-FU.[111] To date, 332 missense, 16 nonsense, 14 frameshift, and 70 splice-site variations have been reported in the *MTHFR* gene.[112] A few of these variants (e.g., c.C677T and A1298C) have been suggested to have a potential role in response to 5-FU.[113-116] Numerous additional studies attempting to link these variants to 5-FU response have reported contradictory conclusions or nonsignificant results.[117] A meta-analysis of C677T failed to demonstrate a significant association with 5-FU response.[106] At present, there are no recommendations from CPIC[83] or others regarding the use of genetic information about this gene to guide either toxicity or antitumor response.

Other Uracil Metabolism Genes

Variability in the conversion of 5-FU to critical nucleotides is theoretically very important in determining response as either tumor efficacy or host toxicity. However, at this point, there is little evidence that monitoring enzyme activity, expression, or genotype of additional genes involved with uracil metabolism has any clinical value.

Thiopurine Drugs (Mercaptopurine, Thioguanine, Azathioprine)

The antimetabolite thiopurine drugs 6-MP and 6-thioguanine (6-TG) have been used for many years in the treatment of acute lymphocytic leukemia (ALL), acute myeloid leukemia (AML), and chronic myeloid leukemia (CML). Azathioprine is a prodrug that is converted to 6-MP by nonenzymatic reduction in the intestinal wall, in the liver, and on the exterior of red blood cells; this process is mediated by glutathione. Azathioprine is not used for cancer treatment, but like 6-MP and 6-TG, it can be used as an immunosuppressive medication in Crohn's disease, ulcerative colitis, rheumatoid arthritis, and organ transplants. Both 6-MP and 6-TG are prodrugs that are converted into thioguanine nucleotides (TGNs) by hypoxanthine-guanine phosphoribosyltransferase (HGPRT, encoded by the *HPRT1* gene). TGNs are incorporated into DNA and inhibit purine nucleotide synthesis, trigger cell cycle arrest, and lead to apoptosis.[98] Despite being used to treat different conditions, all three thiopurine drugs share common pharmacologic effects and pathways of anabolism/catabolism. All three drugs have been recognized to be associated with a pharmacogenomic syndrome. The pathways of thiopurine drug metabolism and action are detailed in Chapter 10 of this textbook.

Thiopurine S-Methyltransferase

Thiopurine catabolism is highly reliant on the activity of thiopurine S-methyltransferase (TPMT, encoded by the *TPMT* gene). TPMT catalyzes the S-methylation of thiopurines in hematopoietic tissues. This decreases the intracellular thiopurine pool and consequently reduces the formation of active TGNs.[118] TPMT activity is inherited as a monogenic codominant trait that displays a trimodal distribution in the general population.[3,119] In a sample of 289 Caucasian blood donors, 89% demonstrated high TPMT enzyme activity, 11% demonstrated intermediate activity, and 0.3% demonstrated undetectable levels of activity.[3] TPMT activity is directly related to TPMT protein expression and is inversely related to TGN circulating concentrations.[120] Children with low levels of TGN and high TPMT activity are at increased risk of cancer relapse.[120-123] It is clear that variability in TPMT is responsible for much of the interindividual variability observed after administration of thiopurines. Individuals deficient for TPMT (i.e., two inactive copies of the *TPMT* gene) universally experience severe myelosuppression.[120,124-126] Most thiopurine recipients that carry one inactive and one active copy of *TPMT* experience moderate-to-severe myelosuppression, and carriers of two functional copies of *TPMT* are at lower risk of myelosuppression.[120,124-126] The endogenous function of this enzyme in the metabolism of natural purine compounds remains unclear.

At present, 107 missense, 5 nonsense, 8 frameshift, and 32 splice-site variants have been reported within the coding region for *TPMT*.[127] Fifteen *TPMT* variants (which comprise 17 *TPMT* haplotypes that are designated by "*" alleles) are associated with reduced TPMT activity and/or thiopurine-induced toxicity.[128-130] Three of these deleterious variants account for greater than 90% of inactivating alleles; therefore, targeted genotype tests are typically highly informative.[119,131] These alleles include rs1800462, rs1800460, and rs1142345. These variants comprise four haplotypes: *2 (rs1800462), *3A (rs1800460 and rs1143245), *3B (rs1800460), and *3C (rs1142345).[128,129] The frequency of *TPMT* variants differs by ethnicity.[4,128,129] Individuals of African and Caucasian ancestry exhibit the highest carrier frequency for individual deleterious *TPMT* haplotypes; *3C is carried by 5.0% of African patients, and *3A is carried by 3.6% of Caucasian patients.[128,129] Lower carrier frequencies for risk haplotypes have been reported for other racial groups.[128,129] This might suggest that expanded genotyping could be of benefit to those with non-African or non-Caucasian ancestry. The trimodal distribution of TGN levels and TPMT activity can largely be explained by the carrier status of the four most common *TPMT* haplotypes (i.e., *2, *3A, *3B, and *3C), with homozygous and compound heterozygous carriers displaying nonexistent TPMT levels, heterozygous carriers displaying intermediate TPMT levels, and noncarriers displaying "normal" TPMT levels. Although present in the general population at a very low frequency,[127] a fourth variant (rs1800584, *4) is also considered to be a strong risk variant for severe thiopurine-induced myelosuppression.[119,131] The additional 11 variants, most of which are extremely rare, exhibit reduced, but not absent, TPMT activity.[128,129]

There is clear evidence that TPMT-deficient individuals (i.e., those carrying homozygous or compound heterozygous deleterious *TPMT* variants) are at significantly increased risk for life-threatening thiopurine toxicity and that toxicity can be minimized by administering a reduced thiopurine dose.[124,125,132–136] Heterozygous carriers of a single deleterious *TPMT* allele/haplotype have also been consistently shown to be at increased risk of thiopurine-related toxicity.[123–125,137] Dose adjustment has likewise been shown to be effective at reducing toxicity and maintaining therapeutic efficacy in heterozygous carriers.[137–139] Current CPIC guidelines for thiopurine dose adjustment by TPMT/*TPMT* status, which were published in 2011 and updated in 2013, are consistent with these findings.[128,129]

Nudix Hydrolase 15

Nudix hydrolase 15 (NUDT15, encoded by the *NUDT15* gene) is a member of the nudix hydrolase superfamily, which catalyzes the hydrolysis of nucleoside triphosphates. NUDT15 acts as a negative regulator of thiopurine activation and toxicity.[140,141] Recent studies have indicated that carriers of loss-of-function alleles of *NUDT15* are unable to tolerate standard thiopurine doses.[140,142,143] These variants are more prevalent in individuals with Asian ancestry and Hispanic ethnicity.[142,143] Specific guidelines for treating patients that carry *NUDT15* variants with thiopurines have not been formulated; however, studies suggest that homozygous variant carriers may only be able to tolerate 10% of the standard dose.[142,143]

Irinotecan

Irinotecan (CPT-11) is a synthetic analog of the naturally occurring compound camptothecin. Irinotecan has been utilized in the treatment of several malignancies, most commonly for advanced metastatic colorectal cancer. Irinotecan is converted to SN-38 by carboxylesterase-mediated hydrolysis. SN-38 is a potent inhibitor of topoisomerase I, with 100 to 1,000× more affinity than the parent drug.[98] Phase II metabolism in the liver inactivates SN-38 via glucuronidation by uridine glucuronosyltransferase 1A1 (UGT1A1, encoded by the *UGT1A1* gene). This enzyme is also involved in bilirubin conjugation, and decreased UGT1A1 expression is thought to be associated with the clinical presentation of Gilbert's syndrome.[98,144,145] Toxicity to irinotecan typically manifests as myelosuppression and/or diarrhea.

UDP-Glucuronosyltransferase Family 1 Member A1

The UDP-glucuronosyltransferase family 1 member A1 (*UGT1A1*) gene is located on chromosome 2q37.1 and is part of a complex locus that encodes several UDP-glucuronosyltransferase enzymes. The coding region for *UGT1A1* contains 493 missense, 27 nonsense, 35 frameshift, and 36 splice-site variants that have been reported to date.[146] The expression of UGT1A1/*UGT1A1* is known to be affected by the number of thymine-adenine (TA) repeats in

the *UGT1A1* promoter at the rs8175347 locus, which is located 52 nucleotides upstream of the start site.[98,144,145] The structure of this promoter region has been shown to contain between 5 (*36 allele) and 8 (*37 allele) TA repeats within the TATA box. The wild-type (*1) allele encodes for 6 TA repeats. The number of TA repeats in the *UGT1A1* promoter is inversely correlated with transcription of the gene and levels of the enzyme.[147] The *28 allele is the most common *UGT1A1* promoter variant and encodes 7 TA repeats. UGT1A1 function is reduced by approximately 70% in patients homozygous for *28 compared to those who are homozygous for the wild-type *1 allele.[144,145,148] In European/Caucasian populations, the genotype frequencies for *28 have been reported to be 8% to 20% for homozygous carriers, 40% to 50% for heterozygous carriers, and 30% to 50% for noncarriers.[149,150] Allele frequencies for *28 vary greatly by region, ethnicity, and/or language groups within individuals of African ancestry (32% to 60%).[149] Whereas the 5-TA repeat variant *36 is exceedingly rare in individuals of European ancestry, the allele is carried at frequencies as high as 16% in individuals with African ancestry.[149] The frequency of repeat expansions has been reported to be lower in Asian populations compared to Caucasian populations, with 27% of Asians carrying *28 or *37 (i.e., 7 or 8 TA repeats) compared to 49% of Caucasians in one study.[148]

Patients with decreased UGT1A1 are more likely to experience diarrhea and myelosuppression during irinotecan therapy due to higher SN-38 levels.[98] Diarrhea is thought to be primarily due to reactivation of SN-38 glucuronide by glucuronidase in the bowel.[151] Four studies that included data from 351 patients demonstrated that *28 homozygous patients (n = 34) experienced 2.5- to 17-fold increased risk for irinotecan toxicity compared to patients homozygous for *1.[152–155] These findings prompted the FDA and producers to change the packaging insert for irinotecan to recommend that patients homozygous for *UGT1A1*28 to receive a lower initial dose of the drug.[156] The FDA has since approved a diagnostic test for *UGT1A1*28.[157] Numerous meta-analyses have evaluated the irinotecan toxicity risk in individuals carrying *28 and have generally concluded that *28 status is significantly associated with increased risk of irinotecan-related severe toxicity.[156,158,159] Two of the analyses indicated that *28 was associated with increased toxicity risk in patients treated with high-to-intermediate doses of irinotecan, but not in patients that received low doses of the drug.[156,158] A third, more recent, meta-analysis demonstrated that grade 3 to 4 neutropenia was significantly more frequent in patients carrying *28 compared to those that do not, irrespective of irinotecan dose.[159]

Two prospective studies have suggested that patients homozygous for *UGT1A1*28 might have significantly higher response rates and progression-free survival when treated with irinotecan-containing therapy than patients that are homozygous for the wild-type *1 allele.[160,161] Heterozygous *28/*1 patients exhibited intermediate responses compared to the two homozygous genotypes. An additional study of the IROX (irinotecan and oxaliplatin) protocol yielded conflicting results, with *28 homozygous patients exhibiting lower response rates, potentially due to poor tolerance to the drug regimen.[162] Meta-analyses reported in 2012 and 2014 failed to identify associations between *28 and response rate, progression-free survival, or overall survival in irinotecan-treated patients.[163,164]

Despite the inconsistent results reported for *UGT1A1*28, there is a general consensus that sufficient evidence exists to reduce the initial irinotecan dose in homozygous carriers of *28, and current FDA guidelines recommend that prescribers consider reducing the starting dose of irinotecan by at least one level in these patients.[165] Prescribers are advised to consider subsequent dose modifications based on individual patient tolerance to treatment.[165] The DPWG recommends a 30% irinotecan dose reduction for regimens containing greater than 250 mg/m[2] in patients that are homozygous for *28, followed by dose titration based on neutrophil count.[46] To minimize the potential for subtherapeutic treatment, the DPWG does not recommend dose reduction for heterozygous carriers of *28.[46] FDA and DPWG guidelines are supported by the joint French workgroup that is composed of the Group of Clinical Oncopharmacology (GPCO-Unicancer) and the National Network of Pharmacogenetics (RNPGx).[166] CPIC has not yet published additional clinical guidance for pharmacogenomics-based dose adjustments for irinotecan in *UGT1A1* variant carriers. The coding region missense variant *UGT1A1*6 (rs4148323), which is most common in Asian populations,[167] has also been linked to an increased risk for neutropenia.[168–170] There is, however, inadequate evidence for irinotecan dose adjustment in *6 carriers at this time. Overall, testing for *UGT1A1* alleles is not a common practice in the clinic because most irinotecan-related toxicities manifest as severe myelosuppression and/or diarrhea, which can be managed by dose reduction in subsequent treatment cycles.

Tamoxifen

Estrogen receptors (ER) or progesterone receptors (PR) are expressed by approximately 65% to 75% of breast cancers.[171] Endocrine therapy has demonstrated effectiveness against ER-positive tumors. Tamoxifen is a selective estrogen receptor modulator (SERM) that has been used as an anticancer agent for over 40 years. Tamoxifen has weak antiestrogen properties itself. However, the compound is extensively metabolized, and certain metabolites exhibit more potent antiestrogenic properties.[172,173] Tamoxifen is subject to extensive primary and secondary metabolism in the liver by cytochrome P450 enzymes. The major metabolic pathway for tamoxifen is demethylation to *N*-desmethyltamoxifen by CYP3A4.[174] The second most predominant pathway is the oxidation to 4-hydroxy-*N*-desmethyltamoxifen (endoxifen) by CYP2D6.[175] Tamoxifen can also be converted to 4-hydroxytamoxifen (4HT) by CYP2D6, CYP3A4, and CYP2C19, which can then be further metabolized to endoxifen.[176,177] The potency of endoxifen and 4HT as antiestrogenic compounds is approximately 100-fold greater than that of tamoxifen.[172,178,179] The metabolism of tamoxifen is described more fully elsewhere in this book (see Chapter 27). Tamoxifen has multiple FDA approvals for the prevention and treatment of premenopausal and postmenopausal breast cancer, and it is the only hormonal agent approved by the FDA for the prevention of premenopausal breast cancer, the treatment of breast ductal carcinoma in situ, and the treatment of premenopausal invasive breast cancer.

Cytochrome P450 Family 2 Subfamily D Member 6

The cytochrome P450 family 2 subfamily D member 6 (CYP2D6) enzyme is encoded by the *CYP2D6* gene on chromosome 22q13.2. Tamoxifen metabolism by CYP2D6 produces highly active hydroxylated metabolites with 100-fold greater potency as ER inhibitors and longer half-lives in plasma than tamoxifen. *CYP2D6* is highly

polymorphic, with 389 missense, 14 nonsense, 36 frameshift, and 79 splice-site variants reported.[180] Commonly studied alleles of *CYP2D6* are generally categorized according to function. Variants including CYP2D6*3, *4, *5, and *6 are classified as "no-function" alleles, whereas *9, *10, *17, and *41 are classified as "decreased function" alleles.[181–184] The initial retrospective study that suggested a link between *4 and breast cancer recurrence found that *4 was carried as a homozygous variant in 6% of the population, making it the most common no-function allele.[185] Additional variants (e.g., *2) are classified as "normal function" alleles, and *1 represents the "wild-type" *UGT1A1* form. *CYP2D6* is also subject to copy number variations, such as deletions and duplications. The *5 allele represents a deletion. Duplications are generally denoted using "xN," where "N" represents the number of copies of a particular allele. For example, *CYP2D6*1/*3x2* would indicate that the patient carried one copy of the wild-type gene and a duplicated copy of the *3 variant-containing gene. Additional details pertaining to the nomenclature used for CYP genes can be obtained from the Pharmacogene Variation Consortium.[186]

Clinical studies of *CYP2D6* genotypes have yielded conflicting results, largely due to variability in treatment regimens, tumor stages, and incomplete genotyping in various studies. "Activity scores" are typically determined for CYP2D6 based on diploid genotypes.[183] The activity score is used to estimate tamoxifen metabolizer status and to identify poor metabolizers, intermediate metabolizers, normal metabolizers, and ultra metabolizers.[183] There is considerable evidence linking *CYP2D6* genotype with endoxifen concentration in tamoxifen-treated patients, with *CYP2D6* genotype accounting for 34% to 52% of variability in endoxifen concentration.[187] Three studies demonstrated that poor metabolizers exhibited two to threefold increased risk of breast cancer recurrence following tamoxifen treatment relative to normal metabolizers.[185,188,189] Additional studies that relied on secondary analyses yielded contradictory findings.[190–192] These discrepant findings prompted a meta-analysis, which concluded that the association was relevant only to disease-free survival in patients receiving adjuvant tamoxifen at a specific dose.[193]

CPIC has recently released updated recommendations for the implementation of *UGT1A1* into tamoxifen therapy.[184] Because of noted extensive biological variability across clinical settings, the guidelines are focused on interpreting *CYP2D6* genotypes in the adjuvant setting for the treatment of ER-positive breast cancer. Poor and intermediate metabolizers are expected to be at increased risk for recurrence and for worse event-free survival compared to normal metabolizers. For partial metabolizers, alternative hormonal therapy with aromatase inhibitors (with or without ovarian function suppression, depending on the clinical case) should be considered. Compounds that are known to affect CYP2D6 function are contraindicated in tamoxifen-treated patients. The DPWG pharmacogenomic guidelines for *CYP2D6*[46] have not been updated since 2011 and are, therefore, largely superseded by the more current CPIC guidelines.[184] The tamoxifen label has been modified to include information pertinent to *CYP2D6* alleles. Clinical diagnostic tests are available; however, due to the number of *CYP2D6* alleles, uncertainty of genetic associations with clinical outcomes, and the potential associations being restricted to specific disease types/ states, testing is not widely used clinically.

Variants in additional CYP genes have been suggested to contribute to altered tamoxifen metabolism and clinical outcomes (e.g.,[194–197]). An analysis of data from the International Tamoxifen Consortium failed to detect correlations with variants within *CYP2C19* as suggested in previous studies.[196,197] Overall, the clinical contribution of variants in additional CYP genes remains unclear.

UDP-Glucuronosyltransferase Family

In addition to the roles described above for UDP-glucuronosyltransferase (UGT) family of enzymes, they can also glucuronidate and inactivate hydroxyl metabolites of tamoxifen. Variants in UGT-encoding genes have been associated with altered tamoxifen metabolism; however, the functional importance of these variants in the clinical setting has not been established.[198]

Sulfotransferase Family 1A Member 1

The sulfotransferase family 1A member 1 (SULT1A1, encoded by the *SULT1A1* gene) *2 allele has been associated with reduced response to breast cancer treatment with tamoxifen.[199–201] Homozygosity for the *2 allele has been associated with a threefold increased risk of death in one study. There are currently no recommendations for the implementation of the *SULT1A1* genotype into the clinical decision-making process.

Platinum Compounds

Cisplatin, carboplatin, and oxaliplatin are platinum analogs that are routinely used in the treatment of non–small cell lung carcinoma and ovarian, breast, gastrointestinal, and testicular cancers.[202] Cisplatin is also one of the most effective agents for the treatment of pediatric neuroblastoma, hepatoblastoma, brain tumors, osteosarcoma, and germ cell tumors. Three-year event-free survival has been reported to be greater than 80% for cisplatin when used as a monotherapy for the treatment of standard-risk hepatoblastoma.[203] However, platinum drugs are rarely administered as a single-agent therapy. The cytotoxic mechanism of platinum compounds involves the inhibition of DNA replication through the formation of inter- and intrastrand DNA adducts.[204] Enhanced DNA repair is an important mechanism of platinum resistance. There has also been considerable interest in determining the biological and therapeutic impact of variants in genes fundamental to DNA repair to both toxicity and efficacy of platinum-containing compounds. Both the nucleotide excision repair (NER) and base excision repair (BER) pathways are involved in repairing platinum-induced DNA adducts. The NER pathway consists of at least nine proteins that excise segments of damaged DNA. As the name implies, the BER pathway is responsible for correcting single base errors in DNA. Platinum-based chemotherapy is often associated with neurological complications, including peripheral neuropathy and/or ototoxicity.

Thiopurine S-Methyltransferase

Variants in the thiopurine S-methyltransferase (*TPMT*) gene, discussed above in regard to thiopurine toxicity, have been associated with cisplatin-induced hearing loss (ototoxicity) in pediatric and adult patients.[205] Cisplatin-induced ototoxicity manifests as permanent and bilateral hearing loss in 10% to 25% of adults and 26% to 90% of children treated with cisplatin.[206,207] Mild ototoxicity in children remains a significant problem because the toxicity can affect speech/language development, affect social development, and increase the risk of learning disabilities.[208,209] CPNDS has published guidelines recommending that pediatric patients who are to receive cisplatin be tested for the *TPMT* *2 (rs1800462), *3A (rs1142345 and rs1800460), *3B (rs1800460), and *3C (rs1142345) variants.[210] These recommendations were based on three cohorts from two studies that contained a total of 317 patients.[211,212] *TPMT* variants failed to significantly associate with ototoxicity in 3 additional studies (4 independent cohorts) that evaluated a total of 390 patients.[213–215] It is noted that differences in length of follow-up and/or criteria used to classify toxicities may have contributed to the observed differences.[216] The U.S. FDA-approved drug label for cisplatin was adjusted in 2015 to reflect the uncertainty in the literature pertaining to *TPMT* variant contributions to cisplatin-induced ototoxicity.

XPC Complex Subunit, DNA Damage Recognition and Repair Factor (XPC)

The XPC complex subunit, DNA damage recognition and repair factor (XPC) protein is encoded by the *XPC* gene on chromosome 3p25.1. XPC is important for damage sensing and DNA binding, with a preference for single-strand DNA, as part of the NER pathway. Mutations in *XPC* can result in xeroderma pigmentosum, a rare autosomal recessive disorder that is characterized by sensitivity to sunlight and early-onset carcinoma. The "G" allele of *XPC* variant rs2228001 has shown evidence for strong association with an increased risk of toxicity, including hearing loss[217] and neutropenia,[218] following treatment with cisplatin. A recent report failed to confirm the association with ototoxicity in a larger cohort consisting of testicular cancer patients that have been treated with cisplatin.[219]

ERCC Excision Repair 1, Endonuclease Non-catalytic Subunit

ERCC excision repair 1, endonuclease non-catalytic subunit (ERCC1, encoded by the *ERCC1* gene) is a component of the NER pathway, and its expression is linked to that of other members of the pathway, including XPA DNA damage recognition and repair factor (XPA), ERCC excision repair 3 TFIIH core complex helicase subunit (ERCC3), and ERCC excision repair 2 TFIIH core complex helicase subunit (ERCC2). The rs11615 variant has been linked with reduced ERCC1 expression at the protein and mRNA levels.[220,221] Patients carrying the "A" allele of rs11615 may be at increased risk for nephrotoxicity, lethal toxicity, poor survival, and poor response to platinum compounds,[222–228] although not all studies concur.[162,229–231] A second common variant (rs3212986, previously named "C8092A") has been suggested to decrease the stability of *ERCC1* mRNA.[232] Early studies linked expression of ERCC1 to platinum drug response in ovarian cancer.[90,233] Overall survival following platinum treatment for lung cancer was improved in homozygous carriers of the minor "C" allele of rs3212986.[232] The "C" allele of rs3212986 was also associated with an increased risk of nephrotoxicity in cisplatin-treated patients.[224] An additional publication has reported that heterozygous carriers of rs3212986 are at increased risk of cisplatin-induced nephrotoxicity[222]; however, a subsequent reanalysis of a subset of this same data set paradoxically failed to identify any association between rs3212986 and cisplatin toxicity.[231]

X-Ray Repair Cross-Complementing Group 1

The x-ray repair cross-complementing group 1 (XRCC1) protein (encoded by the *XRCC1* gene) is involved in the repair of single-strand DNA breaks formed by ionizing radiation and alkylating agents. XRCC1 is part of the BER pathway. The rs25487 "C" variant in *XRCC1* is relatively common, with allele frequencies greater than 10% in all HapMap populations. This variant causes a reduction in DNA repair capacity.[234] There is no consensus regarding the contribution of rs25487 to platinum drug response and/or toxicity. The "C" variant has been associated with increased progression-free[223,235] and overall[223,230,235] survival in some studies, but it has also failed to show correlation in other studies.[162,236] The rs25487 variant does not appear to contribute to platinum-induced toxicity.[162]

ERCC Excision Repair 2, TFIIH Core Complex Helicase Subunit

ERCC excision repair 2, TFIIH core complex helicase subunit (ERCC2, encoded by the *ERCC2* gene), also known as XPD, is part of the NER pathway as described for ERCC1, above. The rs11615 variant of *ERCC2* has been the subject of numerous studies pertaining to platinum response and toxicity. Generally, these studies show an association for the minor "A" allele with increased risk of toxicity,[222,224] increased risk of death,[226,227] and poorer response[223,225,226,237] following platinum therapy. It is notable that the largest reported study to test rs11615 association with platinum drug toxicity did not detect a significant association for the variant with toxicity or response.[162] The lack of association with toxicity[230,231] and response[229–231] has also been observed for rs11615 in other studies. Additional studies have suggested that the "G" allele of rs11615 may associate with improved response to platinum therapy.[228,238] The "C" allele of rs3212986 in *ERCC2* has been associated with an increased risk of nephrotoxicity following cisplatin treatment.[224] Another study has suggested that heterozygous carriers of the "A" and "C" alleles of rs3212986 may have longer progression-free survival and be at increased risk for severe neutropenia (but not nephrotoxicity).[222]

Methotrexate

Methotrexate is a mainstay of childhood leukemia therapy that acts as a competitive inhibitor of dihydrofolate reductase (DHFR, encoded by the *DHFR* gene) with an affinity that is approximately 1,000-fold that of folate.[239] Thymidine synthesis is dependent on folic acid; as a result, inhibition of DHFR by methotrexate blocks DNA synthesis. Methotrexate is also used as an immune system suppressant for the treatment of autoimmune disorders, including rheumatoid arthritis, Crohn's disease, and psoriasis, although additional mechanisms of action besides DHFR inhibition are thought to be involved. The pathways of methotrexate metabolism and action are detailed elsewhere in this book (see Chapter 7). The genetic differences in methotrexate uptake and metabolism, along with variation in *DHFR*, have been identified as possible modulators of methotrexate efficacy.[98] Solute carrier family 19 member 1 (SLC19A1, also known as reduced folate carrier 1, RFC1) transports methotrexate into cells, and decreased transport is a mechanism of resistance.[240] Variations in the genes encoding each of the proteins involved in methotrexate transport, metabolism, and

target have been shown to potentially influence the response and toxicity profiles of methotrexate therapy.

Methylenetetrahydrofolate Reductase

Folate metabolism is involved in the function of both 5-FU (discussed above) and methotrexate; therefore, methylenetetrahydrofolate reductase (MTHFR, encoded by the *MTHFR* gene) is potentially relevant to the efficacy/toxicity of both drugs. This section will focus on the role of MTHFR pharmacogenomics in the context of methotrexate. To date, two *MTHFR* variants have been potentially linked to methotrexate efficacy and/or toxicity—rs1801133 (c.665C>T, often erroneously referenced as c.677C>T throughout the literature due to numbering/naming differences) and rs1801131 (c.1286A>C, often erroneously referenced as c.1298A>C). Both variants decrease enzyme activity, with rs1801133 having a greater impact on function.[241,242] Carriers of the minor allele of rs1801133 may have poorer response to treatment, may be at increased risk of toxicity, may require a reduced dose of methotrexate, and/or may be at increased risk of folate deficiency.[204,243–250] Numerous studies have also produced conflicting results, including a lack of association with toxicity.[244,251–258] Additional studies showed no effect for rs1801133 on cancer relapse.[256,259,260] A 2013 meta-analysis of 24 studies concluded that patients homozygous for the minor allele are not at significantly increased risk of drug toxicity.[261] The evidence for rs1801131 is also largely discrepant, with a number of studies showing either association or lack of association with outcome and/or toxicity.[248,250,253–255,262] No genotype-guided dosing guidelines are provided for methotrexate/*MTHFR*.

ATP Binding Cassette Subfamily B Member 1

ATP binding cassette subfamily B member 1 (ABCB1, encoded by the *ABCB1* gene) is also known as multidrug resistance gene 1 (MDR1). ABCB1 is a membrane-associated protein that is part of the ABC superfamily of proteins, which function to transport various compounds across cellular membranes. ABCB1 is involved in the development of multidrug resistance in tumor cells due to alterations in ATP-dependent drug efflux pumps. The "A" allele of rs1045642 has been associated with increased circulating concentrations of methotrexate and increased risk of toxicity.[263–265] Recent studies have failed to confirm these associations and suggest that the rs1045642 genotype does not affect neural or mucosal toxicity[266,267] nor does it correlate with methotrexate exposure levels or response in adult precursor cell lymphoblastic leukemia-lymphoma.[267]

Solute Carrier Organic Anion Transporter Family Member 1B1 (SLCO1B1)

The membrane-bound sodium-independent organic anion transporter protein SLCO1B1 (previously referred to as OATP1B1 or SLC21A6) is encoded by the *SLCO1B1* gene and is involved in cellular influx of numerous compounds, including xenobiotics. The "C" allele of rs11045879 in *SLCO1B1* has recently been shown to be associated with decreased methotrexate clearance[268–270] and an increased risk of toxicity.[268,271] An additional study failed to demonstrate an association between rs11045879 and methotrexate levels in plasma following initiation of methotrexate therapy in pediatric ALL.[267]

Dihydrofolate Reductase

Dihydrofolate reductase (DHFR, encoded by the *DHFR* gene) acts to reduce dihydrofolate to tetrahydrofolate and is a primary target of methotrexate. Alterations in DHFR levels or reduced binding to methotrexate potentially contributes to therapeutic resistance.[272] Promoter variants that increase *DHFR* transcription have been suggested to be associated with reduced event-free survival in ALL.[273,274] A variant located at a microRNA-binding site in the *DHFR* 3′-untranslated region has been suggested to increase DHFR expression and promote resistance to methotrexate; however, no link to toxicity was noted in a limited study of 37 patients.[275,276] At present, there is no guidance for *DHFR* genotype-guided dosage.

Solute Carrier Family 19 Member 1

Solute carrier family 19 member 1 (SLC19A1, encoded by the *SLC19A1* gene, also known as reduced folate carrier 1) transports methotrexate into cells. *SLC19A1* is located on chromosome 21, and Down syndrome or hyperdiploidy that carries a duplication of chromosome 21 is more sensitive to methotrexate.[277,278] Variants in *SLC19A1* have the potential to affect the efficiency of the transporter[241]; however, there is inadequate conclusive evidence for *SLC19A1* genotype-guided methotrexate dosage at this time.

Anthracyclines

Anthracyclines (e.g., doxorubicin and daunorubicin) are among the most commonly used chemotherapeutics for the treatment of leukemia, lymphoma, a variety of solid tumors (including breast, lung, ovarian, and uterine cancers), and sarcomas. Anthracyclines inhibit topoisomerase II enzymes, which, in turn, block DNA transcription and replication. These effects are most prevalent in rapidly dividing cancer cells. Anthracyclines can also function by intercalating between DNA and RNA, creating DNA-damaging iron-mediated free oxygen radicals, and catalyzing the removal of histones from chromatin. The primary toxicity of concern when prescribing anthracyclines is cardiotoxicity. Cardiotoxicity has been shown to manifest as an asymptomatic cardiac dysfunction in as many as 57% of anthracycline-treated patients[279–282] and as cardiomyopathy resulting in congestive heart failure (CHF) in as many as 20% of anthracycline-treated patients.[280,283,284] Anthracycline-induced CHF is generally resistant to therapeutic intervention and is associated with mortality in up to 79% of cases.[280,283,284] There is evidence that variants in additional genes (*RARG*, *SLC28A3*, and *UGT1A6*) may help to identify individuals at low, moderate, and high risk for anthracycline-induced cardiotoxicity, as described below and detailed in clinical pharmacogenomic guidelines provided by CPNDS.[285] The action and metabolism of anthracyclines are detailed elsewhere in this book (Chapter 14). It should be noted that there is limited information available at present to provide specific dose alterations by genetic risk group.[285]

Retinoic Acid Receptor Gamma (RARγ)

A GWAS using 280 patients treated for childhood cancer identified the rs2229774 variant in the retinoic acid receptor gamma (*RARγ*) gene as significantly associated with anthracycline-induced cardiotoxicity.[285] The authors validated this strong association in two separate smaller patient populations (*n* = 96 and *n* = 80).[285] The rs2229774 variant was shown to alter the function of RARG, which

led to derepression of DNA topoisomerase II beta (TOP2B).[285] TOP2B is one of the direct targets of anthracycline therapy.[286] Mouse models have demonstrated that TOP2B is necessary for the development of anthracycline-induced cardiotoxicity.[287] The strong genetic and mechanistic data linking rs2229774 with anthracycline-induced cardiotoxicity have prompted CPNDS to recommend pharmacogenomics testing for this variant in all pediatric cancer patients that are to receive doxorubicin or daunorubicin.[285] Carriers of this variant should be considered to be at high risk of cardiotoxicity.

UDP-Glucuronosyltransferase Family 1 Member A6 (UGT1A6)

A synonymous variant in the UDP-glucuronosyltransferase family 1 member A6 gene (*UGT1A6*; rs17863783) has demonstrated strong evidence for association with increased cardiotoxicity risk to anthracyclines in pediatric patients.[288,289] This variant is a tag marker of the *UGT1A6*4* haplotype, which has been suggested to reduce UGT1A6 enzyme function by as much as 30% to 100%.[290,291] Reduced glucuronidation of anthracycline metabolites is believed to cause the accumulation of toxic metabolites that contribute to cardiotoxicity in carriers of *UGT1A6*4*/rs17863783.[292] CPNDS recommends pharmacogenomics testing for *UGT1A6*4*/rs17863783 in pediatric cancer patients that are to receive doxorubicin or daunorubicin.[285] Pediatric carriers of the risk allele ("T" allele for rs17863783) should be considered at high risk of cardiotoxicity with anthracycline therapy.[285]

Solute Carrier Family 28 Member 3 (SLC28A3)

Two variants in the solute carrier family 28 member 3 gene (*SLC28A3*; rs7853758 and rs885004) have consistently shown association with a reduced risk of cardiotoxicity in anthracycline studies. These studies have included three independent well-characterized pediatric cohorts in two separate reports.[288,289] Notably, the effects of these two variants are seemingly specific to pediatric patients; studies of adult patients have failed to detect a (protective) cardiotoxicity association.[293,294] The synonymous rs7853758 and intronic rs885004 variants are in strong LD, the minor allele of rs7853758 has been shown to affect *SLC28A3* mRNA levels.[295] As such, the minor allele of rs7853758 is likely "causal" for the protective effect; therefore, clinical recommendations focus on this variant. CPNDS recommends pharmacogenomics testing for *SLC28A3* rs7853758 in childhood cancer patients that are to be treated with doxorubicin or daunorubicin.[285] Because the available data suggest that rs7853758 is protective against cardiotoxicity, patients lacking either the toxicity-associated *RARG* rs2229774 or *UGT1A6*4* variants may be considered at low risk for anthracycline-induced cardiotoxicity.[285] Therefore, patients carrying the major allele of rs7853758 (but not *RARG* rs2229774 or *UGT1A6*4*) would be considered to be at moderate risk for anthracycline-induced cardiotoxicity.[285]

Additional Pathways

There is evidence of varying levels of strength that additional variants may increase the risk of anthracycline-induced cardiotoxicity. Variants in additional solute carrier transporter genes (e.g., *SLC22A17* and *SLC22A7*) have been linked with cardiotoxicity in large, well-characterized pediatric patient populations.[296] Variants in the ATP-binding cassette (ABC) genes *ABCB1*, *ABCB4*, *ABCC1*,

ABCC2, and *ABCC5* have been suggested to be associated with cardiotoxicity in various studies[289,293,297–299]; however, associations have been independently replicated only for rs246221 in *ABCC1*, the rs8187694/rs8187710 haplotype in *ABCC2*, and rs7627754 in *ABCC5*.[285,293,294,300] Weaker and/or inconsistent evidence for cardiotoxicity association has been noted for numerous variants in other genes/pathways. These variants, as well as their potential impact on patient care, have been detailed in recent CPNDS guidelines.[285]

References

1. The Pharmacogenomics Knowledge Base (PharmGKB). Available at https://www.pharmgkb.org/. Accessed December 21, 2017.
2. Einhorn M, Davidsohn I. Hepatotoxicity of mercaptopurine. *JAMA.* 1964;188: 802-806.
3. Weinshilboum RM, Sladek SL. Mercaptopurine pharmacogenetics: monogenic inheritance of erythrocyte thiopurine methyltransferase activity. *Am J Hum Genet.* 1980;32(5):651-662.
4. McLeod HL, Siva C. The thiopurine S-methyltransferase gene locus—implications for clinical pharmacogenomics. *Pharmacogenomics.* 2002;3(1):89-98.
5. Salonga D, et al. Colorectal tumors responding to 5-fluorouracil have low gene expression levels of dihydropyrimidine dehydrogenase, thymidylate synthase, and thymidine phosphorylase. *Clin Cancer Res.* 2000;6(4):1322-1327.
6. Chamary JV, Parmley JL, Hurst LD. Hearing silence: non-neutral evolution at synonymous sites in mammals. *Nat Rev Genet.* 2006;7(2):98-108.
7. Komar AA, Genetics. SNPs, silent but not invisible. *Science.* 2007;315(5811): 466-467.
8. Kimchi-Sarfaty C, et al. A "silent" polymorphism in the MDR1 gene changes substrate specificity. *Science.* 2007;315(5811):525-528.
9. Lander ES, et al. Initial sequencing and analysis of the human genome. *Nature.* 2001;409(6822):860-921.
10. Venter JC, et al. The sequence of the human genome. *Science.* 2001;291(5507): 1304-1351.
11. Sachidanandam R, et al. A map of human genome sequence variation containing 1.42 million single nucleotide polymorphisms. *Nature.* 2001; 409(6822):928-933.
12. Database of Single Nucleotide Polymorphisms (dbSNP), Build 150. Available at https://www.ncbi.nlm.nih.gov/projects/SNP/snp_summary.cgi?view +summary=view+summary&build_id=150. Accessed October 11, 2017.
13. Schork NJ, et al. Common vs. rare allele hypotheses for complex diseases. *Curr Opin Genet Dev.* 2009;19(3):212-219.
14. Halushka MK, et al. Patterns of single-nucleotide polymorphisms in candidate genes for blood-pressure homeostasis. *Nat Genet.* 1999;22(3):239-247.
15. Kryukov GV, Pennacchio LA, Sunyaev SR. Most rare missense alleles are deleterious in humans: implications for complex disease and association studies. *Am J Hum Genet.* 2007;80(4):727-739.
16. Gorlov IP, et al. Shifting paradigm of association studies: value of rare single-nucleotide polymorphisms. *Am J Hum Genet.* 2008;82(1):100-112.
17. Ramsey LB, et al. Rare versus common variants in pharmacogenetics: SLCO1B1 variation and methotrexate disposition. *Genome Res.* 2012;22(1):1-8.
18. Zhu Q, et al. A genome-wide comparison of the functional properties of rare and common genetic variants in humans. *Am J Hum Genet.* 2011;88(4):458-468.
19. Offer SM, et al. Comparative functional analysis of DPYD variants of potential clinical relevance to dihydropyrimidine dehydrogenase activity. *Cancer Res.* 2014;74(9):2545-2554.
20. Offer SM, et al. A DPYD variant (Y186C) in individuals of African ancestry is associated with reduced DPD enzyme activity. *Clin Pharmacol Ther.* 2013;94(1):158-166.
21. Elraiyah T, et al. Novel deleterious dihydropyrimidine dehydrogenase variants may contribute to 5-fluorouracil sensitivity in an East African population. *Clin Pharmacol Ther.* 2017;101(3):382-390.
22. Zhu M, Zhao S. Candidate gene identification approach: progress and challenges. *Int J Biol Sci.* 2007;3(7):420-427.
23. Evans WE, McLeod HL. Pharmacogenomics—drug disposition, drug targets, and side effects. *N Engl J Med.* 2003;348(6):538-549.
24. Alving AS, et al. Enzymatic deficiency in primaquine-sensitive erythrocytes. *Science.* 1956;124(3220):484-485.
25. Lehmann H, Ryan E. The familial incidence of low pseudocholinesterase level. *Lancet.* 1956;268(6934):124.
26. Kalow W. Familial incidence of low pseudocholinesterase level. *Lancet.* 1956;268(6942):576-577.
27. Evans DA, Manley KA, Mc KV. Genetic control of isoniazid metabolism in man. *Br Med J.* 1960;2(5197):485-491.
28. Ulrich CM, Robien K, McLeod HL. Cancer pharmacogenetics: polymorphisms, pathways and beyond. *Nat Rev Cancer.* 2003;3(12):912-920.
29. Slatkin M. Linkage disequilibrium—understanding the evolutionary past and mapping the medical future. *Nat Rev Genet.* 2008;9(6):477-485.
30. International HapMap C. A haplotype map of the human genome. *Nature.* 2005;437(7063):1299-1320.
31. Goldstein DB. Common genetic variation and human traits. *N Engl J Med.* 2009;360(17):1696-1698.
32. Goeman JJ, Solari A. Multiple hypothesis testing in genomics. *Stat Med.* 2014;33(11):1946-1978.
33. Risch N, Merikangas K. The future of genetic studies of complex human diseases. *Science.* 1996;273(5281):1516-1517.
34. Lillie EO, et al. The n-of-1 clinical trial: the ultimate strategy for individualizing medicine? *Per Med.* 2011;8(2):161-173.
35. Grant DM, et al. Acetylation pharmacogenetics. The slow acetylator phenotype is caused by decreased or absent arylamine N-acetyltransferase in human liver. *J Clin Invest.* 1990;85(3):968-972.
36. Wolkenstein P, et al. A slow acetylator genotype is a risk factor for sulphonamide-induced toxic epidermal necrolysis and Stevens-Johnson syndrome. *Pharmacogenetics.* 1995;5(4):255-258.
37. Innocenti F, Iyer L, Ratain MJ. Pharmacogenetics of anticancer agents: lessons from amonafide and irinotecan. *Drug Metab Dispos.* 2001;29(4 Pt 2): 596-600.
38. Heggie GD, et al. Clinical pharmacokinetics of 5-fluorouracil and its metabolites in plasma, urine, and bile. *Cancer Res.* 1987;47(8):2203-2206.
39. Diasio RB, Beavers TL, Carpenter JT. Familial deficiency of dihydropyrimidine dehydrogenase. Biochemical basis for familial pyrimidinemia and severe 5-fluorouracil-induced toxicity. *J Clin Invest.* 1988;81(1):47-51.
40. Whirl-Carrillo M, et al. Pharmacogenomics knowledge for personalized medicine. *Clin Pharmacol Ther.* 2012;92(4):414-417.
41. Clinical Pharmacogenetics Implementation Consortium (CPIC). Available at https://cpicpgx.org/. Accessed December 21, 2017.
42. Relling MV, Klein TE. CPIC: Clinical Pharmacogenetics Implementation Consortium of the Pharmacogenomics Research Network. *Clin Pharmacol Ther.* 2011;89(3):464-467.
43. Caudle KE, et al. Incorporation of pharmacogenomics into routine clinical practice: the Clinical Pharmacogenetics Implementation Consortium (CPIC) guideline development process. *Curr Drug Metab.* 2014;15(2):209-217.
44. Caudle KE, et al. Standardizing terms for clinical pharmacogenetic test results: consensus terms from the Clinical Pharmacogenetics Implementation Consortium (CPIC). *Genet Med.* 2017;19(2):215-223.
45. Swen JJ, et al. Pharmacogenetics: from bench to byte. *Clin Pharmacol Ther.* 2008;83(5):781-787.
46. Swen JJ, et al. Pharmacogenetics: from bench to byte—an update of guidelines. *Clin Pharmacol Ther.* 2011;89(5):662-673.
47. Canadian Pharmacogenomics Network for Drug Safety. Available at http://cpnds.ubc.ca/. Accessed December 21, 2017.
48. United State Food & Drug Administration (FDA) Table of Pharmacogenomic Biomarkers in Drug Labeling. Available at https://www.fda.gov/Drugs/ScienceResearch/ucm572698.htm. Accessed December 21, 2017.
49. Diasio RB. Clinical implications of dihydropyrimidine dehydrogenase on 5-FU pharmacology. *Oncology (Williston Park).* 2001;15(1 Suppl 2):21-26; discussion 27.
50. Heidelberger C, et al. Fluorinated pyrimidines, a new class of tumour-inhibitory compounds. *Nature.* 1957;179(4561):663-666.
51. Kessel D, Hall TC, Wodinsky I. Nucleotide formation as a determinant of 5-fluorouracil response in mouse leukemias. *Science.* 1966;154(3751): 911-913.

52. Sommer H, Santi DV. Purification and amino acid analysis of an active site peptide from thymidylate synthetase containing covalently bound 5-fluoro-2′-deoxyuridylate and methylenetetrahydrofolate. *Biochem Biophys Res Commun.* 1974;57(3):689-695.

53. Santi DV, McHenry CS, Sommer H. Mechanism of interaction of thymidylate synthetase with 5-fluorodeoxyuridylate. *Biochemistry.* 1974;13(3):471-481.

54. Sommadossi JP, et al. Rapid catabolism of 5-fluorouracil in freshly isolated rat hepatocytes as analyzed by high performance liquid chromatography. *J Biol Chem.* 1982;257(14):8171-8176.

55. Diasio RB. Improving fluorouracil chemotherapy with novel orally administered fluoropyrimidines. *Drugs.* 1999;58 suppl 3:119-126.

56. Judson IR, et al. A human capecitabine excretion balance and pharmacokinetic study after administration of a single oral dose of 14C-labelled drug. *Invest New Drugs.* 1999;17(1):49-56.

57. Lu Z, Zhang R, Diasio RB. Dihydropyrimidine dehydrogenase activity in human peripheral blood mononuclear cells and liver: population characteristics, newly identified deficient patients, and clinical implication in 5-fluorouracil chemotherapy. *Cancer Res.* 1993;53(22):5433-5438.

58. Wei X, et al. Molecular basis of the human dihydropyrimidine dehydrogenase deficiency and 5-fluorouracil toxicity. *J Clin Invest.* 1996;98(3):610-615.

59. Lu Z, et al. Decreased dihydropyrimidine dehydrogenase activity in a population of patients with breast cancer: implication for 5-fluorouracil-based chemotherapy. *Clin Cancer Res.* 1998;4(2):325-329.

60. Etienne MC, et al. Population study of dihydropyrimidine dehydrogenase in cancer patients. *J Clin Oncol.* 1994;12(11):2248-2253.

61. National Center for Biotechnology Information (NCBI)—Gene (DPYD). 2017. Available at https://www.ncbi.nlm.nih.gov/gene/1806. Accessed December 21, 2017.

62. Johnson MR, et al. Structural organization of the human dihydropyrimidine dehydrogenase gene. *Cancer Res.* 1997;57(9):1660-1663.

63. Lu ZH, Zhang R, Diasio RB. Purification and characterization of dihydropyrimidine dehydrogenase from human liver. *J Biol Chem.* 1992;267(24):17102-17109.

64. Johnson MR, Wang K, Diasio RB. Profound dihydropyrimidine dehydrogenase deficiency resulting from a novel compound heterozygote genotype. *Clin Cancer Res.* 2002;8(3):768-774.

65. Database of Single Nucleotide Polymorphisms (dbSNP), DPYD Gene. Available at https://www.ncbi.nlm.nih.gov/SNP/snp_ref.cgi?locusId=1806. Accessed December 21, 2017.

66. Johnson MR, Diasio RB. Importance of dihydropyrimidine dehydrogenase (DPD) deficiency in patients exhibiting toxicity following treatment with 5-fluorouracil. *Adv Enzyme Regul.* 2001;41:151-157.

67. Ridge SA, et al. Dihydropyrimidine dehydrogenase pharmacogenetics in patients with colorectal cancer. *Br J Cancer.* 1998;77(3):497-500.

68. Lee AM, et al. DPYD variants as predictors of 5-fluorouracil toxicity in adjuvant colon cancer treatment (NCCTG N0147). *J Natl Cancer Inst.* 2014;106(12).

69. van Kuilenburg AB, et al. Lethal outcome of a patient with a complete dihydropyrimidine dehydrogenase (DPD) deficiency after administration of 5-fluorouracil: frequency of the common IVS14+1G>A mutation causing DPD deficiency. *Clin Cancer Res.* 2001;7(5):1149-1153.

70. Johnson MR, et al. Life-threatening toxicity in a dihydropyrimidine dehydrogenase-deficient patient after treatment with topical 5-fluorouracil. *Clin Cancer Res.* 1999;5(8):2006-2011.

71. Offer SM, et al. Phenotypic profiling of DPYD variations relevant to 5-fluorouracil sensitivity using real-time cellular analysis and in vitro measurement of enzyme activity. *Cancer Res.* 2013;73(6):1958-1968.

72. van Kuilenburg AB, et al. Clinical implications of dihydropyrimidine dehydrogenase (DPD) deficiency in patients with severe 5-fluorouracil-associated toxicity: identification of new mutations in the DPD gene. *Clin Cancer Res.* 2000;6(12):4705-4712.

73. Amstutz U, et al. Dihydropyrimidine dehydrogenase gene variation and severe 5-fluorouracil toxicity: a haplotype assessment. *Pharmacogenomics.* 2009;10(6):931-944.

74. van Kuilenburg AB, et al. Intragenic deletions and a deep intronic mutation affecting pre-mRNA splicing in the dihydropyrimidine dehydrogenase gene as novel mechanisms causing 5-fluorouracil toxicity. *Hum Genet.* 2010;128(5):529-538.

75. Lee AM, et al. Association between DPYD c.1129-5923 C>G/hapB3 and severe toxicity to 5-fluorouracil-based chemotherapy in stage III colon cancer patients: NCCTG N0147 (Alliance). *Pharmacogenet Genomics.* 2016;26(3):133-137.

76. Nie Q, et al. Quantitative Contribution of rs75017182 to Dihydropyrimidine Dehydrogenase mRNA Splicing and Enzyme Activity. *Clin Pharmacol Ther.* 2017;102(4):662-670.

77. Offer SM, Diasio RB. Response to "A case of 5-FU-related severe toxicity associated with the P.Y186C DPYD variant". *Clin Pharmacol Ther.* 2014;95(2):137.

78. Saif MW, et al. A DPYD variant (Y186C) specific to individuals of African descent in a patient with life-threatening 5-FU toxic effects: potential for an individualized medicine approach. *Mayo Clin Proc.* 2014;89(1):131-136.

79. Zaanan A, et al. A case of 5-FU-related severe toxicity associated with the p.Y186C DPYD variant. *Clin Pharmacol Ther.* 2014;95(2):136.

80. Froehlich TK, et al. Clinical importance of risk variants in the dihydropyrimidine dehydrogenase gene for the prediction of early-onset fluoropyrimidine toxicity. *Int J Cancer.* 2015;136(3):730-739.

81. Kuilenburg AB, et al. Phenotypic and clinical implications of variants in the dihydropyrimidine dehydrogenase gene. *Biochim Biophys Acta.* 2016;1862(4):754-762.

82. Shrestha S, et al. Gene-specific variant classifier (DPYD-Varifier) to identify deleterious alleles of dihydropyrimidine dehydrogenase. *Clin Pharmacol Ther.* 2018.

83. Amstutz U, et al. Clinical Pharmacogenetics Implementation Consortium (CPIC) Guideline for dihydropyrimidine dehydrogenase genotype and fluoropyrimidine dosing: 2017 update. *Clin Pharmacol Ther.* 2018;103(2):210-216.

84. Caudle KE, et al. Clinical Pharmacogenetics Implementation Consortium guidelines for dihydropyrimidine dehydrogenase genotype and fluoropyrimidine dosing. *Clin Pharmacol Ther.* 2013;94(6):640-645.

85. Morel A, et al. Clinical relevance of different dihydropyrimidine dehydrogenase gene single nucleotide polymorphisms on 5-fluorouracil tolerance. *Mol Cancer Ther.* 2006;5(11):2895-2904.

86. Schwab M, et al. Role of genetic and nongenetic factors for fluorouracil treatment-related severe toxicity: a prospective clinical trial by the German 5-FU Toxicity Study Group. *J Clin Oncol.* 2008;26(13):2131-2138.

87. Watters JW, McLeod HL. Cancer pharmacogenomics: current and future applications. *Biochim Biophys Acta.* 2003;1603(2):99-111.

88. Chu E, et al. Autoregulation of human thymidylate synthase messenger RNA translation by thymidylate synthase. *Proc Natl Acad Sci U S A.* 1991;88(20):8977-8981.

89. Dolnick BJ. Thymidylate synthase and the cell cycle: what should we believe? *Cancer J.* 2000;6(4):215-216.

90. Metzger R, et al. ERCC1 mRNA levels complement thymidylate synthase mRNA levels in predicting response and survival for gastric cancer patients receiving combination cisplatin and fluorouracil chemotherapy. *J Clin Oncol.* 1998;16(1):309-316.

91. Westra JL, et al. Predictive value of thymidylate synthase and dihydropyrimidine dehydrogenase protein expression on survival in adjuvantly treated stage III colon cancer patients. *Ann Oncol.* 2005;16(10):1646-1653.

92. Database of Single Nucleotide Polymorphisms (dbSNP), TYMS Gene. Available at https://www.ncbi.nlm.nih.gov/SNP/snp_ref.cgi?locusId=7298. Accessed December 21, 2017.

93. Copur MS, Chu E. Thymidylate Synthase Pharmacogenetics in Colorectal Cancer. *Clin Colorectal Cancer.* 2001;1(3):179-180.

94. Marsh S, et al. Novel thymidylate synthase enhancer region alleles in African populations. *Hum Mutat.* 2000;16(6):528.

95. Mandola MV, et al. A novel single nucleotide polymorphism within the 5′ tandem repeat polymorphism of the thymidylate synthase gene abolishes USF-1 binding and alters transcriptional activity. *Cancer Res.* 2003;63(11):2898-2904.

96. Pullarkat ST, et al. Thymidylate synthase gene polymorphism determines response and toxicity of 5-FU chemotherapy. *Pharmacogenomics J.* 2001;1(1):65-70.

97. Villafranca E, et al. Polymorphisms of the repeated sequences in the enhancer region of the thymidylate synthase gene promoter may predict downstaging after preoperative chemoradiation in rectal cancer. *J Clin Oncol.* 2001;19(6):1779-1786.

98. Relling MV, Dervieux T. Pharmacogenetics and cancer therapy. *Nat Rev Cancer.* 2001;1(2):99-108.

99. Aschele C, et al. Immunohistochemical quantitation of thymidylate synthase expression in colorectal cancer metastases predicts for clinical outcome to fluorouracil-based chemotherapy. *J Clin Oncol.* 1999;17(6):1760-1770.

100. Johnston PG, et al. The role of thymidylate synthase expression in prognosis and outcome of adjuvant chemotherapy in patients with rectal cancer. *J Clin Oncol.* 1994;12(12):2640-2647.

101. Kornmann M, et al. Thymidylate synthase is a predictor for response and resistance in hepatic artery infusion chemotherapy. *Cancer Lett.* 1997;118(1):29-35.

102. Lenz HJ, et al. Thymidylate synthase mRNA level in adenocarcinoma of the stomach: a predictor for primary tumor response and overall survival. *J Clin Oncol.* 1996;14(1):176-182.

103. Pestalozzi BC, et al. Increased thymidylate synthase protein levels are principally associated with proliferation but not cell cycle phase in asynchronous human cancer cells. *Br J Cancer.* 1995;71(6):1151-1157.

104. Marsh S, et al. Polymorphism in the thymidylate synthase promoter enhancer region in colorectal cancer. *Int J Oncol.* 2001;19(2):383-386.

105. Lecomte T, et al. Thymidylate synthase gene polymorphism predicts toxicity in colorectal cancer patients receiving 5-fluorouracil-based chemotherapy. *Clin Cancer Res.* 2004;10(17):5880-5888.

106. Jennings BA, et al. Functional polymorphisms of folate metabolism and response to chemotherapy for colorectal cancer, a systematic review and meta-analysis. *Pharmacogenet Genomics.* 2012;22(4):290-304.

107. Rosmarin D, et al. A candidate gene study of capecitabine-related toxicity in colorectal cancer identifies new toxicity variants at DPYD and a putative role for ENOSF1 rather than TYMS. *Gut.* 2015;64(1):111-120.

108. Mandola MV, et al. A 6 bp polymorphism in the thymidylate synthase gene causes message instability and is associated with decreased intratumoral TS mRNA levels. *Pharmacogenetics.* 2004;14(5):319-327.

109. Ulrich CM, et al. Searching expressed sequence tag databases: discovery and confirmation of a common polymorphism in the thymidylate synthase gene. *Cancer Epidemiol Biomarkers Prev.* 2000;9(12):1381-1385.

110. Balboa-Beltran E, et al. Long survival and severe toxicity under 5-fluorouracil-based therapy in a patient with colorectal cancer who harbors a germline codon-stop mutation in TYMS. *Mayo Clin Proc.* 2015;90(9):1298-1303.

111. De Mattia E, Toffoli G. C677T and A1298C MTHFR polymorphisms, a challenge for antifolate and fluoropyrimidine-based therapy personalisation. *Eur J Cancer.* 2009;45(8):1333-1351.

112. Database of Single Nucleotide Polymorphisms (dbSNP), MTHFR Gene. Available at https://www.ncbi.nlm.nih.gov/SNP/snp_ref.cgi?locusId=4524. Accessed December 21, 2017.

113. Cohen V, et al. Methylenetetrahydrofolate reductase polymorphism in advanced colorectal cancer: a novel genomic predictor of clinical response to fluoropyrimidine-based chemotherapy. *Clin Cancer Res.* 2003;9(5):1611-1615.

114. Jakobsen A, et al. Thymidylate synthase and methylenetetrahydrofolate reductase gene polymorphism in normal tissue as predictors of fluorouracil sensitivity. *J Clin Oncol.* 2005;23(7):1365-1369.

115. Terrazzino S, et al. A haplotype of the methylenetetrahydrofolate reductase gene predicts poor tumor response in rectal cancer patients receiving preoperative chemoradiation. *Pharmacogenet Genomics.* 2006;16(11):817-824.

116. Derwinger K, et al. A study of the MTHFR gene polymorphism C677T in colorectal cancer. *Clin Colorectal Cancer.* 2009;8(1):43-48.

117. Ruzzo A, et al. Pharmacogenetic profiling in patients with advanced colorectal cancer treated with first-line FOLFOX-4 chemotherapy. *J Clin Oncol.* 2007;25(10):1247-1254.

118. Weinshilboum R, Wang L. Pharmacogenomics: bench to bedside. *Nat Rev Drug Discov.* 2004;3(9):739-748.

119. Schaeffeler E, et al. Comprehensive analysis of thiopurine S-methyltransferase phenotype-genotype correlation in a large population of German-Caucasians and identification of novel TPMT variants. *Pharmacogenetics.* 2004;14(7):407-417.

120. Lennard L, et al. Genetic variation in response to 6-mercaptopurine for childhood acute lymphoblastic leukaemia. *Lancet.* 1990;336(8709):225-229.

121. Stanulla M, et al. Thiopurine methyltransferase (TPMT) genotype and early treatment response to mercaptopurine in childhood acute lymphoblastic leukemia. *JAMA.* 2005;293(12):1485-1489.

122. Schmiegelow K, et al. Thiopurine methyltransferase activity is related to the risk of relapse of childhood acute lymphoblastic leukemia: results from the NOPHO ALL-92 study. *Leukemia.* 2009;23(3):557-564.

123. Lennard L, et al. Thiopurine pharmacogenetics in leukemia: correlation of erythrocyte thiopurine methyltransferase activity and 6-thioguanine nucleotide concentrations. *Clin Pharmacol Ther.* 1987;41(1):18-25.

124. Black AJ, et al. Thiopurine methyltransferase genotype predicts therapy-limiting severe toxicity from azathioprine. *Ann Intern Med.* 1998;129(9):716-718.

125. Relling MV, et al. Mercaptopurine therapy intolerance and heterozygosity at the thiopurine S-methyltransferase gene locus. *J Natl Cancer Inst.* 1999;91(23):2001-2008.

126. Lennard L, Van Loon JA, Weinshilboum RM. Pharmacogenetics of acute azathioprine toxicity: relationship to thiopurine methyltransferase genetic polymorphism. *Clin Pharmacol Ther.* 1989;46(2):149-154.

127. Database of Single Nucleotide Polymorphisms (dbSNP), TPMT Gene. Available at https://www.ncbi.nlm.nih.gov/SNP/snp_ref.cgi?locusId=7172. Accessed December 21, 2017.

128. Relling MV, et al. Clinical pharmacogenetics implementation consortium guidelines for thiopurine methyltransferase genotype and thiopurine dosing: 2013 update. *Clin Pharmacol Ther.* 2013;93(4):324-325.

129. Relling MV, et al. Clinical Pharmacogenetics Implementation Consortium guidelines for thiopurine methyltransferase genotype and thiopurine dosing. *Clin Pharmacol Ther.* 2011;89(3):387-391.

130. Schaeffeler E, et al. Highly multiplexed genotyping of thiopurine s-methyltransferase variants using MALD-TOF mass spectrometry: reliable genotyping in different ethnic groups. *Clin Chem.* 2008;54(10):1637-1647.

131. Yates CR, et al. Molecular diagnosis of thiopurine S-methyltransferase deficiency: genetic basis for azathioprine and mercaptopurine intolerance. *Ann Intern Med.* 1997;126(8):608-614.

132. Schwab M, et al. Azathioprine therapy and adverse drug reactions in patients with inflammatory bowel disease: impact of thiopurine S-methyltransferase polymorphism. *Pharmacogenetics.* 2002;12(6):429-436.

133. Schutz E, et al. Azathioprine-induced myelosuppression in thiopurine methyltransferase deficient heart transplant recipient. *Lancet.* 1993;341(8842):436.

134. McLeod HL, Miller DR, Evans WE. Azathioprine-induced myelosuppression in thiopurine methyltransferase deficient heart transplant recipient. *Lancet.* 1993;341(8853):1151.

135. Kaskas BA, et al. Safe treatment of thiopurine S-methyltransferase deficient Crohn's disease patients with azathioprine. *Gut.* 2003;52(1):140-142.

136. Evans WE, et al. Altered mercaptopurine metabolism, toxic effects, and dosage requirement in a thiopurine methyltransferase-deficient child with acute lymphocytic leukemia. *J Pediatr.* 1991;119(6):985-989.

137. Evans WE, et al. Preponderance of thiopurine S-methyltransferase deficiency and heterozygosity among patients intolerant to mercaptopurine or azathioprine. *J Clin Oncol.* 2001;19(8):2293-2301.

138. Stocco G, et al. Genetic polymorphism of inosine triphosphate pyrophosphatase is a determinant of mercaptopurine metabolism and toxicity during treatment for acute lymphoblastic leukemia. *Clin Pharmacol Ther.* 2009;85(2):164-172.

139. Meggitt SJ, Gray JC, Reynolds NJ. Azathioprine dosed by thiopurine methyltransferase activity for moderate-to-severe atopic eczema: a double-blind, randomised controlled trial. *Lancet.* 2006;367(9513):839-846.

140. Yang SK, et al. A common missense variant in NUDT15 confers susceptibility to thiopurine-induced leukopenia. *Nat Genet.* 2014;46(9):1017-1020.

141. Carter M, et al. Crystal structure, biochemical and cellular activities demonstrate separate functions of MTH1 and MTH2. *Nat Commun.* 2015;6:7871.

142. Yang JJ, et al. Inherited NUDT15 variant is a genetic determinant of mercaptopurine intolerance in children with acute lymphoblastic leukemia. *J Clin Oncol.* 2015;33(11):1235-1242.

143. Moriyama T, et al. NUDT15 polymorphisms alter thiopurine metabolism and hematopoietic toxicity. *Nat Genet.* 2016;48(4):367-373.

144. Bosma PJ, et al. Mechanisms of inherited deficiencies of multiple UDP-glucuronosyltransferase isoforms in two patients with Crigler-Najjar syndrome, type I. *FASEB J.* 1992;6(10):2859-2863.

145. Monaghan G, et al. Genetic variation in bilirubin UPD-glucuronosyltransferase gene promoter and Gilbert's syndrome. *Lancet.* 1996;347(9001):578-581.

146. Database of Single Nucleotide Polymorphisms (dbSNP), UGT1A1 Gene. Available at https://www.ncbi.nlm.nih.gov/SNP/snp_ref.cgi?locusId=54658. Accessed December 21, 2017.

147. Beutler E, Gelbart T, Demina A. Racial variability in the UDP-glucuronosyltransferase 1 (UGT1A1) promoter: a balanced polymorphism for regulation of bilirubin metabolism? *Proc Natl Acad Sci U S A.* 1998;95(14):8170-8174.

148. Lampe JW, et al. UDP-glucuronosyltransferase (UGT1A1*28 and UGT1A6*2) polymorphisms in Caucasians and Asians: relationships to serum bilirubin concentrations. *Pharmacogenetics.* 1999;9(3):341-349.

149. Horsfall LJ, et al. Prevalence of clinically relevant UGT1A alleles and haplotypes in African populations. *Ann Hum Genet.* 2011;75(2):236-246.

150. Mercke Odeberg J, et al. UGT1A polymorphisms in a Swedish cohort and a human diversity panel, and the relation to bilirubin plasma levels in males and females. *Eur J Clin Pharmacol.* 2006;62(10):829-837.

151. Schulz C, et al. UGT1A1 gene polymorphism: impact on toxicity and efficacy of irinotecan-based regimens in metastatic colorectal cancer. *World J Gastroenterol.* 2009;15(40):5058-5066.

152. Ando Y, et al. Polymorphisms of UDP-glucuronosyltransferase gene and irinotecan toxicity: a pharmacogenetic analysis. *Cancer Res.* 2000;60(24):6921-6926.

153. Innocenti F, et al. Genetic variants in the UDP-glucuronosyltransferase 1A1 gene predict the risk of severe neutropenia of irinotecan. *J Clin Oncol.* 2004;22(8):1382-1388.

154. Marcuello E, et al. UGT1A1 gene variations and irinotecan treatment in patients with metastatic colorectal cancer. *Br J Cancer.* 2004;91(4):678-682.

155. Rouits E, et al. Relevance of different UGT1A1 polymorphisms in irinotecan-induced toxicity: a molecular and clinical study of 75 patients. *Clin Cancer Res.* 2004;10(15):5151-5159.

156. Hoskins JM, et al. UGT1A1*28 genotype and irinotecan-induced neutropenia: dose matters. *J Natl Cancer Inst.* 2007;99(17):1290-1295.

157. Hasegawa Y, et al. Rapid detection of UGT1A1 gene polymorphisms by newly developed Invader assay. *Clin Chem.* 2004;50(8):1479-1480.

158. Hu ZY, et al. Dose-dependent association between UGT1A1*28 genotype and irinotecan-induced neutropenia: low doses also increase risk. *Clin Cancer Res.* 2010;16(15):3832-3842.

159. Liu X, et al. Association of UGT1A1*28 polymorphisms with irinotecan-induced toxicities in colorectal cancer: a meta-analysis in Caucasians. *Pharmacogenomics J.* 2014;14(2):120-129.

160. Toffoli G, et al. The role of UGT1A1*28 polymorphism in the pharmacodynamics and pharmacokinetics of irinotecan in patients with metastatic colorectal cancer. *J Clin Oncol.* 2006;24(19):3061-3068.

161. Cecchin E, et al. Predictive role of the UGT1A1, UGT1A7, and UGT1A9 genetic variants and their haplotypes on the outcome of metastatic colorectal cancer patients treated with fluorouracil, leucovorin, and irinotecan. *J Clin Oncol.* 2009;27(15):2457-2465.

162. McLeod HL, et al. Pharmacogenetic predictors of adverse events and response to chemotherapy in metastatic colorectal cancer: results from North American Gastrointestinal Intergroup Trial N9741. *J Clin Oncol.* 2010;28(20):3227-3233.

163. Dias MM, McKinnon RA, Sorich MJ. Impact of the UGT1A1*28 allele on response to irinotecan: a systematic review and meta-analysis. *Pharmacogenomics.* 2012;13(8):889-899.

164. Dias MM, et al. The effect of the UGT1A1*28 allele on survival after irinotecan-based chemotherapy: a collaborative meta-analysis. *Pharmacogenomics J.* 2014;14(5):424-431.

165. U.S. Food & Drug Administration (FDA) Labeling-Package Insert for Camptosar (Irinotecan Hydrochloride). Available at https://www.accessdata.fda.gov/drugsatfda_docs/label/2014/020571s048lbl.pdf. Accessed December 21, 2017.

166. Etienne-Grimaldi MC, et al. UGT1A1 genotype and irinotecan therapy: general review and implementation in routine practice. *Fundam Clin Pharmacol.* 2015;29(3):219-237.

167. Akaba K, et al. Neonatal hyperbilirubinemia and mutation of the bilirubin uridine diphosphate-glucuronosyltransferase gene: a common missense mutation among Japanese, Koreans and Chinese. *Biochem Mol Biol Int.* 1998;46(1):21-26.

168. Takano M, et al. Clinical significance of UDP-glucuronosyltransferase 1A1*6 for toxicities of combination chemotherapy with irinotecan and cisplatin in gynecologic cancers: a prospective multi-institutional study. *Oncology.* 2009;76(5):315-321.

169. Han JY, et al. Comprehensive analysis of UGT1A polymorphisms predictive for pharmacokinetics and treatment outcome in patients with non-small-cell lung cancer treated with irinotecan and cisplatin. *J Clin Oncol.* 2006;24(15):2237-2244.

170. Cheng L, et al. UGT1A1*6 polymorphisms are correlated with irinotecan-induced toxicity: a system review and meta-analysis in Asians. *Cancer Chemother Pharmacol.* 2014;73(3):551-560.

171. Li CI, Daling JR, Malone KE. Incidence of invasive breast cancer by hormone receptor status from 1992 to 1998. *J Clin Oncol.* 2003;21(1):28-34.

172. Wu X, et al. The tamoxifen metabolite, endoxifen, is a potent antiestrogen that targets estrogen receptor alpha for degradation in breast cancer cells. *Cancer Res.* 2009;69(5):1722-1727.

173. Jordan VC. New insights into the metabolism of tamoxifen and its role in the treatment and prevention of breast cancer. *Steroids.* 2007;72(13):829-842.

174. Tseng E, et al. Relative contributions of cytochrome CYP3A4 versus CYP3A5 for CYP3A-cleared drugs assessed in vitro using a CYP3A4-selective inactivator (CYP3cide). *Drug Metab Dispos.* 2014;42(7):1163-1173.

175. Desta Z, et al. Comprehensive evaluation of tamoxifen sequential biotransformation by the human cytochrome P450 system in vitro: prominent roles for CYP3A and CYP2D6. *J Pharmacol Exp Ther.* 2004;310(3):1062-1075.

176. Murdter TE, et al. Activity levels of tamoxifen metabolites at the estrogen receptor and the impact of genetic polymorphisms of phase I and II enzymes on their concentration levels in plasma. *Clin Pharmacol Ther.* 2011;89(5):708-717.

177. Sanchez Spitman AB, et al. Effect of CYP3A4*22, CYP3A5*3, and CYP3A combined genotypes on tamoxifen metabolism. *Eur J Clin Pharmacol.* 2017;73(12):1589-1598.

178. Jordan VC, et al. A monohydroxylated metabolite of tamoxifen with potent antioestrogenic activity. *J Endocrinol.* 1977;75(2):305-316.

179. Stearns V, et al. Active tamoxifen metabolite plasma concentrations after coadministration of tamoxifen and the selective serotonin reuptake inhibitor paroxetine. *J Natl Cancer Inst.* 2003;95(23):1758-1764.

180. Database of Single Nucleotide Polymorphisms (dbSNP), CYP2D6 Gene. Available at https://www.ncbi.nlm.nih.gov/SNP/snp_ref.cgi?locusId=1565. Accessed December 21, 2017.

181. Crews KR, et al. Clinical Pharmacogenetics Implementation Consortium (CPIC) guidelines for codeine therapy in the context of cytochrome P450 2D6 (CYP2D6) genotype. *Clin Pharmacol Ther.* 2012;91(2):321-326.

182. Crews KR, et al. Clinical Pharmacogenetics Implementation Consortium guidelines for cytochrome P450 2D6 genotype and codeine therapy: 2014 update. *Clin Pharmacol Ther.* 2014;95(4):376-382.

183. Gaedigk A, et al. The CYP2D6 activity score: translating genotype information into a qualitative measure of phenotype. *Clin Pharmacol Ther.* 2008;83(2):234-242.

184. Goetz MP, et al. *Clinical Pharmacogenetics Implementation Consortium (CPIC) Guideline for CYP2D6 and Tamoxifen Therapy.* Available at https://cpicpgx.org/guidelines/cpic-guideline-for-tamoxifen-based-on-cyp2d6-genotype/. Accessed January 26, 2018.

185. Schroth W, et al. Association between CYP2D6 polymorphisms and outcomes among women with early stage breast cancer treated with tamoxifen. *JAMA.* 2009;302(13):1429-1436.

186. Pharmacogene Variation Consortium (PharmVar). Available at https://www.pharmvar.org/. Accessed December 21, 2017.

187. Schroth W, et al. Improved Prediction of Endoxifen Metabolism by CYP2D6 Genotype in Breast Cancer Patients Treated with Tamoxifen. *Front Pharmacol.* 2017;8:582.

188. Goetz MP, et al. Pharmacogenetics of tamoxifen biotransformation is associated with clinical outcomes of efficacy and hot flashes. *J Clin Oncol.* 2005;23(36):9312-9318.

189. Schroth W, et al. Breast cancer treatment outcome with adjuvant tamoxifen relative to patient CYP2D6 and CYP2C19 genotypes. *J Clin Oncol.* 2007;25(33):5187-5193.

190. Rae JM, et al. CYP2D6 and UGT2B7 genotype and risk of recurrence in tamoxifen-treated breast cancer patients. *J Natl Cancer Inst.* 2012;104(6):452-460.

191. Regan MM, et al. CYP2D6 genotype and tamoxifen response in postmenopausal women with endocrine-responsive breast cancer: the breast international group 1-98 trial. *J Natl Cancer Inst.* 2012;104(6):441-451.

192. Goetz MP, et al. CYP2D6 metabolism and patient outcome in the Austrian Breast and Colorectal Cancer Study Group trial (ABCSG) 8. *Clin Cancer Res.* 2013;19(2):500-507.

193. Province MA, et al. CYP2D6 genotype and adjuvant tamoxifen: meta-analysis of heterogeneous study populations. *Clin Pharmacol Ther.* 2014;95(2):216-227.

194. Ruiter R, et al. CYP2C19*2 polymorphism is associated with increased survival in breast cancer patients using tamoxifen. *Pharmacogenomics.* 2010;11(10):1367-1375.

195. van Schaik RH, et al. The CYP2C19*2 genotype predicts tamoxifen treatment outcome in advanced breast cancer patients. *Pharmacogenomics.* 2011;12(8):1137-1146.

196. Powers JL, et al. Multigene and drug interaction approach for tamoxifen metabolite patterns reveals possible involvement of CYP2C9, CYP2C19, and ABCB1. *J Clin Pharmacol.* 2016;56(12):1570-1581.

197. Bai L, et al. Association of CYP2C19 polymorphisms with survival of breast cancer patients using tamoxifen: results of a meta-analysis. *Asian Pac J Cancer Prev.* 2014;15(19):8331-8335.

198. Blevins-Primeau AS, et al. Functional significance of UDP-glucuronosyltransferase variants in the metabolism of active tamoxifen metabolites. *Cancer Res.* 2009;69(5):1892-1900.

199. Wegman P, et al. Genotype of metabolic enzymes and the benefit of tamoxifen in postmenopausal breast cancer patients. *Breast Cancer Res.* 2005;7(3):R284-R290.

200. Nowell S, et al. Association between sulfotransferase 1A1 genotype and survival of breast cancer patients receiving tamoxifen therapy. *J Natl Cancer Inst.* 2002;94(21):1635-1640.

201. Wegman P, et al. Genetic variants of CYP3A5, CYP2D6, SULT1A1, UGT2B15 and tamoxifen response in postmenopausal patients with breast cancer. *Breast Cancer Res.* 2007;9(1):R7.

202. Goetz MP, Ames MM, Weinshilboum RM. Primer on medical genomics. Part XII: Pharmacogenomics—general principles with cancer as a model. *Mayo Clin Proc.* 2004;79(3):376-384.

203. Perilongo G, et al. Cisplatin versus cisplatin plus doxorubicin for standard-risk hepatoblastoma. *N Engl J Med.* 2009;361(17):1662-1670.

204. Ulrich CM, et al. Pharmacogenetics of methotrexate: toxicity among marrow transplantation patients varies with the methylenetetrahydrofolate reductase C677T polymorphism. *Blood.* 2001;98(1):231-234.

205. Kling J. US FDA contemplates collection of pharmacogenomic data. *Nat Biotechnol.* 2003;21(6):590.

206. Li Y, Womer RB, Silber JH. Predicting cisplatin ototoxicity in children: the influence of age and the cumulative dose. *Eur J Cancer.* 2004;40(16):2445-2451.

207. Skinner R, et al. Ototoxicity of cisplatinum in children and adolescents. *Br J Cancer.* 1990;61(6):927-931.

208. Khairi Md Daud M, et al. The effect of mild hearing loss on academic performance in primary school children. *Int J Pediatr Otorhinolaryngol.* 2010;74(1):67-70.

209. Blair JC, Peterson ME, Vieweg SH. The effects of mild sensorineural hearing loss on academic performance of young school age children. *Volta Rev.* 1985;87(2):87-93.

210. Lee JW, et al. Clinical Practice recommendations for the management and prevention of cisplatin-induced hearing loss using pharmacogenetic markers. *Ther Drug Monit.* 2016;38(4):423-431.

211. Ross CJ, et al. Genetic variants in TPMT and COMT are associated with hearing loss in children receiving cisplatin chemotherapy. *Nat Genet.* 2009;41(12):1345-1349.

212. Pussegoda K, et al. Replication of TPMT and ABCC3 genetic variants highly associated with cisplatin-induced hearing loss in children. *Clin Pharmacol Ther.* 2013;94(2):243-251.

213. Yang JJ, et al. The role of inherited TPMT and COMT genetic variation in cisplatin-induced ototoxicity in children with cancer. *Clin Pharmacol Ther.* 2013;94(2):252-259.

214. Lanvers-Kaminsky C, et al. Evaluation of pharmacogenetic markers to predict the risk of Cisplatin-induced ototoxicity. *Clin Pharmacol Ther.* 2014;96(2):156-157.

215. Hagleitner MM, et al. Influence of genetic variants in TPMT and COMT associated with cisplatin induced hearing loss in patients with cancer: two new cohorts and a meta-analysis reveal significant heterogeneity between cohorts. *PLoS One.* 2014;9(12):e115869.

216. Carleton BC, et al. Response to "evaluation of pharmacogenetic markers to predict the risk of Cisplatin-induced ototoxicity". *Clin Pharmacol Ther.* 2014;96(2):158.

217. Caronia D, et al. Common variations in ERCC2 are associated with response to cisplatin chemotherapy and clinical outcome in osteosarcoma patients. *Pharmacogenomics J.* 2009;9(5):347-353.

218. Sakano S, et al. Nucleotide excision repair gene polymorphisms may predict acute toxicity in patients treated with chemoradiotherapy for bladder cancer. *Pharmacogenomics.* 2010;11(10):1377-1387.

219. Drogemoller BI, et al. Association between SLC16A5 genetic variation and cisplatin-induced ototoxic effects in adult patients with testicular cancer. *JAMA Oncol.* 2017;3(11):1558-1562.

220. Shen MR, Jones IM, Mohrenweiser H. Nonconservative amino acid substitution variants exist at polymorphic frequency in DNA repair genes in healthy humans. *Cancer Res.* 1998;58(4):604-608.

221. Yu JJ, et al. A nucleotide polymorphism in ERCC1 in human ovarian cancer cell lines and tumor tissues. *Mutat Res.* 1997;382(1-2):13-20.

222. Khrunin AV, et al. Genetic polymorphisms and the efficacy and toxicity of cisplatin-based chemotherapy in ovarian cancer patients. *Pharmacogenomics J.* 2010;10(1):54-61.

223. Huang MY, et al. Multiple genetic polymorphisms in the prediction of clinical outcome of metastatic colorectal cancer patients treated with first-line FOLFOX-4 chemotherapy. *Pharmacogenet Genomics.* 2011;21(1):18-25.

224. Tzvetkov MV, et al. Pharmacogenetic analyses of cisplatin-induced nephrotoxicity indicate a renoprotective effect of ERCC1 polymorphisms. *Pharmacogenomics.* 2011;12(10):1417-1427.

225. Bradbury PA, et al. Cisplatin pharmacogenetics, DNA repair polymorphisms, and esophageal cancer outcomes. *Pharmacogenet Genomics.* 2009;19(8):613-625.

226. Yan L, et al. Association between polymorphisms of ERCC1 and survival in epithelial ovarian cancer patients with chemotherapy. *Pharmacogenomics.* 2012;13(4):419-427.

227. Stoehlmacher J, et al. A multivariate analysis of genomic polymorphisms: prediction of clinical outcome to 5-FU/oxaliplatin combination chemotherapy in refractory colorectal cancer. *Br J Cancer.* 2004;91(2):344-354.

228. Tibaldi C, et al. Correlation of CDA, ERCC1, and XPD polymorphisms with response and survival in gemcitabine/cisplatin-treated advanced non-small cell lung cancer patients. *Clin Cancer Res.* 2008;14(6):1797-1803.

229. Zucali PA, et al. Thymidylate synthase and excision repair cross-complementing group-1 as predictors of responsiveness in mesothelioma patients treated with pemetrexed/carboplatin. *Clin Cancer Res.* 2011;17(8):2581-2590.

230. Giovannetti E, et al. Association between DNA-repair polymorphisms and survival in pancreatic cancer patients treated with combination chemotherapy. *Pharmacogenomics.* 2011;12(12):1641-1652.

231. Khrunin A, et al. Pharmacogenomics of cisplatin-based chemotherapy in ovarian cancer patients of different ethnic origins. *Pharmacogenomics.* 2012;13(2):171-178.

232. Zhou W, et al. Excision repair cross-complementation group 1 polymorphism predicts overall survival in advanced non-small cell lung cancer patients treated with platinum-based chemotherapy. *Clin Cancer Res.* 2004;10(15):4939-4943.

233. Dabholkar M, et al. Messenger RNA levels of XPAC and ERCC1 in ovarian cancer tissue correlate with response to platinum-based chemotherapy. *J Clin Invest.* 1994;94(2):703-708.

234. Hughes HB, et al. Metabolism of isoniazid in man as related to the occurrence of peripheral neuritis. *Am Rev Tuberc.* 1954;70(2):266-273.

235. Goricar K, Kovac V, Dolzan V. Clinical-pharmacogenetic models for personalized cancer treatment: application to malignant mesothelioma. *Sci Rep.* 2017;7:46537.

236. Zhang L, et al. Pharmacogenetics of DNA repair gene polymorphisms in non-small-cell lung carcinoma patients on platinum-based chemotherapy. *Genet Mol Res.* 2014;13(1):228-236.
237. Kalikaki A, et al. DNA repair gene polymorphisms predict favorable clinical outcome in advanced non-small-cell lung cancer. *Clin Lung Cancer.* 2009;10(2):118-123.
238. Sullivan I, et al. Pharmacogenetics of the DNA repair pathways in advanced non-small cell lung cancer patients treated with platinum-based chemotherapy. *Cancer Lett.* 2014;353(2):160-166.
239. Gorlick R, et al. Intrinsic and acquired resistance to methotrexate in acute leukemia. *N Engl J Med.* 1996;335(14):1041-1048.
240. Gorlick R, et al. Defective transport is a common mechanism of acquired methotrexate resistance in acute lymphocytic leukemia and is associated with decreased reduced folate carrier expression. *Blood.* 1997;89(3):1013-1018.
241. Aplenc R, Lange B. Pharmacogenetic determinants of outcome in acute lymphoblastic leukaemia. *Br J Haematol.* 2004;125(4):421-434.
242. Frosst P, et al. A candidate genetic risk factor for vascular disease: a common mutation in methylenetetrahydrofolate reductase. *Nat Genet.* 1995;10(1):111-113.
243. He HR, et al. Association between methylenetetrahydrofolate reductase polymorphisms and the relapse of acute lymphoblastic leukemia: a meta-analysis. *Pharmacogenomics J.* 2014;14(5):432-438.
244. Imanishi H, et al. Genetic polymorphisms associated with adverse events and elimination of methotrexate in childhood acute lymphoblastic leukemia and malignant lymphoma. *J Hum Genet.* 2007;52(2):166-171.
245. Spyridopoulou KP, et al. Methylene tetrahydrofolate reductase gene polymorphisms and their association with methotrexate toxicity: a meta-analysis. *Pharmacogenet Genomics.* 2012;22(2):117-133.
246. Ongaro A, et al. Gene polymorphisms in folate metabolizing enzymes in adult acute lymphoblastic leukemia: effects on methotrexate-related toxicity and survival. *Haematologica.* 2009;94(10):1391-1398.
247. Krajinovic M, et al. Role of polymorphisms in MTHFR and MTHFD1 genes in the outcome of childhood acute lymphoblastic leukemia. *Pharmacogenomics J.* 2004;4(1):66-72.
248. Aplenc R, et al. Methylenetetrahydrofolate reductase polymorphisms and therapy response in pediatric acute lymphoblastic leukemia. *Cancer Res.* 2005;65(6):2482-2487.
249. Chiusolo P, et al. Preponderance of methylenetetrahydrofolate reductase C677T homozygosity among leukemia patients intolerant to methotrexate. *Ann Oncol.* 2002;13(12):1915-1918.
250. Nuckel H, et al. Methylenetetrahydrofolate reductase (MTHFR) gene 677C>T and 1298A>C polymorphisms are associated with differential apoptosis of leukemic B cells in vitro and disease progression in chronic lymphocytic leukemia. *Leukemia.* 2004;18(11):1816-1823.
251. Kishi S, et al. Homocysteine, pharmacogenetics, and neurotoxicity in children with leukemia. *J Clin Oncol.* 2003;21(16):3084-3091.
252. Dorababu P, et al. Genetic variants of thiopurine and folate metabolic pathways determine 6-MP-mediated hematological toxicity in childhood ALL. *Pharmacogenomics.* 2012;13(9):1001-1008.
253. Huang L, et al. Polymorphisms in folate-related genes: association with side effects of high-dose methotrexate in childhood acute lymphoblastic leukemia. *Leukemia.* 2008;22(9):1798-1800.
254. Kishi S, et al. Ancestry and pharmacogenetics of antileukemic drug toxicity. *Blood.* 2007;109(10):4151-4157.
255. Pakakasama S, et al. Genetic polymorphisms of folate metabolic enzymes and toxicities of high dose methotrexate in children with acute lymphoblastic leukemia. *Ann Hematol.* 2007;86(8):609-611.
256. Seidemann K, et al. MTHFR 677 (C-->T) polymorphism is not relevant for prognosis or therapy-associated toxicity in pediatric NHL: results from 484 patients of multicenter trial NHL-BFM 95. *Ann Hematol.* 2006;85(5):291-300.
257. Costea I, et al. Folate cycle gene variants and chemotherapy toxicity in pediatric patients with acute lymphoblastic leukemia. *Haematologica.* 2006;91(8):1113-1116.
258. Jabeen S, et al. Impact of genetic variants of RFC1, DHFR and MTHFR in osteosarcoma patients treated with high-dose methotrexate. *Pharmacogenomics J.* 2015;15(5):385-390.
259. Rocha JC, et al. Pharmacogenetics of outcome in children with acute lymphoblastic leukemia. *Blood.* 2005;105(12):4752-4758.
260. Timuragaoglu A, et al. Methylenetetrahydrofolate reductase C677T polymorphism in adult patients with lymphoproliferative disorders and its effect on chemotherapy. *Ann Hematol.* 2006;85(12):863-868.
261. Lopez-Lopez E, et al. A systematic review and meta-analysis of MTHFR polymorphisms in methotrexate toxicity prediction in pediatric acute lymphoblastic leukemia. *Pharmacogenomics J.* 2013;13(6):498-506.
262. Robien K, et al. Methylenetetrahydrofolate reductase genotype affects risk of relapse after hematopoietic cell transplantation for chronic myelogenous leukemia. *Clin Cancer Res.* 2004;10(22):7592-7598.
263. Zgheib NK, et al. Genetic polymorphisms in candidate genes predict increased toxicity with methotrexate therapy in Lebanese children with acute lymphoblastic leukemia. *Pharmacogenet Genomics.* 2014;24(8):387-396.
264. Suthandiram S, et al. Effect of polymorphisms within methotrexate pathway genes on methotrexate toxicity and plasma levels in adults with hematological malignancies. *Pharmacogenomics.* 2014;15(11):1479-1494.
265. Gregers J, et al. Polymorphisms in the ABCB1 gene and effect on outcome and toxicity in childhood acute lymphoblastic leukemia. *Pharmacogenomics J.* 2015;15(4):372-379.
266. Tsujimoto S, et al. Influence of ADORA2A gene polymorphism on leukoencephalopathy risk in MTX-treated pediatric patients affected by hematological malignancies. *Pediatr Blood Cancer.* 2016;63(11):1983-1989.
267. Liu SG, et al. Polymorphisms in methotrexate transporters and their relationship to plasma methotrexate levels, toxicity of high-dose methotrexate, and outcome of pediatric acute lymphoblastic leukemia. *Oncotarget.* 2017;8(23):37761-37772.
268. Trevino LR, et al. Germline genetic variation in an organic anion transporter polypeptide associated with methotrexate pharmacokinetics and clinical effects. *J Clin Oncol.* 2009;27(35):5972-5978.
269. Goricar K, et al. Influence of the folate pathway and transporter polymorphisms on methotrexate treatment outcome in osteosarcoma. *Pharmacogenet Genomics.* 2014;24(10):514-521.
270. Ramsey LB, et al. Genome-wide study of methotrexate clearance replicates SLCO1B1. *Blood.* 2013;121(6):898-904.
271. Stocco G, et al. PACSIN2 polymorphism influences TPMT activity and mercaptopurine-related gastrointestinal toxicity. *Hum Mol Genet.* 2012;21(21):4793-4804.
272. Saikawa Y, et al. Decreased expression of the human folate receptor mediates transport-defective methotrexate resistance in KB cells. *J Biol Chem.* 1993;268(7):5293-5301.
273. Dulucq S, et al. DNA variants in the dihydrofolate reductase gene and outcome in childhood ALL. *Blood.* 2008;111(7):3692-3700.
274. Al-Shakfa F, et al. DNA variants in region for noncoding interfering transcript of dihydrofolate reductase gene and outcome in childhood acute lymphoblastic leukemia. *Clin Cancer Res.* 2009;15(22):6931-6938.
275. Mishra PJ, et al. A miR-24 microRNA binding-site polymorphism in dihydrofolate reductase gene leads to methotrexate resistance. *Proc Natl Acad Sci U S A.* 2007;104(33):13513-13518.
276. Goto Y, et al. A novel single-nucleotide polymorphism in the 3'-untranslated region of the human dihydrofolate reductase gene with enhanced expression. *Clin Cancer Res.* 2001;7(7):1952-1956.
277. Belkov VM, et al. Reduced folate carrier expression in acute lymphoblastic leukemia: a mechanism for ploidy but not lineage differences in methotrexate accumulation. *Blood.* 1999;93(5):1643-1650.
278. Taub JW, Ge Y. Down syndrome, drug metabolism and chromosome 21. *Pediatr Blood Cancer.* 2005;44(1):33-39.
279. Kremer LC, et al. Frequency and risk factors of anthracycline-induced clinical heart failure in children: a systematic review. *Ann Oncol.* 2002;13(4):503-512.
280. Lefrak EA, et al. A clinicopathologic analysis of adriamycin cardiotoxicity. *Cancer.* 1973;32(2):302-314.
281. Von Hoff DD, et al. Risk factors for doxorubicin-induced congestive heart failure. *Ann Intern Med.* 1979;91(5):710-717.
282. Hershman DL, Shao T. Anthracycline cardiotoxicity after breast cancer treatment. *Oncology (Williston Park).* 2009;23(3):227-234.

283. Lipshultz SE, Alvarez JA, Scully RE. Anthracycline associated cardiotoxicity in survivors of childhood cancer. *Heart.* 2008;94(4):525-533.

284. Felker GM, et al. Underlying causes and long-term survival in patients with initially unexplained cardiomyopathy. *N Engl J Med.* 2000;342(15):1077-1084.

285. Aminkeng F, et al. A coding variant in RARG confers susceptibility to anthracycline-induced cardiotoxicity in childhood cancer. *Nat Genet.* 2015;47(9):1079-1084.

286. Minotti G, et al. Anthracyclines: molecular advances and pharmacologic developments in antitumor activity and cardiotoxicity. *Pharmacol Rev.* 2004;56(2):185-229.

287. Zhang S, et al. Identification of the molecular basis of doxorubicin-induced cardiotoxicity. *Nat Med.* 2012;18(11):1639-1642.

288. Visscher H, et al. Validation of variants in SLC28A3 and UGT1A6 as genetic markers predictive of anthracycline-induced cardiotoxicity in children. *Pediatr Blood Cancer.* 2013;60(8):1375-1381.

289. Visscher H, et al. Pharmacogenomic prediction of anthracycline-induced cardiotoxicity in children. *J Clin Oncol.* 2012;30(13):1422-1428.

290. Nagar S, Zalatoris JJ, Blanchard RL. Human UGT1A6 pharmacogenetics: identification of a novel SNP, characterization of allele frequencies and functional analysis of recombinant allozymes in human liver tissue and in cultured cells. *Pharmacogenetics.* 2004;14(8):487-499.

291. Krishnaswamy S, et al. UDP glucuronosyltransferase (UGT) 1A6 pharmacogenetics: II. Functional impact of the three most common nonsynonymous UGT1A6 polymorphisms (S7A, T181A, and R184S). *J Pharmacol Exp Ther.* 2005;313(3):1340-1346.

292. Bock KW, Kohle C. UDP-glucuronosyltransferase 1A6: structural, functional, and regulatory aspects. *Methods Enzymol.* 2005;400:57-75.

293. Vulsteke C, et al. Clinical and genetic risk factors for epirubicin-induced cardiac toxicity in early breast cancer patients. *Breast Cancer Res Treat.* 2015;152(1):67-76.

294. Reichwagen A, et al. Association of NADPH oxidase polymorphisms with anthracycline-induced cardiotoxicity in the RICOVER-60 trial of patients with aggressive CD20(+) B-cell lymphoma. *Pharmacogenomics.* 2015;16(4):361-372.

295. Zeller T, et al. Genetics and beyond—the transcriptome of human monocytes and disease susceptibility. *PLoS One.* 2010;5(5):e10693.

296. Visscher H, et al. Genetic variants in SLC22A17 and SLC22A7 are associated with anthracycline-induced cardiotoxicity in children. *Pharmacogenomics.* 2015;16(10):1065-1076.

297. Wojnowski L, et al. NAD(P)H oxidase and multidrug resistance protein genetic polymorphisms are associated with doxorubicin-induced cardiotoxicity. *Circulation.* 2005;112(24):3754-3762.

298. Semsei AF, et al. ABCC1 polymorphisms in anthracycline-induced cardiotoxicity in childhood acute lymphoblastic leukaemia. *Cell Biol Int.* 2012;36(1):79-86.

299. Wang X, et al. Hyaluronan synthase 3 variant and anthracycline-related cardiomyopathy: a report from the children's oncology group. *J Clin Oncol.* 2014;32(7):647-653.

300. Armenian SH, et al. Genetic susceptibility to anthracycline-related congestive heart failure in survivors of haematopoietic cell transplantation. *Br J Haematol.* 2013;163(2):205-213.

Delivering Anticancer Drugs to Brain Tumors

K. Ina Ly, Maciej M. Mrugala, Jeffrey G. Supko, and Tracy T. Batchelor

The average annual age-adjusted incidence rate for primary brain and nervous system tumors in the United States was 22.6 per 100,000 persons between 2010 and 2014.[1] It is expected that approximately 79,000 new cases of primary central nervous system (CNS) tumors will be diagnosed in the United States in 2018.[1] In addition, the incidence of brain metastases—the most common brain tumors overall—is on the rise, given the increasing number of cancer survivors in the era of new therapeutic agents such as targeted and immunotherapy. The most common primary malignant brain tumors are glioblastomas (GBMs), a type of malignant or high-grade glioma. The standard treatment for GBM patients consists of concomitant radiation and daily temozolomide (TMZ), followed by adjuvant monthly TMZ.[2] In the initial landmark trial, this regimen prolonged median overall survival (OS) from 12.1 months with radiation alone to 14.6 months.[2] Preliminary data from a phase III randomized trial of standard radiation + TMZ versus standard radiation + TMZ + lomustine in patients with O[6]-methylguanine methyltransferase (*MGMT*)–methylated newly diagnosed GBMs (a subgroup of patients with a more favorable prognosis compared to those whose tumors lack the *MGMT* methylation) demonstrated a survival of 46.9 months in the lomustine/TMZ arm versus 30.4 months in the TMZ arm ($P = 0.049$).[3] In addition to standard therapy, locally delivered chemotherapy in the form of 1,3-bis (2-chloroethyl)-1-nitrosourea (carmustine; BCNU) polymers has been shown to extend survival slightly in patients with malignant gliomas when applied at the time of the initial debulking procedure.[4] In 2015, the U.S. Food and Drug Administration (FDA) approved the addition of NovoTTF (tumor-treating fields) to standard therapy in patients with newly diagnosed GBM. NovoTTF is a portable medical device applied to the shaved scalp that potentially disrupts cell division by delivering alternating electric fields. In a planned interim analysis of a phase III trial, NovoTTF improved progression-free survival and OS when added to adjuvant TMZ.[5] However, its use has not been widely adopted at this point.[6] The FDA also approved aminolevulinic acid hydrochloride (ALA HCl) in 2017 as an adjunctive optical imaging agent to visualize malignant tissue during surgery in patients with suspected WHO grade III and IV gliomas, with the goal to improve the degree of tumor resection.[7] Despite these treatment options, however, prognosis for GBM patients remains poor with a median OS of less than 20 months. While promising phase II results[8,9] raised initial enthusiasm for the addition of bevacizumab, a humanized monoclonal antibody against vascular endothelial growth factor (VEGF), to the treatment regimen for malignant glioma patients, two placebo-controlled phase III trials comparing bevacizumab plus standard of care versus standard of care alone failed to prolong survival in plus standard of care versus standard of care alone in newly diagnosed GBM patients failed to demonstrate a difference in OS between the two groups.[10,11] Bevacizumab, however, remains approved as monotherapy for the treatment of recurrent glioblastoma.

Recently, interest in the field of neuro-oncology has shifted toward novel targeted agents and immunotherapy. Immunotherapy has demonstrated success in the treatment of specific systemic cancers, including melanoma and non–small cell lung cancer.[12,13] Various immunotherapy agents have recently entered clinical trials for patients with newly diagnosed and recurrent high-grade gliomas as well as brain metastases.[14,15] In addition, the relatively recent identification of the isocitrate dehydrogenase (*IDH*) gene and its prognostic role in diffuse gliomas[16–18] has motivated the development of targeted inhibitors of the *IDH* gene. A number of these inhibitors have also entered clinical trials.[19] Preliminary data suggest that these new targeted and immunotherapy agents produce responses in some patients. Preliminary results from a randomized phase II trial of patients with recurrent GBM (ReACT)[20] showed a survival advantage when rindopepimut, a peptide vaccine against the EGFRvIII protein, was combined with bevacizumab. However, randomized trials have failed to demonstrate improvement in survival in newly diagnosed and recurrent GBM patients treated with rindopepimut[21] and nivolumab,[22] respectively. Therefore, while it remains important to identify appropriate drug targets in the brain, understanding the challenges of drug delivery to the CNS and how to assess target engagement in both the preclinical and clinical phases of drug development are critical to the development of successful therapies.

Drug failure can be a result of multiple mechanisms, including multidrug resistance and increased efficiency of DNA damage repair systems in the tumor.[23] However, brain tumors represent a unique challenge given the presence of the blood-brain barrier (BBB), a physiologic impediment between the circulatory system of the brain and that of the body. The accessibility of many anticancer drugs to brain tumors is at least partially constrained by the BBB. Therefore, difficulty in achieving adequate and sufficiently sustained levels of the cytotoxic moiety at the tumor site is a significant factor contributing to the failure of systemic chemotherapy for malignant brain tumors.[24,25] Accordingly, the development of treatment strategies for brain tumors has emphasized techniques that are intended to overcome this barrier and improve drug delivery to CNS tumors. In addition, the multiplicity of ancillary agents used in the medical management of brain tumor patients, particularly corticosteroids and enzyme-inducing antiepileptics (AEDs), increases the risk for drug interactions that may impact the efficacy or toxicity of chemotherapy. This chapter reviews the current status of approaches for delivering anticancer drugs to CNS tumors, the various techniques that are available for assessing drug distribution to brain tumors, and the important pharmacologic interactions that may affect both the accessibility of anticancer drugs to the CNS and the systemic pharmacokinetics of the anticancer agent.

Blood-Brain Barrier

Three main factors influence the extent to which a systemically administered anticancer agent distributes into the brain and brain tumors: (a) the plasma concentration-time profile of the drug, (b) regional blood flow, and (c) transport of the agent through the BBB and blood-tumor barrier (BTB). The two former considerations are common to all solid tumors, whereas the latter is specific to brain tumors.[24] Ehrlich was the first to propose the concept of the BBB at the end of the nineteenth century. On administering the

dye trypan blue to rats by intravenous injection, he observed that all body organs were stained except for the brain and spinal cord.[26] The anatomic basis of the BBB was determined decades ago with the introduction of the electron microscope. It results from modification of the normal vascular endothelium whereby a sheet of cells is connected by a network of proteins (tight junctions) on a basement membrane (Fig. 6.1B). The BBB has a number of important roles, including maintaining a constant biochemical content of the interstitial milieu and protecting the brain from toxic molecules (including xenobiotics).[27] Low hydraulic conductance, low ionic permeability, and high electrical resistance make it difficult for hydrophilic nonelectrolytes to penetrate the BBB in the absence of a membrane carrier.[28] These properties, together with the lack of intracellular fenestrations and pinocytotic vesicles and the presence of a thicker basal lamina, create a physiologic barrier that is relatively impermeable to many water-soluble compounds.[29,30]

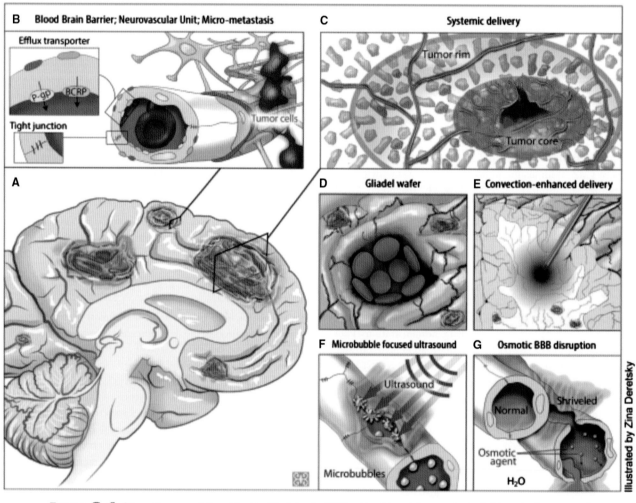

FIGURE **6.1** Schematic representation of the blood-brain barrier (BBB) and local drug delivery methods. **A.** Primary brain tumors and metastases can be located both supra- and infratentorially. **B.** The BBB limits delivery of most systemically administered drugs by means of tight junctions and the presence of efflux transporters on the luminal surface of brain capillary endothelial cells. **C.** Systemically administered drugs typically result in higher drug delivery to the tumor core where the BBB is leaky and lower drug concentrations in the tumor rim. **D–G.** Local drug delivery methods rely on diffusion through the brain parenchyma. Gliadel or BCNU wafers are implanted at the time of surgery and release drug into surrounding tissue with limited penetration into the brain parenchyma **(D)**. With convection-enhanced delivery (CED), a drug is infused through a catheter by exploiting a hydrostatic pressure gradient **(E)**. Focused ultrasound microbubble disruption loosens the tight junctions and transiently opens the paracellular space **(F)**. Osmotic BBB disruption uses hyperosmolar solutions to transiently increase BBB permeability **(G)**. (From Parrish KE, Sarkaria JN, Elmquist WF. Improving drug delivery to primary and metastatic brain tumors: strategies to overcome the blood-brain barrier. *Clin Pharmacol Ther.* 2015; 97(4):336-346. Copyright © 2015 American Society for Clinical Pharmacology and Therapeutics. Reprinted by permission of John Wiley & Sons, Inc.)

Some drugs utilize specific transport mechanisms present in the endothelial cell to traverse the BBB.[31] However, most cytotoxic drugs that gain access to the CNS cross the BBB by passive diffusion. Aside from pharmacokinetic properties, the main factors that influence the extent to which these compounds distribute into the CNS include lipid solubility, molecular mass, charge, and plasma protein binding. Specifically, small organic compounds with a molecular weight less than 200 that are lipid soluble, neutral at physiologic pH, and not highly bound to plasma proteins readily cross the BBB.[28]

In addition to tight junctions, the BBB expresses active efflux proteins on the luminal surface of brain capillary endothelial cells (Fig. 6.1B). These efflux proteins have wide substrate specificity and prevent entry of foreign molecules by actively transporting them back into the systemic circulation. They include adenosine triphosphate (ATP)–binding cassette (ABC) transporters such as P-glycoprotein (P-gp), multidrug resistance–associated proteins (MRPs), and breast cancer resistance proteins (BCRP).[32,33] The presence of P-gp has been implicated in impairing the efficacy of various chemotherapy agents, including vinca alkaloids, doxorubicin, and TMZ.[34] Expression of P-gp has also been reported in malignant gliomas and may contribute to chemotherapy resistance.[35,36] Importantly, MRP1 and P-gp may be differentially expressed in high- and low-grade gliomas: MRP1 overexpression appears to be more common in high-grade gliomas (WHO grade IV), while P-gp expression is observed more often in low-grade tumors (WHO grade II). These findings may have potential therapeutic implications.[37] Agents that reverse the function of P-gp or alter the expression of other signaling molecules involved in the regulation of BBB permeability may represent potential targets to increase drug delivery to brain tumor cells. Multiple P-gp inhibitors, including verapamil, cyclosporin A, and tariquidar, have been evaluated in early-phase clinical trials but did not progress to larger-scale trials due to problems with pharmacokinetic and pharmacodynamic interactions and toxicities.[38] More recent work has suggested that activation of adenosine receptor (AR) signaling may enhance drug delivery. AR signaling is thought to up-regulate BBB permeability by changing VE-cadherin and claudin-5 expression.[39] Activation of the A2A AR with Lexiscan (an FDA-approved A2A AR agonist) decreased P-gp expression in a reversible manner and resulted in higher P-gp substrate levels in rodent brains and human brain endothelial cells.[40] Further exploration of these concepts in a brain tumor model may shed more light on whether or not targeting of AR signaling may improve drug delivery in a disease state.

A common misconception is that breakdown of the BBB and disruption of the tumor vasculature facilitate and do not impair drug delivery. While this may hold true for the central tumor mass or tumor core, which typically demonstrates contrast enhancement on T1-weighted postcontrast MR sequences, this does not apply to the infiltrating tumor edge and peritumoral area (Fig. 6.1C). In fact, the highly infiltrating tumor cells of diffuse gliomas are protected by an intact BBB.[41] From an imaging perspective, the increased permeability of the BBB is reflected by leakage of contrast agent and resultant contrast enhancement on CT and MRI. Consequently, imaging can provide information about the tumor core but does not visualize the infiltrating tumor edges or nonenhancing tumor regions, as seen in the majority of low-grade and some high-grade gliomas. In fact, approximately 30% of anaplastic astrocytomas do not enhance.[42] Perfusion-weighted MR imaging (including T1-weighted dynamic

contrast-enhanced MRI [DCE-MRI] and T2- or T2*-weighted dynamic susceptibility contrast MRI [DSC MRI]) and PET imaging support the notion that conventional gadolinium-enhanced MRI does not fully capture tumor extent and that addition of these imaging techniques provides more accurate visualization of metabolically active tumor.[43-46] Importantly, certain drugs, including antiangiogenic agents targeting VEGF (including bevacizumab and cediranib), can normalize an initially abnormal BBB and BTB[47] and influence drug delivery (see next section). Normalization of the BBB is reflected by partial or complete resolution of contrast enhancement on MRI, which is referred to as "pseudoresponse" (Fig. 6.2).

Vascular Normalization

The vascular network formed by high-grade brain tumors is highly heterogeneous and characterized by dilated and tortuous vessels, increased permeability, heterogeneous cerebral vascular perfusion, and abnormally thickened basement membranes.[48-50] These morphologic changes are associated with the formation of vasogenic cerebral edema and contribute to the hypoxic tumor microenvironment and increased interstitial fluid pressure (IFP).[51] Elevated IFP itself compresses blood vessels, leading to impaired delivery of cytotoxic chemotherapy and oxygen (which is needed for genotoxic radiation and

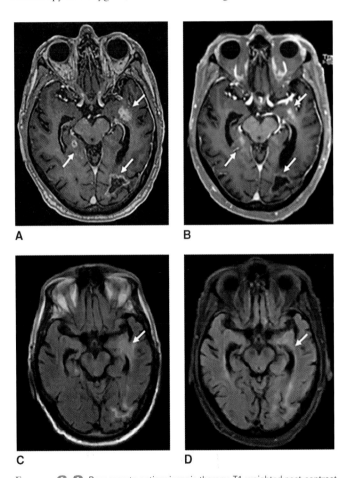

FIGURE 6.2 Response to antiangiogenic therapy. T1-weighted post-contrast (**A**) and T2-weighted FLAIR (**C**) MRI sequences from a patient with multifocal glioblastoma prior to initiation of bevacizumab. Multiple enhancing lesions are seen in the bilateral temporal lobes and left occipital lobe (*white arrows*, **A**) with associated vasogenic edema (*white arrow*, **C**). Two months after starting bevacizumab, there is reduction in the degree of enhancement (**B**) as well as T2/FLAIR hyperintensity (**D**) as a result of vascular normalization.

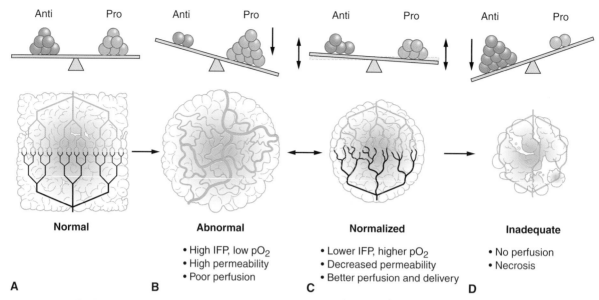

FIGURE **6.3** Schematic diagram to illustrate the process of vascular normalization. **A.** In healthy organs, there is a balance of proangiogenic and antiangiogenic molecules, which maintains an organized and efficient vascular supply. **B.** Tumors produce proangiogenic factors (*various shades of green*) that induce an abnormal, inefficient vascular network. **C.** Judiciously administered anti-VEGF therapy can restore the balance of proangiogenic and antiangiogenic signals and normalize the vascular network, potentially improving drug delivery and efficacy. **D.** However, if anti-VEGF therapy is continued, it can destroy the network totally, impeding delivery of oxygen and nutrients, and ultimately depriving the tumor of essential molecules for growth. In preclinical models, **panel C** usually progresses toward **panel D** (*single arrow*) with currently approved anti-VEGF agents. However, in human tumors, **panel C** commonly reverts to **panel B** after a "window of normalization" (*double arrow*). Anti, antiangiogenic molecules; IFP, interstitial fluid pressure; pO₂, tissue oxygen level; Pro, proangiogenic molecules. (Reprinted by permission from Nature: Jain RK, di Tomaso E, Duda DG, et al. Angiogenesis in brain tumours. *Nat Rev Neurosci.* 2007;8(8):610-622. Copyright © 2007 Springer Nature.)

chemotherapy to be effective) to the tumor. In addition, vasogenic edema can cause significant neurologic morbidity. Many brain tumor patients are thus treated with corticosteroids, which contributes to down-regulation of VEGF,[52] and can relieve edema and neurologic symptoms. However, corticosteroids are associated with significant side effects. Anti-VEGF agents such as bevacizumab and cediranib also have potent antiedema properties but lack the toxicity seen with corticosteroids and are an alternative treatment option in patients who require long-term corticosteroids. Anti-VEGF agents reduce vessel permeability and "normalize" the brain tumor vascular network (Fig. 6.2). According to the vascular normalization hypothesis, this reduces the hypoxic fraction within the tumor and improves oxygenation and drug delivery to the tumor in a subset of patients (Fig. 6.3).[53] Additionally, vascular normalization shifts the immunosuppressive tumor microenvironment to an immunosupportive phenotype, which enables activated tumor-associated macrophages to target tumor cells and suppress their growth.[53–56] However, prolonged anti-VEGF therapy can aggravate hypoxia, resulting in up-regulation of other proangiogenic factors and promotion of a protumorigenic inflammatory state.[49,57] Therefore, it appears that there is a window of normalization during which administration of anti-VEGF therapy may be beneficial while improved cerebral perfusion may not be seen at later treatment time points.

Drug Delivery Methods

Following the administration of an anticancer drug via intravenous or oral routes, the BBB can effectively impede the distribution of drug molecules from the systemic circulation into the CNS. Consequently, considerable effort has been devoted to developing drug delivery strategies that either entirely bypass the BBB or modulate the permeability of the BBB to enhance drug distribution into the brain from systemic circulation. These strategies can either entail systemic or local delivery of drugs. Systemic delivery includes high-dose chemotherapy (HDCT) via the intravenous route, intra-arterial administration of drugs, and BBB disruption with hyperosmolar solutions or biomolecules. Local delivery to the cerebrospinal fluid (CSF) space and/or tumor includes intrathecal (IT) injection, direct intratumoral injection of free drug, or implantation of drug embedded in a controlled-release biodegradable delivery system. However, even when drugs cross the BBB, their migration to tumor cells may be hindered by increased intercapillary distances, greater interstitial pressure, lower microvascular pressure, and the *sink effect* exerted by normal brain tissue.[58] The *sink effect* refers to the selective achievement of higher concentrations of a drug in areas of disrupted BBB in the tumor compared to the rest of the brain. As a result of this concentration gradient, the drug rapidly diffuses out of the tumor into the surrounding brain and compromises tumor exposure time.

Systemic Drug Delivery

High-Dose Chemotherapy with Autologous Stem Cell Rescue

Considering that the BBB is a major factor in brain tumor resistance to chemotherapy and that diffusion across this barrier depends on the concentration-time profile of the free fraction of drug (i.e., drug that is not bound to plasma proteins), the assumption has been that increasing the administered dose would drive more drug across the BBB.[24] The rationale for HDCT was derived from the relatively linear *in vitro* dose-response curve exhibited by classic alkylating agents and the assumption that intrinsic cellular resistance could be overcome by increasing the dose. In the context of treating brain tumors, HDCT could overcome the aforementioned sink effect and provide higher drug concentrations in the tumor for sustained periods. To rescue the myelosuppressive effects associated with HDCT, patients typically undergo autologous stem cell rescue (ASCR).

HDCT with ASCR has demonstrated modest responses in selected pediatric neuro-oncology patients with embryonal tumors, including recurrent medulloblastomas, neuroblastomas, and primitive neuroectodermal tumors (PNETs).[59-62] For instance, in one retrospective study, only 3 of 19 patients who received HDCT had durable disease control (disease-free at 34 to 116 months).[62] Toxicity with this approach can be significant in this patient population: In one study, all patients required blood product transfusions for pancytopenia, broad-spectrum antibiotics for fever and neutropenia, and total parenteral nutrition given the presence of severe oropharyngeal mucositis after treatment with high-dose carboplatin, thiotepa, and etoposide and ASCR.[59] Three of twenty-five patients (12%) died due to multiorgan and infectious complications.[59] The data regarding the role of HDCT and ASCR are limited in adults. Patients with recurrent embryonal tumors appear to have prolonged OS and progression-free survival (PFS) compared to historical controls treated with conventional-dose chemotherapy.[63] In addition, patients with medulloblastomas tend to respond better than those with malignant gliomas.[64] As in children, transplant-related toxicity can be substantial, particularly in those older than 30 years of age.[64] Long-term data from a phase II study of adult patients with newly diagnosed anaplastic oligodendroglioma treated with intensive PCV followed by high-dose thiotepa and ASCR revealed a median PFS of 78 months; mOS had not been reached.[65] A similar phase II study evaluated the use of TMZ, high-dose myeloablative chemotherapy with thiotepa and busulfan, and ASCR in patients with anaplastic oligodendrogliomas and oligoastrocytomas and demonstrated 2- and 5-year PFS of 86% and 60%, respectively.[66] Median PFS and OS had not been reached after a median follow-up of 66 months. The safety and efficacy of HDCT and ASCR were also established in the treatment of recurrent CNS germinomas,[67] but validation studies in randomized trials and long-term data are lacking.

With regard to gliomas, a phase I study demonstrated the feasibility and efficacy of administering genetically engineered hematopoietic stem cells to patients with MGMT-unmethylated GBMs to protect the bone marrow from chemotherapy-induced hematopoietic toxicity.[68] *MGMT*-unmethylated GBMs typically display a poorer response to treatment with alkylating agents such as TMZ, given that chemotherapy-induced DNA breaks are reversed by MGMT. Coadministration of O^6-benzylguanine (O^6BG) can restore tumor cell sensitivity to TMZ but results in off-target myelosuppression, thus limiting the amount of TMZ that can be safely administered. In this study,[68] seven patients with newly diagnosed *MGMT*-unmethylated GBMs were administered autologous gene-modified hematopoietic stem cells, followed by O^6BG/TMZ chemotherapy. This resulted in a significantly higher mean number of O^6BG/TMZ cycles being administered compared to historical controls without gene therapy and translated into a median PFS of 9 months and OS of 20 months.

Notably, HDCT has proven to be effective in patients with primary CNS lymphoma (PCNSL),[69-73] and high-dose (HD-) MTX has been adapted as the cornerstone of induction treatment in this disease population. Two studies using different HD-MTX–based induction regimens, followed by thiotepa-based ASCR as consolida-

tion, have demonstrated objective response rates greater than 90% and prolonged PFS (>74 months).[74,75] In addition, a randomized phase II study using a HD-MTX–based induction regimen, followed by consolidation with either whole-brain radiotherapy or carmustine-/thiotepa-based ASCR, showed no difference in 2-year PFS between the two consolidation groups.[76] A randomized phase II trial (NCT01511562) is ongoing to compare the efficacy of consolidation treatment with HDCT-ASCR versus etoposide/cytarabine after induction with HD-MTX, rituximab, and TMZ.

In summary, HDCT in combination with ASCR warrants further exploration for tumors that are chemosensitive, including embryonal tumors, certain types of gliomas, and CNS lymphomas.

Intra-arterial Administration

The theoretical advantage for delivering anticancer drugs via the intra-arterial (IA) route is related to the ratio of systemic to regional blood flow. Compared to intravenous (IV) injections, a considerably higher local drug concentration can be achieved with IA injection, thereby increasing the concentration gradient that drives the drug across the BBB. In animal models, there was a two- to threefold increase in tumor concentration of cisplatin and a chloroethylnitrosourea, respectively, after IA administration compared to intravenous administration.[77] With this technique, sufficient local drug concentrations can be achieved with smaller doses, which can minimize systemic side effects.[78] The pharmacokinetic advantages of IA administration occur only during the first passage through the CNS because the drug then enters the venous circulation and the plasma profile becomes indistinguishable from that afforded by IV administration.

IA administration has been evaluated in various clinical settings, including neoadjuvant and adjuvant therapy and recurrent malignant gliomas.[79,80] Thus far, clinical trials of IA chemotherapy for malignant gliomas have not demonstrated improved survival compared to conventional IV therapy. A phase III study involving 315 patients with malignant gliomas failed to show any advantages of adjuvant IA BCNU over intravenous infusion of the same drug.[81] Moreover, subjects in the IA BCNU arm of this trial experienced significant treatment-related toxicities. 10% developed leukoencephalopathy and 15% experienced ipsilateral blindness. Two randomized clinical trials compared IA and IV ACNU (nimustine) and found no significant difference in PFS and OS between treatment arms. However, toxicity associated with IA ACNU was modest. No cases of leukoencephalopathy and only one case of transient visual impairment were reported.[82,83]

Potential disadvantages of the IA route include local complications related to catheterization (thrombosis, bleeding, infection) and neurological sequelae (orbital and cranial pain, retinal toxicity, leukoencephalopathy, or cortical necrosis).[79,81,84] In addition, prodrugs requiring hepatic activation, such as cyclophosphamide, procarbazine, and irinotecan, are not suitable for use by the IA route. One factor that partly explains the unique toxicities associated with IA administration is the "streaming" effect.[85] Infusion of drug into the high pressure, rapidly moving arterial bloodstream, results in incomplete mixing of the drug and plasma and great variability in the amount of drug reaching different regions of the vascular territory. Depending on the characteristics of the distribution pattern, higher concentrations of drug might be achieved in the normal brain, whereas lower amounts reach the tumor. Different strategies have been attempted to minimize the streaming effect, including rapid infusion,[85] super selective cannulation of the feeding artery,[84,86] diastole-phased pulsatile infusion,[87,88] and local blood flow–adjusted dosage.[86] All of these techniques were combined in a phase I trial involving 21 brain tumor patients treated with IA carboplatin. The neurologic side effects were minor, and a twofold escalation of the dose beyond the conventional IA dose was achieved.[86]

Despite its serious limitations, there have been a few reports of promising results in patients receiving IA therapy for primary brain tumors. IA carboplatin and etoposide were shown to be safe and useful in the treatment of progressive optic-hypothalamic gliomas in children.[89] In addition, multiple phase I and II studies have evaluated the safety and efficacy of IA chemotherapy in conjunction with osmotic disruption of the BBB in primary and metastatic brain tumor patients.[90–92] These include IA melphalan and carboplatin for primary brain tumors and methotrexate for CNS lymphoma.[91–93]

Osmotic Blood-Brain Barrier Disruption

Osmotic BBB disruption involves the use of hyperosmolar solutions or biomolecules to increase the permeability of the BBB and improve drug delivery to brain tumors (Fig. 6.1G). It is thought that a hyperosmotic environment causes endothelial cell shrinkage with resultant separation of tight junctions.[94] In addition, osmotic stress releases biologically active molecules from endothelial cells, including serine proteases, that could potentially degrade the collagen matrix of the endothelial basement membrane. Finally, cellular shrinkage may also trigger second messenger signals and calcium influx, which could affect the integrity of tight junctions.[27] In addition to potentially improved drug delivery, other advantages include lack of systemic drug toxicity and avoidance of the sink effect. Because BBB disruption theoretically affects the endothelium of both normal brain and brain tumor, a nonselective increase in drug delivery into both areas occurs, and no concentration gradient is established.

From a procedural standpoint, osmolar BBB disruption requires transfemoral angiography and general anesthesia. Most commonly, one major artery (left or right carotid, left or right vertebral) is cannulated and treated. Some have also advocated for BBB disruption with iodinated contrast agents before chemotherapy administration. Given the technical requirements and invasiveness of this procedure, it has not been widely adopted and should only be performed at specialized centers with sufficient expertise. Moreover, an attendant risk of stroke and seizures is associated with this method, further limiting the application of this technique.[94,95]

Both IV and IA administrations of hyperosmolar agents have been tested in brain tumor patients.[94] In a single-arm multi-institutional study of 149 patients with newly diagnosed PCNSL, IA administration of 25% mannitol and methotrexate on 2 consecutive days every 4 weeks apart resulted in an overall response rate of 82% and a median OS of 3.1 years.[96] These results were at least comparable to data from PCNSL trials involving chemotherapy alone or combined chemo- and radiation therapy, but the lack of randomization precludes definitive conclusions on the superiority of this treatment modality to treatment regimens without osmolar BBB disruption. Furthermore, IA bevacizumab with BBB disruption has been explored in case series of GBM patients. These studies demonstrated treatment responses for 3.5 to 4 months after a single dose of bevacizumab[97] and reduction in tumor volume on MRI in

the absence of significant adverse events.[98] Larger validation studies are clearly needed to establish the efficacy profile for delivery of bevacizumab via this route. By contrast, the safety data on IA TMZ with BBB disruption are very limited and conflicting. In one case study, no toxicity was noted after the procedure,[99] while another patient experienced hemodynamic abnormalities and a diffuse skin rash after receiving a second course of treatment.[100]

There is also interest in evaluating the use of biological agents to increase permeability of the BBB. Experimental data have demonstrated the effectiveness of vasoactive compounds, including histamine, leukotriene C4, β-interferon, tumor necrosis factor-α, and bradykinin. In animal xenograft models, the bradykinin analog RMP-7 selectively increased delivery of radiolabeled carboplatin to the brain tumor and improved survival. However, in a randomized double-blind, placebo-controlled phase II study RMP-7 did not improve the efficacy of carboplatin in patients with recurrent malignant glioma.[101]

Intravenously Delivered Nanoparticles

Polymeric nanoparticles are solid colloidal particles that have active drug attached to it. After IV injection, they are transported across the BBB via endocytosis mediated by brain capillary endothelial cells.[102] Ideal nanoparticles are rapidly biodegradable (i.e., within a few days); materials with proven efficacy are poly(butyl cyanoacrylate) (PBCA) and poly(lactic acid) (PLA).

Various nanoparticle-bound anticancer agents, including doxorubicin, BCNU, camptothecin, gemcitabine, methotrexate, paclitaxel, and TMZ, have been tested successfully in rodent models.[102] For instance, administration of pegylated liposomal doxorubicin in tumor-bearing mice resulted in a 20-fold higher sum total area under the curve (AUC) compared to nonliposomal doxorubicin.[103] The addition of a targeted ligand, such as glutathione, may further improve drug delivery.[104] A small number of phase I/II trials in patients with brain metastases and recurrent high-grade gliomas have found that pegylated liposomal doxorubicin was safe and demonstrated moderate efficacy.[105,106] Delivery of nanoparticles has also been explored for a variety of other methods, including in combination with ultrasound-induced BBB opening (see below).

Local Drug Delivery

Intrathecal Administration

Intrathecal (IT) chemotherapy involves the direct injection of drug into the CSF and is an obvious way to bypass the BBB. The rationale is that the cells lining the fluid spaces of the brain are permeable, which results in free exchange of molecules from extracellular fluid (ECF) to CSF and vice versa. Relatively small doses of a drug given by IT injection can achieve high local concentrations, due to the low volume of the CSF compartment (approximately 150 mL), which thereby minimizes systemic toxicity. Furthermore, because of the intrinsically low levels of metabolizing enzymes in the CSF, agents that are subject to rapid metabolism in blood, such as cytosine arabinoside (Ara-C), remain in the active form in CNS for longer periods of time.

IT chemotherapy is administered either via lumbar puncture (LP) into the subarachnoid space or via an intraventricular Rickham or Ommaya reservoir (a port catheter system) implanted

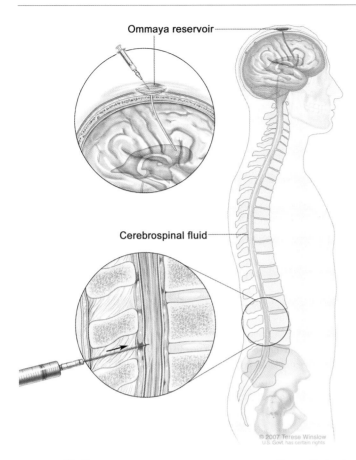

Ommaya reservoir

Cerebrospinal fluid

© 2007 Terese Winslow
U.S. Govt. has certain rights

FIGURE **6.4** Different approaches to IT delivery of drugs. (For the National Cancer Institute © 2007 Terese Winslow, U.S. Govt. has certain rights.)

by a neurosurgeon (Fig. 6.4).[107] Placement of a reservoir is associated with a small risk of hemorrhage and infection related to the surgical procedure. Moreover, the catheter may malfunction over time and require replacement.[108] However, intraventricular injection results in higher CSF drug levels and better dissemination of the drug throughout the CSF axis than after an LP[109] and has been shown to be associated with improved progression-free survival for short-acting agents such as MTX.[110]

The three most commonly administered drugs via the IT route are methotrexate sodium, Ara-C (often administered in its liposomal form), and thiotepa (thiotriethylene phosphoramide). These agents are primarily indicated for the treatment of leptomeningeal metastases from systemic cancer.[107] A small number of studies have compared the efficacy of IT MTX and liposomal Ara-C in patients with leptomeningeal metastases from solid and hematologic malignancies and found conflicting results.[110,111] The efficacy of IT thiotepa is less clear compared to that of IT MTX and Ara-C.[112–114] In addition, certain investigational IT agents have been reported to have some activity and include topotecan,[115,116] etoposide,[117] trastuzumab,[118–123] and rituximab.[124,125] A phase I/II study of IT trastuzumab for leptomeningeal metastases in Her2-positive breast cancer is ongoing (NCT01325207), with phase I results suggesting more activity at the highest doses.[126]

IT drug administration has numerous pharmacokinetic limitations. Among these, the drug must overcome the bulk flow of CSF to penetrate the cisterns and ventricles (Fig. 6.5). In addition, the

flow of interstitial fluid produced by brain cells and microvessels from ECF to CSF counteracts the diffusion of drug from CSF to ECF. CSF undergoes complete renewal every 6 to 8 hours, therefore leading to continuous dilution and turnover of drug concentrations in the CSF. This dilution can only be overcome by a continuous infusion or a sustained-release system to maintain a clinically relevant concentration. For instance, liposomal Ara-C permits sustained release of the drug into the CSF. After a single injection of 50 mg, adequate CSF drug levels can be detected for at least 14 days,[127] which facilitates its administration to once every 14 days, compared to IT MTX and thiotepa, which have to be injected twice weekly.[107] Of note, as of 2017, production of liposomal Ara-C was discontinued by the manufacturer.[128]

Another pharmacologic disadvantage is the fact that production of CSF by the choroid plexus and its elimination into the venous circulation may be altered by the tumor itself, which disturbs bulk flow and modifies drug distribution and diffusion. For example, the clearance of methotrexate from CSF is decreased in the presence of leukemic meningitis.[129,130] Moreover, diffusion in the ventricular space is heterogeneous[109] and may result in uncertain and potentially toxic local concentrations in CSF, even if continuous infusion devices are used.[131] Finally, and importantly, brain tumors are often in locations not adjacent to the ventricular system and may require diffusion of drug from CSF to tumor over a distance of several centimeters, which impairs the ability to achieve cytotoxic concentrations of the drug at the site of the tumor. In the case of methotrexate, the drug concentration is estimated to be no more than 0.1% of the CSF concentration 1 cm from the ependymal edge 48 hours after IT administration.[132] However, the relationship is quite complex. While compounds with greater lipophilicity will access the ECF more effectively, they will also be subject to a higher rate of removal by the vascular and cellular compartments, thus limiting the extent of drug penetration into brain tissue.[133]

Therefore, at this point in time, IT chemotherapy is not feasible for tumors located in the brain parenchyma and is restricted to the treatment and prevention of leptomeningeal metastases.[134] Importantly, even in cases of leptomeningeal metastases, IT chemotherapy is not generally effective for nodular lesions with a diameter greater than 2 to 4 mm, given the inability of the drug to penetrate sufficiently into the nodule.[135]

Intratumoral Administration

The simplest and most direct way to guarantee drug delivery to its target is direct administration into the tumor or the postresection cavity. As with IT injection, this bypasses most of the obstacles pertaining to systemic drug administration for treating brain tumors. Systemic toxicity may also be reduced because substantially lower doses of the drug may be given, and only a relatively small amount of drug distributes from the CNS to the bloodstream. A particularly attractive advantage of this strategy is that anticancer drugs (hydrophilic, high molecular weight molecules) that are normally impeded by the BBB may be used. Conceptually, the low permeability of the BBB to such compounds should promote their retention within the CNS by inhibiting distribution into the bloodstream. Due to the high local drug concentrations that can be achieved, better distribution of drug may be provided within the tumor by diffusion and convection driven by the hydrostatic pressure of the

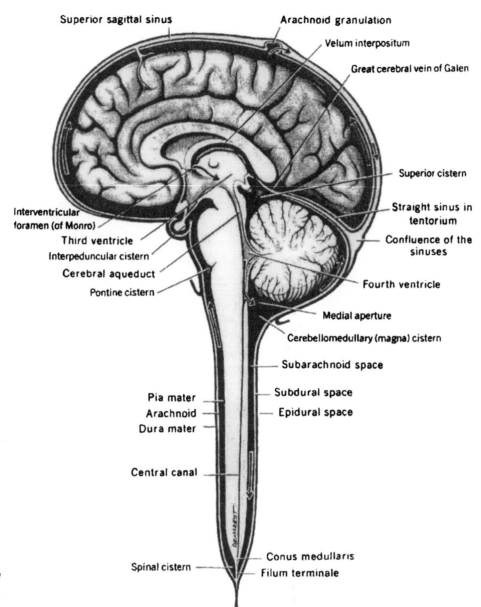

Superior sagittal sinus

Arachnoid granulation

Velum interpositum

Great cerebral vein of Galen

Superior cistern

Straight sinus in tentorium

Confluence of the sinuses

Fourth ventricle

Medial aperture

Cerebellomedullary (magna) cistern

Subarachnoid space

Subdural space

Epidural space

Interventricular foramen (of Monro)

Third ventricle

Interpeduncular cistern

Cerebral aqueduct

Pontine cistern

Pia mater

Arachnoid

Dura mater

Central canal

Spinal cistern

Conus medullaris

Filum terminale

FIGURE **6.5** The subarachnoid spaces and cisterns of the brain and spinal cord. Schematic representation of cerebrospinal fluid pathways (*arrows*). (Reprinted from Fix J. *High-Yield Neuroanatomy*. 2nd ed. Lippincott Williams & Wilkins; 2000:9, with permission.)

tumor. The two techniques that have been most commonly used for directly introducing chemotherapeutic agents into brain tumors are (a) parenteral delivery as either a bolus injection or continuous infusion through a cannula and (b) controlled-release methods by means of implantation of a drug embedded in a slow-release carrier system. It should be noted that, even if intratumoral infusion does avoid some obstacles to drug delivery, it does not circumvent the sink effect or problems associated with drug stability. Indeed, drug molecules released into the ECF must penetrate the brain parenchyma to reach tumor cells.[58] Before reaching its target, the compound could be inactivated by binding to normal tissue, by metabolism, by chemical degradation, or by elimination via the microvascular circulation.[136] In addition, tissue debris may obstruct the catheter.[136,137]

The feasibility of intratumoral infusion has been demonstrated in a number of clinical trials involving multiple different anticancer agents.[137] These studies, however, have not shown a clear survival advantage or direct evidence of increased drug delivery within the tumor. Furthermore, toxicity has been observed with this tech-

nique, including nervous system injury and infection.[137] Over the past decade, multiple primarily phase I trials evaluating the efficacy of injection of genetically engineered oncolytic viruses into the tumor itself or into the walls of the resection cavity have been conducted.[138] Overall, these studies have affirmed the safe administration of oncolytic viruses in humans and revealed treatment responses in select patients.[138] However, many questions remain unanswered, including whether or not and to what extent the viral genotype matters in eliciting an appropriate immune response. Additionally, there is interest in combining oncolytic viruses with checkpoint inhibitors to increase intratumoral immune response; one such trial in melanoma patients is underway (NCT02263508).[138] Lastly, engineered neural stem cells (NSCs) have been explored as vehicles to enhance drug delivery, given their inherent ability to traffic to the site of tumors and cross the BBB. Based on promising rodent studies,[139] cytosine deaminase–expressing clonal NSCs were injected intracranially in a phase I trial of 15 patients with recurrent high-grade glioma at the time of surgery and before administration of the prodrug 5-fluorocytosine.[140] Intracerebral microdialysis data revealed that the NSCs converted 5-fluorocytosine to its active form 5-fluorouracil (a drug with relatively poor CNS penetration). In addition, no dose-limiting toxicities related to NSCs were observed.

Controlled-release methods using polymer, microsphere, and liposomal carriers have been studied extensively *in vitro* and *in vivo*.[25] The goal of this strategy is to provide constant delivery of a cytotoxic drug into the tumor using a matrix that also protects the unreleased drug from hydrolysis and metabolism. A solid polymeric matrix facilitates the delivery of chemotherapeutic agents directly to brain tumors and has potential advantages. Biodegradable carriers have been developed that are unaffected by interstitial pH and provide near zero-order release of drug, with minimal inflammatory response.[141] Potential disadvantages include (a) drug release cannot be controlled once the device has been implanted, (b) unpredictable diffusion, (c) stability of the device and drug in the aqueous milieu, and (d) the possibility that the polymer may not release the drug as intended.

A biodegradable polyanhydride solid matrix, poly[bis(*p*-carboxyphenoxy)propane-sebacic acid] or p(CPP-SA), has been developed that releases drug by a combination of diffusion and hydrolytic polymer degradation.[142] Preclinical studies demonstrated that this system is biocompatible and results in reproducible and sustained continuous release of BCNU (Fig. 6.1D). More than 300 patients with recurrent[143,144] and newly diagnosed[4,145–147] malignant gliomas have been treated with the BCNU polymer in phase I to III clinical studies. A phase III study in patients with recurrent malignant glioma demonstrated that intratumoral implantation of a 3.85% BCNU polymer was safe and resulted in minimal systemic side effects from BCNU. Median survival was longer in subjects with GBM who received the active polymer than in those who did not, even after adjustment for known prognostic factors.[144] A phase III randomized placebo-controlled trial examining BCNU polymer application in malignant glioma patients at the time of primary surgical resection also showed survival benefit.[4,145] A phase I study designed to increase the amount of BCNU in the polymer (up to 20%) demonstrated that at the highest doses, BCNU plasma levels were significantly (500-fold) lower than those associated with systemic BCNU toxicity. As a result, no BCNU-related systemic toxicity was observed.[148] However, the risk of local neurotoxicity may be increased at higher BCNU concentrations in the polymer. Other studies of this delivery strategy have assessed the use of the BCNU polymer in combination with systemic chemotherapy, including the standard TMZ and radiation protocol, and are reviewed in detail elsewhere.[149] To date, several studies, mostly retrospective, have demonstrated an acceptable safety profile and encouraging survival rates. However, the limitations of these trials include potential patient selection bias and lack of randomization.[149]

Delivery of other agents with p(CPP-SA) wafers has been explored in rodent models, including paclitaxel,[150] camptothecin,[151] hydroperoxycyclophosphamide,[152] tirapazamine,[153] and 5-iodo-2V deoxyuridine.[154,155] These studies revealed tumoricidal activity and improved survival in animal models. Similarly, animal models using TMZ-containing biodegradable polymers revealed a threefold increase in intracranial TMZ concentrations compared to orally delivered TMZ, which also correlated with improved survival.[156] However, the majority of these studies have not been advanced to

human clinical trials, partly because of dampened enthusiasm for this technology in light of new emerging local delivery therapies.[149] The exception is a randomized, multicenter phase II trial that compared the efficacy of intratumoral implantation of 5-fluorouracil–releasing biodegradable microspheres followed by radiation therapy versus radiation therapy alone.[157] Median OS was 2.9 months longer in the group that received microspheres, but this did not reach statistical significance.

Convection-Enhanced Delivery

In addition to the physical limitations imposed by the BBB, diffusion barriers intrinsic to the CNS, such as the hydrostatic pressure of brain tissue, can also limit drug delivery to tumors. Convection-enhanced delivery (CED) is a pressure gradient–dependent method that exploits the hydrostatic pressure gradient to deliver drug concentrations via convective flow (Fig. 6.1E). Theoretically, this pressure gradient permits homogeneous distribution of a drug over large distances by displacing interstitial fluid with the infusate. The drug is directly infused through a catheter that is surgically implanted in the brain tumor.[41,158] The path of drug delivery is dependent on the anatomic site of the catheter: Infusion into gray matter results in spherical distribution of the drug, whereas infusion into white matter results in distribution along white matter fiber pathways.[158] Therefore, the specific anatomic location of the brain tumor may be an important determinant of drug delivery. In addition, inherent drug properties may influence the efficacy of drug distribution by CED. For instance, drugs with high passive permeability or those that undergo active efflux from the brain parenchyma to the blood may not reach sufficient concentrations at tumor sites distant from the site of catheter placement.[41] Other factors that can substantially impact drug delivery are catheter design and positioning.[159–161]

While *in vitro* and animal *in vivo* data have demonstrated effective drug delivery via CED, results in humans have been disappointing thus far. Multiple phase I and II trials have evaluated the delivery of various agents, including chemotherapeutics, viral-based agents, targeted toxins,[159,162–167] and immunotherapy,[168,169] in GBMs and diffuse intrinsic pontine glioma (DIPG), but results are difficult to interpret. For instance, in a phase I clinical trial, patients with recurrent malignant gliomas received a CED-delivered recombinant chimeric protein containing a genetically modified form of *Pseudomonas* exotoxin (TP-38), which was targeted against the epidermal growth factor receptor (EGFR). Median OS after TP-38 therapy was 28 weeks.[160] However, in most patients, SPECT imaging demonstrated significant leaks of infusate into the subarachnoid or intraventricular CSF space, thus limiting the amount of intraparenchymal drug concentrations and precluding accurate assessment of the efficacy and safety of the drug. Another phase I study using CED of the protein MR1(Fv)-PE38 (scFV MR1 fused to *Pseudomonas* exotoxin PE-38) directed against EGFRvIII was closed early due to low accrual.[170] The only phase III trial compared a glioma toxin (a fusion protein consisting of interleukin-13 linked to a mutated form of *Pseudomonas* exotoxin [IL-13 PE38QQR]) to BCNU wafers, and there were no differences in OS.[165] Ongoing trials include a phase I/II study of another recombinant protein targeting both wild-type EGFR and the mutated EGFRvIII variant, both of which are frequently overexpressed in GBMs.[171] In addition, preliminary data from a phase I trial of PVS-RIPO, a recombinant oncolytic poliovirus delivered intratumorally by CED, in recurrent GBM patients demonstrated a survival advantage compared to historical controls.[172]

Based on results to date, future directions in CED research should include optimization of infusion catheter designs and infusion parameters. It will also be important to verify appropriate target engagement, for instance, by coinfusion of imaging tracers.[160,161]

Ultrasound-Induced BBB Opening

Ultrasound-induced BBB opening for glioma therapy is a novel technique in the field of drug delivery (Fig. 6.1F). Prior to exposing the target brain area to focused ultrasound, preformed microbubbles (2 to 6 μm in diameter) are injected intravenously. In addition to inducing pressure oscillations over the target area, focused ultrasound causes a phenomenon called "cavitation."[173] On a microscopic level, cavitation leads to rapid growth and collapse (inertial cavitation) or sustained oscillation (stable cavitation) of these microbubbles. These events then produce transient BBB opening via different mechanisms: (a) the sudden collapse of microbubbles leads to the formation of shock waves (>10,000 atmospheres depending on bubble size), which are capable of disrupting tissues, and (b) oscillations generate velocities, which inflict shear stresses on cells and tissues and result in their disruption.[173]

A number of *in vitro* and animal *in vivo* studies have demonstrated the potential efficacy of ultrasound-induced BBB opening in tumor models. In a murine model of brain metastases secondary to breast cancer, selected mice that were exposed to focused ultrasound and anti-HER2 antibodies had a decreased tumor growth rate compared to animals who did not undergo focused ultrasound.[174] In addition, multiple studies using focused ultrasound in conjunction with liposomal doxorubicin have demonstrated improved survival and some tumor regression in rats.[175,176] Another study explored the potential of MRI-guided focused ultrasound with cisplatin-loaded "brain-penetrating" nanoparticles in two rat glioma models and revealed a 6- to 28-fold improvement in drug delivery. These nanoparticles are covered in a dense poly(ethylene glycol (PEG)) coat that provides a nonadhesive surface and permits these particles to spread within normal brain and brain tumors.[177] Consistent with this, higher and more homogenous drug distributions within the tumor parenchyma were seen. Clinically, these findings translated into delayed tumor growth and prolonged animal survival.[177] Interestingly, MRI performed after ultrasound-induced microbubble activation revealed increased intensity and extent of contrast enhancement, indicating enhanced tumor permeability. The concept of increased tissue permeability after exposure to focused ultrasound is also supported by recent dynamic contrast-enhanced (DCE) MRI data that showed an increase in the transfer coefficient K^{trans}—a measure of tissue permeability—after provision of focused ultrasound and doxorubicin.[178]

Future efforts may include correlative studies of drug uptake with perfusion imaging to characterize the impact of a heterogeneous tumor vasculature and increased IFP (both of which are frequently observed in malignant brain tumors) on the efficacy of focused ultrasound. Ultimately, early-phase studies of this method will need to be performed in humans to confirm its safety and feasibility.

Assessing Drug Delivery to the Brain

Characterizing the exposure of brain tumors to chemotherapeutic agents presents an extremely challenging problem. As is the case with any organ or tissue, the time course of the concentration of a drug or active metabolite within a tumor cannot be discerned from experimental data derived from measurements in plasma, serum, or whole blood. Although some temporal relationship undoubtedly exists between drug concentrations in plasma and in tumor, elucidating the tumor concentration-time profile eventually requires measuring drug levels within the tumor itself.

Determining whether adequate concentrations of the active form of a drug reach the target tissue is extremely important in the context of phase I trials. Because objective antitumor responses occur rarely in phase I studies, data on whether or not a drug reaches the tumor would rationalize further clinical evaluation. In this section, we will discuss principal techniques that are less invasive and potentially more informative than tissue biopsy studies to assess the pharmacokinetics of anticancer drugs in the CNS and brain tumors. These include CSF sampling, microdialysis, and noninvasive imaging. Although no single method can be uniformly applied to monitor drugs in human tissues in vivo, these techniques are nonetheless becoming increasingly important to the clinical development of anticancer drugs for the treatment of brain tumors.

Direct Measurement in Tumor Tissue

Direct measurement of drug concentrations in tumor tissue has numerous shortcomings. Subjecting brain cancer patients to the risks of an intracranial surgical procedure that may have little or no direct benefit to the treatment of their disease raises ethical concerns. It may be possible to circumvent this problem by obtaining tissue when a biopsy is indicated for diagnostic reasons or during a tumor-debulking procedure. Nevertheless, measuring the concentration of drug in a single biopsy specimen provides limited information unless the tissue is obtained while drug is being given in a manner that provides continuous systemic exposure to the agent. Otherwise, the most appropriate time to obtain a single biopsy specimen relative to drug administration is speculative, at best, as the presence or absence of a measurable drug concentration has little interpretive value. Acquiring serial tumor specimens from the same patient presents even greater practical constraints, and the effect of prior procedures on altering the transport of drug to and from the tumor represents a significant confounding factor. Multiple studies have attempted to evaluate antineoplastic drug concentrations from surgical tissues using liquid or gas chromatography, mass spectrometry, or atomic absorption spectrometry,[179] but the data are difficult to interpret, given the variability in sampling sites (which is particularly relevant in heterogeneous tumors like high-grade gliomas), sampling times, dosing regimen, reported parameters (e.g., area under the concentration-time curve versus peak concentration versus tissue-to-blood ratios), and patient population. A systematic study should thus consist of the prospective and longitudinal collection of biopsy data from tumor and peritumoral tissue in a moderately sized cohort of patients with comparable disease characteristics who are treated with the same dose of drug. In a number of clinical trials, patients now receive an anticancer drug several days before surgery, followed by measurement of intratumoral drug concentration, drug metabolites, and target molecules from surgical specimens (e.g., NCT02101905, NCT02576665, NCT01849146).

Lastly, despite the above logistical constraints, emerging spectrometry techniques may facilitate the direct measurement of drug concentrations in tumor tissue in the future. In rodent models, matrix-assisted laser desorption ionization mass spectrometry imaging (MALDI MSI) is a potential technique to image drug permeability through the BBB but will require further testing and validation in humans.[180,181]

Cerebrospinal Fluid

Pharmacologic studies of CSF drug or drug metabolite levels are frequently performed as a surrogate marker of tumor drug levels and as a measure of drug delivery beyond the BBB. In this context, it is important to understand the composition and normal physiology of CSF. The most distinct difference between CSF and plasma is the substantially lower concentration of proteins in CSF. As a result, the total concentration of poorly soluble compounds or compounds that bind avidly to proteins is expected to be lower in CSF than in plasma or brain tissue although the free concentration may be increased. In addition, CSF is slightly more acidic than plasma (pH of 7.32 versus 7.40), which could conceivably influence the transport and retention of a drug in the CSF. For compounds that have a functional group with a pK_a in the 7 to 8 range, the pH difference could also impact the drug's chemical stability relative to that in plasma.

Figure 6.5 depicts the normal process involved in CSF formation and flow. The volume of CSF contained within the ventricles, cisterns, and subarachnoid space of a normal adult is approximately 150 mL.[182] Approximately 500 mL of CSF is produced every 24 hours, predominantly by the choroid plexus within the cerebral ventricles; therefore, the entire CSF volume is replenished three times during the course of a day. CSF formed in the lateral ventricles flows into the third ventricle and then to the fourth ventricle. Upon exiting from the fourth ventricle, it passes into the basal cisterns and the cerebral and spinal subarachnoid spaces, descending through the posterior aspect of the spinal cord and returning through the anterior aspect. Ascending CSF passes over the cerebral hemispheres toward the major dural sinuses, where absorption of CSF into the venous system occurs at the arachnoid villi. The presence of a brain tumor can significantly diminish both the formation and flow of CSF.[30]

Concentration gradients between the ventricular and lumbar regions exist for endogenous constituents of CSF as well as for xenobiotics that have gained access to the CSF. The concentration of systemically administered drugs is generally higher in CSF collected from the ventricles than from the lumbar region as drug distribution in the CNS follows CSF flow.[183] Because drug levels are often determined in CSF acquired by LP, this may significantly underestimate the concentrations in the ventricular region. Similarly, drug administered directly into lumbar CSF is poorly distributed to the ventricles.[109,184] Although patients cannot be subjected to frequently repeated LPs, ventricular access devices, such as Ommaya reservoirs, may be used to facilitate serial acquisition of CSF specimens for drug level monitoring. Therefore, the specific space from which

CSF samples were collected must be taken into account whenever drug concentrations are compared. Furthermore, when collecting CSF specimens, the fluid balance or bulk volume of CSF could be significantly altered, which would affect pressure equilibrium and flow between the various CSF compartments, as well as the concentration gradients between CSF and plasma.

The presence of drug in the CSF represents a strong, but not definitive, indication that the compound has gained access to brain tissue, inclusive of tumors. Some level of uncertainty exists because the vascular supply to the choroid plexus, hypophysis, and pineal gland is not protected by the BBB. Although it comprises a comparably small exchange surface, this does provide a direct pathway for the transport of compounds into the CSF. To further complicate matters, the absence of measurable drug or metabolite levels in the CSF does not absolutely imply that the agent has failed to reach a brain tumor. Conceivably, the majority of a compound reaching brain tissue could be trapped in the intracellular space, extensively bound to tissue protein, subject to chemical or enzymatic conversion to unknown products, or effluxed back into the bloodstream before migrating from interstitial spaces to the CSF. Accordingly, many drugs have been found to achieve higher concentrations in a brain tumor than would have been predicted from plasma and CSF data.[185,186] Despite the limitations of CSF as an indirect measure of drug delivery to a brain tumor, it is an accessible compartment, and CSF sampling remains an important method for screening drug access to the CNS.

Microdialysis

Microdialysis is a technique that enables continuous and serial *in vivo* measurement of the concentration of an amenable compound in ECF within a tumor or normal tissues.[187–189] Commercially available microdialysis catheters consist of a chamber that is less than 1 mm in diameter fitted with a semipermeable membrane, which has a molecular weight cutoff ranging from 20 to 100 kd. Two sections of microcatheter are fused into the membrane. The device is stereotactically implanted such that the membrane resides within the desired area of the brain or tumor and the microcatheters are externalized. One of the microcatheters is connected to a syringe pump containing perfusion fluid, while the other microcatheter collects the dialysate (i.e., the solution exiting the probe). Perfusion fluid is similar in composition to ECF and is pumped through the inlet tubing of the catheter at flow rates ranging from 0.1 to 5 µL/min. In theory, microdialysis mimics the passive function of a capillary blood vessel.[188,190,191] The exiting dialysate contains water, inorganic ions, and small hydrophilic organic molecules that freely diffuse across the membrane of the probe. By contrast, proteins, protein-bound compounds, and lipophilic organic compounds cannot diffuse across the membrane.

Due to the low flow rate at which the perfusion solution is delivered, the perfusate must generally be collected over intervals ranging from 5 to 30 minutes in order to obtain a sufficient volume for chemical analysis. Consequently, microdialysis may not be suitable for studying systems in which the concentration of the compound of interest is changing rapidly relative to this time frame. The perfusate obtained by microdialysis can be analyzed directly by methods such as reversed-phase high-performance liquid chromatography, liquid chromatography/mass spectrometry, or capillary electrophoresis without the need for any preliminary sample preparation to remove macromolecules, as is generally required for assays performed on plasma.[187,192,193] Due to the dynamic nature of the system, in which the concentration of compounds in the ECF may be constantly changing while the perfusion fluid within the dialysis probe is continually flowing, steady-state conditions between the sampled fluid and dialysis fluid are not achieved. Nevertheless, it has been conclusively established that the *in vivo* recovery of an analyte, defined as its concentration in the dialysate relative to that in the sampled fluid, is independent of the concentration in the sampled fluid. Because the drug concentration in the dialysate is generally much lower than in ECF, the diluting effect of the technique demands a very sensitive analytical method to enable the detection of low concentrations of an analyte in very small sample volumes.[187]

Insertion and removal of the dialysis probe result in minimal injury to normal brain tissue, alteration of fluid balance, or disruption of the BBB.[187,194,195] Although it can be performed safely, microdialysis is nevertheless an invasive surgical procedure with a small risk of bleeding at the site of insertion and discomfort for the patient.

Considerable experience has been gained with the use of microdialysis, in both animal models and human subjects since the technique was first introduced in the 1970s.[196] Microdialysis has been thoroughly evaluated in head injury patients for monitoring lactic acid, glucose, glutamic acid, γ-aminobutyric acid, oxygen partial pressure, and pH, both for diagnostic purposes and to assess the effect of therapeutic interventions.[187,197–199] Microdialysis was first described as a tool to monitor the distribution of an anticancer drug in a brain tumor by de Lange, who measured the concentration of methotrexate in a rodent brain tumor model.[200] The results obtained with microdialysis were comparable to those in previous studies of intratumoral methotrexate distribution based on the classic methods of autoradiography and tissue excision.[201] Subsequently, the technique has been used to define the concentration-time profile of camptothecin and topotecan in rodent brain tumor models,[202,203] as well as of other antineoplastic agents in various preclinical tumor models.[188,191,204,205] Microdialysis has also been used to measure intratumoral TMZ levels after administration of antiangiogenic agents in rodent models.[206,207]

The feasibility and safety of microdialysis in humans have been demonstrated in numerous studies.[208–211] A pilot study investigated the use of microdialysis to assess intratumoral methotrexate concentration in patients with recurrent high-grade gliomas.[211] Another study evaluated intracerebral microdialysis to monitor the pharmacokinetics of systemically administered TMZ in patients with resectable primary and metastatic brain tumors.[210] TMZ concentrations in the brain interstitium were consistent with published data obtained from preclinical models and those from clinical studies of CSF. The time needed to achieve maximum TMZ concentrations in the brain tissue was longer than previously believed (2.0 ± 0.8 hours), which may have clinical implications for combination studies in which TMZ is paired with radiation.[210] Another study used microdialysis catheters to study the levels of inflammatory markers before and during radiation therapy in high-grade glioma patients and observed a positive correlation between baseline IL-8 and IL-6 levels from microdialysis measurements and survival.[208] Since inflammation and immune reactivity play key roles in tumor

progression and regression, microdialysis may thus be a valuable tool to study delivery of immunotherapy agents and help elucidate why some patients respond better to immunotherapy than others. Importantly, microdialysis studies may be useful in the preclinical setting to prevent drugs with little or no brain penetration from entering phase I trials.[209]

Noninvasive Imaging

The emergence of an increasing number of advanced imaging methods and potential imaging biomarkers has led to heightened efforts to improve imaging-based *in vivo* assessment of target engagement, drug biodistribution, and real-time monitoring of treatment outcome. In addition, there is increased interest in developing imaging-based *in vivo* tracking methods of tumor cells or cells located in the tumor microenvironment (e.g., tumor-infiltrating lymphocytes) as their fate during a patient's treatment course may provide important insights into drug delivery and efficacy. In this section, we discuss two of the most well-established methods to accomplish these goals: MR spectroscopy (MRS) and PET imaging.

Water is the most abundant molecule in brain tissue and generates the strongest signal on MR imaging. However, other less abundant protons bound to macromolecules also produce signals and demonstrate small variations in the Larmor frequency. These variations are expressed in parts per million (ppm) in relation to a known frequency (tetramethylsilane).[212] MRS is a technique that detects these frequency peaks by suppressing the large water peak and thus provides information about the chemical composition of the brain.[212] The isotopes of atoms amenable to detection by MRS that are of greatest interest with regard to drug level monitoring include ^{1}H, ^{2}H (deuterium), ^{11}B, ^{13}C, ^{15}N, ^{19}F, and ^{31}P. In general, ^{1}H and ^{31}P cannot be used to monitor xenobiotics *in vivo* due to their ubiquitous presence in bio-organic molecules and the resultant intensity of their natural background signals. The exception is when a compound has nuclei with chemical shifts that differ substantially from the resonance frequencies arising from these endogenous molecules. Examples of this include the detection of iproplatin by ^{1}H MRS and ifosfamide by ^{31}P MRS.[213,214]

By contrast, many *in vivo* studies have been performed with drugs that contain fluorine in their native structure, such as 5-fluorouracil.[215–218] The ^{19}F nucleus represents an ideal object for *in vivo* MRS studies since it offers high intrinsic sensitivity, a large range of chemical shifts, and lack of a natural background signal from endogenous fluorinated organic compounds.[219] An MRS study involving 103 patients with extraneural malignancies demonstrated that the therapeutic response to 5-fluorouracil significantly correlated with the half-life of the drug within tumors.[215,217,220] Gemcitabine hydrochloride is another fluorinated anticancer agent for which ^{19}F MRS has been successfully used for *in vivo* pharmacokinetic studies.[221]

Hyperpolarization of molecules with NMR-visible nuclei, such as ^{13}C and ^{15}N, has emerged as a potential tool to increase the MRS signal of less abundant isotopes. For instance, the natural abundance of ^{13}C is only 1.1%, thus necessitating long acquisition times and limiting its application in the clinical setting.[222] Hyperpolarization is accomplished by a process termed dissolution dynamic nuclear polarization. Briefly, the labeled compound (e.g., ^{13}C-pyruvate) is mixed with a free radical and exposed to low temperatures (<2 Kelvin) and a high magnetic field (approximately 3 to 5 T).

Microwave irradiation saturates the electron spin resonance, and polarization is transferred from the radical electron to the labeled nucleus, which results in an increase in polarization by 10% to 50%.[222] Notably, hyperpolarized ^{13}C MRS may increase the MRS signal by greater than 10,000-fold compared to conventional ^{13}C MRS[223] and may become an important tool to study cancer metabolism. For instance, hyperpolarized [1-^{13}C]-pyruvate has been used to monitor the production of [1-^{13}C]-lactate and [^{13}C]-bicarbonate. In cancer, the upregulation of aerobic glycolysis (known as the Warburg effect) channels pyruvate metabolism into lactate production and decreases the amount of bicarbonate. Using hyperpolarized [1-^{13}C]-pyruvate MRS in animal GBM models, increased conversion to [1-^{13}C]-lactate and decreased conversion to [^{13}C]-bicarbonate have been observed.[222] Conversely, a decrease in [1-^{13}C]-lactate production was seen after exposure to various anticancer drugs, including everolimus, voxtalisib, and TMZ.[222] Other hyperpolarized probes, including [2-^{13}C]-pyruvate and [1-^{13}C]-alpha-ketoglutarate, have also been evaluated in high- and low-grade gliomas.[222] Further work will need to establish the potential of hyperpolarized MRS to directly study drug delivery to brain tumors.

The main advantage of MRS compared to PET is that the drugs used for MRS are stable compounds with unlimited shelf lives. In addition, patients are not subjected to ionizing radiation.[219] The major disadvantage is the relatively poor sensitivity of MRS compared to PET (10^{-5} to 10^{-3} mol/L [low millimolar range] with MRS compared to approximately 10^{-12} mol/L [picomolar range] with PET).[219] Many anticancer agents in clinical trials tend to be increasingly potent, with maximum tolerated doses that provide peak plasma concentrations in the nanomolar to low micromolar range in patients, and therefore may not be detected by MRS. The detection limits of MRS can be improved to some degree by increasing the data acquisition time. However, this sacrifices temporal resolution, which may be extremely important for pharmacokinetic studies. MRS also does not permit the determination of the absolute concentration of a drug *in vivo* although changes in relative concentration during the course of a single experiment can be readily followed.[215]

Dynamic PET imaging involves administration of tracer quantities (typically in the nanomolar range) of a radiolabeled compound that is specific and selective for the target of interest. From a physical standpoint, the radiolabel ("radionuclide") undergoes positive beta decay by emitting a positron, which travels in tissue until it interacts with an electron. This results in annihilation of both the positron and electron and subsequent emission of a pair of high-energy gamma photons, which are approximately 180° apart and registered by a detector ring configured in the PET camera.[224,225] These registered events are then reconstructed into a three-dimensional image, which reflects the spatial distribution of radioactivity as a function of time.[226] PET is frequently combined with CT or MRI to provide better resolution and anatomic information. Importantly, the half-lives of the radioisotopes should match the pharmacokinetics of the drug carrier used.[225] Compared to MRS, PET enables detection of radiolabeled compounds with 10^6 to 10^9 times greater sensitivity and superior temporal resolution due to shorter data acquisition time.[227] Furthermore, while MRS is effectively limited to monitoring the relative change in concentration of a compound during the course of a study, PET provides a quantitative measurement of radioactivity.[228]

Typically, the drug of interest is labeled with a radioactive form of one of the atoms already present in its native structure such as carbon, nitrogen, fluorine, or oxygen.[219] Thus, ^{11}C, ^{18}F, and ^{13}N have been studied extensively in PET pharmacokinetic studies.[183] Of note, because these radionuclides have very short half-lives (10 minutes for ^{13}N, 20 minutes for ^{11}C, and 110 minutes for ^{18}F), a cyclotron and remote-controlled radiochemical synthesis facility are required for on-site generation of the radionuclide and immediate preparation of the labeled drug.[228,229] The most informative application of PET to pharmacokinetic studies entails the simultaneous acquisition of two sets of data as follows. A series of tomographic images are acquired for a total of 1 to 2 hours after bolus IV administration of a tracer dose of the radiolabeled drug, which typically ranges from 100 to 1,000 MBq, together with the usual dose of unlabeled drug. The time over which individual images are measured generally increases during the course of the experiment and can range from 5 seconds to 10 minutes, as dictated by the combined rates of radioactive decay of the tracer and elimination of the drug from the body. The time-averaged concentration of radiotracer in discrete regions of interest within the image is used to construct time-activity curves. Arterial blood is also serially collected from the patient throughout the experiment for independent measurement of the radiotracer concentration in whole blood or plasma by solid scintillation counting. The empirical kinetic model that best relates the time course of radiotracer in tissue to its concentration in plasma is then identified.[230]

Dynamic PET imaging has been used to study the distribution of the radiolabeled forms of several clinically approved and investigational anticancer agents to human brain tumors, including ^{11}C]-BCNU,[231,232] [13]N]-cisplatin,[233] 5-^{18}F]-fluorouracil,[227] and ^{11}C]-TMZ.[230] The initial uptake of radioactivity originating from ^{11}C]-TMZ in plasma was seven times greater in brain tumors than in normal brain tissue, with the kinetic behavior in these two regions becoming almost indistinguishable by 30 minutes after dosing.[230] Considering these results, the markedly greater accumulation of radiolabeled agent in the tumor than in normal brain tissue, clearly evident in the PET images, was attributed to increased drug delivery due to a breakdown of the BBB within the tumor. The suggestion that the initial uptake of TMZ from plasma could be an important determinant of its efficacy against human brain tumors has potential clinical significance.

Other research in the field of PET imaging–guided drug delivery has focused on studying novel radionuclides (e.g., ^{64}Cu, ^{68}Ga, and [89]Zr) in combination with improved drug delivery methods such as nanocarriers,[226] with the goal to enable simultaneous targeted drug delivery and *in vivo* tracking of the drug. The process of generating these radioisotope-bound nanocarriers is complex. An example of such a molecule is shown in Figure 6.6. In essence, the anticancer drug is bound to a polymer complex that is conjugated to a peptide group and chelators. The peptides target integrin $\alpha_v\beta_3$, which is overexpressed on tumor cells and the tumor vasculature,[234–236] while the chelators serve as a ligand for radioisotope labeling with [64]Cu. As an example, *in vivo* PET imaging and biodistribution studies in a U87MG mouse model demonstrated higher cellular uptake of conjugated micelles compared to nontargeted micelles, which is mediated by increased integrin $\alpha_v\beta_3$–mediated endocytosis.[237] The use of these theranostic agents, that is, a pharmaceutical that

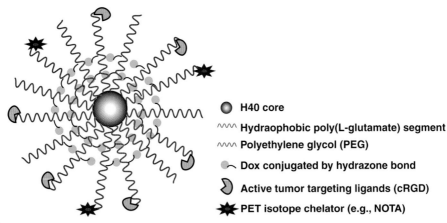

H40 core

Hydraophobic poly(L-glutamate) segment

Polyethylene glycol (PEG)

Dox conjugated by hydrazone bond

Active tumor targeting ligands (cRGD)

PET isotope chelator (e.g., NOTA)

FIGURE **6.6** Schematic illustration of a multifunctional nanocarrier for *in vivo* tumor-targeted drug delivery and PET imaging. An amphiphilic block copolymer consisting of Boltorn® H40 poly(L-glutamate-hydrazone-doxorubicin)-*b*-poly(ethylene glycol) is conjugated to cyclo(*Arg-Gly-Asp-d-Phe-Cys*) peptides (cGRD) and macrocyclic chelators (NOTA) for ^{64}Cu labeling and PET imaging. The H40 core (*gray dot*) is a hyperbranched aliphatic polyester with suitable properties (biodegradability, biocompatibility, and large number of functional groups) for micelle design. Doxorubicin (*green dots*) is conjugated to the hydrophobic segments of the copolymer arms via pH-labile hydrazone linkages, which enable pH-controlled drug release. The cRGD peptides (*yellow half-moon shapes*) enable targeting of integrin $\alpha_v\beta_3$ on tumor cells and vasculature. Complexation of ^{64}Cu onto the micelles via NOTA permits PET imaging. (Reprinted from Xiao Y, Hong H, Javadi A, et al. Multifunctional unimolecular micelles for cancer-targeted drug delivery and positron emission tomography imaging. *Biomaterials.* 2012;33(11):3071-3082. Copyright © 2012 Elsevier. With permission.)

is capable of drug delivery and has targeted diagnostic imaging features, is a rapidly emerging area. It has been studied using different drug classes, including nanocarriers and biologicals, and PET radiolabels.[238–240]

In the era of immunotherapy (including anti-CTLA4, anti-PD1, and anti–PD-L1 agents), there has been strong interest in developing strategies for *in vivo* tracking of the location and viability of immune cells.[241–243] For instance, using CD3- or CD8-specific PET probes, it may now be possible to track subpopulation of T cells in murine systemic cancer models.[244,245] Furthermore, high uptake values of these PET tracers in mice treated with an anti–CTLA-4 agent at day 14 demonstrated potential as a predictive biomarker.[244] Similarly, PET probes targeting PD-1, PD-L1, and CTLA-4—the three primary targets of immune checkpoint inhibition—have been developed and tested successfully in mouse models.[242] Although these cell tracking techniques are in early development and require translation into clinical studies, they provide an exciting framework to potentially improve our understanding of patient response to immunotherapy.

In addition to its inherent expense and technical complexities, PET has a number of other limitations. The time period over which a radiolabeled drug can be monitored after administration of a tracer dose is effectively limited to three to four times the half-life of radioactive decay. The maximum duration of an experiment is therefore only 90 minutes and 6 to 8 hours for a ^{11}C-labeled or ^{18}F-labeled drug, respectively. For some drugs, this may not be enough time to adequately define the time course of the uptake or decline of radiotracer in the tumor. Lastly, PET measures total radioactivity without distinguishing alterations in the chemical structure of the labeled molecule. Because PET cannot distinguish the parent drug from metabolites that retain the label, or free versus protein-bound drug, it may not be suitable for studying the distribution of drugs that are extensively metabolized or highly protein bound. These factors need to be taken into consideration for each individual agent when analyzing and interpreting kinetic data from PET studies.[230] Nevertheless, PET can provide highly informative insights and answer the critical question of whether radiotracer originating from the drug accumulates within a tumor.

Drug Interactions Affecting Brain Tumor Therapy

Patients with primary or metastatic brain tumors are generally excluded from phase I clinical trials of investigational new anticancer drugs because of difficulties in differentiating between potential drug-related neurotoxicities and complications associated with the tumor itself. In addition, the use of other medications in the clinical management of brain tumor patients, especially antiseizure drugs and corticosteroids, could suppress neurologic symptoms related to drug toxicity. In the past, the maximum tolerated dose of an investigational chemotherapeutic agent in adult patients with systemic solid tumors was used directly in phase II trials to assess clinical activity against brain tumors, without provisions to further refine the dose. It has become recognized that this practice often resulted in significantly undertreating patients with CNS malignancies, given pharmacokinetic interactions with concurrent medications that result in increased elimination of anticancer drugs from the systemic circulation and impaired delivery to the CNS.[246,247]

Interactions Affecting the Elimination of Anticancer Agents

It is well known that certain classes of compounds can induce or suppress the expression of CYP450 enzymes and thereby alter the extent to which anticancer drugs are metabolized by these pathways.[246,247] In addition, competitive inhibition could result from concurrent administration of two or more drugs that are substrates for the same CYP450 isozyme. These effects may not result in clinically significant alterations in the pharmacokinetic behavior of most drugs. However, anticancer agents are typically administered at relatively high doses—close to the threshold of tolerability—which may consequently utilize a greater capacity of the elimination pathways than drugs given for other indications. Accordingly, the potential for clinically significant pharmacokinetic interactions is greater for chemotherapeutic agents than for other classes of drugs.[248]

Antiseizure drugs such as phenytoin, carbamazepine, and phenobarbital are sometimes administered on a long-term basis to brain tumor patients and are potent inducers of many of the most important CYP450 enzymes involved in drug metabolism, such as CYP2C8, CYP2C9, and CYP3A4.[249] Patients treated with these medications exhibit increased systemic clearance of epipodophyllotoxins,[250] vinca alkaloids,[251] taxanes,[252] and the camptothecins.[253–255] Administering standard doses of these chemotherapeutic agents together with enzyme-inducing antiseizure drugs (EIASDs) results in lower plasma concentrations of the anticancer drug and reduced systemic toxicity. Considering the potential for these pharmacokinetic interactions, EIASDs are usually avoided in neuro-oncologic patients and substituted with non–enzyme-inducing antiepileptics such as levetiracetam or lacosamide. Table 6.1 lists approved anticancer drugs and their interactions with EIASD, based on clinical studies in brain cancer patients.

In addition to EIASDs, corticosteroids are known to affect the CYP450 system. Dexamethasone, the most commonly used corticosteroid in brain tumor patients, induces CYP3A4 by a pretranslational mechanism involving a glucocorticoid-responsive sequence in the promoter of the gene encoding the enzyme.[256] In addition, dexamethasone is a potent inducer of CYP2C8 and CYP2C9. Preclinical studies have shown that the pharmacokinetic behavior of cyclophosphamide and ifosfamide is markedly affected by pretreatment with corticosteroids.[257–259] Docetaxel metabolism is also induced by dexamethasone in vitro, and decreased plasma concentrations

have been demonstrated in a rodent model.[260,261] Corticosteroids appear to have little or no effect on the pharmacokinetics of the chloroethylnitrosourea alkylating agents.[262] In addition to interactions related to induction of drug-metabolizing enzymes, there is also a risk of diminished elimination of an anticancer agent due to competitive inhibition of a major drug-metabolizing enzyme by a supporting medication.

Therapies That Modulate Drug Distribution to the Brain

Corticosteroids are well known to decrease the permeability of the BBB and BTB to a number of molecules. Preclinical studies have shown that dexamethasone significantly reduces the transport through the BBB of water,[263] small organic molecules with molecular weights in the 100 to 350 range,[264,265] and macromolecules such as horseradish peroxidase.[266] Treatment with corticosteroids diminishes the permeability of experimental brain tumors, brain tissue immediately adjacent to tumor, and normal brain tissue distant to tumor, but the effect is most pronounced within the tumor itself.[267] These findings have been corroborated in studies of brain tumor patients. A marked reduction in the permeability of tumor and normal brain tissue to [82]Rb, as measured by PET imaging, was evident within 6 hours after the administration of dexamethasone by bolus injection to patients, with the effect persisting for at least 24 hours.[268] The magnitude of the decreased uptake of [82]Rb ranged from 6% to 48%.[269] Similar results have been observed in other studies using CT[270] and MRI.[271,272] The effect of corticosteroids on the uptake of systemically administered chemotherapeutic agents has been evaluated in nude mice bearing intracranially implanted xenografts of human glioma. Steroid administration decreased the amount of carboplatin,[273] cisplatin,[274] and methotrexate[275] in the tumor and surrounding brain tissue by 20% to 40%. The extent to which the distribution of an anticancer agent to brain tumors is affected by corticosteroids in humans, however, remains to be determined.

Antiangiogenic agents can also modulate drug delivery and distribution (see section "Vascular Normalization"). While initial

TABLE

6.1   *Influence of enzyme-inducing antiseizure drugs (EIASDs) on the total body clearance of intravenously administered chemotherapeutic agents in cancer patients*

Anticancer Agent	Infusion Time (h)	Dose (mg/m²)		Total Body Clearance[a] (L/h/m²)		Difference (%)	Reference
		−EIASD	+EIASD	−EIASD	+EIASD		
Etoposide	6.0	320–500	320–500	0.80	1.42	76.9	[251]
Irinotecan	1.5	112–125	411	18.8	29.7	58.0	[255]
Paclitaxel	3.0	240	240	4.76	9.75	104.8	[253]
Teniposide	4.0	200	200	0.78	1.92	146.2	[250]
Topotecan	0.5	2.0	2.0	20.8	30.6	47.1	[254]
Vincristine[b]	0.25	2.0	2.0	34.1	55.5	62.6	[252]

[a]Mean or median values.
[b]Dose and clearance values are not normalized to body surface area.

phase II studies suggested that concurrent administration of an antiangiogenic agent and a cytotoxic chemotherapy, such as lomustine and irinotecan[8,9,276], may result in greater efficacy and improve clinical outcome, randomized phase III trials did not corroborate this.[10,11] An improved understanding of how to effectively use the vascular normalization window to enhance cytotoxic drug delivery could help in the design of appropriate clinical trials.

The effect of radiotherapy on the integrity of the BBB and consequent penetration of drug into brain tumors remains an open area of investigation. Preclinical studies indicate that the BBB in normal tissue becomes more permeable shortly after delivery of radiation.[277] Consistent with this, P-gp labeling has been shown to decrease by 60% in the rodent endothelial cells of brain vessels after irradiation.[278] Furthermore, the CSF-to-plasma ratio of trastuzumab in breast cancer patients was shown to be higher in those who had received prior radiation, suggesting that radiation-induced disruption of the BBB may have facilitated drug delivery into the CSF space.[279] In addition, hypoxic tumor cells or tumor volumes display a poorer response to radiation therapy compared to normoxic tumor tissue.[280–282] Eventually, however, slowly progressive changes in the microvasculature of the irradiated tissue result in decreased permeability.

The optimal schedule for delivering chemotherapy concurrently with radiotherapy to treat brain tumors has not been conclusively established. Methotrexate accumulation in a murine brain tumor model was impaired by delivering radiation either before or concurrently with the drug and resulted in shorter survival times, suggesting that chemotherapy should be given before radiation treatments.[283] In contrast, clinical observations indicating that a 30- to 40-Gy dose of radiation increased the permeability of the BBB within the irradiated tumor by 74%, but only by 24% in normal surrounding tissue, formed the basis for advocating for administration of anticancer drugs after radiotherapy.[284] Another study involving pediatric leukemia patients found no difference in the CSF-to-plasma concentration ratio of chemotherapeutic agents when given before, during, or after radiotherapy.[285] Finally, concurrent administration of TMZ and radiotherapy in patients with newly diagnosed glioblastoma extends progression-free survival and OS, implying that concurrent administration may have clinical benefit.[2]

Conclusion

An increasing number of novel investigational agents have entered clinical trials for malignant brain tumors over the past decade. While some success has been achieved in identifying new drugs for certain types of brain metastases (e.g., erlotinib for metastases from EGFR-mutant non–small cell lung cancer and immunotherapy for melanoma-associated metastases), little progress has been made for patients with malignant gliomas. While drug target identification and selection are critical, ensuring adequate delivery of the drug to its target is equally important. The past decade has seen a rise in the design of nanoparticles, which could substantially improve drug delivery and be combined with sophisticated noninvasive imaging-based tracking techniques. Further evaluation of these nanocarriers in humans will be critical to assess their clinical

efficacy. In addition, with the emergence of new targets and therapeutic agents, appropriate biomarkers of response assessment need to be identified. While conventional contrast-enhanced MRI forms the basis for response assessment,[286] it does not provide information on drug penetration and fails to fully capture areas of metabolically active tumor. In addition, the introduction of immunotherapy has been accompanied by challenges associated with the interpretation of imaging findings in response to treatment since treatment-induced inflammation can appear similar to tumor progression. Advanced MR imaging techniques, including diffusion- and perfusion-weighted imaging and 2-hydroxyglutarate MR spectroscopy (which detects the oncometabolite of the *IDH* mutation), as well as novel PET tracers may be more equipped to distinguish between true tumor progression and treatment-related changes. Finally, drug interactions have assumed great importance in brain tumor clinical trials with the recognition that many common supporting medications used in this patient population affect the metabolism of cytotoxic drugs through induction of the CYP450 enzyme family. The development of noninvasive methods to facilitate evaluation of drug distribution and accumulation in local tissue and tumor is a fundamental challenge for the future. The availability of such techniques will allow efficient assessment of promising agents for the treatment of malignant brain tumors.

References

1. Ostrom QT, Gittleman H, Liao P, et al. CBTRUS Statistical Report: primary brain and other central nervous system tumors diagnosed in the United States in 2010–2014. *Neuro Oncol.* 2017;19(suppl 5):v1-v88.
2. Stupp R, Mason WP, van den Bent MJ, et al. Radiotherapy plus concomitant and adjuvant temozolomide for glioblastoma. *N Engl J Med.* 2005;352(10):987-996.
3. Herrlinger U, Tzaridis T, Mack F, et al. Phase III trial of CCNU/temozolomide (TMZ) combination therapy vs. standard TMZ therapy for newly diagnosed MGMT-methylated glioblastoma patients: the CeTeg/NOA-09 trial. Paper presented at: Society for Neuro-Oncology Annual Meeting 2017; San Francisco.
4. Westphal M, Hilt DC, Bortey E, et al. A phase 3 trial of local chemotherapy with biodegradable carmustine (BCNU) wafers (Gliadel wafers) in patients with primary malignant glioma. *Neuro Oncol.* 2003;5(2):79-88.
5. Stupp R, Taillibert S, Kanner AA, et al. Maintenance therapy with tumor-treating fields plus temozolomide vs temozolomide alone for glioblastoma: a randomized clinical trial. *JAMA.* 2015;314(23):2535-2543.
6. Sampson JH. Alternating electric fields for the treatment of glioblastoma. *JAMA.* 2015;314(23):2511-2513.
7. Administration USFaD. Aminolevulinic acid hydrochloride, known as ALA HCl (Gleolan, NX Development Corp.) as an optical imaging agent indicated in patients with gliomas. 2017. Available at: https://www.fda.gov/Drugs/InformationOnDrugs/ApprovedDrugs/ucm562645.htm. Accessed November 25, 2017.
8. Friedman HS, Prados MD, Wen PY, et al. Bevacizumab alone and in combination with irinotecan in recurrent glioblastoma. *J Clin Oncol.* 2009;27(28):4733-4740.
9. Kreisl TN, Kim L, Moore K, et al. Phase II trial of single-agent bevacizumab followed by bevacizumab plus irinotecan at tumor progression in recurrent glioblastoma. *J Clin Oncol.* 2009;27(5):740-745.
10. Chinot OL, Wick W, Mason W, et al. Bevacizumab plus radiotherapy-temozolomide for newly diagnosed glioblastoma. *N Engl J Med.* 2014;370(8):709-722.
11. Gilbert MR, Dignam JJ, Armstrong TS, et al. A randomized trial of bevacizumab for newly diagnosed glioblastoma. *N Engl J Med.* 2014;370(8):699-708.

12. Luke JJ, Flaherty KT, Ribas A, Long GV. Targeted agents and immunotherapies: optimizing outcomes in melanoma. *Nat Rev Clin Oncol.* 2017;14(8):463-482.

13. Herzberg B, Campo MJ, Gainor JF. Immune checkpoint inhibitors in non-small cell lung cancer. *Oncologist.* 2017;22(1):81-88.

14. Maxwell R, Jackson CM, Lim M. Clinical trials investigating immune checkpoint blockade in glioblastoma. *Curr Treat Options Oncol.* 2017;18(8):51.

15. Tan AC, Heimberger AB, Menzies AM, Pavlakis N, Khasraw M. Immune checkpoint inhibitors for brain metastases. *Curr Oncol Rep.* 2017;19(6):38.

16. Parsons DW, Jones S, Zhang X, et al. An integrated genomic analysis of human glioblastoma multiforme. *Science.* 2008;321(5897):1807-1812.

17. Yan H, Parsons DW, Jin G, et al. IDH1 and IDH2 mutations in gliomas. *N Engl J Med.* 2009;360(8):765-773.

18. Hartmann C, Hentschel B, Wick W, et al. Patients with IDH1 wild type anaplastic astrocytomas exhibit worse prognosis than IDH1-mutated glioblastomas, and IDH1 mutation status accounts for the unfavorable prognostic effect of higher age: implications for classification of gliomas. *Acta Neuropathol.* 2010;120(6):707-718.

19. Dang L, Yen K, Attar EC. IDH mutations in cancer and progress toward development of targeted therapeutics. *Ann Oncol.* 2016;27(4):599-608.

20. Reardon DA, Desjardins A, Schuster J, et al. ReACT: Long-term survival from a randomized phase II study of rindopepimut (CDX-110) plus bevacizumab in relapsed glioblastoma. Paper presented at: Society for Neuro-Oncology Annual Meeting 2015; San Antonio, TX.

21. Weller M, Butowski N, Tran DD, et al. Rindopepimut with temozolomide for patients with newly diagnosed, EGFRvIII-expressing glioblastoma (ACT IV): a randomised, double-blind, international phase 3 trial. *Lancet Oncol.* 2017;18(10):1373-1385.

22. Reardon DA, Omuro A, Brandes AA, et al. Randomized Phase 3 study evaluating the efficacy and safety of nivolumab vs. bevacizumab in patients with recurrent glioblastoma: CheckMate 143. Paper presented at: 5th Quadrennial Meeting of the World Federation of Neuro-Oncology Societies (WFNOS) 2017; Zurich, Switzerland.

23. Phillips PC. Antineoplastic drug resistance in brain tumors. *Neurol Clin.* 1991;9(2):383-404.

24. Greig NH. Optimizing drug delivery to brain tumors. *Cancer Treat Rev.* 1987;14(1):1-28.

25. Sipos EP, Brem H. New delivery systems for brain tumor therapy. *Neurol Clin.* 1995;13(4):813-825.

26. Ehrlich P. *Das Sauerstoff-Beduerfnis des Organismus: eine farbenanalytische Studie.* Berlin, Germany: Hirschwand; 1885.

27. Zlokovic BV, Apuzzo ML. Strategies to circumvent vascular barriers of the central nervous system. *Neurosurgery.* 1998;43(4):877-878.

28. Crone C. The blood-brain barrier: a modified tight epithelium. In: Suckling AJ, Rumsby MG, Bradbury MWB, eds. *The Blood-brain Barrier in Health and Disease.* Chichester, UK: Ellis Horwood; 1986.

29. Muldoon LL, Pagel MA, Kroll RA, Roman-Goldstein S, Jones RS, Neuwelt EA. A physiological barrier distal to the anatomic blood-brain barrier in a model of transvascular delivery. *AJNR Am J Neuroradiol.* 1999;20(2):217-222.

30. Fishman R. *Cerebrospinal Fluid in Diseases of the Nervous System.* Vol 43. Philadelphia, PA: WB Saunders; 1992.

31. Greig NH, Momma S, Sweeney DJ, Smith QR, Rapoport SI. Facilitated transport of melphalan at the rat blood-brain barrier by the large neutral amino acid carrier system. *Cancer Res.* 1987;47(6):1571-1576.

32. Henson JW, Cordon-Cardo C, Posner JB. P-glycoprotein expression in brain tumors. *J Neurooncol.* 1992;14(1):37-43.

33. Uchida Y, Ohtsuki S, Katsukura Y, et al. Quantitative targeted absolute proteomics of human blood-brain barrier transporters and receptors. *J Neurochem.* 2011;117(2):333-345.

34. Munoz JL, Walker ND, Scotto KW, Rameshwar P. Temozolomide competes for P-glycoprotein and contributes to chemoresistance in glioblastoma cells. *Cancer Lett.* 2015;367(1):69-75.

35. Fenart L, Buee-Scherrer V, Descamps L, et al. Inhibition of P-glycoprotein: rapid assessment of its implication in blood-brain barrier integrity and drug transport to the brain by an in vitro model of the blood-brain barrier. *Pharm Res.* 1998;15(7):993-1000.

36. Tsuji A. P-glycoprotein-mediated efflux transport of anticancer drugs at the blood-brain barrier. *Ther Drug Monit.* 1998;20(5):588-590.

37. de Faria GP, de Oliveira JA, de Oliveira JG, Romano Sde O, Neto VM, Maia RC. Differences in the expression pattern of P-glycoprotein and MRP1 in low-grade and high-grade gliomas. *Cancer Invest.* 2008;26(9):883-889.

38. Coley HM. Overcoming multidrug resistance in cancer: clinical studies of P-gp inhibitors. *Multi-drug Resistance in Cancer.* 2009.

39. Kim DG, Bynoe MS. A2A adenosine receptor regulates the human blood-brain barrier permeability. *Mol Neurobiol.* 2015;52(1):664-678.

40. Kim DG, Bynoe MS. A2A adenosine receptor modulates drug efflux transporter P-glycoprotein at the blood-brain barrier. *J Clin Invest.* 2016;126(5):1717-1733.

41. Parrish KE, Sarkaria JN, Elmquist WF. Improving drug delivery to primary and metastatic brain tumors: strategies to overcome the blood-brain barrier. *Clin Pharmacol Ther.* 2015;97(4):336-346.

42. Chamberlain MC, Murovic JA, Levin VA. Absence of contrast enhancement on CT brain scans of patients with supratentorial malignant gliomas. *Neurology.* 1988;38(9):1371-1374.

43. Di Costanzo A, Scarabino T, Trojsi F, et al. Multiparametric 3T MR approach to the assessment of cerebral gliomas: tumor extent and malignancy. *Neuroradiology.* 2006;48(9):622-631.

44. Durst CR, Raghavan P, Shaffrey ME, et al. Multimodal MR imaging model to predict tumor infiltration in patients with gliomas. *Neuroradiology.* 2014;56(2):107-115.

45. Pafundi DH, Laack NN, Youland RS, et al. Biopsy validation of 18F-DOPA PET and biodistribution in gliomas for neurosurgical planning and radiotherapy target delineation: results of a prospective pilot study. *Neuro Oncol.* 2013;15(8):1058-1067.

46. Munck Af Rosenschold P, Costa J, Engelholm SA, et al. Impact of [18F]-fluoro-ethyl-tyrosine PET imaging on target definition for radiation therapy of high-grade glioma. *Neuro Oncol.* 2015;17(5):757-763.

47. Ott RJ, Brada M, Flower MA, Babich JW, Cherry SR, Deehan BJ. Measurements of blood-brain barrier permeability in patients undergoing radiotherapy and chemotherapy for primary cerebral lymphoma. *Eur J Cancer.* 1991;27(11):1356-1361.

48. Folkman J. Tumor angiogenesis: therapeutic implications. *N Engl J Med.* 1971;285(21):1182-1186.

49. Carmeliet P, Jain RK. Molecular mechanisms and clinical applications of angiogenesis. *Nature.* 2011;473(7347):298-307.

50. Jain RK, di Tomaso E, Duda DG, Loeffler JS, Sorensen AG, Batchelor TT. Angiogenesis in brain tumours. *Nat Rev Neurosci.* 2007;8(8):610-622.

51. Boucher Y, Salehi H, Witwer B, Harsh GR IV, Jain RK. Interstitial fluid pressure in intracranial tumours in patients and in rodents. *Br J Cancer.* 1997;75(6):829-836.

52. Heiss JD, Papavassiliou E, Merrill MJ, et al. Mechanism of dexamethasone suppression of brain tumor-associated vascular permeability in rats. Involvement of the glucocorticoid receptor and vascular permeability factor. *J Clin Invest.* 1996;98(6):1400-1408.

53. Gerstner ER, Emblem KE, Sorensen GA. Vascular magnetic resonance imaging in brain tumors during antiangiogenic therapy—are we there yet? *Cancer J.* 2015;21(4):337-342.

54. Tong RT, Boucher Y, Kozin SV, Winkler F, Hicklin DJ, Jain RK. Vascular normalization by vascular endothelial growth factor receptor 2 blockade induces a pressure gradient across the vasculature and improves drug penetration in tumors. *Cancer Res.* 2004;64(11):3731-3736.

55. Winkler F, Kozin SV, Tong RT, et al. Kinetics of vascular normalization by VEGFR2 blockade governs brain tumor response to radiation: role of oxygenation, angiopoietin-1, and matrix metalloproteinases. *Cancer Cell.* 2004;6(6):553-563.

56. Lee CG, Heijn M, di Tomaso E, et al. Anti-vascular endothelial growth factor treatment augments tumor radiation response under normoxic or hypoxic conditions. *Cancer Res.* 2000;60(19):5565-5570.

57. Keunen O, Johansson M, Oudin A, et al. Anti-VEGF treatment reduces blood supply and increases tumor cell invasion in glioblastoma. *Proc Natl Acad Sci U S A.* 2011;108(9):3749-3754.

58. Jain RK. Transport of molecules in the tumor interstitium: a review. *Cancer Res.* 1987;47(12):3039-3051.

59. Dunkel IJ, Gardner SL, Garvin JH Jr, Goldman S, Shi W, Finlay JL. High-dose carboplatin, thiotepa, and etoposide with autologous stem cell rescue for patients with previously irradiated recurrent medulloblastoma. *Neuro Oncol.* 2010;12(3):297–303.

60. Dunkel IJ, Boyett JM, Yates A, et al. High-dose carboplatin, thiotepa, and etoposide with autologous stem-cell rescue for patients with recurrent medulloblastoma. Children's Cancer Group. *J Clin Oncol.* 1998;16(1):222-228.

61. Sung KW, Yoo KH, Cho EJ, et al. High-dose chemotherapy and autologous stem cell rescue in children with newly diagnosed high-risk or relapsed medulloblastoma or supratentorial primitive neuroectodermal tumor. *Pediatr Blood Cancer.* 2007;48(4):408-415.

62. Gururangan S, Krauser J, Watral MA, et al. Efficacy of high-dose chemotherapy or standard salvage therapy in patients with recurrent medulloblastoma. *Neuro Oncol.* 2008;10(5):745-751.

63. Gill P, Litzow M, Buckner J, et al. High-dose chemotherapy with autologous stem cell transplantation in adults with recurrent embryonal tumors of the central nervous system. *Cancer.* 2008;112(8):1805-1811.

64. Abrey LE, Rosenblum MK, Papadopoulos E, Childs BH, Finlay JL. High dose chemotherapy with autologous stem cell rescue in adults with malignant primary brain tumors. *J Neurooncol.* 1999;44(2):147-153.

65. Abrey LE, Childs BH, Paleologos N, et al. High-dose chemotherapy with stem cell rescue as initial therapy for anaplastic oligodendroglioma: long-term follow-up. *Neuro Oncol.* 2006;8(2):183-188.

66. Thomas AA, Abrey LE, Terziev R, et al. Multicenter phase II study of temozolomide and myeloablative chemotherapy with autologous stem cell transplant for newly diagnosed anaplastic oligodendroglioma. *Neuro Oncol.* 2017;19(10):1380-1390.

67. Modak S, Gardner S, Dunkel IJ, et al. Thiotepa-based high-dose chemotherapy with autologous stem-cell rescue in patients with recurrent or progressive CNS germ cell tumors. *J Clin Oncol.* 2004;22(10):1934-1943.

68. Adair JE, Johnston SK, Mrugala MM, et al. Gene therapy enhances chemotherapy tolerance and efficacy in glioblastoma patients. *J Clin Invest.* 2014;124(9):4082-4092.

69. Colombat P, Lemevel A, Bertrand P, et al. High-dose chemotherapy with autologous stem cell transplantation as first-line therapy for primary CNS lymphoma in patients younger than 60 years: a multicenter phase II study of the GOELAMS group. *Bone Marrow Transplant.* 2006;38(6):417-420.

70. Soussain C, Hoang-Xuan K, Taillandier L, et al. Intensive chemotherapy followed by hematopoietic stem-cell rescue for refractory and recurrent primary CNS and intraocular lymphoma: Societe Francaise de Greffe de Moelle Osseuse-Therapie Cellulaire. *J Clin Oncol.* 2008;26(15):2512-2518.

71. Abrey LE, Moskowitz CH, Mason WP, et al. Intensive methotrexate and cytarabine followed by high-dose chemotherapy with autologous stem-cell rescue in patients with newly diagnosed primary CNS lymphoma: an intent-to-treat analysis. *J Clin Oncol.* 2003;21(22):4151-4156.

72. Soussain C, Suzan F, Hoang-Xuan K, et al. Results of intensive chemotherapy followed by hematopoietic stem-cell rescue in 22 patients with refractory or recurrent primary CNS lymphoma or intraocular lymphoma. *J Clin Oncol.* 2001;19(3):742-749.

73. Illerhaus G, Marks R, Ihorst G, et al. High-dose chemotherapy with autologous stem-cell transplantation and hyperfractionated radiotherapy as first-line treatment of primary CNS lymphoma. *J Clin Oncol.* 2006;24(24):3865-3870.

74. Illerhaus G, Kasenda B, Ihorst G, et al. High-dose chemotherapy with autologous haemopoietic stem cell transplantation for newly diagnosed primary CNS lymphoma: a prospective, single-arm, phase 2 trial. *Lancet Haematol.* 2016;3(8):e388-e397.

75. Omuro A, Chinot O, Taillandier L, et al. Methotrexate and temozolomide versus methotrexate, procarbazine, vincristine, and cytarabine for primary CNS lymphoma in an elderly population: an intergroup ANOCEF-GOELAMS randomised phase 2 trial. *Lancet Haematol.* 2015;2(6):e251-e259.

76. Ferreri AJM, Cwynarski K, Pulczynski E, et al. Whole-brain radiotherapy or autologous stem-cell transplantation as consolidation strategies after high-dose methotrexate-based chemoimmunotherapy in patients with primary CNS lymphoma: results of the second randomisation of the International Extranodal Lymphoma Study Group-32 phase 2 trial. *Lancet Haematol.* 2017;4(11):e510-e523.

77. Yamada K, Ushio Y, Hayakawa T, et al. Distribution of radiolabeled 1-(4-amino-2-methyl-5-pyrimidinyl)methyl-3-(2-chloroethyl)-3-nitrosourea hydrochloride in rat brain tumor: intraarterial versus intravenous administration. *Cancer Res.* 1987;47(8):2123-2128.

78. Bullard DE, Bigner SH, Bigner DD. Comparison of intravenous versus intracarotid therapy with 1,3-bis(2-chloroethyl)-1-nitrosourea in a rat brain tumor model. *Cancer Res.* 1985;45(11 Pt 1):5240-5245.

79. Fine HA, Dear KB, Loeffler JS, Black PM, Canellos GP. Meta-analysis of radiation therapy with and without adjuvant chemotherapy for malignant gliomas in adults. *Cancer.* 1993;71(8):2585-2597.

80. Larner JM, Phillips CD, Dion JE, Jensen ME, Newman SA, Jane JA. A phase 1-2 trial of superselective carboplatin, low-dose infusional 5-fluorouracil and concurrent radiation for high-grade gliomas. *Am J Clin Oncol.* 1995;18(1):1-7.

81. Shapiro WR, Green SB, Burger PC, et al. A randomized comparison of intra-arterial versus intravenous BCNU, with or without intravenous 5-fluorouracil, for newly diagnosed patients with malignant glioma. *J Neurosurg.* 1992;76(5):772-781.

82. Imbesi F, Marchioni E, Benericetti E, et al. A randomized phase III study: comparison between intravenous and intraarterial ACNU administration in newly diagnosed primary glioblastomas. *Anticancer Res.* 2006;26(1B):553-558.

83. Kochii M, Kitamura I, Goto T, et al. Randomized comparison of intra-arterial versus intravenous infusion of ACNU for newly diagnosed patients with glioblastoma. *J Neurooncol.* 2000;49(1):63-70.

84. Tamaki M, Ohno K, Niimi Y, et al. Parenchymal damage in the territory of the anterior choroidal artery following supraophthalmic intracarotid administration of CDDP for treatment of malignant gliomas. *J Neurooncol.* 1997;35(1):65-72.

85. Blacklock JB, Wright DC, Dedrick RL, et al. Drug streaming during intra-arterial chemotherapy. *J Neurosurg.* 1986;64(2):284-291.

86. Cloughesy TF, Gobin YP, Black KL, et al. Intra-arterial carboplatin chemotherapy for brain tumors: a dose escalation study based on cerebral blood flow. *J Neurooncol.* 1997;35(2):121-131.

87. Gobin YP, Cloughesy TF, Chow KL, et al. Intraarterial chemotherapy for brain tumors by using a spatial dose fractionation algorithm and pulsatile delivery. *Radiology.* 2001;218(3):724-732.

88. Saris SC, Blasberg RG, Carson RE, et al. Intravascular streaming during carotid artery infusions. Demonstration in humans and reduction using diastole-phased pulsatile administration. *J Neurosurg.* 1991;74(5):763-772.

89. Osztie E, Varallyay P, Doolittle ND, et al. Combined intraarterial carboplatin, intraarterial etoposide phosphate, and IV Cytoxan chemotherapy for progressive optic-hypothalamic gliomas in young children. *AJNR Am J Neuroradiol.* 2001;22(5):818-823.

90. Doolittle ND, Miner ME, Hall WA, et al. Safety and efficacy of a multicenter study using intraarterial chemotherapy in conjunction with osmotic opening of the blood-brain barrier for the treatment of patients with malignant brain tumors. *Cancer.* 2000;88(3):637-647.

91. Fortin D, Desjardins A, Benko A, Niyonsega T, Boudrias M. Enhanced chemotherapy delivery by intraarterial infusion and blood-brain barrier disruption in malignant brain tumors: the Sherbrooke experience. *Cancer.* 2005;103(12):2606-2615.

92. Guillaume DJ, Doolittle ND, Gahramanov S, Hedrick NA, Delashaw JB, Neuwelt EA. Intra-arterial chemotherapy with osmotic blood-brain barrier disruption for aggressive oligodendroglial tumors: results of a phase I study. *Neurosurgery.* 2010;66(1):48-58; discussion 58.

93. Fortin D, Gendron C, Boudrias M, Garant MP. Enhanced chemotherapy delivery by intraarterial infusion and blood-brain barrier disruption in the treatment of cerebral metastasis. *Cancer.* 2007;109(4):751-760.

94. Kroll RA, Neuwelt EA. Outwitting the blood-brain barrier for therapeutic purposes: osmotic opening and other means. *Neurosurgery.* 1998;42(5):1083-1099; discussion 1099-1100.

95. Neuwelt EA, Howieson J, Frenkel EP, et al. Therapeutic efficacy of multiagent chemotherapy with drug delivery enhancement by blood-brain barrier modification in glioblastoma. *Neurosurgery.* 1986;19(4):573-582.

96. Angelov L, Doolittle ND, Kraemer DF, et al. Blood-brain barrier disruption and intra-arterial methotrexate-based therapy for newly diagnosed primary CNS lymphoma: a multi-institutional experience. *J Clin Oncol.* 2009;27(21):3503-3509.

97. Chakraborty S, Filippi CG, Burkhardt JK, et al. Durability of single dose intra-arterial bevacizumab after blood/brain barrier disruption for recurrent glioblastoma. *J Exp Ther Oncol.* 2016;11(4):261-267.

98. Boockvar JA, Tsiouris AJ, Hofstetter CP, et al. Safety and maximum tolerated dose of superselective intraarterial cerebral infusion of bevacizumab after osmotic blood-brain barrier disruption for recurrent malignant glioma. Clinical article. *J Neurosurg.* 2011;114(3):624-632.

99. Shin BJ, Burkhardt JK, Riina HA, Boockvar JA. Superselective intra-arterial cerebral infusion of novel agents after blood-brain disruption for the treatment of recurrent glioblastoma multiforme: a technical case series. *Neurosurg Clin N Am.* 2012;23(2):323-329, ix-x.

100. Muldoon LL, Pagel MA, Netto JP, Neuwelt EA. Intra-arterial administration improves temozolomide delivery and efficacy in a model of intracerebral metastasis, but has unexpected brain toxicity. *J Neurooncol.* 2016;126(3):447-454.

101. Prados MD, Schold SJS, Fine HA, et al. A randomized, double-blind, placebo-controlled, phase 2 study of RMP-7 in combination with carboplatin administered intravenously for the treatment of recurrent malignant glioma. *Neuro Oncol.* 2003;5(2):96-103.

102. Kreuter J. Drug delivery to the central nervous system by polymeric nanoparticles: what do we know? *Adv Drug Deliv Rev.* 2014;71:2-14.

103. Anders CK, Adamo B, Karginova O, et al. Pharmacokinetics and efficacy of PEGylated liposomal doxorubicin in an intracranial model of breast cancer. *PLoS One.* 2013;8(5):e61359.

104. Gaillard PJ, Appeldoorn CC, Dorland R, et al. Pharmacokinetics, brain delivery, and efficacy in brain tumor-bearing mice of glutathione pegylated liposomal doxorubicin (2B3-101). *PLoS One.* 2014;9(1):e82331.

105. Hau P, Fabel K, Baumgart U, et al. Pegylated liposomal doxorubicin-efficacy in patients with recurrent high-grade glioma. *Cancer.* 2004;100(6):1199-1207.

106. Kerklaan BM. Phase 1/2a study of glutathione pegylated liposomal doxorubicin (2B3-101) in breast cancer patients with brain metastases (BCBM) or recurrent high-grade gliomas (HGG). Paper presented at: Society for Neuro-oncology Annual Meeting 2014; Miami.

107. Mack F, Baumert BG, Schafer N, et al. Therapy of leptomeningeal metastasis in solid tumors. *Cancer Treat Rev.* 2016;43:83-91.

108. Chamberlain MC, Kormanik PA, Barba D. Complications associated with intraventricular chemotherapy in patients with leptomeningeal metastases. *J Neurosurg.* 1997;87(5):694-699.

109. Shapiro WR, Young DF, Mehta BM. Methotrexate: distribution in cerebrospinal fluid after intravenous, ventricular and lumbar injections. *N Engl J Med.* 1975;293(4):161-166.

110. Glantz MJ, Van Horn A, Fisher R, Chamberlain MC. Route of intracerebrospinal fluid chemotherapy administration and efficacy of therapy in neoplastic meningitis. *Cancer.* 2010;116(8):1947-1952.

111. Glantz MJ, Jaeckle KA, Chamberlain MC, et al. A randomized controlled trial comparing intrathecal sustained-release cytarabine (DepoCyt) to intrathecal methotrexate in patients with neoplastic meningitis from solid tumors. *Clin Cancer Res.* 1999;5(11):3394-3402.

112. Grossman SA, Finkelstein DM, Ruckdeschel JC, Trump DL, Moynihan T, Ettinger DS. Randomized prospective comparison of intraventricular methotrexate and thiotepa in patients with previously untreated neoplastic meningitis. Eastern Cooperative Oncology Group. *J Clin Oncol.* 1993;11(3):561-569.

113. Comte A, Jdid W, Guilhaume MN, et al. Survival of breast cancer patients with meningeal carcinomatosis treated by intrathecal thiotepa. *J Neurooncol.* 2013;115(3):445-452.

114. Fisher PG, Kadan-Lottick NS, Korones DN. Intrathecal thiotepa: reappraisal of an established therapy. *J Pediatr Hematol Oncol.* 2002;24(4):274-278.

115. Groves MD, Glantz MJ, Chamberlain MC, et al. A multicenter phase II trial of intrathecal topotecan in patients with meningeal malignancies. *Neuro Oncol.* 2008;10(2):208-215.

116. Gammon DC, Bhatt MS, Tran L, Van Horn A, Benvenuti M, Glantz MJ. Intrathecal topotecan in adult patients with neoplastic meningitis. *Am J Health Syst Pharm.* 2006;63(21):2083-2086.

117. Chamberlain MC, Tsao-Wei DD, Groshen S. Phase II trial of intracerebrospinal fluid etoposide in the treatment of neoplastic meningitis. *Cancer.* 2006;106(9):2021-2027.

118. Stemmler HJ, Schmitt M, Harbeck N, et al. Application of intrathecal trastuzumab (Herceptintrade mark) for treatment of meningeal carcinomatosis in HER2-overexpressing metastatic breast cancer. *Oncol Rep.* 2006;15(5):1373-1377.

119. Stemmler HJ, Mengele K, Schmitt M, et al. Intrathecal trastuzumab (Herceptin) and methotrexate for meningeal carcinomatosis in HER2-overexpressing metastatic breast cancer: a case report. *Anticancer Drugs.* 2008;19(8):832-836.

120. Ferrario C, Davidson A, Bouganim N, Aloyz R, Panasci LC. Intrathecal trastuzumab and thiotepa for leptomeningeal spread of breast cancer. *Ann Oncol.* 2009;20(4):792-795.

121. Zagouri F, Sergentanis TN, Bartsch R, et al. Intrathecal administration of trastuzumab for the treatment of meningeal carcinomatosis in HER2-positive metastatic breast cancer: a systematic review and pooled analysis. *Breast Cancer Res Treat.* 2013;139(1):13-22.

122. Oliveira M, Braga S, Passos-Coelho JL, Fonseca R, Oliveira J. Complete response in HER2+ leptomeningeal carcinomatosis from breast cancer with intrathecal trastuzumab. *Breast Cancer Res Treat.* 2011;127(3):841-844.

123. Platini C, Long J, Walter S. Meningeal carcinomatosis from breast cancer treated with intrathecal trastuzumab. *Lancet Oncol.* 2006;7(9):778-780.

124. Rubenstein JL, Fridlyand J, Abrey L, et al. Phase I study of intraventricular administration of rituximab in patients with recurrent CNS and intraocular lymphoma. *J Clin Oncol.* 2007;25(11):1350-1356.

125. Antonini G, Cox MC, Montefusco E, et al. Intrathecal anti-CD20 antibody: an effective and safe treatment for leptomeningeal lymphoma. *J Neurooncol.* 2007;81(2):197-199.

126. Lu NT, Raizer J, Gabor EP, et al. Intrathecal trastuzumab: immunotherapy improves the prognosis of leptomeningeal metastases in HER-2+ breast cancer patient. *J Immunother Cancer.* 2015;3:41.

127. Kim S. Liposomes as carriers of cancer chemotherapy. Current status and future prospects. *Drugs.* 1993;46(4):618-638.

128. Administration USFaD. *Current and resolved drug shortages and discontinuation reported to FDA.* 2017. Available at: https://www.accessdata.fda.gov/scripts/drugshortages/dsp_ActiveIngredientDetails.cfm?AI=Cytarabine%20Liposome%20(DepoCyt)%20Injection&st=d. Accessed November 27, 2017.

129. Ettinger LJ, Chervinsky DS, Freeman AI, Creaven PJ. Pharmacokinetics of methotrexate following intravenous and intraventricular administration in acute lymphocytic leukemia and non-Hodgkin's lymphoma. *Cancer.* 1982;50(9):1676-1682.

130. Bleyer WA, Drake JC, Chabner BA. Neurotoxicity and elevated cerebrospinal-fluid methotrexate concentration in meningeal leukemia. *N Engl J Med.* 1973;289(15):770-773.

131. Bakhshi S, North RB. Implantable pumps for drug delivery to the brain. *J Neurooncol.* 1995;26(2):133-139.

132. Blasberg RG, Patlak C, Fenstermacher JD. Intrathecal chemotherapy: brain tissue profiles after ventriculocisternal perfusion. *J Pharmacol Exp Ther.* 1975;195(1):73-83.

133. Blasberg RG. Methotrexate, cytosine arabinoside, and BCNU concentration in brain after ventriculocisternal perfusion. *Cancer Treat Rep.* 1977;61(4):625-631.

134. Chamberlain MC. Leptomeningeal metastases: a review of evaluation and treatment. *J Neurooncol.* 1998;37(3):271-284.

135. Berg SL, Chamberlain MC. Systemic chemotherapy, intrathecal chemotherapy, and symptom management in the treatment of leptomeningeal metastasis. *Curr Oncol Rep.* 2003;5(1):29-40.

136. Mak M, Fung L, Strasser JF, Saltzman WM. Distribution of drugs following controlled delivery to the brain interstitium. *J Neurooncol.* 1995;26(2):91-102.

137. Walter KA, Tamargo RJ, Olivi A, Burger PC, Brem H. Intratumoral chemotherapy. *Neurosurgery.* 1995;37(6):1128-1145.

138. Foreman PM, Friedman GK, Cassady KA, Markert JM. Oncolytic Virotherapy for the Treatment of Malignant Glioma. *Neurotherapeutics.* 2017;14(2):333-344.

139. Aboody KS, Najbauer J, Metz MZ, et al. Neural stem cell-mediated enzyme/prodrug therapy for glioma: preclinical studies. *Sci Transl Med.* 2013;5(184):184ra159.

140. Portnow J, Synold TW, Badie B, et al. Neural stem cell-based anticancer gene therapy: a first-in-human study in recurrent high-grade glioma patients. *Clin Cancer Res.* 2017;23(12):2951-2960.

141. Wu MP, Tamada JA, Brem H, Langer R. In vivo versus in vitro degradation of controlled release polymers for intracranial surgical therapy. *J Biomed Mater Res.* 1994;28(3):387-395.

142. Leong KW, D'Amore PD, Marletta M, Langer R. Bioerodible polyanhydrides as drug-carrier matrices. II. Biocompatibility and chemical reactivity. *J Biomed Mater Res.* 1986;20(1):51-64.

143. Brem H, Mahaley MS Jr, Vick NA, et al. Interstitial chemotherapy with drug polymer implants for the treatment of recurrent gliomas. *J Neurosurg.* 1991;74(3):441-446.

144. Brem H, Piantadosi S, Burger PC, et al. Placebo-controlled trial of safety and efficacy of intraoperative controlled delivery by biodegradable polymers of chemotherapy for recurrent gliomas. The Polymer-brain Tumor Treatment Group. *Lancet.* 1995;345(8956):1008-1012.

145. Westphal M, Ram Z, Riddle V, Hilt D, Bortey E; Executive Committee of the Gliadel Study G. Gliadel wafer in initial surgery for malignant glioma: long-term follow-up of a multicenter controlled trial. *Acta Neurochir (Wien).* 2006;148(3):269-275; discussion 275.

146. Brem H, Ewend MG, Piantadosi S, Greenhoot J, Burger PC, Sisti M. The safety of interstitial chemotherapy with BCNU-loaded polymer followed by radiation therapy in the treatment of newly diagnosed malignant gliomas: phase I trial. *J Neurooncol.* 1995;26(2):111-123.

147. Valtonen S, Timonen U, Toivanen P, et al. Interstitial chemotherapy with carmustine-loaded polymers for high-grade gliomas: a randomized double-blind study. *Neurosurgery.* 1997;41(1):44-48; discussion 48-49.

148. Olivi A, Barker F, Tatter S. Toxicities and pharmacokinetics of interstitial BCNU administered via wafers: results of phase I study in patients with recurrent malignant glioma. Paper presented at: Proc Am Soc Clin Oncol 1999.

149. Wait SD, Prabhu RS, Burri SH, Atkins TG, Asher AL. Polymeric drug delivery for the treatment of glioblastoma. *Neuro Oncol.* 2015;17(suppl 2):ii9-ii23.

150. Walter KA, Cahan MA, Gur A, et al. Interstitial taxol delivered from a biodegradable polymer implant against experimental malignant glioma. *Cancer Res.* 1994;54(8):2207-2212.

151. Storm PB, Moriarity JL, Tyler B, Burger PC, Brem H, Weingart J. Polymer delivery of camptothecin against 9L gliosarcoma: release, distribution, and efficacy. *J Neurooncol.* 2002;56(3):209-217.

152. Judy KD, Olivi A, Buahin KG, et al. Effectiveness of controlled release of a cyclophosphamide derivative with polymers against rat gliomas. *J Neurosurg.* 1995;82(3):481-486.

153. Yuan X, Tabassi K, Williams JA. Implantable polymers for tirapazamine treatments of experimental intracranial malignant glioma. *Radiat Oncol Investig.* 1999;7(4):218-230.

154. Yuan X, Dillehay LE, Williams JR, Williams JA. Synthetic, implantable polymers for IUdR radiosensitization of experimental human malignant glioma. *Cancer Biother Radiopharm.* 1999;14(3):187-202.

155. Williams JA, Dillehay LE, Tabassi K, Sipos E, Fahlman C, Brem H. Implantable biodegradable polymers for IUdR radiosensitization of experimental human malignant glioma. *J Neurooncol.* 1997;32(3):181-192.

156. Brem S, Tyler B, Li K, et al. Local delivery of temozolomide by biodegradable polymers is superior to oral administration in a rodent glioma model. *Cancer Chemother Pharmacol.* 2007;60(5):643-650.

157. Menei P, Capelle L, Guyotat J, et al. Local and sustained delivery of 5-fluorouracil from biodegradable microspheres for the radiosensitization of malignant glioma: a randomized phase II trial. *Neurosurgery.* 2005;56(2):242-248; discussion 242-248.

158. Groothuis DR. The blood-brain and blood-tumor barriers: a review of strategies for increasing drug delivery. *Neuro Oncol.* 2000;2(1):45-59.

159. Lonser RR, Sarntinoranont M, Morrison PF, Oldfield EH. Convection-enhanced delivery to the central nervous system. *J Neurosurg.* 2015;122(3):697-706.

160. Sampson JH, Raghavan R, Provenzale JM, et al. Induction of hyperintense signal on T2-weighted MR images correlates with infusion distribution from intracerebral convection-enhanced delivery of a tumor-targeted cytotoxin. *AJR Am J Roentgenol.* 2007;188(3):703-709.

161. Sampson JH, Archer G, Pedain C, et al. Poor drug distribution as a possible explanation for the results of the PRECISE trial. *J Neurosurg.* 2010;113(2):301-309.

162. Sampson JH, Akabani G, Archer GE, et al. Intracerebral infusion of an EGFR-targeted toxin in recurrent malignant brain tumors. *Neuro Oncol.* 2008;10(3):320-329.

163. Vogelbaum MA, Sampson JH, Kunwar S, et al. Convection-enhanced delivery of cintredekin besudotox (interleukin-13-PE38QQR) followed by radiation therapy with and without temozolomide in newly diagnosed malignant gliomas: phase 1 study of final safety results. *Neurosurgery.* 2007;61(5):1031-1037; discussion 1037-1038.

164. Weaver M, Laske DW. Transferrin receptor ligand-targeted toxin conjugate (Tf-CRM107) for therapy of malignant gliomas. *J Neurooncol.* 2003;65(1):3-13.

165. Kunwar S, Chang S, Westphal M, et al. Phase III randomized trial of CED of IL13-PE38QQR vs Gliadel wafers for recurrent glioblastoma. *Neuro Oncol.* 2010;12(8):871-881.

166. Laske DW, Youle RJ, Oldfield EH. Tumor regression with regional distribution of the targeted toxin TF-CRM107 in patients with malignant brain tumors. *Nat Med.* 1997;3(12):1362-1368.

167. Weber F, Asher A, Bucholz R, et al. Safety, tolerability, and tumor response of IL4-Pseudomonas exotoxin (NBI-3001) in patients with recurrent malignant glioma. *J Neurooncol.* 2003;64(1-2):125-137.

168. Carpentier A, Laigle-Donadey F, Zohar S, et al. Phase 1 trial of a CpG oligodeoxynucleotide for patients with recurrent glioblastoma. *Neuro Oncol.* 2006;8(1):60-66.

169. Carpentier A, Metellus P, Ursu R, et al. Intracerebral administration of CpG oligonucleotide for patients with recurrent glioblastoma: a phase II study. *Neuro Oncol.* 2010;12(4):401-408.

170. Bigner DD. *Study of Immunotoxin, MR1-1 (MR1-1).* 2015. Available at: https://clinicaltrials.gov/ct2/show/record/NCT01009866. Accessed August 25, 2017.

171. Bigner DD. *D2C7 for Adult Patients With Recurrent Malignant Glioma.* 2017. Available at: https://clinicaltrials.gov/ct2/show/NCT02303678?term=NCT02303678&rank=1. Accessed August 25, 2017.

172. Desjardins A, Sampson JH, Peters KB, et al. Patient survival on the dose escalation phase of the Oncolytic Polio/Rhinovirus Recombinant (PVSRIPO) against WHO grade IV malignant glioma (MG) clinical trial compared to historical controls. Paper presented at: American Society for Clinical Oncology Meeting 2015; Chicago, IL.

173. Mitragotri S. Healing sound: the use of ultrasound in drug delivery and other therapeutic applications. *Nat Rev Drug Discov.* 2005;4(3):255-260.

174. Kobus T, Zervantonakis IK, Zhang Y, McDannold NJ. Growth inhibition in a brain metastasis model by antibody delivery using focused ultrasound-mediated blood-brain barrier disruption. *J Control Release.* 2016;238:281-288.

175. Aryal M, Vykhodtseva N, Zhang YZ, Park J, McDannold N. Multiple treatments with liposomal doxorubicin and ultrasound-induced disruption of blood-tumor and blood-brain barriers improve outcomes in a rat glioma model. *J Control Release.* 2013;169(1-2):103-111.

176. Aryal M, Vykhodtseva N, Zhang YZ, McDannold N. Multiple sessions of liposomal doxorubicin delivery via focused ultrasound mediated blood-brain barrier disruption: a safety study. *J Control Release.* 2015;204:60-69.

177. Timbie KF, Afzal U, Date A, et al. MR image-guided delivery of cisplatin-loaded brain-penetrating nanoparticles to invasive glioma with focused ultrasound. *J Control Release.* 2017;263:120-131.

178. Park J, Aryal M, Vykhodtseva N, Zhang YZ, McDannold N. Evaluation of permeability, doxorubicin delivery, and drug retention in a rat brain tumor model after ultrasound-induced blood-tumor barrier disruption. *J Control Release.* 2017;250:77-85.

179. Pitz MW, Desai A, Grossman SA, Blakeley JO. Tissue concentration of systemically administered antineoplastic agents in human brain tumors. *J Neurooncol.* 2011;104(3):629-638.

180. Liu X, Ide JL, Norton I, et al. Molecular imaging of drug transit through the blood-brain barrier with MALDI mass spectrometry imaging. *Sci Rep.* 2013;3:2859.

181. Sun Y, Alberta JA, Pilarz C, et al. A brain-penetrant RAF dimer antagonist for the noncanonical BRAF oncoprotein of pediatric low-grade astrocytomas. *Neuro Oncol.* 2017;19(6):774-785.

182. Cserr HF. Physiology of the choroid plexus. *Physiol Rev.* 1971;51(2):273-311.

183. Zamboni WC, Gajjar AJ, Mandrell TD, et al. A four-hour topotecan infusion achieves cytotoxic exposure throughout the neuraxis in the nonhuman primate model: implications for treatment of children with metastatic medulloblastoma. *Clin Cancer Res.* 1998;4(10):2537-2544.

184. Blaney SM, Poplack DG, Godwin K, McCully CL, Murphy R, Balis FM. Effect of body position on ventricular CSF methotrexate concentration following intralumbar administration. *J Clin Oncol.* 1995;13(1):177-179.

185. Donelli MG, Zucchetti M, D'Incalci M. Do anticancer agents reach the tumor target in the human brain? *Cancer Chemother Pharmacol.* 1992;30(4):251-260.

186. Stewart DJ. A critique of the role of the blood-brain barrier in the chemotherapy of human brain tumors. *J Neurooncol.* 1994;20(2):121-139.

187. de Lange EC, Danhof M, de Boer AG, Breimer DD. Methodological considerations of intracerebral microdialysis in pharmacokinetic studies on drug transport across the blood-brain barrier. *Brain Res Brain Res Rev.* 1997;25(1):27-49.

188. Johansen MJ, Newman RA, Madden T. The use of microdialysis in pharmacokinetics and pharmacodynamics. *Pharmacotherapy.* 1997;17(3):464-481.

189. Muller M, Mader RM, Steiner B, et al. 5-fluorouracil kinetics in the interstitial tumor space: clinical response in breast cancer patients. *Cancer Res.* 1997;57(13):2598-2601.

190. Groth L. Cutaneous microdialysis. Methodology and validation. *Acta Derm Venereol Suppl (Stockh).* 1996;197:1-61.

191. Mary S, Muret P, Makki S, Kantelip JP, Humbert P. [A new technique for study of cutaneous biology, microdialysis]. *Ann Dermatol Venereol.* 1999;126(1):66-70.

192. Hogan BL, Lunte SM, Stobaugh JF, Lunte CE. On-line coupling of in vivo microdialysis sampling with capillary electrophoresis. *Anal Chem.* 1994;66(5):596-602.

193. Chen A, Lunte CE. Microdialysis sampling coupled on-line to fast microbore liquid chromatography. *J Chromatogr A.* 1995;691(1-2):29-35.

194. Major O, Shdanova T, Duffek L, Nagy Z. Continuous monitoring of blood-brain barrier opening to Cr51-EDTA by microdialysis following probe injury. *Acta Neurochir Suppl (Wien).* 1990;51:46-48.

195. Westergren I, Nystrom B, Hamberger A, Johansson BB. Intracerebral dialysis and the blood-brain barrier. *J Neurochem.* 1995;64(1):229-234.

196. Ungerstedt U, Pycock C. Functional correlates of dopamine neurotransmission. *Bull Schweiz Akad MedWiss.* 1974;30(1-3):44-55.

197. Hamani C, Luer MS, Dujovny M. Microdialysis in the human brain: review of its applications. *Neurol Res.* 1997;19(3):281-288.

198. Landolt H, Langemann H. Cerebral microdialysis as a diagnostic tool in acute brain injury. *Eur J Anaesthesiol.* 1996;13(3):269-278.

199. Benveniste H, Hansen AJ, Ottosen NS. Determination of brain interstitial concentrations by microdialysis. *J Neurochem.* 1989;52(6):1741-1750.

200. de Lange EC, Bouw MR, Mandema JW, Danhof M, de Boer AG, Breimer DD. Application of intracerebral microdialysis to study regional distribution kinetics of drugs in rat brain. *Br J Pharmacol.* 1995;116(5):2538-2544.

201. Devineni D, Klein-Szanto A, Gallo JM. In vivo microdialysis to characterize drug transport in brain tumors: analysis of methotrexate uptake in rat glioma-2 (RG-2)-bearing rats. *Cancer Chemother Pharmacol.* 1996;38(6):499-507.

202. El-Gizawy SA, Hedaya MA. Comparative brain tissue distribution of camptothecin and topotecan in the rat. *Cancer Chemother Pharmacol.* 1999;43(5):364-370.

203. Zamboni WC, Houghton PJ, Hulstein JL, et al. Relationship between tumor extracellular fluid exposure to topotecan and tumor response in human neuroblastoma xenograft and cell lines. *Cancer Chemother Pharmacol.* 1999;43(4):269-276.

204. Ekstrom O, Andersen A, Warren DJ, Giercksky KE, Slordal L. Evaluation of methotrexate tissue exposure by in situ microdialysis in a rat model. *Cancer Chemother Pharmacol.* 1994;34(4):297-301.

205. Palsmeier RK, Lunte CE. Microdialysis sampling in tumor and muscle: study of the disposition of 3-amino-1,2,4-benzotriazine-1,4-di-N-oxide (SR 4233). *Life Sci.* 1994;55(10):815-825.

206. Grossman R, Rudek MA, Brastianos H, et al. The impact of bevacizumab on temozolomide concentrations in intracranial U87 gliomas. *Cancer Chemother Pharmacol.* 2012;70(1):129-139.

207. Grossman R, Tyler B, Rudek MA, et al. Microdialysis measurement of intratumoral temozolomide concentration after cediranib, a pan-VEGF receptor tyrosine kinase inhibitor, in a U87 glioma model. *Cancer Chemother Pharmacol.* 2013;72(1):93-100.

208. Tabatabaei P, Visse E, Bergstrom P, Brannstrom T, Siesjo P, Bergenheim AT. Radiotherapy induces an immediate inflammatory reaction in malignant glioma: a clinical microdialysis study. *J Neurooncol.* 2017;131(1):83-92.

209. Portnow J, Badie B, Liu X, et al. A pilot microdialysis study in brain tumor patients to assess changes in intracerebral cytokine levels after craniotomy and in response to treatment with a targeted anti-cancer agent. *J Neurooncol.* 2014;118(1):169-177.

210. Portnow J, Badie B, Chen M, Liu A, Blanchard S, Synold TW. The neuropharmacokinetics of temozolomide in patients with resectable brain tumors: potential implications for the current approach to chemoradiation. *Clin Cancer Res.* 2009;15(22):7092-7098.

211. Blakeley JO, Olson J, Grossman SA, et al. Effect of blood brain barrier permeability in recurrent high grade gliomas on the intratumoral pharmacokinetics of methotrexate: a microdialysis study. *J Neurooncol.* 2009;91(1):51-58.

212. Pope WB, Djoukhadar I, Jackson A. Neuroimaging. *Handb Clin Neurol.* 2016;134:27-50.

213. He Q, Bhujwalla ZM, Maxwell RJ, Griffiths JR, Glickson JD. Proton NMR observation of the antineoplastic agent Iproplatin in vivo by selective multiple quantum coherence transfer (Sel-MQC). *Magn Reson Med.* 1995;33(3):414-416.

214. Rodrigues LM, Maxwell RJ, McSheehy PM, et al. In vivo detection of ifosfamide by 31P-MRS in rat tumours: increased uptake and cytotoxicity induced by carbogen breathing in GH3 prolactinomas. *Br J Cancer.* 1997;75(1):62-68.

215. Wolf W, Waluch V, Presant CA. Non-invasive 19F-NMRS of 5-fluorouracil in pharmacokinetics and pharmacodynamic studies. *NMR Biomed.* 1998;11(7):380-387.

216. Findlay MP, Leach MO. In vivo monitoring of fluoropyrimidine metabolites: magnetic resonance spectroscopy in the evaluation of 5-fluorouracil. *Anticancer Drugs.* 1994;5(3):260-280.

217. Presant CA, Wolf W, Waluch V, et al. Association of intratumoral pharmacokinetics of fluorouracil with clinical response. *Lancet.* 1994;343(8907):1184-1187.

218. Maxwell RJ. New techniques in the pharmacokinetic analysis of cancer drugs. III. Nuclear magnetic resonance. *Cancer Surv.* 1993;17:415-423.

219. Fischman AJ, Alpert NM, Rubin RH. Pharmacokinetic imaging: a non-invasive method for determining drug distribution and action. *Clin Pharmacokinet.* 2002;41(8):581-602.

220. Presant CA, Wolf W, Albright MJ, et al. Human tumor fluorouracil trapping: clinical correlations of in vivo 19F nuclear magnetic resonance spectroscopy pharmacokinetics. *J Clin Oncol.* 1990;8(11):1868-1873.

221. Kristjansen PE, Quistorff B, Spang-Thomsen M, Hansen HH. Intratumoral pharmacokinetic analysis by 19F-magnetic resonance spectroscopy and cytostatic in vivo activity of gemcitabine (dFdC) in two small cell lung cancer xenografts. *Ann Oncol.* 1993;4(2):157-160.

222. Najac C, Ronen SM. MR molecular imaging of brain cancer metabolism using hyperpolarized 13C magnetic resonance spectroscopy. *Top Magn Reson Imaging.* 2016;25(5):187-196.

223. Ardenkjaer-Larsen JH, Fridlund B, Gram A, et al. Increase in signal-to-noise ratio of > 10,000 times in liquid-state NMR. *Proc Natl Acad Sci U S A.* 2003;100(18):10158-10163.

224. Goel S, England CG, Chen F, Cai W. Positron emission tomography and nanotechnology: a dynamic duo for cancer theranostics. *Adv Drug Deliv Rev.* 2017;113:157-176.

225. Chakravarty R, Hong H, Cai W. Positron emission tomography image-guided drug delivery: current status and future perspectives. *Mol Pharm.* 2014;11(11):3777-3797.

226. Ametamey SM, Honer M, Schubiger PA. Molecular imaging with PET. *Chem Rev.* 2008;108(5):1501-1516.

227. Kissel J, Brix G, Bellemann ME, et al. Pharmacokinetic analysis of 5-[18F] fluorouracil tissue concentrations measured with positron emission tomography in patients with liver metastases from colorectal adenocarcinoma. *Cancer Res.* 1997;57(16):3415-3423.

228. Tilsley DW, Harte RJ, Jones T, et al. New techniques in the pharmacokinetic analysis of cancer drugs. IV. Positron emission tomography. *Cancer Surv.* 1993;17:425-442.

229. Rubin RH, Fischman AJ. Positron emission tomography in drug development. *Q J Nucl Med.* 1997;41(2):171-175.

230. Meikle SR, Matthews JC, Brock CS, et al. Pharmacokinetic assessment of novel anti-cancer drugs using spectral analysis and positron emission tomography: a feasibility study. *Cancer Chemother Pharmacol.* 1998;42(3):183-193.

231. Tyler JL, Yamamoto YL, Diksic M, et al. Pharmacokinetics of superselective intra-arterial and intravenous [11C]BCNU evaluated by PET. *J Nucl Med.* 1986;27(6):775-780.

232. Diksic M, Sako K, Feindel W, et al. Pharmacokinetics of positron-labeled 1,3-bis(2-chloroethyl)nitrosourea in human brain tumors using positron emission tomography. *Cancer Res.* 1984;44(7):3120-3124.

233. Ginos JZ, Cooper AJ, Dhawan V, et al. [13N]cisplatin PET to assess pharmacokinetics of intra-arterial versus intravenous chemotherapy for malignant brain tumors. *J Nucl Med.* 1987;28(12):1844-1852.

234. Nasongkla N, Shuai X, Ai H, et al. cRGD-functionalized polymer micelles for targeted doxorubicin delivery. *Angew Chem Int Ed Engl.* 2004;43(46):6323-6327.

235. Ruoslahti E, Pierschbacher MD. New perspectives in cell adhesion: RGD and integrins. *Science.* 1987;238(4826):491-497.

236. Chen X. Integrin targeted imaging and therapy. *Theranostics.* 2011;2011(1):28-29.

237. Xiao Y, Hong H, Javadi A, et al. Multifunctional unimolecular micelles for cancer-targeted drug delivery and positron emission tomography imaging. *Biomaterials.* 2012;33(11):3071-3082.

238. Zhou J, Patel TR, Sirianni RW, et al. Highly penetrative, drug-loaded nanocarriers improve treatment of glioblastoma. *Proc Natl Acad Sci U S A.* 2013;110(29):11751-11756.

239. Lanza GM, Moonen C, Baker JR Jr, et al. Assessing the barriers to image-guided drug delivery. *Wiley Interdiscip Rev Nanomed Nanobiotechnol.* 2014;6(1):1-14.

240. Weissleder R, Schwaiger MC, Gambhir SS, Hricak H. Imaging approaches to optimize molecular therapies. *Sci Transl Med.* 2016;8(355):355ps316.

241. Rashidian M, Keliher EJ, Bilate AM, et al. Noninvasive imaging of immune responses. *Proc Natl Acad Sci U S A.* 2015;112(19):6146-6151.

242. Ehlerding EB, England CG, McNeel DG, Cai W. Molecular imaging of immunotherapy targets in cancer. *J Nucl Med.* 2016;57(10):1487-1492.

243. Kircher MF, Gambhir SS, Grimm J. Noninvasive cell-tracking methods. *Nat Rev Clin Oncol.* 2011;8(11):677-688.

244. Larimer BM, Wehrenberg-Klee E, Caraballo A, Mahmood U. Quantitative CD3 PET imaging predicts tumor growth response to anti-CTLA-4 therapy. *J Nucl Med.* 2016;57(10):1607-1611.

245. Tavare R, Escuin-Ordinas H, Mok S, et al. An effective immuno-PET imaging method to monitor CD8-dependent responses to immunotherapy. *Cancer Res.* 2016;76(1):73-82.

246. van Meerten E, Verweij J, Schellens JH. Antineoplastic agents. Drug interactions of clinical significance. *Drug Saf.* 1995;12(3):168-182.

247. McLeod HL. Clinically relevant drug-drug interactions in oncology. *Br J Clin Pharmacol.* 1998;45(6):539-544.

248. Kivisto KT, Kroemer HK, Eichelbaum M. The role of human cytochrome P450 enzymes in the metabolism of anticancer agents: implications for drug interactions. *Br J Clin Pharmacol.* 1995;40(6):523-530.

249. Tanaka E. Clinically significant pharmacokinetic drug interactions between antiepileptic drugs. *J Clin Pharm Ther.* 1999;24(2):87-92.

250. Baker DK, Relling MV, Pui CH, Christensen ML, Evans WE, Rodman JH. Increased teniposide clearance with concomitant anticonvulsant therapy. *J Clin Oncol.* 1992;10(2):311-315.

251. Rodman JH, Murry DJ, Madden T, Santana VM. Altered etoposide pharmacokinetics and time to engraftment in pediatric patients undergoing autologous bone marrow transplantation. *J Clin Oncol.* 1994;12(11):2390-2397.

252. Villikka K, Kivisto KT, Maenpaa H, Joensuu H, Neuvonen PJ. Cytochrome P450-inducing antiepileptics increase the clearance of vincristine in patients with brain tumors. *Clin Pharmacol Ther.* 1999;66(6):589-593.

253. Chang SM, Kuhn JG, Rizzo J, et al. Phase I study of paclitaxel in patients with recurrent malignant glioma: a North American Brain Tumor Consortium report. *J Clin Oncol.* 1998;16(6):2188-2194.

254. Zamboni WC, Gajjar AJ, Heideman RL, et al. Phenytoin alters the disposition of topotecan and N-desmethyl topotecan in a patient with medulloblastoma. *Clin Cancer Res.* 1998;4(3):783-789.

255. Gilbert MR, Supko JG, Batchelor T, et al. Phase I clinical and pharmacokinetic study of irinotecan in adults with recurrent malignant glioma. *Clin Cancer Res.* 2003;9(8):2940-2949.

256. Liddle C, Goodwin BJ, George J, Tapner M, Farrell GC. Separate and interactive regulation of cytochrome P450 3A4 by triiodothyronine, dexamethasone, and growth hormone in cultured hepatocytes. *J Clin Endocrinol Metab.* 1998;83(7):2411-2416.

257. Chang TK, Yu L, Maurel P, Waxman DJ. Enhanced cyclophosphamide and ifosfamide activation in primary human hepatocyte cultures: response to cytochrome P-450 inducers and autoinduction by oxazaphosphorines. *Cancer Res.* 1997;57(10):1946-1954.

258. Brain EG, Yu LJ, Gustafsson K, Drewes P, Waxman DJ. Modulation of P450-dependent ifosfamide pharmacokinetics: a better understanding of drug activation in vivo. *Br J Cancer.* 1998;77(11):1768-1776.

259. Yu LJ, Drewes P, Gustafsson K, Brain EG, Hecht JE, Waxman DJ. In vivo modulation of alternative pathways of P-450-catalyzed cyclophosphamide metabolism: impact on pharmacokinetics and antitumor activity. *J Pharmacol Exp Ther.* 1999;288(3):928-937.

260. Marre F, Sanderink GJ, de Sousa G, Gaillard C, Martinet M, Rahmani R. Hepatic biotransformation of docetaxel (Taxotere) in vitro: involvement of the CYP3A subfamily in humans. *Cancer Res.* 1996;56(6):1296-1302.

261. Kamataki T, Yokoi T, Fujita K, Ando Y. Preclinical approach for identifying drug interactions. *Cancer Chemother Pharmacol.* 1998;42(suppl):S50-S53.

262. Levin VA, Stearns J, Byrd A, Finn A, Weinkam RJ. The effect of phenobarbital pretreatment on the antitumor activity of 1,3-bis(2-chloroethyl)-1-nitrosourea (BCNU), 1-(2-chloroethyl)-3-cyclohexyl-1-nitrosourea (CCNU) and 1-(2-chloroethyl)-3-(2,6-dioxo-3-piperidyl)-1-nitrosourea (PCNU), and on the plasma pharmacokinetics and biotransformation of BCNU. *J Pharmacol Exp Ther.* 1979;208(1):1-6.

263. Reid AC, Teasdale GM, McCulloch J. The effects of dexamethasone administration and withdrawal on water permeability across the blood-brain barrier. *Ann Neurol.* 1983;13(1):28-31.

264. Ziylan YZ, LeFauconnier JM, Bernard G, Bourre JM. Effect of dexamethasone on transport of alpha-aminoisobutyric acid and sucrose across the blood-brain barrier. *J Neurochem.* 1988;51(5):1338-1342.

265. Ziylan YZ, Lefauconnier JM, Bernard G, Bourre JM. Regional alterations in blood-to-brain transfer of alpha-aminoisobutyric acid and sucrose, after chronic administration and withdrawal of dexamethasone. *J Neurochem.* 1989;52(3):684-689.

266. Hedley-Whyte ET, Hsu DW. Effect of dexamethasone on blood-brain barrier in the normal mouse. *Ann Neurol.* 1986;19(4):373-377.

267. Shapiro WR, Hiesiger EM, Cooney GA, Basler GA, Lipschutz LE, Posner JB. Temporal effects of dexamethasone on blood-to-brain and blood-to-tumor transport of 14C-alpha-aminoisobutyric acid in rat C6 glioma. *J Neurooncol.* 1990;8(3):197-204.

268. Jarden JO, Dhawan V, Moeller JR, Strother SC, Rottenberg DA. The time course of steroid action on blood-to-brain and blood-to-tumor transport of 82Rb: a positron emission tomographic study. *Ann Neurol.* 1989;25(3):239-245.

269. Jarden JO, Dhawan V, Poltorak A, Posner JB, Rottenberg DA. Positron emission tomographic measurement of blood-to-brain and blood-to-tumor transport of 82Rb: the effect of dexamethasone and whole-brain radiation therapy. *Ann Neurol.* 1985;18(6):636-646.

270. Yeung WT, Lee TY, Del Maestro RF, Kozak R, Bennett J, Brown T. Effect of steroids on iopamidol blood-brain transfer constant and plasma volume in brain tumors measured with X-ray computed tomography. *J Neurooncol.* 1994;18(1):53-60.

271. Andersen C, Astrup J, Gyldensted C. Quantitation of peritumoural oedema and the effect of steroids using NMR-relaxation time imaging and blood-brain barrier analysis. *Acta Neurochir Suppl (Wien).* 1994;60:413-415.

272. Ostergaard L, Hochberg FH, Rabinov JD, et al. Early changes measured by magnetic resonance imaging in cerebral blood flow, blood volume, and blood-brain barrier permeability following dexamethasone treatment in patients with brain tumors. *J Neurosurg.* 1999;90(2):300-305.

273. Matsukado K, Nakano S, Bartus RT, Black KL. Steroids decrease uptake of carboplatin in rat gliomas—uptake improved by intracarotid infusion of bradykinin analog, RMP-7. *J Neurooncol.* 1997;34(2):131-138.

274. Straathof CS, van den Bent MJ, Ma J, et al. The effect of dexamethasone on the uptake of cisplatin in 9L glioma and the area of brain around tumor. *J Neurooncol.* 1998;37(1):1-8.

275. Neuwelt EA, Barnett PA, Bigner DD, Frenkel EP. Effects of adrenal cortical steroids and osmotic blood-brain barrier opening on methotrexate delivery to gliomas in the rodent: the factor of the blood-brain barrier. *Proc Natl Acad Sci U S A.* 1982;79(14):4420-4423.

276. Taal W, Oosterkamp HM, Walenkamp AM, et al. Single-agent bevacizumab or lomustine versus a combination of bevacizumab plus lomustine in patients with recurrent glioblastoma (BELOB trial): a randomised controlled phase 2 trial. *Lancet Oncol.* 2014;15(9):943-953.

277. d'Avella D, Cicciarello R, Angileri FF, Lucerna S, La Torre D, Tomasello F. Radiation-induced blood-brain barrier changes: pathophysiological mechanisms and clinical implications. *Acta Neurochir Suppl.* 1998;71:282-284.

278. Mima T, Toyonaga S, Mori K, Taniguchi T, Ogawa Y. Early decrease of P-glycoprotein in the endothelium of the rat brain capillaries after moderate dose of irradiation. *Neurol Res.* 1999;21(2):209-215.

279. Stemmler HJ, Schmitt M, Willems A, Bernhard H, Harbeck N, Heinemann V. Ratio of trastuzumab levels in serum and cerebrospinal fluid is altered in HER2-positive breast cancer patients with brain metastases and impairment of blood-brain barrier. *Anticancer Drugs.* 2007;18(1):23-28.

280. Brizel DM, Light K, Zhou SM, Marks LB. Conformal radiation therapy treatment planning reduces the dose to the optic structures for patients with tumors of the paranasal sinuses. *Radiother Oncol.* 1999;51(3):215-218.

281. Stadler P, Becker A, Feldmann HJ, et al. Influence of the hypoxic subvolume on the survival of patients with head and neck cancer. *Int J Radiat Oncol Biol Phys.* 1999;44(4):749-754.

282. Nordsmark M, Overgaard M, Overgaard J. Pretreatment oxygenation predicts radiation response in advanced squamous cell carcinoma of the head and neck. *Radiother Oncol.* 1996;41(1):31-39.

283. Remsen LG, McCormick CI, Sexton G, Pearse HD, Garcia R, Neuwelt EA. Decreased delivery and acute toxicity of cranial irradiation and chemotherapy given with osmotic blood-brain barrier disruption in a rodent model: the issue of sequence. *Clin Cancer Res.* 1995;1(7):731-739.

284. Qin DX, Zheng R, Tang J, Li JX, Hu YH. Influence of radiation on the blood-brain barrier and optimum time of chemotherapy. *Int J Radiat Oncol Biol Phys.* 1990;19(6):1507-1510.

285. Riccardi R, Riccardi A, Lasorella A, Servidei T, Mastrangelo S. Cranial irradiation and permeability of blood-brain barrier to cytosine arabinoside in children with acute leukemia. *Clin Cancer Res.* 1998;4(1):69-73.

286. Wen PY, Chang SM, Van den Bent MJ, Vogelbaum MA, Macdonald DR, Lee EQ. Response assessment in neuro-oncology clinical trials. *J Clin Oncol.* 2017;35(21):2439-2449.

Antifolates

Bruce A. Chabner and Carmen J. Allegra

The folate-dependent enzymes represent attractive targets for antitumor chemotherapy because of their critical role in the synthesis of the nucleotide precursors of DNA. In 1948, Farber et al.[1] reported that aminopterin, a 4-amino analogue of folic acid, could inhibit the proliferation of leukemic cells and produce remissions in acute leukemia cases. Their findings ushered in the era of antimetabolite chemotherapy and generated great interest in the antifolate class. Huennekens identified dihydrofolate reductase (DHFR) as the primary site of inhibition by methotrexate (MTX), a well-tolerated successor molecule. Since then, multiple new antifolate compounds have become valuable in the treatment of malignancies as well as and infectious diseases.[2] High-dose regimens have further expanded the role of MTX in treating acute lymphocytic leukemia (ALL), primary central nervous system (CNS) lymphomas, osteogenic sarcomas, and for prevention of meningeal leukemia,[3] where it has replaced cranial irradiation in children with low-risk ALL. A newer antifolate, pemetrexed, which potently inhibits thymidylate synthase (TS), was introduced in 2004 for treating mesothelioma and subsequently lung adenocarcinoma.[4] At this time, the antifolates are one of the best understood and most versatile of all the chemotherapeutic drug classes. The key features of MTX, pemetrexed, and the newest antifolate, pralatrexate, are presented in Figure 7.1.

Mechanism of Action

Substitution of an amino group for the hydroxyl at the 4-N position of the pteridine ring of folic acid critically changes the structure of folate compounds, leading to their enzyme inhibitory and antitumor activities (Fig. 7.1). For MTX, this change transforms the molecule from a substrate to a tight-binding inhibitor of DHFR, a key enzyme in intracellular folate homeostasis. The critical importance of DHFR stems from the fact that folic acid compounds are active as coenzymes only in their fully reduced, tetrahydrofolate, form. Two specific tetrahydrofolates play essential roles as one-carbon carriers in the synthesis of DNA precursors. The cofactor 10-formyltetrahydrofolate provides its one-carbon group for the de novo synthesis of purines in reactions mediated by glycinamide ribonucleotide transformylase (GART) and aminoimidazole carboxamide ribonucleotide transformylase (AICART). A second cofactor, 5,10-methylenetetrahydrofolate (CH_2-FH_4), donates its one-carbon group to the reductive methylation reaction that converts deoxyuridylate (dUMP) to thymidylate (TMP) (Fig. 7.2). In this reaction, CH_2FH_4 is oxidized to dihydrofolate (FH_2), which must then be reduced to tetrahydrofolate by the enzyme DHFR to enable it to rejoin the pool of active reduced folate cofactors. In actively proliferating

tumor cells, inhibition of DHFR by MTX or other 2,4-diamino antifolates leads to an accumulation of folates in the inactive FH_2 form, with depletion of the pool of reduced folates.[2,5] Folate depletion, however, does not fully account for the metabolic inhibition associated with MTX. MTX and other antifolates (pemetrexed and pralatrexate) are converted to polyglutamated derivatives which potently inhibit TS[6] and the purine synthetic pathway[7] (see Table 7.1). Dihydrofolate polyglutamates (PGs) accumulate as a consequence of DHFR inhibition and may add to the action of direct inhibitors of TS and purine biosynthesis.[8] Thus, inhibition of DNA biosynthesis by 2,4-diamino folates is a multifactorial process consisting of both depletion of reduced folate substrates and direct inhibition of folate-dependent enzymes. The relative roles of each of these mechanisms in determining antifolate-associated metabolic inhibition may depend on factors specific to various cancer cell lines and tumors.

The anti-inflammatory and immunosuppressive properties of MTX may result from alternative sites of action, such as inhibition of the JAK-STAT pathway,[9] an effect not counteracted by folic acid, or by inhibition of methionine biosynthesis.[10]

Chemical Structure

The physiological folate structure, as shown in Figure 7.1, consists of a pteridine ring, which connects via a para-amino N-10 bridge to benzoic acid and thence to a terminal glutamic acid. Various heterocyclic compounds with the 2,4-diamino configuration may bind to DHFR and have antifolate activity. Anti-infective 2,4-diaminopyrimidine analogues such as pyrimethamine and trimethoprim are in general weak inhibitors of the mammalian DHFR and have modest marrow suppressive effect. Antifolates with near stoichiometric DHFR inhibitory activity conserve the 2,4-diamino configuration but have structural features of folates; these compounds include classical pteroyl glutamates such as aminopterin and MTX; compounds with an altered pteridine ring, such as those with replacement of the 5- or 8-N position, or both nitrogens, with a carbon atom (the pyrrolopyrimidines and quinazolines); lipid-soluble derivatives lacking a terminal glutamate (trimetrexate); or folate-like compounds with a substitution linked to the N-10 bridge, such as pralatrexate.[4,10] Each of these changes alters the pharmacological properties (transport, enzyme binding, and polyglutamation) of the folate inhibitory molecule, as described below. Other antifolates have specificity for enzymes other than DHFR, such as those folate-dependent enzymes required for the de novo synthesis of purines (lometrexol) and TS (raltitrexed), but failed in clinical trials. Potent

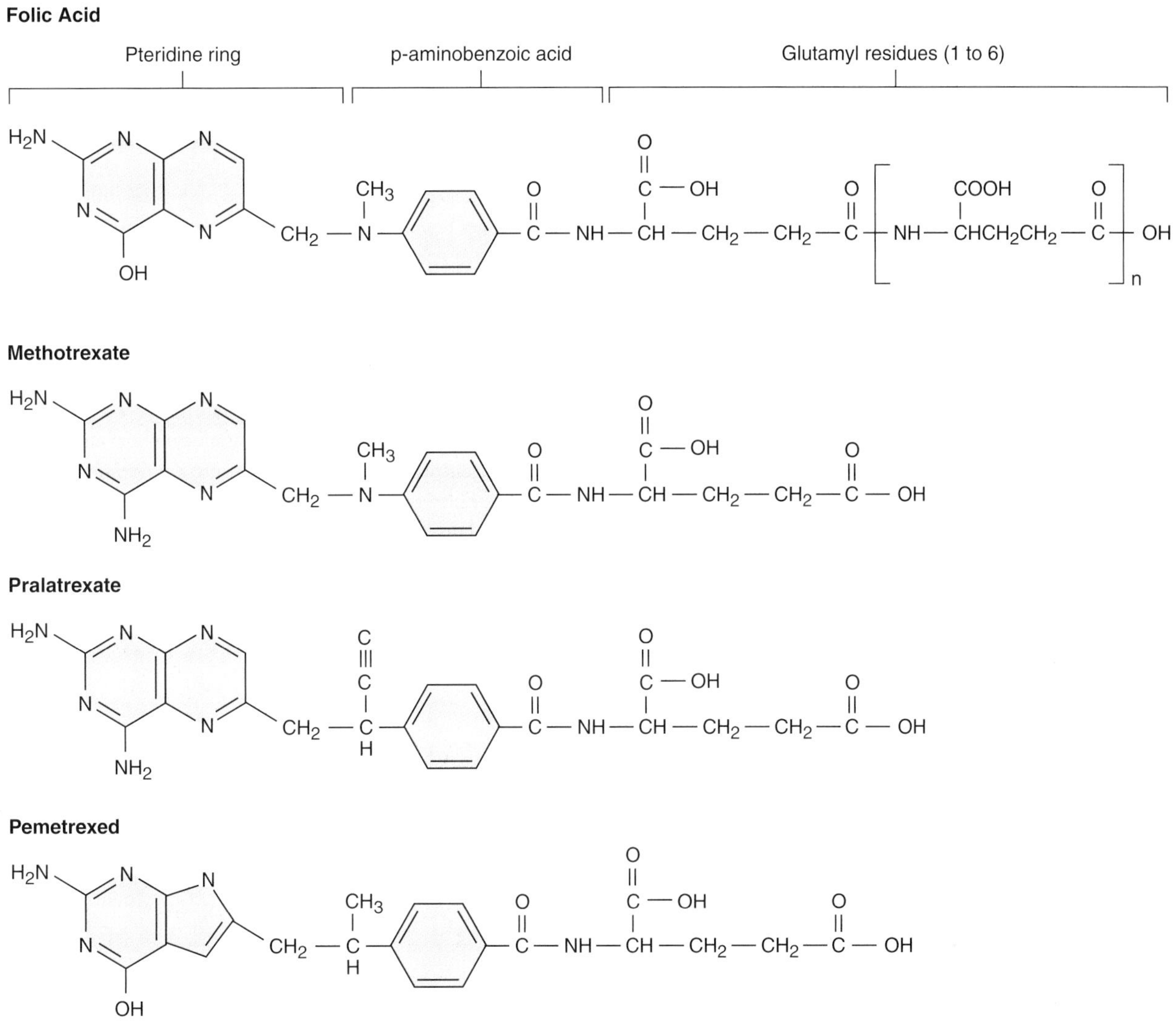

Folic Acid

Methotrexate

Pralatrexate

Pemetrexed

FIGURE **7.1** Structure of folic acid PG, showing its component subgroups (pteroic acid, para-amino benzoic acid, glutamate). Also shown are the analogues methotrexate, pralatrexate, and pemetrexed, which preserve many of the essential features of folates and are readily converted to polyglutamates (PGs) within cells. MTX and pralatrexate contain the critical 2,4-diamino configuration that inhibits DHFR. Pemetrexed inhibits TS and GARTF (see text).

TS inhibitors, which utilize physiological folate pathways for transport and polyglutamation, such as Tomudex and pemetrexed (LY231514, Alimta) conserve the 2-amino, 4-hydroxy configuration of physiological folates, and weakly inhibit DHFR.[4]

Cellular Pharmacology and Mechanisms of Resistance

In this section, the sequence of events that leads to the cytotoxic action of MTX is considered, beginning with drug movement across the cell membrane, followed by its intracellular metabolism to the PG derivatives, binding to DHFR and other folate-dependent enzymes, effects on intracellular folates, and, finally, inhibition of DNA synthesis.

Transmembrane Transport

Folate influx into mammalian cells proceeds via three distinct transport systems: (a) the reduced folate carrier (RFC) system, (b) the folate-receptor (FR) system (Table 7.2),[11,12] and (c) a low–pH-sensitive transporter first identified in the intestinal epithelium and found in most tissues and in selected tumor cells[13] (see Table 7.2). The proliferative or kinetic state of tumor cells, as well as the temperature and pH of the extracellular environment, influences the rate of folate and antifolate transport. In general, rapidly dividing cells have a greater rate of folate and antifolate uptake and a lower rate of drug efflux than cells that are either in the stationary phase or that are slowly growing. The RFC system, with its large transport capacity, imports folic acid inefficiently (K_t [transport coefficient] = 200 μmol/L) and is a primary transport mechanism of the reduced folates, including the rescue agent 5-formyltetrahydrofolate (leucovorin); it is the predominant inward carrier with greater affinity for pemetrexed and pralatrexate, as compared to transport of the affinity for MTX (K_t = 0.7 to 6.0 μmol/L)[14] Mutations in the RFC, affecting glutamic acid residue 45 and other sites, have been associated with MTX resistance.[15,16]

A second folate transport system is mediated by the FR, which internalizes folates and analogues via a high-affinity membrane-bound 38 to 45-kD glycoprotein.[17] The FR gene family encodes

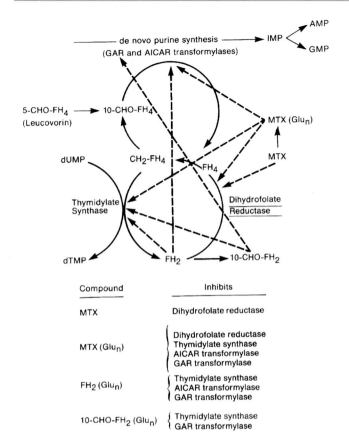

FIGURE 7.2 Sites of action of methotrexate (MTX), its polyglutamated metabolites (MTX[Glu$_n$]), and folate byproducts of the inhibition of DHFR, including dihydrofolate (FH$_2$) and 10-formyldihydrofolate (10-CHO-FH$_2$). Also shown are 5,10-methylenetetrahydrofolate (CH$_2$-FH$_4$), the folate cofactor required for thymidylate synthesis and 10-formyltetrahydrofolate (10-CHO-FH$_4$), the required intermediate in the synthesis of purine precursors. AICAR; aminoimidazole carboxamide ribonucleotide; AMP, adenosine monophosphate; dUMP, deoxyuridylate; dTMP, thymidylate; GAR; glycinamide ribonucleotide; GMP, guanosine monophosphate. (Adapted from DeVita VT, Hellman S, Rosenberg SA, eds. *Cancer: Principles and Practice of Oncology.* Philadelphia, PA: JB Lippincott, 1989:349-397.)

homologous glycoproteins that share a similar folate-binding site. The α and β FRs are anchored to the plasma membrane by a carboxyl-terminal glycosylphosphatidylinositol tail and transport the reduced folates and MTX at a lower capacity than the RFC system. The functions of the FR-γ and FR-γ are unknown. The FR of major current interest is the alpha isoform, which is expressed at high levels in embryonic tissues and on the apical surface of kidney tubules, intestine, and the choroid plexus. It is found in higher levels in epithelial tumors such as lung and ovarian adenocarcinomas, where it may have signaling and transcriptional activity in addition to its transport function. It has become the target for experimental anticancer antibodies and toxin loaded folate analogues (Fig. 7.3).[17,18]

The FR system has a higher affinity for folic acid and the reduced folates (1 nM) and for pemetrexed than for MTX (5 to 10 nM). Variation in exogenous folate concentrations and normal physiologic conditions, such as pregnancy, can alter the tissue expression of FR. Intracellular levels of homocysteine, which increase under folate-deficient conditions, are a critical modulator of the translational up-regulation of FRs.[19] Under conditions of relative folate deficiency, elevated levels of homocysteine stimulate the

interaction between heterogeneous nuclear ribonucleoprotein E1 and an 18–base-pair region in the 5′-untranslated region of the FR mRNA resulting in increased translational efficiency and therefore elevated cellular levels of FR protein. This mechanism of transcriptional regulation through protein binding to its message is operative in DHFR and TS protein synthesis as well.

The FR isoforms (α, β, γ) are independently expressed in mammalian cells and normal human tissues. FR-α is expressed on the apical and luminal surfaces of placenta, choroid plexus, renal tubules, and alveolar cells and in human epithelial neoplasms (ovarian cancer, papillary serous endometrial cancer, renal cell cancers, and non–small cell lung cancers).[20] FR-α is up-regulated by folate depletion and down-regulated in folate-replete medium. FR-γ, found in hematopoietic and lymphatic cells and tissues, lacks a glycosylphosphatidylinositol membrane anchor and is secreted. Although human FR-α, FR-β, and FR-γ share 70% amino acid sequence homology, they differ in binding affinities for stereoisomers of folates.[21]

The precise mechanism of FR-mediated folate uptake remains controversial: two separate pathways for FR-mediated folate uptake have been reported: (a) the classic receptor-mediated internalization of the ligand-receptor complex through clathrin-coated pits with subsequent formation of secondary lysosomes, and (b) a mechanism of small molecule uptake, termed potocytosis,[22] in which receptor complexes accumulate within distinct subdomains of the plasma membrane known as caveolae that internalize to form intracellular vesicles. Once internalization has occurred, acidification within the vesicle causes the FR complex to dissociate and translocate across the cell membrane.

The third transporter for folates and analogues, the low-pH, proton-coupled transporter, was first identified in intestinal cells, but is found in many normal tissues as well as tumors, and mediates folate transport into the CNS.[13] It utilizes an inwardly directed H$^+$ gradient to move folates and analogues into cells and its absence leads to an inherited folate malabsorption disorder. It efficiently transports pemetrexed ($K_m = 0.2$ to 0.8 mM) but has a lower affinity for MTX, pralatrexate, and reduced folates. At this writing, the RFC system appears to be the more relevant transporter of MTX in most mammalian cells and tumors.

Role of Transporters in Resistance to MTX

Both in vitro and in vivo experimental systems and limited clinical studies have identified decreased transport as a common mechanism of intrinsic or acquired resistance to MTX.[23,24] An MTX-resistant human lymphoblastic CCRF-CEM/MTX cell line maintained in physiologic (micromolar) concentrations of folate (2 nmol/L) lacked the RFC protein but retained the FR, however, and maintained growth even in nanomolar concentrations of folic acid, but was resistant to MTX.[23]

A mutated murine RFC (RFC1) with increased affinity for folic acid and decreased affinity for MTX contained an amino acid substitution at glutamic acid residue 45. This region of the RFC is also a cluster site for mutations that occur when cells are placed under selective pressure with antifolates that use RFC1 as the major route of entry into mammalian cells.[25] However, none of 121 samples of ALL cells from drug-resistant patients contained a mutation of glutamic acid residue 45.[26]

TABLE

7.1   Key features of methotrexate, pemetrexed, and pralatrexate

	Methotrexate	Pemetrexed	Pralatrexate
Mechanism of action	Inhibition of DHFR leads to depletion of reduced folates. PGs of MTX and dihydrofolate inhibit purine and thymidylate biosynthesis	Inhibition of TS > GAR.	Inhibition of DHFR
Metabolism	Converted to PGs in normal and malignant tissues. 7-Hydroxylation in liver	Converted to PGs	Converted to PGs
Pharmacokinetics	$t_{1/2} \alpha$ = 2 to 3 h; $t_{1/2} \beta$ = 8 to 10 h	$t_{1/2}$ = 4 h	$t_{1/2}$ = 4 to 6 h
Elimination	Primarily as intact drug through renal secretion and excretion	Same	Same
Drug interactions	Toxicity to normal tissues rescued by leucovorin calcium	Pretreatment with folic acid and B12 prevents myelosuppression	Pretreatment with folic acid and B12 Prevents myelosuppression
	L-Asparaginase blocks toxicity and antitumor activity	—	—
	Pretreatment with MTX increases 5-fluorouracil and cytosine arabinoside nucleotide formation	—	—
	Nonsteroidal anti-inflammatory agents decrease renal clearance and increase toxicity	—	—
Toxicity	Myelosuppression	Same	Same
	Mucositis, gastrointestinal epithelial denudation	Same	Same
	Renal tubular obstruction and injury	With doses of 600 mg/m^2, may cause serum creatinine increase	Not observed
	Hepatotoxicity (enzyme elevations). Chronic dosing in nononcologic settings may lead to fibrosis.	Same enzyme elevations	Same enzyme elevations
	Pneumonitis	Same	—
	Hypersensitivity reactions	Rash	—
	Neurotoxicity (seizures, altered mental status) with high dose or intrathecal regimens	—	—
Precaution	Reduce dose in proportion to creatinine clearance	Creatine clearance >40 mL/min required	Dose adjustment not defined, but likely should be reduced in proportion to decreased creatinine clearance
	Do not administer high-dose MTX to patients with abnormal renal function	—	—
	Monitor plasma concentrations of drug, hydrate patients during high-dose therapy (see Tables 7.3 and 7.4)	—	—

$t_{1/2}$, half-life in plasma.

Other studies provide suggestive evidence for a role of transport deficiency in MTX resistance in both ALL and in osteosarcoma.[27-29] In patients with newly diagnosed ALL, low RFC expression at diagnosis correlated with a significantly reduced event-free survival.[27] In osteosarcoma treatment, 17 of 26 posttreatment tumor samples (65%) derived from high-grade tumors and with poor response to chemotherapy had low RFC expression.[28] Poor response to MTX-based chemotherapy was also observed in tumor samples with low levels of RFC at diagnosis.[29]

TABLE 7.2	*Folate transporters and their substrates*				
	Substrate				
Transporter	**Folic Acid**	**Reduced folates**	**MTX**	**PMD**[a]	**PRTX**[b]
Reduced folate carrier	+	++++	+++	++++	+++++
Folate receptor	+++	+++ (5-methyl THF)	+	+++	?
Proton-coupled transporter	+++	+++	++	++++	+

Pluses (+) indicate relative affinity.
[a]Pemetrexed.
[b]Pralatrexate.
Source: Mauritz R, Peters GJ, Kathmann I, et al. Dynamics of antifolate transport via the reduced folate carrier and the membrane folate receptor in murine leukemia cells in vitro and in vivo. *Cancer Chemother Pharmacol*. 2008;62:937-948.

Newer antifolate analogues have improved transport properties. Pralatrexate, approved for cutaneous T-cell lymphomas, is a 10-deaza-aminopterin with a 10-fold greater efficiency as a substrate for the reduced folate transporter.[30] Other antifolate inhibitors (CB3717, raltitrexed, lometrexol, and BW1843U89) that rely on the FR for transport have proven ineffective in the clinic. Because pemetrexed is efficiently transported by both FR and proton-coupled folate transport systems, it may be less susceptible to clinical resistance resulting from decreased RFC.[31]

Low folate conditions may increase the toxicity of antifolates as a consequence of the up-regulations of FR in normal tissues in response to folate starvation. Based on evidence of a deficiency of folate or B12 in a subset of patients at highest risk for toxicity, folic acid and B12 are supplemented pretreatment, effectively reducing the incidence of severe myelosuppression related to pralatrexate and pemetrxed.[32]

MTX Efflux Mechanisms

Early studies suggested the presence of active efflux mechanisms for folates and analogues[33] due to the multidrug resistance–associated

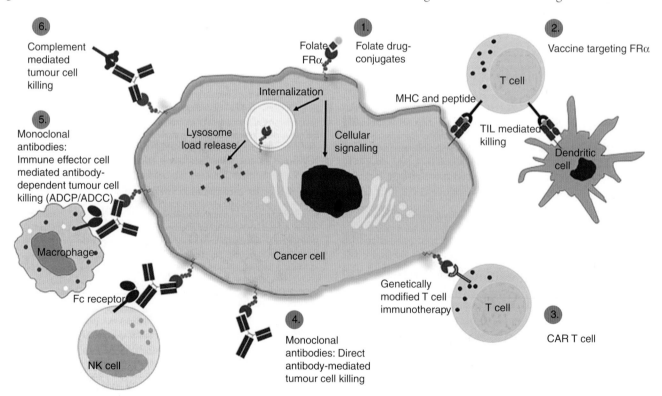

FIGURE 7.3 New approaches to antifolate therapy targeting the folate receptor. Shown are the multiple avenues for killing tumor cells that express the folate receptor alpha. These tactics utilize naked antibodies that fix complement or depend on cell killing; CAR-T cells that recognize FR and kill cells; vaccines; antibodies armed with toxins or radionuclides, or that link to macrophages or NK cells; and folate analogues coupled to toxic molecules. (From Cheung A, Bax HJ, Illeva KM, et al. Targeting folate receptor alpha for cancer treatment. *Oncotarget*. 2016;7(32):52553-52574. doi: 10.18632/oncotarget.9651, with permission.)

protein family of ATP-binding cassette transporters, particularly MRP-1, MRP-2, and MRP-3 and the breast cancer resistance protein (BCRP), which actively extrude MTX in both normal and tumor cells.[34,35] MRP-2 and BRCP or ABCG2 excrete MTX from liver cells into the bile and efflux drug into the intestinal lumen and urine in mice. Knockout-of BCRP produces increased MTX levels in the systemic circulation in mice as a consequence of decreased biliary and urinary excretion.

Intracellular Transformation

Naturally occurring folates exist within cells predominately in a polyglutamated form (Fig. 7.1). The polyglutamation of folate and antifolate substrates is directed by folylpolyglutamyl synthetase (FPGS), an enzyme that adds up to eight glutamyl groups in γ peptide linkage. Separate isoforms of the enzyme exist in the cytosol, where folates are crucial for purine and TMP synthesis, and in mitochondria, in which folates mediate one-carbon transfers from serine and glycine. The folate PG compartments in cytosol and mitochondria are not in free exchange.[36] Alternative splicing of the cytosolic FPGS RNA has been implicated in resistance to MTX in childhood ALL, where exon 6 skipping and intron 8 partial retention terminate transcription of the protein and decrease accumulation of the antifolate PGs; specific mutations of the FPGS gene have been identified in MTX-resistant ALL.[37] Polyglutamation facilitates the accumulation of intracellular folates in a form selectively retained in vast excess of a monoglutamate pool, which is otherwise freely transported out of cells. It prolongs the intracellular half-life of folates under conditions of reduced folate availability. The addition of each glutamate enhances folate cofactor affinity 10-fold for some folate-dependent enzymes, especially GARF, AICARF, and TS. The same effects are seen with antifolates. The PGs of MTX and pemetrexed are slightly more potent inhibitors of DHFR than the parent drug, but significantly more potent antagonists of TS and the transformylases as compared to the parent drugs. The other glutamyl-terminal analogues also undergo polyglutamation in normal liver cells and bone marrow myeloid precursors,[38] likely enhancing their toxicity. Polyglutamation occurs in most tumors to varying degrees and influences antitumor response.[39]

The efficiency of the polyglutamation reaction for various folate substrates and antifolates varies considerably. Pralatrexate is 10-fold more avidly polyglutamated than MTX.[40] The polyglutamation of MTX occurs progressively over several hours of exposure; after 24 hours, 80% or more of intracellular drug exists in the PG form.[40,41] Human liver retains MTX PGs for several months after drug administration.[42] Thus, selective retention of PGs in excess of free monoglutamate, as seen with physiologic folates, characterizes MTX PGs as well.

FPGS is a 62-kD magnesium-, adenosine triphosphate-, and potassium-dependent protein.[42-44] The FPGS gene is located on chromosome region 9q34.11 and produces two proteins, the major one having 537-amino acids; a second with 579 amino acids is found in mitochondria. The most avid substrate for this enzyme is dihydrofolate (K_m [binding affinity] = 2 μmol/L), with the following folates and analogues in descending order of affinity: tetrahydrofolate (K_m = 6 μmol/L) > 10-formyltetrahydrofolate or 5-methyltetrahydrofolate > aminopterin > leucovorin > MTX. Pralatrexate and pemetrexed have greater affinity for FPGS than MTX. Because of the slow rate of formation of antifolate PGs compared with the naturally occurring folate PGs, reductions in FPGS activity or cellular glutamate levels

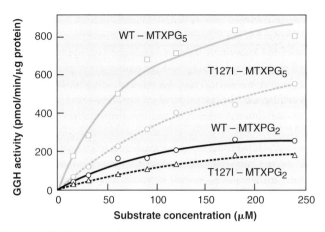

FIGURE **7.4** Catalytic activity of T127I variant gamma-glutamylhydrolase (GGH) on MTX PG substrates, as compared to wild-type (WT) enzyme. Enzymes were incubated with MTX PGs with chain length of 2 and 5 glutamyl groups. A 2.7-fold increase in K_m was observed for the variant enzyme. (From Cheng Q, Wu B, Kager L, et al. A substrate specific functional polymorphism of human gamma-glutamyl hydrolase alters catalytic activity and methotrexate polyglutamate accumulation in acute lymphoblastic leukemia cells. *Pharmacogenetics.* 2004;14(8):557-567. With permission.)

may have little effect on folate PG pools but may critically reduce MTX PG formation and decrease cytotoxicity of antifolates.

The intracellular content of PG derivatives represents a balance between the activities of two different enzymes[45]: FPGS, which synthesizes PGs, and γ-glutamyl hydrolase (GGH, conjugase), a γ-glutamyl-specific peptidase that removes terminal glutamyl groups and returns MTX PGs to their monoglutamate form.[46] The cloned complementary DNA for GGH codes for an enzyme of 318 amino acids with molecular weight of 36 kD.

While the functional importance of GGH in determining response to MTX is not known, the St. Jude group has found a substrate specific polymorphism (C452T) of the enzyme, present in 10% of Caucasian patients, that reduces catalytic activity and allows greater accumulation of MTX PGs in leukemic cells (Fig. 7.4).[47] Although it may be expected that overexpression of hydrolase may result in MTX resistance, particularly with brief drug exposures, such was not the case in several human cell line models in which hydrolase was overexpressed.[48]

MTX PGs exist primarily within cells and cross membranes sparingly. The diglutamate form has an uptake velocity of one-fifteenth that of MTX,[49] whereas higher glutamates are transported at slower rates, leading to their selective retention as extracellular levels of MTX fall.

Cellular activity of FPGS correlates directly with the rate of cell growth and inversely with the level of intracellular folates.[50] Enhancement of cell proliferation with growth factors such as insulin, dexamethasone, tocopherol, and estrogen in hormone-responsive cells increases polyglutamation, whereas deprivation of essential amino acids inhibits polyglutamation.[51] MTX and L-asparaginase are frequently used in treatment of acute leukemia. Conversion of MTX to PG forms can be markedly inhibited by pretreatment with L-asparaginase, presumably through growth arrest due to amino acid depletion. Increasing intracellular folate pools through exposure of cells to high concentrations of leucovorin or 5-methyltetrahydrofolate suppresses MTX polyglutamation,[50] while a folate-free medium enhances PG formation.

An important factor in the selective nature of MTX cytotoxicity may derive from modest PG formation in normal tissues relative to that in malignant tissues. Although little metabolism to PGs is observed in normal murine intestinal cells in vivo, most murine leukemias and Ehrlich ascites tumor cells efficiently convert MTX to higher PG forms in tumor-bearing animals.[52] Additionally, normal human and murine myeloid progenitor cells form relatively small amounts of MTX PGs compared with leukemic cells.[38]

In addition to increasing its retention within cells, polyglutamation of MTX and pemetrexed enhances markedly their inhibitory effects on TS, AICART, and GART, but not on DHFR. The pentaglutamates have a slightly slower dissociation rate from DHFR than does MTX[53] but a markedly enhanced inhibitory potency for TS ($K_i = 50$ nmol/L), AICAR transformylase ($K_i = 57$ nmol/L), and, to a lesser extent, GAR transformylase ($K_i = 2$ µmol/L). Pemetrexed pentaglutamates inhibit the purine synthetic enzymes in the low nanomolar range and TS with a subnanomolar K_i.[54] The well-described incomplete depletion of physiologic folate cofactors by MTX suggests that direct enzymatic inhibition of multiple folate-dependent sites by MTX PGs must contribute to MTX cytotoxicity. These effects may also explain the competitive nature of rescue by leucovorin posttreatment, in that leucovorin and its derived tetrahydrofolates suppress antifolate PG formation and compete with PGs at enzymatic sites.

The ability of antifolate analogues to undergo polyglutamation is one of several properties that influence cytotoxic potency. Aminopterin is a better substrate for FPGS than is MTX and is a more potent cytotoxic agent Pemetrexed and particularly pralatrexate are more efficient substrates than MTX. The ability of tumor cells to generate PGs appears to be a prerequisite for response to MTX antifolates polyglutamation and is defective in some drug-resistant human and murine tumor cell lines[55] and in human ALL of B- and T-cell-type ALL.[56,57] The low level of PG formation in human tumors has been ascribed in various studies to a relative increase in GGH activity,[58] defective FPGS splicing and exon skipping,[59] and a decreased enzyme affinity for MTX in acute myelogenous leukemia (AML).

Leukemic cells differ greatly in their expression of FPGS. Hyperdiploid status in childhood ALL is a good prognostic feature; cells with hyperdiploidy show higher levels of synthesis of cytotoxic MTX PGs than cells of diploid lymphoblasts. A higher concentration of MTX long-chain PGs, and a better outcome of therapy, is found in lymphoid leukemia and in B- versus T-cell lymphoblasts.[57,60]

PG formation is only one of several factors affecting outcome of treatment for ALL with MTX. A study involving 52 children with B-cell ALL did not confirm that MTX accumulation and polyglutamation have prognostic significance in patients receiving prolonged oral MTX therapy.[61] This finding supports the notion that, under the conditions of continuous low–dose drug exposure, the activity of MTX may not depend on cellular polyglutamation to sustain intracellular levels and antitumor effect. The role of PG formation in solid tumor therapy is also unclear. Small cell carcinoma resistant to MTX contained low levels of PGs.[56] In specimens from patients with soft-tissue sarcoma, 12 of 15 tumors exhibited impaired polyglutamation, although the relationship to clinical response was uncertain.[62]

Genetic variants may also influence the function of FPGS, as suggested by the finding that two variants (R424C and S457F) slow the rate of PG formation for both folates and MTX and decrease cytotoxicity of MTX when the variants are expressed in Aux B1 cells.[63]

In summary, limited experimental and clinical evidence suggests a relationship between clinical response and PF formation. The role of genomic variation in contributing to FPGS and GGH activities and PG formation is still unresolved.

Binding to Dihydrofolate Reductase

The physical characteristics of binding of NADPH (reduced form of nicotinamide adenine dinucleotide phosphate [NADP]) and MTX to DHFR of various species have been established by x-ray crystallographic studies and nuclear magnetic resonance spectroscopy of native and chemically modified enzyme, and enzyme modified by site-directed mutagenesis[64,65]; strong amino acid sequence homology is found among mammalian species at positions involved in substrate cofactor and inhibitor binding. In general, a long hydrophobic pocket binds folates and analogues and is formed in part by the isoleucine-5, alanine-7, aspartate-27, phenylalanine-31 (Phe-31) and phenylalanine-34 (Phe-34), and other amino acid residues. Several particularly important interactions contribute to the binding potency of the 4-amino antifolates: (a) hydrogen bonding of the carbonyl oxygen of isoleucine-5 to the 4-amino group of the inhibitor; (b) a salt bridge between aspartate and the N-1 position of MTX, which is not involved in binding to the physiologic substrates; (c) hydrophobic interactions of the inhibitor with DHFR, particularly with Phe-31 and Phe-34; (d) hydrogen bonding of the 2-amino group to aspartate-27 and to a consistent bound water molecule; and (e) hydrogen binding of the terminal glutamate to an invariant arginine-70 residue. Interactions of MTX with Phe-31 and Phe-34 appear to be essential because mutations in these positions result in a 100-fold and 80,000-fold decrease in MTX affinity for the enzyme, respectively.[66] Mutation of arginine-70 results in a decrease in MTX affinity by greater than 22,000-fold but does not alter the binding affinity of trimetrexate, a nonglutamate antifolate.[67] Mutations outside the folate-binding site also may result in marked reductions in folate and antifolate affinities. In fact the binding of 2,4-di-amino-folate analogues is inverted in the substrate pocket, as compared to the folates. The reader is referred to more detailed reviews of substrate and cofactor binding characteristics of native and mutated DHFR.[68,69]

Optimal binding of MTX to DHFR depends on the concentration of NADPH. NADH (reduced form of nicotinamide adenine dinucleotide) may also act as a cosubstrate for DHFR but, unlike NADPH, it does not promote binding of MTX to the enzyme.[70] Thus, the intracellular ratios of NADPH/NADP and NADPH/NADH may play an important role in the selective action of MTX to the extent that the cosubstrate ratios may differ in malignant and in normal tissues. In the presence of excess NADPH, the binding affinity of MTX for DHFR has been estimated to lie between 10 and 200 pM.[71] This affinity is significantly affected by pH, salt concentration, and the status of enzyme sulfhydryl groups. Under conditions of low pH and with a low ratio of inhibitor to enzyme, binding is essentially stoichiometric, that is, one molecule of MTX is bound to one molecule of DHFR.

Binding of MTX to DHFR isolated from parasitic, bacterial, and mammalian sources in the presence of NADPH generates a slowly formed ternary complex. The overall process has been termed slow, tight-binding inhibition and involves an initial rapid but weak enzyme-inhibitor interaction followed by a slow but extremely tight-binding isomerization to the final complex.[69] The final isomerization step probably involves a conformational change of the enzyme with subsequent binding of the para-aminobenzoyl moiety to the enzyme.[59] Other folate analogues, such as aminopterin, follow the same slow, tight-binding kinetic process, in contrast to the pteridines and pyrimethamine, which behave as classic single step inhibitors of bacterial DHFR.

In the therapeutic setting, and in intact cells, MTX acts as a tight-binding but reversible inhibitor. Under conditions of high concentrations of competitive substrate (dihydrofolate) and at neutral intracellular pH, an excess of free drug is required to fully inhibit the enzyme. As drug concentration falls below 10^{-8} M in tissue culture and at lower concentrations in cell-free systems, enzyme activity resumes, and tritium-labeled MTX bound to intracellular enzyme can be displaced by unlabeled drug or dihydrofolate.[72,73]

MTX PGs have similar potency in their tight-binding inhibition of mammalian DHFR but exhibit a slower rate of dissociation from the enzyme than MTX. In pulse-chase experiments using intact human breast cancer cells, MTX pentaglutamate dissociated from DHFR with a half-life of 120 minutes compared to 12 minutes for the parent compound. In experiments using purified mammalian enzyme, MTX PGs had a modest twofold to sixfold greater inhibition of DHFR catalytic activity versus parent drug.[69] As with MTX, enzyme-bound MTX PGs may also be displaced by reduced folates and dihydrofolate,[74] albeit at a slower rate than displacement of MTX.

These observations indicate that, in the absence of excess free drug, a small fraction of intracellular DHFR, either through new synthesis or through dissociation from the inhibitor, becomes available for catalytic activity and allows for continued intracellular metabolism. The requirement for free drug to inhibit enzyme activity completely is important in understanding the clinical effects and toxicity of this agent and is fundamental to the relationship between pharmacokinetics and pharmacodynamics.

Resistance to MTX as a result of decreased DHFR binding affinity for MTX has been described in experimental cell lines.[75,76] These mutant enzymes may have several 1,000-fold reduced binding affinity for MTX and, in general, are less efficient in catalyzing the reduction of dihydrofolate than is wild-type DHFR.

DHFR with reduced affinity for MTX may represent a clinically important mechanism of MTX resistance, as this phenomenon was observed in the leukemic cells of 4 of 12 patients with resistant AML.[77] Transfection of MTX-resistant, mutant DHFR has become a tool for creating drug-resistant hematopoietic progenitor cells.[78]

A common finding in both laboratory and clinical studies of MTX is an increase in the expression of DHFR protein within hours of exposure to MTX. This acute and transient increase in DHFR has been attributed to altered regulation of translation (see below). A persistent elevations in DHFR occur through drug selection of DHFR-amplified cells. In murine and human tumor cells, DHFR gene amplification, is readily promoted by exposure to stepwise increases in the concentration of MTX.[79-81] Gene duplication appear as a long homogeneously staining region (HSR) inserted into a chromosome or nonintegrated pieces of DNA known as double-minute chromosomes (DMs). While HSRs appear to confer stable resistance to the cell, DMs are unequally distributed during cell division,[81] and in the absence of the continued selective pressure of drug exposure, the cells may revert to the original low-DHFR genotype. Evidence exists that gene amplification occurs initially in the form of DMs.[82-84] Other investigations suggest the opposite sequence wherein chromosomal breaks result in HSRs, which are then processed to DMs or not, depending on how different cell types handle extra chromosomal sequences. Experimentally, DMs appear following drug exposure in cell overexpressing nonhomologous end joining capability for DNA repair, while cell showing no change in NHEJ seem to express gene amplification through HSRs.[83]

MTX resistance through DHFR gene amplification becomes apparent only after the prolonged selective pressure of drug exposure to MTX alone, but highly MTX-resistant cells, may be generated more rapidly by simultaneous treatment with hydroxyurea during a single cell cycle.[84] Early S-phase cells exposed transiently to hydroxyurea, which stops DNA synthesis, may undergo reduplication of multiple genes synthesized during early S phase, including DHFR, after removal of the DNA synthetic inhibitor. This finding has broad implications for the rapid development of drug resistance in patients treated with MTX and other inhibitors of DNA synthesis. Exposure of cells to a variety of chemical and physical agents unrelated to MTX including hypoxia, chemotherapy, and carcinogens may increase the frequency of MTX resistance through DHFR mutation or gene amplification with subsequent increases in DHFR protein.[85,86] The induction of MTX resistance by toxic exposures may explain de novo MTX resistance in certain human tumors, given the constant presence of a host of environmental mutagens. Unlike in malignant cells, amplification of DNA has not been reported in normal cells of patients undergoing therapy with antifolates or in cell lines of normal cells.[87]

In addition to gene amplification, more subtle mechanisms regulate DHFR expression, including autoregulation on DHFR message by the unbound enzyme, variants in gene sequence, and microRNAs.[88] Exposure of human breast cancer cells to MTX results in an acute increase (up to fourfold) in the cellular DHFR content. The expression of DHFR protein in this setting appears to be controlled at the level of mRNA translation, as no acute associated change occurs in the amount of DHFR mRNA or DHFR gene copy number after MTX exposure nor are alterations seen in DHFR enzyme stability. Using an RNA gel mobility shift assay, human recombinant DHFR protein was shown to specifically bind to its corresponding DHFR mRNA.[89] Incubation of DHFR protein either with the normal substrates dihydrofolate or NADPH, or with MTX, completely represses its binding to the target DHFR mRNA. In an in vitro translation system, this specific interaction between DHFR and its message is associated with inhibition of translation. These studies provide evidence for a translational autoregulatory mechanism underlying the control of DHFR expression. The presence of either excess MTX or dihydrofolate prevents DHFR protein from performing its normal autoregulatory function, thereby allowing for increased DHFR protein synthesis.[90]

Although various in vitro and in vivo model systems have clearly demonstrated an association between DHFR gene amplification and MTX resistance, the clinical importance of gene amplification among the various possible resistance mechanisms remains uncertain. A few studies have found tumor samples from patients resistant to MTX in association with elevated levels of DHFR enzyme and DHFR gene amplification. A small cell lung carcinoma cell line isolated from a patient clinically resistant to high-dose MTX had amplification of the DHFR gene in DMs and increased expression of DHFR protein.[91]

Consequences of Dihydrofolate Reductase Enzyme Inhibition

The critical cellular events associated with MTX inhibition of DHFR are illustrated in Figure 7.2. TS catalyzes the sole biochemical reaction resulting in the oxidation of tetrahydrofolates. Continued activity of this enzymatic reaction in the presence of DHFR inhibition results in rapid increases in intracellular levels of dihydrofolate

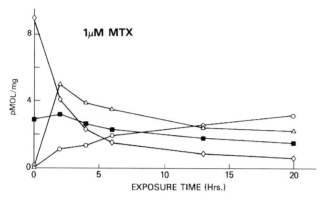

<figure>**FIGURE 7.5** Effects of 1 µmol/L MTX on intracellular folate pools in human breast cancer cells (MCF-7). △, dihydrofolate; ○, 10-formyldihydrofolate; ■, 10-formyltetrahydrofolate; ◇, 5-methyltetrahydrofolate. (Reprinted with permission from Allegra CJ, Fine RL, Drake JC, et al. The effect of methotrexate on intracellular folate pools in human MCF-7 breast cancer cells. Evidence for direct inhibition of purine synthesis. *J Biol Chem.* 1986;261(14):6478-6485. Copyright © 1986 The American Society for Biochemistry and Molecular Biology.)</figure>

PGs and depletion of critical reduced folate pools, including notably 5-methyltetrahydrofolate. In vitro studies indicate that the reduced folate cofactors required for de novo purine and TMP synthesis (10-formyltetrahydrofolate and 5,10-methylenetetrahydrofolate) are relatively preserved in the presence of cytotoxic concentrations of MTX[7-12] (Fig. 7.5) adding credence to the postulated importance of direct inhibition of the various folate-dependent enzymes in the metabolic inhibition associated with MTX exposure.[92]

Leucovorin rescue of MTX-treated cells causes an accumulation of reduced folates that compete with MTX PGs for transport, polyglutamation, and occupancy of enzymatic binding sites, thereby overcoming the block in nucleotide production. These considerations may, in large part, explain the competitive nature of leucovorin rescue observed in vitro and clinically. The selectivity of the cytotoxic effects of MTX and selectivity of leucovorin rescue on normal and malignant cells may depend on their ability to transport and polyglutamate folate and MTX PGs.

An additional factor that influences the folate pool changes associated with MTX exposure and, hence, cellular sensitivity to MTX is the level of activity of TS. Inhibition of TS by 5-fluorodeoxyuridylate or by depletion of its substrate dUMP diminishes sensitivity to MTX. Low levels of TS in experimental tumor settings are usually associated with MTX resistance.[56] In cells with low levels of TS, the slow rate of oxidation of 5,10-methylenetetrahydrofolate to dihydrofolate creates less dependence on DHFR to regenerate tetrahydrofolates. Under conditions of low cellular TS activity, a block in DHFR by MTX exposures produces minimal accumulation of inhibitory dihydrofolate and minimal depletion of tetrahydrofolates.

Mechanisms of Cell Death

As a consequence of the multiple effects of antifolates on nucleotide biosynthesis, several mechanisms of cell death are possible. Inhibition of TMP and purine synthesis leads to a cessation of DNA synthesis Deoxythymidine triphosphate and deoxypurine nucleotides are required for both the synthesis of DNA and its repair. A close correlation is found between DNA strand breaks, resulting from nucleotide depletion or misincorporation of dUMP for dTMP, and cell death in Ehrlich ascites tumor cell exposed to MTX.[93] This work is supported by similar experimental findings in a mutant murine cell line lacking TS activity and grown in thymidine-deplete media. The

high concentrations of dUMP resulting from a failure of dTMP synthesis may ultimately lead to misincorporation of dUMP into cellular DNA. An enzyme, uracil-DNA-glycosylase, specifically excises uracil bases from DNA, a process that may be responsible for the fragments of DNA observed in antifolate-treated cells.[94,95] Deoxyuridine triphosphatase activity may also regulate the size of dUMP pools and thereby influence dUMP incorporation into DNA and MTX toxicity. Although the induction of DNA strand breaks is central to the activity of MTX, it is the cellular response to these breaks, mediated by p53 and the apoptotic pathway, that ultimately determines whether a cell incurring a given level of DNA damage dies.[96]

Pharmacokinetic and Cytokinetic Determinants of Cytotoxicity

At least two pharmacokinetic factors—drug concentration and duration of cell exposure—are critical determinants of cytotoxicity. In tissue culture and in intact animals, extracellular drug concentrations of 10 nmol/L are required to stop DNA synthesis in normal bone marrow. This same drug concentration is associated with depletion of bone marrow cellularity when maintained for 24 hours or longer. The rate of cell loss from murine bone marrow increases with increasing drug concentrations up to 10 µmol/L[97] (Fig. 7.6). Similar findings have been reported in studies with murine tumor cells, in which cytotoxicity is both time and drug concentration dependent. Compared with drug concentration, the duration of exposure to MTX is a more critical factor in determining cell death, provided the minimal threshold concentration for cytotoxicity is exceeded. For a given concentration of drug, cytotoxicity for human leukemic cells in culture is directly proportional to the time period of exposure but doubles only with a 10-fold increase in drug concentration.[97] This relationship is likely the result of the S-phase specificity of MTX. With longer duration of exposure, more cells are allowed to enter the vulnerable DNA-synthetic phase of the cell cycle.

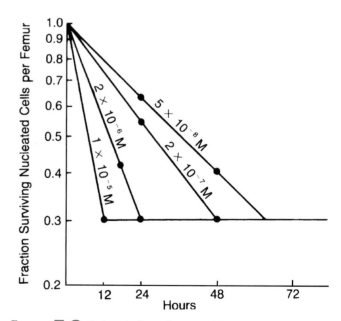

<figure>**FIGURE 7.6** Nucleated cells per femur remaining after constant infusion of MTX sodium into mice to achieve indicated drug concentration for various periods. (Reprinted from Pinedo HM, Zaharko DS, Bull J, et al. The relative contribution of drug concentration and duration of exposure to mouse bone marrow toxicity during continuous methotrexate infusion. *Cancer Res.* 1977;37(2):445-450. Copyright © 1977 American Association for Cancer Research. With permission from AACR.)</figure>

In addition to pharmacokinetic and cytokinetic factors, physiologic compounds in the cellular environment may profoundly affect the cytotoxicity of MTX. Most prominent among these factors are the naturally occurring purine bases, purine nucleosides, and thymidine. In bone marrow and intestinal epithelium, the de novo synthesis of both TMP and purines is inhibited by concentrations of MTX above 10 nmol/L, but cells can survive this block when bone marrow is supplied with 10 mM thymidine and a purine source (adenosine, inosine, or hypoxanthine) at similar concentrations. Thymidine alone is incapable of completely reversing the cytotoxic effect of MTX.[98] As a more specific inhibitor of TS, pemetrexed is substantially rescued by thymidine, but at thymidine concentrations above 1 μM.[4] The purine salvage pathways in normal bone marrow appear to be more efficient, and the endogenous concentrations of purines in this tissue are high.[99] Plasma thymidine levels in humans are approximately 0.2 μmol/L, whereas the concentration of the purine bases and nucleosides in the systemic circulation is higher (0.5 μmol/L) but still below rescue levels.[100] Pharmacologic interventions, such as allopurinol treatment (which elevates circulating hypoxanthine concentrations) and chemotherapy, with subsequent tumor lysis, may further raise levels of the circulating nucleosides and ameliorate toxicity to tumor or host tissues.

A third determinant of antifolate cytotoxic action is the concentration of reduced folate in the circulation and in the cell. Methyltetrahydrofolate (the predominant circulating folate cofactor), when present in sufficient concentration in vitro, can readily reverse MTX toxicity, as can leucovorin. Circulating levels of 5-methyltetrahydrofolate are approximately 0.01 μmol/L and of little pharmacologic relevance. Exogenous administration of reduced folates, however, is able to reverse MTX toxicity in a competitive manner. Leucovorin is commonly used after MTX administration to reduce or prevent toxicity and is effective when given within 24 to 36 hours after MTX treatment. The concentration of leucovorin required to prevent MTX toxicity increases as the drug concentration increases (Fig. 7.7),[98] related to competition for transport, pG formation, or enzyme inhibition. An additional factor affecting competition of folates and antifolates

is the adequacy of vitamin B12, which is required in the methionine synthase reaction for conversion of 5-methyl tetrahydrofolate to tetrahydrofolate, the usable precursor of the reactive reduced folate cofactor. B12 induces methionine synthase activity, which in turn elevates tetrahydrofolate, the precursor of usable reduced folates, and experimentally is known to protect against antifolate cytotoxicity.[101] Pretreatment of patients with B12 and folate effectively mitigates pemetrexed and pralatrexate toxicity without impairing antitumor activity. A full explanation for this differential rescue of host versus tumor is not apparent.

In clinical practice, (see below), while the actual locus of competition (transport, enzyme target, polyglutamation) is unclear, the dose of reduced folate required to prevent antifolate toxicity varies directly with the opposing concentration of antifolate and the duration of exposure to unopposed antifolate.[98,102] Because leucovorin is capable of reversing the cytotoxic effects of MTX on host and malignant cells, the minimum dose of leucovorin needed to rescue host cells should be used. Careful consideration must be given to the dose and timing of leucovorin when used in combination with MTX to avoid rescue of both cancerous and normal tissues. Periods of unopposed MTX for up to 36 hours are tolerated by mice and humans, after which toxicity to bone marrow and intestinal epithelium is not averted by leucovorin.

Methotrexate Assay

MTX levels in plasma, first measured by an enzyme inhibition assay, by a radioimmunoassay, or by competitive enzyme binding of labeled drug, are now routinely determined by high-pressure liquid chromatography (HPLC)-based assays, which provide extremely sensitive measurement of MTX levels greater than 10 nmol/L in biologic fluids. The competitive enzyme-binding assay and the HPLC assay offer the greatest specificity.

Radioimmuno assays cross-react with one MTX metabolite, 2,4-diamino-N_{10}-methyl pteroic acid (DAMPA) (40%), which lacks the terminal glutamate group, but not with 7-hydroxymethotrexate (7-OH-MTX) (1%). At later time points after drug administration,

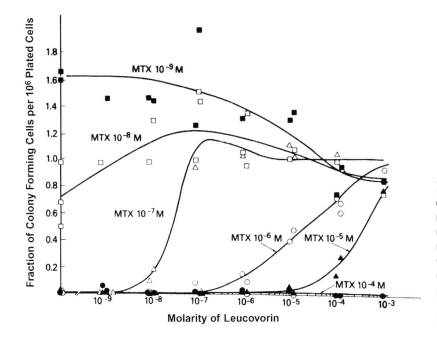

FIGURE **7.7** Effect of various combinations of leucovorin calcium and MTX on formation of granulocyte colonies in vitro by mouse bone marrow. Values are normalized to control value for marrow incubated without either drug. MTX concentrations: ■, 10^{-9} mol/L; □, 10^{-8} mol/L; △, 10^{-7} mol/L; ○, 10^{-6} mol/L; ▲, 10^{-5} mol/L; ●, 10^{-4} mol/L. (Reprinted from Pinedo HM, Zaharko DS, Bull JM, et al. The reversal of methotrexate cytotoxicity to mouse bone marrow cells by leucovorin and nucleosides. *Cancer Res.* 1976;36(12):4418-4424. Copyright © 1976 American Association for Cancer Research. With permission from AACR.)

DAMPA is found in plasma in relatively high concentrations (equal to or greater than that of MTX), and thus, these assays produce spuriously elevated values for the parent compound[103] that are on average twofold to fourfold higher than HPLC or DHFR competitive binding.

Monitoring of MTX pharmacokinetics takes place primarily in the context of high-dose regimens, where delays in renal elimination of parent drug may lead to serious toxicity or death. HPLC can be used to separate and quantitate MTX and its various metabolites. Although the sensitivity of HPLC is primarily limited by the ultraviolet detection systems commonly used (0.2 μmol/L), its sensitivity may be markedly enhanced by a preliminary drug concentration step, electrochemical detection, postcolumn derivatization and fluorescence detection, or mass spectrometry.[104] Although HPLC technology may be cumbersome for routine clinical monitoring, its use is required when high sensitivity and specificity along with an ability to measure individual MTX metabolites are required. Two more commonly used assay techniques, enzyme-multiplied immunoassay and fluorescence-polarization immunoassay HPLC, in over 100 patient plasma samples tested give high concordance with HPLC, although the immunoassays cross-react with 7-OH-MTX and thus may be less useful for research studies and at later time points.[105] The final selection of an assay to be used in the clinical setting may ultimately depend on the requirements for sensitivity, specificity, identification of specific MTX metabolites, and cost and time constraints.

Assays for pemetrexed and pralatrexate utilize HPLC, but are not used in routine practice (see below).

Pharmacokinetics

Exploitation of the pharmacologic properties of MTX for patient treatment depends on a detailed understanding of the time profile of drug concentration in extracellular and intracellular spaces and the complex relationship of drug levels to toxicities and antitumor effects.

The first attempts to define the distribution and disposition of MTX in a comprehensive manner were reported by Zaharko et al.[106] They developed a detailed model for MTX pharmacokinetics that accurately predicted drug-derived radioactivity in various tissue compartments for a 4-hour period after drug administration. The primary elements of that model were (a) elimination of MTX by renal excretion, (b) an active enterohepatic circulation, (c) metabolism of at least a small fraction of drug within the gastrointestinal tract by intestinal flora (and later by the liver), and (d) multiple phases of drug disappearance in plasma, the longest of which was found to be approximately 3 hours. Each of these elements has been observed in humans, although an additional terminal 8-hour half-life in plasma is now appreciated.

Absorption

MTX is administered as a daily oral dose in treating autoimmune disease, psoriasis and as a maintenance therapy of acute leukemia. It is absorbed from the gastrointestinal tract by a proton-coupled transporter.[13] Absorption is variable and incomplete at higher doses (15 mg). Bioavailability (BA) for doses of 50 mg/m² or greater may be improved by subdividing the dose. In one study, for doses greater than 12 mg/m², peak drug levels in plasma were reached in 2.5 hours, with 51% oral BA, as compared to a shorter time to peak levels (1.5 hours) and great BA (87%) for doses less than 12 mg/m².[107]

In first pass of oral drug through the hepatic circulation, hepatocellular uptake, metabolism to PGs and 7-OH-MTX, and storage as PGs occur, and oral drug is further subject to degradation (deglutamylation) by intestinal flora to the inactive metabolite (DAMPA). In cancer patients, drugs taken orally are also subject to the variable absorption resulting from drug-induced epithelial damage, motility changes, and alterations in flora. MTX pharmacokinetics may be quite variable in children receiving even small oral doses of MTX (20 mg/m²).[108] Larger doses of MTX are usually given IV.

Pemetrexed and pralatrexate are administered intravenously on intermittent schedules.

Distribution

The volume of distribution of MTX approximates that of total body water. The drug is loosely bound (60%) to serum albumin at concentrations at or above 1 μmol/L in plasma.[109] Weak organic acids such as aspirin[110] can displace MTX from plasma proteins, but the clinical significance of this displacement is unknown.

MTX penetrates slowly into third-space fluid collection, such as pleural or joint effusions or ascites.[111] It exits slowly from these compartments, producing a concentration gradient of severalfold in favor of the loculated fluid at time points 6 hours after administration. The clearance of MTX from peritoneal fluid is approximately 5 mL/min, substantially less than its clearance from the plasma compartment (120 mL/min), which equals or exceeds glomerular filtration. The mechanism responsible for drug accumulation in closed fluid spaces results from the limited permeability of tissue surfaces to high molecular weight, charged compounds.

Drug either not retained by tissue or metabolized in the liver remains in the systemic circulation and greater than 80% of a given dose is excreted in the urine.

Third-space retention of intravenously administered drug leads to a prolonged terminal drug half-life in plasma, as sequestered drug slowly re-enters the bloodstream.[111] This effect must be considered when treating patients with ascites or pleural effusions. It is advisable to evacuate third-space fluid before treatment and to monitor plasma drug levels in such patients. Likewise, unexpectedly high levels of MTX are reported in patients with bladder cancer who had previously undergone cystectomy and ileal conduit diversion, presumably due to drug resorption from the ileal conduit.[112] Dose reduction is advised in this setting.

MTX distributes modestly well into the CNS. CSF levels at steady state are usually 3% or less than simultaneous levels in plasma, but high-dose systemic therapy produces CSF concentrations above 1 μM for 24 to 48 hours, and is an effective treatment for preventing CNS relapse in patients with good prognosis ALL, and is the treatment of choice for CNS lymphomas. Direct installation of 12 mg into the CSF is the preferred treatment for meningeal leukemia.

Plasma Pharmacokinetics

Typical graphs of MTX pharmacokinetics in plasma are shown in Figure 7.8. After the initial distribution phase, which lasts a relatively few minutes, at least two phases of drug disappearance from plasma are evident in laboratory animals and humans. Conventional doses of 25 to 100 mg/m² produce peak plasma concentrations of 1 to 10 μmol/L, whereas high-dose infusion regimens using 1.5 g/m² or more yield peak levels of 100 μmol/L or greater.[107] The initial phase of drug disappearance from plasma has a half-life of 2 to 3 hours,

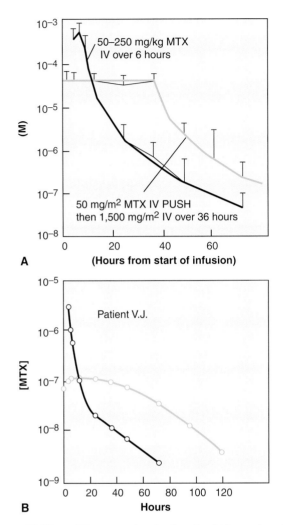

FIGURE 7.8 A. MTX concentrations (median of multiple samples taken at each time point) in plasma during and following infusion of 50 to 250 mg/kg MTX over 6 hours, and 40 mg/kg over 36 hours. Note the lower peak drug concentration and the more extended exposure to drug concentrations above 10 mM with the more prolonged drug infusion. The terminal $t_{1/2}$ in both schedules of infusion is the same: 8 to 10 hours. **B.** Simultaneous MTX levels in plasma and ascites, during intravenous bolus infusion of 25 mg/m² in a patient with ovarian cancer, demonstrating the delayed uptake and clearance from a third-space fluid collection.

with little variation as doses are increased to the high-dose range. This phase extends for the first 12 to 24 hours after drug administration and is largely determined by the rate of renal excretion of MTX. The half-life of this phase, as well as of the terminal phase of drug disappearance from plasma, is significantly greater in patients with renal dysfunction and increases in proportion to the serum creatinine.[113] In moderate renal insufficiency, MTX elimination half-life correlates inversely with the degree of renal impairment. In patients with normal creatinine clearance, the half-life of the initial phase of drug disappearance increases with advancing age of the patient, adding variability to plasma levels, disappearance kinetics, and toxicity in the elderly.

The final phase of drug disappearance represents the cumulative effects of renal clearance and to a lesser extent hepatic metabolism, enterohepatic recirculation, and drug re-entry into plasma from tissue compartments and has a longer half-life of 8 to 10 hours: This half-life may greatly lengthen in patients with renal dysfunction or with third-space fluid such as ascites.[111] After conventional doses of

25 to 200 mg/m², this terminal phase begins at drug concentrations above the threshold for toxicity to bone marrow and gastrointestinal epithelium. Thus, any prolongation of the terminal half-life is likely to be associated with significant toxicity.

The use of constant-infusion MTX has received increasing consideration because it offers the advantage of providing predictable blood and cerebrospinal fluid (CSF) concentrations for a specific period of time. Bleyer[114] has used the following formulas for achieving a desired plasma concentration in pediatric patients with normal renal function:

1. Priming dose (in mg/m²) = 15 × target plasma MTX concentration (in μmol/L)
2. Infusion rate (in mg/m²/h) = 3 × target plasma MTX concentration (in μmol/L)

An approximate correction for renal function may be made by reducing the infusion doses in proportion to the reduction in creatinine clearance based on a normal creatinine clearance of 60 mL/min/m².

The plasma pharmacokinetics of MTX may independently predict relapse in children treated during the maintenance phase of ALL with intermediate drug doses (1 g/m²). In a study of 108 children, a rapid drug clearance (84 to 132 mL/min/m²) was associated with a 40% risk of relapse, whereas those children with relatively slow drug clearance (45 to 72 mL/min/m²) had a significantly decreased ($P_2 = 0.01$) risk of relapse (25%).[115] In children receiving prolonged infusions of MTX, steady-state MTX concentrations of less than 16 μmol/L were also associated with a higher probability of relapse ($P < 0.05$) than concentrations in excess of 16 μmol/L.[116] Systemic clearance averaged 123 mL/min/m² in 25 children who relapsed with ALL versus 72 mL/min/m² in 33 children who remained in continuous remission.[117] These results suggest that dose should be adjusted to differences in drug clearance to achieve target MTX levels.

Renal Excretion

The bulk of drug is excreted in the urine in the first 12 hours after administration, with renal excretion varying from 44% to virtually 100% of the administered dose.[112] The higher figure is likely to be true for patients with normal renal function. MTX clearance by the kidney has exceeded creatinine clearance in some patients studied, suggesting tubular secretion.[118]

During high-dose infusion, rapid drug excretion may lead to high MTX concentrations in renal tubular fluid. These concentrations, approaching 10 mmol/L, exceed the solubility of the drug at pHs below 7.0 and may lead to precipitation of drug renal failure. Thus, in high-dose regimens, hydration and alkalinization of the urine are necessary to avoid renal toxicity (Table 7.3). To ensure adequate intrarenal dissolution of MTX during high-dose therapy (0.7 to 8.4 g/m²), a 20-fold greater urine flow is required at pH 5.0 (2 to 42 mL/min/m²) than at pH 7.0 (0.1 to 1.2 mL/min/m²).[119] *Thus maintenance of a neutral urine pH is by far the most important factor in assuring protection from renal damage.* Intensive hydration does not affect the clearance of MTX or the plasma pharmacokinetics, aside from its effects on the prevention of renal damage.[120]

The exact mechanism of MTX excretion by the human kidney has not been fully elucidated. In dog and monkey models, active

TABLE
7.3 *Aqueous solubility of MTX and metabolites*

Agent	Solubility (mg/mL)		
	pH 5.0	**pH 6.0**	**pH 7.0**
Methotrexate	0.39	1.55	9.04
7-Hydroxy MTX	0.13	0.37	1.55
2,4-Diamino-N_{10}-methyl pteroic acid	0.05	0.10	0.85

secretion of MTX takes place in the proximal renal tubule, with reabsorption in the distal tubule. MTX excretion is inhibited by weak organic acids such as aspirin, penicillins, and ciprofloxacin.[121] The cephalosporins and sulfamethoxazole enhance the renal elimination of MTX, probably through competition for tubular reabsorption.[122] Simultaneous folic acid administration blocks MTX reabsorption, which suggests that leucovorin might accelerate MTX excretion in high-dose rescue regimens.

In high-dose MTX therapy, despite interindividual variation in pharmacokinetics, blood levels of drug may be accurately predicted by a preliminary determination of drug clearance using a small test dose (10 to 50 mg/m²).[123] Pharmacokinetic measurements made after delivery of this test dose provide a basis for calculating high-dose infusion rates according to the following formula (units of conversion must be carefully considered):

$$\text{Clearance (mL/min)} = \text{infusion rate (mg/min)}/\text{AUC (mg/ml)} \times \text{min}$$

$$\text{Infusion rate (mg/min)} = \text{target drug concentration (in mg/mL)} \times \text{clearance}$$

Thus, the desired infusion rate is the product of the target steady-state concentration multiplied by the MTX clearance rate, as determined from the test dose.

Extrapolation from the test dose of 50 mg/m² to a high-dose infusion schedule has proven to be reliable as long as renal function remains normal during the infusion period. The test dose technique has also been used to identify the subset of patients with impaired MTX elimination who are at increased risk for toxicity.[124]

The pharmacokinetics of pemetrexed and pralatrexate are considered below in sections related to their specific clinical properties.

Hepatic Uptake and Biliary Excretion

The glutamated antifolates are actively transported into hepatocytes by the RFC and converted to PG forms that persist for several months after drug administration.[125] As described previously, MTX undergoes active excretion into the biliary tract by the BCRP and MRP transporters and is reabsorbed into the systemic circulation from the small intestine. In the liver, MTX impairs methionine synthesis, an effect counteracted by choline and by betaine (methyl group donors).[126]

The unconjugated bile salt deoxycholate and the conjugated salt taurocholate significantly diminished MTX absorption in the small

intestine. Folic acid, 5-methyltetrahydrofolate, and the organic anions, rose bengal and sulfobromophthalein, also inhibited intestinal transport and likely diminish enterohepatic circulation of antifolates. Estimates of biliary excretion vary widely (<1% to 20%),[127] and less than 10% of an intravenous dose is found in the feces. Activated charcoal or cholestyramine may prevent reabsorption of MTX.[128]

Methotrexate Metabolism

Two MTX metabolites have been identified in subjects receiving high-dose MTX[129]: 7-OH-MTX and DAMPA. 7-OH-MTX constituted a minor percentage of material in the urine in the first 12 hours of infusion but 20% to 46% of material in the urine in the interval between 12 and 24 hours and as much as 86% in the period from 24 to 48 hours. A second metabolite, DAMPA, has also been identified in plasma and urine, and only at later times does this metabolite become an important fraction of drug-derived material (25% of material excreted in the interval from 24 to 48 hours).[103] Both of these metabolites are known to accumulate in plasma, and at 48 hours after high-dose MTX, they account for most of the MTX-derived material in plasma and may give spuriously high MTX values measured by immunoassays.

In the liver, aldehyde oxidase inactivates a small portion of the MTX dose to 7-OH-MTX, an inactive metabolite which is excreted in the bile. Levels of the 7-OH-MTX metabolite are 700-fold higher in bile than in serum.[130] The extent to which polyglutamated 7-OH-MTX is formed in malignant but not in normal cells may be important in the selective action of MTX because the 7-OH PGs are modest inhibitors of AICAR transformylase and TS. These metabolites are weak inhibitors ($K_i = 9$ nM) of DHFR.[131] No dose adjustment of MTX is necessary for patients with mild hepatic dysfunction. The drug is contraindicated in patients with cirrhosis or biliary obstruction because of its intrinsic hepatotoxicity.

The pteroic acid metabolite DAMPA is probably formed by the action of bacterial carboxypeptidases in the gastrointestinal tract. Enzymes specific for cleaving the glutamate terminal peptide bonds have been characterized.[132] DAMPA is also produced by the enzymatic cleavage of MTX in a rescue regimen with glucarpidase (see below).[2]

While the metabolites play no proven role in producing MTX toxicity or therapeutic activity, 7-OH-MTX and DAMPA are both less soluble than the parent drug. 7-OH-MTX constituted more than 50% of precipitated intrarenal material in study of MTX-induced renal failure in monkeys.[129] The role of either metabolite in the clinical syndrome of MTX-associated nephrotoxicity in humans is unproven.

Toxicity

The toxic side effects of pralatrexate and pemetrexed are described in a separate section.

Primary Toxic Effects of MTX

The primary toxic effects of folate antagonists are myelosuppression and gastrointestinal mucositis. The incidence and severity of these and other toxicities depend on the specific dose, schedule, and route of drug administration. The intestinal and oral epithelia are more sensitive than granulocyte and platelet precursors in drug schedules using prolonged, low-dose infusion. In mice, the threshold plasma concentration of MTX required to inhibit DNA synthesis in bone marrow has been estimated to be 10 nM, whereas gastrointestinal epithelium is inhibited at 5 nM plasma MTX.[133] This differential sensitivity is believed to result from greater accumulation and persistence of MTX PGs in intestinal epithelium as compared to bone marrow. Mucositis usually appears 3 to 7 days after drug administration and precedes the onset of a fall in white blood count or platelet count by several days. In patients with compromised renal function, small doses (25 mg or less) may provide cytotoxic blood levels for up to 3 to 5 days and may result in serious bone marrow toxicity. Myelosuppression and mucositis usually peak at 5 to 7 days and return to baseline within 14 days.

The introduction of high-dose MTX regimens (>500 mg/m^2) with leucovorin rescue[134] has been associated with a spectrum of toxicities that may become overwhelming or fatal. Careful attention to pretreatment hydration and urine alkalinization and routine monitoring of drug pharmacokinetics have largely prevented serious toxicity. High-dose MTX regimens use otherwise lethal doses in a 4- to 36-hour infusion, followed by a 24- to 48-hour period of multiple leucovorin doses to terminate the toxic effect of MTX. Several of the more commonly used high-dose regimens and their related pharmacokinetics are presented in Table 7.4. For each regimen, successful rescue by leucovorin depends on the rapid elimination of MTX by the kidneys. Early experience with high-dose regimens, however, indicated that MTX itself may have acute toxic effects on renal function during the period of drug infusion, leading to delayed drug clearance, inappropriately high drug levels in plasma, ineffective rescue by leucovorin, and a host of secondary toxicities, including severe myelosuppression, mucositis, and desquamation. In early clinical trials of high-dose MTX, many toxic deaths were recorded.[135]

Drug-induced renal dysfunction is usually manifested as an abrupt rise in serum blood urea nitrogen and creatinine and a corresponding fall in urine output. It arises from the precipitation of MTX and possibly its less soluble metabolites, 7-OH-MTX and DAMPA, in the acidic environment of the renal tubules.[129,135] A direct toxic effect of antifolates on the renal tubule, however, has been suggested by the observation that aminopterin, an equally soluble compound that is used at one-tenth the dose of MTX, is also associated with renal toxicity, as is pemetrexed; however, a direct nephrotoxic role of MTX has not been substantiated in clinical investigations.[136] The syndrome of MTX-induced renal failure with drug precipitation in the renal tubules, first shown in a monkey model system, has been demonstrated in renal biopsies in a patient treated with high-dose MTX.[135]

To prevent precipitation, most centers use vigorous hydration (e.g., 2.5 to 3.5 L of fluid per square meter per 24 hours, beginning 12 hours before MTX infusion and continuing for 24 to 48 hours), with alkalinization of the urine (45 to 50 mEq of sodium bicarbonate per liter of intravenous fluid). The MTX infusion should not begin until urine flow exceeds 100 mL/h and urine pH is 7.0 or higher, and these parameters should be carefully monitored during the course of drug infusion.

With hydration and alkalinization of urine, the incidence of renal failure and myelosuppression has been markedly reduced. No change in the rate of MTX excretion or alteration of plasma pharmacokinetics results from the intense hydration used in the preparatory regimen previously described[120]; thus, these safety measures should have no deleterious effect on the therapeutic efficacy of the regimen. However, despite careful attention to the details of hydration and alkalinization, 1% to 5% of patients develop renal dysfunction and are at risk for serious or even fatal toxicity. In these patients, delayed MTX clearance from plasma and can be predicted by routine monitoring of drug concentration in plasma at appropriate times after drug infusion.[137] In an analysis of 790 patients treated with high-dose MTX for osteosarcoma, the incidence of delayed MTX clearance (plasma level >5 μM at 24 hours postinfusion) was 1.6% per cycle of treatment.[137] The specific time for monitoring, and the guidelines for distinguishing between normal and dangerously elevated levels, must be determined for each regimen and for each assay method. In general, a time point for monitoring well into the final phase of drug disappearance, 24 to 48 hours after the start of infusion, is chosen. Nonsteroidal anti-inflammatory drugs (NSAIDs) decrease glomerular filtration and inhibit MTX exporters, delaying MTX excretion, and have been associated with severe MTX toxicity.[138]

Early detection of elevated concentrations of MTX allows institution of specific clinical measures. Leucovorin in increased doses is required in these patients and must be continued until plasma MTX concentration falls below 100 nmol/L. Because of the competitive relationship between MTX and leucovorin, the leucovorin dose must be increased in proportion to the plasma concentration of MTX. Small doses of leucovorin are unable to prevent toxicity in patients with markedly elevated drug levels, even when leucovorin is continued beyond 48 hours.[136] A reasonable course is to treat with leucovorin at a dosage of 100 mg/m^2 every 6 hours for patients with MTX levels of 1 μmol/L and to increase this dosage in proportion to the MTX level above 1 μM up to a maximum of 500 mg/m^2 leucovorin. These doses of calcium leucovorin may elevate serum calcium levels, particularly in patients with renal dysfunction. An alternative is to use levofolinate, the L-isomer, allowing a dose reduction of 50%. Subsequent leucovorin dosage adjustments should be based on repeated plasma MTX levels taken at 24-hour intervals. In vitro studies indicate that leucovorin alone may not rescue patients with plasma MTX above 10 μmol/L.

The absorption of oral leucovorin is saturable such that the bioavailability of the compound is limited above total doses of 40 mg. The fractional absorption of a 40-mg dose is 0.78, whereas that of 60- and 100-mg doses is 0.62 and 0.42, respectively. For this reason, leucovorin is usually administered intravenously to assure its absorption in high-risk settings.

Because of the variable effectiveness of leucovorin in preventing toxicity in patients with levels of 10 μmol/L or greater at 48 hours, alternative methods of rescue have been developed. Hemodialysis has been effective in reducing plasma MTX concentration and preventing toxicity in patients with MTX-induced renal failure.[139] Clearance of MTX from plasma with continuous flow, high-flux hemodialysis approached 0.77 mL/min/kg, very close to the value of 1 mL/min/kg found in patients with normal renal function.

TABLE

7.4 *High-dose methotrexate (HD MTX) therapy*

Hydration and urinary alkalinization

Administer a total of 2.5 to 3.5 L/m^2/d of IV fluids starting 12 h before and continuing for 24 to 48 h after administration of MTX drug infusion. Sodium bicarbonate 45 to 50 mEq/L of IV fluid to keep urine pH > 7.0.

Commonly used drug infusion regimens

MTX dose	Duration (h)	Fluid (L/24 h)	Bicarbonate (mEq/24 h)	Leucovorin calcium rescue	Onset of rescue (h after start of MTX)
1.5 to 7.5 g/m^2	6.0	3/m^2	NS	15 mg IV q3h × 3, then 15 mg PO q6h × 7	18
8 to 12 g/m^2	4.0	1.5 to 2.0/m^2	2 to 3/kg	10 mg PO q6h × 10	20
3.0 to 7.5 g/m^2	0.3	3/m^2	288	10 mg/m^2 IV × 1, then 10 mg/m^2 PO q6h × 12	24
1 g/m^2	24.0	2.4/m^2	48/m^2	15 mg/m^2 IV q6h × 2, then 3 mg/m^2 PO q12h × 3	36
1.0 to 7.5 g/m^2	0.5	3/m^2	288	10 mg/m IV × 1, then 10 mg/m^2 PO q6h × 11	24

IV, intravenously; NS, not specified; PO, per os.
Adapted from Ackland SP, Schilsky RL. High-dose methotrexate: a critical reappraisal. *J Clin Oncol.* 1987;5(12):2017-2031. Reprinted with permission. Copyright © 1987 American Society of Clinical Oncology. All rights reserved.

Suggested Monitoring Points

MTX drug levels above 5 × 10^{-7} mol/L at 48 h after the start of MTX infusion require continued leucovorin rescue.[a] A general guideline for leucovorin rescue is as follows:

MTX level	Leucovorin dosage
5 × 10^{-7} mol/L	15 mg/m^2 q6h × 8
1 × 10^{-6} mol/L	100 mg/m^2 q6h × 8
2 × 10^{-6} mol/L	200 mg/m^2 q6h × 8

[a]MTX drug levels should be measured every 24 h and the dosage of leucovorin adjusted until the MTX level is <5 × 10^{-8} mol/L.

A bacterial enzyme, carboxypeptidase G2, which inactivates MTX by removal of its terminal glutamate, producing the (4-deoxy-4-amino pteroic acid) DAMP metabolite, instantly destroys circulating MTX when infused intravenously.[132] A recombinant form, glucarpidase (G2), is now approved for rescue in high-dose MTX patients in renal failure. DeAngelis et al.[140] conducted a pilot study to determine the efficacy of G2 rescue after high-dose MTX in patients with recurrent cerebral lymphoma. All patients had at least a 2-log decline in plasma MTX levels within 5 minutes of CPDG2 administration, whereas CSF MTX concentrations remained elevated for 4 hours after CPDG2. No G2-related toxicity was observed, and anti-CPDG2 activity antibodies were not detected in any patient. Additional work has established that G2 rescue is a safe and effective antidote for high-risk patients (drug levels above 1 μM 24 to 48 hours after infusion, with associated renal failure) after high-dose MTX chemotherapy.[141] Following G2

administration, MTX levels disappear rapidly, but often rebound to 1 to 5 μM levels 24 to 28 hours after G2, as drug re-enters the plasma compartment from tissues and as enzyme levels fall. The major metabolic product, 7-OH-MTX, has a half-life in plasma of 10 hours and will cross-react in immunoassays for the parent drug. An HPLC assay is specific for MTX and can be used to follow drug disappearance after G2. The enzyme has a half-life in plasma of 6 to 9 hours. It readily cleaves natural folates, including leucovorin. Therefore, leucovorin rescue should be restarted no sooner than 2 hours after G2 and probably would not survive in plasma until the enzyme has proceeded through several half-lives. The dosage of leucovorin should be based on the residual MTX level in plasma.

Additional analysis indicates that G2 rescue is indicated and effective for patients who have received high-dose MTX for up to 24 hours and have plasma MTX concentrations above 30 μM at 36 hours, 10 μM at 42 hours, or 5 μM at 48 hours, in association with elevated creatinine. The dose of G2, 50 units/kg, as approved by the FDA, may be unnecessarily high. Capping the dose at 2,000 units provides equivalent rescue, regardless of patients' weight, and reduces the considerable cost of G2.[142]

Other Toxicities

Hepatotoxicity

In addition to its inhibitory effects on rapidly dividing tissues, MTX has toxic effects on nondividing tissues not explained by its primary action on DNA synthesis. High-dose MTX commonly causes rapidly reversible hepatic enzyme elevations but rarely significant long-term damage. In chronic MTX therapy for psoriasis or rheumatoid arthritis, elevated liver enzymes were detected in 13% of patients over the course of a year, but only 4% or less stopped treatment because of liver toxicity. Less than 3% are found to have portal fibrosis on biopsy, and on rare occasions, this lesion may progress to frank cirrhosis.[143]

Acute elevations of liver enzymes after high-dose MTX administration usually return to normal within 10 days. The frequency and severity of liver enzyme elevations appear to be directly related to the number of MTX doses received.[144] Liver biopsy reveals fatty infiltration but no evidence of hepatocellular necrosis or periportal fibrosis. The late occurrence of cirrhosis in patients treated with high-dose MTX has not been reported.

Pneumonitis

MTX causes a poorly understood, and in most cases self-limited pneumonitis, with fever, cough, and an interstitial pulmonary infiltrate.[145] Eosinophilia has not been a consistent finding, either in the peripheral blood or in open lung biopsy specimens. Lung biopsies reveal interstitial edema, and an inflammatory infiltrate, rarely with noncaseating granulomas. The failure of some patients to react to reinstitution of MTX therapy suggests that the cause may not be hypersensitivity, but infectious or related to tissue damage. In patient on long-term weekly low-dose MTX therapy for rheumatoid arthritis, approximately 5% develop MTX-associated lung toxicity.[146] Clinical symptoms of MTX toxicity in the cohort included the subacute development of shortness of breath (93%), cough (82%), and fever (69%); 5 of 27 patients experienced a fatal outcome. Early symptom recognition and the cessation of MTX administration will avoid the serious and sometimes fatal outcome of this MTX-associated toxicity. Corticosteroids have been used with apparent benefit in a small number of patients who ultimately recovered.

Induction of EBV-Related Lymphoproliferative Disorder

Patients on long-term MTX for immunosuppression are prone to develop a *lymphoproliferative disorder* (LPD) related to reactivation of Epstein-Barr virus (EBV). A spectrum of presentations have been reported, including benign mononucleosis like illness, malignant lymphomas, and vasculitis with lymphoid infiltration of the skin. With pulmonary involvement, it may present with chest pain and shortness of breath and nodular opacities on chest x-ray. These changes usually regress with drug discontinuation. In most cases,

biopsy shows no organisms, but central necrosis surrounded by lymphocytes and epithelioid cells. Serological studies may reveal evidence of EBV infection.[147] In patients with a biopsy showing frank malignant lymphoma, appropriate chemotherapy may be required. Skin ulcerations independent of LPD have been described as a toxic adverse effect of MTX.

Hypersensitivity

Acute hypersensitivity reaction to MTX occurs rarely.[148] Symptoms may range from urticaria and wheezing to acute cardiovascular collapse, which may recur on rechallenge of such patients. Patients receiving bacille Calmette-Guérin or other immune stimulants may be at increased risk. In a few instances, patients had hypersensitivity to folic acid as well. The cross-reactivity to folic acid would not affect the major circulating forms of the vitamin, which are found in a reduced form in tissues and in the systemic circulation. In the authors' limited experience, desensitization in patients with mild initial reactions, using small incremental doses of MTX with corticosteroids and antihistamines, enabled retreatment at full doses of MTX.

Reversible oligospermia with testicular failure has been reported in men treated with high-dose MTX.[149] No alterations in follicle-stimulating hormone, luteinizing hormone, estradiol, or progesterone have been observed in women exposed to MTX. MTX is a potent abortifacient, probably related to its effects on the placenta.

Pharmacokinetics and Toxicity of Methotrexate in the Central Nervous System

Because of its high degree of ionization at physiological pH, MTX penetrates into the CSF with difficulty. During a constant intravenous drug infusion, the ratio of venous MTX concentration to CSF concentration is approximately 30:1 at equilibrium.[150] Thus, plasma levels in excess of 30 μmol/L would be required to achieve the concentration of 1 μmol/L that is thought to be necessary for killing of leukemic cells. Protocols for prophylaxis against meningeal leukemia and lymphoma using systemic high-dose infusions of MTX have demonstrated that high-dose MTX infusions are a reasonable treatment alternative to intrathecal prophylaxis. Overt meningeal leukemia increases the CSF: plasma ratio and experience supports the use of MTX at a loading dose of 700 mg/m² followed by a 23-hour infusion of 2,800 mg/m², with leucovorin rescue as an alternative to intrathecal treatment for patients with carcinomatous meningitis. This regimen achieves the requisite CSF levels of 1 μmol/L.[67] In children with ALL, a diminished CSF:plasma ratio increases the risk of CNS relapse.[151]

Direct intrathecal injection of MTX is the standard measure for the treatment and prophylaxis of meningeal malignancy.[152] Drug injected into the intrathecal space distributes in a total volume of approximately 120 mL for patients over 3 years of age. Thus, a maximal total dose of 12 mg is advised for all patients over 3 years, with lower doses indicated for younger children. Based on pharmacokinetic studies, Bleyer[153] has recommended a dose of 6 mg for age 1 or younger, 8 mg for ages 1 to 2, and 10 mg for ages 2 to 3. The peak CSF concentration achieved by this schedule is approximately 100 µmol/L. Lumbar CSF drug concentrations decline in a biphasic pattern with a terminal half-life of 7 to 16 hours. This terminal phase of disappearance may be considerably prolonged in patients with active meningeal disease and in older-age patients.[152] MTX is cleared from spinal fluid with bulk resorption of spinal fluid (i.e., "bulk flow"), a process that may be prolonged by increases in intracranial pressure. A second component of resorption involves the active transport of this organic anion from the CSF by the choroid plexus. A prolongation of the terminal half-life has been described in patients who develop drug-related neurotoxicity, although a causal relationship between abnormal pharmacokinetics and neurotoxicity has not been firmly established.[152]

MTX administered into the lumbar space distributes poorly over the cerebral convexities and into the ventricular spaces.[150] The concentration gradient between lumbar and ventricular CSF may exceed 10:1. Although this uneven distribution has no documented role in determining clinical relapse of patients treated for meningeal leukemia, awareness of this potential problem has led to clinical trials using direct intraventricular injection of MTX via an Ommaya reservoir for treatment of leukemia and other malignancies involving the subdural space. A regimen in which 1 mg MTX is injected into the Ommaya reservoir every 12 hours for 3 days yields continuous CSF levels above 0.5 µM, and achieved therapeutic results in pediatric ALL equivalent to those with the conventional intralumbar injection.[153] Moreover, this concentration × time regimen was associated with a considerable reduction in neurotoxic side effects, presumably owing to the avoidance of high peak levels of drug associated with 12 mg MTX doses.

Three different neurotoxic syndromes have been observed after treatment with intrathecal MTX. The most common and most immediate side effect is an acute chemical arachnoiditis manifested as severe headache, nuchal rigidity, vomiting, fever, and inflammatory cell pleocytosis of the spinal fluid. This constellation of symptoms appears to be a function of the frequency and dose of drug administered and may be ameliorated either by reduction in dose or by a change in therapy to intrathecal cytosine arabinoside. A less acute but more serious neurotoxic syndrome has been observed in approximately 10% of patients treated with intrathecal MTX. This subacute toxicity appears during the 2nd or 3rd week of treatment, usually in adult patients with active meningeal leukemia, and is manifested as motor paralysis of the extremities, cranial nerve palsy, seizures, or coma. Readministration of MTX, in some cases with a reduction in dose, is well tolerated in most cases.[154] Because MTX pharmacokinetics are abnormal in these patients, particularly in those with active meningeal leukemia, the suspicion is that this subacute neurotoxicity may be the result of extended exposure to toxic drug concentrations. Other risk factors for acute and subacute neurotoxicity are concomitant high-dose MTX, given during the consolidation phase of ALL treatment, and concomitant intrathecal cytosine arabinoside.[154] Finally, a more chronic demyelinating encephalopathy has been observed in children months or years after intrathecal MTX therapy or less commonly after high-dose MTX alone.[155] The primary symptoms of this toxicity are dementia, limb spasticity, and, in more advanced cases, coma. Computerized axial tomography (CT) has revealed ventricular enlargement, white matter changes, cortical thinning, and diffuse intracerebral calcification in children who have received prophylactic intrathecal MTX. Most of these patients had

also received cranial irradiation (>2,000 rad), and all had received systemic chemotherapy, including high-dose MTX.

Also associated with high-dose systemic MTX is an acute transient cognitive dysfunction, which occurs in 4% to 15% of treated patients.[155] The syndrome consists of any combination of paresis, aphasia, behavioral abnormalities, and seizures. The neurologic events occur on an average of 6 days after the MTX dose, and in most cases, completely resolve, usually within 48 to 72 hours. Patients may have received any number of MTX doses before the onset of this neurotoxic event, and some patients may have repeat episodes with subsequent MTX doses. In general, CSF and CT scans of the brain are normal, but low-density lesions have been noted in some cases.[156] The electroencephalogram may represent the only abnormal study and shows a diffuse or focal slowing. No clinical evidence exists to support the use of leucovorin.

A comparison of neurologic toxicities was undertaken in a prospective trial involving 49 children with acute leukemia treated with either intrathecal MTX plus radiation or high-dose systemic MTX for CNS prophylaxis.[157] Long-term toxicities were similar with either treatment option, and overall decreases in intelligence quotients were found to be clinically significant in 61% of the children. In addition, 58% of the patients treated with systemic therapy had abnormal electroencephalograms and 57% of those treated with intrathecal MTX and radiation experienced a somnolence syndrome.

The etiology of the MTX-associated neurotoxicity is unknown. Vascular events in the form of vasospasm or emboli have been proposed to explain these neurologic abnormalities, and studies have suggested alterations in brain glucose metabolism after MTX treatment.[158] One study found that, in children treated for acute leukemia with MTX, seizures were associated with acute elevations in serum homocysteine levels following MTX treatment and discussed evidence that homocysteine metabolites are neurotoxic.[159] These investigators looked at a possible association between neurotoxicity and MTHFR genotype, in view of evidence that MTHFR variants cause a deficiency of 5-methyltetrahydrofolate, the cofactor required for the conversion of homocysteine to methionine, but they found no evidence to support that theory.

Inadvertent overdose of intrathecal MTX generally has a fatal outcome. Immediate lumbar puncture with CSF removal along with ventriculolumbar perfusion has been successfully used to avert catastrophe in such situations.[160]

In clinical practice, for patients with meningeal carcinomatosis, intrathecal MTX and intrathecal cytosine arabinoside (see Chapter 9) give equivalent results in terms of alleviation of acute symptoms and a 4- to 5-month median survival.[161] Prognosis is determined by the ability to alter the course of systemic disease.

Pharmacogenomic Determinants of Drug Toxicity and Response

Despite analyses of multiple genetic variants for the enzymes of folate metabolism, the folate transporters involved in drug excretion and metabolism, the findings implicating specific variants as determinants of toxicity or response have not been consistent, perhaps due to different antifolate regimens (low versus high dose), and diverse populations studied (children versus adults).[162] A variant of the reduced folate carrier (RFC1) (G80A) impairs uptake and has been implicated in resistance[163] in pediatric ALL and in osteosarcoma, but further studies failed to show the same association. Other variants affecting drug clearance by MTX exporters have been linked to high drug levels and toxicity,[164] while variants affecting the conversion of reduced folates to 5-methyltetrahydroflate by methylenetetrahydrofolate reductase (MTHFR) (C677T and A1298C) have been associated with hepatic and other toxicity, and with relapse in ALL.[165] However, polymorphisms of MTHFR (or RFC1) were not correlated with toxicity of high-dose MTX in children with ALL (see Chapter 5 for further discussion).[166]

Clinical Dosage Schedules

A variety of dosage schedules and routes of administration are used clinically, including high-dose therapy with the addition of leucovorin rescue. The selection of an appropriate schedule depends largely on the specific disease being treated, on other antineoplastic agents or radiation to be used in combination regimens, on the patient's tolerance for host toxicity, and on other factors that might alter pharmacokinetics. Parenteral schedules are preferred for induction therapy regimens in which maximal concentrations and duration of exposure are desirable in an effort to achieve complete remission. High-dose MTX regimens and leucovorin rescue offer the advantage of minimal bone marrow toxicity. This regimen, however, can safely be used only in patients with normal renal and hepatic function and under conditions in which no large extracellular accumulations of fluid are present. Patients of advanced age tend to experience slower drug clearance and a higher incidence of renal toxicity. As emphasized previously, high-dose regimens should be instituted only when plasma monitoring is available to determine the adequacy of drug clearance and the risk of serious toxicity. Furthermore, because leucovorin may rescue tumor cells as well as normal cells, the optimal dose, schedule, and clinical utility of high-dose MTX with leucovorin rescue need to be carefully defined.

Clinical Pharmacology and Toxicity of Other Antifolates

Pemetrexed

TS represents a logical target for new drug development using folate analogues. Of the many antifolates synthesized as TS antagonists, pemetrexed (LY231514), a pyrrolo(2,3-D)pyrimidine-based antifolate analogue (see Fig. 7.1), is the most effective. Its key features are shown in Table 7.1. Pemetrexed is readily transported into cells via the RFC and by the proton-coupled carrier described earlier.[167]

As noted above, it is a primary inhibitor of TS, with lesser potency for other folate-dependent enzymes.

Its antitumor efficacy against human tumor cell lines is modulated by external folate concentrations such that folate or reduced folate (RF) supplementation inhibits its effects.[168] Pretreatment with folic acid in mice protected normal tissues from pemetrexed while preserving the antitumor activity, but at drug doses that would not be tolerated in humans due to renal toxicity. In patients, severe myelosuppression due to pemetrexed correlates with high pretreatment serum concentrations of homocysteine, an indicator of folate deficiency and/or B12 deficiency, and in patients with pretreatment elevation of methylmalonic acid, an indicator of B12

deficiency. Addition of vitamin B_{12} (1 mg intramuscularly every 9 weeks) and folic acid (400 μg/mg/d beginning 1 week prior to each course of pemetrexed and continuing through treatment) resulted in an improved and predictable toxicity profile, without diminishing antitumor efficacy, in patients with mesothelioma treated with pemetrexed.[169] The primary toxicities of pemetrexed are myelosuppression, diarrhea, peripheral edema, and a frequent and bothersome rash, which is effectively suppressed by pretreatment dexamethasone, 4 mg on days −1, 0, and +1. At the doses commonly used, 500 mg/m² every 3 weeks, the drug is well tolerated. Resistance to pemetrexed in the clinical setting is poorly understood but, in experimental systems, has been attributed to mutations in FPGS, increased TS, or loss of RFC transport.[167]

Clinical Pharmacokinetics and Toxicity

Pemetrexed is eliminated as parent drug, primarily (70% to 90%) by renal tubular secretion and glomerular filtration. It has a serum half-life of approximately 4 hours in patients with normal renal function, but the half-life increases markedly in subjects who have a creatinine clearance of 30 mL/min or less.[170,171] At doses above 500 mg/m², the drug causes a decrease in creatinine clearance in a fraction of patients and greater toxicity in those with diminished renal function.[171] Drug clearance correlates with glomerular filtration rate. At approved doses, and with vitamin supplementation, the drug can be given safely to patients with a glomerular filtration rate of at least 40 mL/min. The drug is poorly absorbed by oral administration and is therefore given as a brief infusion of 500 mg/m² once every 3 weeks. There is no proven therapeutic benefit of escalating dose above the approved dose and schedule. TS, FPGS, and RFC expression have all been implicated in resistance to pemetrexed, but there is no consensus regarding these mechanisms in clinical trials.[172]

Pemetrexed, in combination with cisplatin, has been approved for treatment of mesothelioma, in combination with cisplatin. Pemetrexed is also approved for treating non–small cell lung cancer, either as a second-line single agent or as first-line therapy with carboplatin. Its activity is primarily confined to the subset of adenocarcinoma.

Pralatrexate

Pralatrexate, (Fig. 7.1), resulted from a series of experiments to develop analogues that had favorable transport properties (see Table 7.2). While its inhibition of DHFR was comparable in potency to MTX,[173] it proved to have 10-fold greater affinity for the RFC transporter than MTX and inhibited tumor cell growth at 30- to 40-fold lower extracellular concentrations than MTX; its increased potency is likely related to its more efficient transport and its more avid polyglutamation. It was only partially cross-resistant with MTX in experimental tumors.[32,172] Clinical trials demonstrated consistent activity against cutaneous T-cell lymphoma and peripheral T-cell lymphoma, for which it is now approved.[173]

The recommended dose of pralatrexate is 30 mg/m²/wk for 6 of 7 weeks, the dose-limiting toxicities being stomatitis, rash, thrombocytopenia, neutropenia, fatigue, and hepatic enzyme elevations. The incidence of stomatitis was reduced by supplementing folic acid (1 mg/d for 10 days prior to treatment and continuing thereafter) and B12 (1,000 mg orally or 1 mg IM every 8 to 10 weeks). The drug is cleared by excretion in the urine and has a plasma $t_{1/2}$ of 12 to 18 hours, although studies are preliminary.[32] No guidelines are available for modifying dose for renal dysfunction, but it is likely that reductions in proportion to abnormalities in creatine clearance will be necessary.

References

1. Farber S, Diamond LK, Mercer RD, et al. Temporary remission in acute leukemia in children produced by folic acid antagonist 4-amethopteroylglutamic acid (aminopterin). *N Engl J Med.* 1948;238:787.

2. Allegra CJ, Fine RL, Drake JC, et al. The effect of methotrexate on intracellular folate pools in human MCF-7 breast cancer cells. Evidence for direct inhibition of purine synthesis. *J Biol Chem.* 1986;261:6478-6485.

3. Pui C-H, Campana D, Pei D, et al. Treating childhood acute lymphoblastic leukemia without cranial irradiation. *N Engl J Med.* 2009;360:2730-2741.

4. Walling J. From methotrexate to pemetrexed and beyond. Review of the pharmacodynamic and clinical properties of antifolates. *Invest New Drugs* 2006;24:37-77.

5. Baram J, Allegra CJ, Fine RL, et al. Effect of methotrexate on intracellular folate pools in purified myeloid precursor cells from normal human bone marrow. *J Clin Invest.* 1987;79:692-697.

6. Allegra CJ, Chabner BA, Drake JC, et al. Enhanced inhibition of thymidylate synthase by methotrexate polyglutamates. *J Biol Chem.* 1985;260:9720-9726.

7. Allegra CJ, Drake JC, Jolivet J, et al. Inhibition of phosphoribosylaminoimidazolecarboxamide transformylase by methotrexate and dihydrofolic acid polyglutamates. *Proc Natl Acad Sci U S A.* 1985;82:4881-4885

8. Allegra CJ, Hoang K, Yeh GC, et al. Evidence for direct inhibition of de novo purine synthesis in human MCF-7 breast cells as a principal mode of metabolic inhibition by methotrexate. *J Biol Chem.* 1987;262:13520-13526.

9. Thomas S, Fisher KH, Snowden JA, et al. Methotrexate is a JAK/STAT pathway inhibitor. *PLoS One.* 2015;10(7):e0130078. doi:10.1371/journal.pone.00130078.

10. Sirotnak FM, DeGraw JI, Schmid FA, et al. New folate analogs of the 10-deaza-aminopterin series. Further evidence for markedly increased antitumor efficacy compared with methotrexate in ascitic and solid murine tumor models. *Cancer Chemother Pharmacol.* 1984;12:26-30.

11. Antony AC, Kane MA, Portillo RM, et al. Studies of the role of a particulate folate-binding protein in the uptake of 5-methyltetrahydrofolate by cultured human KB cells. *J Biol Chem.* 1985;260:14911-14917.

12. Fan J, Vitols KS, Huennekens FM. Biotin derivatives of methotrexate and folate. Synthesis and utilization for affinity purification of two membrane-associated folate transporters from L1210 cells. *J Biol Chem.* 1991;266:14862-14865.

13. Zhao R, Qui A, Tsai E, et al. The proton-coupled folate transporter: impact on pemetrexed Transport and on antifolates activities compared with the reduced folate carrier. *Mol Pharmacol.* 2008;74:854-862.

14. Goldman ID, Zhao R. Molecular, biochemical and cellular pharmacology of pemetrexed. *Semin Oncol.* 2002;(suppl 18):3-17.

15. Zhao R, Wang PJ, Gao F, et al. Residues 45 and 404 in the murine reduced folate carrier may interact to alter carrier binding and mobility. *Biochim Biophys Acta.* 2003;1613(1-2):49-56.

16. Sharina IG, Zhao R, Wang Y, et al. Mutational analysis of the functional role of conserved arginine and lysine residues in transmembrane domains of the murine reduced folate carrier. *Mol Pharmacol.* 2001;59(5):1022-1028.

17. Elwood PC, Kane MA, Portillo RM, et al. The isolation, characterization, and comparison of the membrane-associated and soluble folate-binding proteins from human KB cells. *J Biol Chem.* 1986;261:15416-15423.

18. Cheung A, Bax HJ, Illeva KM, et al. Targeting folate receptor alpha for cancer treatment. *Oncotarget.* 2016;7(32):52553-52574. doi: 10.18632/oncotarget.9651.

19. Shen F, Ross JF, Wang X, et al. Identification of a novel folate receptor, a truncated receptor, and receptor type beta in hematopoietic cells: cDNA cloning, expression, immunoreactivity, and tissue specificity. *Biochemistry.* 1994;33:1209-1215.

20. Allard JE, Risinger JI, Morrison C, et al. Overexpression of folate binding protein is associated with shortened progression-free survival in uterine adenocarcinomas. *Gynecol Oncol.* 2007;107:52-55.

21. Shen F, Zheng X, Wang J, et al. Identification of amino acid residues that determine the differential ligand specificities of folate receptors alpha and beta. *Biochemistry.* 1997;36:6157-6163.

22. Anderson RG, Kamen BA, Rothberg KG, et al. Potocytosis: sequestration and transport of small molecules by caveolae. *Science.* 1992;255:410-411.

23. Schuetz JD, Matherly LH, Westin EH, et al. Evidence for a functional defect in the translocation of the methotrexate transport carrier in a methotrexate-resistant murine L1210 leukemia cell line. *J Biol Chem.* 1988;263:9840-9847.

24. Jansen G, Westerhof GR, Kathmann I, et al. Identification of a membrane-associated folate-binding protein in human leukemic CCRF-CEM cells with transport-related methotrexate resistance [published erratum appears in Cancer Res. 1995;55(18):4203]. *Cancer Res.* 1989;49:2455-2459.

25. Zhao R, Assaraf YG, Goldman ID. A mutated murine reduced folate carrier (RFC1) with increased affinity for folic acid, decreased affinity for methotrexate, and an obligatory anion requirement for transport function. *J Biol Chem.* 1998;273:19065-19071.

26. Gifford AJ, Haber M, Witt TL, et al. Role of the E45K-reduced folate carrier gene mutation in methotrexate resistance in human leukemia cells. *Leukemia.* 2002;16(12):2379-2387.

27. Trippett T, Schlemmer S, Elisseyeff Y, et al. Defective transport as a mechanism of acquired resistance to methotrexate in patients with acute lymphoblastic leukemia. *Blood.* 1992;80:1158-1162.

28. Guo W, Healey JH, Meyers PA, et al. Mechanisms of methotrexate resistance in osteosarcoma. *Clin Cancer Res.* 1999;5:621-627.

29. Ifergan I, Meller I, Issakov J, et al. Reduced folate carrier protein expression in osteosarcoma: implications for the prediction of tumor chemosensitivity. *Cancer.* 2003;98(9):1958-1966.

30. Sirotnak FM, DeGraw JI. A new analogue of 10-deazaanimopterin with markedly enhanced curative effects against human tumor xenografts in mice. *Cancer Chemother Pharmacol.* 1998;42:313-318.

31. Zhao R, Hanscom M, Chattopadhyay S, et al. Selective Preservation of pemetrexed pharmacological activity in HeLa cells lacking the reduced folate carrier: association with the presence of a secondary transport pathway. *Cancer Res.* 2004;64(9):3313-3319.

32. Molina JR. Pralatrexate, a dihydrofolate reductase inhibitor for the potential treatment of several malignancies. *Drugs.* 2008;11:508-521.

33. Henderson GB, Tsuji JM. Methotrexate efflux in L1210 cells. Kinetic and specificity properties of the efflux system sensitive to bromosulfophthalein and its possible identity with a system which mediates the efflux of 3′,5′-cyclic AMP. *J Biol Chem.* 1987;262:13571-13578.

34. Vlaming MLH, Pala Z, van Esch A, et al. Functionally overlapping roles of Abcg2 (Bcrp1) and Abcc2 (Mrp2) in the elimination of methotrexate and its main toxic metabolite 7-hydroxymethotrexate in vivo. *Clin Cancer Res.* 2009;15:3084-3093.

35. Kitamura Y, Hirouchi M, Kusuhara H, et al. Increasing systemic exposure of methotrexate by active efflux mediated by multidrug resistance-associated protein 3 (Mrp3/Abcc3). *J Pharmacol Exp Ther.* 2008;327:465-473.

36. Lawrence SA, Titus SA, Ferguson J, et al. Mammalian mitochondrial and cytosolic folylpolyglutamate synthase maintain the subcellular compartmentalization of folates. *J Biol Chem.* 2014;289:29386-29396.

37. Wojtuszkiewicz A, Raz S, Stark M, et al. Folylpolyglutamate synthetase splicing alterations in acute lymphoblastic leukemia are provoked by methotrexate and other chemotherapeutics and mediate chemoresistance. *Int J Cancer.* 2016;138:1645-1656.

38. Koizumi S, Curt GA, Fine RL, et al. Formation of methotrexate polyglutamates in purified myeloid precursor cells from normal human bone marrow. *J Clin Invest.* 1985;75:1008-1014.

39. Schilsky RL, Bailey BD, Chabner BA. Methotrexate polyglutamate synthesis by cultured human breast cancer cells. *Proc Natl Acad Sci U S A.* 1980;77:2919-2922.

40. Visentin M, Unal ES, Zhao R, Goldman ID. The membrane transport and polyglutamation of pralatrexate: a new-generation dihydrofolate reductase inhibitor. *Cancer Chemother Pharmacol.* 2013;72:597-605.

41. Jolivet J, Chabner BA. Intracellular pharmacokinetics of methotrexate polyglutamates in human breast cancer cells. Selective retention and less dissociable binding of 4-NH2-10-CH3-pteroylglutamate4 and 4-NH2–10-CH3-pteroylglutamate5 to dihydrofolate reductase. *J Clin Invest.* 1983;72:773-778.

42. Clarke L, Waxman DJ. Human liver folylpolyglutamate synthetase: biochemical characterization and interactions with folates and folate antagonists. *Arch Biochem Biophys.* 1987;256:585-596.

43. Cichowicz DJ, Shane B. Mammalian folylpoly-gamma-glutamate synthetase. 1. Purification and general properties of the hog liver enzyme. *Biochemistry.* 1987;26:504-512.

44. Cichowicz DJ, Shane B. Mammalian folylpoly-gamma-glutamate synthetase. 2. Substrate specificity and kinetic properties. *Biochemistry.* 1987;26:513-521.

45. Panetta JC, Wall A, Pui CH, et al. Methotrexate intracellular disposition in acute lymphoblastic leukemia: a mathematical model of gamma-glutamyl hydrolase activity. *Clin Cancer Res.* 2002;8(7):2423-2429.

46. Kager L, Cheok M, Yang W, et al. Folate pathway gene expression differs in subtypes of acute lymphoblastic leukemia and influences methotrexate pharmacodynamics. *J Clin Invest.* 2005;115:110-117.

47. Yao R, Schneider E, Ryan TJ, et al. Human gamma-glutamyl hydrolase: cloning and characterization of the enzyme expressed in vitro. *Proc Natl Acad Sci U S A.* 1996;93:10134-10138.

48. Cole PD, Kamen BA, Gorlick R, et al. Effects of overexpression of gamma-glutamyl hydrolase on methotrexate metabolism and resistance. *Cancer Res.* 2001;61(11):4599-4604.

49. Sirotnak FM, Chello PL, Piper JR, et al. Growth inhibitory, transport and biochemical properties of the gamma-glutamyl and gamma-aspartyl peptides of methotrexate in L1210 leukemia cells in vitro. *Biochem Pharmacol.* 1978;27:1821-1825.

50. Galivan J, Nimec Z, Balinska M. Regulation of methotrexate polyglutamate accumulation in vitro: effects of cellular folate content. *Biochem Pharmacol.* 1983;32:3244-3247.

51. Jolivet J, Cole DE, Holcenberg JS, et al. Prevention of methotrexate cytotoxicity by asparaginase inhibition of methotrexate polyglutamate formation. *Cancer Res.* 1985;45:217-220.

52. Matherly LH, Fry DW, Goldman ID. Role of methotrexate polyglutamylation and cellular energy metabolism in inhibition of methotrexate binding to dihydrofolate reductase by 5-formyltetrahydrofolate in Ehrlich ascites tumor cells in vitro. *Cancer Res.* 1983;43:2694-2699.

53. Allegra CJ, Drake JC, Jolivet J, et al. Inhibition of folate-dependent enzymes by methotrexate polyglutamates. In: Goldman ID, ed. *Proceedings of the Second Workshop on Folyl and Antifolyl Polyglutamates.* New York, NY: Praeger; 1985:348-359.

54. Shih C, Habeck LI, Mendelsohn LG, et al. Multiple folate enzyme inhibition: mechanisms of a novel pyrrolopyrimidines based antifolate LY231514 (MTA). *Adv Enzyme Regul.* 1998;135:152.

55. Samuels LL, Moccio DM, Sirotnak FM. Similar differential for total polyglutamylation and cytotoxicity among various folate analogues in human and murine tumor cells in vitro. *Cancer Res.* 1985;45:1488-1495.

56. Curt GA, Jolivet J, Carney DN, et al. Determinants of the sensitivity of human small-cell lung cancer cell lines to methotrexate. *J Clin Invest.* 1985;76:1323-1329.

57. Longo GS, Gorlick R, Tong WP, et al. Gamma-glutamyl hydrolase and folylpolyglutamate synthetase activities predict polyglutamylation of methotrexate in acute leukemias. *Oncol Res.* 1997;9:259-263.

58. Galpin AJ, Schuetz JD, Masson E, et al. Differences in folylpolyglutamate synthetase and dihydrofolate reductase expression in human B-lineage versus T-lineage leukemic lymphoblasts: mechanisms for lineage differences in methotrexate polyglutamylation and cytotoxicity. *Mol Pharmacol.* 1997;52:155-163.

59. Stark M, Wichman C, Avivi I, Assaraf YG. Aberrant splicing of folylpolyglutamate synthetase as a novel mechanism of antifolate resistance in leukemia. *Blood.* 2008;113:4362-4369.

60. Panetta JC, Yanishevski Y, Pui CH, et al. A mathematical model of in vivo methotrexate accumulation in acute lymphoblastic leukemia. *Cancer Chemother Pharmacol.* 2002;50(5):419-428.

61. Mantadakis E, Smith AK, Hynan L, et al. Methotrexate polyglutamation may lack prognostic significance in children with B-cell precursor acute lymphoblastic leukemia treated with intensive oral methotrexate. *J Pediatr Hematol Oncol.* 2002;24(8):736-642.

62. Li WW, Lin JT, Schweitzer BI, et al. Intrinsic resistance to methotrexate in human soft tissue sarcoma cell lines. *Cancer Res.* 1992;52:3908-3913.

63. Leil TA, Endo C, Adjei AA, et al. Identification and characterization of genetic variation in the folylpolyglutamate synthase gene. *Cancer Res.* 2007;67:8772-8782.

64. Matthews DA, Alden RA, Bolin JT, et al. Dihydrofolate reductase: x-ray structure of the binary complex with methotrexate. *Science.* 1977;197:452-455.

65. Lamb KM, G-Dayandandan N, Wright DL, Anderson A. Elucidating features that drive the design of selective antifolates using crystal structures of human dihydrofolate reductase. *Biochemistry.* 2013;52:7318-7326. doi:10.102/bi400852h.

66. Schweitzer BI, Srimatkandada S, Gritsman H, et al. Probing the role of two hydrophobic active site residues in the human dihydrofolate reductase by site-directed mutagenesis. *J Biol Chem.* 1989;264:20786-20795.

67. Thompson PD, Freisheim JH. Conversion of arginine to lysine at position 70 of human dihydrofolate reductase: generation of a methotrexate-insensitive mutant enzyme. *Biochemistry.* 1991;30:8124-8130.

68. Mareya SM, Sorrentino BP, Blakley RL. Protection of CCRF-CEM human lymphoid cells from antifolates by retroviral gene transfer of variants of murine dihydrofolate reductase. *Cancer Gene Ther.* 1998;5:225-235.

69. Appleman JR, Prendergast N, Delcamp TJ, et al. Kinetics of the formation and isomerization of methotrexate complexes of recombinant human dihydrofolate reductase. *J Biol Chem.* 1988;263:10304-10313.

70. Kamen BA, Whyte-Bauer W, Bertino JR. A mechanism of resistance to methotrexate. NADPH but not NADH stimulation of methotrexate binding to dihydrofolate reductase. *Biochem Pharmacol.* 1983;32:1837-1841.

71. Kumar P, Kisliuk RL, Gaumont Y, et al. Interaction of polyglutamyl derivatives of methotrexate, 10-deazaaminopterin, and dihydrofolate with dihydrofolate reductase. *Cancer Res.* 1986;46:5020-5023.

72. Allegra CJ, Boarman D. Interaction of methotrexate polyglutamates and dihydrofolate during leucovorin rescue in a human breast cancer cell line (MCF-7). *Cancer Res.* 1990;50:3574-3578.

73. White JC, Loftfield S, Goldman ID. The mechanism of action of methotrexate. III. Requirement of free intracellular methotrexate for maximal suppression of (14C)formate incorporation into nucleic acids and protein. *Mol Pharmacol.* 1975;11:287-297.

74. Boarman DM, Baram J, Allegra CJ. Mechanism of leucovorin reversal of methotrexate cytotoxicity in human MCF-7 breast cancer cells. *Biochem Pharmacol.* 1990;40:2651-2660.

75. Melera PW, Davide JP, Oen H. Antifolate-resistant Chinese hamster cells. Molecular basis for the biochemical and structural heterogeneity among dihydrofolate reductases produced by drug-sensitive and drug-resistant cell lines. *J Biol Chem.* 1988;263:1978-1990.

76. McIvor RS, Simonsen CC. Isolation and characterization of a variant dihydrofolate reductase cDNA from methotrexate-resistant murine L5178Y cells. *Nucleic Acids Res.* 1990;18:7025-7032.

77. Dedhar S, Hartley D, Fitz-Gibbons D, et al. Heterogeneity in the specific activity and methotrexate sensitivity of dihydrofolate reductase from blast cells of acute myelogenous leukemia patients. *J Clin Oncol.* 1985;3:1545-1552.

78. Bertino JR. Transfer of drug resistance genes into hematopoietic stem cells for marrow protection. *Oncologist.* 2009;13:1036-1042.

79. Haber DA, Schimke RT. Unstable amplification of an altered dihydrofolate reductase gene associated with double-minute chromosomes. *Cell.* 1981;26:355-362.

80. Hamlin JL, Biedler JL. Replication pattern of a large homogenously staining chromosome region in antifolate-resistant Chinese hamster cell lines. *J Cell Physiol.* 1981;107:101-114.

81. Brown PC, Beverley SM, Schimke RT. Relationship of amplified dihydrofolate reductase genes to double minute chromosomes in unstably resistant mouse fibroblast cell lines. *Mol Cell Biol.* 1981;1:1077-1083.

82. Haber DA, Schimke RT. Unstable amplification of an altered dihydrofolate reductase gene associated with double-minute chromosomes. *Cell.* 1981;26:355-362.

83. Meng X, Qi X, Guo H, et al. Novel role for non-homologous end joining in the formation of double minutes in methotrexate-resistant colon cancer cells. *J Med Genet.* 2015;52:135-144.

84. Hoy CA, Rice GC, Kovacs M, et al. Over-replication of DNA in S phase Chinese hamster ovary cells after DNA synthesis inhibition. *J Biol Chem.* 1987;262:11927-11934.

85. Fanin R, Banerjee D, Volkenandt M, et al. Mutations leading to antifolate resistance in Chinese hamster ovary cells after exposure to the alkylating agent ethylmethanesulfonate. *Mol Pharmacol.* 1993;44:13-21.

86. Sharma RC, Schimke RT. Enhancement of the frequency of methotrexate resistance by gamma-radiation in Chinese hamster ovary and mouse 3T6 cells. *Cancer Res.* 1989;49:3861-3866.

87. Wright JA, Smith HS, Watt FM, et al. DNA amplification is rare in normal human cells. *Proc Natl Acad Sci U S A.* 1990;87:1791-1795.

88. Mishra PJ, Humeniuk R, Mishra PJ, et al. An miR-24 microRNA binding-site polymorphism in dihydrofolate reductase gene leads to methotrexate resistance. *PNAS.* 2007;104:13513-13518.

89. Chu E, Takimoto CH, Voeller D, et al. Specific binding of human dihydrofolate reductase protein to dihydrofolate reductase messenger RNA in vitro. *Biochemistry.* 1993;32:4756-4760.

90. Ercikan-Abali EA, Banerjee D, Waltham MC, et al. Dihydrofolate reductase protein inhibits its own translation by binding to dihydrofolate reductase mRNA sequences within the coding region. *Biochemistry.* 1997;36:12317-12322.

91. Curt GA, Carney DN, Cowan KH, et al. Unstable methotrexate resistance in human small-cell carcinoma associated with double minute chromosomes. *N Engl J Med.* 1983;308:199-202.

92. Rhee MS, Coward JK, Galivan J. Depletion of 5,10-methylenetetrahydrofolate and 10-formyltetrahydrofolate by methotrexate in cultured hepatoma cells. *Mol Pharmacol.* 1992;42:909-916.

93. Li JC, Kaminskas E. Accumulation of DNA strand breaks and methotrexate cytotoxicity. *Proc Natl Acad Sci U S A.* 1984;81:5694-5698.

94. Curtin NJ, Harris AL, Aherne GW. Mechanism of cell death following thymidylate synthase inhibition: 2′-deoxyuridine-5′-triphosphate accumulation, DNA damage, and growth inhibition following exposure to CB3717 and dipyridamole. *Cancer Res* 1991;51:2346-2352.

95. Jacobs AC, Calkins MJ, Jadhay A, et al. Inhibition of DNA glycosylases via small molecule purine analogs. *PLoS One.* 2013;8:e81667.

96. Goker E, Waltham M, Kheradpour A, et al. Amplification of the dihydrofolate reductase gene is a mechanism of acquired resistance to methotrexate in patients with acute lymphoblastic leukemia and is correlated with p53 gene mutations. *Blood.* 1995;86:677-684.

97. Pinedo HM, Zaharko DS, Bull J, et al. The relative contribution of drug concentration and duration of exposure to mouse bone marrow toxicity during continuous methotrexate infusion. *Cancer Res.* 1977;37:445-450.

98. Pinedo HM, Zaharko DS, Bull JM, et al. The reversal of methotrexate cytotoxicity to mouse bone marrow cells by leucovorin and nucleosides. *Cancer Res.* 1976;36:4418-4424.

99. Howell SB, Mansfield SJ, Taetle R. Thymidine and hypoxanthine requirements of normal and malignant human cells for protection against methotrexate cytotoxicity. *Cancer Res.* 1981;41:945-950.

100. Rustum YM. High-pressure liquid chromatography. I. Quantitative separation of purine and pyrimidine nucleosides and bases. *Anal Biochem.* 1978;90:289-299.

101. McLean G, Pathare PM, Wilbur CS, et al. Cobalamin analogues modulate the growth of leukemia cells *in vitro*. *Cancer Res.* 1997;57:4013-4022.

102. Matherly LH, Barlowe CK, Goldman ID. Antifolate polyglutamylation and competitive drug displacement at dihydrofolate reductase as important elements in leucovorin rescue in L1210 cells. *Cancer Res.* 1986;46:588-593.

103. Donehower RC, Hande KR, Drake JC, et al. Presence of 2,4-diamino-N10-methylpteroic acid after high-dose methotrexate. *Clin Pharmacol Ther.* 1979;26:63-72.

104. So N, Chandra DP, Alexander IS, et al. Determination of serum methotrexate and 7-hydroxymethotrexate concentrations. Method evaluation showing advantages of high-performance liquid chromatography. *J Chromatogr.* 1985;337:81-90.

105. Slordal L, Prytz PS, Pettersen I, et al. Methotrexate measurements in plasma: comparison of enzyme multiplied immunoassay technique, TDx fluorescence polarization immunoassay, and high pressure liquid chromatography. *Ther Drug Monit.* 1986;8:368-372.

106. Zaharko DS, Dedrick RL, Bischoff KB, et al. Methotrexate tissue distribution: prediction by a mathematical model. *J Natl Cancer Inst.* 1971;46:775-784.

107. Balis FM, Savitch JL, Bleyer WA. Pharmacokinetics of oral methotrexate in children. *Cancer Res.* 1983;43:2342-2345.

108. Balis FM, Holcenberg JS, Poplack DG, et al. Pharmacokinetics and pharmacodynamics of oral methotrexate and mercaptopurine in children with lower risk acute lymphoblastic leukemia: a joint children's cancer group and pediatric oncology branch study. *Blood.* 1998;92:3569-3577.

109. Steele WH, Lawrence JR, Stuart JF, et al. The protein binding of methotrexate by the serum of normal subjects. *Eur J Clin Pharmacol.* 1979;15:363-366.

110. Liegler DG, Henderson ES, Hahn MA, et al. The effect of organic acids on renal clearance of methotrexate in man. *Clin Pharmacol Ther.* 1969;10:849-857.

111. Chabner BA, Stoller RG, Hande K, et al. Methotrexate disposition in humans: case studies in ovarian cancer and following high-dose infusion. *Drug Metab Rev.* 1978;8:107-117.

112. Fossa SD, Heilo A, Bormer O. Unexpectedly high serum methotrexate levels in cystectomized bladder cancer patients with an ileal conduit treated with intermediate doses of the drug. *J Urol.* 1990;143:498-501.

113. Kristenson L, Weismann K, Hutters L. Renal function and the rate of disappearance of methotrexate from serum. *Eur J Clin Pharmacol.* 1975;8:439-444.

114. Bleyer WA. The clinical pharmacology of methotrexate: new applications of an old drug. *Cancer.* 1978;41:36-51.

115. Evans WE, Crom WR, Stewart CF, et al. Methotrexate systemic clearance influences probability of relapse in children with standard-risk acute lymphocytic leukaemia. *Lancet.* 1984;1:359-362.

116. Evans WE, Crom WR, Abromowitch M, et al. Clinical pharmacodynamics of high-dose methotrexate in acute lymphocytic leukemia. Identification of a relation between concentration and effect. *N Engl J Med.* 1986;314:471-477.

117. Borsi JD, Moe PJ. Systemic clearance of methotrexate in the prognosis of acute lymphoblastic leukemia in children. *Cancer.* 1987;60:3020-3024.

118. Monjanel S, Rigault JP, Cano JP, et al. High-dose methotrexate: preliminary evaluation of a pharmacokinetic approach. *Cancer Chemother Pharmacol.* 1979;3:189-196.

119. Sasaki K, Tanaka J, Fujimoto T. Theoretically required urinary flow during high-dose methotrexate infusion. *Cancer Chemother Pharmacol.* 1984;13:9-13.

120. Romolo JL, Goldberg NH, Hande KR, et al. Effect of hydration on plasma-methotrexate levels. *Cancer Treat Rep.* 1977;61:1393-1396.

121. Iven H, Brasch H. Influence of the antibiotics piperacillin, doxycycline, and tobramycin on the pharmacokinetics of methotrexate in rabbits. *Cancer Chemother Pharmacol.* 1986;17:218-222.

122. Iven H, Brasch H. Cephalosporins increase the renal clearance of methotrexate and 7-hydroxymethotrexate in rabbits. *Cancer Chemother Pharmacol.* 1990;26:139-143.

123. Kerr IG, Jolivet J, Collins JM, et al. Test dose for predicting high-dose methotrexate infusions. *Clin Pharmacol Ther.* 1983;33:44-51.

124. Favre R, Monjanel S, Alfonsi M, et al. High-dose methotrexate: a clinical and pharmacokinetic evaluation. Treatment of advanced squamous cell carcinoma of the head and neck using a prospective mathematical model and pharmacokinetic surveillance. *Cancer Chemother Pharmacol.* 1982;9:156-160.

125. Jacobs SA, Derr CJ, Johns DG. Accumulation of methotrexate diglutamate in human liver during methotrexate therapy. *Biochem Pharmacol.* 1977;26:2310-2313.

126. Barak AJ, Tuma D, Bechenhauer HC. Methotrexate hepatotoxicity. *J Am Coll Nutr.* 1884;3:93-96.

127. Lerne PR, Creaven PJ, Allen LM, et al. Kinetic model for the disposition and metabolism of moderate and high-dose methotrexate in man. *Cancer Chemother Rep.* 1975;59:811-817.

128. Erttmann R, Landbeck G. Effect of oral cholestyramine on the elimination of high-dose methotrexate. *J Cancer Res Clin Oncol.* 1985;110:48-50.

129. Jacobs SA, Stoller RG, Chabner BA, et al. 7-Hydroxymethotrexate as a urinary metabolite in human subjects and rhesus monkeys receiving high dose methotrexate. *J Clin Invest.* 1976;57:534-538.

130. Bremnes RM, Slordal L, Wist E, et al. Formation and elimination of 7-hydroxymethotrexate in the rat in vivo after methotrexate administration. *Cancer Res.* 1989;49:2460-2464.

131. Sholar PW, Baram J, Seither R, et al. Inhibition of folate-dependent enzymes by 7-OH-methotrexate. *Biochem Pharmacol.* 1988;37:3531-3534.

132. McCullough JL, Chabner BA, Bertino JR. Purification and properties of carboxypeptidase G1. *J Biol Chem.* 1971;246:7207-7213.

133. Chabner BA, Young RC. Threshold methotrexate concentration for in vivo inhibition of DNA synthesis in normal and tumorous target tissues. *J Clin Invest.* 1973;52:1804-1811.

134. Ackland SP, Schilsky RL. High-dose methotrexate: a critical reappraisal. *J Clin Oncol.* 1987;5:2017-2031.

135. Garneau AP, Riopel J, Isenring P. Acute methotrexate-Induced crystal nephropathy. *N Engl J Med.* 2015;373:2691-2693.

136. Stoller RG, Hande KR, Jacobs SA, et al. Use of plasma pharmacokinetics to predict and prevent methotrexate toxicity. *N Engl J Med.* 1977;297: 630-634.

137. Bacci G, Ferrari S, Longhi A, et al. Delayed methotrexate clearance in osteosarcoma patients treated with multiagent regimens of neoadjuvant chemotherapy. *Oncol Rep.* 2003;10(4):851-857.

138. Nozaki Y, Kusuhara H, Endou H, et al. Quantitative evaluation of the drug-drug interactions between methotrexate and nonsteroidal anti-inflammatory drugs in the renal uptake process based on the contribution of organic anion transporters and reduced folate carrier. *J Pharmacol Exp Ther.* 2004;309(1):226-234.

139. Murashima M, Adamski J, Milone MC, et al. Methotrexate clearance by high-flux hemodialysis and peritoneal dialysis: a case report. *Am J Kidney Dis.* 2009;53:871-874.

140. DeAngelis LM, Tong WP, Lin S, et al. Carboxypeptidase G2 rescue after high-dose methotrexate. *J Clin Oncol.* 1996;14:2145-2149.

141. Ramsey LB, Balis FM, O'Brien MM, et al. Consensus guideline for the use of glucarpidase in patients with high-dose methotrexate induced acute kidney injury and delayed methotrexate clearance. *Oncologist.* 2017;22:1-10.

142. Widemann BC. Using a lower dose of glucarpidase to reduce plasma levels of methotrexate. *Clin Adv Hematol Oncol.* 2013;11:324-326.

143. Salliot C, van der Heijde D. Long-term safety of methotrexate monotherapy in patients with rheumatoid arthritis: a systematic literature research. *Ann Rheum Dis.* 2009;68:1100-1104.

144. Weber BL, Tanyer G, Poplack DG, et al. Transient acute hepatotoxicity of high-dose methotrexate therapy during childhood. *J Natl Cancer Inst Monogr.* 1987;5:207-212.

145. Sostman HD, Matthay RA, Putman CE, et al. Methotrexate-induced pneumonitis. *Medicine (Baltimore).* 1976;55:371-388.

146. Alarcon GS, Kremer JM, Macaluso M, et al. Risk factors for methotrexate-induced lung injury in patients with rheumatoid arthritis. A multicenter, case-control study. Methotrexate Lung Study Group. *Ann Intern Med.* 1997;127:356-364.

147. Suemori K, Hasegawa H, Ishizaki J, et al. Methotrexate-associated lymphoproliferative disease with multiple pulmonary nodules in a patient with rheumatoid arthritis. *Intern Med.* 2015;54:1421-1425.

148. Nishitani N, Adachi A, Fukumoto T, et al. Folic acid-induced anaphylaxis showing cross-reactivity with methotrexate: a case report and review of the literature. *Int J Dermatol.* 2009;48:522-524.

149. Shamberger RC, Rosenberg SA, Seipp CA, et al. Effects of high-dose methotrexate and vincristine on ovarian and testicular functions in patients undergoing postoperative adjuvant treatment of osteosarcoma. *Cancer Treat Rep.* 1981;65:739-746.

150. Shapiro WR, Young DF, Mehta BM. Methotrexate: distribution in cerebrospinal fluid after intravenous, ventricular and lumbar injections. *N Engl J Med.* 1975;293:161-166.

151. Bleyer WA, Drake JC, Chabner BA. Neurotoxicity and elevated cerebrospinal-fluid methotrexate concentration in meningeal leukemia. *N Engl J Med.* 1973;289:770-773.

152. Blaney SM, Balis FM, Poplack DG. Current pharmacological treatment approaches to central nervous system leukaemia. *Drugs.* 1991;41: 702-716.

153. Bleyer WA, Poplack DG, Simon RM. "Concentration × time" methotrexate via a subcutaneous reservoir: a less toxic regimen for intraventricular chemotherapy of central nervous system neoplasms. *Blood.* 1978;51:835-842.

154. Badke C, Fleming A, Iqbal A, et al. Rechallenging with intrathecal methotrexate after developing subacute neurotoxicity in children with hematologic malignancies. *Pediatr Blood Cancer.* 2016;63:723-726.

155. Walker RW, Allen JC, Rosen G, et al. Transient cerebral dysfunction secondary to high-dose methotrexate. *J Clin Oncol.* 1986;4:1845-1850.

156. Kubo M, Azuma E, Arai S, et al. Transient encephalopathy following a single exposure of high-dose methotrexate in a child with acute lymphoblastic leukemia. *Pediatr Hematol Oncol.* 1992;9:157-165.

157. Ochs J, Mulhern R, Fairclough D, et al. Comparison of neuropsychologic functioning and clinical indicators of neurotoxicity in long-term survivors of childhood leukemia given cranial radiation or parenteral methotrexate: a prospective study. *J Clin Oncol.* 1991;9:145-151.

158. Phillips PC, Dhawan V, Strother SC, et al. Reduced cerebral glucose metabolism and increased brain capillary permeability following high-dose methotrexate chemotherapy: a positron emission tomographic study. *Ann Neurol.* 1987;21:59-63.

159. Kishi S, Griener J, Cheng C, et al. Homocysteine, pharmacogenetics, and neurotoxicity in children with leukemia. *J Clin Oncol.* 2003;21(16):3084-3091.

160. Spiegel RJ, Cooper PR, Blum RH, et al. Treatment of massive intrathecal methotrexate overdose by ventriculolumbar perfusion. *N Engl J Med.* 1984;311:386-388.

161. Didani S, Mazzzarello S, Hilton J, et al. Optimal management of leptomeningeal carcinomatosis in breast cancer patients—a systematic review. *Clin Breast Cancer.* 2016;16(6):456-470.

162. Mei L, Evelena P, Griffiths E, et al. Pharmacogenetics predictive of response and toxicity in acute lymphoblastic leukemia therapy. *Blood Rev.* 2015;29:243-249.

163. Chango A, Emery-Fillon N, de Courcy GP, et al. A polymorphism (G80A) in the reduced folate carrier gene and its associations with folate status and homocysteinemia. *Mol Genet Metab.* 2000;70:310-315.

164. Ramsey LB, Bruun GH, Yang W, et al. Rare versus common variants in pharmacogenetics: SLCO1B1 variation and methotrexate disposition. *Genome Res.* 2012;22:1-8.

165. Toffoli G, Russo A, Innocenti F, et al. Effect of methyltetrahydrofolate reductase C677T polymorphism on toxicity and homocysteine plasma level after chronic methotrexate treatment of ovarian cancer patients. *Int J Cancer.* 2003;103:294-299.

166. Chiusolo P, Reddiconto G, Casorelli I, et al. Preponderance of methylene-tetrahydrofolate reductase C677T homozygosity among leukemia patients intolerant to methotrexate. *Ann Oncol.* 2002;13:1915-1918.

167. Chattopadhyay S, Moran RD, Goldman ID. Pemetrexed: biochemical and cellular pharmacology, mechanisms and clinical applications. *Mol Cancer Ther.* 2007;6:404-417.

168. Worzalla JF, Shih C, Schultz RM. Role of folic acid in modulating the toxicity and efficacy of the multitargeted antifolate, LY231514. *Anticancer Res.* 1998;18:3235-3239.

169. Vogelzang NJ, Rusthoven JJ, Symanowski J, et al. Phase III study of pemetrexed in combination with cisplatin versus cisplatin alone in patients with malignant pleural mesothelioma. *J Clin Oncol.* 2003;21(14):2636-2644.

170. Mita AC, Sweeney CJ, Baker SD, et al. Phase I and pharmacokinetic study of pemetrexed administered every 3 weeks to advance cancer patients with normal and impaired renal function. *J Clin Oncol.* 2006;24: 552-562.

171. Takimoto CH, Hammond-Thelin LA, Latz JE, et al. Phase I and pharmacokinetic study of pemetrexed with high-dose folic acid supplementation of multivitamin supplementation in patients with locally advanced or metastatic cancer. *Clin Cancer Res.* 2007;13:2675-2683.

172. Ozasa H, Oguri T, Uemura T, et al. Significance of thymidylate synthase for resistance to pemetrexed in lung cancer. *Cancer Sci.* 2010;101:161-166.

173. O'Connor OA, Horwitz S, Hamlin P, et al. Phase II-I-II study of two different doses and schedules of pralatrexate, a high-affinity substrate for the reduced folate carrier, in patients with relapsed or refractory lymphoma reveals marked activity in T-Cell malignancies. *J Clin Oncol.* 2009;27:4357-4364.

5-Fluoropyrimidines

David P. Ryan, Jean Grem, and Bruce A. Chabner

The 5-fluorinated pyrimidines play a central role in the chemotherapy of epithelial tumors. 5-Fluorouracil (5-FU) was the first effective agent for treating colon cancer, and despite its six decades of use, it and other fluoropyrimidine analogues continue to find no applications in tumors of the gastrointestinal tract. This chapter will review the basic and clinical pharmacology of these drugs and will provide a context of understanding their use in clinical treatment regimens.

The 5-fluoropyrimidine analogues were synthesized by Heidelberger et al.[1] on the basis of the observation that rat hepatomas avidly incorporate radiolabeled uracil into nucleic acids, perhaps creating a therapeutic advantage for treatment. Enhancement of 5-FU activity by leucovorin (LV) and synergistic interaction of fluoropyrimidines with other antitumor agents and with irradiation have further broadened its effectiveness and value in cancer treatment.

Structure and Cellular Pharmacology

The chemical structures of the intravenous preparations of 5-fluoropyrimidines in clinical use in the United States are shown in Figure 8.1. The simplest derivative, 5-FU (molecular weight [MW] = 130), has the slightly bulkier fluorine atom substituted at the carbon-5 position of the pyrimidine ring in place of hydrogen.

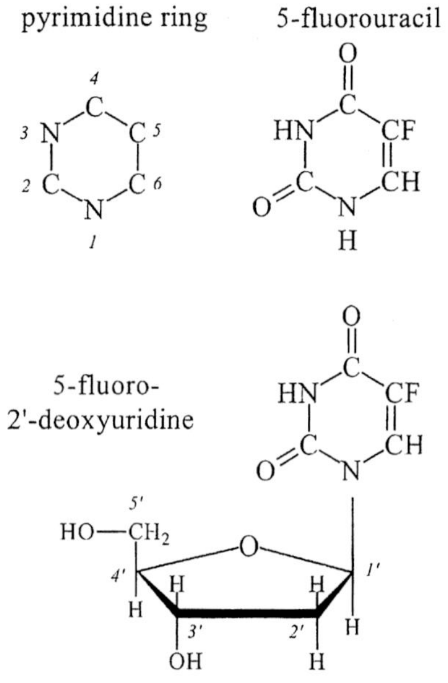

FIGURE **8.1** Structures of pyrimidine ring, 5-FU, and FdUrd.

The key features of 5-FU are outlined in Table 8.1. Activation to the nucleotide level is essential to antitumor activity. The deoxyribonucleoside 5-fluoro-2′-deoxyuridine (FdUrd, MW = 246) is commercially available (floxuridine, FUDR) but only sporadically employed for hepatic arterial infusion.

Transport

5-FU shares the same facilitated transport system that imports uracil, adenine, and hypoxanthine. The system is neither temperature dependent nor energy dependent,[2] although entry is limited by ionization of the hydroxyl substitution on the fourth carbon of the pyrimidine ring. 5-FU permeation reaches a steady status in 3 to 5 minutes.

FdUrd is a deoxynucleoside and enters cells via multiple systems that vary in substrate specificity, sodium dependence, and sensitivity to nitrobenzylthioinosine.[3] Two basic classes of human nucleoside transport systems are present: equilibrative (bidirectional) and concentrative (sodium dependent, unidirectional). Human equilibrative nucleoside transport (hENT-1) and concentrative nucleoside transport (CNT-1) systems are selective for pyrimidines; the former is present in most cell types, including cancer cells, while the latter is present in liver, kidney, intestine, choroid plexus, and some tumor cells. Intracellular drug concentrations reach equilibrium with extracellular drug within seconds. Total intracellular drug continues to accumulate thereafter from rate-limiting phosphorylation to form fluorodeoxyuridylate (5-fluoro-2′-deoxyuridine-5′monophosphate, FdUMP) and other nucleotides.

Metabolic Activation

Activation of 5-FU to the (deoxy)ribonucleotide level may occur through three pathways, as outlined in Figure 8.2[4-6]: direct transfer of a ribose phosphate to 5-FU from 5-phosphoribosyl-1-pyrophosphate (PRPP) as catalyzed by orotic acid phosphoribosyltransferase (OPRTase) and the addition of a ribose or deoxyribose moiety by uridine (Urd) phosphorylase or deoxyribose by thymidine phosphorylase, followed by phosphorylation by Urd kinase. Sequential action of uridine/cytidine monophosphate (UMP/CMP) kinase and pyrimidine diphosphate kinase results in the formation of fluorouridine diphosphate (FUDP) and fluorouridine triphosphate (FUTP); the latter is incorporated into RNA by the action of RNA polymerase.

The pathway, catalyzed by OPRTase, may be of primary importance for 5-FU activation in healthy tissues because its inhibition diminishes toxicity to bone marrow and GI mucosa,[5] but it is also the dominant route of 5-FU activation in many murine leukemias.[4] Other cancer cell lines appear to activate the drug by the action of Urd phosphorylase and Urd kinase.[7] Although one activation

TABLE 8.1 *Key features of 5-FU*

Mechanism of action	Incorporation of 5-FdUMP into RNA interferes with RNA processing and function
	5-FdUMP inhibits TS, depletes dThd nucleotides
	Incorporation of fluorouridine and Urd nucleotides into DNA triggers DNA repair and strand breaks, apoptosis
Metabolism	Converted to active nucleotides by multiple pathways intracellularly
Pharmacokinetics	Plasma $t_{1/2}$ 8 to 14 min after IV bolus
	Saturable catabolism leads to nonlinear pharmacokinetics: total body clearance decreases with increasing doses; clearance is faster with infusional schedules
	Volume of distribution slightly exceeds extracellular fluid space
Elimination	DPD catalyzes the initial, rate-limiting step in 5-FU catabolism and clearance. 90% eliminated by metabolism (catabolism/anabolism)
	<10% unchanged drug excreted by kidneys after infusion or bolus
Drug interactions	Pharmacologic inhibitors of DPD: see Table 8.7
	Cimetidine (but not ranitidine) may decrease the clearance of 5-FU
	LV increases intracellular folates, enhances ternary TS complex with 5-FdUMP
	Oxaliplatin down-regulates expression of TS
Toxicity	GI epithelial ulceration
	Myelosuppression
	Dermatologic: rash, palmar-plantar dysesthesia
	Conjunctival irritation, keratitis
	Neurotoxicity (cognitive dysfunction and cerebellar ataxia)
	Cardiac (coronary spasm)
	Biliary sclerosis (after hepatic arterial infusion)
Precautions	Nonlinear pharmacokinetics: difficulty in predicting plasma concentrations and toxicity at high doses. Pharmacokinetic monitoring, with adjustment of drug infusion, may increase response rate and decrease toxicity
	Patients with deficiency of DPD may have life-threatening or fatal toxicity if treated with 5-fluoropyrimidines
	Patients receiving sorivudine should not receive concurrent 5-fluoropyrimidines (4-wk washout period recommended)
	Older, female, and poor-performance–status patients have greater risk of toxicity
	Closely monitor prothrombin time and INR in patients receiving concurrent warfarin DPD

pathway may appear to predominate in a given cancer cell under certain conditions, multiple pathways are often available.

In the presence of a 2′-deoxyribose-1-phosphate (dR-1-P) donor, 5-FU is converted to FdUrd by a third activation pathway involving thymidine (dThd) phosphorylase.[8] dThd kinase then forms 5-FdUMP, a potent inhibitor of thymidylate synthase (TS). 5-FdUMP may also be produced from 5-FUMP by a several-step pathway in which 5-FUDP in reduced to 5-fluorodeoxyuridine diphosphate (5-FdUDP), followed by dephosphorylation to 5-FdUMP. 5-FdUMP and 5-FdUDP are substrates for dThd monophosphate and diphosphate kinases, respectively, resulting in the formation of 5-fluorodeoxyuridine triphosphate (5-FdUTP), which is a substrate for DNA polymerase and is incorporated into DNA.

Physiologic Urd metabolites are largely present in vivo as nucleotide sugars that are necessary for the glycosylation of proteins and lipids and become incorporated into membrane. 5-FU nucleotide sugars, such as 5-FUDP-glucose, 5-FUDP-hexose, 5-FUDP-*N*-acetylglucosamine, and 5-FdUDP-*N*-acetylglucosamine, have been detected in mammalian cells.[9] The extent to which 5-FU nucleotide sugars are incorporated into proteins and lipids and any possible metabolic consequences is unclear.

The 5-FU nucleotides are subject to degradation by several different phosphatase enzymes, as are the nucleotides of physiological pyrimidines. Acid and alkaline phosphatases and 5′-nucleotidases, including the SAMHD1 nucleotidase, have a yet to be determined role in drug response. The pyrimidine phosphorylases catalyze the important *reversible* conversion from 5-FUrd and 5-FdUrd and back to 5-FU, as noted above.

Mechanism of Action

Inhibition of Thymidylate Synthase

At least two primary mechanisms of action appear capable of causing cell injury: inhibition of TS and incorporation into RNA. Of these, the preponderance of evidence suggests that TS inactivation is the primary mechanism.[10] 5-FdUMP binds tightly to TS and prevents formation of thymidylate (thymidine 5′-monophosphate, dTMP), the essential precursor of thymidine 5′-triphosphate (dTTP), a component of DNA.

The functional TS enzyme comprises a dimer of two identical subunits, each of MW approximately 30 kDa (bacterial) or approximately 36 kDa (human). Each subunit has a nucleotide-binding site and two distinct folate-binding sites, one for 5,10-methylenetetrahydrofolate (5,10-CH_2 FH_4) monoglutamate or polyglutamate, and an inhibitory site for dihydrofolate polyglutamates. 5-FdUMP

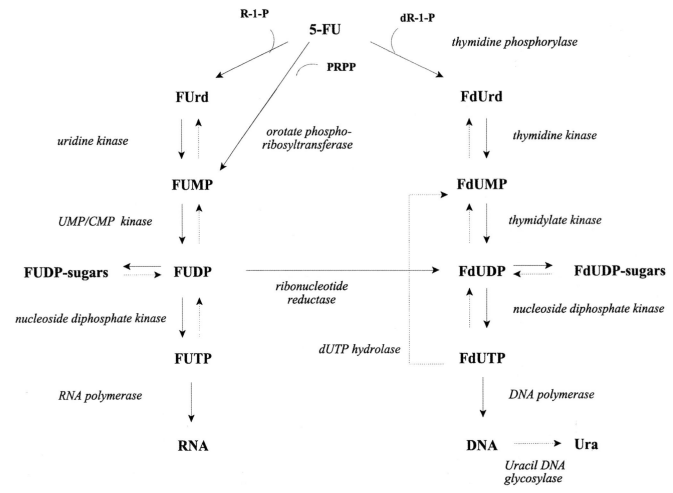

FIGURE **8.2** Intracellular activation of 5-FU, 5-fluorouracil; dUTP, deoxyuridine triphosphate; 5-FdUDP, 5-fluorodeoxyuridine diphosphate; 5-FdUMP, fluorodeoxyuridylate; 5-FdUrd, 5-fluoro-2'-deoxyuridine; 5-FdUTP, fluorodeoxyuridine triphosphate; 5-FUDP, fluorouridine diphosphate; 5-FUMP, fluorouridine monophosphate; 5-FUrd, 5-fluorouridine triphosphate; PPRP, phosphoribosyl phosphate.

competes with the natural substrate 2′-deoxyuridine monophosphate (dUMP) for the TS catalytic site.[11] During methylation of dUMP, transfer of the folate methyl group to dUMP occurs by elimination of hydrogen attached to the pyrimidine carbon-5 position (Fig. 8.3A). This elimination cannot occur with the more tightly bound fluorine atom of 5-FdUMP, and the enzyme is trapped in a virtually irreversible ternary complex with FdUMP and folate (Fig. 8.3B). The "thymineless state" that ensues is toxic to actively dividing cells. Toxicity can be circumvented by salvage of dThd released into the bloodstream from degradation of DNA. Salvage of thymidine requires dThd kinase. The circulating concentrations of dThd in humans are not thought to be sufficient (approximately 0.1 μmol/L) to afford protection from TS inhibition for actively dividing cells.[12] The plasma levels of dThd are approximately 10-fold higher in rodents, which complicates preclinical evaluation of the antitumor activity of various TS inhibitors.

A reduced folate cofactor is required for tight binding of the inhibitor to TS. The natural cofactor for the TS reaction, 5,10-CH$_2$ FH$_4$, in its monoglutamate and polyglutamate forms, binds through its methylene group to the carbon-5 position of 5-FdUMP. The polyglutamates of 5,10-CH$_2$ FH$_4$ are much more effective in stabilizing the 5-FdUMP-TS-folate ternary complex.[13] Other naturally occurring folates promote 5-FdUMP binding to the enzyme but

form a more readily dissociable complex. Polyglutamated forms of dihydrofolic acid (FH$_2$) promote extremely tight binding of 5-FdUMP to the enzyme.[14]

FH$_2$ accumulates in cells exposed to methotrexate (MTX). Although MTX is a relatively weak inhibitor of TS in cell-free experiments, MTX polyglutamates are more potent inhibitors, as are FH$_2$ polyglutamates. MTX polyglutamates inhibit the formation of the 5-FdUMP-TS-folate ternary complex.[14]

In the presence of folate cofactor, 5-FdUMP binds avidly to the mammalian enzyme, with a dissociation half-life ($t_{1/2}$) of 6.2 hours.[15] Elucidation of the crystal structure of TS has permitted a complex kinetic and thermodynamic description of ternary complex formation.[16] The interaction proceeds by an ordered mechanism with initial nucleotide binding followed by 5,10-CH$_2$ FH$_4$ binding to form a rapidly reversible noncovalent ternary complex (Fig. 8.4). Enzyme-catalyzed conversions result in the formation of a covalent bond between carbon-5 of FdUMP and the methylene of the folate cofactor. The binding constant of 5,10-CH$_2$ FH$_4$ from the covalent complex is approximately 1×10^{-11} mol/L.

Despite the high specificity and potency of TS inhibition by 5-FdUMP and the well-established lethality of dTMP and dTTP depletion, inhibition of TS may not be the sole cause of 5-FU toxicity. If 5-FU toxicity results from dTTP depletion, then dThd

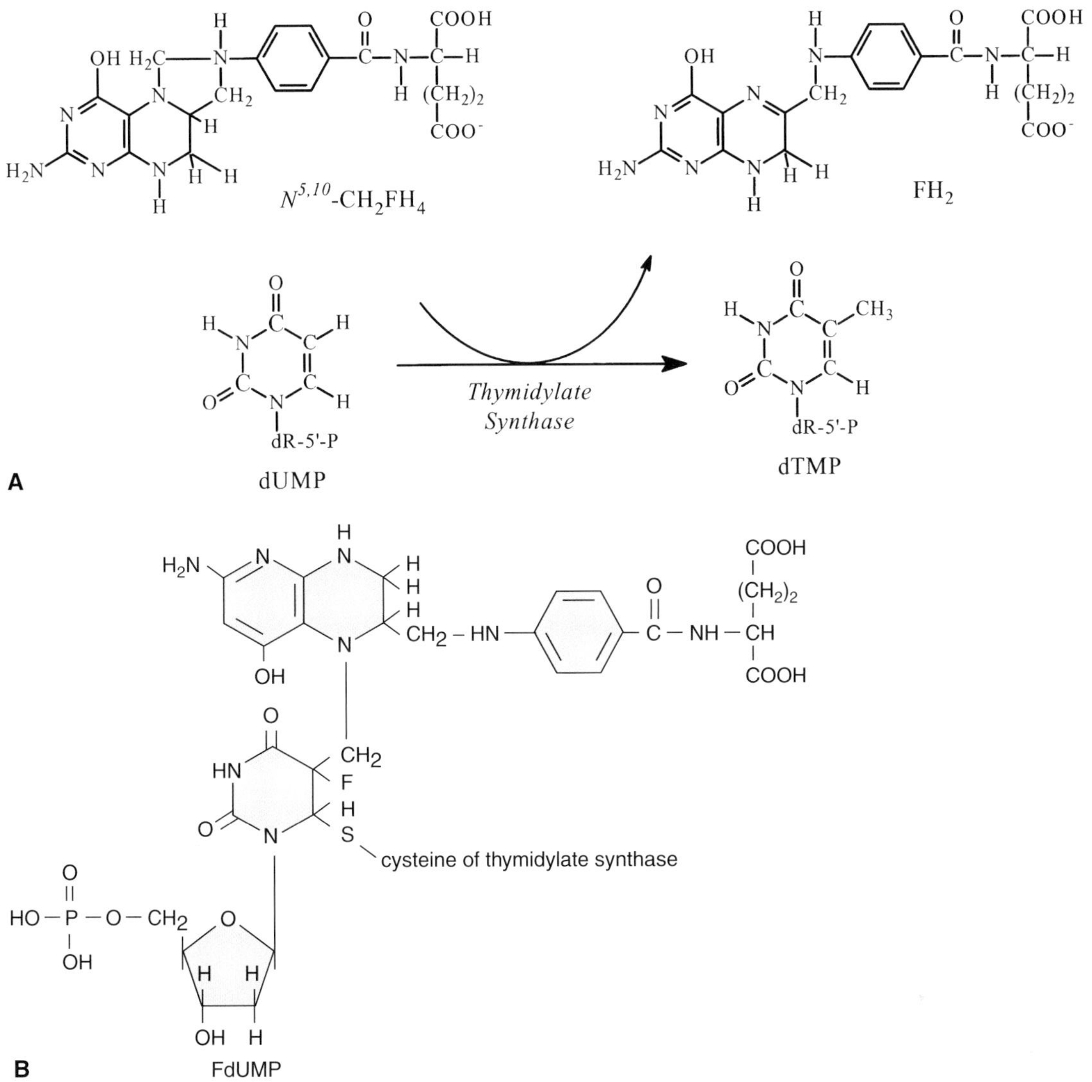

FIGURE **8.3** **A.** Thymidylate synthase reaction, with cofactor 5,10-methylenetetrahydrofolate, converting deoxyuridylate (dUMP) to deoxythymidylate (dTMP). **B.** Interaction of 5-fluorodeoxyuridylate (5-FdUMP) with thymidylate synthase and N^{5-10} CH_2 FH_4 to form an essentially irreversible complex.

should reverse the toxic effects. But dThd shows variable effectiveness in rescuing cells exposed to 5-FU.[17] Depending on the target cell, drug concentration, and ability of cells to salvage dThd, 5-FU toxicity may be fully dependent on thymidylate depletion. Coadministration of 5-FU and dThd may increase 5-FU toxicity to healthy tissues in animal experiments and may increase the antitumor effect of 5-FU against certain animal tumors and increase [³H]5-FUrd incorporation into RNA, a second potential mechanism of toxicity.[18]

RNA-Directed Effects

5-FU is rapidly converted to 5-FUTP, and extensively incorporated into nuclear and cytoplasmic RNA fractions, inhibiting the processing of initial pre-rRNA transcripts to the cytoplasmic rRNA species in a dose- and time-dependent manner.[19-21] Substantial amounts of [³H] 5-FU accumulate in low-MW (4S) RNA at lethal drug concentrations.[20,22] While the analog replaces only a small percentage of uracil residues in RNA, it persists in RNA for many days after drug exposure.[23]

Net RNA synthesis is reduced during and after fluoropyrimidine exposure in a concentration- and time-dependent fashion. In some cancer cell lines, a highly significant relationship exists between 5-FU incorporation into total cellular RNA and the loss of clonogenic survival. 5-FU is incorporated into all species of RNA.

5-FU exposure affects mRNA processing, splicing, and translation.[24-29] Polyadenylation of mRNA and methylation of tRNA are inhibited at relatively low concentrations of 5-FU,[27] and altered translation of precursor RNAs of specific proteins such as dihydrofolate reductase (DHFR) has been reported.[24,25] Incorporation of 5-FU into RNA may affect quantitative and qualitative aspects of protein synthesis.

In summary, the changes in certain key mRNAs resulting from 5-FU exposure may be relevant to its cytotoxicity, but the specific alterations that lead to toxicity are not known and may include effects on splicing, rates of translation, and specific errors in coding. For example, 5-FU mediates inhibition of expression of RNA coding for the important DNA repair protein, ERCC-1, in cancer cells, a property that could enhance response to DNA damaging agents.[30]

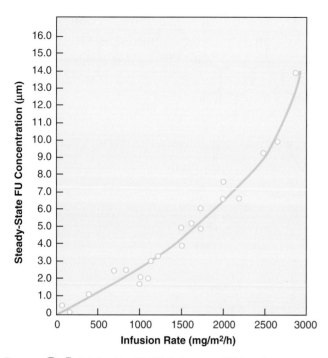

FIGURE 8.4 Relationship of 5-FU infusion rate to 5-FU steady-state concentration in plasma. (Adapted from data in Table 7-6, 4th ed. *Principles and Practice of Cancer Chemotherapy and Biological Response Modifiers.*)

DNA-Directed Mechanisms of Potential Toxicity

The biochemical consequences of TS inhibition and the potential effects on DNA integrity have been extensively studied, but their relationship to cytotoxicity is incompletely understood. Inhibition of TS results in depletion of dTMP and dTTP, thus leading to inhibition of DNA synthesis and interference with DNA repair. Accumulation of dUMP occurs behind the blockade of TS, and its further metabolism to the deoxyuridine triphosphate (dUTP) level leads to its misincorporation into DNA.[31] FdUTP and dUTP are both substrates for DNA polymerase, and their incorporation may contribute to cytotoxicity.[32,33] 5-FU cytotoxicity in some models correlates with the level of 5-FU-DNA. Two mechanisms prevent incorporation of FdUTP and dUTP into DNA. The enzyme dUTP pyrophosphatase or dUTP hydrolase catalyzes the hydrolysis of 5-FdUTP to 5-FdUMP and inorganic pyrophosphate.[34] The DNA repair enzyme uracil-DNA-glycosylase (UDG) hydrolyzes the 5-FU-deoxyribose glycosyl bond of the 5-FdUMP residues in DNA, thereby creating an apyrimidinic site.[35] The base deoxyribose 5′-monophosphate is subsequently removed from the DNA backbone by an AP (apurinic/apyrimidinic) endonuclease, creating a single-strand break, which must be repaired. With dTTP depletion, however, the efficiency of the repair process is impaired.

UDG is a cell cycle–dependent enzyme with maximal levels of activity at the G1 and S interface, such that excision of the fraudulent bases occurs before DNA replication. The activity of UDG inversely correlates with the level of 5-FdUMP incorporation into DNA in human lymphoblastic cells. Because the affinity of human UDG is much lower for 5-FU than for uracil, 5-FU is removed more slowly from DNA by this mechanism.[35] 5-FdUTP itself inhibits the activity of UDG.[36] Accumulation of deoxyadenosine triphosphate (dATP) accompanies TS inhibition.[37] The combined effects of

deoxyribonucleotide imbalance (high dATP, low dTTP, high dUTP) and misincorporation of 5-FdUTP and dUTP into DNA may have deleterious consequences affecting DNA synthesis and the integrity of nascent DNA and may induce apoptosis.

5-FU produces extensive alterations in DNA including strand breaks, decreases in the average DNA chain length,[38] and single- and double-stranded DNA strand breaks, the patterns of which differ from that created by simple thymidine depletion.[39] Resistance to 5-FU in SW620 tumor cells correlates best with the failure to accumulate dUTP in DNA; thus, the role of dUTP and its incorporation into DNA are possibly important as well.

Factors that regulate recognition of and response to DNA damage likely contribute to 5-FU lethality. The oncogene *p53* plays a pivotal role in the regulation of cell cycle progression and induction of apoptosis, and its mutation decreases the sensitivity of cells to 5-FU in some experimental systems[40] but remains controversial as a predictor for 5-FU response. Transfection and expression of the *bcl-2* oncogene in a human lymphoma cell line render it resistant to 5-FdUrd. Bcl-2 expression, which inhibits apoptosis, protects cells against 5-FU damage.[41]

Genotoxic stress resulting from TS inhibition activates programmed cell-death pathways, resulting in induction of DNA fragmentation. Depending on the cell line, different patterns of DNA damage may be noted: internucleosomal DNA laddering, the hallmark of classical apoptosis, and high-MW DNA fragmentation with segments ranging from approximately 50 kb to 1 to 3 Mb. Differences in the type and activity of endonucleases and DNA-degradative enzymes triggered in a given cell line most likely explain these disparate patterns of parental DNA fragmentation. In "apoptosis-competent" cancer cell lines, such as HL60 promyelocytic leukemia cells, genotoxic stress results in rapid (within hours) induction of programmed cell death, with classic DNA laddering. In contrast, many cancer cell lines derived from epithelial tumors, including colon cancer, appear to undergo delayed programmed cell death. This phenomenon may reflect a "postmitotic" cell death, in which one or more rounds of mitosis are needed before cell death occurs.[42] In such cell lines, the duration of the genotoxic insult may determine whether induction of cytostasis or programmed cell death occurs. One possible explanation for delayed apoptosis is that sublethal damage to genes, essential for cell survival, may ultimately lead to cell death with subsequent rounds of DNA replication.

Factors operating downstream from TS clearly influence the cellular response to genotoxic stress, such as overexpression of the cellular oncoproteins *bcl-2* and mutant *p53*. Disruption of the signal pathways that sense genotoxic stress or lead to induction of programmed cell death, or both, may render a cancer cell inherently resistant to 5-FU. In some cancer cell lines, thymineless death may be mediated by Fas and Fas-ligand interactions.[43] Cancer cell lines insensitive to Fas-mediated apoptosis are insensitive to 5-FU, suggesting that modulation of their expression may influence sensitivity to 5-FU. As previously mentioned, base excision repair (BER) plays an essential role in removing incorporated 5-FU and uracil residues from DNA, resulting in single-strand DNA breaks. BER recognizes the mispairing of 5-FU with guanine in DNA and excises the fluoropyrimidine. Because BER involves multiple proteins, deficiencies in one of the components, such as UDG, XRCC1, or

DNA polymerase-β, may reduce the toxic effects of TS inhibitors. Abrogation of UDG protects against cytotoxicity in some, but not all, cell lines.[44]

Microsatellite instability (MSI) is a manifestation of genomic instability in human cancers that have a decreased overall ability to faithfully replicate DNA and is a surrogate phenotypic marker of underlying functional inactivation of the human DNA mismatch repair (MMR) family of genes. In vitro studies suggest that MMR recognizes DNA breaks resulting from 5-FU incorporated into DNA and signals cell cycle (G2M) arrest. Functional loss of a MMR gene results from inactivation of both alleles via some combination of coding region mutations, loss of heterozygosity, and/or promoter methylation. In vitro studies suggest that *MMR-proficient* cells are more sensitive to 5-FU or FdUrd than *MMR-deficient* cells.[45,46] The loss of MMR proficiency leads to fluoropyrimidine resistance in some cell lines, but not others.[47]

The MSI phenotype has been associated with a better prognosis in stage-for-stage matched tumors in primary colorectal cancer,[48] but data are conflicting as to whether MSI status influences benefit from 5-FU–based adjuvant therapy. Additionally, it is unclear whether sporadic MSI-high tumors from gene methylation, including the BRAF mutant tumors, behave in a manner similar to tumors from patients with germ-line mismatch repair defects (Lynch syndrome).[49] Given the small numbers of patients with MSI-high tumors resulting from gene silencing or from germ-line mutations, it is unlikely that clear answers to the question of MSI and therapeutic response to fluoropyrimidines will emerge from current trials.

Relative Importance of RNA Versus DNA-Directed Effects

The relative contributions of DNA- and RNA-directed mechanisms to the cytotoxicity of 5-FU are influenced by the specific patterns of intracellular drug metabolism, which vary among different healthy and tumor tissues. 5-FU concentration and duration of exposure play pivotal roles in determining the basis of cytotoxicity. The improved response rates observed with LV modulation of bolus 5-FU therapy, the correlation between high TS expression in tumor tissue and insensitivity to 5-FU–based therapy, and the clinical activity of the antifolate-based TS inhibitors provide strong evidence that TS is the most important therapeutic target. In most human tumors, RNA-directed effects, which are not dependent on active cell division, may play a greater role in regimens with low level, but continuous drug exposure. DNA-directed effects have been important during short-term exposure of cells in S phase.[50]

Determinants of Sensitivity and Resistance to Fluoropyrimidines

Multiple factors contribute to tumor sensitivity to 5-FU (Table 8.2). Diminished or total loss of activity of the various activating enzymes (OPRTase, thymidine, and Urd phosphorylases) may result in resistance to 5-FU.[51,52]

In addition to the importance of these activating enzymes, the availability of ribose-1-phosphate, dR-1-P, and PRPP may influence activation and response.[52] Guanine nucleotides augment 5-FU activation to the ribonucleotide and deoxyribonucleotide levels by serving as a source of ribose-1-phosphate and dR-1-P.

TABLE 8.2	*Determinants of sensitivity to 5-FU*

5-FU anabolism to FdUMP and triphosphate nucleotides
- Activity of anabolic enzymes
- Activity of catabolic pathway, especially DPD

Catabolism of 5-FU and its nucleosides and nucleotides (including 5-FdUMP, dUTP, TTP)
- Activity of DPD
- Activity of thymidine phosphorylase
- Activity of 5-nucleotidase and other phosphatases

Inhibition of thymidylate synthase
- Baseline activity of TS and amplification after drug exposure
- Mutation of TS
- Availability of reduced folate cofactor LV
- Polyglutamation of folate cofactor
- Concentration of competitive dUMP

Extent of 5-FUTP incorporation into RNA
- Competitive pool of UTP

Extent of dUTP and 5-FdUTP incorporation into DNA
- Competitive pools of TTP through salvage pathway
- Uracil-DNA glycosylase activity

DNA strand breaks and their repair

Cellular response to genotoxic stress (apoptosis versus persistence)

5-FdUrd, 5-fluoro-2'-deoxyuridine; 5-FUrd, 5-fluoro-uridine; dUMP, deoxyuridine monophosphate; 5-FdUMP, 5-fluoro-2'deorguridine monophosphate; TS, thymidylate synthase; 5-FU, 5-flurouracil; dUTP, deoxyuridine triphosphate; 5-FdUTP, dUTP deoxyuridine triphosphate; UTP, uridine triphosphate; DPD, dihydropyrimidine dehydrogenase; 5-FU, 5-fluorouracil; LV, leucovorin.

The formation of 5-fluoropyrimidine nucleotides within target cells and the size of the competitive physiologic pools of UTP and dTTP also influence 5-FU cytotoxicity.[53] The extent of 5-FU incorporation into RNA depends on 5-FUTP formation and the size of the competing pool of UTP. Strategies that increase 5-FUTP formation generally increase incorporation of FUTP into RNA and enhance 5-FU toxicity.

While the various factors affecting sensitivity have been extensively studied in animal tumors, there are few such studies in human experiments. In one study, RNA and DNA incorporation in tumor biopsy specimens taken 2, 24, or 48 hours from patients receiving bolus 5-FU (500 mg/m^2) was measured using gas chromatography/mass spectrometry (GC/MS) after complete degradation of isolated RNA and DNA to bases. Maximal incorporation occurred 24 hours after 5-FU administration: 1.0 pmol/mg RNA ($n = 59$) and 127 pmol/mg DNA ($n = 46$). Incorporation into RNA, but not DNA, significantly correlated with intratumoral 5-FU levels. The extent of TS inhibition, but not RNA or DNA incorporation, correlated with response to 5-FU therapy.[54] Results of such studies in clinical samples from patients receiving various infusional schedules of 5-FU are needed for a fuller understanding of determinants of response.

Determinants of Thymidylate Synthase Inhibition

The ability of 5-FdUMP to inhibit TS is influenced by several variables, including the concentration of enzyme, the amount of 5-FdUMP formed and its rate of breakdown, the levels of the competing healthy substrate (dUMP) and 5,10-CH$_2$ FH$_4$ cofactor, and the latter's extent of polyglutamation. The degree and persistence of TS inhibition are crucial determinants of cytotoxicity. Blockade of TS can lead to a gradual expansion of the intracellular dUMP pool; resumption of DNA synthesis is a function of three factors: the availability of intracellular 5-FdUMP versus the rate of increase in dUMP, which competes with 5-FdUMP for newly synthesized TS and for enzyme that has dissociated from the ternary complex, and the rate of synthesis of new TS protein.

Determination of TS activity in tumor tissue now appears to determine the response to 5-FU. High levels of TS gene expression in tumor biopsies correlate with insensitivity to 5-FU–based regimens.[55,56] Immunohistochemical detection of nuclear TS has provided further evidence that high TS expression is correlated with decreased survival in patients with metastatic disease.

Studies of TS activity, the ternary complex, and free 5-FdUMP in tissue samples have provided a profile of the kinetics of TS inhibition. Sequential biopsies of liver metastases obtained 20 to 240 minutes after 500 mg/m^2 5-FU among 21 patients undergoing elective surgery revealed that maximal TS inhibition occurred within 90 minutes and averaged 70% to 80% in tumor tissue.[57] Large variations in TS binding and catalytic activity were noted in primary colon tumors, but the overall enzyme levels were significantly higher than in adjacent healthy colonic tissue.[58]

Quantitative and qualitative changes in TS have been identified in cells with innate or acquired resistance to fluoropyrimidines. Amplification of the TS gene, with corresponding elevation of enzyme content, has been found in lines resistant to 5-FU or 5-FdUrd.[59] Resistant cell lines may have an altered TS protein with either decreased binding affinity for 5-FdUMP or decreased affinity for 5,10-CH$_2$ FH$_4$.[60] Adequate reduced folate pools are required to form and maintain a stable ternary complex. Administration of exogenous reduced folates enhances the cytotoxicity of 5-FU and 5-FdUrd in preclinical models, and clinical administration of LV elevates the reduced folate content in the cancer cell.[61]

In summary, to inhibit TS, 5-FU must be converted to 5-FdUMP to inhibit TS. Sensitivity is determined by tumor cell ability to form 5-FdUMP, the tumor's TS enzyme activity, mutations affecting TS binding, and folate cofactor concentration. The tumor cell must enter the vulnerable DNA synthetic phase of the cell cycle during drug exposure. A final factor, the ratio of endogenous dUMP, which rises during TS inhibition, to 5-FdUMP, can affect the duration of TS inhibition.

Regulation of Thymidylate Synthase

TS is required for DNA replication; its activity is higher in rapidly proliferating cells than in noncycling cells. In proliferating cancer cells, TS activity varies by fourfold to eightfold from resting to synthetic phase.[62] Increased expression of the TS gene at the G1-S boundary is controlled by both transcriptional and posttranscriptional events.

In both experimental and clinical observations, 5-FU exposure may be accompanied by an acute increase in TS content, which may in turn permit recovery of enzymatic activity, and the magnitude of the increase is influenced by drug concentration and duration of exposure. In NCI-H630 colon cancer cells,[63] TS content increases up to 5.5-fold during 5-FU exposure and is regulated at the translational level.[64] TS protein binds to specific regions in its

corresponding TS-mRNA, inhibiting its own translation.[65] Reduced folate content also decreases TS expression, whereas TS activity was induced by LV.[65]

Importance of Schedule of Administration in Preclinical Models

Drug concentration and duration of exposure in vitro are important determinants of response to 5-FU.[66] High drug concentrations (above 100 μmol/L) are generally required for cytotoxicity if the duration of exposure is brief (<6 hours), whereas prolonged exposure (>72 hours) to concentrations between 1 and 10 μmol/L effectively kills many tumors in culture. As set forth below, schedules designed to provide extended exposure via continuous drug infusion are currently favored in clinical practice.

Clinical Pharmacology of 5-Fluorouracil

The pharmacokinetics of 5-FU are an important consideration in the choices of routes and schedules of administration. Regional approaches, such as hepatic arterial infusion, permit selective exposure of specific tumor-bearing sites to high local concentrations of drug, but are infrequently used.

Assay Methods

5-FU has been assayed in biologic fluids using high-performance liquid chromatography (HPLC) coupled with mass spectroscopy and detect 0.6 μM or higher drug concentrations in plasma.[67] In general, an initial deproteination step is performed by chemical or filtration techniques. HPLC methods without MS and using ultraviolet detection are typically associated with limits of detection in the range of 0.2 to 1.0 μmol/L. The nucleotide metabolites of intracellular FU, particularly 5-FUTP, can be measured with HPLC-MS,[68] although methods are of limited sensitivity for 5-FdUMP and 5-FdUTP. 5-FdUMP is also measurable by an enzyme competitive binding assay for research purposes. Fluorine-19 magnetic resonance imaging (MRI) can be used to monitor the pharmacokinetics and tissue uptake of 5-FU in patients.[69]

5-FU is unstable in whole blood and plasma at room temperature. Catabolism by dihydropyrimidine dehydrogenase (DPD) is much more rapid in whole blood than in plasma.[70] Blood samples should be placed on ice immediately; plasma should be quickly isolated. 5-FU is stable in plasma at 4°C for up to 24 hours and is stable for prolonged periods at −20°C.

Absorption and Distribution

Bioavailability of 5-FU by the oral route is highly variable. Less than 75% of a dose reaches the systemic circulation.[71] When administered by intravenous bolus or infusion, 5-FU readily penetrates the extracellular space, cerebrospinal fluid (CSF), and extracellular "third spaces" such as effusions. The volume of distribution (V_d) ranges from 13 to 18 L (8 to 11 L/m^2) after intravenous bolus doses of 370 to 720 mg/m^2. The V_d exceeds extracellular fluid space.

Plasma Pharmacokinetics

The pharmacokinetic profile of 5-FU varies according to dose and schedule of administration. After intravenous bolus injection of 370 to 720 mg/m^2, peak plasma concentrations (C_p) of 5-FU primarily lie in the range of 300 to 1,000 µmol/L.[72] Rapid metabolic elimination accounts for a primary $t_{1/2}$ of 8 to 14 minutes; 5-FU levels fall to 1 µmol/L or lower in 2 hours.

The most sensitive assays have found triphasic $t_{1/2}$ values in plasma of 2 (distribution) and 12 (metabolism) minutes,[73] and a prolonged third phase, noted by GC-MS, of 2 to 5 hours: 5-FU plasma concentration fell to 36 to 136 nmol/L 4 to 8 hours after intravenous bolus doses of 500 to 720 mg/m². The slower phase may reflect the combined effects of metabolism and tissue release. The area under the C × T curve (AUC) ranges between about 4,000 and 16,000 µM (x) minutes, after doses in the range of 370 to 720 mg/m².

The clearance of 5-FU is rapid during continuous drug infusion. Clearance rates decrease as the dose rate increases[71,74-76] and lie in the range of 1,000 to 3,000 mL/min/m². As the duration of 5-FU infusion increases, the tolerated daily dose decreases. A recommended starting dose of single-agent 5-FU given by protracted (>14 days) CI is 300 mg/m²/d, achieving a C_{ss} in the submicromolar range. With CI over a shorter interval of 96 to 120 hours, a daily dose of 1 g/m² produces a C_{ss} in the 1 to 3 µmol/L range, and an intermittent administration schedule is necessary to avoid toxicity. CI of 2 to 2.6 g/m² 5-FU daily given either for 72 hours every 3 weeks or for 24 hours weekly yields a C_{ss} in the range of 5 to 10 µmol/L.

5-FU clearance varies considerably between individuals. The AUC and C_{ss} vary at least 10-fold for any sizeable cohort of patients receiving continuous infusion 5-FU in either single agent or in combinations such as FOLFOX6. The elimination kinetics of 5-FU are nonlinear.[74-78]

The following are noted with increasing oral doses: a decrease in hepatic extraction ratio, an increase in oral bioavailability, an increase in plasma $t_{1/2}$, a decrease in total-body clearance, and a disproportionate increase in 5-FU area under the curve (AUC). This nonlinear behavior represents saturation of metabolic processes at higher drug concentrations, leading to difficulty in predicting plasma levels or toxicity at higher dosages. 5-FU pharmacokinetics has been reported to vary up to fivefold according to time of day but with no consistent pattern between studies.[77]

5-FU pharmacokinetics have correlated with toxicity[67,72,79] as reflected in the total AUC with bolus injection or with plasma steady-state concentration (C_{ss}) of drug or AUC in patients receiving treatment by CI.[67,79] Therapeutic drug monitoring has been employed to adjust drug levels to optimal C_{ss} or AUC values and has consistently improved response rates and decreased toxicity in nonrandomized trials.[67,80-82] Studies of continuous infusion regimens, such as the 46-hour infusion of 2,500 mg/m² in FOLFOX6/7,[81] established an AUC of 20 to 24 mg h/L, as a safe and maximally effective target for dose adjustment,[67] and found that up to 50% of patients will require upward adjustment, while 10% or less will need a lower dose to achieve this target.

5-FdUrd is given by CI. The achieved C_{ss} with protracted schedules have not been well defined because the predicted C_p is below the detection limits of HPLC assays; analysis by GC-MS has been hampered by the difficulty in preparing stable, volatile derivatives of 5-FdUrd. With intravenous bolus 5-FdUrd given weekly, the AUC of 5-FU is twofold to threefold greater than 5-FdUrd, but the levels of 5-FU may not be pharmacologically significant.[83]

Regional Administration of 5-Fluorouracil

The administration of 5-FU and 5-FdUrd by intrahepatic arterial infusion (HAI) maximizes regional exposure while limiting systemic toxicity. Twenty to fifty percent of infused 5-FU is cleared in its first pass through the liver, whereas 5-FdUrd first-pass clearance exceeds 94%. Systemic and hepatic metabolic clearances and extraction ratios decrease progressively with increasing 5-FU dose rates. Systemic exposure (AUC) to 5-FU after HAI ranges from 12% to 52% of that after intravenous administration of dose rates equivalent to doses of 0.37 to 10 g/m²; the regional advantage relative to systemic exposure varies from sixfold at the lowest 5-FU doses to twofold at the highest doses.[78] Portal venous perfusion was based on the premise that although most large metastases obtain their blood supply predominantly from the arterial circulation, early, and perhaps clinically undetected, metastases may be fed by the portal circulation. Mean tumor uptake of 5-FdUrd in patients with established metastases was 15.5-fold greater after bolus administration of [³H]5-FdUrd into the hepatic artery compared with portal vein, whereas the uptake into healthy liver is similar.[84] However, clinical trials have failed to demonstrate consistent benefit from portal venous infusion, and similar trials of hepatic arterial infusion at the time of resection of liver metastases from colorectal cancer have not shown survival benefit, in part due to extrahepatic recurrence.

Low MW compounds such as 5-FU and FdUrd injected into the peritoneal cavity are absorbed primarily through the portal circulation, passing through the liver before reaching the systemic circulation. The rates of absorption and clearance from the peritoneal cavity depend on the drug's lipid solubility and MW, as well as the surface area of the peritoneum (which may be altered by tumor, adhesions, or other pathologic changes). Intraperitoneal drug concentrations up to 5 mmol/L 5-FU maintained by intermittent exchanges of fluid are tolerated for up to 5 days. One report found that mean 5-FU clearance from the peritoneal cavity was 840 mL/min, about fivefold slower than systemic clearance; the ratio of intraperitoneal to systemic 5-FU levels was 300.[85] Higher intraperitoneal drug concentrations (>5 mmol/L) saturate hepatic clearance mechanisms, leading to increased systemic levels and significant myelosuppression. Between dialysate concentrations of 5 and 24 mmol/L, the mean peritoneal levels of 5-FU ranged from 2.2 to 12.5 mmol/L (much higher than levels achieved in plasma in systemic 5-FU therapy), and peak plasma levels, which occurred 1 hour after intraperitoneal instillation, ranged from 6 to 60 µmol/L, in the range of peak levels with conventional systemic treatment. Mild-to-moderate abdominal pain and chemical peritonitis may occur, particularly with repeated dosing. 5-FU is given intraperitoneally in escalating concentrations for 4 hours along with a fixed dose of cisplatin (90 mg/m²) every 28 days. This regimen led to dose-limiting neutropenia with 5-FU concentrations of greater than 20 mmol/L; other toxicities included nausea, vomiting, and diarrhea.[86] There are no conclusive therapeutic trials of intraperitoneal 5-FU, an approach now confined to intraperitoneal *cis*-platinum.

Topical 5-FU, 2% to 5% in a hydrophilic cream base or propylene glycol, is used by dermatologists for the treatment of multiple actinic keratoses of the face, intraepidermal carcinomas, superficial basal cell carcinoma, vaginal intraepithelial neoplasia, and genital

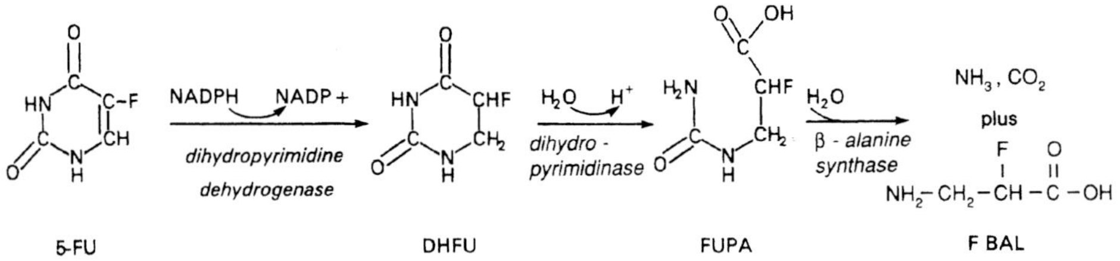

FIGURE 8.5 Catabolism of 5-FU. DHFU, dihydrofluorouracil; FBAL, fluoro-*β*-alanine; FUPA, *α*-fluoroureido-propionic acid; NADP, nicotinamide adenine dinucleotide; NADPH, nicotinamide adenine dinucleotide phosphate.

condylomas. Local application of 5-FU has also been used after trabeculectomy in patients with uncontrolled glaucoma to improve intraocular pressure control.

Mechanisms of Drug Elimination

After bolus dosing of 5-FU, about 90% is eliminated by metabolism (catabolism > > anabolism) and less than 10% is excreted intact in the urine. With CI of 5-FU 2.3 g/m^2, less than 2% of 5-FU was excreted in the urine.[87] The initial rate-limiting step in 5-FU catabolism is reduction of the pyrimidine ring by DPD (Fig. 8.5), forming dihydrofluorouracil [DHFU]). Mammalian-purified DPD has equal affinity for uracil and 5-FU (K_m ranging from 1.8 to 5.5 µmol/L).[88] Saturation of DPD accounts for the dose-dependent 5-FU pharmacokinetics. DPD is widely distributed in tissues throughout the body, including the liver, GI mucosa, and peripheral blood mononuclear cells (PBMCs).[89] Because of its size, the liver has the highest total content of DPD in the body and is the major site of 5-FU catabolism.

The clearance of 5-FU during CI exceeds hepatic blood flow (1,000 mL/min) by several fold, suggesting that a substantial portion of 5-FU metabolism occurs in extrahepatic tissue. While the dose of 5-FU need not be reduced for hepatic dysfunction, a conservative approach may be prudent in jaundiced patients with a poor performance status.

DH5-FU appears rapidly after intravenous bolus 5-FU. The pyrimidine ring is subsequently opened by dihydropyrimidinase forming 5-fluoroureido-propionic acid (FUPA); FUPA is then converted by *β*-alanine synthase to fluoro-*β*-alanine (FBAL), with the release of ammonia from the nitrogen-3 position and CO^2 from the carbon-2 of the pyrimidine ring. In 10 subjects receiving 500 to 700 mg/m^2 [3H]5-FU, peak DHFU C_p of 10 to 30 µmol/L was seen 30 to 90 minutes later. FUPA reached maximum C_p (C_{max}) of 13 µmol/L at 90 minutes; FBAL C_{max} occurred between 60 and 90 minutes (60 µmol/L). In these subjects, the excretion of unchanged drug, FBAL, and FUPA in the urine occurred within the 6 hours; FBAL was the major metabolite. FBAL accumulates in high concentrations in normal tissues and in bile (as a cholic acid conjugate), but it has unknown effects, if any, on toxicity or antitumor response.[71]

Dihydropyrimidine Dehydrogenase Activity and 5-Fluorouracil Toxicity

The genetics and polymorphisms related to 5-FU toxicity are discussed in detail in Chapter 5 (Pharmacogenetics), to which the reader is referred for further detail. About 1% of patients have significant DPD variants that lead to severe toxicity. Several different genetic variant changes have been described in DPD-deficient kindreds, including point mutations and deletions caused by exon skipping, and have been associated with a high risk of toxicity; the advantages and results of pretreatment assessment of DPD status are discussed in Chapter 5.

Human DPD protein has been purified and its crystal structure has been elucidated.[88,90] DPD enzymatic activity has often been measured by a complex assay that has generally limited its availability to research laboratories. Although there appears to be a relationship between DPD activity and 5-FU clearance, the correlation is inexact in clinical studies.[74,75,91] In contrast, profound DPD deficiency has been identified in patients who have experienced excessive toxicity with a 5-FU–based therapy (see Chapter 5). Measurement of DPD activity in human PBMCs suggests a Gaussian distribution.[92,93] It is clear that DPD deficiency is only one of many factors that contribute to 5-FU toxicity (pharmacokinetics being a significant player). In one study of 47 British patients with severe toxicity on various 5-FU–containing regimens, only 9 of 47 (19%) had variants of DPD gene sequence possibly associated with deficiency, while others estimate that up to 50% of severe 5-FU toxicities are related to DPD variants or gene methylation.[92-94] In addition to polymorphism of the DPD gene, methylation of promoter regions may contribute to low levels of gene expression.[94]

As an alternative to DPD variant analysis, plasma uracil levels and the ratio of uracil to dihydrouracil in plasma has been proposed as a predictor of DPD deficiency and toxicity.[95] Pretreatment uracil levels greater than 16 ng/mL predicted severe toxicity in a retrospective study of patients treated with a variety of fluoropyrimidines and regimens, but requires confirmation. Other factors, such as variable numbers of tandem repeats at the 5′-UTR of the TS gene as well as deletions in this region, may affect TS enzymatic activity and 5-FU toxicity. No single clinical study has taken into account the multiplicity of pharmacokinetic and genetic factors that likely contribute to 5-FU toxicity.

Pharmacokinetic interactions between 5-FU and several compounds, including dThd, other pyrimidine bases and their nucleosides, and cimetidine (an H-2 receptor antagonist) produce interference with 5-FU catabolism by DPD.[96,97] The antiviral agent and Urd analog sorivudine form a metabolite that inactivates DPD and, when used with oral 5-FU, caused the death of patients in Japan due to extreme 5-FU toxicity. It is advisable not to use 5-FU in combination with antiviral or anticancer pyrimidine bases or nucleosides unless clinical trials have established the safety of the regimen.[98]

Clinical Toxicities

Impact of Schedule of 5-FU

The main toxic effects of 5-FU and FdUrd occur in rapidly dividing tissues (primarily GI mucosa and bone marrow). The spectrum of toxicity associated with 5-FU and FdUrd varies according to dose, schedule, and route. In general, bolus administration produces more myelosuppression than infusional schedules. The toxicity of infusional 5-FU depends on dose and duration of infusion.

For the first three decades of its use, 5-FU was administered as either a daily times five bolus infusion every 4 weeks (the "Mayo" regimen) or as a single weekly bolus (the "Roswell Park" regimen). Mucositis and diarrhea are dose limiting with bolus 5-FU given intravenous daily for 5 days every 4 weeks, although neutropenia may also be problematic.[99] A single intravenous bolus dose given weekly is associated with myelosuppression, diarrhea, and mucositis.[100]

In order to avoid acute myelosuppression and to extend the duration of drug exposure, CI of 5-FU has been given over durations ranging from 24 hours to several weeks.[101,102] With infusion durations of 72 to 120 hours, 5-FU is generally given at 3- to 4-week intervals. The tolerated daily dosage decreases as the duration of infusion increases. Mucositis is usually dose limiting with CI of 1,000 or 750 mg/m^2/d for 4 or 5 days, respectively, although diarrhea and dermatitis occur; myelosuppression is generally mild to moderate.[75,101] With a 48- to 72-hour CI, 2,000 to 2,300 mg/m^2/d is tolerated. Mucositis and hand-foot syndrome (HFS) are dose limiting in long-term infusions, whereas diarrhea is less common.

An every 2-week schedule of LV-modulated 5-FU, given by combined bolus and CI, exploits the potential for lesser myelosuppression and prolonged drug exposure as compared to bolus administration and has been incorporated into combination regimens with oxaliplatin (FOLFOX) or irinotecan (FOLFIRI). These regimens in general employ a loading dose of 400 mg/m^2 of 5-FU given as an IV bolus, LV 400 mg/m^2, and then 5-FU by a CI for 22 hours (1,200 mg/m^2/d) or 2,400 mg/m^2 over 46 to 48 hours.[103] An advantage of the infusion schedules is the decreased risk of severe toxicity in DPD-deficient subjects compared to the toxicity of the weekly bolus schedule or daily for a 5-day schedule.

FdUrd Schedules

The highest tolerated dose of 5-FdUrd administered as a 14-day CI is 0.125 to 0.15 mg/kg/d (4.6 to 5.6 mg/m^2/d).[104] Diarrhea predominates, whereas mucositis is less common. Severe myelosuppression is uncommon with prolonged CI of either 5-FU or FdUrd. The tolerated doses of FdUrd given by CI for either 5 or 14 days are 90- and 50-fold lower than comparable 5-FU for the respective schedules.[83,105]

Myelosuppression

Serious myelosuppression is more common with intravenous bolus schedules of 5-FU and FdUrd. The greatest impact is on leukocytes and neutrophils, although anemia may also be problematic after multiple cycles of treatment. Clinically relevant thrombocytopenia occurs with the high-dose loading schedules but is uncommon with prolonged infusion. The acute megaloblastic changes seen with this bolus loading schedule likely result from inhibition of TS.

Gastrointestinal Toxicity

5-FU–associated GI toxicity can be severe and life-threatening. In clinical practice, the dosage of 5-FU is not usually reduced in the presence of hepatic dysfunction. Full-dose 5-FU has been given by HAI to patients with extensive liver replacement and jaundice; improvement or resolution of jaundice may occur in some patients without undue systemic toxicity. Patients with severe hepatic dysfunction in general have been excluded from randomized trials of HAI 5-FdUrd and systemic 5-FU. Mucositis may be preceded by a sensation of dryness that is followed by erythema, formation of a white, patchy membrane, ulceration, and necrosis. Similar lesions have been observed throughout the GI tract and in the stoma of colostomies. Enteric lesions may occur at any level, resulting in clinical symptoms of dysphagia, retrosternal burning, watery diarrhea, abdominal pain, and proctitis. The diarrhea can be bloody. Nausea, vomiting, and profuse diarrhea can lead to dehydration and hypotension. Disruption of the integrity of the gut lining permits access of enteric organisms into the bloodstream, with the potential for overwhelming sepsis, particularly if the neutrophil nadir coincides with diarrhea. Imaging of the small bowel may show extensive or segmental narrowing and effacement of the mucosal folds in the distal ileum.[106]

Before each dose, it is essential to question whether the patient has experienced mouth soreness, watery stools, or both. 5-FU should be withheld in cases of ongoing moderate-to-severe diarrhea. Subsequent dosages should be reduced when the patient has fully recovered. If diarrhea occurs, supportive care and vigorous hydration should be given as dictated by the severity of the toxic reaction. Antidiarrheal agents may provide symptomatic relief from secretory diarrhea. Loperamide is a standard therapy for uncomplicated diarrhea, but it is less effective in the setting of severe diarrhea. Aggressive management of complicated or prolonged diarrhea requires intravenous fluids, octreotide, administration of antibiotics, and stool workup for blood, fecal leukocytes, and infectious causes of colitis such as *Clostridium difficile*.[107]

In severe episodes of mucositis, diarrhea, and neutropenia with the initial cycle or dose of 5-FU, the care team must suspect a polymorphism in DPD. Clinical tests for DPD deficiency are available commercially (Molecular Diagnostics Labs, Cincinnati, Ohio, 45219-2374). The utility of these tests for all polymorphisms of severe DPD deficiency is not clear. If DPD deficiency is suspected, a drastic reduction of 5-FU dose or a change of regimen should be considered.

Skin Toxicity

Dermatologic toxicity occurs with bolus and CI schedules.[108] Loss of hair, occasionally progressing to total alopecia, nail changes (onycholysis and pigmentation), dermatitis, and increased pigmentation and atrophy of the skin may occur. Manifestations vary from erythema alone to a maculopapular erythematous rash. 5-FU enhances the cutaneous toxicity of radiation; reactions typically occur within 7 days of radiation. Erythema followed by dry desquamation occurs, with vesicle formation in severe cases. Photosensitivity reactions, while uncommon, may occur and can result in exaggerated sunburn reactions, residual tanning, or both, in the distribution of sunlight exposure. Hyperpigmentation may develop over the veins into which 5-FU has been administered. Allergic contact dermatitis may result from application of topical 5-FU. Actinic keratoses appear as an erythematous inflammatory reaction with systemic 5-FU. Hand-foot syndrome, an erythematous, painful reaction over palms and soles, may progress to trunk desquamation and ulceration and can limit doses for CI regimens and for capecitabine.

Neurotoxicity

5-FU may produce acute neurologic symptoms. A cerebellar syndrome has been most frequently reported, but ataxia, global motor weakness, bulbar palsy, bilateral oculomotor nerve palsy, upper motor neuron signs, and cognitive impairment have been occasionally associated with systemic 5-FU.[109] These symptoms are usually reversible after drug discontinuation. Neurologic toxicity is more prominent on schedules that feature high daily doses (bolus and 24- to 48-hour infusions) or with carotid artery infusion. Severe neurotoxic reactions, including coma, have been reported in patients with previously unrecognized complete deficiency of DPD after receiving conventional doses of 5-FU, and the time to recovery may be longer than in non–DPD-deficient patients.[110]

5-FU alone or in combination regiments is rarely associated with cerebral demyelination reminiscent of multifocal leukoencephalopathy.[111] The symptoms occur after several months of adjuvant therapy and include a decline in mental status, ataxia, and loss of consciousness. MRI scans with gadolinium enhancement show prominent multifocal-enhancing white matter lesions, and cerebral biopsy shows morphologic features of an active, demyelinating disease. Occasional patients may recover after cessation of therapy and administration of corticosteroids.

Cardiotoxicity

5-FU therapy may be complicated by cardiac toxicity characterized by chest pain, arrhythmia, and changes in electrocardiograms (ECGs) with bolus and infusional schedules.[112] Chest pain generally occurs in temporal association with 5-FU administration. The chest discomfort is often accompanied by ECG and serum enzyme changes indicative of myocardial ischemia. Some of these episodes have occurred in patients with a prior history of chest irradiation or cardiac disease, but coronary angiography performed subsequently showed no evidence of atherosclerotic disease, suggesting that coronary vasospasm might be involved. Cardiogenic shock and sudden death have also been reported. In a prospective multicenter cohort study of 483 patients receiving CI 5-FU, the incidence of suspected or documented cardiotoxic events was 1.9%; preexisting cardiac disease appeared to be a risk factor.[113] There is no unequivocally effective prophylaxis or treatment for this syndrome. Once 5-FU administration is discontinued, symptoms are usually reversible, although fatal outcomes have been reported. There is a high risk of recurrent cardiac symptoms when patients are re-exposed to this drug; therefore, it seems prudent to discontinue 5-FU after the first episode. The cause of vasospasm is unknown.

Ocular Toxicity

5-FU may cause significant ocular toxicity, such as ocular irritation, tearing, epiphora, blepharitis, conjunctivitis, keratitis, eyelid dermatitis, cicatricial ectropion, tear duct stenosis, punctal-canalicular stenosis, and blurred vision.[114] Excessive lacrimation is the most frequent ocular symptom, followed by pruritus and burning. Conjunctivitis is reversible with discontinuation of 5-FU early in the patient's course, but progression of the inflammatory response may require surgical correction of dacryostenosis and ectropion. An ocular ice pack during drug infusion may lessen 5-FU–induced ocular toxicity.[115] Ocular toxicity often improves with dose reduction. Early ophthalmologic evaluation of symptoms should be considered to avoid potentially permanent damage from fibrosis.

Toxicity of Hepatic Arterial Infusion

HAI of 5-FU or 5-FdUrd, often used in patients with liver-only metastases from colorectal cancer, has largely been supplanted by more convenient and less toxic systemic combination therapy. Systemic toxicities (leukopenia and diarrhea) are usually dose limiting with HAI of 5-FU. Chemical hepatitis is mild. In contrast, systemic toxicities are uncommon with 5-FdUrd, whereas hepatic toxicity is dose limiting.[116,117] Peptic ulcers, gastritis, and duodenitis occurred in up to 25% of patients in older studies, but the incidence has been substantially reduced with improved surgical and radiographic technique that allow selective infusion in right and left branches of the hepatic artery.

Chemical hepatitis, evidenced by elevations of alkaline phosphatase, transaminases, and bilirubin, occurs commonly with HAI 5-FdUrd. Cholestatic jaundice is a serious complication, and may progress to biliary sclerosis, and is believed to result from diminished vascular perfusion via small vessel injury for the gallbladder and upper bile duct. In more severely affected patients, cholangiograms reveal narrowing of the common hepatic duct and the lobar ducts and intrahepatic ductal stricture, but sparing of the common bile duct. Liver biopsy discloses canalicular cholestasis and focal pericholangitis. The hepatocytes appear normal, although inflammatory infiltrate changes are present. Some patients require cholecystectomy for acalculous cholecystitis; at surgery, the gallbladder appears shrunken, hypovascular, and densely fibrotic. The onset of biliary sclerosis can be delayed by decreasing the initial dose (median time to toxicity at 0.2 or 0.3 mg/kg/d is three or five cycles). Although 5-FdUrd may be reinstituted at a lower dose after normalization of liver enzymes, most patients became progressively intolerant. The clinical picture may not improve after interruption of therapy. LV given with HAI increases biliary sclerosis, while dexamethasone, added to the infusion, decreased the incidence to only 3%.[117]

Catheter-related complications include arterial thrombosis, hemorrhage or infection at the arterial puncture site, and slippage of the catheter into the arterial supply of the duodenum or stomach, with necrosis of the intestinal epithelium, hemorrhage, and perforation. The occurrence of epigastric pain or vomiting should alert the clinician to promptly reassess the catheter position. In some patients, HAI may be impossible because of difficulties in catheter placement, thrombosis of the portal vein, or variations in vascular anatomy.

Age and Gender as Prognostic Factors for 5-Fluorouracil Clinical Toxicity

A number of clinical studies have reported greater frequency and severity of toxicity in female and older patients treated with 5-FU–based therapy.[118,119] The Meta-Analysis Group in Cancer, using individual data from six randomized trials comparing infusional with bolus 5-FU, found that female patients, older patients, and those with poorer performance had a significantly higher risk of diarrhea, mucositis, nausea, and vomiting.[119] Hand-foot syndrome (HFS) was 2.6-fold more common in patients receiving infusional 5-FU versus bolus drug (34% versus 13%, $P < 0.0001$). Female patients and older patients also had a higher risk of HFS. Grade 3 to 4 hematologic toxicity, mainly neutropenia, was sevenfold more common with bolus 5-FU therapy (31% versus 4%, $P < 0.0001$). Poor performance status was a prognostic factor for serious hematologic toxicity. Pooled analyses of multiple trials of single-agent 5-FU with or without LV showed no significant difference in toxicity or response rates in patients older than 70 versus young than 70.[120,121] It is unclear whether age or gender affects rates of drug clearance.

It seems prudent to closely monitor blood counts and symptoms in older and female patients, particularly in those with poor-performance status, during 5-FU–based therapy, with appropriate dose adjustments according to toxicity. The dose should not be lowered a priori in these subsets.

Randomized Trials Comparing Various Fluoropyrimidine Routes and Schedules

A series of meta-analyses, performed by the Advanced Colorectal Cancer Meta-Analysis Group,[122-124] reached the following conclusions: (a) CI yields superior response rate as compared to intravenous bolus 5-FU (22% versus 11%) when given as a single agent; (b) HFS is more common with CI (34% versus 13%); and (c) diarrhea and hematologic toxicity are much less frequent with HAI (4% versus 31%). HAI of 5-FU or 5-FdUrd produced higher response rates in patients with liver metastases compared with systemic single-drug regimens, although evidence for improved survival is inconclusive, and LV enhanced response rates of single-agent bolus 5-FU (13.6% versus 22.5%).[122] Many of these conclusions are no longer relevant, as continuous 26-hour infusion regimens of systemic 5-FU and LV with oxaliplatin +/− irinotecan dominate the chemotherapy landscape for gastrointestinal tumors.

Modulation of Fluoropyrimidines

The multiple enzymatic steps in the activation and catabolism of 5-FU offered opportunities for enhancing cytotoxicity or decreasing host toxicity by combining 5-FU with second agents that affect its metabolism. Many such combinations have reached the stage of clinical trial, but with the exception of LV enhancement, none has become a standard regimen. Modulation of alternative fluoropyrimidines has yielded S-1 and TAS-102, which will be discussed separately.

The combinations explored for host protection included (a) allopurinol, and its active metabolite, oxypurinol, which inhibits orotidylate decarboxylase, expanding the pool of orotidylate, an inhibitor of OPRTase[125]; (b) Urd, which expands cellular pools of dUTP and UTP, decreases 5-FU incorporation into nucleic acids, and seems to provide selective rescue of bone marrow or intestinal epithelium in mouse tumor models, but has unsuccessful in clinical trials[126]; and (c) thymidine, discussed above, which rescues from TS inhibition but enhances RNA incorporation, and in clinical trials markedly reduces FU clearance and caused unacceptable toxicity. None of these modifications have proven to be useful in clinical practice.

Leucovorin Modulation

The most successful approach to enhancing 5-FU antitumor activity resulted from tissue culture and animal experiments showing that LV (5-formyl tetrahydrofolate) could enhance 5-FU killing (Fig. 8.6).[127] LV is a stable and transportable precursor of the active folate cofactors, $5–10~CH_2~FH_4$, required in thymidylate synthesis, and 10-formyl FH_4, used in purine synthesis. One micrometer or

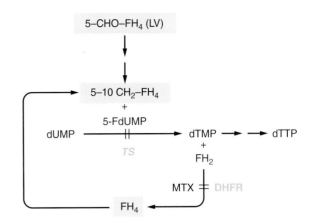

FIGURE 8.6 Interaction of folate and thymidylate synthesis pathways. 5-FdUMP and $5–10~CH_2~FH_4$ (5–10-methylenetetrahydrofolate) form a ternary complex with thymidylate synthase (TS), blocking formation of thymidylate (dTMP) and inhibiting DNA synthesis. Exogenous folate, in the form of LV (5-formyl tetrahydrofolate, 5-CHO FH_4), is converted in a multistep reaction to $5–10~CH_2~FH_4$ and expands the cellular pool of the required cofactor. Dihydrofolate (FH_2) generated in any residual TS catalytic activity must be recycled to tetrahydrofolate reductase, a step which is inhibited by methotrexate (MTX). Complete inhibition of TS negates the generation of FH_2 and renders MTX ineffective.

greater concentrations of LV in plasma are optimal for forming the tight ternary complex of folate, 5-FdUMP with TS, and need to be maintained throughout the period of 5-FU exposure.[127,128] The optimal conditions for LV administration, before or during 5-FU, may vary among cell lines and in clinical treatment.[129,130] Pretreatment for up to 18 hours with LV allows an optimal buildup of folate polyglutamates, while longer exposures of drug likely require lower concentrations of continuous LV.

LV is available through chemical synthesis, the clinical material consisting of equal amounts of the R- (or D-) and S- (or L-) isomers. The active or S-isomer must be converted to the active $5–10~CH_2$ FH_4 in a multistep process.[131] There appears to be no advantage to using the active isomer, as opposed to the racemic mixture. Tumor cells with impaired ability to transport and polyglutamate folates (see Chapter 7) will also become insensitive to LV modulation of 5-FU.

Various combinations of 5-FU and LV are used in clinical regimens. With intravenous bolus doses of 50 mg LV, plasma concentrations of reduced folate remain above 1 µM for 1 hour, With a 2-hour infusion of 500 mg LV, peak levels of reduced folate exceed 40 µM.[132] Oral absorption of LV, as with other folates, is saturable, and therefore, this route is less reliable for 5-FU enhancement.

LV has become a standard component of most 5-FU regimens, but it is not used with capecitabine, as there is no evidence for enhancement of 5-FU efficacy, either improved survival or higher response rates, associated with schedules using prolonged infusion of 5-FU or with oral administration of capecitabine. The addition of LV to oral fluoropyrimidines is associated with increased toxicity.

5-FU in Combination with Other Cytotoxics and Irradiation

In clinical practice, 5-FU is rarely used as a single agent. In most regimens, it is combined with LV and with other cytotoxic agents, particularly cisplatin or oxaliplatin, irinotecan, and cyclophosphamide,

TABLE

8.3 *Commonly used fluoropyrimidine-based combination therapy regimens and indications*

Combination Regimen	Clinical Indications
5-FU or capecitabine with irradiation	Many carcinomas of the aerodigestive tract and genitourinary tract
FOLFOX (5-FU, leucovorin, oxaliplatin)	Colorectal cancer: Adjuvant and metastatic
CAPOX (capecitabine/oxaliplatin)	Gastric cancer: Adjuvant and metastatic
S-1/oxaliplatin	Pancreatic cancer: Adjuvant (single-agent S-1) and metastatic
	Bile duct cancer: Adjuvant (single-agent capecitabine) and metastatic
S-1/cisplatin	Lung cancer: Metastatic
Capecitabine/lapatinib	Breast cancer: Metastatic
Capecitabine/docetaxel	Breast cancer: Metastatic
Capecitabine/gemcitabine	Pancreatic cancer: Adjuvant and metastatic
FOLFIRI (5-FU/irinotecan)	Colorectal cancer: Metastatic
	Gastroesophageal cancer: Metastatic
FOLFIRINOX (5-FU/leucovorin/oxaliplatin/irinotecan)	Colorectal cancer: Metastatic
	Pancreatic cancer: Metastatic

and, in breast cancer treatment, with MTX and anthracyclines. These combinations of drugs are more successful than single-agent therapy, and there is strong clinical evidence to support specific drug combinations (Table 8.3).

Of greatest importance are the combinations of 5-FU and cisplatin with irradiation in head and neck cancer, cervical cancer, endometrial cancer, bladder cancer, and other epithelial cancers. Preclinical studies have demonstrated that 5-FU enhances the cytotoxicity of cisplatin,[133,134] probably by its depletion of thymidylate nucleotides or by its incorporation into DNA. The effect of dTTP depletion is to inhibit repair of radiation-induced DNA strand breaks.

The combination of 5-FU/LV and oxaliplatin (FOLFOX) has become standard and highly effective for both adjuvant therapy of colorectal cancer and for metastatic disease.[135,136] Oxaliplatin differs from cisplatin in several aspects of its mechanism of action, including its lack of dependence on mismatch repair for recognition of DNA breaks and apoptosis, and alternative mechanisms of repair of its adducts (see Chapter 13). One noteworthy feature of oxaliplatin is its down-regulation of TS in colon cancer cell lines.[134]

5-FU/LV is commonly combined with irinotecan in an alternative regimen (FOLFIRI) for colon cancer and for pancreatic cancer in a regimen that combines these drugs with oxaliplatin (FOLFIRINOX). Irinotecan exerts its tumor-killing effects when it creates single-strand DNA breaks, which are converted to lethal double-strand breaks when the complex is encountered by a replication fork. In experimental systems, the combination is most effective when irinotecan precedes 5-FU/L, as irinotecan cytotoxicity is inhibited when DNA synthesis is blocked by earlier 5-FU.[137] In clinical practice, sequencing of drug administration is inconvenient.

Interaction with Radiation

Early in its clinical development, 5-FU was found to sensitize cells to irradiation.[138] Continuous 5-FU exposure of cells for a period longer than cell doubling time during irradiation produces the greatest cell kill (a finding confirmed by the superior results of continuous drug infusion in rectal cancer trials).[139] Thus, in clinical practice, 5-FU is often administered by continuous intravenous infusion with daily- or twice daily irradiation for tumors of the aerodigestive tracts.

Oral Fluoropyrimidines

Two oral preparations of fluoropyrimidines, capecitabine and TAS-102, have been approved for cancer treatment in the United States and are available abroad, while a third, S-1, is under active investigation. The key features of capecitabine, S-1, and TAS-102 are presented in Table 8.4. The structures of these oral fluoropyrimidines are shown in Figure 8.7.

Capecitabine

Capecitabine (N4-pentoxycarbonyl-5′-deoxy-5-fluorocytidine, Xeloda) is the first oral 5-FU prodrug marketed in the United States, on the basis of its activity in patients with metastatic breast cancer, either alone[140] or with docetaxel[141] or with lapatinib for trastuzumab-resistant breast cancer.[142] It is also a component of regimens for adjuvant and metastatic colon cancer (XELOX),[143] for which it appears to be equally as active as 5-FU/oxaliplatin-containing regimens. This agent is absorbed intact as the parent drug and then undergoes a three-step enzymatic conversion to 5-FU (Fig. 8.8). In the liver, 5′-deoxy-5-fluorocytidine (5′-dFCyd) formation is catalyzed by microsomal or cytosolic carboxylesterase (CES).[144] In a second step, cytidine deaminase, an enzyme in the liver, plasma, and tissues, produces 5′-deoxyFUrd, and thirdly, thymidine phosphorylase, found in the liver and tumor, then removes the 5′-deoxy sugar and generates 5-FU. Clinical studies have documented rapid GI absorption of the parent drug with efficient conversion to 5′-deoxyFUrd; 5-FU concentrations in plasma are low.[145]

Preclinical and clinical studies suggest that capecitabine administration leads to preferential accumulation of 5-FU in tumor tissue compared with healthy tissue.[146-148] With capecitabine, the

TABLE

8.4   *Key features of capecitabine, TAS-102, and S-1*

	Capecitabine	TAS-102	S-1
Mechanism of action	Metabolically activated to 5-FU by removal of ester and by deamination and removal of furan	Activated by thymidine kinase	Activated by removal of furan sugar
	5-FdUMP inhibits TS	TFT (trifluorothymidine) inhibits TS	5-FdUMP inhibits TS
	Incorporated into RNA and DNA	Incorporated into DNA	Incorporated into RNA and DNA
Metabolism: activation	Three-step activation (see Fig. 8.8) Carboxyl esterase Cytidine deaminase dThd phosphorylase	One step, see above	One step, removal of furan by CPY2A4 or by nucleoside phosphorylases
Clearance	5-FU is eliminated by DPD		5-FU eliminated by DPD
Pharmacokinetics	Plasma $t_{1/2}$ of 5-FU: 8 to 14 min	$t_{1/2}$ of TFT 2 h: urinary excretion of both components (TFT and tipiracil) < 10%	As 5-FU, $t_{1/2}$ = 8 to 14 min
	Nonlinear 5-FU PK with dose increase		Nonlinear 5-FU PK
Toxicity	Myelosuppression	Myelosuppression	Myelosuppression
	GI epithelial ulceration	G-I toxicity mild	G-I
	Palmar-plantar dysesthesia		
Precautions	Patients with DPD deficiency may experience extreme toxicity	Not known	CYP2A4 variants may lead to toxicity
			DPD variant predispose to toxicity
	May increase INR in patients on Coumadin	Not known	Likely but not known
	Radiation sensitizer	Not know	Likely but not known

median AUC of 5-FU in tumor tissue was 250 nmol/h/g, 120-fold higher than the plasma AUC. After 5-FU, the median 5-FU AUC in tumor tissue was 12.2 nmol/h/g, a twofold increase over the plasma AUC.

Pharmacokinetics

The pharmacokinetics of capecitabine and metabolites, as measured by LC/MS[68,149] after an initial dose of 1,255 mg/m^2, indicated peak plasma levels of parent drug approaching 10 µM about 1 hour after ingestion, and the peak levels of de-esterified nucleoside metabolites and 5-FU are reached 1 to 2 hours after dosing. The de-esterified metabolite and the deaminated product have plasma $t_{1/2}$ of 1 hour. The AUC of 5′-deoxyFUrd is the greatest of the metabolites and exceeds the AUC (units = microgram × hour per milliliter) of 5-FU by 12-fold. Thus, it appears that 5′deoxyFUrd may serve as the primary vehicle for delivery of drug to tumor. Over the clinical dosage range, pharmacokinetic parameters are linearly correlated with dose. No appreciable accumulation of either parent drug or metabolites is noted when comparing pharmacokinetic values from days 1 and 14, other than a 22% higher 5-FU AUC on day 14, suggesting a small decrease in 5-FU clearance or increased rate of 5-FU formation with time. The low concentration of 5-FU in plasma supports the notion that its formation primarily occurs within cells. Intracellular 5-FUTP peaks at about 0.4 µM in PBMCs,[68] and has a $t_{1/2}$ of 3.5 hours.[68]

The drug is administered within 30 minutes after food ingestion. Comparison of capecitabine pharmacokinetics before and after food intake indicates a significant increase (1.5-fold) of the AUC of capecitabine when taken before food; a moderate effect is also noted for 5′-dFCyd, a 1.26-fold higher AUC before food, but only a minor influence of food on the AUC of the other metabolites.[150] Hepatic dysfunction had minor effects on drug clearance and no discernable effect on toxicity; it is recommended that full doses can be administered in the presence of mild hepatic dysfunction (normal bilirubin levels).[151] In a small study, the AUC of 5′-deoxyFUrd was higher in those patients with impaired renal function, and this increase correlated with an excess risk of severe toxicity.[152] Based on these results, the sponsor recommends that patients with severe renal dysfunction (creatinine clearance < 30 mL/min) should not be treated with capecitabine. Information from the clinical safety database supports the recommendation that patients with moderate renal impairment (creatinine clearance of 30 to 50 mL/min) should be treated with 75% of the standard starting dose to achieve systemic exposure comparable to that in patients with normal renal function.

Two schedules for capecitabine administration have been evaluated in the clinic: a continuous schedule for 28 days (MTD 1,600 mg/m^2 orally daily) and a daily for 14 days every 3-week schedule (2,500 mg/m^2/d).[145] The daily dose of capecitabine is split into two equal doses approximately 12 hours apart, taken within 30 minutes after a meal. The toxicity profile favors the daily for 14- of

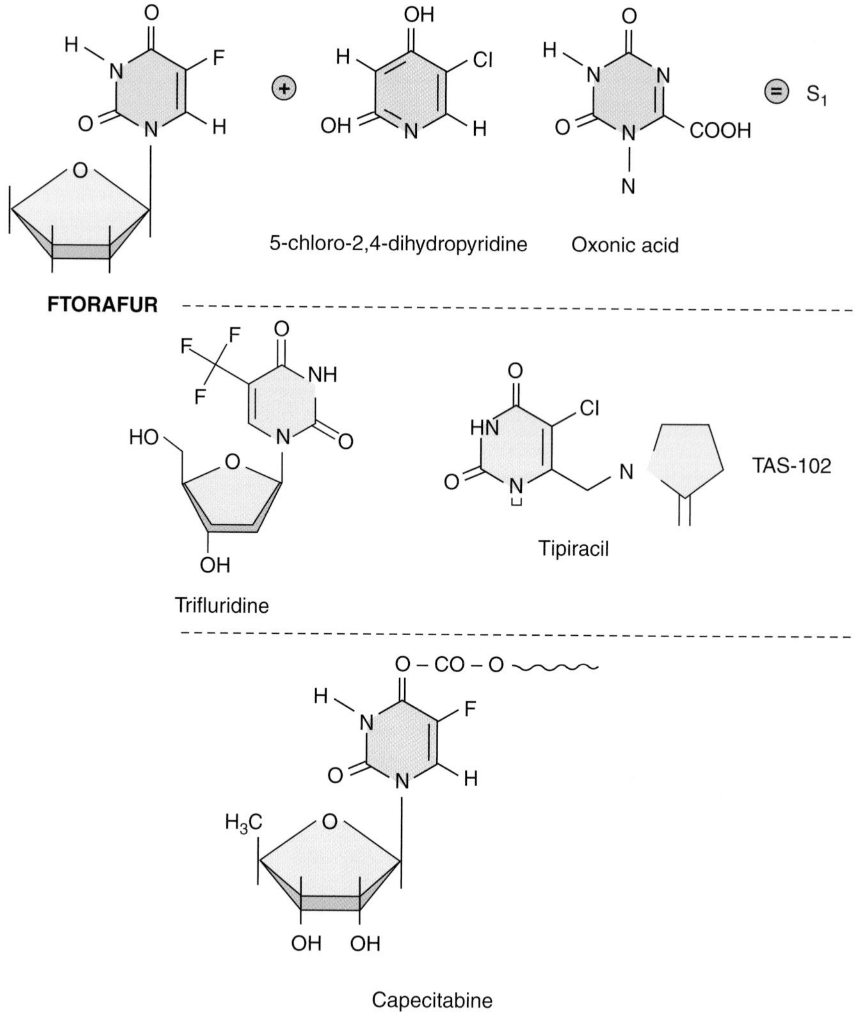

FIGURE **8.7** Structures of oral fluoropyrimidine preparations. Ftorafur is combined with 5-chloro-2,4-dihydropyridine (a highly potent DPD inhibitor also known as gimeracil) and with oxonic acid (an inhibitor of OPRTase, also known as oteracil) in S-1. TAS-102 is composed of a thymidine analogue (trifluorothymidine or trifluridine), combined with a DPD inhibitor, tipiracil. Capecitabine, a 5-FU prodrug, is activated as shown in Figure 8.8. (Modified from Figure 9.8 of fifth edition.)

21-day schedule. Dose-limiting toxicities include diarrhea, nausea, vomiting, fatigue, and HFS; severe myelosuppression is uncommon. Ocular and neurologic toxicities have also been reported.[153,154] HFS, also known as palmar plantar erythrodysesthesia, is associated with erythema, swelling, pain, paresthesias, and occasionally blisters, ulceration, or desquamation on the palms and soles. The median incidence of HFS in clinical trials was 54%, with 16% to 24% of patients experiencing severe symptoms.[144,155]

Although the mechanism of HFS remains unknown, one study of healthy volunteers demonstrated elevated dThd-phosphorylase

levels in palmar skin compared to the skin of the torso.[156] Alternatively, the reduced incidence and severity of HFS in patients treated with DPD inhibitors in combination with 5-FU or ftorafur suggest an etiologic role for 5-FU catabolites.[156,157]

Phase 2 studies suggest that daily administration of 2,000 mg/m[2] is associated with a more acceptable toxicity profile and comparable efficacy,[158] but no randomized trials of standard versus dose-reduced capecitabine have been reported. The reduced dose is commonly used in the United States, where excess toxicity may be due in part to increased dietary folate (leading to more available

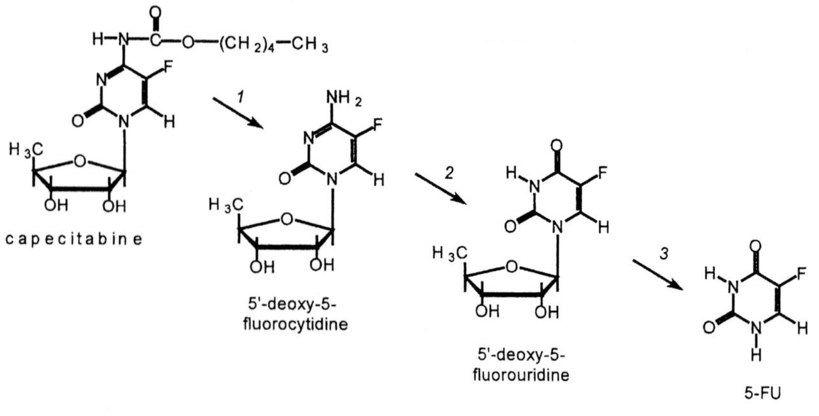

FIGURE **8.8** Pathway for activation of capecitabine. The enzymes are *1*, carboxylesterase; *2*, cytidine deaminase; and *3*, deoxythymidine phosphorylase (dTP).

5,10-CH$_2$ FH$_4$ for binding to TS). Pharmacogenetic studies have not revealed a consistent cause for individual variation in toxicity or pharmacokinetics.[159]

There are reports of severe toxicity to capecitabine in patients with DPD deficiency.[160] In addition, capecitabine toxicity may be greater in women and the elderly due to reduced clearance. The AUC and plasma levels of FBAL are modestly higher (10% to 20%) in women compared to men and increase with age in adults.[158] In a minor fraction of patients (<3%), capecitabine causes cardiotoxicity manifesting as chest pain. Less than 1% of patients develop congestive heart failure, cardiogenic shock, ventricular tachycardia, or sudden death, about the same incidence as with 5-FU.[161] Pretreatment with calcium channel blockers or nitrates in patients experiencing chest pain in prior infusions allowed for successful retreatment in most subjects. While chest pain is most commonly attributed to coronary vasospasm, in some cases, failure to document coronary vasospasm during angiography suggests alternative explanations, such as endothelial dysfunction.[162]

Large randomized trials have compared capecitabine and 5-FU/LV in patients with metastatic colorectal cancer and have found comparable or slightly improved response rates with capecitabine[155,163] either as single-agent therapy or combined with oxaliplatin.[164] No pharmacokinetic interaction occurs with oxaliplatin. Capecitabine is also effective with oxaliplatin in adjuvant therapy for stage III colorectal cancer[165] and with radiation in neoadjuvant therapy for rectal cancer.[166] In randomized trials comparing the fluoropyrimidines, thrombocytopenia, diarrhea, and HFS were more common in patients who received capecitabine, while neutropenia was more common among those who received 5-FU. Capecitabine is ineffective in patients with metastatic disease resistant to 5-FU.[167]

Capecitabine has significant activity in cancers of the upper digestive tract, similar to 5-FU, and is also extensively used in metastatic breast cancer, where it is FDA approved either with docetaxel or in HER 2+ tumors with trastuzumab.[168] It decreases recurrences when used after neoadjuvant chemotherapy and surgery for patients with primary breast cancer.[169]

Multiple studies have sought to determine biomarkers for capecitabine response. For example, lower TS and higher ratios of dTP/DPD protein and mRNA levels predicted better outcomes in patients with metastatic colon and breast cancer treated with capecitabine.[170,171] A high ratio of dTP/DPD correlated with a clinical response and disease-free survival in patients with breast and colon cancer treated with capecitabine.[172]

Alternative strategies focus on combining capecitabine with agents that might induce thymidine phosphorylase (dTP) in tumor tissue, such as cytokines and ionizing radiation.[173] A phase III trial comparing 5-FU/radiation with capecitabine/radiation in rectal cancer showed no advantage for capecitabine.[166] Capecitabine is considered equivalent to infusional 5-FU as a radiation sensitizer.

Interference of Warfarin and Phenytoin Metabolism by 5-Fluorouracil and Capecitabine

Retrospective series have described significant drug interactions in patients treated with fluoropyrimidines and warfarin or phenytoin.[174,175] In 95 patients on warfarin, 1 mg/d, that received

infusional 5-FU, the anticoagulant elevated the institutional normalized ratio (INR) to more than 1.5 in 33% of patients; the INR was greater than 3.0 in 19%, and bleeding complications were observed in 8%.[176] In a prospective study, the pharmacokinetics of a 20-mg dose of warfarin were significantly altered by concurrent capecitabine. Changes noted were a 57% increase in plasma AUC, a 51% prolongation of the elimination half-life, and a 36% reduction in apparent clearance of the more active S-warfarin enantiomer, an interaction likely due to fluoropyrimidine-induced inhibition of CYP2C, a key enzyme in warfarin metabolism.[177] CYP2C also metabolizes other drugs, especially phenytoin and paclitaxel, and may delay their clearance, leading to unexpected toxicity.[174] Prothrombin time (INR) or phenytoin level should be monitored closely in patients receiving warfarin with a 5-fluoropyrimidine, with appropriate dose adjustments.

S-1

The newest fluoropyrimidine-containing preparation, S-1, has well-established activity against colorectal, gastric, and pancreatic cancers.[178] S-1 is a three-drug preparation containing ftorafur, a prodrug of 5-FU; gimeracil (5-chloro-2,4-dihydroxypyridine), a competitive, reversible, and more potent inhibitor of DPD; and oteracil (oxonic acid), which strongly inhibits the anabolism of 5-FU to 5-UMP by OPRTase, a predominant anabolic route in normal tissues (Fig. 8.7). The molar ratio is 1.0:0.4:1.0.

The active antitumor agent in S-1 is ftorafur [1-(2-tetrahydrofuranyl)-5-FU, tegafur; MW = 200], a furan nucleoside prodrug, which was the first orally administered analogue of 5-FU approved in Japan; it is now a component of S-1. It is slowly metabolized to 5-FU by two major metabolic pathways (Fig. 8.9). In the less active pathway, microsomal cytochrome P450 oxidation at the 5′-carbon of the tetrahydrofuran moiety results in the formation of a labile intermediate (5′-hydroxyftorafur) that spontaneously cleaves to produce succinaldehyde and 5-FU.[179] This process occurs predominantly in the liver, which is the major source of CYP2A4, and to a lesser extent in the GI tract and brain. The second pathway to 5-FU is mediated by dTP, an enzyme found in high concentrations in tumor cells. It removes the furan sugar, yielding 5-FU.[180] Levels of 5-FU in plasma are in low μM range, suggesting that most metabolic conversion to 5-FU occurs in peripheral tissues and in tumors.[181] Oral administration of ftorafur primarily causes GI toxicities.[178]

Ftorafur has been a component of several other pharmaceutical preparations, including UFT, which combined ftorafur with uracil, a competitive inhibitor of DPD, in a molar ratio of 4:1, and Orzel, which combined UFT with LV. Neither drug proved equivalent to 5-FU, and their development has halted.

With a standard dose of the S-1 mixture, the AUC of 5-FU ranges from 8 to 10 μM × hour.[181] Ftorafur is metabolized by Cyp2A4 and subject to variable pharmacokinetics based upon variant genotypes of Cyp2A4, which may be responsible for some cases of severe diarrhea.[182] Gimeracil is cleared by the kidneys and leads to increased toxicity in renal dysfunction due to higher levels of ftorafur. Liver dysfunction does not seem to alter the pharmacokinetic profile of S-1 components. In a phase I/II study of S-1 in patients with hepatocellular carcinoma, there was no difference in pharmacokinetic profile between the patient Childs A and Childs B/C cirrhosis.[183] Oteracil was included in the S-1 formulation to reduce the GI toxicity of

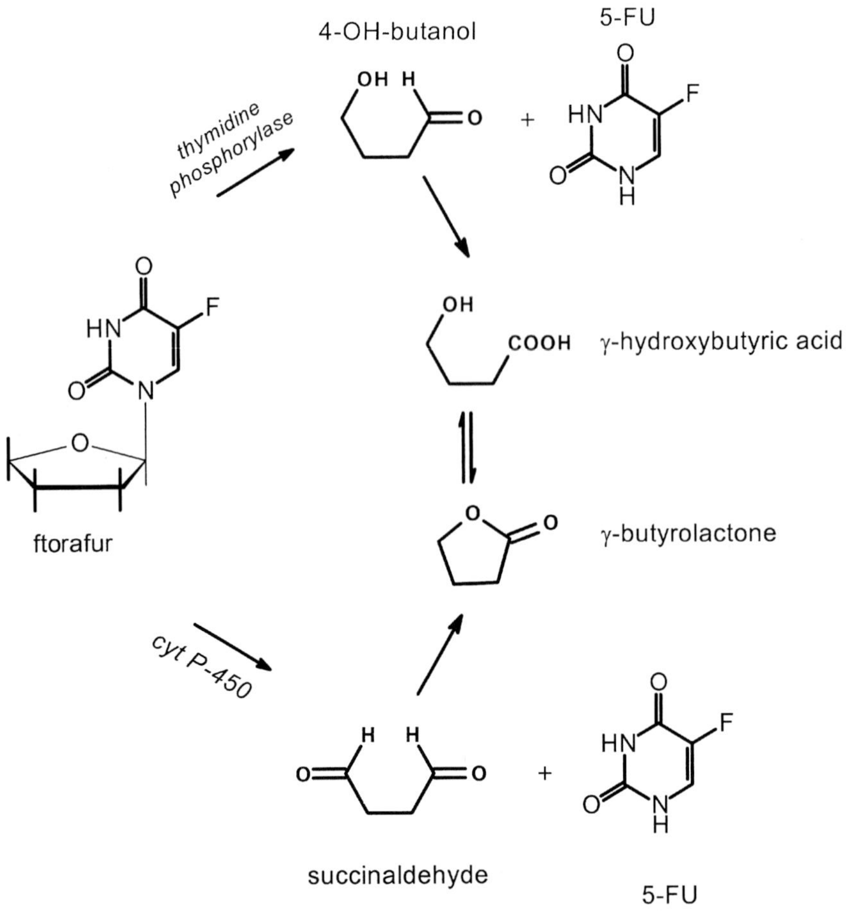

FIGURE 8.9 Pathway for activation of ftorafur.

5-FU by reducing the conversion to 5-FdUMP in gastrointestinal mucosa. However, 5-FU can by phosphorylated by Urd phosphorylase and thymidine phosphorylase into 5-FdUMP, and thus, the protective effect against diarrhea has not been well established.

S-1 is used extensively outside the United States as it is not FDA approved for use in the United States and has replaced intravenous 5-FU as the standard therapy for gastrointestinal malignancies in many Asian countries and appears to have equivalent activity as to standard fluoropyrimidines.

Investigators from the Dutch Colorectal Cancer Study Group randomized patients with stage 4 colorectal cancer to single-agent capecitabine versus single-agent S-1 and demonstrated equivalent efficacy and less hand-foot syndrome with the use of S-1.[184] Japanese investigators randomized patients with stage 2/3 rectal cancer to 1 year of UFT or S-1 and demonstrated superior relapse-free survival in the patients receiving S-1.[185] Korean investigators performed a noninferiority phase III study in patients with metastatic colon cancer comparing CAPOX (capecitabine 1,000 mg/m^2 twice daily on days 1 to 14 and oxaliplatin 130 mg/m^2 on day 1) with SOX (S-1 40 mg/m^2 twice daily on days 1 to 14 and oxaliplatin 130 mg/m^2 on day 1).[186] There was no difference in progression-free survival. In Japan, SOX plus bevacizumab was noninferior to FOLFOX plus bevacizumab in patients with metastatic colorectal cancer.[187] S-1 was compared with gemcitabine as adjuvant therapy for resected pancreatic cancer and demonstrated improved overall survival.[188] A randomized phase III study of patients with stage 2 or 3 gastric cancer demonstrated that S-1 improves survival when administered for 1 year as adjuvant therapy.[189]

S-1 has also demonstrated efficacy in multiple nongastrointestinal cancers, including breast and non–small cell lung cancers.[190,191]

TAS-102

TAS-102 is a combination of trifluorothymidine (trifluridine, TFT) and tipiracil hydrochloride (Fig. 8.7), a thymidine phosphorylase inhibitor.[192] TFT, a deoxynucleoside, the active cytotoxic component of TAS-102, is converted by thymidine kinase to the monophosphate, TFTMP, and its triphosphate is a substrate for DNA polymerase, leading to its incorporation into DNA. TFTMP inhibits TS reversibly, but its modest TS inhibition declines much more rapidly than the inhibition of TS by 5-FdUMP.[193] TFT triphosphate is resistant to dUPTase degradation and is incorporated into DNA at a much higher rate than 5-FdUTP, resulting in single- and double-strand breaks,[194] It also resists removal from DNA by glycosylases. The antitumor activity of TFT in xenografts correlates best with the degree of incorporation into DNA. It induces single- and double-strand breaks, that latter requiring repair by homologous recombination pathways.[194] Tipiracil hydrochloride selectively inhibits thymidine phosphorylase (K_i = 1.7 μM), the enzyme that degrades TFT to trifluoro-2,4(1H, 3H)-pyrimidinedione, and this catabolic reaction is found in high activity in the intestinal mucosa, liver, and tumor.[195] Combined with TFT in the oral form of TAS-102, tipiracil inhibits intestinal degradation and improves the bioavailability of TFT and maintains adequate plasma levels of the active drug. In a phase I study of TFT alone or in combination with tipiracil, the TFT area under the curve (AUC$_{0\text{-last}}$) and maximum observed plasma concentrations (C_{max}) were approximately 37- and 22-fold higher, respectively, with tipiracil than without.[196] The combination produced a TFT C_{max} of approximately 4 µM. The plasma $t_{1/2}$ of TFT is about 1.5 to 2.5 hours, with little evidence of accumulation over a course of treatment, and both TFT and tipiracil undergo extensive metabolism, with only less than 10% excreted in the urine unchanged.[192]

The recommended dose is 35 mg/m² twice daily on days 1 to 5 and 8 to 12 on a 28-day cycle. When compared with placebo in 800 patients with metastatic colon cancer refractory to standard therapy, it improved overall survival by 1.8 months, $P < 0.001$, leading to its approval by the FDA.[196] The major toxicity is grade 3 to 4 neutropenia in about 40% of patients. Severe nonhematologic toxicities occur in less than 5% of individuals and include fatigue, diarrhea, and nausea. Polymorphisms in genes responsible for homologous recombination repair of DNA double-strand breaks, specifically ATM and XRCC3, may be associated with improved efficacy.[197]

References

1. Heidelberger C, Chaudhuari NK, Daneberg P, et al. Fluorinated pyrimidines. A new class of tumor inhibitory compounds. *Nature*. 1957;179:663-666.
2. Domin BA, Mahony WB, Zimmerman TP. Transport of 5-fluorouracil and uracil into human erythrocytes. *Biochem Pharmacol*. 1993;46:503-510.
3. Pastor-Anglada M, Felipe A, Casado FJ. Transport and mode of action of nucleoside derivatives used in chemical and antiviral therapies. *Trends Pharmacol Sci*. 1998;19:424-430.
4. Kessel D, Deacon J, Coffey B, et al. Some properties of a pyrimidine phosphoribosyltransferase from murine leukemia cells. *Mol Pharmacol*. 1972;8:731-739.
5. Houghton JA, Houghton PJ. Elucidation of pathways of 5-fluorouracil metabolism in xenografts of human colorectal adenocarcinoma. *Eur J Cancer Clin Oncol*. 1983;19:807-815.
6. Finan PJ, Kiklitis PA, Chisholm EM, et al. Comparative levels of tissue enzymes concerned in the early metabolism of 5-fluorouracil in normal and malignant human colorectal tissue. *Br J Cancer*. 1984;50:711-715.
7. Schwartz PM, Moir RD, Hyde CM, et al. Role of uridine phosphorylase in the anabolism of 5-fluorouracil. *Biochem Pharmacol*. 1987;34:3585-3589.
8. Niedzwicki JG, El Kouni MH, Chu SH, et al. Structure activity relationship of ligands of the pyrimidine nucleoside phosphorylases. *Biochem Pharmacol*. 1983;32:399-415.
9. Peterson MS, Ingraham HA, Goulian M. 2′-Deoxyribosyl analogues of UDP-N-acetylglucosamine in cells treated with methotrexate or 5-fluorodeoxyuridine. *J Biol Chem*. 1983;258:10831-10834.
10. Santi DV, McHenry CS, Sommer A. Mechanisms of interactions of thymidylate synthetase with 5-fluorodeoxyuridylate. *Biochemistry*. 1974;13:471-480.
11. Sommer A, Santi DV. Purification and amino acid analysis of an active site peptide from thymidylate synthetase containing covalently bound 5′-fluoro-2′-deoxyuridylate and methylene tetrachloride. *Biochem Biophys Res Commun*. 1974;57:689-696.
12. Howell SB, Mansfield SJ, Taetle R. Significance of variation in serum thymidine concentration for the marrow toxicity of methotrexate. *Cancer Chemother Pharmacol*. 1981;5:221-226.
13. Dolnick BJ, Cheng Y-C. Human thymidylate synthase: II. Derivatives of pteroylmono- and polyglutamates as substrates and inhibitors. *J Biol Chem*. 1978;253:3563-3567.
14. Allegra CJ, Chabner BA, Jolivet J. Enhanced inhibition of thymidylate synthase by methotrexate polyglutamates. *J Biol Chem*. 1986;230:9720-9726.
15. Washtien WL, Santi DV. Assay of intracellular free and macromolecular-bound metabolites of 5-fluorodeoxyuridine and 5-fluorouracil. *Cancer Res*. 1979;39:3397-3404.
16. Hardy LW, Finer-Moore JS, Montfort WR, et al. Atomic structure of thymidylate synthase: target for rational drug design. *Science*. 1987;235:448-455.
17. Evans RM, Laskin JD, Hakala MT. Assessment of growth-limiting events caused by 5-fluorouracil in mouse cells and in human cells. *Cancer Res*. 1980;40:4113-4122.
18. Spiegelman S, Sawyer R, Nayak R, et al. Improving the antitumor activity of 5-fluorouracil by increasing its incorporation into RNA via metabolic modulation. *Proc Natl Acad Sci U S A*. 1980;77:4966-4970.
19. Herrick D, Kufe DW. Lethality associated with incorporation of 5-fluorouracil into preribosomal RNA. *Mol Pharmacol*. 1984;26:135-140.
20. Greenhalgh DA, Parish JH. Effect of 5-fluorouracil combination therapy on RNA processing in human colonic carcinoma cells. *Br J Cancer*. 1990;61:415-419.
21. Ghoshal K, Jacob ST. Specific inhibition of pre-ribosomal RNA processing in extracts from the lymphosarcoma cells treated with 5-fluorouracil. *Cancer Res*. 1994;54:632-636.
22. Kufe DW, Major PP. 5-Fluorouracil incorporation into human breast carcinoma RNA correlates with cytotoxicity. *J Biol Chem*. 1981;256:9802-9805.
23. Spears CP, Shani J, Shahinian AH, et al. Assay and time course of 5-fluorouracil incorporation into RNA of L1210/0 ascites cells in vivo. *Mol Pharmacol*. 1985;27:302-307.
24. Will CL, Dolnick BJ. 5-Fluorouracil inhibits dihydrofolate reductase precursor mRNA processing and/or nuclear mRNA stability in methotrexate-resistant KB cells. *J Biol Chem*. 1989;264:21413-21421.
25. Takimoto CH, Voeller DB, Strong JM, et al. Effects of 5-fluorouracil substitution on the RNA conformation and in vitro translation of thymidylate synthase messenger RNA. *J Biol Chem*. 1993;28:21438-21442.
26. Schmittgen TD, Danenberg KD, Horikoshi T, et al. Effect of 5-fluoro- and 5-bromouracil substitution on the translation of human thymidylate synthase mRNA. *J Biol Chem*. 1994;269:16269-16275.
27. Carrico CK, Glazer RI. The effect of 5-fluorouracil on the synthesis and translation of poly(A) RNA from regenerating liver. *Cancer Res*. 1979;39:3694-3701.
28. Doong SL, Dolnick BJ. 5-Fluorouracil substitution alters pre-mRNA splicing in vitro. *J Biol Chem*. 1988;263:4467-4473.
29. Santi DV, Hardy LW. Catalytic mechanism and inhibition of tRNA (uracil-5-)methyltransferase: evidence for covalent catalysis. *Biochemistry*. 1987;26:8599-8606.
30. Fujishima H, Niho Y, Kondo T, et al. Inhibition by 5-fluorouracil of ERCC1 and gamma-glutamylcysteine synthetase messenger RNA expression in a cisplatin-resistant HST-1 human squamous carcinoma cell line. *Oncol Res*. 1997;9:167-172.
31. Grem JL, Mulcahy RT, Miller EM, et al. Interaction of deoxyuridine with fluorouracil and dipyridamole in a human colon cancer cell line. *Biochem Pharmacol*. 1989;38:51-59.
32. Kufe DW, Scott P, Fram R, et al. Biologic effect of 5-fluoro-2′-deoxyuridine incorporation in L1210 deoxyribonucleic acid. *Biochem Pharmacol*. 1983;32:1337-1340.
33. Caradonna DJ, Cheng YC. The role of deoxyuridine triphosphate nucleotidohydrolase, uracil-DNA glycosylase, and DNA polymerase alpha in the metabolism of FUdR in human tumor cells. *Mol Pharmacol*. 1980;18:513-520.
34. Harris JM, McIntosh EM, Muscat GE. Structure/function analysis of a dUTPase: catalytic mechanism of a potential chemotherapeutic target. *J Mol Biol*. 1999;2:275-287.
35. Mauro DJ, De Riel JK, Tallarida RJ, et al. Mechanisms of excision of 5-fluorouracil by uracil DNA glycosylase in normal human cells. *Mol Pharmacol*. 1993;43:854-857.
36. Wurzer JC, Tallarida RJ, Sirover MA. New mechanism of action of the cancer chemotherapeutic agent 5-fluorouracil in human cells. *J Pharmacol Exp Ther*. 1994;269:39-43.
37. Houghton JA, Tillman DM, Harwood FG. Ratio of 2′-deoxyadenosine-5′-triphosphate/thymidine-5′-triphosphate influences the commitment of human colon carcinoma cells to thymineless death. *Clin Cancer Res*. 1995;1:723-730.
38. Jones S, Willmore E, Durkacz BW. The effects of 5-fluoropyrimidines on nascent DNA synthesis in Chinese hamster ovary cells monitored by pH-step alkaline and neutral elution. *Carcinogenesis*. 1994;15:2435-2438.
39. Canman CE, Tang H-Y, Normolle DP, et al. Variations in patterns of DNA damage induced in human colorectal tumor cells by 5-fluorodeoxyuridine. Implications for mechanisms of resistance and cytotoxicity. *Proc Natl Acad Sci U S A*. 1992;89:10474-10478.

40. Kandioler D, Mittlbock M, Kappel S, et al. *TP53* mutational status and prediction of benefit from adjuvant 5-fluorouracil in stage III colon Cancer Patients. *EBioMedicine.* 2015;2:825-830.

41. Fisher TC, Milner AE, Gregory CD, et al. Bcl-2 modulation of apoptosis induced by anticancer drugs: resistance to thymidylate stress is independent of classical resistance pathways. *Cancer Res.* 1993;53:3321-3326.

42. Darzynkiewicz Z. Methods in analysis of apoptosis and cell necrosis. In: Parker J, Stewart C, eds. *The Purdue Cytometry CD-ROM.* vol. 3. West Lafayette, IN: Purdue University, 1997.

43. Longley DB, Allen WL, McDermott U, et al. The roles of thymidylate synthase and p53 in regulating Fas-mediated apoptosis in response to antimetabolites. *Clin Cancer Res.* 2004;10:3562-3571.

44. Luo Y, Walla M, Wyatt MD. Uracil incorporation into genomic DNA does not predict toxicity caused by chemotherapeutic inhibition of thymidylate synthase. *DNA Repair.* 2008;7:162-169.

45. Meyers M, Wagner MW, Hwang HS, et al. Role of the hMLH1 DNA mismatch repair protein in fluoropyrimidine-mediated cell death and cell cycle responses. *Cancer Res.* 2001;61(13):5193-5201.

46. Arnold CN, Goel A, Boland CR. Role of hMLH1 promoter hypermethylation in drug resistance to 5-fluorouracil in colorectal cancer cell lines. *Int J Cancer.* 2003;106(1):66-73.

47. Liu A, Yoshioka K-I, Salerno V, et al. The mismatch repair-mediated cell cycle checkpoint response to fluorodeoxyuridine. *J Cell Biochem.* 2008;105:245-254.

48. Gryfe R, Kim H, Hsieh ET, et al. Tumor microsatellite instability and clinical outcome in young patients with colorectal cancer. *N Engl J Med.* 2000;342:69-77.

49. Saradaki Z, Souglakos J, Georgoulias V. Prognostic and predictive significance of MSI in stages II/III colon cancer. *World J Gastroenterol* 2014;20:6809-6814.

50. Ren Q-F, Van Groeningen CJ, Geoffroy F, et al. Determinants of cytotoxicity with prolonged exposure to fluorouracil in human colon cancer cells. *Oncol Res.* 1997;9:77-88.

51. Mulkins MA, Heidelberger C. Biochemical characterization of fluoropyrimidine-resistant murine leukemic cell lines. *Cancer Res.* 1982;42:965-973.

52. Peters GJ, Laurensse E, Leyva A, et al. Sensitivity of human, murine and rat cells to 5-fluorouracil and 5-deoxy-5-fluorouridine in relation to drug-metabolizing enzymes. *Cancer Res.* 1986;46:20-28.

53. Berger SH, Hakala MT. Relationship of dUMP and free FdUMP pools to inhibition to thymidylate synthase by 5-fluorouracil. *Mol Pharmacol.* 1984;25:303-309.

54. Noordhuis P, Holwerda U, Van Der Wilt CL, et al. 5-Fluorouracil incorporation into RNA and DNA in relation to thymidylate synthase inhibition of human colorectal cancers. *Ann Oncol.* 2004;15(7):1025-1032.

55. Leichman CG, Lenz H-J, Leichman L, et al. Quantitation of intratumoral thymidylate synthase expression predicts for disseminated colorectal cancer response and resistance to protracted-infusion fluorouracil and weekly leucovorin. *J Clin Oncol.* 1997;15:3223-3229.

56. Wong, NA, Brett L, Leitch SM, et al. Nuclear thymidylate synthase expression, p53 expression and 5FU response in colorectal cancer. *Br J Cancer.* 2001;55:1937-1943.

57. Spears CP, Gustavsson BG, Mitchell MS, et al. Thymidylate synthetase inhibition in malignant tumors and normal liver of patients given intravenous 5-fluorouracil. *Cancer Res.* 1984;44:4144-4150.

58. Peters GJ, van Groeningen CJ, Leurensse EJ, et al. Thymidylate synthase from untreated human colorectal cancer and colonic mucosa: enzyme activity and inhibition by 5-fluoro-2-deoxyuridine-5-monophosphate. *Eur J Cancer.* 1991;27:263-267.

59. Berger SH, Jenh C-H, Johnson LF, et al. Thymidylate synthase overproduction and gene amplification in fluorodeoxyuridine-resistant human cells. *Mol Pharmacol.* 1985;28:461-467.

60. Kawate H, Landis DM, Loeb LA. Distribution of mutations in human thymidylate synthase yielding resistance to 5-fluorodeoxyuridine. *J Biol Chem.* 2002;277(39):36304-36311.

61. Grem JL, Hoth DF, Hamilton JM, et al. Overview of current status and future direction of clinical trials with 5-fluorouracil in combination with folinic acid. *Cancer Treat Rep.* 1987;71:1249-1264.

62. Cadman E, Heimer R. Levels of thymidylate synthetase during normal culture growth of L1210 cells. *Cancer Res.* 1986;46:1195-1198.

63. Chu E, Voeller DM, Johnston PG, et al. Regulation of thymidylate synthase in human colon cancer cells treated with 5-fluorouracil and interferon-gamma. *Mol Pharmacol.* 1993;43:527-533.

64. Chu E, Voeller D, Koeller DM, et al. Identification of an RNA binding site for human thymidylate synthase. *Proc Natl Acad Sci U S A.* 1993;90:517-521.

65. Houghton PJ, Rahman A, Will CL, et al. Mutations of the thymidylate synthase gene of human adenocarcinoma cells causes a thymidylate synthase-negative phenotype that can be attenuated by exogenous folates. *Cancer Res.* 1992;52:558-565.

66. Moran RG, Scanlon KL. Schedule-dependent enhancement of the cytotoxicity of fluoropyrimidines to human carcinoma cells in the presence of folinic acid. *Cancer Res.* 1991;51:4618-4623.

67. Lee JJ, Beumer JH, Chu E. Therapeutic drug monitoring of 5-fluorouracil. *Cancer Chemother Pharmacol.* 2016;75:447-464.

68. Derissen EJ, Jacobs BA, Huitema AD, et al. Exploring the intracellular pharmacokinetics of the 5-fluorouracil nucleotides during capecitabine treatment. *Br J Pharmacol.* 2016;81:949-957.

69. Martino R, Malet-Martino M, Gilarad V. Fluorine nuclear magnetic resonance, a privileged tool for metabolic studies of fluoropyrimidine drugs. *Curr Drug Metab.* 2000;1:271-303.

70. Murphy RF, Balis FM, Poplack DG. Stability of 5-fluorouracil in whole blood and plasma. *Clin Chem.* 1987;33:2299-2300.

71. Heggie GD, Sommadossi J-P, Cross DS, et al. Clinical pharmacokinetics of 5-fluorouracil and its metabolites in plasma, urine, and bile. *Cancer Res.* 1987;47:2203-2206.

72. Grem JL, McAtee N, Murphy RF, et al. Phase I and pharmacokinetic study of recombinant human granulocyte-macrophage colony-stimulating factor given in combination with fluorouracil plus calcium leucovorin in metastatic gastrointestinal adenocarcinoma. *J Clin Oncol.* 1994;12:560-568.

73. McDermott BJ, van der Berg HW, Murphy RF. Nonlinear pharmacokinetics for the elimination of 5-fluorouracil after intravenous administration in cancer patients. *Cancer Chemother Pharmacol.* 1982;9:173-178.

74. Yoshida T, Araki E, Iigo M, et al. Clinical significance of monitoring serum levels of 5-fluorouracil by continuous infusion in patients with advanced colonic cancer. *Cancer Chemother Pharmacol.* 1990;26:352-354.

75. Petit E, Milano G, Levi F, et al. Circadian rhythm-varying plasma concentration of 5-fluorouracil during a five-day continuous venous infusion at a constant rate in cancer patients. *Cancer Res.* 1988;48:1676-1680.

76. Fleming RF, Milano G, Thyss A, et al. Correlation between dihydropyrimidine dehydrogenase activity in peripheral mononuclear cells and systemic clearance of fluorouracil in cancer patients. *Cancer Res.* 1982;52:2899-2902.

77. Collins JM, Dedrick RL, King FG, et al. Nonlinear pharmacokinetic models for 5-fluorouracil in man: intravenous and intraperitoneal routes. *Clin Pharmacol Ther.* 1980;28:235-246.

78. Wagner JG, Gyves JW, Stetson PL, et al. Steady-state nonlinear pharmacokinetics of 5-fluorouracil during hepatic arterial and intravenous infusions in cancer patients. *Cancer Res.* 1986;46:1499-1506.

79. Fety R, Rolland F, Barberi-Heyob M. Clinical impact of pharmacokinetically-guided dose adaptation of 5-fluorouracil: results from a multicentric randomized trial in patients with locally advanced head and neck carcinomas. *Clin Cancer Res.* 1998;4:2039-2045.

80. Gamelin E, Delva R, Jacob J, et al. Individual fluorouracil dose adjustment based on pharmacokinetic follow-up compared with conventional dosage: results of a multicenter randomized trial of patients with metastatic colorectal cancer. *J Clin Oncol.* 2008;26:2099-2105.

81. Capitain O, Asevoaia A, Boisdron-Celic M, et al. Individual fluorouracil dose adjustment in FOLFOX based on pharmacokinetic follow-up compared with conventional body-area-surface dosing: a phase II proof-of-concept study. *Clin Colorectal Cancer.* 2012;11:263-267.

82. Di Paolo A, Lencioni M, Amatori F, et al. 5-Fluorouracil pharmacokinetics predicts disease-free survival in patients administered adjuvant chemotherapy for colorectal cancer. *Clin Cancer Res.* 2008;14:2749-2755.

83. Creaven PJ, Rustum YM, Petrelli NJ, et al. Phase I and pharmacokinetic evaluation of floxuridine/leucovorin given on the Roswell Park weekly regimen. *Cancer Chemother Pharmacol.* 1994;34:261-265.

84. Sigurdson ER, Ridge JA, Kemeny N. Tumor and liver drug uptake following hepatic artery and portal vein infusion. *J Clin Oncol.* 1987;5:1836-1840.

85. Speyer JL, Collins JM, Dedrick RL, et al. Phase I and pharmacologic studies of 5-fluorouracil administered intraperitoneally. *Cancer Res.* 1980;40:567-572.

86. Schilsky RL, Choi KE, Grayhack J, et al. Phase I clinical and pharmacologic study of intraperitoneal cisplatin and fluorouracil in patients with advanced intra-abdominal cancer. *J Clin Oncol.* 1990;8:2054-2061.

87. Grem JL, Harold N, Shapiro J, et al. A phase I and pharmacokinetic trial of weekly oral 5-fluorouracil given with eniluracil and low-dose leucovorin. *J Clin Oncol.* 2000;18:3952-3963.

88. Lu Z, Zhang R, Diasio RB. Purification and characterization of dihydropyrimidine dehydrogenase from human liver. *J Biol Chem.* 1992;267:17102-17109.

89. Naguib FN, El Kouni MH, Cha S. Enzymes of uracil catabolism in normal and neoplastic tissues. *Cancer Res.* 1985;45:5405-5412.

90. Dobritzsch D, Schneider G, Schnackerz KD, et al. Crystal structure of dihydropyrimidine dehydrogenase, a major determinant of the pharmacokinetics of the anti-cancer drug 5-fluorouracil. *EMBO J.* 2001;20(4):650-660.

91. Etienne MC, Lagrange JL, Dassonville O, et al. Population study of dihydropyrimidine dehydrogenase in cancer patients. *J Clin Oncol.* 1994;12:2248-2253.

92. Lu A, Zhang R, Diasio RB. Dihydropyrimidine dehydrogenase activity in human peripheral blood mononuclear cells and liver: population characteristics, newly identified deficient patients, and clinical implication in 5-fluorouracil chemotherapy. *Cancer Res.* 1993;53:5433-5438.

93. Loganayagam A, Arenas-Hernandez M, Fairbanks L, et al. The contribution of deleterious DPYD gene sequence variants to fluoropyrimidine toxicity in British cancer patients. *Cancer Chemother Pharmacol.* 2010;65(2):403-406.

94. Meulendijks D, Henricks LM, Sonke GS, et al. Clinical relevance of DPYD variants c.1679T.G, c.1236G>A/HapB3, and c.1601G>A as predictors of severe fluoropyrimidine-associated toxicity: a systematic review and meta-analysis of individual patient data. *Lancet Oncol.* 2015;16:1639-1650.

95. Ezzeldin HH, Diasio RB. Predicting fluorouracil toxicity: can we finally do it? *J Clin Oncol.* 2008;26:2080-2082.

96. Meulendijks D, Henricks LM, Jacobs BAW, et al. Pretreatment serum uracil concentration as a predictor of severe and fatal fluoropyrimidine-associated toxicity. *Br J Cancer.* 2017;116:1415-1424.

97. Au JL-S, Rustum YM, Ledesma EJ, et al. Clinical pharmacological studies of concurrent infusion of 5-fluorouracil and thymidine in treatment of colorectal carcinomas. *Cancer Res.* 1982;42:2930-2937.

98. Diasio RB. Sorivudine and 5-fluorouracil; a clinically significant drug-drug interaction due to inhibition of dihydropyrimidine dehydrogenase. *Br J Clin Pharmacol.* 1998;46:1-4.

99. Poon MA, O'Connell MJ, Moertel CG, et al. Biochemical modulation of fluorouracil: evidence of significant improvement of survival and quality of life in patients with advanced colorectal carcinoma. *J Clin Oncol.* 1989;7:1407-1418.

100. Petrelli N, Douglass HD, Herrera L, et al. The modulation of fluorouracil with leucovorin in metastatic colorectal carcinoma: a prospective randomized phase III trial. *J Clin Oncol.* 1991;7:1419-1426.

101. Seifert P, Baker L, Reed ML, et al. Comparison of continuously infused 5-fluorouracil with bolus injection in treatment of patients with colorectal adenocarcinoma. *Cancer.* 1975;36:123-128.

102. Erlichman C, Fine S, Elkakim T. Plasma pharmacokinetic of 5-FU given by continuous infusion with allopurinol. *Cancer Treat Rep.* 1986;70:903-904.

103. de Gramont A, Bosset JF, Milan C, et al. Randomized trial comparing monthly low-dose leucovorin and fluorouracil bolus with bimonthly high-dose leucovorin and fluorouracil bolus plus continuous infusion for advanced colorectal cancer: a French intergroup study. *J Clin Oncol.* 1997;15:808-815.

104. Kemeny N, Daly J, Reichman B, et al. Intrahepatic or systemic infusion of fluorodeoxyuridine in patients with liver metastases from colorectal carcinoma. *Ann Intern Med.* 1987;107:459-465.

105. Anderson N, Lokich J, Bern M, et al. A phase I clinical trial of combined fluoropyrimidines with leucovorin in a 14-day infusion. Demonstration of biochemical modulation. *Cancer.* 1989;63:233-237.

106. Kelvin FM, Gramm HF, Gluck WL, et al. Radiologic manifestations of small-bowel toxicity due to floxuridine therapy. *AJR Am J Roentgenol.* 1986;146:39-43.

107. Benson AB III, Ajana JA, Catalano RB, et al. Recommended guidelines for the treatment of cancer treatment-induced diarrhea. *J Clin Oncol.* 2004;22:2918-2926.

108. DeSpain JD. Dermatologic toxicity of chemotherapy. *Semin Oncol.* 1992;19:501-507.

109. Moore DH, Fowler WC Jr, Crumpler LS. 5-Fluorouracil neurotoxicity. *Gynecol Oncol.* 1990;36:152-154.

110. Diasio RB, Beavers TL, Carpenter T. Familial deficiency of dihydropyrimidine dehydrogenase: biochemical basis for familial pyrimidinemia and severe 5-fluorouracil-induced toxicity. *J Clin Invest.* 1998;81:47-51.

111. Hook CC, Kimmel DW, Kvols LK, et al. Multifocal inflammatory leukoencephalopathy with 5-fluorouracil and levamisole. *Ann Neurol.* 1992;31:262-267.

112. Tsavaris N, Kosmas C, Vadiaka M, et al. Cardiotoxicity following different doses and schedules of 5fluorouracil administration for malignancy—a survey of 427 patients. *Med Sci Monit.* 2002;8:151-157.

113. Meyer CC, Calis KA, Burke LB, et al. Symptomatic cardiotoxicity associated with 5-fluorouracil. *Pharmacotherapy.* 1997;17:729-736.

114. Eiseman AS, Flanagan JC, Brooks AB, et al. Ocular surface, ocular adnexal, and lacrimal complications associated with the use of systemic 5-fluorouracil. *Ophthal Plast Reconstr Surg.* 2003;19:216-224.

115. Loprinzi CL, Wender DB, Veeder MH, et al. Inhibition of 5-fluorouracil-induced ocular irritation by ocular ice packs. *Cancer.* 1994;74:945-948.

116. Kemeny N, Seiter K, Conti JA, et al. Hepatic arterial floxuridine and leucovorin for unresectable liver metastases from colorectal carcinoma. New dose schedules and survival update. *Cancer.* 1994;73:1134-1142.

117. Kemeny N, Conti JA, Cohen A, et al. Phase II study of hepatic arterial floxuridine, leucovorin, and dexamethasone for unresectable liver metastases from colorectal carcinoma. *J Clin Oncol.* 1994;12:2288-2295.

118. Meta-Analysis Group in Cancer. Toxicity of fluorouracil in patients with advanced colorectal cancer. Effect of administration schedule and prognostic factors. *J Clin Oncol.* 1988;16:3537-3541.

119. Sloan JA, Goldberg RM, Sargent DJ, et al. Women experience greater toxicity with fluorouracil-based chemotherapy for colorectal cancer *J Clin Oncol.* 2002;20:1491-1498.

120. Popescu RA, Norman A, Ross PJ, et al. Adjuvant or palliative chemotherapy for colorectal cancer in patients 70 years or older. *J Clin Oncol.* 1999;17:2412-2418.

121. Etienne MC, Chatelut E, Pivot X, et al. Co-variables influencing 5-fluorouracil clearance during continuous venous infusion. A NONMEM analysis. *Eur J Cancer.* 1998;34:92-97.

122. The Advanced Colorectal Cancer Meta-Analysis Project. Modulation of fluorouracil by leucovorin in patients with advanced colorectal cancer. Evidence in terms of response rate. *J Clin Oncol.* 1992;10:896-903.

123. Meta-Analysis Group in Cancer. Efficacy of intravenous continuous infusion of fluorouracil compared with bolus administration in advanced colorectal cancer. *J Clin Oncol.* 1998;16:301-308.

124. Meta-Analysis Group in Cancer. Reappraisal of hepatic arterial infusion in the treatment of nonresectable liver metastases from colorectal cancer. *J Natl Cancer Inst.* 1996;88:252-258.

125. Loprinzi CL, Ciafione SG, Dose AM, et al. A controlled evaluation of allopurinol mouthwash as prophylaxis against 5-fluorouracil stomatitis. *Cancer.* 1990;65:1879-1882.

126. Peters GJ, van Dijk J, Laurensse E, et al. In vitro biochemical and in vivo biological studies of the uridine "rescue" of 5-fluorouracil. *Br J Cancer.* 1988;57:259-265.

127. Drake JC, Voeller DM, Allegra CJ, et al. The effect of dose and interval between 5-fluorouracil and leucovorin on the formation of thymidylate synthase ternary complex in human cancer cells. *Br J Cancer.* 1995;71:1145-1150.

128. Cao S, Frank C, Rustum YM. Role of fluoropyrimidine schedule and (6R,S) leucovorin dose in a preclinical animal model of colorectal carcinoma. *J Natl Cancer Inst.* 1996;88:430-436.

129. Radparvar S, Houghton PJ, Houghton JA. Effect of polyglutamylation of 5,10-methylenetetrahydrofolate on the binding of 5-fluoro-2-deoxyuridylate to thymidylate synthase purified from a human colon adenocarcinoma xenograft. *Biochem Pharmacol.* 1989;38:335-342.

130. Houghton JA, Williams LG, Cheshire PJ, et al. Influence of dose of [6RS]-leucovorin on reduced folate pools and 5-fluorouracil-mediated thymidylate synthase inhibition in human colon adenocarcinoma xenografts. *Cancer Res.* 1990;50:3940-3946.

131. Bertrand R, Jolivet J. Lack of interference by the unnatural isomer of 5-formyltetrahydrofolate with the effects of the natural isomer in leucovorin preparations. *J Natl Cancer Inst.* 1989;81:1175-1178.

132. Priest DG, Schmitz JC, Bunni MA, et al. Pharmacokinetics of leucovorin metabolites in human plasma as a function of dose administered orally and intravenously. *J Natl Cancer Inst.* 1991;83:1806-1812.

133. Scanlon KJ, Newman EM, Lu Y, et al. Biochemical basis for cisplatin and 5-fluorouracil synergism in human ovarian carcinoma cells. *Proc Natl Acad Sci U S A.* 1986;83:8923-8925.

134. Johnston PG, Geoffroy F, Drake J, et al. The cellular interaction of 5-fluorouracil and cisplatin in a human colon carcinoma cell line. *Eur J Cancer.* 1996;32A:2148-2154.

135. de Gramont A, Figer A, Seymour M, et al. Leucovorin and fluorouracil with or without oxaliplatin as first-line treatment in advanced colorectal cancer. *J Clin Oncol.* 2000;18:2938-2947.

136. Andre T, Boni C, Mounedji-Boudiaf L, et al. Oxaliplatin, fluorouracil, and leucovorin as adjuvant treatment for colon cancer. *N Engl J Med.* 2004;350:2343-2351.

137. Azrak RG, Cao S, Slocum HK, et al. Therapeutic synergy between irinotecan and 5-fluorouracil against human tumor xenografts. *Clin Cancer Res.* 2004;10:1121-1129.

138. Heidelberger C, Griesvach L, Montag BJ, et al. Studies on fluorinated pyrimidines. II. Effects on transplanted tumors. *Cancer Res.* 1958;18:305-317.

139. O'Connell MJ, Martenson JA, Wieand HS, et al. Improving adjuvant therapy for rectal cancer by combining protracted infusion fluorouracil with radiation therapy after curative surgery. *N Engl J Med.* 1994;33:502-507.

140. Dooley M, Goa KL. Capecitabine. *Drugs.* 1999;58(1):69-76.

141. O'Shaughnessy J, Miles D, Vukelja S, et al. Superior survival with capecitabine plus docetaxel combination therapy in anthracycline-pretreated patients with advanced breast cancer: phase III trial results. *J Clin Oncol.* 2002;20:2812-2823.

142. Geyer CE, Forster J, Lindquist D, et al. Lapatinib plus capecitabine for HER2-positive advanced breast cancer. *N Engl J Med.* 2006;355:2733-2743.

143. Cassidy J, Clarke S, Díaz-Rubio E, et al. Randomized phase III study of capecitabine plus oxaliplatin compared with fluorouracil/folinic acid plus oxaliplatin as first-line therapy for metastatic colorectal cancer. *J Clin Oncol.* 2008;26:2006-2012.

144. Tabata T, Katoh M, Tokudome S, et al. Identification of the cytosolic carboxylesterase catalyzing the 5′-deoxy-5-fluorocytidine formation from capecitabine in human liver. *Drug Metab Dispos.* 2004;32:1103-1110.

145. Budman DR, Meropol NJ, Reigner B, et al. Preliminary studies of a novel oral fluoropyrimidine carbamate. Capecitabine. *J Clin Oncol.* 1998;16:1795-1802.

146. Miwa M, Ura M, Nishida M, et al. Design of a novel oral fluoropyrimidine carbamate, capecitabine, which generates 5-fluorouracil selectively in tumours by enzymes concentrated in human liver and cancer tissue. *Eur J Cancer.* 1998;34:1274-1281.

147. Ishikawa T, Utoh M, Sawada N, et al. Tumor selective delivery of 5-fluorouracil by capecitabine, a new oral fluoropyrimidine carbamate, in human cancer xenografts. *Biochem Pharmacol.* 1998;55:1091-1097.

148. Schuller J, Cassidy J, Dumont E, et al. Preferential activation of capecitabine in tumor following oral administration to colorectal cancer patients. *Cancer Chemother Pharmacol.* 2000;45:291-297.

149. Reigner B, Blesch K, Weidekamm E. Clinical pharmacokinetics of capecitabine. *Clin Pharmacokinet.* 2001;40:85-104.

150. Reigner B, Verweij J, Dirix L, et al. Effect of food on the pharmacokinetics of capecitabine and its metabolites following oral administration in cancer patients. *Clin Cancer Res.* 1998;4:941-948.

151. Twelves C, Glynne-Jones R, Cassidy J, et al. Effect of hepatic dysfunction due to liver metastases on the pharmacokinetics of capecitabine and its metabolites. *Clin Cancer Res.* 1999;5:1696-1702.

152. Poole C, Gardiner J, Twelves C, et al. Effect of renal impairment on the pharmacokinetics and tolerability of capecitabine (Xeloda) in cancer patients. *Cancer Chemother Pharmacol.* 2002;49:225-234.

153. Walkhorm B, Fraunfelder FT. Severe ocular irritation and corneal deposits associated with capecitabine use. *N Engl J Med.* 2004;343:740-741.

154. Couch LS, Groteluschen DL, Stewart JA, et al. Capecitabine-related neurotoxicity presenting as trismus. *Clin Colorectal Cancer.* 2003;3:121-123.

155. Van Cutsem E, Twelves C, Cassidy J, et al. Oral capecitabine compared with intravenous fluorouracil plus leucovorin in patients with metastatic colorectal cancer: results of a large phase III study. *J Clin Oncol.* 2001;19:4097-4106.

156. Milano G, Etienne-Grimaldi MC, Mari M, et al. Candidate mechanisms for capecitabine-related hand-foot syndrome. *Br J Clin Pharmacol.* 2008;66:88-95.

157. Yen-Revollo JL, Goldberg RM, McLeod HL. Can inhibiting dihydropyrimidine dehydrogenase limit hand-foot syndrome caused by fluoropyrimidines? *Clin Cancer Res.* 2008;14:8-13.

158. Midgley R, Kerr DJ, Capecitabine: have we got the dose right? *Nat Clin Pract Oncol.* 2009;6:17-24.

159. Largillier R, Etienne-Grimaldi MC, Formento JL, et al. Pharmacogenetics of capecitabine in advanced breast cancer patients. *Clin Cancer Res.* 2006;12(18):5496-5502.

160. Saif MW, Diasio R. Is capecitabine safe in patients with gastrointestinal cancer and dihydropyrimidine dehydrogenase deficiency? *Clin Colorectal Cancer.* 2006;5:359-362.

161. Ng M, Cunningham D, Norman AR. The frequency and pattern of cardiotoxicity observed with capecitabine used in conjunction with oxaliplatin in patients treated for advanced colorectal cancer (CRC). *Eur J Cancer.* 2005;41:1542-1546.

162. Goldsmith YB, Roistacher N, Baum MS. Capecitabine-induced coronary vasospasm. *J Clin Oncol.* 2008;26:3802-3804.

163. Hoff PM, Ansari R, Batist G, et al. Comparison of oral capecitabine versus intravenous fluorouracil plus leucovorin as first-line treatment in 606 patients with metastatic colorectal cancer: results of a randomized phase III study. *J Clin Oncol.* 2001;19:2282-2292.

164. Arkenau HT, Arnold D, Cassidy J, et al. Efficacy of oxaliplatin plus capecitabine or infusion fluorouracil/leucovorin in patients with metastatic colorectal cancer: a pooled analysis of randomized trials. *J Clin Oncol.* 2008;26:5910-5919.

165. Twelves C, Wong A, Nowacki MP, et al. Capecitabine as adjuvant treatment for stage III colon cancer. *N Engl J Med.* 2005;352:2696-2704.

166. Allegra CJ, Yothers G, O'Connell MJ, et al. Neoadjuvant 5-FU or capecitabine plus radiation with or without oxaliplatin in rectal cancer patients: a phase III randomized clinical trial. *J Natl Cancer Inst.* 2015;107: doi: 10.1093/jnci/djv248.

167. Cameron D, Casey M, Press M, et al. A phase III randomized comparison of lapatinib plus capecitabine versus capecitabine alone in women with advanced breast cancer that has progressed on trastuzumab: updated efficacy and biomarker analyses. *Breast Cancer Res Treat.* 2008;112:533-543.

168. Masoda N, Lee SJ, Ohtani S, et al. Adjuvant capecitabine for breast cancer after pre-operative chemotherapy. *N Engl J Med.* 2017;376:2147-2159.

169. Saltz LB, Clarke S, Díaz-Rubio E, et al. Bevacizumab in combination with oxaliplatin-based chemotherapy as first-line therapy in metastatic colorectal cancer: a randomized phase III study. *J Clin Oncol.* 2008;26:2013-2019.

170. Puglisi F, Cardellino GG, Crivellari D, et al. Thymidine phosphorylase expression is associated with time to progression in patients receiving low-dose, docetaxel-modulated capecitabine for metastatic breast cancer. *Ann Oncol.* 2008;19:1541-1546.

171. Uchida K, Danenberg PV, Danenberg KD, et al. Thymidylate synthase, dihydropyrimidine dehydrogenase, ERCC1, and thymidine phosphorylase gene expression in primary and metastatic gastrointestinal adenocarcinoma tissue in patients treated on a phase I trial of oxaliplatin and capecitabine. *BMC Cancer.* 2008;8:386.

172. Honda J, Sasa M, Moriya T, et al. Thymidine phosphorylase and dihydropyrimidine dehydrogenase are predictive factors of therapeutic efficacy of capecitabine monotherapy for breast cancer-preliminary results. *J Med Invest.* 2008;55:54-60.

173. Blanquicett C, Gillespie GY, Nabors LB, et al. Induction of thymidine phosphorylase in both irradiated and shielded, contralateral human U87MG glioma xenografts: implications for a dual modality treatment using capecitabine and irradiation. *Mol Cancer Ther.* 2002;1:1139-1145.

174. Brickell K, Porter D, Thompson P. Phenytoin toxicity due to fluoropyrimidines (5FU/capecitabine): three case reports. *Br J Cancer.* 2003;89:615-616.

175. Shah HR, Ledbetter L, Diasio R, et al. A retrospective study of coagulation abnormalities in patients receiving concomitant capecitabine and warfarin. *Clin Colorectal Cancer.* 2006;5:354-358.

176. Masci G, Magagnoli M, Zucali PA, et al. Minidose warfarin prophylaxis for catheter-associated thrombosis in cancer patients: can it be safely associated with fluorouracil-based chemotherapy? *J Clin Oncol.* 2003;21:736-739.

177. Camidge R, Reigner B, Cassidy J, et al. Significant effect of capecitabine on the pharmacokinetics and pharmacodynamics of warfarin in patients with cancer. *J Clin Oncol.* 2005;23:4719-4725.

178. Mahlberg R, Lrenzen S, Thuss-Patience P, et al. New perspectives in the treatment of advanced gastric cancer: S-1 as a novel oral 5-FU therapy in combination with cisplatin. *Chemotherapy.* 2017;62:62-70.

179. Shewach DS, Lawrence TS. Antimetabolite radiosensitizers. *J Clin Oncol.* 2007;25:4043-4050.

180. Komatsu T, Yamazaki H, Shimada N, et al. Involvement of microsomal P450 and cytosolic thymidine phosphorylase in 5-fluorouracil formation from tegafur in human liver. *Clin Cancer Res.* 2001;7:675-681.

181. Antilla MI, Sotaniemi EA, Kaiaralcoma MI, et al. Pharmacokinetics of ftorafur after intravenous and oral administration. *Cancer Chemother Pharmacol.* 1983;10:150-153.

182. Yang L, Zou S, Song Y, et al. CEP2A6 polymorphisms associate with outcomes of S-1 plus oxaliplatin chemotherapy in Chinese gastric cancer patients. *Genomics Proteomics Bioinformatics.* 2017;15:255-262.

183. Furuse J, Okusaka T, Keneko S, et al. Phase I/II study of the pharmacokinetics, safety, and efficacy of S-1 in patients with advanced hepatocellular carcinoma. *Cancer Sci.* 2010;101:2606-2611.

184. Aoyama T, Nichiikawa K, Fujitani K, et al. Early results of a randomized two-by-two factorial phase II trial comparing neoadjuvant chemotherapy with two and four courses of cisplatin/S-1 and docetaxel/cisplatin/S-1 as neoadjuvant chemotherapy for locally advanced gastric cancer. *Ann Oncol.* 2017;28:1876-1881.

185. Oki E, Murata A, Yoshida K, et al. A randomized phase III trial comparing S-1 versus UFT as adjuvant chemotherapy for Stage II/III rectal cancer (JFMC35-C1: ACTS-RC). *Ann Oncol.* 2016;27:1266-1272.

186. Kim ST, Hong YS, Lim HY, et al. S-1 plus oxaliplatin versus capecitabine plus oxaliplatin for the first line treatment of patients with metastatic colorectal cancer: updated results from a phase 3 trial. *BMC Cancer.* 2014;14:883.

187. Yamada T, Takahari D, Matsumoto H, et al. Leucovorin, fluorouracil, and oxaliplatin plus bevacizumab versus S-1 and oxaliplatin plus bevacizumab in patients with metastatic colorectal cancer (SOFT): an open-label, non-inferiority, randomised phase 3 trial. *Lancet Oncol.* 2013;14:1278-12836

188. Uesaka K, Boku N, Fukutomi A, et al. Adjuvant chemotherapy of S-1 versus gemcitabine for resected pancreatic cancer: a phase 3, open-label, randomised, non-inferiority trial (JASPAC01). *Lancet.* 2016;388:248-257.

189. Sakuramoto S, Sasako M, Yamaguchi T, et al. Adjuvant chemotherapy for gastric cancer with S-1 an oral fluoropyrimidine. *N Engl J Med.* 2007;357:1810-1820.

190. Takashima T, Mukai H, Hara F, et al. Taxanes versus S-1 as the first-line chemotherapy for metastatic breast cancer (SELECTBC): an open-label, non-inferiority randomized phase 3 trial. *Lancet Oncol.* 2016;17:190-198.

191. Kubota K, Sakai H, Katakami N, et al. A randomized phase III trial of oral S-1 plus cisplatin versus docetaxel plus cisplatin in Japanese patients with advanced non-small C-cell lung cancer: TCOG0701 CATS trial. *Ann Oncol.* 2015;26:1401-1408.

192. Lenz H-J, Stintzing S, Loupakis F. TAS-102, a novel antitumor agent; a review of the mechanism of action. *Cancer Treat Rev.* 2015;41:777-783.

193. Suzuki N, Nakagawa F, Nukatsuka M, Fukushima M. Trifluorothymidine exhibits potent antitumor activity via the induction of DNA double-strand breaks. *Exp Ther Med.* 2011;2:393-397.

194. Tanaka N, Sakamoto K, Okabe H, et al. Repeated oral dosing of TAS-102 confers high trifluridine incorporation into DNA and sustained antitumor activity in mouse models. *Oncol Rep.* 2014;32:2319-2326.

195. Fukushima M, Suzuki N, Emura T, et al. Structure and activity of specific inhibitors of thymidine phosphorylase to potentiate the function of antitumor 2′-deoxyribonucleosides. *Biochem Pharmacol.* 2000;59:1227-1236.

196. Clearly JM, Rosen LS, Yoshida K, et al. A phase I study of the pharmacokinetics of nucleoside analog trifluridine and thymidine phosphorylase inhibitor tipiracil (components of TAS-102) vs. trifluridine alone. *Invest New Drugs.* 2017;20:189-197.

197. Suenaga M, Schirripa M, Cao S, et al. Genetic variants of DNA repair-related genes predict efficacy of TAS-102 in patients with refractory metastatic colorectal cancer. *Ann Oncol.* 2017;28:1015-1022.

Cytidine Analogues

Bruce A. Chabner, Christopher S. Nabel, and Andrew M. Brunner

Cytosine Arabinoside (Cytarabine, ara-C)

Nucleoside analogues have earned an important place in the treatment of acute leukemia. Through modification of the base or sugar component, chemists have created molecules that inhibit aspects of DNA synthesis or function. Among these analogues are the arabinose nucleosides, a unique class of antimetabolites first isolated from the sponge *Cryptotethya crypta*[1] but now produced synthetically.[2] They differ from the physiologic deoxyribonucleosides in the presence of a 2'-OH group, rather than a simple hydrogen bond, in the *cis* configuration relative to the N-glycosyl bond between cytosine and the arabinose sugar (Fig. 9.1). Several arabinose nucleosides, including cytosine arabinoside (ara-C, cytarabine), 2-fluoro-ara-adenosine monophosphate (an adenosine analogue), and nelarabine (a guanine analogue), have become important agents for treating hematological cancers.

Ara-C is a standard component of regimens for treatment of acute myelogenous leukemia (AML). For emission induction, it is typically combined with an anthracycline (daunorubicin hydrochloride or idarubicin hydrochloride), and during consolidation, it is given in high (3 g/m^2) doses.[3] High-dose ara-C confers particular benefit in AML patients with cytogenetic abnormalities resulting in translocations of core binding factor genes that regulate hematopoiesis (t8:21, inv 16, del 16, t16:16).[4] Ara-C is also active against other hematologic malignancies, including Burkitt's lymphoma and acute lymphocytic leukemia, but has little value as a single agent against solid tumors. This limited spectrum of activity has been attributed to the lack of metabolic activation of this agent in solid tumors and its selective action against rapidly dividing cells. The essential features of ara-C pharmacology are described in Table 9.1.

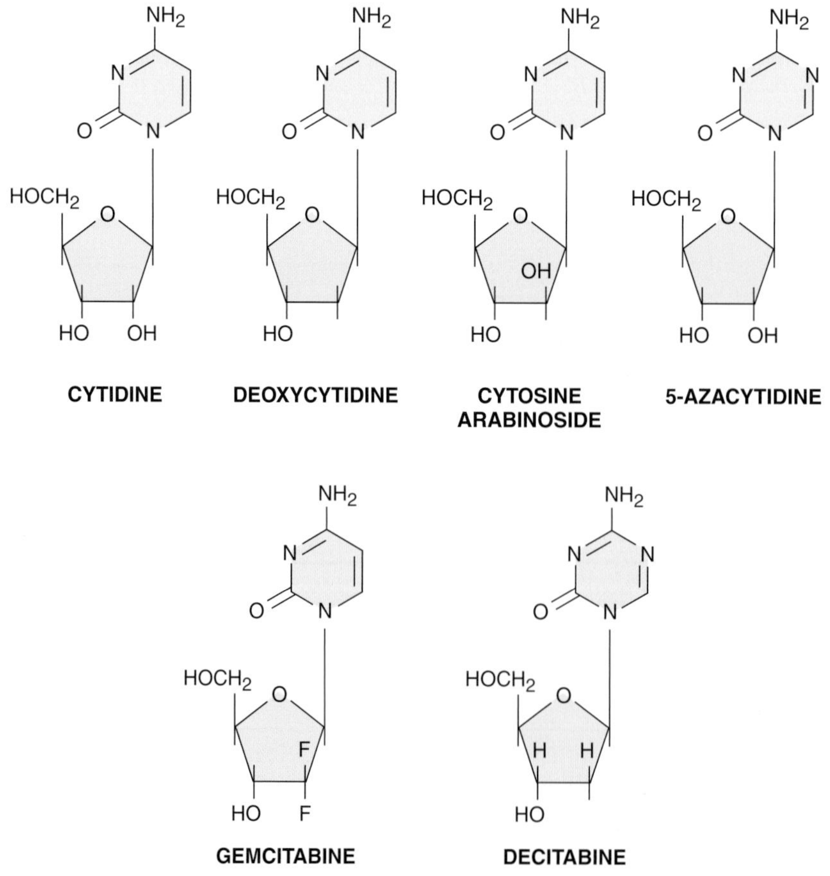

CYTIDINE   DEOXYCYTIDINE   CYTOSINE ARABINOSIDE   5-AZACYTIDINE

GEMCITABINE   DECITABINE

FIGURE 9.1 Structure of cytidine analogs.

TABLE

9.1   *Key features of ara-C pharmacology*

Factor	Result
Mechanism of action	Inhibits DNA polymerase α, is incorporated into DNA, and terminates DNA chain elongation
Metabolism	Activated to triphosphate in tumor cells. Degraded to inactive ara-U by deamination
	Converted to ara-CDP choline derivative
Pharmacokinetics	Plasma: $t_{1/2\alpha}$ 7 to 20 min, $t_{1/2\beta}$ 2 h; CSF: $t_{1/2}$ 2 h
Elimination	Deamination by cytidine deaminase in liver, plasma, and peripheral tissues—100%
Drug interactions	Methotrexate increases ara-CTP formation
	THU inhibits deamination
	Fludarabine phosphate increases ara-CTP formation
	Ara-C blocks DNA repair, enhances activity of alkylating agents
Toxicity	Myelosuppression
	Gastrointestinal epithelial ulceration
	Intrahepatic cholestasis, pancreatitis
	Cerebellar and cerebral dysfunction (high dose)
	Conjunctivitis (high dose)
	Hidradenitis
	Noncardiogenic pulmonary edema
Precautions	Increased incidence of cerebral-cerebellar toxicity with high-dose ara-C in the elderly, especially in those with compromised renal function

ara-CDP, arabinosylcytosine diphosphate; ara-CTP, arabinosylcytosine triphosphate; ara-U, uracil arabinoside; CSF, cerebrospinal fluid; $t_{1/2}$, half-life; THU, tetrahydrouridine; ara-C, cytosine arabinoside.

Mechanism of Action

Ara-C acts as an analogue of deoxycytidine (CdR) and has multiple effects on DNA synthesis. Ara-C crosses cell membranes via the hENT1 nucleoside transporter and undergoes intracellular phosphorylation to form arabinosylcytosine triphosphate (ara-CTP), which competitively inhibits DNA polymerase α in opposition to the normal substrate deoxycytidine 5′-triphosphate (dCTP).[5] Ara-CTP has an affinity for human leukemia cell DNA polymerase α in the range of 1×10^{-6} M.[6] Ara-CTP inhibits DNA polymerase β with lesser potency.[7] The effects of ara-C on DNA polymerase activity extend not only to DNA replication but also to DNA repair.[8] In addition to inhibiting DNA synthesis, however, it becomes incorporated into DNA, a feature that correlates closely with cytotoxicity[9] (Fig. 9.2). A preponderance of evidence suggests that this is the major cytotoxic lesion in ara-C–treated cells. Drugs that prevent ara-C incorporation into DNA, such as aphidicolin, block its cytotoxicity.[10] In cell culture experiments, a linear relationship exists between the picomoles of ara-C incorporated into DNA and the log of cell survival for a wide range of drug concentrations and durations of exposure. Incorporation into DNA varies directly with drug concentration and duration of exposure.[11] Once incorporated into DNA, ara-C is excised slowly,[12] and the incorporated ara-C inhibits template function and chain elongation.[10,12] In experiments with purified enzyme and calf thymus DNA, the consecutive incorporation of two ara-C or two arabinosyl-5-azacytidine nucleotide residues effectively stops chain elongation.[5] At high concentrations of ara-C, one finds a greater than expected proportion of ara-C residues at the 3′-terminus, a finding that implies potent chain termination.[13] These observations support the hypothesis that ara-C incorporation into DNA is a prerequisite for drug action and is responsible for cytotoxicity.

Ara-C also causes an unusual reiteration of DNA segments.[14] Human lymphocytes exposed to ara-C in culture synthesize small reduplicated segments of DNA, which results in multiple copies of limited portions of DNA. These reduplicated segments increase the possibility of recombination, crossover, and gene amplification; gaps and breaks are observed in karyotype preparations after ara-C treatment. The same mechanism, reiteration of DNA synthesis after its inhibition by an antimetabolite, may also explain the high frequency of gene reduplication induced by methotrexate, 5-fluorouracil, and hydroxyurea (Chapters 7 to 9).

Other biochemical actions of ara-C include a relatively weak inhibition of ribonucleotide reductase[15] and formation of arabinosylcytosine diphosphate (ara-CDP-choline). The latter functions as an analogue of cytidine 5′-diphosphocholine (CDP-choline) and inhibits synthesis of membrane glycoproteins and glycolipids.[16] Ara-C also has the interesting property of promoting differentiation of leukemic cells in tissue culture, an effect that is accompanied by decreased c-*myc* oncogene expression.[17] These changes in morphology and oncogene expression occur at concentrations above the threshold for cytotoxicity and may simply represent terminal injury of cells. After exposure to ara-C, both normal and malignant cells undergo apoptosis in experimental models.[18]

The mechanism by which ara-C induces apoptosis is uncertain. Cell death may be triggered by p53 in response to DNA breaks and by futile attempts to excise incorporated ara-C nucleotides.

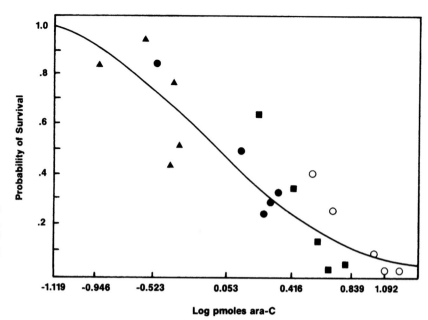

 Fɪɢᴜʀᴇ **9.2** Relationship between AML blast clonogenic survival and incorporation of tritium-labeled ara-C into DNA at ara-C concentrations of 10^{-7} mol/L (▲), 10^{-6} mol/L (●), 10^{-5} mol/L (■), and 10^{-4} mol/L (○) during periods of 1, 3, 6, 12, and 24 hours. (Reprinted from Kufe DW, Spriggs DR. Biochemical and cellular pharmacology of cytosine arabinoside. *Semin Oncol.* 1985;12(2 Suppl 3):34-48. Copyright © 1985 Grune & Stratton, Inc. With permission.)

However, ara-C also stimulates the formation of ceramide, a potent inducer of apoptosis.[19] Cells exposed to ara-C display marked alterations in transcription factor expression. Ara-C induces AP-1 (a dimer of jun-fos or jun-jun proteins) and NF-kB, and AP-1 induction has been temporally associated with apoptosis.[20] PKC inhibitors promote ara-C–induced apoptosis despite their antagonizing c-jun up-regulation, calling into question the involvement of c-jun expression in apoptosis secondary to ara-C.[21] Ara-C induces pRb phosphatase activity, another possible mechanism responsible for p53-independent G_1 arrest and apoptosis.[22] The resulting hypophosphorylated Rb binds to and inactivates the E2F transcription factor, thereby inhibiting the transcription of genes responsible for cell cycle progression.

Cellular Pharmacology and Metabolism

Ara-C penetrates cells by a carrier-mediated process shared by physiologic nucleosides.[23] Several classes of nucleoside transporters in mammalian cells may be responsible for influx; the most extensively characterized in human tumors is hENT1, the equilibrative transporter, identified by its binding to nitrobenzylthioinosine (NBMPR). The number of transport sites on the cell membrane, enumerated by NBMPR binding, is greater in AML cells than in acute lymphocytic leukemia cells[24] and is highly up-regulated in biphenotypic leukemia associated with the 11q23 MLL gene (4:11) translocation.[24] Increased expression of the FLT3 membrane protein correlates with hENT1 expression, and may be involved in the regulation of the transporter.[25] Uptake by hENT1 occurs rapidly. A steady-state level of intracellular drug is achieved within 90 seconds at 37°C.[26] Studies of Wiley et al.[23] and others[26] suggest that the NBMPR-sensitive transporter protein expression correlates with the formation of ara-CTP, the ultimate toxic metabolite (Fig. 9.3). A point mutation in the hENT1 carrier confers resistance in selected leukemic cell lines in vitro.[27] At drug concentrations above 10 μM, the transport process becomes saturated, and further entry takes place by passive diffusion. hENT1 is strongly inhibited by various receptor tyrosine kinase inhibitors, an interaction that could limit ara-C use with targeted drugs.[28] OCTN1, a second high-affinity nucleoside carrier, also mediates ara-C transport, is

present in AML cell membrane, and its low expression correlates with AML resistance to ara-C and poor overall survival.[29]

Ara-C and ara-CMP efflux may be dependent on ABCC4 (MRP4), an ATP-dependent active transporter found in AML cells, although the clinical relevance of this finding is uncertain.[30]

As shown in Figure 9.4, ara-C must be converted to its active form, ara-CTP, through the sequential action of three enzymes: (a)

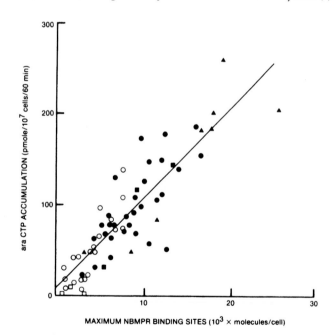

Fɪɢᴜʀᴇ **9.3** Correlation between accumulation of ara-CTP and nucleoside transport capacity measured by the maximal number of NBMPR binding sites on leukemic cells ($r = 0.87$; $P < 0.0001$). Ara-CTP accumulation was measured after incubation of cells with 1 μM of tritium-labeled ara-C for 60 minutes. ●, acute myelogenous leukemia; ○, non–T-cell acute lymphoblastic leukemia; ▲, T-cell leukemia/lymphoma, lymphoblastic leukemia; ■, chronic lymphocytic leukemia. (From Wiley JS, Taupin J, Jamieson GP, et al. Cytosine arabinoside transport and metabolism in acute leukemias and T-cell lymphoblastic lymphoma. *J Clin Invest.* 1985;75(2):632-642. Copyright © 1985 The American Society for Clinical Investigation. Reproduced with permission of American Society for Clinical Investigation in the format Book via Copyright Clearance Center.)

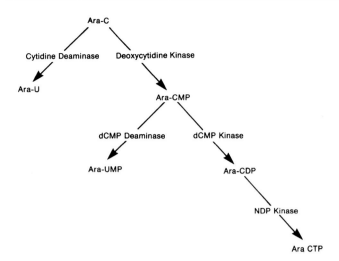

FIGURE **9.4** Metabolism of ara-C by tumor cells. The conversion of ara-UMP to a triphosphate has not been demonstrated in mammalian cells. Ara-CMP, arabinosylcytosine monophosphate; ara-CDP, arabinosylcytosine diphosphate; ara-CTP, arabinosylcytosine triphosphate; ara-U, uracil arabinoside; dCMP, deoxycytidine monophosphate; NDP, nucleoside diphosphate.

CdR kinase, (b) deoxycytidine monophosphate (dCMP) kinase, and (c) nucleoside diphosphate (NDP) kinase. Ara-C is subject to degradation by cytidine deaminase, forming the inactive product uracil arabinoside (ara-U); arabinosylcytosine monophosphate (ara-CMP) is likewise degraded by dCMP deaminase to the inactive arabinosyluracil monophosphate (ara-UMP). Each of these enzymes, with the exception of NDP kinase, has been studied regarding its potential role in ara-C resistance.

CdR kinase, the first activating enzyme, is found in the lowest concentration (Table 9.2) of the pathway enzymes and is rate limiting in ara-CTP formation. The enzyme is a 30.5-kDa protein that phosphorylates ara-C and many other cytidine and purine nucleosides and their analogues.[27] The rate-limiting role of CdR kinase in ara-C activation is illustrated by transfection of malignant cell lines with retroviral vectors containing CdR kinase cDNA, a maneuver that substantially increases the susceptibility of cells to ara-C, gemcitabine (GEM), and purine analogues,[31] and by knockdown with siRNA, which leads to ara-C resistance.[32]

CdR kinase activity is highest during the S phase of the cell cycle. The K_m, or affinity constant, for ara-C is 20 μM, compared with the higher affinity or 7.8 μM for the physiologic substrate CdR.[33] This enzyme is strongly inhibited by dCTP but weakly inhibited by ara-CTP. This weak "feedback" inhibition allows accumulation of ara-C nucleotides to higher concentrations. The second activating enzyme, dCMP kinase,[34] is found in several hundredfold higher concentration than CdR kinase. Its affinity for ara-CMP is low (K_m = 680 μmol/L) but greater than the affinity for the competitive physiologic substrate dCMP. Because of its relatively poor affinity for ara-CMP, this enzyme could become rate limiting at low ara-CMP concentrations. The third activating enzyme, the diphosphate kinase, appears not to be rate limiting because it is present in very high concentration, and the intracellular pool of ara-CDP is only a fraction of the ara-CTP pool.[35]

Opposing the activation pathway are two deaminases found in high concentration in some tumor cells and normal tissues. Cytidine deaminase (CD) is widely distributed in mammalian tissues, including intestinal mucosa, liver, plasma, and granulocytes.[36] Its concentration in granulocyte precursors and in leukemic myeloblasts is much lower than in mature granulocytes, but even in these immature cells, the deaminase level exceeds the activity of CdR kinase, the initial activating enzyme.[33,36]

The second degradative enzyme, dCMP deaminase (Fig. 10.4), diverts the flow of physiologic deoxycytidine nucleotides from dCMP into the deoxyuridine monophosphate (dUMP) pool, and thence into deoxythymidine 5′-phosphate (dTMP) via the action of thymidylate synthase. The enzyme dCMP deaminase is strongly activated by intracellular dCTP (K_m = 0.2 μmol/L) and strongly inhibited by dTTP in concentrations of 0.2 μmol/L or greater. Ara-CTP weakly activates this enzyme (K_m = 40 μM)[37] and, thus,

TABLE

9.2 *Kinetic parameters of enzymes that metabolize ara-C*

Enzyme	Substrate	K_m (mol/L)	Activity in AML cells (nmol/h/mg protein at 37°C)
CdR kinase	Ara-C	2.6×10^{-5}	15.4 ± 16
	CdR	7.8×10^{-6}	
dCMP kinase	Ara-CMP	6.8×10^{-4}	$1,990 \pm 1,500$
	dCMP	1.9×10^{-3}	
dCDP kinase	Ara-CDP	Not determined	Not determined
	Other NDPs	Not determined	Not determined
CR deaminase	Ara-C	8.8×10^{-5}	372 ± 614
	CdR	1.1×10^{-5}	
dCMP deaminase	Ara-CMP	Ara-CMP has higher K_m than	$1,250$ (five patients)
	dCMP	dCMP; exact K_m not determined	

AML, acute myelogenous leukemia; Ara-C, cytosine arabinoside; ara-CDP, arabinosylcytosine diphosphate; ara-CMP, arabinosylcytosine monophosphate; CdR, deoxycytidine; CR, cytidine; dCDP, deoxycytidine diphosphate; dCMP, deoxycytosine monophosphate; NDPs, nucleoside diphosphates.

would not promote degradation of its own precursor nucleotide, ara-CMP. The affinity of dCMP deaminase for ara-CMP is somewhat higher than the affinity of dCMP kinase for the same substrate, but the activity of these competitive enzymes depends greatly on their degree of activation or inhibition by regulatory triphosphates (dCTP), and dCMP deaminase concentration in leukemic myeloblasts is lower than that of dCMP kinase (Table 9.2).

Thus, the balance between activating and degrading enzymes is crucial in determining the quantity of drug converted to the active intermediate, ara-CTP. This enzymatic balance varies greatly among cell types.[34] CdR kinase activity is higher and cytidine deaminase activity is lower in ALL than in AML. Enzyme activities vary also with cell maturity; deaminase increases dramatically with maturation of granulocyte precursors, whereas kinase activity decreases correspondingly.[36] Admixture of normal granulocyte precursors with leukemic cells in human bone marrow samples complicates the interpretation of enzyme measurements unless normal and leukemic cells are separated. In general, cytidine deaminase (CD) activity greatly exceeds kinase (CdK). The CdK/CD ratio averages 0.03 in human AML, whereas the enzyme activities are approximately equal in acute lymphoblastic leukemia and Burkitt's lymphoma. The biochemical setting seems to favor drug activation by lymphoblastic leukemia cells if these initial enzymes play a rate-limiting role. However, Chou et al. found the opposite; specifically, human AML cells formed 12.8 ng of ara-CTP per 10^6 cells after 45 minutes of incubation with 1×10^{-5} mol/L ara-C while acute lymphoblastic leukemia cells formed less ara-CTP, 6.3 ng/10^6 cells.[35] The likelihood is that other factors, such as transport and regulatory effects of intracellular dNTPs, may limit ara-CTP formation.

Polymorphisms of the ara-C metabolic enzymes may affect enzyme activity, altering toxicity to both normal and neoplastic cells. The limited investigations of this aspect of ara-C pharmacology point toward a poorer therapeutic outcome (shorter overall survival and a shorter duration of first remission) in normal AML karyotype patients with the 79 A>C variant, which is associated, paradoxically, with decreased enzyme activity, perhaps the result of greater toxicity to normal blood precursors.[38] A second study of AML patients found a similar poorer outcome for patients with a variant of the deoxycytidylate deaminase gene, as well as variants of cytidine triphosphate synthetase.[39] These and other studies of variants are compromised by the small numbers of patients analyzed, a lack of information on variant enzyme function, and reasons for clinical failure other than lack of response.

In addition to its activation to ara-CTP, ara-C is converted intracellularly to ara-CDP-choline,[40] an analogue of the physiologic CDP-choline lipid precursor. However, ara-C does not inhibit incorporation of choline into phospholipids of normal or transformed hamster embryo fibroblasts. Ara-CMP does inhibit the transfer of galactose, N-acetylglucosamine, and sialic acid to cell surface glycoproteins. Further, high concentrations (approaching 1 mM) of ara-CTP inhibit the synthesis of cytidine monophosphate (CMP)-acetylneuraminic acid, an essential substrate in sialylation of glycoproteins.[41] Thus, ara-C treatment could alter membrane structure, antigenicity, and function.

The precise mechanism of cell death related to ara-C is not well understood (see below). Inhibition of DNA elongation likely produces stalled replication forks and strand breaks, which induce attempts at repair and apoptosis. Ara-C is modestly mutagenic, inducing base errors in TpCpT and TpGpA triplicates at the C or G locus postchemotherapy.[42]

Biochemical Determinants of Cytosine Arabinoside Resistance

The foregoing consideration of ara-C metabolism and transport makes it clear that a number of factors could affect ara-C response. Not surprisingly, many of these factors have been implicated in various preclinical models of ara-C resistance. The most frequent abnormality found in resistant leukemic cells recovered from mice treated with ara-C has been decreased activity of CdR kinase.[43] As mentioned previously, specific mutations and deletions in the CdR kinase gene from resistant cells have been described.[27,30]

The role of cytidine deaminase in experimental models of resistance is less clear. Retrovirus-mediated transfer of the cytidine deaminase cDNA into 3T3 murine fibroblast cells significantly increased drug resistance to ara-C and other cytidine analogues, 5-aza-2′-CdR and GEM. Tetrahydrouridine, a potent CD inhibitor, reversed resistance in this model system. The relevance of transporter activity, and CD and CdK activity to resistance in human leukemia, is less certain. Clinical studies have disclosed isolated instances of deletion of CdR kinase,[44] increased CD, decreased nucleoside transport,[45] and increased dCTP pools.[46] Other clinical investigators have not found a correlation of resistance with either CdR kinase or cytidine deaminase or their ratio.[47] All studies have shown extreme variability in enzyme levels among patients with leukemia. Thus, no agreement exists as to the specific changes responsible for resistance in human leukemia.

Although *specific biochemical lesions* associated with resistance in humans are unclear, the current understanding of ara-C action suggests that intracellular levels of ara-CTP and the duration of its persistence in leukemic cells determine response.[35,48] Preisler et al. and others[49,50] found that the duration of remission induced by ara-C–containing regimens was strongly correlated with the ability of cells to *retain* ara-CTP in vitro after removal of ara-C from the medium. The mechanism by which ara-CTP is degraded is uncertain. Two groups have identified a deoxynucleoside triphosphate phosphorylase, SAMHD1, which hydrolyzes the terminal phosphate of both physiologic and pharmacological triphosphates.[51,52]

Not all attempts to monitor ara-CTP formation in leukemic cells taken from patients during therapy have disclosed useful correlations of ara-CTP levels or intracellular persistence with response.[53] Ara-CTP has an intracellular half-life of about 3 to 4 hours. Again, considerable variability has been observed in the rates of formation of ara-CTP, and this rate does not correlate well with plasma ara-C pharmacokinetics in individual patients (Fig. 9.5).

The cellular response to ara-C–mediated DNA damage also governs whether the genotoxic insult results in cell death. Ara-C incorporation into DNA stalls the replication fork for cells in active DNA synthesis, activating ATR and Chk 1; these checkpoint kinases block cell cycle progression and allow for removal of ara-C from DNA. Absence of either of these checkpoints sensitizes cells to apoptosis. Levels of expression of apoptotic proteins influence response. Overexpression of the antiapoptotic proteins Bcl-2 and Bcl-X$_L$ in leukemic blasts causes in vitro resistance to ara-C–mediated apoptosis. The intracellular metabolism of ara-C and its initial effects on DNA are not modified by Bcl-2 expression, which suggests that Bcl-2 primarily regulates the more distal steps in the ara-C–induced

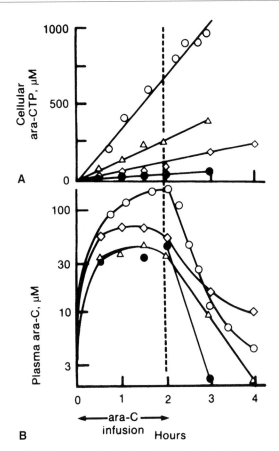

greatest cytotoxic effects during the S phase of the cell cycle perhaps because of the requirement for its incorporation into DNA and the greater activity of anabolic enzymes during S phase. The duration of exposure of cells to ara-C is directly correlated with cell kill because the longer exposure period allows ara-C to be incorporated into the DNA of a greater percentage of cells as they pass through S phase. The cytotoxic action of ara-C is not only cell cycle phase–dependent but is influenced by the rate of DNA synthesis. That is, cell kill in tissue culture is greatest if cells are exposed during periods of maximal rates of DNA synthesis, as in the recovery period after exposure to another cytotoxic agent. In experimental situations, sequential doses of ara-C that coincide with the peak in recovery of DNA synthesis seem to improve the therapeutic results.[56]

In humans, the influence of tumor cell kinetics on response is unclear. Although earlier studies showed that the complete remission rate seems to be *higher* in patients who have a high percentage of cells in S phase, remissions are *longer* in patients with leukemias that have long cell cycle time.[57]

Clinical Pharmacokinetics

The preferred method for assay of ara-C and its primary metabolite ara-U is high-pressure liquid chromatography, which has the requisite specificity and adequate (0.1 µM) sensitivity.[58] An alternative method using gas chromatography-mass spectrometry combines high specificity with greater sensitivity (4 nM) but requires derivatization of samples and thus prolonged performance time.[59] Because of the presence of cytidine deaminase in plasma, the deaminase inhibitor THU must be added to plasma samples immediately after blood samples are obtained.

Pharmacokinetics

The important factors that determine ara-C pharmacokinetics are its high aqueous solubility and its susceptibility to deamination in liver, plasma, and other tissues. Ara-C is amenable to use by multiple schedules and routes of administration and has shown clinical activity in dosages ranging from 20 mg/m² subcutaneously twice daily times 10 to 3 g/m² intravenously every 12 hours days 1, 3, and 5. Remarkably, over this wide dosage range, its pharmacokinetics remains quite constant and predictable.

Distribution

As a nucleoside, ara-C is highly soluble and distributes rapidly into total body water.[60] It then crosses into the central nervous system (CNS) with surprising facility for a water-soluble compound and reaches steady-state levels at 20% to 40% of those found simultaneously in plasma during constant intravenous infusion. At conventional doses of ara-C (100 mg/m² by 24-hour infusion), spinal fluid levels reach 0.2 µM, which is probably above the cytotoxic threshold for leukemic cells. Higher doses of ara-C yield proportionately higher ara-C levels in the spinal fluid.[61]

Plasma Pharmacokinetics

The pharmacokinetics of ara-C is characterized by rapid disappearance from plasma owing to deamination.[60] Peak plasma concentrations reach 10 µM after bolus doses of 100 mg/m² and are proportionately higher (up to 150 µM) for doses up to 3 g/m² given

FIGURE 9-5 Pharmacokinetics of ara-CTP in leukemia cells **(A)** and of ara-C in plasma **(B)**. Blood samples were drawn at the indicated times during and after infusion of ara-C, 3 g/m², to patients with acute leukemia in relapse. Symbols for each analysis are the same for individual patients. (Reprinted from Plunkett W, Liliemark JO, Estey E, et al. Saturation of ara-CTP accumulation during high-dose ara-C therapy: pharmacologic rationale for intermediate-dose ara-C. *Semin Oncol.* 1987;14[2 (Suppl 1)]:159-166. Copyright © 1987 Grune & Stratton, Inc. With permission.)

cell death pathway. Although the precise mechanism by which these proteins prevent ara-C–induced cytotoxicity remains to be elucidated, Bcl-2 and Bcl-X_L antagonize ara-C–mediated apoptosis.[54] The fact that patients whose blasts express high levels of Bcl-2 respond poorly to ara-C–containing regimens,[55] further supports the pivotal role of Bcl-2 in ara-C response and resistance.

Clinical studies of determinants of ara-C response are complicated by the fact that ara-C is almost always given in combination with an anthracycline. Thus, a complete response or long remission duration does not necessarily imply sensitivity to ara-C. A lack of response does imply resistance to both agents in the combination, except for the not infrequent cases in which failure can be attributed to infection or inability to administer full dosages of drug. With these limitations, the duration of complete response is probably the most appropriate and most important single yardstick of drug sensitivity because it reflects the fractional cell kill during induction therapy, but no single factor has emerged as a determinant of remission duration.

Cell Kinetics and Cytosine Arabinoside Cytotoxicity

In addition to biochemical factors that determine response, cell kinetic properties exert an important influence on the results of ara-C treatment. As an inhibitor of DNA synthesis, ara-C has its

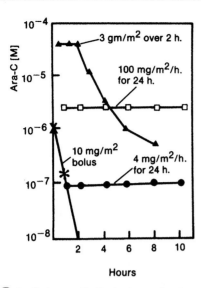

FIGURE **9.6** Ara-C pharmacokinetics in plasma after doses of 3 g/m² given over 2 hours, 100 mg/m²/h by continuous infusion for 24 hours, 4 mg/m²/h (a conventional antileukemic dose) by continuous intravenous infusion, and 10 mg/m² subcutaneously or intravenously as a bolus.

over a 1- or 2-hour infusion[62] (Fig. 9.6). Thereafter, the plasma concentration of ara-C declines, with a half-life of 7 to 20 minutes. A second phase of drug disappearance has been detected after high-dose ara-C infusion, with a terminal half-life of 30 to 150 minutes, but the drug concentration during this second phase has cytotoxic potential only in patients treated with high-dose ara-C.[63] Seventy to eighty percent of a given dose is excreted in the urine as ara-U,[63] which, within minutes of drug injection, becomes the predominant compound found in plasma. Ara-U has a longer half-life in plasma (3.2 to 5.8 hours) than does ara-C and may enhance the activation of ara-C through feedback inhibition of ara-C deamination in leukemic cells. The steady-state level of ara-C in plasma achieved by constant intravenous infusion remains proportional to dose for dose rates up to 2 g/m²/d. At this dose, steady-state plasma levels approximate 5 μM. Above this rate of infusion, the deamination reaction is saturated and ara-C plasma levels rise unpredictably, which may lead to severe toxicity. To accelerate the achievement of a steady-state concentration, one may give a bolus dose of three times the hourly infusion rate before infusion.[64] Equivalent drug exposure (area under the curve [AUC]) is achieved by subcutaneous or intravenous infusion of ara-C.

Owing to the presence of high concentrations of cytidine deaminase in the gastrointestinal mucosa and liver, orally administered ara-C provides much lower plasma levels than does direct intravenous administration. Threefold to tenfold higher doses must be given in animals to achieve a biologic effect equivalent to that produced by intravenous drug. The oral route, therefore, is not routinely used in humans.

Ara-C has been administered by intraperitoneal infusion for treatment of ovarian cancer.[65] After instillation of 100 μM of drug, ara-C levels fall in the peritoneal cavity with a half-life of approximately 2 hours. Simultaneous plasma levels are 100- to 1,000-fold lower, presumably because of deamination of ara-C in liver before it reaches the systemic circulation. In 21-day continuous exposure to IP ara-C, patients tolerated up to 100 μM intraperitoneal concentrations but developed peritonitis at higher concentrations.[66]

Cerebrospinal Fluid Pharmacokinetics

After intravenous administration of 100 mg/m² of ara-C, parent drug levels reach 0.1 to 0.3 μM in the cerebrospinal fluid (CSF). Thereafter, levels decline with a half-life of 2 hours. Proportionately higher CSF levels are reached by intravenous high-dose ara-C regimens; for example, a 3 g/m² infusion intravenously over 1 hour yields peak CSF concentrations of 4 μM,[61] whereas the same dose over 24 hours yields peak CSF ara-C concentrations of 1 μM.[63]

Ara-C is effective when administered intrathecally for the treatment of metastatic neoplasms. A number of dosing schedules for giving intrathecal ara-C have been recommended, but twice weekly or weekly schedules of administration are the most often used. The dose of ara-C ranges from 30 to 50 mg/m². The dose is generally adjusted in pediatric patients according to age (15 mg for children below 1 year of age, 20 mg for children between 1 and 2 years, 30 mg for children between 2 and 3 years, and 40 mg for children older than 3 years). The clinical pharmacology of ara-C in the CSF following intrathecal administration differs considerably from that seen in the plasma following a parenteral dose. Systematically administered ara-C is rapidly eliminated by biotransformation to the inactive metabolite ara-U. In contrast, little conversion of ara-C to ara-U takes place in the CSF following an intrathecal injection. The ratio of ara-U to ara-C is only 0.08, a finding that is consistent with the very low levels of cytidine deaminase present in the brain and CSF. Following an intraventricular administration of 30 mg of ara-C, peak levels exceed 1 to 2 mM in the CSF, and levels decline slowly, with the terminal half-life of approximately 3.4 hours.[67] Concentrations above the threshold for cytotoxicity (0.1 μg/mL, or 0.4 μM) are maintained in the CSF for 24 to 48 hours. The CSF clearance is 0.42 mL/min, which is similar to the CSF bulk flow rate. This finding suggests that drug elimination occurs primarily by this route. Plasma levels following intrathecal administration of 30 mg/m² of ara-C are less than 1 μM, which illustrates the advantage of intracavitary therapy with a drug that is rapidly cleared once it reaches the systemic circulation.

Depot cytarabine (DCT or DepoCyt) is a depot formulation of ara-C encapsulated in microscopic Gelfoam particles (DepoFoam) and provides sustained release of drug into the CSF, thus reducing the number of lumbar punctures. DCT results in a 55-fold increase in drug half-life in CSF after intraventricular administration in rats, from 2.7 hr for unbound ara-C to 148 hours for DCT. In patients with leptomeningeal metastasis receiving a dose of 50 mg of DTC, ara-C concentrations were maintained above the cytotoxic threshold for 12 ± 3 days. The maximum tolerated dosage was 75 mg administered every 3 weeks, and the dose-limiting toxicity was headache, and arachnoiditis.[68] A randomized study involving patients with lymphomatous meningitis demonstrated a possible prolongation of time to neurologic progression in patients treated with 50 mg of DTC every 2 weeks compared with patients treated with standard intrathecal ara-C.[69] DTC gave equivalent results to standard intrathecal methotrexate, given every 4 days for treatment of carcinomatous meningitis.[70] Prophylactic DCT, 50 mg, prevented lymphomatous meningitis in 24 high-risk patients.[71] About 15% of patients receiving DCT experience arachnoiditis or symptoms of cauda equina dysfunction including lower limb paresis and urinary retention.[72]

Alternate Schedules of Administration

Although ara-C is used most commonly in regimens of 100 to 200 mg/m^2/d for 7 days, other high-dose and low-dose schedules have been used in treating leukemia. The more effective of these newer regimens have been high-dose schemes, usually 2 to 3 g/m^2 every 12 hours for six doses on days 1, 3, and 5.[73] High-dose ara-C is typically used during the consolidation phase of treatment for AML.[3] The rationale for the higher-dose regimen initially rested on the assumption that ara-C phosphorylation is the rate-limiting intracellular step in the drug's activation and could be promoted by raising intracellular concentrations to the K_m of CdR kinase for ara-C, or approximately 20 µmol/L. Above this level, further increases in ara-C do not lead to increased ara-CTP because the phosphorylation pathways enzymes become saturated.

Others have examined the clinical activity of low-dose ara-C, particularly in older patients with myelodysplastic syndromes.[74] These regimens have used dosages in the range of 3 to 20 mg/m^2/d or bid, for up to 3 weeks, with the expectation that low doses would produce less toxicity and promote leukemic cell differentiation (or apoptosis). Chromosomal markers for the leukemic cell line persist in remission granulocytes, findings that support DAC causing the induction of differentiation.[75] In general, myelosuppression often supervenes in patients on low-dose ara-C, and less than 20% of patients achieve any meaningful improvement in blood counts.

Toxicity

The primary determinants of ara-C toxicity are drug concentration and duration of exposure. Because ara-C is cell cycle phase specific, the duration of cell exposure to the drug is critical in determining the fraction of cells killed. In humans, single-bolus doses of ara-C as large as 4.2 g/m^2 are well tolerated because of the rapid inactivation of the parent compound and the brief period of exposure, whereas constant infusion of drug for 48 hours using total doses of 1 g/m^2 produces severe myelosuppression.[76]

Myelosuppression and gastrointestinal epithelial injury are the primary toxic side effects of ara-C. With conventional 5- to 7-day courses of treatment, the period of maximal toxicity begins during the 1st week of treatment and lasts 14 to 21 days. Ara-C severely depresses platelet production and granulopoiesis, although anemia also occurs. Little acute effect is seen on the lymphocyte count, although cell-mediated immunity is depressed in patients receiving ara-C.[77] Both white and red cell precursors become megaloblastic, as the result of suppression of DNA synthesis.

Gastrointestinal symptoms, including nausea, vomiting, and diarrhea, are frequent complaints during drug administration but subside quickly after treatment. Severe gastrointestinal lesions occur in patients treated with ara-C as part of complex chemotherapy regimens, and the specific contribution of ara-C is difficult to ascertain in these cases. All parts of the gastrointestinal tract can be affected. Oral mucositis may be severe and prolonged in patients receiving more than 5 days of continuous treatment. Clinical symptoms of diarrhea, ileus, and abdominal pain may be accompanied by gastrointestinal bleeding, electrolyte abnormalities, and protein-losing enteropathy. Radiologic evidence of dilatation of the terminal ileum, associated with neutropenia, and termed typhlitis, may be associated with progressive abdominal pain and may lead to bowel perforation. Pathologic findings in the gastrointestinal tract include denudation of the epithelial surface and loss of crypt cell mitotic activity.

Reversible intrahepatic cholestasis with jaundice occurs frequently in patients receiving ara-C for induction therapy but discontinuation of therapy is necessary in fewer than 25% of patients.[78] Hepatotoxicity is manifested primarily as an asymptomatic increase in hepatic enzymes in the serum, together with mild jaundice, and rapidly reverses after treatment. Ara-C treatment may be infrequently associated with pancreatitis.[79]

Toxicity of High-Dose Cytosine Arabinoside

High-dose ara-C significantly increases the incidence and severity of bone marrow and gastrointestinal toxic effects.[3] Hospitalization for fever and neutropenia is required in 71% of the treatment courses in patients receiving 3 g/m^2 per 12 hours given on alternative days for six doses, and platelet transfusions are required in 86%. Patients on high-dose ara-C become neutropenic ($<0.5 \times 10^6$/mL) 10 to 14 days after treatment, depending on dose and schedule. Treatment-related deaths, primarily the result of infection, occur in approximately 5% of the patients treated with this schedule. In addition, high-dose ara-C produces pulmonary toxicity, including noncardiogenic pulmonary edema, in approximately 10% of patients, and a surprisingly high incidence of *Streptococcus viridans* pneumonia is seen, especially in pediatric populations.[80] The pulmonary edema syndrome presents 1 to 2 weeks after drug administration with fever, dyspnea, and pulmonary infiltrates and is fatal in 10% to 20% of patients with this toxicity.

High-dose regimens frequently cause cholestatic jaundice and elevation of serum transaminases and alkaline phosphatase.[81] These changes are in general reversible. A more dangerous toxicity involving cerebral and cerebellar dysfunction occurs in 10% of patients receiving 3 g/m^2 for 6 doses[4] and in two thirds of patients receiving 4.5 g/m^2 for 12 doses.[82] Age over 40 years, abnormal alkaline phosphatase activity in serum, and compromised renal function are risk factors associated with an increased susceptibility to CNS toxicity, which is manifested as slurred speech, unsteady gait, dementia, and coma. Symptoms of neurologic toxicity resolve within several weeks in approximately 60% of patients; however, a permanent disability is present in the remaining 40%, and occasionally, patients have died of CNS toxicity.[3] Progressive brainstem dysfunction[83] and an ascending peripheral neuropathy[84] also have been reported.

Other bothersome toxicities complicate high-dose ara-C. Conjunctivitis, responsive to topical steroids, is a frequent side effect. Rarely, skin rash occurs. Neutrophilic eccrine hidradenitis, an unusual febrile cutaneous reaction manifested as plaques or nodules during the second week after chemotherapy, may also be seen after high-dose ara-C.[85]

Finally, sporadic reports of cardiac toxicity (arrhythmias, pericarditis, congestive heart failure) have been associated with ara-C treatment, generally in patients receiving high-dose therapy. These cases involve multidrug regimens and do not represent conclusive evidence for a cause-and-effect relationship with ara-C.

Although ara-C causes chromosomal breaks in cultured cells and an increased rate of point mutation in circulating white cells of patients receiving therapy, it is not an established carcinogen in humans. In cultured cells, and in acute leukemia cells from patients treated with Ara-C, it produces mutations preferentially in G:C base pair sequences (TpGpA/TpCpA), and most frequently in mismatch repair deficient cells.[86] The drug is teratogenic in animals.

Cytidine-deaminase deficiency due to polymorphisms of the CD gene may underlie instances of severe toxicity after ara-C gemcitabine, or 5-azacytidine.[87] The C79A genotype has been associated with slower metabolism of cytidine analogues, while rapid deamination variants may lead to a poor response.[88]

Toxicity of Intrathecal Cytosine Arabinoside

Intrathecal Ara-C is frequently (20% of patients) associated with fever and headache and, less commonly, seizures may occur within 1 to 7 days of intrathecal ara-C administration.[6] Rarely, ara-C causes a progressive brainstem toxicity that may be fatal.[89] Intrathecal ara-C should be used with caution in patients receiving systemic high-dose methotrexate, or those with a history of methotrexate neurotoxicity.

Drug Interactions

Ara-C has synergistic antitumor activity with a number of other antitumor agents in animal tumor models (cyclophosphamide, cisplatin, purine analogs, methotrexate, and etoposide). The basis for ara-C potentiation of alkylating agents and cisplatin is thought to be inhibition of repair of DNA-alkylator adducts.[90] THU, a potent transition state inhibitor of cytidine deaminase (CD) ($K_i = 3 \times 10^{-8}$ mol/L), enhances ara-CTP formation in acute myelocytic leukemia cells in vitro.[91] Clinical evaluation of the combination indicated that THU in intravenous doses of 50 mg/m^2 markedly prolongs the plasma half-life of ara-C from 10 to 120 minutes and causes a corresponding enhancement of toxicity to bone marrow.[92] In combination with THU, the tolerable dosage of ara-C is reduced at least 30-fold to 0.1 mg/kg/d for 5 days. Whether the combination has greater therapeutic effects, ara-C alone is unclear.

Inhibitors of ribonucleotide reductase such as hydroxyurea and fludarabine[93] decrease dCTP pools and increase ara-CTP formation several fold. A decrease in dCTP should enhance ara-CTP incorporation into DNA by increasing ara-CTP pools and decreasing its competitor, dCTP.

The favorable effects of fludarabine on ara-CTP concentration have not led to improvement of clinical therapy outcome in patients with AML,[94] perhaps due to their additive toxicity. Combinations of ara-C, daunorubicin, and cladribine have entered clinical trial for AML, with promising early results and no obvious additive toxicity.[95]

Ara-C is commonly used in combination with daunorubicin or idarubicin for the treatment of AML. In experimental systems, minute (0.01 µM) concentrations of ara-C cause an increase in levels of topoisomerase II, the necessary enzymatic target of anthracyclines. Ara-C enhances the number of protein-associated DNA strand breaks induced by etoposide, a topo II inhibitor, and increases etoposide cytotoxicity.[96]

The period of Ara-C myelosuppression is shortened by hematopoietic growth factors (HGFs) following ara-C. However, there was a theoretical concern that these growth factors might stimulate leukemia cell proliferation but there is no evidence for higher relapse rates in patients receiving G-CSF. It was proposed that giving HGFs before ara-C would recruit leukemia cells into the susceptible S phase of the cell cycle, and would thereby enhance leukemic cytotoxicity, but randomized clinical trials have shown no advantage in response rate or survival in patients with AML treated with HGFs in combination with ara-C.[97]

Vyxeos (daunorubicin and cytarabine) Liposome for Injection

Vyxeos, or CPX-351, is a liposomal formulation of daunorubicin (see Chapter 14, "topoisomerase inhibitors") and ara-C that contains a 5:1 molar ratio of ara-C to daunorubicin. The liposomes are composed of distearylphosphatidylcholine, distearoylphosphatidylglycerol, and cholesterol in a 7:2:1 molar ratio, with a mean diameter of 100 ± 20 nm.[98] This formulation has been studied primarily in the treatment of poor risk AML, both among older untreated patients as well as patients with relapsed AML.

Pharmacology, Metabolism, and Mechanism of Action

The rationale for liposomal delivery of cytarabine and daunorubicin is based upon the variability of the relative concentrations of these agents when administered intravenously. Data suggest that combination chemotherapies are more effective when given at ratios which have the highest synergy; at other ratios, multiple agents may not have an additive antitumor effect or may even antagonize one another.[99] The liposomal formulation of vyxeos was based on studies in P388 murine lymphocytic leukemia and HL60 human acute promonomyelocytic leukemia cells and the drug-dependent synergy and antagonism at various molar ratios of cytarabine and daunorubicin; a ratio of 5:1 was found to have the most favorable.[98] Vyxeos was shown to maintain this 5:1 ratio in the plasma and has first-order monoexponential clearance with accumulation with sequential doses and results in a mean half-life of daunorubicin of 31.5 hours and cytarabine of 40.4 hours.[100] Nearly all of drug remains encapsulated in the plasma, and the liposomal formulation of cytarabine and daunorubicin has preferential uptake within AML cells compared to normal cells, resulting in preferential leukemic cytotoxicity.[101]

Clinical Indications

Vyxeos was FDA approved in 2017 for the treatment of adults with newly diagnosed therapy-related AML or AML with myelodysplasia-related changes. A phase II study comparing vyxeos to conventional 7+3 showed a signal for improved response in the subgroup of patients with secondary AML.[102] A subsequent phase III study randomized 309 patients age 60 to 75 with untreated secondary AML to receive either vyxeos ($n = 153$) or conventional 7+3 induction chemotherapy ($n = 156$); patients receiving vyxeos had an improved rate of complete remission or complete remission with incomplete count recovery (47.7% versus 33.3%), and lower 60-day mortality (13.7% versus 21.2%).[103] The complete response rate was 38% versus 26% with standard 7+3, and the median overall survival was improved at 9.6 months compared to 5.9 months (FDA label). Survival both among patients age 60 to 69 (HR 0.68) and 70 to 75 (HR 0.55) improved in the vyxeos arm, possibly related in part to improved rates of undergoing transplantation.[104]

Azacytidine Analogs

5-Aza-analogs of cytidine have become important therapeutic agents and unique tools for investigating epigenetic modification of DNA. Although first discovered and tested in high doses against AML, 5-azacytidine (5-azaC) and more recently, 2′-deoxy-5-azacytidine (DEC) (decitabine) have become standard agents in lower dose regimens for management of myelodysplasia (MDS), a preleukemic state characterized by defective maturation of cells and affecting all bone marrow hematopoietic lineages. MDS is characterized by cytopenias and carries the risk of progression to bone marrow failure or AML. The drugs normalize bone marrow morphology in up to 10% of these patients and reduce red blood cell and platelet transfusion requirements in more than one third of such patients; 5-azaC treatment leads to an increase in survival of MDS patients as compared to best supportive care.[105] Both drugs are also approved for treatment of AML patients with low leukemic blast counts (20% to 30% bone marrow infiltration), otherwise not candidates for intensive induction therapy.

Both analogues are incorporated into DNA and inhibit methylation of CpG islands in DNA (Fig. 9.7), thereby modifying gene expression and promoting differentiation of both normal and malignant cells in experimental systems.[106] 5-AzaC is also incorporated into RNA, a property that may contribute to its antitumor activity. DEC is exclusively incorporated into DNA and is a more effective inducer of erythroid differentiation than 5-aza, with less acute toxicity. Both analogues continue to be investigated in various types of acute leukemia, and as modifiers of gene expression in other cancers, but their primary use is in the treatment of MDS.[107]

5-Azacytidine

5-AzaC, an analog of cytidine, was synthesized by Sorm and colleagues in 1963,[108] who characterized it as an inhibitor of DNA synthesis. In clinical trials, its most notable activity was exerted in cytotoxic doses against myeloid leukemias and in lower dose regimens against MDS, an approved indication.[109] Aside from its anticancer activity, the drug induces synthesis of fetal hemoglobin by red cell precursors in sickle cell anemia, an effect believed to be mediated by hypomethylation of the γ-globin gene.[110] Its value as a treatment for hemoglobinopathies has been limited by its bone marrow toxicity and by concerns about carcinogenesis. More recently, the ability of low doses of 5-azaC and DEC to induce expression

of tumor-associated antigens and endogenous retroviral genes, and stimulate antitumor immune responses has led to great interest in their use with immune checkpoint inhibitors and antitumor vaccines.[111] The important features of the pharmacokinetics and clinical effects of 5-azacytidine are summarized in Table 9.3.

Structure and Mechanism of Action of Azacytidine Analogues

The biochemistry and pharmacology of 5-azaC[112] derive from its close structural analogy to cytidine, with the important difference of its nitrogen at the 5-position of the heterocyclic ring (Fig. 9.1). This substitution renders the ring chemically unstable and leads to spontaneous decomposition of the compound in neutral or alkaline solution, with a half-life of approximately 4 hours. The product of this ring opening, N-formylamidinoribofuranosylguanylurea, may recyclize to form the parent compound but also spontaneously degrades to ribofuranosylurea. Spontaneous decomposition of the ring may contribute to its cytotoxicity, once incorporated into DNA or RNA, but poses the more practical consideration that the clinical formulation must be administered within several hours of its dissolution in dextrose and water or in saline. In buffered solutions such as Ringer's lactate and at acidic pH, the agent is considerably more stable, with a half-life of 65 hours at 25°C and 94 hours at 20°C.

5-AzaC has multiple molecular and biological effects that may contribute to its antitumor activity. As a triphosphate, it competes with CTP for incorporation into RNA and alters RNA methylation and processing.[113] It inhibits formation of ribosomal 28 S and 18 S RNA from higher molecular-weight species, decreases RNA methylation, blocks the acceptor function of transfer RNA, disassembles polyribosomes, and markedly inhibits protein synthesis.[114]

Other effects of 5-azaC, however, are likely more relevant to its antitumor activity at low concentrations. This analogue is incorporated into DNA, although to a lesser extent than into RNA, and thereby inhibits DNA methylation of daughter cells following replication of DNA. As shown in Figure 9.7, inhibition of DNA methyltransferase by the 5-azaC occurs through formation of a covalent bond between the azacytidine base and a prolylcysteine dipeptide group on the enzyme,[115] as proposed by Santi et al.[116] based on his studies with unmodified cytidine. Abstraction of the proton at the 5-position of cytidine is required for beta-elimination of the reactive sulfhydryl at the 6-position to separate methylated cytidine and active DNA methyltransferase (DNMT1). Substitution

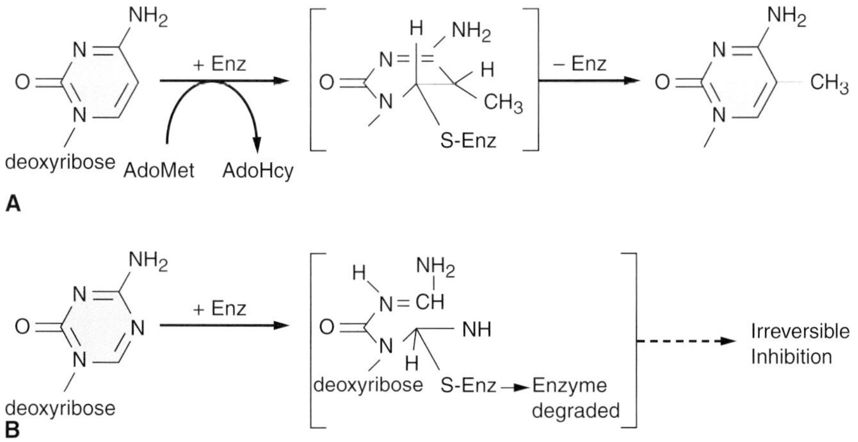

FIGURE 9.7 Formation of a dihydropyrimidine intermediate during methylation of a target DNA containing **(A)** deoxycytidine (CdR). In **(B)**, the enzyme forms a covalent bond with the 5-azacytidine nucleotide in a CpG sequence. In the enzymatic reaction **(A)**, adenosylmethionine (AdoMet) donates the methyl group and is converted to adenosylhomocysteine (AdoHC). (Adapted by permission from Nature: Christman JK. 5-Azacytidine and 5-aza-2′-deoxycytidine as inhibitors of DNA methylation: mechanistic studies and their implications for cancer therapy. *Oncogene.* 2002;21(35):5483–5495. Copyright © 2002 Springer Nature.)

TABLE **9.3**	Key features of 5-azacytidine (5-azaC) and decitabine (DEC) pharmacology
Factor	**Result**
Mechanism of action	5-AzaC incorporated into DNA and RNA; DEC incorporated into DNA. Primary effect of both is to inhibit DNA methyl transferase (DNMT1)
Metabolism	Both drugs are activated to a deoxytriphosphate. Uridine-cytidine kinase activates 5-azaC; CdR kinase activates DEC
	Both drugs are degraded to inactive metabolites by cytidine deaminase
Pharmacokinetics and elimination	5-AzaC: $t_{1/2}$ 20 to 40 min
	DEC: $t_{1/2}$ 20 min
Drug interactions	THU inhibits deamination
Toxicity	Myelosuppression
	Nausea, vomiting after bolus dose
	Hepatocellular dysfunction (5-azaC, high dose)
	Muscle tenderness, weakness (5-azaC, high dose)
	Lethargy, confusion, coma (5-azaC, high dose)
Precautions	Hepatic failure may occur in patients with underlying liver dysfunction (5-azaC)
	Use high-dose 5-azaC with caution in patients with altered mental status

of a nitrogen for carbon at the 6 position removes this proton, and beta elimination cannot proceed, resulting a trapped, covalent TNA-DNMT adduct. The same chemistry is applicable to the 5-fluoro–substituted pyrimidines in their bonding to thymidylate synthase (Chapter 8). The first evidence for this mechanism was published in 1984 when it was reported that bacterial DNA treated with 5-azaC eluted in a covalent complex with Hpall methyltransferase.[117] Through covalent binding to DNA, the DNMTs become tethered and have diminished ability to methylate the genome. The decreased genomic methylation has been thus invoked as responsible for the ability of 5-azaC to induce gene expression and differentiation in cell culture. DEC blocks DNA methylation in an identical fashion.

Methylation of promoter sequences in DNA leads to loss of expression of these genes. It has been well established that unusually, dense clusters of the CpG dinucleotide, sequence known as CpG islands, are found in a hypomethylated state in normal tissue but acquire excessive methylation in malignancies,[118] a finding that likely reflects a broader pattern of epigenetic dysregulation. The consequence of CpG methylation is a silencing of promoter function and gene expression. Methylation of promoter sequences for tumor suppressor genes such as P53 and BRCA 1 and 2 is a relatively common finding cyin human tumors. 5-AzaC leads to enhanced expression of a multitude of genes, depending on the cell type

studied.[14] The specific genes activated by DNA demethylation and responsible for the antineoplastic effects of 5-azaC and DEC activity have yet to be fully elucidated.[119]

Alternatively, the antitumor action of 5-azaC and DEC could result from formation of bulky DNA-DNMT adducts, possibly leading to stalled replication forks and strand breaks. There existed an underappreciated body of evidence that DNA damage results from the covalent trapping of DNMT. The Jaenisch laboratory found that DEC toxicity correlated with the level of enzyme in cell culture.[120] Embryonic stem cells had decreased survival when wild-type DNMT1 was retained relative to a hypomorphic DNMT1 variant. Intrauterine DEC treatment of wild-type mice but not the heterozygous littermates led to a remarkable growth defect in the offspring.

Early clinical experience with 5-azaC indicated that the drug may have actions beyond inhibiting gene methylation. Karyotypes normalized before global demethylation in patients with MDS.[121] Increased gamma-H2AX staining, ATM, and p53 activation were observed in cultured cells exposed to high concentrations of 5-azaC.[122] These markers of DNA damage response (DDR) correlated with DNMT expression levels in cultured cells. Further, it was reported that DEC-induced DNA damage is reduced by aphidicolin, which inhibits replication, leading to the conclusion that DEC induces fork stalling.[123] Aza-analogue toxicity is accentuated in isogenic FANCC and XRCC-1 knockout cell lines, indicating a role for homologous recombination and base excision repair, respectively, in resolving DEC-induced lesions.[124] Treatment with the PARP inhibitor olaparib potentiates DEC-induced DNA damage and decreased leukemic cell survival *in vitro*. While these in vitro studies used suprapharmacological concentrations of the analogues, further analysis of patient tumor samples is needed to explore the role of DNA damage and repair in the clinical activity of these drugs. The sequence of covalent binding of DNMTs to DEC incorporated into DNA, leading to strand breaks and apoptosis, represents a plausible alternative or complimentary explanation for azacytidine action.

Cellular Pharmacology

5-AzaC readily enters mammalian cells by hENT1, an equilibrative nucleoside transporter.[125] It is then converted to a monophosphate by uridine-cytidine kinase (U-C kinase), which is found in low concentration in human AML cells,[126] has low affinity for the drug (K_m = 0.2 to 11 mM), and probably represents the rate-limiting step in its activation.

Further activation of 5-aza-CMP to a triphosphate probably occurs by the enzyme dCMP kinase and nucleoside NDP kinase. It is converted to a deoxynucleotide by RNR and thence to deoxy-5-azaCTP, which is incorporated into DNA. One hour after exposure of cells to the radiolabeled drug, 60% to 70% of acid-soluble radioactivity in cells was identified as 5-azaCTP,[127] while a smaller fraction is found as the deoxytriphosphate.

DEC follows a somewhat different path of activation to a triphosphate. Like ara-C, its first phosphorylation is accomplished by CdR kinase, an enzyme lost in drug-resistant cell lines. Thereafter, it follows the same activation pathway as ara-C. Its clearance depends on deamination. When used as cytotoxics, drug concentration and duration of exposure are important determinants of cell killing by both aza analogues, a finding consistent with a preferential action on rapidly dividing cells and effects on DNA.[112]

At submicromolar drug concentrations, however, the aza analogues induce differentiation, likely through expression of specific genes. Demethylation of promoter sites affects expression of a multitude of genes,[115] including β- and γ-globin and histocompatibility proteins,[128] and tumor suppressor genes. Of particular interest are its effects on the immune system, as it activates cytotoxic T-cells,[129] increases expression of tumor antigens such as testes antigens, and stimulates expression of a host of immune response genes (the "AZA immune gene set"), checkpoint receptors and ligands, inflammatory cytokines, and interferon response elements.[111] Additional effects on the immune response, including up-regulation of PD-1 in T cells by 5-azaC in MDS patients,[130] and stimulation of endogenous retroviral gene sequences and a potent beta-interferon response,[131] have evoked great interest in the combination of aza-analogues and checkpoint immune therapies. The aza-analogues have mutagenic and teratogenic effects[132] but are not known to be carcinogens.

Cells respond to the incorporation of azacytidine analogues into DNA by removal through base excision repair, which is antagonized by poly-adenosylribosylation inhibitors and by activation of CHK1, CHK2, and Rad51 in the DDR pathway. The importance of DDR responses in determining cell differentiation and cell death is not yet understood.

Resistance to Aza Analogues

Deletion of U-C kinase has been observed in cells resistant to cytotoxic concentrations of 5-azaC, and deletion of deoxycytidine kinase was found in nonresponders to DEC.[105] Cytidine deaminase, found in 10- to 30-fold higher concentration than the activating kinases in leukemic cells, and the ratio of kinase to deaminase activities appear to predict response to DEC.[126] Other factors may determine sensitivity to both aza analogues in lower dose regimens, as approved for MDS. TET-2 mutations, found in 20% of MDS, have been associated with a somewhat higher response rate,[133] while resistance has been

attributed to incomplete depletion of DNMT1 in clinical studies and to increase expression of DNMT1[134] and of tyrosine kinases (c-KIT) in cell culture experiments.[135] DEC seems highly active in the p53 mutant subset of MDS and AML.[136] All 21 patients with mutant p53 tumors, in a trial of 20 mg/m² for 10 consecutive days per month, achieved clearance of bone marrow blasts, as compared to 32/78 (41%) with wild-type p53.

Assay Methods and Pharmacokinetics

5-AzaC and DEC are assayed by high-performance liquid chromatography with tandem mass spectrometry,[137,138] which has the requisite sensitivity and specificity for clinical studies.

After subcutaneous injection, [14C]5-azaC rapidly distributes into a volume approximately equal to or greater than total body water (0.58 to 1.15 L/kg) with little plasma protein binding. Isolated measurements of radioactivity in the CSF indicate poor penetration of drug, with a CSF:plasma ratio of less than 0.1.

For treatment of MDS, 5-azaC is given subcutaneously, typically in doses of 75 mg/m²/d for 7 days in a 28-day cycle. After either subcutaneous (89% bioavailability) or intravenous bolus administration of 75 mg/m², the drug reaches a C_{max} of approximately 2 to 10 µM and has an AUC of 4 µmol h/mL. Its volume of distribution is approximately 75 L.[133,139] It undergoes rapid deamination,[140–142] with a clearance from plasma of 146 to 167 L/h and a plasma half-life of 20 to 40 minutes.[140] An unquantified fraction undergoes renal excretion, and the package insert advises discontinuing treatment if serum creatinine or BUN is elevated, waiting for renal function to return to normal and then using a 50% reduction in dose. A longer $t_{1/2}$ of 1.2 hours was reported in a patient in renal failure who received a subcutaneous dose of 45 mg/m².[141]

DEC has a plasma $t_{1/2}$ of 20 minutes. It may be used safely in patients with renal insufficiency. Estimated plasma concentrations reach 1 µM during infusion[138] (Fig 9.8).

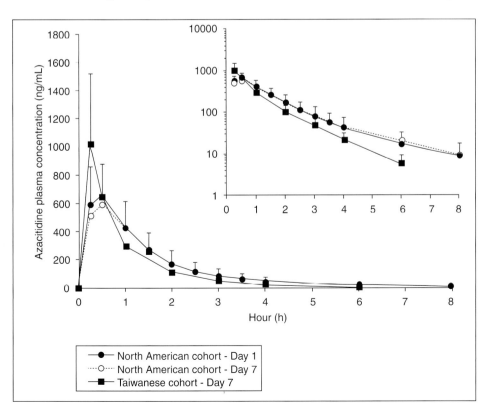

FIGURE 9.8 Decitabine plasma pharmacokinetics,[132] plotted on an arithmetic scale and on a log scale.

The identity of metabolites is unclear in humans.[112] 5-AzaC is known to undergo spontaneous ring opening in vitro, generating metabolites previously described in this chapter, and is also subject to deamination by cytidine deaminase, as also occurs with DEC.

Clinical Regimens and Toxicity

In patients with AML, a number of schedules of administration have been used for 5-azacytidine,[143] including single weekly intravenous doses of up to 750 mg/m², daily doses of 150 to 200 mg/m² for 5 to 10 consecutive days, and continuous infusion of similar daily doses for up to 5 days. With each regimen, the primary toxicity was leukopenia, although nausea and vomiting were prominent symptoms after higher doses and bolus administration. The relatively low response rate to high-dose 5-azaC in previously treated patients, 17% to 36%, and its differentiating effects in tissue culture[144] led to exploration of low-dose regimens.

In patients with MDS, a lower dose of 5-azaC, 75 mg/m²/d for 7 days repeated every 28 days, yields a best response, usually after the fifth cycle of therapy.[109] After an initial decrease in WBC counts, mature WBCs containing molecular evidence of the original tumor steadily increase in responding patients. Platelet counts increase and transfusion requirements abate in responding patients. Oral 5-azaC has a bioavailability approaching 20% and produces a similar profile of responses in MDS and AML at doses of 480 mg daily for 7 days. Further trials of this more convenient route of administration are underway.[145]

In treating AML with higher doses of 5-azaC, occasional patients have developed hepatic enzyme elevations and hyperbilirubinemia.[146] A syndrome of neuromuscular toxicity was observed in patients receiving 200 mg/m²/d by intravenous bolus injection. Neurotoxicity has been reported only sporadically.[147] Several less worrisome acute toxic reactions have been associated with 5-azaC, including transient fever, a pruritic skin rash, and, rarely, hypotension during or immediately after bolus intravenous administration. These toxicities are uncommon with low-dose regimens, which are primarily limited by myelosuppression.

Clinical Application of 5-Azacytidine Analogues

5-AzaC was approved for treatment of patients with intermediate- or high-risk MDS in 2004, based on improved survival in a randomized phase III trial comparing the drug to best supportive care. Thirty-five percent of patients achieved either a clear improvement in blood counts or decreased transfusion requirements, the transfusion benefits lasting a median of more than 330 days.[109] In an overview of MDS trials, 6% achieved a complete response in bone marrow and peripheral blood.[148]

Subsequently, the AZA-001 phase II study showed a survival benefit among MDS patients and patients with AML with 20% to 30% blasts. The study compared 5-azaC to investigator's choice.[149] On the conventional therapy arm, patients with intermediate-2 or high-risk MDS or AML received best supportive care, low-dose cytarabine, or intensive chemotherapy, according to their physician's choice. The 5-azaC arm reached a median survival of 24.5 months as compared to 15 months on the conventional care arm. Additional studies have tested a combination of 5-azaC and other epigenetic modifying agents, including a histone deacetylase inhibitor, and in another trial, in combination with lenalidomide, which is active against del(5q) MDS, but without positive results.[150]

DEC was approved by the FDA for treatment of MDS using a regimen of 15 mg/m² intravenously three times daily for 3 days every 6 weeks, based on improved time to progression. Subsequent trials established the equal efficacy of a more convenient regimen of 20 mg/m²/d for 5 days every 4 weeks, given intravenously.[107] Its toxicity includes most prominently myelosuppression and gastrointestinal symptoms, although neutropenia may prevent its use beyond a limited number of cycles of therapy. An alternative regimen of 0.1 to 0.2 mg/kg 2 to 3 days per week, given for an indefinite period for responders, appears to deplete DNA methyltransferase and induce a fraction of long-term remissions[134] but has not been compared to the approve regimen. DEC has also been evaluated in AML patients with greater than 30% blasts. A randomized phase III trial compared conventional care to DEC and found only a small, but nonstatistically significant advantage in favor of DEC (10.4- vs 6.5-month survival).[151]

Gemcitabine

GEM (2,2-difluorodeoxycytidine, dFdC) is the most important cytidine analog to enter clinical trials since ara-C (Fig. 9.1). It has become a standard first-line therapy for patients with pancreatic cancer, and it is also used for non–small cell lung cancer, ovarian cancer, and transitional cell cancer of the bladder.[152–154] The drug was selected for development on the basis of its impressive activity against murine solid tumors and human xenografts in nude mice. In tissue culture, it is generally more potent than ara-C; the 50% inhibition concentration values for human leukemic cells range from 3 to 10 nM for 48-hour exposure compared with 26 to 52 nM for ara-C. Although its metabolism to triphosphate status and its effects on DNA in general mimic those of ara-C, differences are found in kinetics of inhibition and additional sites of action of the newer compound, and in its spectrum of clinical activity.

Cellular Pharmacology, Metabolism, and Mechanism of Action

GEM retains many of the characteristics of ara-C. Its key features are shown in Table 9.4. Influx of GEM through the cell membrane occurs via the hENT1 equilibrative nucleoside transporter. A concentrative transporter may also participate in its uptake.[155] CdR kinase phosphorylates GEM intracellularly to produce its monophosphate (dFdCMP), from which point it is converted to its diphosphate and triphosphate difluorodeoxycytidine (dFdCDP, dFdCTP).[156] Its affinity for CdR kinase is threefold lower than the affinity of the natural substrate, CdR, whereas it has a 50% lower affinity (95 μM) for cytidine deaminase than for CdR.[157] Cytidine deaminase conversion of GEM to difluorodeoxyuridine (dFdU) represents the main catabolic pathway and is responsible for its brief 15-minute half-life in the systemic circulation. Its monophosphate is subject to cleavage by deoxycytidylate deaminase, yielding difluorodeoxyuridine monophosphate, a weak inhibitor of thymidylate synthase. To a lesser extent, pyrimidine nucleoside phosphorylase clears GEM by cleaving the pyrimidine base from the furanose ring.

As with ara-C, in vitro studies of GEM suggest potent inhibition of DNA synthesis as a major component of its mechanism of action,[158] but kinetic studies indicate that the killing effects of GEM are not confined to the S phase of the cell cycle, and the

TABLE

9.4   *Key features of gemcitabine*

Factor	Result
Mechanism of action	Incorporation into DNA terminates chain elongation
	Inhibits ribonucleotide reductase, depletes physiological deoxynucleotides
"Metabolism"	Converted to a triphosphate
	Deaminated to inactive 2'-2' di fluorouridine
Pharmacokinetics	Plasma $t_{1/2}$ 8 min
Elimination	Deamination in liver, plasma, and peripheral tissues
	Reduce doses in patients with elevated serum bilirubin
Drug interactions	Radiosensitizer
	Sensitizes cells to platinum-induced DNA damage
Toxicity	Myelosuppression
	Gastrointestinal epithelial ulceration
	Flu-like symptoms
	Abnormal liver function tests
	Microangiopathic anemia-uremia
	Pulmonary infiltrates

drug is as effective against confluent cells as it is against cells in log-phase growth.[159] The cytotoxic activity may be a result of several actions on DNA synthesis: dFdCTP competes with dCTP as a weak inhibitor of DNA polymerase[158]; dFdCDP is a potent inhibitor of ribonucleotide reductase, which results in depletion of deoxyribonucleotide pools necessary for DNA synthesis,[160,161] and dFdCTP becomes a weak substrate for DNA polymerase, becoming incorporated and chain terminating the growing DNA strand. The mechanism of inhibition of RNR proceeds via formation of a tight complex between the difluoro sugar of GEM, six catalytic

alpha subunits of RNR, and ATP. In addition, dFdCTP is a substrate for incorporation of the monophosphate into DNA and, after the incorporation of one more other nucleotide, leads to DNA strand termination. This "extra" nucleotide may be important in hiding the dFdCMP from DNA excision-repair enzymes.[162] Incorporation of dFdCTP into DNA, as facilitated by RNR inhibition, is the critical event leading to apoptosis.

Deamination of dFdCMP by dCMP deaminase requires activation by dCTP. As dCTP pools become depleted by the effect of GEM on ribonucleotide reductase, less deamination of GEM monophosphate occurs and intracellular accumulation of GEM deoxynucleotides increases. Furthermore, high intracellular concentration of dFdCTP appears to inhibit dCMP deaminase directly.

The kinetics of intracellular nucleotide metabolism differs between ara-C and GEM. dFdCTP has a slower, biphasic elimination from leukemic cells with α half-life ($t_{1/2\alpha}$) of 3.9 hours and β half-life ($t_{1/2\beta}$) of 16 hours, whereas ara-CTP has a monophasic elimination with $t_{1/2}$ = 0.7 to 3.5 hours[163] (Fig. 9.9). Also, dFdCDP is a much stronger inhibitor of RNR (IC_{50} of 4 μM) and blocks incorporation of labeled cytidine into the competitive cellular pool of dCTP. Further, dFdC causes a decrease in all intracellular deoxynucleotide triphosphates, consistent with inhibition of RNR.[160]

The RNR inhibition and reduction of deoxynucleotides likely contribute to its potent radiosensitization, by blocking repair of DNA, and by reducing the availability of nucleotides for repair. Cell lines selected for resistance to other RNR inhibitors, such as hydroxyurea and deoxyadenosine analogues, do not show cross-resistance to dFdC, likely because their differing mechanisms of inhibiting RNR[160] and the mutant and resistant forms of RNR generated by the other inhibitors remain sensitive to GEM.[163,164]

The activity of dFdCTP on DNA repair mechanisms increases the cytotoxicity of other chemotherapeutic agents, particularly platinum compounds. Cisplatin creates interstrand and intrastrand cross-links, which are removed by nucleotide excision repair (NER). Preclinical studies of tumor cell lines show that cisplatin-DNA adduct formation is enhanced in the presence of GEM. In cisplatin-resistant tumor cell lines, which have increased expression of NER, the addition of GEM inhibited the repair of cisplatin-induced DNA lesions and increased cytotoxic.[165] Combinations of GEM and

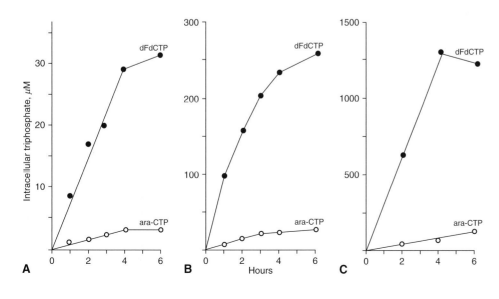

FIGURE 9.9 Accumulation of difluorodeoxycytidine triphosphate (dFdCTP) and ara-CTP as a function of time after incubation of cells with either GEM or ara-C at drug concentrations of 1 μM **(A)**, 10 μM **(B)**, and 100 μM **(C)**. (Adapted from Heinemann V, Hertel LW, Grindey GB, et al. Comparison of the cellular pharmacokinetics and toxicity of 2',2'-difluorodeoxycytidine and 1-beta-D-arabinofuranosylcytosine. *Cancer Res.* 1988;48(14):4024-4031. Copyright © 1988 American Association for Cancer Research. With permission from AACR.)

cisplatin are used in the treatment of non–small cell lung cancer, transitional cell carcinoma of the bladder, and pancreatic cancer.

Mechanisms of Resistance

Multiple mechanisms of resistance to GEM are known, but it is uncertain which of these is responsible for clinical drug resistance. In vitro studies have suggested several possible mechanisms. GEM resistance has been correlated with low tumor levels of CdR kinase.[166] Induction of cytidine deaminase,[167] increased concentrations of stromal-derived insulin-like growth factors as secreted by macrophages and myelofibroblasts,[168] and activation of the JAK-STAT pathway[169] have been implicated in GEM resistance. Preclinical studies have also demonstrated that increased expression or mutation of RNR may be associated with GEM resistance in pancreatic cancer and lung cancer trials.[164,170] The absence of transporters, especially hENT1 was associated with decreased overall survival,[171,172] and further a lack of hENT1 localized to plasma membrane have been associated with reduced disease-free survival in patients with pancreatic cancer.[173] Lastly, high activity of cytidine deaminase, found in 15% of Caucasian adults, appeared to be associated with milder drug toxicity and earlier disease progression in pancreatic cancer patients.[88] On the other hand, profound deficiency of deaminase activity, associated with genomic variants (the CDA2* allele), may lead to increased toxicity but higher response rates. The effect of these and other CDA variants on enzyme activity, toxicity, and efficacy of cytidine analogues is controversial.

Pharmacokinetics

In animals and humans, GEM pharmacokinetics ($t_{1/2}$ 8 to 15 minutes) is largely determined by its rapid cleavage by cytidine deaminase.[174] The predominant elimination product is dFdU, an inactive metabolite which undergoes renal excretion. In cell lines and in cells taken from patients during treatment, maximal accumulation of dFdCTP occurs in cells when plasma (or tissue culture) drug concentrations are in the range of 10 to 20 µM, a level achieved during 3-hour infusions of 300 mg/m^2.[175]

In a phase I study of GEM as a 30-minute infusion on days 1, 8, and 15, followed by a 1-week rest in patients with refractory solid tumors, the maximum tolerated dose (MTD) was 1,000 mg/m^2/wk. The dose-limiting toxicity was myelosuppression characterized by thrombocytopenia with relative sparing of granulocytes. Pharmacokinetic analysis showed a $t_{1/2}$ of 8 minutes for the parent compound and a biphasic elimination of dFdU, with $t_{1/2\alpha} = 27$ minutes and $t_{1/2\beta} = 14$ hours. No relationship was found between degree of myelosuppression and any pharmacokinetic parameter. The AUC of plasma dFdC was proportional to the dose over a range of 10 to 1,000 mg/m^2/wk. Clearance was dose independent but varied widely among individuals (39 to 1,239 L/h/m^2 at a dose of 1,000 mg/m^2).[176]

A higher GEM dose of 2,200 mg/m^2 administered over 30 minutes on days 1, 8, and 15 can be safely given to less heavily treated or chemo-naive patients. Plasma levels rise linearly with dose up to that level, and peak at about 75 µM, but become nonlinear above 3,650 mg/m^3.[177] The question remains unanswered as to whether cells generate higher concentration of the active metabolite as the dose rate increases. A similar series of studies with GEM have demonstrated that activation of GEM by CdR kinase to dFdCTP is saturated at infusion rates of approximately 10 mg/m^2/min. This "dose-rate infusion" produced steady-state dFdC levels of 15 to 20 µM in plasma. Based on these data, a phase I study using constant dose-rate infusion of increasing duration was carried out in patients with metastatic solid tumors.[178] Although the first-cycle MTD was estimated to be 2,250 mg/m^2 over 225 minutes, the recommended phase II dose of GEM administered as a dose-rate infusion was 1,500 mg/m^2 over 150 minutes because of the occurrence of cumulative neutropenia and thrombocytopenia at higher doses. Tempero et al.[179] performed a randomized phase II study of constant dose-rate infusion at 10 mg/m^2/min for 150 minutes versus dose-intense infusion of 2,200 mg/m^2 over 30 minutes in patients with advanced pancreatic cancer. Constant dose-rate infusion resulted in a two-fold increase in intracellular GEM triphosphate in peripheral blood mononuclear cells compared with the standard 30-minute infusion. However, no improvement in therapeutic outcome was seen.

GEM has been studied in children, and the MTD of GEM given as a 30-minute infusion weekly for 3 of 4 weeks is 1,200 mg/m^2. Myelosuppression is the dose-limiting toxicity, and pharmacokinetics in pediatric patients is similar to those in the adult population.[180]

Toxicity

The dose-limiting toxicity of GEM is invariably hematologic, and the maximum tolerated dose differs according to schedule. In general, the longer duration infusions lead to greater myelosuppression. The weekly dose schedule is the standard regimen and is implemented as a 30-minute infusion for 3 of 4 weeks. The MTD for chemo-naive patients is 2,200 mg/m^2/wk, and the MTD for pretreated patients is 800 to 1,000 mg/m^2/wk.[175,176] A dose of 1,000 mg/m^2/wk, for 3 to 4 weeks, given over 30 minutes, is recommended for treatment of pancreatic cancer and other solid tumors, and in other tumor types, it is often given in combination with cis- or carboplatin. The safety of GEM has been evaluated in a database including 22 studies using the once-weekly treatment regimen.[181] In treating 979 patients, grade 3 and 4 neutropenia occurred in 19.3% and 6% of patients, respectively. Grade 3 and 4 thrombocytopenia occurred in 4.1% and 1.1% of patients, respectively. Among nonhematologic toxicities, flu-like symptoms including fever, headache, back pain, and myalgias occur in approximately 45% of patients. The duration of these symptoms was short, and rarely led to drug discontinuation. A transient, mild elevation in liver function tests was detected in 41% of cycles.

Although severe nonhematologic reactions are rare, several specific syndromes complicating GEM therapy have emerged from its expanding clinical experience. Thrombotic microangiopathy, leading to progressive anemia and renal failure, is a late complication of multiple cycles of GEM therapy[182,183]; a review of the manufacturer's database estimated an overall incidence rate of 0.015%. In most patients, the syndrome abates with drug discontinuation, but in patients with progressive anemia and renal failure, plasmapheresis has been used with inconsistent results, while rituximab has effectively terminated this potentially lethal side effect in a few patients.[184] Severe pulmonary toxicity, presenting as acute respiratory distress associated with interstitial pneumonitis, occurs in 0.1% in patients treated with GEM.[185] GEM may exacerbate the pulmonary toxicity of bleomycin. A study substituting GEM for etoposide in the BEACOPP regimen in Hodgkin's lymphoma led to severe pulmonary toxicity, possibly as a result of GEM interaction with bleomycin.[186] Rare cases of posterior reversible encephalopathy, with altered mental status, have been attributed to GEM.[187]

A multicenter study evaluated the role of GEM in patients with hepatic or renal dysfunction.[188] Patients with elevated bilirubin experienced increased toxicity and should receive reduced doses, whereas elevated transaminases without bilirubin abnormality did not lead to increase toxicity. Patients with elevated creatinine appeared to be more sensitive to GEM, perhaps due to dFdU retention, but there are no guidelines for dose reduction for these patients.

Radiation Sensitization

Because of its inhibition of RNR and, incorporation into DNA, GEM has strong radiosensitizing effects. Preclinical studies of GEM have shown potent radiosensitization in human epithelial cancer cell lines.[189,190] These effects parallel the intracellular depletion of deoxyadenosine triphosphate and are most prominent when the drug is administered before radiation therapy. Radiation recall reactions may occur when GEM is administered after irradiation. Maximal enhancement of radiation sensitization occurs when GEM is administered before radiation. DNA damage is most pronounced when this time interval is 24 to 60 hours. Radiosensitization is most evident in mismatch repair-deficient cells[191] and depends on the presence of intact homologous recombination.[192] These studies suggest that DNA damage results from depletion of nucleotide pools and mismatch incorporation of deoxynucleotides into DNA.

Despite the radiosensitization seen in preclinical studies, the initial phase I and II studies of GEM and radiation therapy have not demonstrated markedly improved clinical activity and are associated primarily with increased toxicity. In a phase I trial of twice-weekly GEM and concurrent radiation in patients with advanced pancreatic cancer, the MTD was 40 mg/m² administered over 30 minutes on Monday and Thursday of each week.[193] The dose-limiting toxicities were grade 3 neutropenia, thrombocytopenia, nausea, and vomiting. This regimen was subsequently evaluated in phase II study for patients with locally advanced pancreatic cancer, and the median survival was 7.9 months.[194] When given once weekly with radiation at doses of 300 to 500 mg/m² to patients with locally advanced pancreatic cancer, the drug caused severe toxicity and no improvement in survival compared to historical controls treated with 5-fluorouracil and radiation therapy.[195] Other trials in head and neck cancer[196] and lung cancer[197] led to unacceptable rates of mucosal and lung toxicity, respectively. A most recent study in glioma patients identified a phase II dose of 750 mg/m²/wk given in the last 4 weeks of a 6-week course of 60-Gy irradiation. Therapeutic efficacy was promising.[198]

References

1. Bergmann W, Feeney R. Contributions to the study of marine products: XXXII. The nucleosides of sponges. *J Org Chem.* 1951;16:981-987.
2. Roberts WK, Dekker CA. A convenient synthesis of arabinosylcytosine (cytosine arabinoside). *J Org Chem.* 1967;32:816-817.
3. Mayer RJ, Davis RB, Schiffer CA, et al. Intensive chemotherapy in adults with acute myeloid leukemia. *N Engl J Med.* 1994;331:896-903.
4. Bloomfield CD, Lawrence D, Byrd JC, et al. Frequency of prolonged remission duration after high-dose cytarabine by cytogenetic subtype. *Cancer Res.* 1998;58:4173-4179.
5. Townsend AJ, Cheng YC. Sequence-specific effects of ara-5-aza-CTP and ara-CTP on DNA synthesis by purified human DNA polymerases in vitro: visualization of chain elongation on a defined template. *Mol Pharmacol.* 1987;32:330-339.
6. Chu MY, Fischer GA. A proposed mechanism of action of 1-β-D-arabinofuranosylcytosine as an inhibitor of the growth of leukemic cells. *Biochem Pharmacol.* 1962;11:423-430.
7. Yoshida S, Yamada M, Masaki S. Inhibition of DNA polymerase-α and -β of calf thymus by 1-β-D-arabinofuranosylcytosine-5′-triphosphate. *Biochim Biophys Acta.* 1977;477:144-150.
8. Fram RJ, Kufe DW. Inhibition of DNA excision repair and the repair of x-ray-induced DNA damage by cytosine arabinoside and hydroxyurea. *Pharmacol Ther.* 1985;31:165-176.
9. Kufe WE, Major PP, Egan EM, et al. Correlation of cytotoxicity with incorporation of araC into DNA. *J Biol Chem.* 1980;255:8997-9000.
10. Kufe DW, Munroe D, Herrick D, et al. Effects of 1-β-D-arabinofuranosylcytosine incorporation on eukaryotic DNA template function. *Mol Pharmacol.* 1984;26:128-134.
11. Kufe DW, Spriggs DR. Biochemical and cellular pharmacology of cytosine arabinoside. *Semin Oncol.* 1985;12:34-48.
12. Mikita T, Beardsley GP. Functional consequences of the arabinosylcytosine structural lesion in DNA. *Biochemistry.* 1988;27:4698-4705.
13. Major P, Egan E, Herrick D, et al. The effects of ara-C incorporation o DNA synthesis. *Biochem Pharmacol.* 1982;31:2937-2940.
14. Woodcock DM, Fox RM, Cooper IA. Evidence for a new mechanism of cytotoxicity of 1-β-D-arabinofuranosylcytosine. *Cancer Res.* 1979;39:418-424.
15. Moore EC, Cohen SS. Effects of arabinonucleotides on ribonucleotide reduction by an enzyme system from rat tumor. *J Biol Chem.* 1967;242:2116-2118.
16. Hawtrey AO, Scott-Burden T, Robertson G. Inhibition of glycoprotein and glycolipid synthesis in hamster embryo cells by cytosine arabinoside and hydroxyurea. *Nature.* 1974;252:58-60.
17. Bianchi Scarra GL, Romani M, Civiello DA, et al. Terminal erythroid differentiation in the K-562 cell line by 1-β-D-arabinofuranosylcytosine: accompaniment by c-myc messenger RNA decrease. *Cancer Res.* 1986;46:6327-6332.
18. Gunji H, Kharbanda S, Kufe D. Induction of internucleosomal DNA fragmentation in human myeloid leukemia cells by 1-β-D-arabinofuranosylcytosine. *Cancer Res.* 1991;51:741-743.
19. Strum JC, Small GW, Pauig SB, et al. 1-β-D-arabinofuranosylcytosine stimulates ceramide and diglyceride formation in HL-60 cells. *J Biol Chem.* 1994;269:15493-15497.
20. Kharbanda S, Datta R, Kufe D. Regulation of c-jun gene expression in HL-60 leukemia cells by 1-β-D-arabinofuranosylcytosine. Potential involvement of a protein kinase C dependent mechanism. *Biochemistry.* 1991;30:7947-7952.
21. Bullock G, Ray S, Reed J, et al. Evidence against a direct role for the induction of c-jun expression in the mediation of drug-induced apoptosis in human acute leukemia cells. *Clin Cancer Res.* 1995;1:559-564.
22. Dou QP, An B, Will P. Induction of a retinoblastoma phosphatase activity by anticancer drugs accompanies p53-independent G₁ arrest and apoptosis. *Proc Natl Acad Sci U S A.* 1995;92:9019-9023.
23. Wiley JS, Jones SP, Sawyer WH, et al. Cytosine arabinoside influx and nucleoside transport sites in acute leukemia. *J Clin Invest.* 1982;69:479-489.
24. Pui CH, Relling MV, Downing JR. Acute lymphoblastic leukemia. *N Engl J Med.* 2004;350:1535-1548.
25. Catala A, Pastor-Anglada M, Caviedas-Cardenas L, et al. FLT3 is implicated in cytarabine transport by human equilibrative nucleoside transporter 1 in pediatric acute leukemia. *Oncotarget.* 2016;7:49786-49799.
26. White JC, Rathmell JP, Capizzi RL. Membrane transport influences the rate of accumulation of cytosine arabinoside in human leukemia cells. *J Clin Invest.* 1987;79:380-387.
27. Cai J, Damaraju VL, Grouix N, et al. Two distinct molecular mechanisms underlying cytarabine resistance in human leukemic cells. *Cancer Res.* 2008;68:2349-2357.
28. Damaraju VL, Damarjus S, Young JD, et al. Nucleoside anticancer drugs: the role of nucleoside transporters in resistance to cancer chemotherapy. *Oncogene.* 2003;22:7524-7536.
29. Drenberg C, Gibson A, Pounds S, et al. OCTN1 is a high-affinity carrier of nucleoside analogues. *Cancer Res.* 2017;77:2102-2111.
30. Drenberg C, Hiu S, Buelow D, et al. ABCC4 is a determinant of cytarabine-induced cytotoxicity and myelosuppression. *Clin Transl Sci.* 2016;9:51-59.

31. Hapke DM, Stegmann APA, Mitchell BS. Retroviral transfer of deoxycytidine kinase into tumor cell lines enhances nucleoside toxicity. *Cancer Res.* 1996;56:2343-2347.

32. Lachmann N, Czarnecki K, Brennig S, et al. Deoxycytidine kinase knockdown as a novel myeloprotective strategy in the context of fludarabine, cytarabine, or cladribine therapy. *Leukemia.* 2015;29:2266-2269.

33. Coleman CN, Stoller RG, Drake JC, et al. Deoxycytidine kinase: properties of the enzyme from human leukemic granulocytes. *Blood.* 1975;46:791-803.

34. Hande KR, Chabner BA. Pyrimidine nucleoside monophosphate kinase from human leukemic blast cells. *Cancer Res.* 1978;38:579-585.

35. Chou T-C, Arlin Z, Clarkson BD, et al. Metabolism of 1-β-D-arabinofuranosylcytosine in human leukemic cells. *Cancer Res.* 1977;37:3561-3570.

36. Chabner B, Johns D, Coleman C, et al. Purification and properties of cytidine deaminase from normal and leukemic granulocytes. *J Clin Invest.* 1974;53:922-931.

37. Ellims P, Kao AH, Chabner BA. Deoxycytidylate deaminase: purification and kinetic properties of the enzyme isolated from human spleen. *J Biol Chem.* 1987;256:6335-6340.

38. Kim L, Cheong H, Koh Y et al. Cytidine deaminase polymorphisms and worse treatment response in normal karyotype AML. *J Hum Genet.* 2015;60:749-754.

39. Amaki J, Onizuka M, Ohmachi K, et al. Single nucleotide polymorphisms of cytarabine metabolic genes influence treatment outcome in acute myeloid leukemia patients receiving high-dose cytarabine therapy. *Int J Hematol.* 2015;101:543-553.

40. Lauzon GJ, Paran JH, Paterson ARP. Formation of 1-β-D-arabinofuranosylcytosine diphosphate choline in cultured human leukemic RPMI 6410 cells. *Cancer Res.* 1978;38:1723-1729.

41. Myers-Robfogel MW, Spatato AC. 1-β-D-Arabinofuranosylcytosine nucleotide inhibition of sialic acid metabolism in WI-38 cells. *Cancer Res.* 1980;40:1940-1943.

42. Fordham SE, Cole M, Irving JA, Allan JM. Cytarabine preferentially induces mutation at specific sequences in the genome which are identifiable in relapsed acute myeloid leukeamia. *Leukemia.* 2015;29:491-494.

43. Chu MY, Fischer GA. Comparative studies of leukemic cells sensitive and resistant to cytosine arabinoside. *Biochem Pharmacol.* 1965;14:333-341.

44. Tattersall MNH, Ganeshaguru K, Hoffbrand AV. Mechanisms of resistance of human acute leukaemia cells to cytosine arabinoside. *Br J Haematol.* 1974;27:39-46.

45. Marin J, Briz O, Rodrigues-Macias G, et al. Role of drug transport and metabolism in the chemoresistance of acute myeloid leukemia. *Blood Rev.* 2016;30:55-64.

46. Chiba P, Tihan T, Szekeres T, et al. Concordant changes of pyrimidine metabolism in blasts of two cases of acute myeloid leukemia after repeated treatment with ara-C in vivo. *Leukemia.* 1990;4:761-765.

47. Smyth JF, Robins AB, Leese CL. The metabolism of cytosine arabinoside as a predictive test for clinical response to the drug in acute myeloid leukaemia. *Eur J Cancer.* 1976;12:567-573.

48. Estey E, Plunkett W, Dixon D, et al. Variables predicting response to high dose cytosine arabinoside therapy in patients with refractory acute leukemia. *Leukemia.* 1987;1:580-583.

49. Estey EH, Keating MJ, McCredie KB, et al. Cellular ara-CTP pharmacokinetics, response, and karyotype in newly diagnosed acute myelogenous leukemia. *Leukemia.* 1990;4:95-99.

50. Preisler HD, Rustum Y, Priore RL. Relationship between leukemic cell retention of cytosine arabinoside triphosphate and the duration of remission in patients with acute non-lymphocytic leukemia. *Eur J Cancer Clin Oncol.* 1985;21:23-30.

51. Schneider C, Oellerich T, Baldauf HM, et al. SAMHD1 is a biomarker for cytarabine response and a therapeutic target in acute myeloid leukemia. *Nat Med.* 2017;2:250.

52. Herold N, Rudd SG, Ljungblad L, et al. Targeting SAMHD1 with the Vpx protein to improve cytarabine therapy for hematological malignancies. *Nat Med.* 2017;2:256.

53. Plunkett W, Iacoboni S, Keating MJ. Cellular pharmacology and optimal therapeutic concentrations of 1-β-D-arabinofuranosylcytosine 5′-triphosphate in leukemic blasts during treatment of refractory leukemia with high-dose 1-β-D-arabinofuranosylcytosine. *Scand J Haematol.* 1986;34:51-59.

54. Ibrado AM, Uang Y, Fang G, et al. Overexpression of Bcl-2 or Bcl-xL inhibits araC-induced CPP32/Yama protease activity and apoptosis of human acute myelogenous leukemia HL-60 cells. *Cancer Res.* 1996;56:4743-4748.

55. Campos L, Rouault J, Sabido O, et al. High expression of bcl-2 protein in acute myeloid leukemia cells is associated with poor response to chemotherapy. *Blood.* 1993;81:3091-3096.

56. Young RC, Schein PS. Enhanced antitumor effect of cytosine arabinoside given in a schedule dictated by kinetic studies in vivo. *Biochem Pharmacol.* 1973;22:277-280.

57. Raza A, Preisler HD, Day R, et al. Direct relationship between remission duration in acute myeloid leukemia and cell cycle kinetics: a leukemia intergroup study. *Blood.* 1990;76:2191-2197.

58. Sinkule JA, Evans WE. High-performance liquid chromatographic assay for cytosine arabinoside, uracil arabinoside, and some related nucleosides. *J Chromatogr.* 1983;274:87-93.

59. Harris AL, Potter C, Bunch C, et al. Pharmacokinetics of cytosine arabinoside in patients with acute myeloid leukaemia. *Br J Clin Pharmacol.* 1979;8:219-237.

60. Van Prooijen R, van der Kleijn E, Haanen C. Pharmacokinetics of cytosine arabinoside in acute leukemia. *Clin Pharmacol Ther.* 1977;21:744-750.

61. Slevin ML, Piall EM, Aherne GW, et al. Effect of dose and schedule on pharmacokinetics of high-dose cytosine arabinoside in plasma and cerebrospinal fluid. *J Clin Oncol.* 1983;1:546-551.

62. Early AP, Preisler HD, Slocum H, et al. A pilot study of high-dose of 1-β-D-arabinofuranosylcytosine for acute leukemia and refractory-lymphoma: clinical response and pharmacology. *Cancer Res.* 1982;42:1587-1594.

63. Donehower RC, Karp JE, Burke PJ. Pharmacology and toxicity of high-dose cytarabine by 72-hour continuous infusion. *Cancer Treat Rep.* 1986;70:1059-1065.

64. Wau SH, Huffman DH, Azarnoff DL, et al. Pharmacokinetics of 1-β-D-arabinofuranosylcytosine in humans. *Cancer Res.* 1974;34:392-397.

65. Markman M. The intracavitary administration of cytarabine to patients with nonhematopoietic malignancies: pharmacologic rationale and results of clinical trials. *Semin Oncol.* 1985;12(suppl 3):177-183.

66. Kirmani S, Zimm S, Cleary SM, et al. Extremely prolonged continuous intraperitoneal infusion of cytosine arabinoside. *Cancer Chemother Pharmacol.* 1990;25:454-458.

67. Ho DHW, Frei EIII. Clinical pharmacology of 1-β-D-arabinofuranosylcytosine. *Clin Pharmacol Ther.* 1971;12:944-954.

68. Chamberlain MC, Khatibi S, Kim JC, et al. Treatment of leptomeningeal metastasis with intraventricular administration of Depot cytarabine (DTC 101). *Arch Neurol.* 1993;50:261-254.

69. Howell SB, Glantz MJ, LaFollette S, et al. A controlled trial of Depocyt™ for the treatment of lymphomatous meningitis [abstract 34]. *Proc Am Soc Clin Oncol.* 1999;18:11a.

70. Cole BF, Glantz MJ, Jaeckle KA, et al. Quality-of-life-adjusted survival comparison of sustained-release cytosine arabinoside versus intrathecal methotrexate for treatment of solid tumor neoplastic meningitis. *Cancer.* 2003;97:3053-3060.

71. Gonzalez-Barca E, Caneales M, Salar A, et al. Central nervous system prophylaxis with intrathecal liposomal cytarabine in a subset of high risk patients with diffuse large B-cell lymphoma receiving first line systemic therapy in a prospective trial. *Ann Hematol.* 2016;95:893-899.

72. Jahn F, Jordan K, Behlendorf T, et al. Safety and efficacy of liposomal cytarabine in the treatment of neoplastic meningitis. *Oncology.* 2015;89:137-142.

73. Capizzi RL, Powell BL, Cooper MR, et al. Dose-related pharmacologic effects of high-dose araC and its use in combination with asparaginase for the treatment of patients with acute nonlymphocytic leukemia. *Scand J Haematol.* 1986;34(suppl 44):17-23.

74. Wisch JS, Griffin JD, Kufe DN. Response of preleukemic syndromes to continuous infusion of low-dose cytarabine. *N Engl J Med.* 1983;309:1599-1602.

75. Tilly H, Bastard C, Bizet M, et al. Low-dose cytarabine: persistence of a clonal abnormality during complete remission of acute nonlymphocytic leukemia. *N Engl J Med.* 1986;314:246-247.

76. Frei E III, Bickers JN, Hewlett JS, et al. Dose schedule and antitumor studies of arabinosyl cytosine (NSC 63878). *Cancer Res.* 1969;29:1325-1332.

77. Mitchell MS, Wade ME, DeConti RC, et al. Immunosuppressive effects of cytosine arabinoside and methotrexate in man. *Ann Intern Med.* 1969;70:535-547.

78. Slavin RE, Dias MA, Saral R. Cytosine arabinoside-induced gastrointestinal toxic alterations in sequential chemotherapeutic protocols. *Cancer.* 1978;42:1747-1759.

79. Altman A, Dinndorf P, Quinn JJ. Acute pancreatitis in association with cytosine arabinoside therapy. *Cancer.* 1982;49:1384-1386.

80. Weisman SJ, Scoopo FJ, Johnson GM, et al. Septicemia in pediatric oncology patients: the significance of viridans streptococcal infections. *J Clin Oncol.* 1990;8:453-459.

81. George CB, Mansour RP, Redmond J, et al. Hepatic dysfunction and jaundice following high-dose cytosine arabinoside. *Cancer.* 1984;54:2360-2362.

82. Rubin EH, Anderson JW, Berg DT, et al. Risk factors for high-dose cytarabine neurotoxicity: an analysis of a cancer and leukemia group B trial in patients with acute myeloid leukemia. *J Clin Oncol.* 1992;10:948-953.

83. Shaw PJ, Procopis PG, Menser MA, et al. Bulbar and pseudobulbar palsy complicating therapy with high-dose cytosine arabinoside in children with leukemia. *Med Pediatr Oncol.* 1991;19:122-125.

84. Paul M, Joshua D, Rahme N, et al. Fatal peripheral neuropathy associated with axonal degeneration after high-dose cytosine arabinoside in acute leukemia. *Br J Haematol.* 1991;79:521-523.

85. Flynn TC, Harris TJ, Murphy GF, et al. Neutrophilic eccrine hidradenitis: a distinctive rash associated with cytarabine therapy and acute leukemia. *J Am Acad Dermatol.* 1984;11:584-590.

86. Fordham SE, Cole M, Irving JA, Allan JM. Cytarabine preferentially induces mutation at specific sequences in the genome which are identifiable in relapsed acute myeloid leukemia. *Leukemia.* 2015;29:491-494.

87. Fanuillino R, Mercier C, Serdjebi C, et al. Lethal toxicity after administration of azacytidine: implication of the cytidine deaminase-deficiency syndrome. *Pharmacogenet Genomics.* 2015;25:317-321.

88. Cicolini J, Serdjebi C, Peters G, Giovannetti E. Pharmacokinetics and pharmacogenetics of gemcitabine as a mainstay in adult and pediatric oncology: an EORTC-PAMM perspective. *Cancer Chemother Pharmacol.* 2016;78:1-12.

89. Kleinschmidt-DeMasters BK, Yeh M. "Locked-in syndrome" after intrathecal cytosine arabinoside therapy for malignant immunoblastic lymphoma. *Cancer.* 1992;70:2504-2507.

90. Kern DH, Morgan CR, Hildebrand-Zanki SU. In vitro pharmacodynamics of 1-β-D-arabinofuranosylcytosine: synergy of antitumor activity with cis-diamminedichloroplatinum(II). *Cancer Res.* 1988;48:117-121.

91. Ho DHW, Carter CJ, Brown NS, et al. Effects of tetrahydrouridine on the uptake and metabolism of 1-β-D-arabinofuranosylcytosine in human normal and leukemic cells. *Cancer Res.* 1980;40:2441-2445.

92. Wong PP, Currie VE, Mackey RW, et al. Phase I evaluation of tetrahydrouridine combined with cytosine arabinoside. *Cancer Treat Rep.* 1979;63:1245-1249.

93. Kemena A, Gandhi V, Shewach DS, et al. Inhibition of fludarabine metabolism by arabinosylcytosine during therapy. *Cancer Chemother Pharmacol.* 1992;31:193-199.

94. Gandhi V, Estey E, Du M, et al. Minimum dose of fludarabine for the maximal modulation of 1-β-D-arabinofuranosylcytosine triphosphate in human leukemia blasts during therapy. *Clin Cancer Res.* 1997;3:1539-1545.

95. Woelich SK, Braun JT, Schoen MW, et al. Efficacy and toxicity of induction therapy with cladribine, idarubicin, and cytarabine (IAC) for acute myeloid leukemia. *Anticancer Res.* 2017;37; 713-717.

96. Bakic M, Chan D, Andersson BS, et al. Effect of 1-β-D-arabinofuranosylcytosine on nuclear topoisomerase II activity and on the DNA cleavage and cytotoxicity produced by 4'-(9-acridinylamino)methanesulfon-m-anisidide and etoposide in m-AMSA-sensitive and -resistant human leukemia cells. *Biochem Pharmacol.* 1987;36:4067-4077.

97. Stone RM, Berg DT, George SL, et al. Granulocyte-macrophage colony-stimulating factor after initial chemotherapy for elderly patients with primary acute myelogenous leukemia. *N Engl J Med.* 1995;332(25):1671-1677.

98. Tardi P, Johnstone S, Harasym N, et al. In vivo maintenance of synergistic cytarabine:daunorubicin ratios greatly enhances therapeutic efficacy. *Leuk Res.* 2009;33:129-139.

99. Mayer LD, Harasym TO, Tardi PG, et al. Ratiometric dosing of anticancer drug combinations: controlling drug ratios after systemic administration regulates therapeutic activity in tumor-bearing mice. *Mol Cancer Ther.* 2006;5:1854-1863.

100. Pharmacokinetics of CPX-351; a nano-scale liposomal fixed molar ratio formulation of cytarabine:daunorubicin, in patients with advanced leukemia—ScienceDirect. Available at http://www.sciencedirect.com.ezp-prod1.hul.harvard.edu/science/article/pii/S0145212612002937#bib0075. Accessed August 31, 2017.

101. Kim HP, Gerhard B, Harasym TO, Mayer LD, Hogge DE. Liposomal encapsulation of a synergistic molar ratio of cytarabine and daunorubicin enhances selective toxicity for acute myeloid leukemia progenitors as compared to analogous normal hematopoietic cells. *Exp Hematol.* 2011;39:741-750.

102. Lancet JE, Cortes JE, Hogge DE, et al. Phase 2 trial of CPX-351, a fixed 5:1 molar ratio of cytarabine/daunorubicin, vs cytarabine/daunorubicin in older adults with untreated AML. *Blood.* 2014;123:3239-3246.

103. Lancet JE, Uy GL, Cortes JE, et al. Final results of a phase III randomized trial of CPX-351 versus 7+3 in older patients with newly diagnosed high risk (secondary) AML. *J Clin Oncol.* 2016;34:7000.

104. Medeiros BC, Lancet JE, Cortes JE, et al. Analysis of efficacy by age for patients aged 60-75 with untreated secondary acute myeloid leukemia (AML) treated with CPX-351 liposome injection versus conventional cytarabine and daunorubicin in a phase III trial. *Blood.* 2016;128:902.

105. Diesch J, Zwick A, Garz A-K, et al. A clinical-molecular update on aza-nucleoside-based therapy for the treatment of hematologic cancers. *Clin Epigenetics.* 2016;8:71-88.

106. Christman JK. 5-Azacytidine and 5-aza-2'-deoxycytidine as inhibitors of DNA methylation: mechanistic studies and their implications for cancer therapy. *Oncogene.* 2002; 21:5483-5495.

107. Steensma DP, Baer MR, Slack JL, et al. Multicenter study of decitabine administered daily for 5 days every 4 weeks to adults with myelodysplastic syndromes: the alternative dosing for outpatient treatment (ADOPT) trial. *J Clin Oncol.* 2009;27:3842-3848.

108. Sorm F, Piskala A, Cihak A, et al. 5-Azacytidine, a new highly effective cancerostatic. *Experientia.* 1964;20:202-203.

109. Silverman LR, Demakos EP, Peterson BL, et al. Randomized controlled trial of azacitidine in patients with the myelodysplastic syndrome: a study of the cancer and leukemia group B. *J Clin Oncol.* 2002;20:2429-2440.

110. Galanello R, Stamatoyannopoulos G, Papayannopoulou T. Mechanism of Hb F stimulation by S-stage compounds: in vitro studies with bone marrow cells exposed to 5-azacytidine, araC, or hydroxyurea. *J Clin Invest.* 1988;81:1209-1216.

111. Wolff F, Leisch M, Greil R, et al. The double-edged sword of (re)expression of genes by hypomethylating agents: from viral mimicry to exploitation as priming agents for targeted immune checkpoint modulation. *Cell Commun Signal.* 2017;15:13-27.

112. Glover AB, Leyland-Jones B. Biochemistry of azacytidine: a review. *Cancer Treat Rep.* 1987;71:959-964.

113. Weiss JW, Pitot HC. Inhibition of ribosomal precursor RNA maturation by 5-azacytidine and 8-azaguanine in Novikoff hepatoma cells. *Arch Biochem Biophys.* 1974;165:588-596.

114. Lee T, Karon MR. Inhibition of protein synthesis in 5-azacytidine-treated HeLa cells. *Biochem Pharmacol.* 1976;25:1737-1742.

115. Issa J-P, Kantarjian HM. Targeting DNA methylation. *Clin Cancer Res.* 2009;15:3938-3946.

116. Santi DV, Garrett CE, Barr PJ, On the mechanism of inhibition of DNA cytosine methyltransferases by cytosine analogs. *Cell.* 1983;33:9-10.

117. Santi DV, Norment A, Garrett CE. Covalent bond formation between a DNA-cytosine methyltransferase and DNA containing 5-azacytosine. *Proc Natl Acad Sci U S A.* 1984;81:6993-6997.

118. Issa JP. CpG island methylator phenotype in cancer. *Nat Rev Cancer.* 2004;4:988-993.

119. Cameron EE, Bachman KE, Myohanen S, et al. Synergy of demethylation and histone deacetylase inhibition in the re-expression of genes silenced in cancer. *Nat Genet.* 1999;21:103-107.

120. Jutterman R, Li E, Jaenisch R. Toxicity of 5-aza-2'-deoxycytidine to mammalian cells is mediated primarily by covalent trapping of DNA methyltransferase rather than DNA demethylation. *Proc Natl Acad Sci U S A.* 1994;91:11797-11801.

121. Mund C, Hackonson B, Stresemann C, Lubbert M, Lyko F. Characterization of DNA demethylation effects induced by 5-Aza-2'-deoxycytidine in patients with myelodysplastic syndrome. *Cancer Res.* 2005;65:7086-7090.

122. Palii SS, Van Emburgh BO, Sankpal UT, Brown KD, Robertson KD. DNA methylation inhibitor 5-Aza-2'-deoxycytidine induces reversible genome wide DNA damage that is distinctly influenced by DNA methyltransferase 1 and 3B. *Mol Cell Biol.* 2007;28:752-771.

123. Orta ML, Calderon-Montano JM, Dominguez I, et al. 5-Aza-deoxycytidine causes replication lesions that require Fanconi anemia dependent homologous recombination for repair. *Nucleic Acids Res.* 2013;41:5827-5836.

124. Orta ML, Hoglund A, Calderon-Montano JM, et al. The PARP inhibitor Olaparib disrupts base excision repair of 5-aza-2′-deoxycytidine lesions. *Nucleic Acids Res.* 2014;42:9108-9120.

125. Streisemann C, Lyko F. Modes of action of the DNA methyltransferase inhibitors azacytidine and decitabine. *Int J Cancer.* 2008;123:8-13.

126. Drake JC, Stoller RG, Chabner BA. Characteristics of the enzyme uridine-cytidine kinase isolated from a cultured human cell line. *Biochem Pharmacol.* 1977;26:64-66.

127. Adams RL, Burdon RH. DNA methylation in eukaryotes. *CRC Crit Rev Biochem.* 1992;13:349-384.

128. Bonal FJ, Pareja E, Martin J, et al. Repression of class I H-2K, H-2D antigens or GR9 methylcholanthrene-induced tumour cell clones is related to the level of DNA methylation. *J Immunogenet.* 1986;13:179-186.

129. Richardson B, Kahl L, Lovett EJ, et al. Effect of an inhibitor of DNA methylation on T cells: I. 5-Azacytidine induces T4 expression on T8+ T cells. *J Immunol.* 1986;137:35-39.

130. Orskov A, Treppandahl M, Skovbo A, et al. Hypomethylation and up-regulation of PD-1 in T cells by azacytidine in MDS/AML patients: a rationale for combined targeting of PD-1 and DNA methylation. *Oncotarget.* 2015;6:9612-9626.

131. Chiappinelli K, Strissel P, Desrichard A, et al. Inhibiting DNA methylation causes an interferon response in cancer via dsRNA including endogenous retroviruses. *Cell.* 2015;162:974-986.

132. Karon M, Benedict W. Chromatid breakage: differential effect of inhibitors of DNA synthesis during G2 phase. *Science.* 1972;178:62-67.

133. Bejar R, Lord A, Stevenson K, et al. TET2 mutations predict response to hypomethylating agents in myelodysplastic syndrome patients. *Blood.* 2014;124:2705-2712.

134. Saunthararajah Y, Sekeres M, Advani A, et al. Evaluation of noncytotoxic DNMT1-depleting therapy in patients with myelodysplastic syndromes. *J Clin Invest.* 2015;125:1043-1055.

135. Yan F, Shen N, Pang J, et al. The DNA methyltransferase DNMT1 and tyrosine-protein KIT cooperatively promote resistance to 5-aza-2′deoxycytidine (decitabine) and midostaurin (PKC4123) in lung cancer cells. *J Biol Chem.* 2015;280:18480-18494.

136. Welch JS, Petti AA, Miller CA, et al. TP53 and decitabine in acute myeloid leukemia and myelodysplastic syndromes. *N Engl J Med.* 2016;375:2023-2036.

137. Chou W-C, Yeh S-P, Hsiao L-T, et al. Efficacy, safety and pharmacokinetics of subcutaneous azacytidine in Taiwanese patients with higher-risk myelodysplastic syndromes. *Asia Pac J Clin Oncol.* 2017;13:e430-e439.

138. Karahoca M, Momparler R. Pharmacokinetic and pharmacodynamic analysis of 5-aza-2′-deoxycytidine (decitabine) in the design of its dose-schedule for cancer therapy. *Clin Epigenetics.* 2013;5:3-19.

139. Qin T, Castoro E, El Ahdab S, et al. Mechanisms of resistance to decitabine in the myelodysplastic syndrome. *PLoS One.* 2011;6:e23372. doi:10.1371/journal.pone.0023372.

140. Zhao M, Rudek MA, He P, et al. Quantification 5-azacytidine in plasma by electrospray tandem mass spectrometry couples with high performance liquid chromatography. *J Chromatogr B Analyt Technol Biomed Life Sci.* 2004;813:81-88.

141. Tsao CF, Dalal J, Peters C, et al. Azacitidine pharmacokinetics in an adolescent patient with renal compromise. *J Pediatr Hematol Oncol.* 2007;29:330-333.

142. Chabner BA, Drake JC, Johns DC. Deamination of 5-azaytidine by a human leukemia cell cytidine deaminase. *Biochem Pharmacol.* 1973;48:331-2765.

143. Vogler WR, Miller DS, Keller JW. 5-Azacytidine (NSC-102816): a new drug for the treatment of myeloblastic leukemia. *Blood.* 1976;48:331-337.

144. Jones PA, Taylor SM, Wilson V. DNA modification, differentiation, and transformation. *J Exp Zool.* 1983;228:287-295.

145. Cogle CR, Scott BL, Boyd T, Garcia-Manero G. Oral azacitidine(CC-486) for the treatment of myelodysplastic syndromes and acute myeloid leukemia. *Oncologist.* 2015;20:1404-1412.

146. Bellet RE, Mastrangelo MJ, Engstrom PF, et al. Hepatotoxicity of 5-azacytidine (NSC-102816): a clinical and pathologic study. *Neoplasma.* 1973;20:303-309.

147. Levi J, Wiernik P. A comparative clinical trial of 5-azacytidine and guanazole in previously treated adults with acute nonlymphocytic leukemia. *Cancer.* 1976;38:36-41.

148. Kaminskas E, Farrell AT, Wang YC, et al. FDA Drug approval summary: azacytidine (5 azacytidine, Vidaza™) for injectable suspension. *Oncologist.* 2005;10:176-182.

149. Fenaux P, Ghulam JM, Hellstrom-Lindberg E, et al. Efficacy of azacytidine compared with that of conventional care regimens in the treatment of higher-risk myelodysplastic syndromes: a randomized, open-label, phase III study. *Lancet Oncol.* 2009;10:223-232.

150. Sekeres MS, Othus M, List AF, et al. Randomized phase II study of azacytidine alone or in combination with lenalidomide and or vorinostat in higher-risk myelodysplastic syndromes and chronic myelomonocytic leukemia: North American Intergroup Study SWOG S1117. *J Clin Oncol.* 2017;36:2745-2753.

151. Dombret J, Seymour JF, Butrym A, et al. International phase 3 study of azacytidine vs conventional care regimens in older patients with newly diagnosed AML with >30% blasts. *Blood.* 2015;126:291-299.

152. Burris HA III, Moore MJ, Andersen J, et al. Improvements in survival and clinical benefit with gemcitabine as first-line therapy for patients with advanced pancreas cancer: a randomized trial. *J Clin Oncol.* 1997;15:2403-2413.

153. von der Maase H, Hansen SW, Robert JT, et al. Gemcitabine and cisplatin versus methotrexate, vinblastine, doxorubicin, and cisplatin in advanced or metastatic bladder cancer: results of a large, randomized, multinational, multicenter phase III study. *J Clin Oncol.* 2000;18:3068-3077.

154. Schiller JH, Harrington D, Belani CP, et al. Comparison of four chemotherapy regimens for advanced non-small cell lung cancer. *N Engl J Med.* 2002;346:92-98.

155. Mackey JR, Mani RS, Selner M, et al. Functional nucleoside transporters are required for gemcitabine influx and manifestation of toxicity in cancer cell lines. *Cancer Res.* 1998;58:4349-4357.

156. Heinemann V, Hertel LW, Grindey GB, et al. Comparison of the cellular pharmacokinetics and toxicity of 2′,2′-difluorodeoxycytidine and 1-beta-D-arabinofuranosylcytosine. *Cancer Res.* 1988;48:4024-4031.

157. Bouffard DY, Laliberte J, Momparler RL. Kinetic studies on 2′,2′-difluorodeoxycytidine (gemcitabine) with purified human deoxycytidine kinase and cytidine deaminase. *Biochem Pharmacol.* 1993;45:1857-1861.

158. Gandhi V, Plunkett W. Modulatory activity of 2′,2′-difluorodeoxycytidine on the phosphorylation and cytotoxicity of arabinosyl nucleosides. *Cancer Res.* 1990;50:3675-3680.

159. Rockwell S, Grindey GB. Effect of 2′,2′-difluorodeoxycytidine on the viability and radiosensitivity of EMT6 cells in vitro. *Oncol Res.* 1992;4:151-155.

160. Heinemann V, Xu YZ, Chubb S, et al. Inhibition of ribonucleotide reduction in CCRF-CEM cells by 2′,2′-difluorodeoxycytidine. *Mol Pharmacol.* 1990;38:567-572.

161. Wang J, Lohman GJS, Stubbe J. Enhanced subunit interactions with gemcitabine-5′-diphosphate inhibit ribonucleotide reductase. *Proc Natl Acad Sci U S A.* 2007;104:14323-14329.

162. Huang P, Plunkett W. Fludarabine- and gemcitabine-induced apoptosis: incorporation of analogs into DNA is a critical event. *Cancer Chemother Pharmacol.* 1995;36:181-188.

163. Cory AH, Hertel LW, Kroin JS, et al. Effects of 2′,2′-difluorodeoxycytidine (gemcitabine) on wild type and variant mouse leukemia L1210 cells. *Oncol Res.* 1993;5:59-63.

164. Goan YG, Zhou B, Hu E, et al. Overexpression of ribonucleotide reductase as a mechanism of resistance to 2′,2′-difluorodeoxycytidine in human KB cancer line. *Cancer Res.* 1999;59:4204-4207.

165. Lang LY, Li L, Jiang H, et al. Expression of ERCC1 Antisense RNA abrogates gemcitabine-mediated cytotoxic synergism with cisplatin in human colon tumor cells defective in mismatch repair but proficient in nucleotide excision repair. *Clin Cancer Res.* 2000;6:773-781.

166. Kroep JR, Loves WJP, van der Wilt CL, et al. Pretreatment deoxycytidine kinase levels predict in vivo gemcitabine sensitivity. *Mol Cancer Ther.* 2002;1:371-376.

167. Neff T, Blau CA. Forced expression of cytidine deaminase confers resistance to cytosine arabinoside and gemcitabine. *Exp Hematol.* 1996;24:1340-1346.

168. Ireland L, Santos A, Ahmed MS, et al. Chemoresistance in pancreatic cancer is driven by stroma-derived insulin-like growth factors. *Cancer Res.* 2016;76:6851-6863.

169. Wormann SM, Song L, Diakopoulos KN, et al. Loss of P53 function activates JAk2-STAT3signaling to promote pancreatic tumor growth, stroma modification, and gemcitabine resistance in mice and is associated with patient survival. *Gastroenterology.* 2016;15:180-193.

170. Davidson JD, Ma L, Flagella M, et al. An increase in the expression of ribonucleotide reductase large subunit 1 is associated with gemcitabine resistance in non-small cell lung cancer cell lines. *Cancer Res.* 2004;64:3761-3766.

171. Spratlin J, Sangha R, Glubrecht D, et al. The absence of human equilibrative nucleoside transporter 1 is associated with reduced survival in patients with gemcitabine treated pancreas adenocarcinoma. *Clin Cancer Res.* 2004;10:6956-6961.

172. Giovannetti E, Del Tacca M, Mey V, et al. Transcription analysis of human equilibrative nucleoside transporter-1 predicts survival in pancreas cancer patients treated with gemcitabine. *Cancer Res.* 2006;66:3928-3935.

173. Brandi G, Derti M, Vasuri F, et al. Membrane localization of human equilibrative nucleoside transporter 1 in tumor cells may predict response to adjuvant gemcitabine in resected cholangiocarcinoma patients. *Oncologist.* 2016;21:600-607.

174. Shipley LA, Brown TJ, Cornpropst JD, et al. Metabolism and disposition of gemcitabine, and oncolytic deoxycytidine analog, in mice, rats, and dogs. *Drug Metab Dispos.* 1992;20:849-855.

175. Grunewald R, Abbruzzese JL, Tarassoff P, et al. Saturation of 2′,2′-difluorodeoxycytidine 5″-triphosphate accumulation by mononuclear cells during a phase I trial of gemcitabine. *Cancer Chemother Pharmacol.* 1991;27:258-262.

176. Abbruzzese JL, Grunewald R, Weeks EA, et al. A phase I clinical, plasma, and cellular pharmacology study of gemcitabine. *J Clin Oncol.* 1991;9:491-498.

177. Fossella FV, Lippman SM, Shin DM, et al. Maximum-tolerated dose defined for single-agent gemcitabine: a phase I dose-escalation study in chemotherapy-naive patients with advanced non-small cell lung cancer. *J Clin Oncol.* 1997;15:310-316.

178. Touroutoglou N, Gravel D, Raber MN, et al. Clinical results of a pharmacodynamically-based strategy for higher dosing of gemcitabine in patients with solid tumors. *Ann Oncol.* 1998;9:1003-1008.

179. Tempero M, Plunkett W, Ruiz van Haperen V, et al. Randomized phase II comparison of dose-intense gemcitabine: thirty minute infusion and fixed dose rate infusion in patients with pancreatic adenocarcinoma. *J Clin Oncol.* 2003;21:3402-3498.

180. Reid JM, Qu W, Safgren S, et al. Phase I trial and pharmacokinetics of gemcitabine in children with advanced solid tumors. *J Clin Oncol.* 2002;22:2445-2451.

181. Appro MS, Martin C, Hatty S. Gemcitabine—a safety review. *Anticancer Drugs.* 1998;9:191-201.

182. Fung MC, Storniolo AM, Nguyen B, et al. A review of hemolytic uremic syndrome in patients treated with gemcitabine therapy. *Cancer.* 1999;85:2023-2332.

183. Humphreys BD, Sharman JP, Henderson JM, et al. Gemcitabine-associated thrombotic microangiopathy. *Cancer.* 2004;100:2664.

184. Ritchie GE, Fernando M, Goldstein D. Rituximab to treat gemcitabine-induced hemolytic-uremic syndrome (HUS) in pancreatic adenocarcinoma: a case series and literature review. *Cancer Chemother Pharmacol.* 2017;79:1-7.

185. Roychowdhury DF, Cassidy CA, Peterson P, et al. A report on serious pulmonary toxicity associated with gemcitabine-based therapy. *Invest New Drugs.* 2002;20:311-315.

186. Bredenfeld H, Franklin J, Nogova L, et al. Severe pulmonary toxicity in patients with advanced stage Hodgkin's disease treated with a modified bleomycin, doxorubicin, cyclophosphamide, vincristine, procarbazine, prednisone, and gemcitabine (BEACOPP) regimen is probably related to the combination of gemcitabine and bleomycin: a report of the German Hodgkin's Lymphoma Study Group. *J Clin Oncol.* 2004;22:2424-2429.

187. Cherniawsky H, Merchant N, Sawyer M, Ho M. A case report of posterior reversible encephalopathy syndrome in a patient receiving gemcitabine and cisplatin. *Medicine (Baltimore).* 2017;96:e5850.

188. Venook AP, Egorin MK, Rosner GL, et al. Phase I and pharmacokinetic trial of gemcitabine in patients with hepatic or renal dysfunction: Cancer and Leukemia Group B 9565. *J Clin Oncol.* 2000;18:2780-2787.

189. Shewach DS, Hahn TM, Chang E, et al. Metabolism of 2′-2′-difluoro-2′-deoxycytidine and radiation sensitization of human colon carcinoma cells. *Cancer Res.* 1994;54:3218-3223.

190. Lawrence TS, Chang EY, Hahn TM, et al. Radiosensitization of pancreatic cancer cells by 2′,2′-difluoro-2′-deoxycytidine. *Int J Radiat Oncol Biol Phys.* 1996;34:867-872.

191. Flanagan SA, Robinson BW, Krokosky CM, et al. Mismatched nucleotides as the lesions responsible for radiosensitization with gemcitabine; a new paradigm for antimetabolite radiosensitizers. *Mol Cancer Ther.* 2007;6:1858-1868.

192. Im MM, Flanagan SA, Ackroyd JJ, et al. Late DNA damage mediated by homologous recombination repair results in radiosensitization with gemcitabine. *Radiat Res.* 2016;186:466-477.

193. Blackstock AW, Bernard SA, Richards F, et al. Phase I trial of twice-weekly gemcitabine and concurrent radiation in patients with advanced pancreatic cancer. *J Clin Oncol.* 1999;17:2208-2812.

194. Blackstock AW, Tempero MA, Niedzwiecki D, et al. Cancer and Leukemia Group B 89805: phase II chemoradiation trial using gemcitabine in patients with locoregional adenocarcinoma of the pancreas (abstract). *Proc Annu Meet Am Assoc Cancer Res.* 2001;A627.

195. Crane CH, Abbruzzese JL, Evans DB, et al. Is the therapeutic index better with gemcitabine-based chemoradiation than with 5-fluorouracil based chemoradiation in locally advanced pancreatic cancer? *Int J Radiat Oncol Biol Phys.* 2002;52:1293-1302.

196. Eisbruch A, Shewach DS, Bradford CR, et al. Radiation concurrent with gemcitabine for locally advanced head and neck cancer: a phase I trial and intracellular drug incorporation study. *J Clin Oncol.* 2001;19:792-799.

197. Van Putten JW, Price A, van der Leest AH, et al. A phase I study of gemcitabine with concurrent radiotherapy in stage III, locally advanced non-small cell lung cancer. *Clin Cancer Res.* 2003;9:2472-2477.

198. Kim MM, Camelo-Piragua S, Schnipper M, et al. Gemcitabine plus radiation therapy for high-grade glioma: long-term results of a Phase 1 dose-escalation study. *Int J Radiat Oncol Biol Phys.* 2018;94:305-311.

Purine Analogs

Kenneth R. Hande and Bruce A. Chabner

6-Mercapotopurine

Over 60 years ago, 6-mercaptopurine (6-MP) and its closely related cousin, 6-thioguanine were synthesized by Elion and Hitchings as analogs of physiological purines found in DNA, and proved to be essential drugs in the early attempts to cure childhood leukemia.[1] 6-MP remains a primary therapy for adults and children with acute lymphoblastic leukemia (ALL). A second product of the Burroughs-Wellcome research, azathioprine, a prodrug of 6-MP, remains the primary agent for immunosuppression, while 6-thioguanine, once a common treatment for acute myeloid leukemia, is no longer in common use. These three drugs are closely related in structure (Fig. 10.1), metabolism, mechanism of action, and toxicity. The key pharmacologic features of 6-MP are summarized in Table 10.1.

Mechanism of Action

6-MP is a structural analog of hypoxanthine, having a thiol substitution in place of the physiological 6-hydroxyl group (Fig. 10.1). 6-MP requires extensive cellular metabolism for activation and elimination.[2] The initial step of its activation is its conversion to thioinosine monophosphate by the enzyme hypoxanthine guanine phosphoribosyltransferase (HGPRT) followed by[1] T-IMP conversion to a guanine nucleotide by IMP dehydrogenase,[2] its reduction to a deoxynucleotide by ribonucleotide reductase (RNR), and[3] further phosphorylation to form dTGTP, which can then be incorporated into DNA (Fig. 10.2). The quantity of 6-MP metabolite present in DNA correlates with cytotoxicity.[3] Incorporation of 6-dTGTP into DNA triggers programmed cell death by a process involving the mismatch repair pathway.[4] Incorporation of 6-TG deoxynucleotide into DNA also leads to mispairing of bases and miscoding during DNA replication. The mispairing is recognized by proteins of the postreplicative mismatch repair system.[5] Loss of mismatch repair competency is associated with resistance to 6-MP. Methylation of 6-MP nucleotides to methyl thioinosine triphosphate may also contribute to the antiproliferative properties of the thioguanines through the inhibition of de novo purine synthesis by methylmercaptopurine nucleotides.[6] (Fig. 10.2).

6-TG follows a somewhat simpler path to its active metabolite, 6-TdGTP. Significantly higher cellular concentrations of thioguanine nucleotides are seen after 6-TG administration than with 6-MP.[7]

Azathioprine (Fig. 10.1) is rapidly cleaved in plasma by nonenzymatic mechanisms to 6-MP and methyl-4-nitro-5-imidazole derivatives (Fig. 10.2). Although incorporation of false nucleotides into DNA and inhibition of purine synthesis by 6-MP ribonucleotides are the probable mechanisms for cytotoxicity, other mechanisms may underlie its suppression of the T-cell response. 6-thioguanine triphosphate (6-TGTP) binds to and inhibits Rac1, a small GTP-binding protein. Rac proteins play a major role in T-cell development, differentiation, and proliferation. The activation of Rac1 targeted genes, such as mitogen-activated protein kinase (MEK), $NF_k B$, and bcl-X_L, is suppressed by azathioprine leading to T-cell apoptosis.[8]

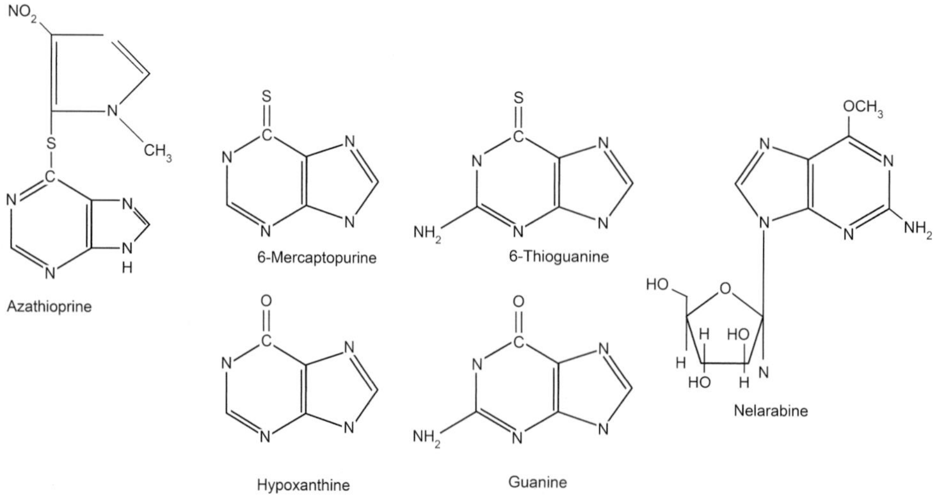

FIGURE **10.1** Structures of the naturally occurring purines, guanine and hypoxanthine, and related *antineoplastic* agents 6-mercaptopurine, 6-thioguanine, and nelarabine, and the immunosuppressant, azathioprine.

<table>
<tr><td colspan="2"></td></tr>
</table>

TABLE 10.1 *Key features of mercaptopurine*

Factor	Results
Mechanism of action	1. Primary: incorporation of metabolites into DNA causes miscoding during DNA replication. Correlates with cytotoxicity 2. Secondary: inhibits de novo purine synthesis; incorporated into RNA
Metabolism	Activation: conversion to thiopurine nucleotides Catabolism: to 6-thiouric acid by xanthine oxidase Catabolism: to 6-methylthiopurine by TPMT (thiopurine methyltransferase)
Pharmacokinetics	$t_{1/2}$: 50 min in plasma Poor (<25%) and variable oral bioavailability
Elimination	Metabolism, by xanthine oxidase and TPMT
Drug interactions	Allopurinol decreases mercaptopurine elimination. Concomitant use of these two drugs requires dose reduction (75%) Mesalamine, sulphasalazine, and olsalazine inhibit TPMT increasing thiopurine toxicity
Toxicity	1. Myelosuppression 2. Mild gastrointestinal (nausea, vomiting) 3. Hepatotoxicity including venoocclusive disease 4. Immunosuppression
Precautions	1. Dose reductions with allopurinol 2. Persons with genetic deficiency of TPMT will have significantly increased toxicity (genetic screening available to test for TPMT deficiency)

Clinical Pharmacology

6-MP is available in 50-mg tablets, and is administered in a dose of 75 mg/m^2 in maintenance therapy of ALL. An intravenous preparation of 6-MP has been formulated for research purposes. 6-MP is relatively insoluble and unstable in alkaline solutions.

Plasma 6-MP and metabolite concentrations as low as 0.1 μM can be measured using high-performance liquid chromatography.[9] Following oral administration of 75 mg/m^2, peak plasma concentrations of 0.3 to 1.8 μM are reached within 2 hours.[10] The volume of distribution exceeds that of total body water (0.9 L/kg). There is little penetration into the cerebrospinal fluid (CSF). With high-dose oral 6-MP (500 mg/m^2), plasma 6-MP concentrations of 5 to 12 μM are achieved.[11] Following intravenous dosing, the half-life of 6-MP is 50 to 100 minutes and plasma concentrations of 6-MP reach 25 μM and CSF concentrations 3.8 μM.[12] 6-MP is weakly protein bound in plasma (20% bound).

Oral absorption of 6-MP is incomplete and highly variable.[13] At a dose of 75 mg/m^2, mean 6-MP bioavailability is 16% (range, 5% to 37%).[14] Clearance occurs primarily through two routes of metabolism. 6-MP is oxidized to the inactive metabolite, 6-thiouric acid, by xanthine oxidase (Fig. 10.2). The intestinal mucosa and liver contain high concentrations of the enzyme xanthine oxidase. The low oral bioavailability of 6-MP is the result of a large first-pass effect as drug is absorbed through the intestinal wall into the portal circulation and metabolized by hepatic xanthine oxidase. Allopurinol (an inhibitor of xanthine oxidase) increases 6-MP bioavailability fivefold.[15] Allopurinol does not alter the plasma kinetics of intravenously administered 6-MP, although more 6-MP and less thiouric acid are excreted in the urine when administered with allopurinol.[16] Methotrexate, often used with 6-MP in maintenance treatment of ALL, is a weak inhibitor of xanthine oxidase and modestly increases the bioavailability of 6-MP.[13]

The plasma concentration versus time profile of 6-MP exhibits intrapatient variability.[17] High-dose, oral 6-MP (500 mg/m^2) has been used in an attempt to saturate the first-pass metabolism of 6-MP, thereby increasing bioavailability. However, even at a dose of 500 mg/m^2 6-MP, xanthine oxidase is not saturated and

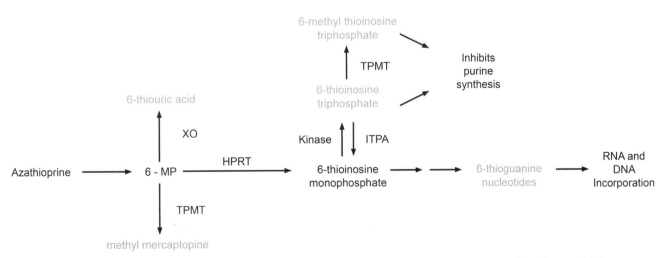

FIGURE 10.2 Mechanism of activation and catabolism of azathioprine and 6-MP. Toxic metabolites are shown in *green*. 6-MP, 6-mercaptopurine; HGPRT, hypoxanthine guanine phosphoribosyltransferase; ITPA, inosine triphosphate pyrophosphatase; XO, xanthine oxidase; TPMT, thiopurine methyltransferase.

bioavailability remains low. Food intake and oral antibiotics reduce the oral absorption of 6-MP.[18] The drug should be taken 1 to 2 hours after a meal.

In addition to the xanthine oxidase catabolic pathway, 6-MP is metabolized by TPMT. Polymorphisms in TPMT activity results in significant interpatient variability in 6-MP metabolism and drug toxicity. As seen in Figure 10.2, TPMT catalyzes the S-methylation of 6-MP to a less active metabolite, 6-methyl mercaptopurine. TMPT also metabolizes thioinosine monophosphate to methyl thioinosine monophosphate, a molecule that inhibits de novo purine biosynthesis. The frequency distribution of TPMT activity in large population studies is trimodal.[19] About 0.5% of subjects have absent enzyme activity; 10% of the population have intermediate activity, and the rest have high enzyme activity. A reciprocal relationship between TPMT activity and the formation of 6-thiopurine nucleotides has been demonstrated.

Over 20 nonsynonymous variations in the TMPT gene have been identified, 17 of which have reduced TMPT activity.[20] (See Chapter 5). Among these genetic variations, three (TPMT*2, TPMT*3A, and TMPT*3C) account for 90% of patients with low or intermediate TMPT activity. The proteins formed by TPMT*2 and TMPT*3A have degradation half-lives of 15 minutes compared to a half-life of 18 hours for wild-type TPMT.[21] Lymphoblasts from individuals homozygous or heterozygous for a variant TMTP gene have lower TMPT activity than do lymphoblasts homozygous for the wild-type gene.[22]

Patients with low TPMT activity are susceptible to greater 6-MP and 6-TG–induced myelosuppression. Genetic testing using PCR-based methods can now identify TPMT-deficient and heterozygous patients.[23] Alternatively, enzyme activity can be measured in circulating red blood cells, although this test may be affected by prior blood transfusions.[24] The FDA has encouraged TMPT testing for pre–B-cell ALL patients who develop myelosuppression while receiving standard dose 6-MP, with subsequent dosage modifications for TMPT-deficient patients.[24] Children with ALL should receive only 5% to 10% of a standard mercaptopurine dose if they are homozygous for a variant TMPT gene and 65% if they are heterozygous.[25]

Several studies,[24,26,27] but not all,[14] have suggested that children with high TPMT activity are at greater risk of disease relapse as a result of drug inactivation. In a large Scandinavian study in children with ALL, the risk of relapse following therapy was 18% for patients with wild-type TPMT versus 6% for patients heterozygous or deficient in TMPT activity ($P = 0.03$). Despite a lower probability of relapse, patients with low TPMT activity did not have superior survival ($P = 0.08$), perhaps due to increased drug toxicity and increased secondary malignancies.[28]

While screening for TMPT variants with decreased enzymatic activity identifies individuals at risk for 6-MP toxicity, the association is not perfect, and other factors, such as variable pharmacokinetics and metabolism, modify toxicity and response. Toxicity still occurs in individuals with wild-type TMPT. Secondly, individuals heterozygous for TPMT*2, *3A, and *3C can have a broad range of TPMT activity. Thirdly, mercaptopurine metabolism is not dependent on a single gene (Fig. 10.2). Inosine triphosphate pyrophosphatase (ITPA) catalyzes the hydrolysis of inosine triphosphate (ITP) to inosine monophosphate, which protects cells from the accumulation

of potentially toxic nucleotides. A polymorphism in the ITPA gene occurring in roughly 10% of individuals results in a 25% decrease in enzyme activity in heterozygous individuals.[29] In children with ALL who have had their mercaptopurine dose adjusted based on TMPT phenotype, the lower activity ITPA allele has been associated with an increase incidence of febrile neutropenia.[30] Relapse in ALL patients on 6-MP in perhaps 60% of cases has been attributed to low adherence to prescribed therapy.[31,32] Biochemical resistance to 6-MP has been ascribed to loss of the initial activating enzyme, HGPRT, and in T-cell ALL, to activating mutations in the 5'nucleotidase II gene, NT5C2, which degrades the monophosphates of 6-MP and 6-TG.[32] This mutation, while found in 20% of T-cell ALL after relapse, occurs in less than 5% of relapsed ALL. Several different point mutations (R367Q, R258W, L375F) significantly increase activity of this enzyme.

Toxicity

The dose-limiting toxicity of 6-MP is myelosuppression, occurring 1 to 4 weeks following the onset of daily oral therapy. Platelets, granulocytes, and erythrocytes are all affected. Weekly monitoring of blood counts during the first 2 months of therapy is recommended. Myelosuppression following 6-MP therapy is related to TPMT phenotype (see above). Most patients (65%) with excessive toxicity following 6-MP or azathioprine administration have TMPT deficiency or heterozygosity.

Like azathioprine, 6-MP is an immunosuppressant. In particular, the T-cell response to infectious agents or vaccines is subnormal in patients receiving 6-MP. Patients are susceptible to fungal and parasitic infection, in addition to bacterial pathogens.

Gastrointestinal mucositis and stomatitis are modest. Approximately one quarter of treated patients experienced nausea, vomiting, and anorexia. Gastrointestinal side effects appear to be more common in adults than in children. Pancreatitis is seen in 3% of patients with long-term therapy. Rash, fever, or joint pains are seen in less than 5%.[28]

Three types of hepatotoxicity may result from thiopurine therapy.[33] A small percentage of patients have transient, asymptomatic elevation in transaminases, which return to normal with follow-up and do not require changes in dose. Thiopurines may induce a several cholestatic jaundice that may not regress, and requires drug discontinuation. Thiopurines may cause endothelial cell injury with raised portal pressures (VOD or venoocclusive disease). The development of hepatotoxicity, in contrast to myelosuppression, is not associated with TPMT polymorphisms[34] but is correlated with the dose of 6-MP given and with the formation of methylated metabolites of 6-MP.[35]

At very high doses (>1,000 mg/m²), the limited solubility of 6-MP can cause precipitation of drug in the renal tubules with hematuria and crystalluria.[36] Children with ALL and with reduced TMPT activity have an increased risk of myelodysplasia or AML following treatment with 6-MP.[37]

Use and Drug Interactions

The only anticancer indication for 6-MP is its use as a standard component of maintenance therapy for ALL. 6-MP is also used to suppress autoimmunity in various noncancer contexts, including inflammatory bowel disease (IBD). As previously mentioned, allopurinol inhibits the catabolism of 6-MP and increases its bioavailability. Oral doses of 6-MP should be reduced by at least 75% in patients also receiving allopurinol.[38] Olsalazine, mesalazine, and sulfasalazine are inhibitors of TPMT and can increase the toxicity of mercaptopurine or azathioprine when used in combination therapy against IBD.[39]

Adenosine Analogs

Adenosine analogs with documented clinical utility are fludarabine, pentostatin, cladribine (2'-chlorodeoxyadenosine), and clofarabine (Fig. 10.3). These drugs have specific indications for subsets of leukemia, either chronic or acute, but several (fludarabine, cladribine, and clofarabine) are also the subject of investigation for high-dose therapies with marrow replacement, and for remission induction in relapsed and high-risk AML.[40] Key pharmacologic features of the adenosine analogs are listed in Tables 10.2 to 10.6.

The original arabinose antipurine, adenosine arabinoside, was cytotoxic in vitro but in man proved ineffective as it was quickly inactivated by the enzyme adenosine deaminase (ADA). Substitution of a halogen (fluorine in fludarabine or chlorine in cladribine) at the two positions of deoxyadenosine produced molecules resistant to ADA.

Fludarabine (Fludara)

Fludarabine (9-β-D-arabinofuranosyl-2-fluoroadenine monophosphate) is a monophosphate analog of adenosine (Fig. 10.3). The monophosphate formulation confers aqueous solubility, allowing intravenous administration,[41] and is quickly hydrolyzed in the bloodstream to the key metabolite, fludarabine. The molecule was designed as an ADA resistant analogue of adenosine, with facile incorporation into DNA, producing chain termination. Key features

TABLE

10.2   *Key features of fludarabine*

Factor	Result
Mechanism of action	1. Incorporation into DNA as a false nucleotide 2. Inhibition of DNA polymerase, DNA primase, and DNA ligase 3. DNA chain termination 4. Inhibition of RNR
Metabolism	1. Rapid dephosphorylation in plasma to 2-fluoro-ara (F-ara-A) 2. Activation of F-ara-A to F-ara-ATP (the active metabolite) within cells. Deoxycytidine kinase is initial step, and rate limiting
Pharmacokinetics	1. Rapid dephosphorylation to 2-F-ara-A 2. $t_{1/2}$ 2-F-ara-A highly variable, 7–33 h in plasma; intracellular $t_{1/2}$ of F-ara-ATP = 15 h
Elimination	Primarily renal excretion of 2-F-ara-A
Drug interactions	Increases cytotoxicity of cytarabine
Toxicity	1. Myelosuppression 2. Immunosuppression with resulting infections 3. Neurotoxicity at high doses 4. Pneumonitis 5. Autoimmune hemolytic anemia and other auto-immune events
Precautions	Dose reduction needed for patients with renal failure (see text)

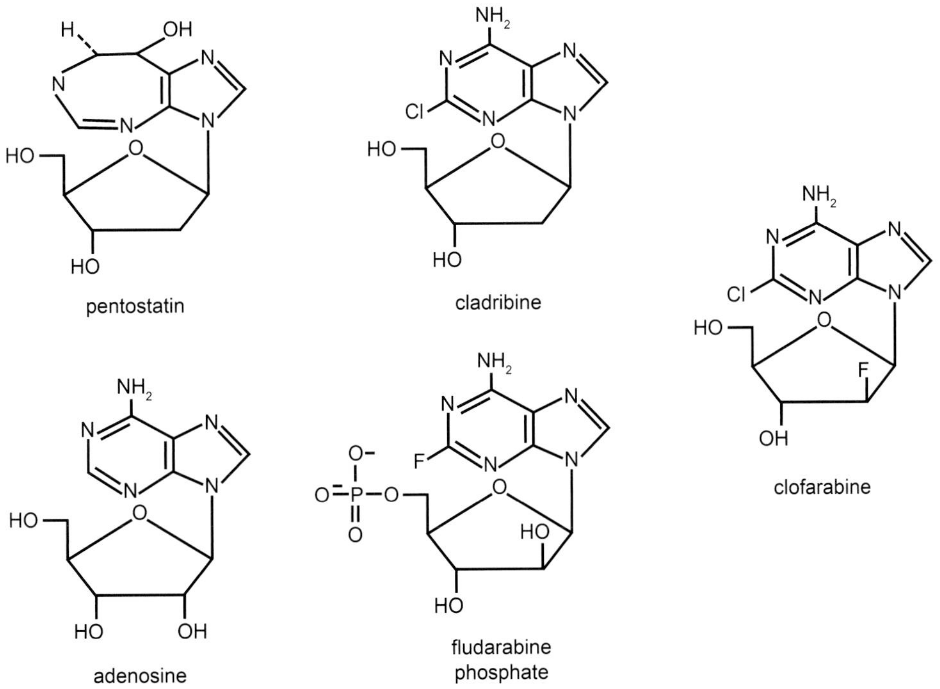

FIGURE **10.3** Chemical structure of adenosine, and adenosine analogues: pentostatin, fludarabine phosphate, cladribine, and clofarabine. Note the ara-configuration of the glycoside in fludarabine. The halogen substitutions in the 2-position on the purine ring in clofarabine, fludarabine, and cladribine render these drugs resistant to adenosine deaminase.

pentostatin

cladribine

clofarabine

adenosine

fludarabine phosphate

TABLE

10.3 *Key features of pentostatin*

Factor	Result
Mechanism of action	1. Inhibits adenosine deaminase (ADA) with subsequent accumulation of dATP pools, which inhibit ribonucleotide reductase, alter pools of other deoxynucleotides
Metabolism	Minimal
Pharmacokinetics	Clearance rate of 8 mL/min/m², which decreases with decreasing creatinine clearance. $t\,\tfrac{1}{2}$ in plasma 6 h
Elimination	Majority of drug is excreted unchanged in the urine
Drug interactions	Increased risk of pulmonary toxicity when continued with fludarabine
Toxicity	1. Well tolerated at low doses 2. At higher doses; nausea, immunosuppression, nephrotoxicity, and CNS disturbances
Precautions	Dose reductions for patients with renal failure

TABLE

10.5 *Key features of clofarabine*

Factor	Result
Mechanism of action	1. Triphosphate metabolites are incorporated into DNA, inhibiting DNA strand elongation 2. Inhibits ribonucleotide reductase lowering deoxynucleotide pools needed for DNA synthesis
Metabolism	Activation to triphosphate metabolite within cells, triphosphate $t\,\tfrac{1}{2}$ 24 h
Pharmacokinetics	50% to 60% renal excretion
Drug interactions	Increases toxicity of cytarabine
Toxicity	1. Myelosuppression 2. Infections 3. Elevated liver function tests 4. Rash

of fludarabine are summarized in Table 10.2. It has a number of different standard indications: first-line therapy for chronic lymphocytic leukemia (CLL), as a component of conditioning regimens for bone marrow transplantation, and occasional use for relapsed low-grade B-cell lymphomas.

TABLE

10.4 *Key features of cladribine (2-chlorodeoxyadenosine)*

Factor	Result
Mechanism of action	1. Incorporated into DNA as a false nucleotide resulting in inhibition of DNA stand elongation 2. Inhibits DNA polymerase 3. Potently inhibits ribonucleotide reductase
Metabolism	Activation to 2-CdATP within cells
Pharmacokinetics	1. Significant variability in cladribine plasma AUC 2. 40% to 50% oral bioavailability 3. 50% urinary excretion
Drug interactions	Increases toxicity of cytarabine Rash when used with allopurinol
Toxicity	1. Myelosuppression 2. Fever 3. Immunosuppression with resulting infection complications 4. Rash

Mechanism of Action

After intravenous administration, fludarabine is rapidly dephosphorylated in plasma to the nucleoside, 9-β-D-arabinofuranosyl-2-fluoroadenine (F-ara-A) (Fig. 10.4).[41] F-ara-A enters cells via the equilibrative carrier, hENT1,[42] and is phosphorylated to its active form, F-ara-ATP. The initial phosphate is added by deoxycytidine kinase. The cytotoxic mechanisms of action of fludarabine require the presence of fludarabine triphosphate (F-ara-ATP). F-ara-ATP inhibits several intracellular enzymes important in DNA replication including DNA polymerase, DNA primase, and DNA ligase I.[43,44] In addition, fludarabine is incorporated into DNA. Once incorporated, F-ara-AMP is an effective DNA chain terminator,[44] primarily at the 3′ end of DNA. The amount of fludarabine incorporated into DNA is linearly correlated with loss of clonogenicity. Once incorporated into DNA, the 3′-terminal F-ara-AMP is not easily excised, and the presence of this false nucleotide leads to apoptosis. F-ara-ADP also inhibits RNR,[45] an action that lowers dATP levels and promotes the incorporation of the inhibitor in place of dAMP into DNA.

The unique mechanism of RNR inhibition by fludarabine, clofarabine, and cladribine nucleotides contrasts with the irreversible binding of gemcitabine dinucleotide to the RNR $\alpha 2\beta 2$ and inactivation of electron transfer, and involves the formation of reversible hexamers of the α subunit bound to the di- and triphosphates of these analogues (Fig. 10.5). The clofarabine nucleotide is 10- to 100-fold more potent than are the nucleotides of fludarabine or cladribine[45] in inhibiting RNR. Mutation of the α subunit at a key oligomer-promoting site (D57N) abolishes binding of these drug nucleotides to RNR and suggests that this might be a source of resistance in tumors.

Although the effects of fludarabine on DNA synthesis account for its activity in dividing cells, fludarabine is also cytotoxic in diseases with very low growth fractions such as CLL or indolent lymphomas. This raises the question as to how an "S-phase" agent is active in nondividing cells[46] and may implicate its ability to

TABLE 10.6	Key features of nelarabine	

Factor	Result
Mechanism of action	1. Triphosphate metabolites are incorporated into DNA inhibiting DNA strand elongation 2. Inhibits ribonucleotide reductase lowering deoxynucleotide pools needed for DNA synthesis
Metabolism	1. Conversion to ara-G by demethylation via adenosine deaminase 2. Activation of ara-G to ara-guanosine triphosphate metabolite within cells. Deoxycytidine kinase responsible for first phosphorylation 3. Degradation to guanine
Pharmacokinetics	1. $t\frac{1}{2}$ of nelarabine in plasma 30 min, ara-G in plasma 3 h 2. 30% of dose excreted in urine as ara-G or parent compound 3. Intracellular $t\frac{1}{2}$ of ara-GTP 10–24 h
Drug interactions	Increased intracellular drug concentrations when used with fludarabine
Toxicity	1. Neurotoxicity (somnolence, neuropathy, myelopathy, encephalopathy) 2. Myelosuppression 3. Fatigue, fever 4. Nausea and vomiting

inhibit RNA polymerases, its depletion of nicotinamide adenine dinucleotide (NAD) with resultant decrease in cellular energy stores, and its interference with normal DNA repair processes, all of which may contribute to triggering apoptosis.[47] Specific subsets of CLL display quite unique responsiveness to fludarabine: those with mutated Ig heavy chain variable gene are much more sensitive than unmutated CLL, while those with del(17p) by karyotype are highly resistant.[48]

Resistance to fludarabine arises through depletion of deoxycytidine kinase, or possibly increased 5′nucleotidase II activity (mutation of NT5C2), which degrades the monophosphate intermediate of purine nucleotides.[32]

Clinical Pharmacology

Following intravenous administration, parent drug (2-F-ara-AMP) undergoes rapid (2 to 4 minutes) and complete conversion to F-ara-A through the action of 5′nucleotidase present in erythrocytes and endothelial cells. With commonly used doses of 25 to 30 mg/m², fludarabine reaches peak plasma F-ara-A concentrations of 1 to 5 μmol/L.[49] Wide variations in terminal drug half-life (7 to 33 hours) and area under the curve (AUC) are found among patients. Drug clearance does not change with repeated doses in individual patients. Peak F-ara-ATP concentrations in circulating leukemic cells are achieved 4 hours after intravenous fludarabine administration. F-ara-ATP has a relatively long intracellular half-life (15 hours), which may account for the efficacy of a daily administration schedule.[50] A direct relationship exists between plasma F-ara-A concentrations and intracellular F-ara-ATP in leukemic cells.[51]

F-ara-A is excreted primarily in the urine (50% to 60%) with no metabolites detected.[45] Patients with renal impairment, compared to patients with normal kidney function, have a significant decrease in clearance of 2-F-ara-A (Cl_T = 51.82 ± 6.70 versus 73.53 ± 3.79 mL/min/m²).[52]

Recommendations for dose reduction in patients with impaired renal function vary: Lichtman et al.[53] have proposed that patients with a creatinine clearance (Cl_{cr}) of greater than 70 mL/min per 1.73 m² should receive 25 mg/m²/d for 5 days of fludarabine, and patients with Cl_{cr} of 30 to 70 mL/min per 1.73 m² should receive 20 mg/m²/d for 5 days, and those with Cl_{cr} of less than 30 mL/min per 1.73 m² should receive 15 mg/m²/d for 5 days. Alternatively, Aronoff et al.[54] suggest a 25% dose reduction for a Cl_{cr} of 10 to 50 mL/min and a 50% dose reduction for a Cl_{cr} less than 10 mL/min. The drug label suggests a 20% dose reduction for Cl_{cr} of 30 to 70 mL/min and avoiding use in patients with a Cl_r less than 30 mL/min.

Oral administration of fludarabine leads to adequate bioavailability of 50% to 55%.[55] The AUC of F-ara-A increases linearly with increasing oral dose. Absorption is not affected by meals.[56] An oral dose of 40 mg/m²/d should provide similar systemic drug exposure to an intravenous dose of 25 mg/m²/d

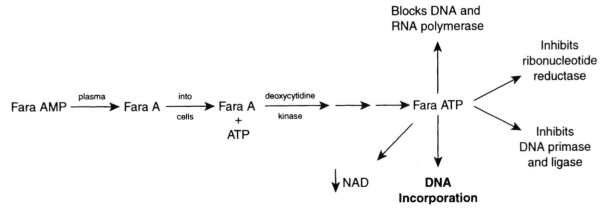

FIGURE **10.4** Activation pathway of fludarabine phosphate. Note multiple antitumor mechanisms related to F-ara-ATP.

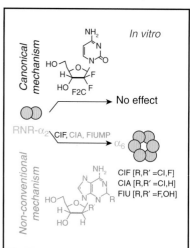
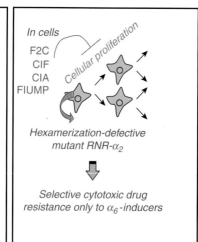

FIGURE 10.5 Mechanisms of inhibition of ribonucleotide reductase by the di-and triphosphates of the purine antimetabolites, cladribine (CIA), fludarabine (FIU), and clofarabine (CIF), which induce hexamer formation of the α subunit, in contrast to the "canonical" mechanism of suicide inhibition of the $\alpha_2\beta_2$ heterodimeric complex by gemcitabine (F2C) diphosphate. (Reprinted with permission from Wisitpittyaha S, Zhao Y, Long M, et al. Cladribine and fludarabine nucleotides induce distinct hexamers defining a common mode of reversible RNR inhibition. *ACS Chem Biol.* 2016;11(7):2021-2032. Copyright © 2016 American Chemical Society.)

Toxicity

The primary dose-limiting toxicities of fludarabine are myelosuppression and infectious complications resulting from immunosuppression.[57] Toxicity is similar with oral and intravenous preparations.[55] Reversible leukopenia and thrombocytopenia have been reported following fludarabine administration with a median time to nadir of 13 days (range, 3 to 25 days) and 16 days (range, 2 to 32 days), respectively. Grade 3 neutropenia (nadir <1,000/mm^3 at standard doses of 25 mg/m^2/d for 5 days) is seen in 25% to 30% of patients with grade 3 thrombocytopenia (platelet nadirs <50,000/mm^3) in 5% to 10%.[58] Myelosuppression is more common and more profound when fludarabine is combined with other chemotherapeutic drugs, including rituximab. Up to 25% of patients treated with fludarabine will have a febrile episode. Many fevers will be unassociated with infection, but one third will have a serious documented infectious cause.[59]

Fludarabine is potently immunosuppressive, inhibiting signal transduction important in lymphocyte activation.[60] Therapy is associated with an increased risk of opportunistic infections. CD4 and CD8 T-lymphocytic subpopulations decrease to levels of 150 to 200/mm^3 after three courses of therapy.[61] Lymphopenia may persist for over 1 year. The most frequent infectious complications are respiratory. Infections with *Cryptococcus*, *Listeria monocytogenes*, *Pneumocystis carinii*, cytomegalovirus, herpes simplex virus, varicella-zoster, and mycobacterial infections.[62] Previous therapy, advanced disease, and neutropenia are risk factors for opportunistic infection, which may occur many months after treatment. The incidence of infectious complications and grade 3 to 4 myelosuppression is significantly greater in patients with a creatinine clearance less than 80 mL/min, again supporting the need for dose modifications for patients with renal insufficiency.[57] Patient age is not an independent risk factor for fludarabine toxicity.

The development of autoimmune hemolytic anemia has been seen with fludarabine, and has been attributed to suppression of T-reg lymphocytes.[62] Hemolysis may occur following any treatment cycle, but it is most common during cycles one through three (71% of cases). A range of autoimmune side effects, including hypothyroidism, red cell aplasia, arthritis, and prolonged neutropenia, have been reported.

Acute tumor lysis is a rare but potentially fatal complication in patients with CLL and indolent lymphomas treated with fludarabine.[63] Other reported fludarabine toxicities include mild nausea and vomiting (30%), rash, peripheral sensorimotor neuropathy, and hepatocellular toxicity with elevations in serum transaminases.

An irreversible neurotoxicity syndrome with cortical blindness, optic neuritis, encephalopathy, generalized seizures, and coma has been described.[64] in patients receiving high drug doses (>40 mg/m^2/d for 5 days). However, mild, reversible neurotoxicity is seen at lower doses, and increases in frequency and severity with older age. Neurotoxicity is reported in 16% of patients. Pulmonary toxicity characterized by fever, cough, hypoxia, and diffuse interstitial pneumonitis has been reported in 5% to 10%[66] of fludarabine-treated patients, and responds to corticosteroids. Although less well studied, oral fludarabine appears to have similar toxicities to the intravenous preparation[66] with a somewhat greater frequency of gastrointestinal side effects (diarrhea). Myelodysplasia and AML may arise as late adverse effects of fludarabine treatment.[67]

Clinical Use

Fludarabine has demonstrated clinical activity in a variety of low-grade lymphoproliferative malignancies including CLL, hairy cell leukemia, Waldenström's macroglobulinemia, and small cell variants of non-Hodgkin's lymphoma. Response rates from 32% to 57% have been reported among patients with refractory CLL treated with single agent fludarabine. The median duration of disease control is 65 to 91 weeks. Among patients with previously untreated CLL, fludarabine has produced responses in more than 70% of patients, including complete responses in one third. A median survival of 63 months has been reported. In CLL, the combination of fludarabine, cyclophosphamide, and rituximab (FCR) for six cycles of treatment has become standard upfront therapy and results in an overall response rate approaching 95% and a complete response rate of 70% with a 6-year survival rate of 77% and a median time to progression of 80 months.[68] Patients with del(17p) chromosomal abnormality had inferior responses and are now treated with ibrutinib. Fludarabine has also been employed as a component of nonmyeloablative stem cell transplantation for lymphoma,[69] and in combination with cytosine arabinoside for AML patients potentially intolerant of anthracyclines[70] or in an intensive multidrug induction regimen.[71]

A pharmacokinetic model for predicting fludarabine clearance, based on renal function and body weight, has found a correlation of renal function and nonrelapse mortality and the incidence of acute graft versus host disease in patients receiving reduced intensity conditioning with fludarabine (40 mg/m²/d for 5 days). Thirty-five percent of clearance was accounted for by renal excretion.[69] The authors provide a formula for predicting safe drug levels (based on a designation of a safe AUC).

Drug Interactions

Fludarabine combined with pentostatin has resulted in a high incidence of fatal pulmonary toxicity.[72] As an immunosuppressant, fludarabine may diminish the effectiveness of vaccine therapy and increase the risk of toxicity of live vaccines.

Pentostatin or Deoxycoformycin (Nipent)

Pentostatin or 2′-deoxycoformycin (dCF) is a purine analog isolated from a *Streptomyces* culture but now chemically synthesized. dCF is a potent inhibitor of ADA,[72] an enzyme present at high concentrations in lymphocytes. dCF failed its initial evaluation as treatment for ALL but produced consistent and long-term complete responses in hairy cell leukemia.[73] Key pharmacologic features of pentostatin are listed in Table 10.3.[72-80]

Mechanism of Action

Inherited deficiency of ADA is associated with lymphopenia and immunodeficiency. dCF binds with nM affinity to ADA with a slow dissociation rate of 60 hours,[72] leading to high levels of deoxyadenosine triphosphate (dATP). Accumulation of dATP inhibits RNR leading to decreased formation of other deoxynucleotides such as dCTP and dGTP. This imbalance slows DNA synthesis and alters DNA replication and repair. dATP also inhibits S-adenosylhomocysteine hydrolase resulting in a fall of cellular S-adenosyl methionine, preventing normal cellular methylation of proteins, including histones.[73] dCF is incorporated into nucleic acids, although the importance of this action is not clear, dCF was originally postulated to be more effective in T-cell lymphocytic tumors with high ADA levels. However, it has subsequently shown activity in both T-and B-cell lymphocytic neoplasms. The antineoplastic activity depends, to a certain extent, on the intracellular ADA activity of the neoplasm. In indolent lymphoid neoplasms in which cellular ADA levels are lower, ADA can be inhibited at low drug concentrations, with minimal systemic side effects.[75]

Clinical Pharmacology

dCF is reasonably stable at neutral pH; however, care must be taken if the drug is extensively diluted with 5% dextrose in water as it becomes unstable at pH ≤ 5.[76] It has a large volume of distribution with little protein binding.[77] The terminal elimination half-life averages 6 hours.[78] Plasma levels 1 hour after administration exceed the ADA inhibitory concentration by a wide margin, supporting the recommendation for an intermittent infusion schedule. Only a small amount of pentostatin is metabolized; 40% to 80% of the drug is excreted in urine unchanged within 24 hours.[78,79] In patients with impaired renal function (creatinine clearance <60 mL/min),

drug half-life is prolonged (approximately 18 hours). Patients with a creatinine clearance greater than 60 mL/min should receive a dose of 4 mg/m² every 14 days, patients with Cl$_{cr}$ of 41 to 60 mL/min should receive 3 mg/m² every 2 weeks, and patients with a Cl$_{cr}$ of 20 to 40 mL/min should receive a 2 mg/m² dose every 14 days.[80] The drug has poor oral bioavailability. It crosses the blood-brain barrier, producing CSF concentrations 10% of simultaneous drug concentrations in plasma.[81]

Toxicity

At commonly used doses (4 mg/m² every 2 weeks), pentostatin toxicity is modest, and therapy is usually well tolerated.[82] In a large intergroup trial of hairy cell leukemia, grade 3 to 4 toxicity was evident, but usually reversible.[83] Twenty-two percent of patients treated at 4 mg/m² every 2 weeks develop grade 3 to 4 neutropenia. Nausea and vomiting (>grade 3) occur in 11% of patients, and may be delayed for 12 to 72 hours after drug administration. Mild-to-moderate lethargy (3% incidence), rash, and reactivation of herpes zoster have been reported. Higher doses (≥10 mg/m²/d) produce immunosuppression, with T-cell function being notably impaired, other toxicities included conjunctivitis, renal impairment, hepatic enzyme elevation, and central nervous system disturbances.[81] Renal toxicity seen in early trials during dose excalation is minimized with the use of lower drug doses and adequate hydration. Cardiac complications have been described in older patients but are rarely seen with the current regimen.[84] Opportunistic fungal and parasitic infections may result from immunosuppression.[85] Initial concerns regarding an increased risk of second malignancies following use of dCF have not been confirmed.[86]

Clinical Use

dCF, delivered in low doses, produces responses in over 90% of patients with hairy cell leukemia with estimated disease-free survival at 5 years of 85% and at 10 years of 65%, respectively.[86] However, most patients have evidence of residual disease upon molecular testing. dCF produces responses in a number of other closely related disorders, including B-cell CLL, Waldenström's macroglobulinemia, refractory multiple myeloma, and adult T-cell lymphomas,[87] but is not a standard or approved agent alone or in combination in these patients. dCF's suppresses graft versus host disease developing after stem cell transplantation,[88] another potential indication.

Cladribine or 2-Chlorodeoxyadenosine (Leustatin)

Cladribine or 2-chlorodeoxyadenosine is a purine nucleoside analog with antineoplastic activity against low-grade lymphoproliferative diseases, especially hairy cell leukemia, but also childhood leukemias, and multiple sclerosis. Its important pharmacologic features are noted in Table 10.4.

Mechanism of Action

Cladribine (2-CdA) (Fig. 10.3) requires intracellular phosphorylation by deoxycytidine kinase for activation.[89] The 5′-triphosphate metabolite (2-chloro-2′-deoxyadenosine 5-triphosphate [2-CdATP]) accumulates in cells rich in deoxycytidine kinase (Fig. 10.6).

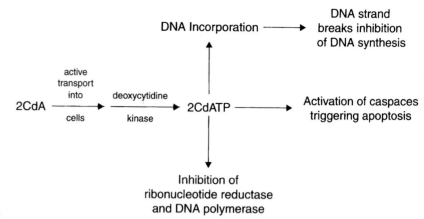

FIGURE **10.6** Activation of cladribine (2 CdA).

2-CdAMP is incorporated into DNA, producing DNA strand breaks. The presence of three successive Cl-d-AMP residues in DNA blocks strand elongation.[90] Cladribine, incorporated into DNA promoter sequences, acts as a transcription antagonist.[91] As Cl-dATP, it is a potent inhibitor of RNR (see above)[92] causing an imbalance in deoxyribonucleotide triphosphate pools with subsequent impairment of DNA synthesis and repair.

Cladribine exposure leads to apoptosis in sensitive cells.[93] 2-CdATP interacts with cytochrome C and protease activating factor-1 (PAF-1) to initiate the caspase cascade leading to DNA degradation, even in the absence of cell division.[94] Cladribine resistance can result from deficiency in deoxycytidine kinase[95] (the initial enzyme in the activation pathway) and p53 mutations.[96]

Clinical Pharmacology

The drug is approved for hairy cell leukemia treatment in doses of 0.1 mg/kg/d given for 7 days. An alternative schedule is 5.6 mg/m[2] for 5 days. Liquid chromatography is used to determine plasma concentrations of cladribine and its primary metabolite, 2-chlorodeoxyadenosine.[97] The parent drug has a t ½ of 9 hours in plasma. Cladribine nucleotides are retained in leukemic cells with an intracellular half-life of 9 to 30 hours. Intracellular concentrations exceed the concentration of free drug in plasma by 100-fold.[98] The long intracellular nucleotide half-life supports the use of intermittent drug administration.[99] Following a 2-hour infusion of 0.12 mg/kg cladribine, peak serum concentrations of roughly 100 nM are achieved. A linear dose-concentration relationship is present up to infusion doses of 2.5 mg/m[2]/h. Cladribine clearance rates of 664 to 978 mL/h/kg have been reported with significant interpatient variability (±50%). The drug is weakly bound to plasma protein (20%). Renal clearance accounts for 50% of total drug clearance, with 20% to 30% of drug excreted as unchanged cladribine within the first 24 hours.[99,100] Little information is available regarding dose adjustments for renal or hepatic insufficiency. However, given the high renal drug clearance, caution should be taken in using cladribine in patients with renal failure. Chloroadenine, the analog base, is the major metabolite formed. Renal excretion of chloroadenine accounts for clearance of 3% of administered cladribine.[99]

Bioavailability of subcutaneously administered cladribine is excellent (100%).[101] An oral preparation has been evaluated with bioavailability of 40% to 50%. Increased metabolism to chloroadenine is seen following oral administration suggesting a first-pass effect.[97,101] Significant patient-to-patient variability (±28%) exists in the AUC achieved following administration of drug by any method.[99] Oral drug is not yet FDA approved. FDA approval is for intravenous drug administration, but several studies suggest that the subcutaneous administration of 3.4 mg/m[2]/d for 7 days is equivalent to intravenous administration of 0.1 mg/kg/d for 7 days.[102] Cladribine penetrates the blood-brain barrier, and CSF concentrations are 25% of those in plasma.[103]

Toxicity

The primary toxicity using a standard dosage of 0.7 mg/kg/cycle of cladribine (usually as a continuous 7-day infusion at 0.1 mg/m[2]/d) is myelosuppression.[104] Nausea, alopecia, hepatic, and renal toxicity rarely occur at this dose. Fever (temperature > 100°F) is seen in two thirds of patients treated with cladribine, mostly during the period of neutropenia but may occur without neutropenia. Only 10% to 15% of febrile patients will have documented infections. Myelosuppression and immunosuppression with development of opportunistic infections are the major adverse events.[99] Grade 3 to 4 neutropenia and lymphopenia occur in half of treated patients. Neutrophil counts decrease 1 to 2 weeks after starting therapy and do not recover for 3 to 4 weeks.[97–104] Twenty percent of patients develop grade 3 to 4 thrombocytopenia. Infections occur in 15% to 40% of patients, often opportunistic infections, such as *Candida* or *Aspergillus*. Betticher et al.[105] have found that reducing the dose of 2CdA from 0.7 to 0.5 mg/kg/cycle decreases the grade 3 myelosuppression rate (33% to 8%) and the infection rate (30% to 7%) without a change in response rate. A weekly schedule of 0.12 mg/kg CdA has been evaluated.[106] Response rates and toxicities were not different from a daily × 7 schedule. Toxicities other than myelosuppression and infections are rare but have been reported. Following high-dose 2-CdA (five to ten times the recommended therapeutic dose), renal failure, motor weakness, and autoimmune hemolytic anemia become significant toxicities.

Clinical Use and Drug Interactions

Cladribine has become the treatment of choice for patients with hairy cell leukemia with remission rate and long-term survival comparable to those of dCF, either alone or with Rituxan, which improves the complete response rate.[107,108] Patients with CLL, low-grade non-Hodgkin's lymphomas, cutaneous T-cell lymphoma, Waldenström's macroglobulinemia, mantle cell lymphoma, mastocytosis, Langerhans cell histiocytosis, and blast-phase chronic myelogenous leukemia (CML) have responded to cladribine therapy.[109–111] Pretreatment of patients with cladribine increases the intracellular accumulation of ara-CTP, the active metabolite of cytarabine, by 40%[112] leading to ongoing trials in combination with daunorubicin and cytosine arabinoside for AML, and promising complete response rates in FLT3-ITD+ AML.[113] An increased frequency of drug rash has been noted when cladribine and allopurinol have been used concomitantly.[114]

Clofarabine (Clolar)

Clofarabine was synthesized in a search for new 2-halo-2′-halo-deoxyarabinofuranosyl adenine analogs with potentially better activity than was fludarabine or cladribine.[115] Clofarabine (Fig. 10.3) retains the 2-chloroadenine aglycone of cladribine making it resistant to inactivation by ADA. It also has a fluorine at the 2′ position of the carbohydrate in the arabinosyl configuration, which is thought to enhance activation of the compound by deoxycytidine kinase. The substitution of the fluorine at the C-2′ position also decreases phosphorolytic cleavage of clofarabine monophosphate by purine nucleoside phosphorylase (PNP).[116] The key features of clofarabine are summarized in Table 10.5.

Mechanism of Action

Following cellular uptake, clofarabine must be converted to the 5′-triphosphate metabolite, in a manner similar to fludarabine and cladribine (Figs. 10.4 and 10.5). Clofarabine is a better substrate for deoxycytidine kinase than either fludarabine or cladribine.[116] The triphosphate form of clofarabine inhibits DNA synthesis and repair. Clofarabine nucleotide is incorporated into DNA, inhibits RNR, inhibits DNA polymerases, depletes intracellular deoxynucleotides, and inhibits elongation of DNA strands.[117,118] It irreversibly binds to the active site of RNR, a self-potentiating action that reduces dATP levels and increases its incorporation into DNA. Clofarabine and fludarabine are superior to cladribine as inhibitors of DNA polymerases. Clofarabine can induce cellular apoptosis via induction of mitochondrial damage, an effect not seen with fludarabine.[119]

Clinical Pharmacology

Clofarabine is approved for treatment of relapsed ALL in children, where the usual dose is 52 mg/m² daily as a 2-hour infusion for five consecutive days. It has also been tested for relapsed AML in doses of 40 mg/m² for 5 days.[120] Plasma concentrations appear to be dose proportional.[121] Clofarabine's plasma half-life is about 5 hours, with 50% to 60% of the drug excreted in the urine unchanged. No data are currently available to make recommendations for dosing in patients with renal or hepatic insufficiency. Intracellular clofarabine triphosphate concentrations are similar to those achieved with cladribine and fludarabine, but persist longer, with an intracellular half-life of over 24 hours.[122]

Toxicity

The primary toxicity with clofarabine, as with fludarabine and cladribine, is myelosuppression resulting in an increased risk of infectious complications.[121,122] Reversible hepatic transaminase elevation is noted in 15% to 25% of patients.[123] Other side effects include nausea, fatigue, edema, and plantar palmar dysesthesia. In children, febrile neutropenia, anorexia, hypotension, and nausea have been the most commonly reported toxicities.[124] A capillary leak syndrome, manifested as hypotension, tachypnea, fever, and pulmonary edema on x-ray, and elevated hepatic enzymes, occurs in a small minority of patients but leads to immediate discontinuation of the drug. Hypokalemia and hypophosphatemia may also be detected during treatment, and warrant electrolyte replacement. Acute renal injury has been reported in 29 cases of refractory or relapsed AML treated with clofarabine, but the mechanism of renal toxicity is unclear.[125]

Clinical Use and Drug Interactions

Clofarabine was approved by the FDA in 2004 for the treatment of pediatric patients with relapsed or refractory ALL following the use of at least two prior therapies. Clofarabine increases the intracellular concentrations of cytosine arabinoside, potentiating ara-C cytotoxicity. The combination of clofarabine and cytarabine, compared to clofarabine alone, is being evaluated against AML.[126]

Nelarabine

Nelarabine is the most recent purine analog approved by the FDA (2005). It is indicated for treatment of patients with T-cell acute leukemia (T-ALL) and T-cell lymphoblastic lymphoma (T-LBL) who have not responded to or have relapsed after at least two prior chemotherapy regimens.[127] The key pharmacologic features of nelarabine are listed in Table 10.6.

Mechanism of Action

Both normal and malignant T cells are sensitive to the inhibitory effects of high concentrations of deoxyguanosine, which becomes phosphorylated within the cell leading to inhibition of DNA synthesis.[128] Deoxyguanosine, however, is not a useful drug as it has a short half-life in plasma due to rapid deamination by PNP, which is present in high concentrations in red blood cells. 9-β-D arabinofuranosyl guanine (ara-G), an analog of deoxyguanine, is resistant to deamination by PNP but is poorly soluble. Nelarabine (Fig 10.1), a 6-O-methylated, soluble prodrug of ara-G, is converted by ADA to ara-G. Ara-G then accumulates in cells in higher concentrations in T cells than in B lymphocytes.[129] Ara-G is phosphorylated to ara-GTP via deoxycytidine kinase and deoxyguanosine kinase. Ara-GTP is then incorporated into DNA where it terminates DNA elongation, leading to inhibition of DNA synthesis and cell death.[90,130] Ara-GTP also inhibits RNR causing depletion of the deoxynucleotides required for DNA synthesis. Avid uptake of nelarabine and accumulation of ara-GTP by leukemic cells are the critical determinants of response to nelarabine therapy.[131]

Clinical Pharmacology

The standard dose for nelarabine is 1,500 mg/m² given as a 2-hour infusion on days 1, 3, and 5 of a 21-day cycle. The dose for children is 650 mg/m² on days one through five every 21 days. Following intravenous administration, nelarabine is converted by removal of the methoxy group to ara-G.[132] The half-life of nelarabine is short (30 minutes). The half-life of the active metabolite, ara-G, is 3 hours with a mean plasma concentration of 115 µM during an infusion of 1,500 mg/m².[133] Pediatric patients have an increased clearance rate of ara-G with a resulting shorter plasma half-life (2 hours).[132] Small quantities of nelarabine (5%) and ara-G (23%) are excreted unchanged in the urine. The drug readily penetrates into the CSF, where it persists in high concentrations.[134]

At present, no dose modifications are recommended for patients with renal insufficiency. Most nelarabine is converted to ara-G, which is subsequently hydrolyzed to guanine, and guanine is in turn converted to xanthine and uric acid.

Intracellular accumulation of ara-GTP has been measured.[135] A median ara-GTP C_{max} of 150 µmol/L is found in T-ALL cells (more than double the concentration found in other normal or malignant cell lineages). The intracellular elimination half-life of ara-GTP varies from 10 to 24 hours. The concomitant use of fludarabine prior to the administration of nelarabine increases intracellular concentrations of ara-GTP by 10%, possibly by up-regulating deoxycytidine and deoxyguanosine kinase concentrations.[135]

Toxicity

In phase I and II trials, the dose-limiting toxicity of nelarabine has been central nervous system (seizures, encephalopathy, obtundation) and peripheral neurotoxicity.[136] There are uncommon but consistent reports of ascending myelopathy, with loss of both sensory and motor function, and associated with posterior column changes on MRI scans.[137,138] The most common adverse events are malaise, fever, headache, somnolence, nausea, peripheral neuropathy, and myelosuppression.[133,139] Grade 3 or 4 neurologic events occur in 10% to 15% of patients.

Clinical Use and Drug Interactions

Nelarabine has been approved exclusively for treatment of patients with T-ALL and T-lymphoblastic lymphoma (LBL). Response rates in patients with relapsed/refractory T-cell malignancies are low (23% in pediatric patients and 31% in adults).[129] Some of these patients have proceeded on to stem cell transplantation. The median survival for adult relapsed T-ALL/LBL patients treated with nelarabine is 20 weeks with 25% alive at 1 year. Results to date are based on phase I and II trials in a small number of patients.

Hydroxyurea (HU)

HU, one of the simplest chemical structures among the anticancer drugs, plays a supportive role in the treatment of leukemia and myeloproliferative disorders (MPDs) because of its ability to suppress proliferation of myeloid, erythroid, and platelet precursors, but its value is limited by its inability to induce bone marrow remission and the equally rapid reversibility of its myelosuppressive effect. It has other notable clinical properties, including its induction of fetal hemoglobin (HbF) synthesis in patients with sickle cell anemia

and thalassemia. It has been an invaluable probe for the laboratory study of its intracellular target, RNR, the rate-limiting step in the de novo synthesis of deoxyribonucleotide triphosphates (dNTPs). Other actions, including the generation of nitric oxide and nitroxyl radicals and radiosensitizing effects, have potential clinical applications. The key features of this drug are shown in Table 10.7.

TABLE 10.7	*Key features of hydroxyurea*
Mechanism of action	Inhibitor of RNR by inactivation of the tyrosyl-free radical on the M-2 subunit, with resultant depletion of deoxynucleotides and inhibition of DNA synthesis and repair
Pharmacokinetics	Nonlinear at high doses
	Bioavailability of essentially 100%, C_{max} 1 h after oral dose
	Elimination half-life of 2–6 h
	Rapid distribution to tissues. Limited penetration of cerebrospinal fluid
Elimination/metabolism	Renal excretion predominates (40% of dose), although interpatient variability is significant.
	Several enzyme systems capable of metabolism of HU exist, but the extent of metabolism in humans is not known
Drug interactions	Increases conversion of ara-C to active metabolite and increases the incorporation of arabinosylcytosine nucleotide into DNA
	Enhances the activation of purine antimetabolites
	Enhances effects of ionizing radiation
Toxicity	Myelosuppression with white blood cells affected to a greater extent than with platelets or red blood cells
	Gastrointestinal effects (nausea, vomiting, changes in bowel habits)
	Dermatologic effects (pigmentation, erythema, rash, leukocytoclastic vasculitis, ulceration, squamous carcinoma of the skin)
	Hepatic enzyme elevations, jaundice
	Acute interstitial lung infiltrates
Precautions	Decrease dosage in renal failure until patient tolerance is demonstrated
	When given with concomitant radiotherapy, anticipate increased tissue reaction, mucosal ulceration.
	May enhance toxicity of ara-C or other antimetabolites
	Use with caution in pregnant or lactating women.

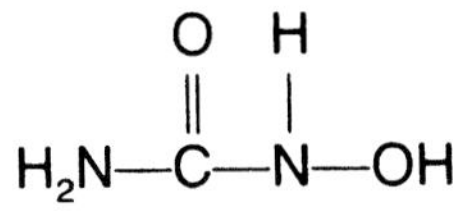

O   H
‖ |
H₂N—C—N—OH

FIGURE **10.7** Structure of hydroxyurea.

HU (Fig. 10.7) was originally synthesized in Germany in 1860[140] and was found to have inhibitory effects on granulocyte production.[141] It displayed antileukemic properties in the National Cancer Institute's screening system,[142] entered clinical trials in the 1960s, and was soon recognized as a potent and acutely myelosuppressive agent with a novel mechanism of action and few side effects, properties that have earned it a limited but constant role in cancer chemotherapy. Other inhibitors of RNR have since been evaluated in the clinic, including compounds of the thiosemicarbazone series[143] and guanazole,[144] but they have no special therapeutic advantage and greater toxicity. The purine analogues inhibit RNR by an alternative mechanism, competition for the dATP regulatory site, but have their primary affect on DNA synthesis. The principal use of HU at present is in suppressing proliferation of bone marrow elements, as it provides excellent control of MPDs.[145–147]

Once a primary agent with interferon-α in first-line therapy against CML, it has been largely replaced by imatinib and related bcr-abl kinase inhibitors, and is now used primarily for acute reduction of white cell count in patients with acute leukemia. In polycythemia vera (PV), it effectively prevents thrombosis resulting from elevated hematocrit and high platelet count,[145] and it similarly lessens the incidence of thrombosis in patients with essential thrombocythemia (ET) and platelet counts above 1.5 million.[146] It is especially useful in controlling white blood cell counts in myeloproliferative diseases (MPDs), such as myelofibrosis.[147] Because both PV and ET are chronic, slowly progressive diseases, there is concern that HU may increase the risk of leukemic conversion, a risk that has not been substantiated thus far.[148] In younger patients with PV, who have the prospect of long-term treatment, prophylactic phlebotomy prevails for initial management, and in patients with ET, anagrelide and interferon-α are alternatives to HU. Newer drugs such as ruxolitinib that attack the mutant Jak-2 kinase (Chapter 24) found in patients with myelofibrosis and other MPDs reduce splenomegaly, improve symptoms, and may displace HU as first line therapy in the future.[147,149]

A major current use of HU is in the prevention of complications of sickle cell anemia and related disorders.[150] In patients with sickle cell anemia, HU increases the production of HbF, ameliorates symptoms, and reduces the incidence of painful crisis and hospitalization.[151,152] In vitro incubation of HU with erythroid progenitors elevates HbF production.[153] Whether the induction of HbF represents a response to inhibition of DNA synthesis in red cell progenitors or a specific alteration of γ-globin gene transcription is uncertain. Nitroxyl radicals produced by decomposition of HU may directly stimulate γ-globin gene transcription through the Sar 1a promoter.[153] HbF maintains its solubility and resists polymerization in hypoxic environments, and prevents the downward spiral of intravascular red cell sickling and endothelial adhesion that leads to thrombosis, pulmonary hypertension and insufficiency, and bone pain. There is considerable evidence that induction of HbF is not the only contributor to the drug's efficacy. The benefit from HU may also be related to its suppression of the neutrophil count and its

inhibition of adhesion of white and red cells to vessel walls.[154] HU reduces adhesion of a patient's blood cells, coincident with a down-regulation of l-selectin on the red cell and white cell surfaces, after 2 weeks of HU therapy, before HbF levels rise. HU inhibits breakdown of nitric oxide, a vasodilator, through inhibition of myeloperoxidase.[155] HU appears to be as effective in children with sickle cell disease[156] and in patients with sickle cell–β-thalassemia and sickle cell–hemoglobin C disease, and in β-thalassemia.[157,158]

Mechanism of Action and Cellular Pharmacology

HU enters cells by passive diffusion. The primary site of cytotoxic action for HU is inhibition of RNR. This highly regulated enzyme converts ribonucleotide diphosphates to the deoxyribonucleotides that can be incorporated into DNA.[159] HU inhibits RNR in vitro,[160] and the extent of inhibition of DNA synthesis observed in HU-treated cells correlates with degree of decrease in deoxyribonucleotide pools.[161] Through its regulation of deoxynucleotide pools, the enzyme becomes the rate-limiting reaction in the regulation of DNA synthesis. RNR consists of two subunits M-1 and M-2.[162] M-1, a dimer with a molecular weight of 170 Kd, contains the binding site for the diphosphate substrates as well as the allosteric nucleotide triphosphate regulatory sites.[163] dATP inhibits the reduction of all substrates, and in the presence of high concentrations of dATP, the enzyme complex dissociates.[164] M-1 is present at a relatively constant level throughout the cell cycle, except in cells in G_0 or those that have undergone terminal differentiation, in which it is markedly decreased.[165] The gene for M-1 is on chromosome 11.

Protein M-2 is the catalytic subunit of the enzyme and exists as a dimer with a molecular weight of 88 kD. This unique protein contains stoichiometric amounts of iron and a stable organic-free radical localized to a tyrosine residue. The tyrosyl radical is essential to enzyme activity and is localized in proximity to and stabilized by the nonheme iron complex.[166] The cellular concentration of M-2 protein is variable throughout the cell cycle; it peaks in S phase, which suggests that functional enzyme activity depends on the concentration of M-2 protein.[167] The M-2 subunit sequences have been mapped to chromosome 2 in human cells and seem to be in the same amplification unit as the gene for ornithine decarboxylase.

The inhibition of RNR occurs through the drug's chelation of iron and its inactivation of the tyrosyl-free radical on the M-2 subunit, with disruption of the enzyme's iron-binding center.[168] The fact that this inhibition can be partially reversed in vitro by ferrous iron and that cytotoxicity can be enhanced by iron-chelating agents[169] emphasizes the importance of chelation of the nonheme iron cofactor in this process.

HU selectively kills rapidly proliferating cells in S phase. The cytotoxic effects of HU correlate with dose or concentration achieved, as well as with duration of drug exposure.[170] Following HU exposure, cells progress normally through the cell cycle until they reach the G_1-S interface. Rather than being prevented from entering S phase, as was once thought, cells enter S phase at a normal rate but are accumulated there as a result of the deficiency of dNTPs.[171] Cells undergo apoptosis in a process mediated by both *p53* and non-*p53* pathways.

HU may be transformed in vivo to nitric oxide (NO), which is also an RNR inhibitor. The possibility, therefore, exists that the inactivation of RNR by HU may result from both chelation of iron and indirectly from inhibition by NO. Indeed, HU-borne NO may be the intermediate effector in other actions of the drug, such as its induction of HbF, pulmonary vasodilation, and decreased vascular adhesion of leukocytes.[172]

Several of the enzymes involved in DNA polymerization and DNA precursor synthesis are assembled in a *replitase complex* during S phase of the cell cycle to channel metabolites to enzymes sequentially during the synthetic process. Replitase contains DNA polymerases, thymidine kinase, dihydrofolate reductase, nucleoside-5′ phosphate kinase, thymidylate synthase, and RNR. Cross inhibition is a phenomenon observed with enzymes of the replitase complex; when one enzyme in the complex is inhibited, other enzymes in the complex shut down. This occurs only in intact cells and only in S phase. Evidence suggests that this cross inhibition is the result of a direct allosteric, structural interactions within the complex, because decreases of dNTP pools do not produce the same effects.[173]

Cell death is triggered by genotoxic stress resulting from gaps and breaks in DNA due to the deficiency of deoxynucleotides. HU exposure leads to DNA strand breaks and stalled replication forks. DNA repair proteins respond to this damage, and influence outcome of HU treatment. Key to the repair of these stalled forks are DNA protein kinase (PK) and PARP 1, which associate with DNA ends and recruit XRCC1, an early and key component of the repair complex. Loss of either DNA PK or PARP1 increases sensitivity to HU in tumor cell lines[174] raising the possibility of synergy with inhibitors of these enzymes. BRCA2, in combination with RAD51, protects stalled replication forks produced by HU and allows restart of replication after repair of the DNA lesion.[175]

A potentially important HU action is the accelerated loss of extrachromosomally amplified genes that are present in double-minute chromosomes.[176] Acentric extrachromosomal elements are common in the gene amplification process. Exposure to HU at clinically achievable concentrations leads to enhanced loss of both amplified oncogenes and drug-resistance genes.[177]

Mechanisms of Cellular Resistance

The principal mechanism by which cells achieve resistance to HU is increased synthesis of cellular RNR.[178] Transfection of the human M-2 gene into drug-sensitive KB cells confers resistance by increasing the enzyme activity.[179] Transfection of the M-1 gene, and elevation of M-1 protein levels, do not decrease sensitivity to HU, although transfected cells resist dNTP inhibition of RNR activity, probably because of the alteration in function of inhibitory binding sites. Several different molecular mechanisms can contribute to the increased RNR activity in HU-resistant cells. A number of cell lines have amplifications of the gene coding for M-2 protein accompanied by an elevation in M-2 messenger RNA and M-2 protein levels.[180] It also seems that posttranscriptional modifications, such as an increase in initiation factor 4E, can occur during drug selection, which results in an increased translational efficiency. An increase in M-2 protein biosynthetic rate can then occur with no further increase in messenger RNA levels.[181]

In most studies, HU resistance has been associated with a parallel decrease in sensitivity to other RNR inhibitors and often to other antimetabolites.[182] Interestingly, inhibitors of the M-2 subunit, including 3-aminopyridine-2-carboxaldehyde thiosemicarbazone, or 3-AP, retain their antitumor effect in HU-resistant cell lines.[143] In addition, some of these cell lines with increased RNR activity display an increased sensitivity to other cytotoxics, particularly analogs such as 6-thioguanine (via increased conversion to the deoxynucleotide and enhancement of its incorporation into DNA)[183] or cytidine analogues (via increased drug uptake by the cells).[184]

Drug Interactions

HU enhances the cytotoxicity of both purine and pyrimidine analogues by reducing the competitive pools of physiologic triphosphates. It causes a significant increase in formation of ara-C triphosphate and ara-C incorporation into DNA[185] and has similar enhancing effect on the antipurines. However, clinical trials have not confirmed synergy of HU in combination with ara-C or other antimetabolites in clinical trials.

The major clinical interest in HU in the treatment of solid tumors has been in combination with 5-fluorouracil. Synergy has been demonstrated in experimental tumor models, presumably based on the ability of HU to lower cellular pools of deoxyuridine monophosphate, the physiologic substrate of thymidylate synthase.[186] Again, clinical trials of the combination of HU and 5-FU have not confirmed conclusive benefit.

HU has been evaluated in both clinical and laboratory studies in combination with chemotherapy agents that produce DNA damage, such as alkylating agents, cisplatin, and inhibitors of topoisomerase II.[186] Although synergy has been observed in preclinical testing, the clinical role for such combinations is uncertain. By depleting deoxynucleotide pools, HU inhibits DNA repair, and increases sensitivity to irradiation. It has been used as a radiosensitizer in cervical cancer and head and neck cancer.

Clinical Pharmacology

Pharmacokinetics

HU is generally administered orally (an intravenous formulation is also available, but rarely used), and doses are titrated in response to changes in peripheral white blood cell counts. Doses range from 80 mg/kg, given to acutely lower leukemic cell counts, to 15 mg/kg/d, the starting dose for patients with sickle cell anemia. In each case, the doses are adjusted to achieve the desired degree of myelosuppression. For sickle cell patients, a neutrophil count of 2,000 cells/mm³ is the lower threshold for holding dosage. Neutrophil counts respond rapidly to discontinuation of drug, the period of myelosuppression lasting 2 weeks or less. Although significant interpatient variability is observed, peak concentrations of 0.1 to 2.0 mmol/L are achieved 1.0 to 1.5 hours after doses of 15 to 80 mg/kg.[187] Oral bioavailability is excellent (80% to 100%), and comparable areas under the C × T curve in plasma are seen after oral and intravenous dosing.[187,188] After attainment of peak plasma concentrations 1 hour after an oral dose, HU disappears rapidly from plasma. The elimination half-life ranges from 2 to 6 hours.

Data available from a comprehensive population pharmacokinetic study of multiple oral and intravenous dosing are best described by a one-compartment model with parallel Michaelis-Menten metabolism and first-order renal excretion.[189] Clearance averages 0.2 L/h/kg. Renal clearance at standard doses is 60 to 90 mL/min in an average patient and 40% of an oral dose is recovered as parent compound in the urine. A liquid formulation for infants gives equivalent pharmacokinetics.[190]

Several high-dose 24- to 120-hour continuous infusion regimens for HU administration, with or without initial loading, have been evaluated.[191,192] Continuous infusion of 1 g/h for 24 hours is capable of sustaining plasma concentrations in excess of 1 mmol/L. Doses of 0.5 g/m^2/d were tolerated for 12 weeks, 1 g/m^2/d was tolerated for 5 weeks, 1.66 g/m^2/d was tolerated for 3 weeks, and 2.5 g/m^2/d was tolerated for 1 week.[193] Based on the available data, from the standpoint of pharmacokinetics and bioavailability, administering HU parenterally has no clear advantages, except in those patients with impaired gastrointestinal function.

Although precise guidelines are not available, the prudent course is to modify dosages for patients with abnormal renal function until individual tolerance can be assessed. Unfortunately, pharmacokinetic studies of patients with altered renal function have not been performed to provide guidelines. The full extent and significance of HU metabolism in humans have not been established.

Animal experiments suggest that the metabolism of HU does occur, but metabolites have not been demonstrated conclusively in humans. HU is degraded by urease, an enzyme found in intestinal bacteria.[194] Hydroxylamine (NH_2OH), a product of this reaction, has not been identified in humans. Acetohydroxamic acid is found in the plasma of patients receiving HU therapy, however, and may represent the product of a reaction between hydroxylamine and acetyl-coenzyme A, a major thioester in mammalian tissues.[195] The conversion of HU to urea in mice has also been reported.[196] An enzyme system capable of this conversion is found in mouse liver, with the greatest activity localized in the mitochondrial subcellular fraction. Similar activity has not been demonstrated in human liver.

HU distributes rapidly to well-perfused tissues.[195] The drug readily enters breast milk. It slowly enters CSF, and third-space collections of fluid such as ascites or pleural effusions. CSF:plasma ratios are 1:4 to 1:9, and plasma:ascites concentrations are 1:2 to 1:7 in the limited time point sampling reported.[197]

Toxicity

The primary toxicity of HU is myelosuppression, which results from inhibition of DNA synthesis in bone marrow, and produces megaloblastic changes in granulocyte and erythroid precursors within 48 hours of the first dose. In patients with nonhematologic malignancies, the peripheral white blood cell count begins to fall in 2 to 5 days, while in patients with leukemia or myeloproliferative syndromes, the white blood cell count falls within 24 to 48 hours. The rapidity of the effect on the circulating leukemia cell population forms basis for the use of HU in patients with acute myelogenous leukemia who present with markedly elevated peripheral blood blast counts, or in patients with dangerously elevated platelet counts, as in cases of ET.

Patients with nonleukemic bone marrow receiving doses of 80 mg/kg/d become leukopenic within 14 days, whereas the incidence is 70% for patients receiving half that dose. Intermittent, doses decrease the severity of hematologic toxicity. Treatment of the myeloproliferative syndromes usually begins with much lower dosages of 0.5 to 2.0 g/d, while sickle cell patients usually begin treatment with 15 mg/kg/d.[150]

The gastrointestinal side effects of nausea, vomiting, anorexia, and either diarrhea or constipation rarely require discontinuation of therapy at the usual doses. Oral mucositis and ulceration of the gastrointestinal tract are less common but become symptomatic in patients receiving concomitant radiation and HU, as compared to those receiving either therapy alone.

Patients who have taken HU for an extended period may develop one of several dermatologic changes, including hyperpigmentation, acral keratosis, erythema of the face and hands, a more diffuse maculopapular rash, or dry skin with atrophy.[198] Evidence of leukocytoclastic vasculitis may be found on biopsy of skin lesions.[199] Changes in the nails may include atrophy or the formation of multiple pigmented nail bands. Skin lesions may ulcerate, and may resemble lichen planus.[200] Painful, extensive skin ulcerations, usually on the legs, may necessitate drug discontinuation in patients undergoing long-term treatment for myeloproliferative diseases.[201] Patients receiving HU seem to have an increased tissue reaction to irradiation and may have a recurrence or "recall" of erythema or hyperpigmentation in previously irradiated areas.[202] There have been scattered single case reports of amyopathic dermatomyositis in patients receiving HU for MDPs. Alopecia rarely occurs.

Other, less frequent, drug-related effects have been reported anecdotally in patients on long-term regimens. Transient abnormalities of renal function have been noted, including elevations of serum urea nitrogen and creatinine, and proteinuria. Liver function test abnormalities may become significant, and occasionally progress to clinical jaundice.[203] Acute interstitial lung disease and alveolitis[204] and drug-induced fever have also been reported, but are rarely seen in patients receiving short-term HU to lower leukemic blood counts.[205]

Of particular concern are potential effects on growth, development, and mutagenesis (teratogenic and carcinogenic sequelae) in patients with nonmalignant diseases, who frequently need long-term drug administration. To date, no growth failures or chronic organ damage has been observed in children with sickle cell disease who are treated with HU.[206] The risk of leukemic transformation does not appear to be increased in myeloproliferative diseases treated with HU. Among sickle cell patients treated with HU, there have been anecdotal case reports of leukemias, but no convincing evidence of an increased risk.[150] Squamous carcinomas of the skin, a known complication of immunosuppression, are seen in patients with malignant disease receiving chronic HU, although a detailed evaluation of immune function and response to vaccines in children on HU disclosed no impairment.[207]

HU is a potent teratogen in all animal species tested thus; it should not be used in women of childbearing age unless interventions to prevent pregnancy are employed. However, a few patients who conceived while receiving HU completed normal pregnancies after discontinuation of the drug.[208]

References

1. Burchenal JH, Murphy ML, Ellison RR, et al. Clinical evaluation of a new antimetabolite, 6-mercaptopurine, in the treatment of leukemia and allied diseases. *Blood.* 1953;8:965-999.

2. Sahasranaman S, Howard D, Roy S. Clinical pharmacology and pharmacogenetics of thiopurines. *Eur J Clin Pharmacol.* 2008;64:753-767.

3. Tidd DM, Patterson ARP. Distinction between inhibition of purine nucleotide synthesis and the delayed cytotoxic reaction of 6-mercaptopurine. *Cancer Res.* 1974;34:733-737.

4. Sommerville L, Krynetski E, Krynetskaia N, et al. Structure and dynamics of thioguanine-modified duplex DNA. *J Biol Chem.* 2003;278:1005-1011.

5. Swann PF, Waters TR, Moulton DC, et al. Role of postreplicative DNA mismatch repair in the cytotoxic action of thioguanine. *Science.* 1996;273:1109-1011.

6. Dervieux T, Blanco JG, Krynetcki EY, et al. Differing contribution of thiopurine methyltransferase to mercaptopurine versus thioguanine effects in human leukemic cells. *Cancer Res.* 2001;61:5810-5816.

7. Erb N, Harms DO, Janka-Schaab G. Pharmacokinetics and metabolism of thiopurines in children with ALL receiving 6-thioguanine versus 6-mercaptopurine. *Cancer Chemother Pharmacol.* 1998;42:266-272.

8. Tiede I, Fritz G, Stand S, et al. C28-dependent RAC activation is the molecular target of azathioprine in primary human CD4 T lymphocytes. *J Clin Invest.* 2003;111:1133-1145.

9. Lavi L, Holcenberg JS. A rapid sensitive high performance liquid chromatography assay for 6-mercaptopurine metabolites in red blood cells. *Anal Biochem.* 1985;144:514-521.

10. Zimm S, Collins JM, Riccardi R, et al. Variable bioavailability of oral mercaptopurine. Is maintenance chemotherapy in ALL being optimally delivered? *N Engl J Med.* 1983;308:1005-1009.

11. Arndt CAS, Balis FM, McCully CL, et al. Bioavailability of low-dose vs high-dose 6-mercaptopurine. *Clin Pharmacol Ther.* 1988;43:588-591.

12. Jacqz-Aigrain E, Nafa S, Medard Y, et al. Pharmacokinetics and distribution of 6-mercaptopurine administered intravenously in children with lymphoblastic leukemia. *Eur J Clin Pharmacol.* 1997;53:71-74.

13. Balis FM, Holcenberg JS, Zimm S, et al. The effect of methotrexate on the bioavailability of oral 6-mercaptopurine. *Clin Pharmacol Ther.* 1987;41:384-387.

14. Balis FM, Holcenberg JS, Poplack DG, et al. Pharmacokinetics and pharmacodynamics of oral methotrexate and mercaptopurine in children with lower risk ALL; a joint Children's Cancer Group and Pediatric Oncology Branch study. *Blood.* 1998;92:3569-3577.

15. Zimm S, Collins JM, O'Neill D, et al. Chemotherapy: inhibition of first-pass metabolism in cancer interaction of 6-mercaptopurine and allopurinol. *Clin Pharmacol Ther.* 1983;34:810-817.

16. Zimm S, Ettinger LJ, Holcenberg JS, et al. Phase I and clinical pharmacological study of mercaptopurine administered as a prolonged intravenous infusion. *Cancer Res.* 1985;45:1869-1873.

17. Lafolie P, Hayder S, Bjork O, et al. Intraindividual variation in 6-mercaptopurine pharmacokinetics during oral maintenance therapy of children with ALL. *Eur J Clin Pharmacol.* 1991;40:599-601.

18. Burton NK, Barnett MJ, Aherne GW, et al. The affect of food on the oral administration of 6-mercaptopurine. *Cancer Chemother Pharmacol.* 1986;18:90-91.

19. Schaeffeler E, Fisher C, Brockmeirer D, et al. Comprehensive analysis of thiopurine S-methyltransferase phenotype-genotype correlation in a large population of German-Caucasians, and identification of novel TMPT variants. *Pharmacogenetics.* 2004;14:407-414.

20. Weinshilboum RM. Methyltransferase pharmacogenetics. *Pharmacol Ther.* 1989;43:77-90.

21. Tai HL, Krynetski EY, Schueta EG, et al. Enhanced proteolysis of thiopurine S-methyltransferase (TMPT) encoded by mutant alleles in humans (TPMT*3a, TPMT*2) mechanisms for the genetic polymorphism of TMPT activity. *Proc Natl Acad Sci.* 1997;94:6444-6449.

22. Coulthard SA, Howell C, Robson J, et al. The relationship between thiopurine methyltransferase activity and genotype in blasts from patients with acute leukemia. *Blood.* 1998;92:2856-2862.

23. Yates CR, Krynetski EY, Loennechen T, et al. Molecular diagnosis of thiopurine 5-methylltransferase deficiency: genetic basis for azathioprine and mercaptopurine intolerance. *Ann Intern Med.* 1997;126:608-614.

24. Schmiegelow K, Forestie E, Kristinsson J, et al. Thiopurine methyltransferase activity is related to the risk of relapse of childhood acute lymphoblastic leukemia. *Leukemia.* 2009;23:557-564.

25. McLeod HL, Siva C. The thiopurine S-methyltransferase gene locus—implication for clinical pharmacogenomics. *Pharmacogenomics.* 2002;3:89-98.

26. Koren G, Ferrazini G, Sulh H, et al. Systemic exposures to mercaptopurine as a prognostic factor in acute lymphocytic leukemia. *N Engl J Med.* 1990;323:17-21.

27. Lennard L, Lilleyman JS, Van Loon JA, et al. Genetic variation in response to 6-mercaptopurine for childhood acute lymphoblastic leukemia. *Lancet.* 1991;336:225-229.

28. Evans WE, Hon YY, Bomgaars L, et al. Preponderance of thiopurine S-methyltransferase deficiency and heterozygosity among patients intolerant to mercaptopurine or azathioprine. *J Clin Oncol.* 2001;19:2293-2301.

29. Marsh S, Van Booven DJ. The increasing complexity of mercaptopurine pharmacogenetics. *Clin Pharmacol Ther.* 2009;85:139-141.

30. Stoco G, Cheok MH, Crews KR, et al. Genetic polymorphism of inosine triphosphate pyrophosphatase is a determinant of mercaptopurine metabolism and toxicity during treatment of acute lymphoblastic leukemia. *Clin Pharmacol Ther.* 2009;85:164-171.

31. Bhatia S, et al. Nonadherence to oral mercaptopurine and risk of relapse in Hispanic and non-Hispanic white children with acute lymphoblastic leukemia: a report from the children's oncology group. *J Clin Oncol.* 2012;30:2094-2101.

32. Tzoneva G, Perez-Garcia A, Carpenter Z, et al. Activating mutations in the NT5C2 nucleotidase gene drive chemotherapy resistance in relapsed ALL. *Nature.* 2013;19:368-373.

33. Gisbert JP, Gonzalez-Lama Y, Mate J. Thiopurine-induced liver injury in patients with inflammatory bowel disease: a systemic review. *Am J Gastroenterol.* 2007;102:1518-1527.

34. Gearry RB, Barclay ML, Burt MJ, et al. Thiopurine 5-methltransferase (TPMT) gene type does not predict adverse drug reactions to thiopurine drugs in patients with inflammatory bowel disease. *Aliment Pharmacol Ther.* 2003;18:395-400.

35. Nygaard U, Toft N, Schmiegelow K. Methylated metabolites of 6-mercaptopurine are associated with hepatotoxicity. *Clin Pharmacol Ther.* 2004;75:274-281.

36. Duttera MJ, Caralla RL, Gallelli JF. Hematuria and crystalluria after high-dose 6-mercaptopurine administration. *N Engl J Med.* 1972;287:292-294.

37. Schmiegelow K, Al-Modhwahi I, Andersen MK, et al. Methotrexate/6-mercaptopurine maintenance therapy influences the risk of a second malignant neoplasm after childhood acute lymphoblastic leukemia: results from the NOPHO ALL-92 study. *Blood.* 2009;113:6077-6084.

38. Kennedy DT, Hayney MS, Lake KD. Azathioprine and allopurinol: the price of an avoidable drug interaction. *Ann Pharmacother.* 1996;30:951-954.

39. Lowry PW, Franklin CL, Weaver AL, et al. Leucopenia resulting from a drug interaction between azathioprine or 6-mercaptopurine and mesalamine, sulphasalazine or balsalazide. *Gut.* 2001;49:656-662.

40. Guolo F, Minetto P, Clavio M, et al. Intensive fludarabine-high dose cytarabine-idarubicin combination as induction therapy with risk-adapted consolidation may improve treatment efficacy in younger acute myeloid leukemia (AML) patients: rational, evidences and future perspectives. *Biosci Trends.* 2017;11:110-114.

41. Adkins JC, Peters DH, Markham A. Fludarabine. an update of its pharmacology and use in the treatment of haematological malignancies. *Drugs.* 1997;53:1005-1037.

42. Molina-Arcas M, Bellosillo B, Casado FJ, et al. Fludarabine uptake mechanisms in B-cell chronic lymphocytic leukemia. *Blood.* 2003;101:2328-2334.

43. Kamiiya K, Huang P, Plunkett W. Inhibition of the 3'-5' exonucleases of human DNA polymerase epsilon by fludarabine-terminated DNA. *J Biol Chem.* 1996;271:19428-19435.

44. Pettitt A. Mechanism of action of purine analogs in chronic lymphocytic leukemia. *Br J Haematol.* 2003;121:692-702.

45. Wisitpittyaha S, Zhao Y, Long M, et al. Cladribine and fludarabine nucleotides induce distinct hexamers defining a common mode of reversible RNR inhibition. *ACS Chem Biol.* 2016;11:2021-2032.

46. Plunkett W, Begleiter A, Liliemark O, et al. Why do drugs work in CLL? *Leuk Lymphoma.* 1996;22(suppl 2):1-11.

47. Sandoval A, Consoli U, Plunkett W. Fludarabine-mediated inhibition of nucleotide excision repair induces apoptosis in quiescent human lymphocytes. *Clin Cancer Res.* 1996;2:1731-1741.

48. Thompson P, Tam C, O'Brien S, et al. Fludarabine, cyclophosphamide, and rituximab treatment achieves long-term disease-free survival in *IGHV*-mutated chronic lymphocytic leukemia. *Blood.* 2016;127:303-309.

49. Danhauser L, Plunkett W, Liliemark J, et al. Comparison between the plasma and intracellular pharmacology of 1-beta-D-arabinofuranosylcytosine and 9-beta-D-arabinofuranosyl-2-fluoroadenine 5′-monophosphate in patients with relapsed leukemia. *Leukemia.* 1987;1:638-643.

50. Gandhi V, Plunkett W. Cellular and clinical pharmacology of fludarabine. *Clin Pharmacokinet.* 2002;41:93-103.

51. Gandhi V, Estey E, Du M, et al. Maximum dose of fludarabine for maximal modulation of arabinosyl-cytosine triphosphate in human leukemic blast cells during therapy. *Clin Cancer Res.* 1997;3:1539-1545.

52. Danhauser L, Plunkett W, Keating M, et al. 9-beta-D-arabinofuranosyl=2-fluoroadenine 5′monophosphate pharmacokinetics in plasma and tumor cells of patients with relapsed leukemia and lymphoma. *Cancer Chemother Pharmacol.* 1986;18:145-152.

53. Lichtman SM, Etcubanas E, Budman D, et al. The pharmacokinetics and pharmacodynamics of fludarabine phosphate in patients with renal impairment: a perspective dose adjustment study. *Cancer Invest.* 2002;20:904-913.

54. Aronoff GR, Bennett WM, Berns JS, et al. *Drug Prescribing in Renal Failure: Dosing Guidelines for Adults and Children.* 5th ed. Philadelphia, PA: American College of Physicians; 2007.

55. Posker GL, Figgitt DP. Oral fludarabine. *Drugs.* 2003;63:2317-2323.

56. Oscier D, Orchard JA, Culligan D, et al. The bioavailability of oral fludarabine phosphate is unaffected by food. *Hematol J.* 2001;2:316-321.

57. Mortell RE, Peterson BL, Cohen HJ, et al. Analysis of age, estimated creatinine clearance and pretreatment hematologic parameters as predictors of fludarabine toxicity in patients treated for chronic lymphocytic leukemia. *Cancer Chemother Pharmacol.* 2002;50:37-45.

58. Byrd JC, Peterson BL, Morrison VA, et al. Randomized Phase II study of fludarabine with concurrent versus sequential treatment with rituximab in symptomatic untreated patients with B-cell chronic lymphocytic leukemia: results from the CALGB 9712. *Blood.* 2003;101:6-14.

59. Anaissie EJ, Kontoyiannis DP, O'Brien S, et al. Infections in patients with chronic lymphocytic leukemia treated with fludarabine. *Ann Intern Med.* 1998;129:559-566.

60. Frank DA, Mahajan S, Ritz J. Fludarabine-induced immunosuppression is associated with inhibitor of STAT 1 signaling. *Nat Med.* 1999;5:444-447.

61. Keating MJ, O'Brien S, Lerner S, et al. Long-term follow-up of patients with chronic lymphocytic leukemia (CLL) receiving fludarabine regimens as initial therapy. *Blood.* 1998;92:1165-1171.

62. Weiss RB, Freiman J, Kweder SL, et al. Hemolytic anemia after fludarabine therapy for chronic lymphocytic leukemia. *J Clin Oncol.* 1998;16:1885-1889.

63. Cheson BD, Frame JN, Vena D, et al. Tumor lysis syndrome: an uncommon complication of fludarabine therapy of chronic lymphocytic leukemia. *J Clin Oncol.* 1998;16:2313-2320.

64. Cheson BD, Vena DA, Foss FM, et al. Neurotoxicity of purine analogs: a review. *J Clin Oncol.* 1994;12:2216-2228.

65. Helman DL, Byrd JL, Alex NC, et al. Fludarabine-related pulmonary toxicity: a distinct clinical entity in chronic lymphoproliferative syndromes. *Chest.* 2002;127:785-790.

66. Ogawa Y, Hotta T, Watanabe K, et al. Phase I and pharmacokinetic study of oral fludarabine phosphate in relapsed indolent B-cell non-Hodgkin's lymphoma. *Ann Oncol.* 2006;17:330-333.

67. Tam CS, O'Brien S, Wierda W, et al. Long-term results of the fludarabine, cyclophosphamide, and rituximab regimen as initial therapy of chronic lymphocytic leukemia. *Blood.* 2008;112:975-980.

68. Bachow S, Lamanna N. Evolving strategies for the treatment of chronic lymphocytic leukemia in the upfront setting. *Curr Hematol Malig Rep.* 2016;11:61-70.

69. Sanghavi K, Wiseman A, Kirstein M, et al. Personalized fludarabine dosing to reduce nonrelapse mortality in hematopoietic stem-cell transplant recipients receiving reduced intensity conditioning. *Transl Res.* 2016;175:103-115.

70. Saini L, Brandwein J, Turner R, et al. The fludarabine, cytarabine, and granulocyte colony-stimulating factor (FLAG) chemotherapy regimen is an alternative to anthracycline-based therapy for the treatment of acute myeloid leukemia for patients with pre-existing cardiac disease. *Eur J Haematol.* 2016;97:471-478.

71. Jabbour E, Short NJ, Ravandi F, et al. A randomized phase 2 study of idarubicin and cytarabine with clofarabine or fludarabine in patients with newly diagnosed acute myeloid leukemia. *Cancer.* 2017;123:4430-4439. doi:10.1002/cncr.30883.

72. Agarwal RP. Inhibitors of adenosine deaminase. *Pharmacol Ther.* 1982;17:399-429.

73. O'Dwyer PJ, Wagner B, Leyland-Jones B, et al. 2′-Deoxycoformycin (Pentostatin) for lymphoid malignancies. *Ann Intern Med.* 1988;108:733-743.

74. Wiley JS, Smith CL, Jamieson GP. Transport of 2′deoxycoformycin in human leukemic and lymphoma cells. *Biochem Pharmacol.* 1991;42:708-710.

75. Johnston JB, Glazer RI, Pugh L, et al. The treatment of hairy-cell leukemia with 2′-deoxycoformycin. *Br J Haematol.* 1986;63:525-534.

76. Al-Razzak KA, Benedetti AE, Waugh WN, et al. Chemical stability of pentostatin (NSC-218321), a cytotoxic and immunosuppressant agent. *Pharm Res.* 1990;7:452-460.

77. Kane BJ, Kuhn JG, Roush MK. Pentostatin: an adenosine deaminase inhibitor for the treatment of hairy cell leukemia. *Ann Pharmacother.* 1992;26:939-946.

78. Major PP, Hgarwal RP, Kufe DW. Clinical pharmacology of deoxycoformycin. *Blood.* 1981;58:91-96.

79. Smyth JF, Paine RM, Jackman AL, et al. The clinical pharmacology of the adenosine deaminase inhibitor 2′deoxycorformycin. *Cancer Chemother Pharmacol.* 1980;5:93-101.

80. Lathia C, Fleming G, Mayer M, et al. Pentostatin pharmacokinetics and dosing recommendations in patients with mild renal impairment. *Cancer Chemother Pharmacol.* 2002;50:121-126.

81. Major PP, Agarwal RP, Kufe DW. Deoxycoformycin: neurological toxicity. *Cancer Chemother Pharmacol.* 1981;5:193-196.

82. Margolis J, Grever MR. Pentostatin; nipent: a review of potential toxicity and its management. *Semin Oncol.* 2000;27(2 suppl 5):9-14.

83. Grever M, Kopecky K, Foucar MK, et al. Randomized comparison of pentostatin versus interferon alfa 2A in previously untreated patients with hairy cell leukemia: an intergroup study. *J Clin Oncol.* 1995;13:974-982.

84. Grem JL, King SA, Chun HG, et al. Cardiac complications observed in elderly patients following 2′deoxycoformycin therapy. *Am J Hematol.* 1991;38:245-247.

85. Samonis G, Kontoyiannis DP. Infectious complications of purine analog therapy. *Curr Opin Infect Dis.* 2001;14:409-413.

86. Flinn IW, Kopecky KJ, Foucar MK, et al. Long-term follow-up of remission duration mortality and second malignancy in hairy cell leukemia patients treated with pentostatin. *Blood.* 2000;96:2981-2986.

87. Ho AD, Hensel M. Pentostatin for the treatment of indolent lymphoproliferative disorders. *Semin Hematol.* 2006;43S:S2-S10.

88. Jacobson DA, Chen AR, Zahurak M, et al. Phase II study of pentostatin in patients with corticosteroid-refractory chronic graft-versus-host disease. *J Clin Oncol.* 2007;25:4255-4261.

89. Kawasaki H, Carrera CJ, Piro LO, et al. Relationship of deoxycytidine kinase and cytoplasmic 5′ nucleotidase to the chemotherapeutic efficacy of 2-chlorodeoxyadenosine. *Blood.* 1993;81:597-601.

90. Parker W. Enzymology of purine and pyrimidine antimetabolites used in the treatment of cancer. *Chem Rev.* 2009;109:2880-2893.

91. Hartman WR, Hantosh P. The antileukemic drug 2-chlorodeoxyadenosine: an intrinsic transcription antagonist. *Mol Pharmacol.* 2004;65:227-234.

92. Hentosh P, Kools R, Blakley RL. Incorporation of 2-halogen-2′-deoxyadenosine 5-triphosphates into DNA during replication by human polymerases alpha and beta. *J Biol Chem.* 1990;265:4033-4040.

93. Ceruti S, Beltrami E, Matarrese P, et al. A key role for caspase-2 and caspase-3 in apoptosis induced by 2′chloro-2-deoxyadenosine (cladribine) and 2-chloro adenosine in human astrocytoma cells. *Mol Pharmacol.* 2003;63:1437-1447.

94. Leoni LM, Chao Q, Cottam HB, et al. Induction of an apoptotic program in cell free extracts by 2-chloro-2′deoxyadenosine 5′ triphosphate and cytochrome C. *Proc Natl Acad Sci U S A.* 1998;95:9567-9571.

95. Mansson E, Spaskoukoskaja T, Sallstrom J, et al. Molecular and biochemical mechanisms of fludarabine and cladribine resistance in a human promyelo-cytic cell line. _Cancer Res._ 1999;59:5956-5963.

96. Galnarini CM, Voorzanger N, Faletten N, et al. Influence of P53 and P21 (WAFI) expression on sensitivity of cancer cells to cladribine. _Biochem Pharmacol._ 2003;65:121-129.

97. Lindemalm S, Lilemark I, Julinsson G, et al. Cytotoxicity and pharmacokinetic of cladribine metabolite 2-chloroadenine in patients with leukemia. _Cancer Lett._ 2004;210:171-177.

98. Liliemark J, Juliusson G. Cellular pharmacokinetics of 2-chloro-2'-deoxyadenosine nucleotides: comparison of intermittent and continuous intravenous infusion and subcutaneous and oral administration in leukemia patients. _Clin Cancer Res._ 1995;1:385-390.

99. Liliemark J. The clinical pharmacokinetics of cladribine. _Clin Pharmacokinet._ 1997;32:120-131.

100. Kearns CM, Blakley RL, Santana VM, et al. Pharmacokinetics of cladrib-ine (2-chlorodeoxyadenosine) in children with acute leukemia. _Cancer Res._ 1994;54:1235-1239.

101. Lilliemark J, Albertioni F, Hansen M, et al. On the bioavailability of oral and subcutaneous 2-chloro2'-deoxyadenosine in humans: alternative routes of administration. _J Clin Oncol._ 1992;10:1514-1518.

102. Zenhausern R, von Rohr A, Rufiback K, et al. Low dose 2-chlordeoxy-adenosine given as a single subcutaneous injection in patients with hairy cell leukemia: a multicentre trial SAKK 32/95. _Leuk Lymphoma._ 2009;50:133-136.

103. Juliusson G, Lilemark J. Purine analogs: rationale for development, mecha-nisms of action and pharmacokinetics in hairy cell leukemia. _Hematol Oncol Clin North Am._ 2006;20:1087-1097.

104. Piro LD, Carrera CJ, Carson DA, et al. Lasting remission in hairy-cell leu-kemia induced by a single infusion of 2-chlorodeoxyadenosine. _N Engl J Med._ 1990;322:1117-1121.

105. Betticher DC, von Rohr A, Ratschiller D, et al. Fewer infections, but main-tained antitumor activity with lower-dose vs standard-dose cladribine in pretreated low-grade non-Hodgkin's lymphoma. _J Clin Oncol._ 1998;16:850-858.

106. Robak T, Jamroziak K, Gore-Tybor J, et al. Cladribine in a weekly ver-sus daily schedule for untreated hairy cell leukemia: final report from the Polish Adult Leukemia Group (PALG) of a prospective, randomized, mul-ticenter trial. _Blood._ 2007;109:3672-3675.

107. Chadha P, Rademaker AW, Mendiratta P, et al. Treatment of hairy cell leu-kemia with 2-cholordeoxyadenosine (2-CdA): long-term follow-up of the Northwestern experience. _Blood._ 2005;106:241-246.

108. Getta B, Park J, Tallman M. Hairy cell leukemia: past present and future. _Best Pract Res Clin Haematol._ 2015;28:269-272.

109. Piro LD. 2-Chlorodeoxyadenosine treatment of lymphoid malignancies. _Blood._ 1992;79:843-845.

110. Inwards DJ, Fishkin PA, Hillman DW, et al. Long-term results of treat-ment of patients with mantle cell lymphoma with cladribine (2-CdA) alone or 2-CdA and rituximab in the North Central Cancer Treatment Group. _Cancer._ 2008;113:108-116.

111. Donadieu J, Bernard F, van Noesel M, et al. Cladribine and cytarabine in refractory multisystem Langerhans cell histiocytosis: results of an interna-tional phase 2 study. _Blood._ 2015;126:1415-1423.

112. Libora M, Giebel S, Platkowska-Jakubas B, et al. Cladribine added to dau-norubicin-cytarabine induction prolongs survival in FLT3-ITD+ normal karyotype AML patients. _Blood._ 2016;127:360-362.

113. Crews KR, Gandhi V, Srivostava DK, et al. Interim comparison of a con-tinuous infusion versus a short daily infusion of cytarabine given in combi-nation with cladribine for pediatric acute myeloid leukemia. _J Clin Oncol._ 2002;20:4217-4224.

114. Chubar Y, Bennett M. Cutaneous reactions in hairy cell leukemia treated with 2-chlorodeoxyadenosine and allopurinol. _Br J Haematol._ 2003;122:768-770.

115. Montgomery JA, Shortnay-Fowler AT, Clayton SD, et al. Synthesis and bio-logic activity of 2' fluoro 2 halo derivative of 9 beta D arabinofuranosylad-enine. _J Med Chem._ 1992;35:397-401.

116. Parker WB, Shaddix SC, Rose LM, et al. Comparison of the mechanisms of 2-choro-9-(2-deoxy-2-fluoro-β-D-arabinofuranosyl) adenine, of 2-chloro-9 (2-deoxy-2-fluoroβ-D ribofuranosyl adenine and of 2-cholor (2-deoxy-2,2difluoro-β-D-arabinosyl adenine in CEM cells. _Mol Pharmacol._ 1999;55:515-520.

117. Parker WB, Shaddix SC, Chang CH, et al. Effects of 2-cholor-9-(2 deoxy-2-fluoro-β-D arabinofuranosyl) adenine on K562 cellular metabolism and the inhibition of human ribonucleotide reductase and DNA polymerases by its 5'-triphosphate. _Cancer Res._ 1991;51:2386-2394.

118. Xie KC, Plunkett W. Deoxynucleotide pool depletion and sustained inhibition of ribonucleotide reductase and DNA synthesis after treat-ment of human lymphoblastoid cells with 2-chlor-(2-deoxy-fluoro-β-D-arabinofuranosyl) adenine. _Cancer Res._ 1996;56:3030-3037.

119. Gemini D, Adachi S, Chao Q, et al. Deoxyadenosine analogs induce pro-grammed cell death in chronic lymphocytes by damaging the DNA and by directly affecting the mitochondria. _Blood._ 2000;96:3537-3543.

120. Cooper T, Kantarjian H, Plunkett W, et al. Clofarabine in adult acute leuke-mias: clinical success and pharmacokinetics. _Nucleosides Nucleotides Nucleic Acids._ 2004;23:1417-1423.

121. Kantajarian H, Gandhi V, Kozuch P, et al. Phase I clinical and pharmaco-logic study of clofarabine in patients with solid tumors and hematologic cancers. _J Clin Oncol._ 2003;21:1167-1173.

122. Gandhi V, Plunkett W, Bonate PL, et al. Clinical and pharmacokinetic study of clofarabine in chronic lymphocytic leukemia: strategy for treatment. _Clin Cancer Res._ 2006;12:4011-4017.

123. Kantarjian H, Jehe S, Gandhi V, et al. Clofarabine: past present and future. _Leuk Lymphoma._ 2007;48:1922-1930.

124. Jeha S, Gaynon P, Razzouk B, et al. Phase II study of clofarabine in pediatric patients with refractory or relapsed acute lymphoblastic leukemia. _J Clin Oncol._ 2006;24:1917-1923.

125. Jhaven K, Chidella S, Allen S, Fishbane S. Clofarabine induced kidney toxic-ity. _J Oncol Pharm Pract._ 2014;20:305-308.

126. Faderk S, Ravandi F, Huang X, et al. A randomized study of clofarabine ver-sus clofarabine plus low-dose cytarabine as front-line therapy for patients aged 60 years and older with acute myeloid leukemia and high risk myelo-dysplasia. _Blood._ 2008;112:1638-1645.

127. Kadia TM, Gandhi V. Nelarabine in the treatment of pediatric and adult patients with T-cell acute lymphoblastic leukemia and lymphoma. _Expert Rev Hematol._ 2017;10:1-8.

128. Cohen A, Lee JW, Gelfand EW. Sensitivity of deoxyguanosine and arabino-syl guanine for T-leukemic cells. _Blood._ 1983;61:660-666.

129. DeAngelo DJ. Nelarabine for the treatment of patients with relapsed or refractory T-cell acute lymphoblastic leukemia or lymphoblastic lym-phoma. _Hematol Oncol Clin North Am._ 2009;23:1121-1135.

130. Rodriguez CO, Strellrecht CM, Gandhi V. Mechanisms for T-cell selective cytotoxicity of arabinosylguanine. _Blood._ 2003;102:1842-1848.

131. Gandhi V, Tam C, Jewel RC, et al. Phase I trial of nelarabine in indolent leukemias. _J Clin Oncol._ 2008;26:1098-1105.

132. Kisor DF, Plunkett W, Kurtzberg J, et al. Pharmacokinetics of nelarabine and 9-β-D-arabinofuranosyl guanine in pediatric and adult patients during a phase I study of nelarabine for the treatment of refractory hematologic malignancies. _J Clin Oncol._ 2000;18:995-1003.

133. Sanford M, Lyseng-Williamson A. Nelarabine. _Drugs._ 2008;68:439-447.

134. Buie LW, Epstein SS, Lindley CM. Nelarabine: a novel purine antimetabo-lite antineoplastic agent. _Clin Ther._ 2007;29:1887-1899.

135. Gandhi V, Plunkett W, Weller S, et al. Evaluation of the combination of nelarabine and fludarabine in leukemias: clinical response, pharmacoki-netics and pharmacodynamics in leukemia cells. _J Clin Oncol._ 2001;19:2142-2152.

136. Kurtzberg J, Ernst TJ, Keating MJ, et al. Phase I study of 506U78 administer on a consecutive 5-day schedule in children and adults with refractory malignancies. _J Clin Oncol._ 2000;18:995-1003.

137. Lalayanni C, Baldoumi E, Papayiannolpoulos S, et al. Nelarabine-associated reversible Guillain-Barre-like syndrome or myelopathy in an adult patient with primary refractory T-lymphoblastic lymphoma. _Curr Probl Cancer._ 2017;41:138-143.

138. Gollard R, Selco S. Irreversible myelopathy associated with nelarabine In T-cell acute lymphoblastic leukemia. _J Clin Oncol._ 2013;19:e327-e331.

139. DeAngelo DJ, Yu D, Johnson JL, et al. Nelarabine induces complete remis-sions in adults with relapsed or refractory T-linage acute lymphoblastic leu-kemia or lymphoblastic lymphoma: a Cancer and Leukemia Group B study. _Blood._ 2007;109:5136-5142.

140. Dresler WFC, Stein R. Uber den Hydroxylharnstoff. _Justus Liebigs Ann Chem._ 1869;150:242-252.

141. Rosenthal F, Wislicki L, Koller L. Uber die Beziehungen von schwersten Blutgiften zu Abbauprodukten des Eiweisses: ein Beitrag zum Entstehungmechanismus der pernizosen Anemie. *Klin Wochenschr.* 1928;7:972-977.

142. Tarnowski GS, Stock CC. Chemotherapy studies on the RC and S790 mouse mammary carcinomas. *Cancer Res.* 1958;18:201.

143. Finch RA, Liu MC, Cory AH, et al. Triapine (3-aminopyridine-2-carboxaldehyde thiosemicarbazone; 3-AP): an inhibitor of ribonucleotide reductase with antineoplastic activity. *Adv Enzyme Regul.* 1999;39:3-12.

144. Yakar D, Holland JF, Ellison RR, et al. Clinical pharmacological trial of guanazole. *Cancer Res.* 1973;33:972-975.

145. Frutchman SM, Mack K, Kaplan ME, et al. From efficacy to safety: a Polycythemia Vera Study Group Report on hydroxyurea in patients with polycythemia vera. *Semin Hematol.* 1997;34:17-23.

146. Cortelazzo S, Finazzi G, Ruggieri M, et al. Hydroxyurea for patients with essential thrombocythemia and a high risk of thrombosis. *N Engl J Med.* 1995;332:1126-1136.

147. Geyer HL, Mesa RA. Therapy for myeloproliferative neoplasms: when, which agent, and how? *Blood.* 2014;124:3529-3537.

148. Murphy S, Peterson P, Iland H, et al. Experience of the Polycythemia Vera Study Group with essential thrombocythemia: a final report on diagnostic criteria, survival, and leukemic transition to treatment. *Semin Hematol.* 1997;34:29-39.

149. Harrison C, Liladjian JJ, Al-Ali HK, et al. JAK inhibition with ruxolitinib versus best available therapy for myelofibrosis. *N Engl J Med.* 2012;366:787-798.

150. Azar S, Wong TE. Sickle cell disease. *Med Clin North Am.* 2017;101:375-393.

151. Platt OS. Hydroxyurea for the treatment of sickle cell anemia. *N Engl J Med.* 2008;358:1362-1369.

152. Charache S, Terrin ML, Moore RD, et al. Effects of hydroxyurea on the frequency of painful crises in sickle cell anemia. *N Engl J Med.* 1995;332:1317-1322.

153. Galanello R, Stamatoyannopoulos G, Papayannopoulou T. Mechanism of Hb F stimulation by S-stage compounds: in vitro studies with bone marrow cells exposed to 5-azacytidine, ARA-C, or hydroxyurea. *J Clin Invest.* 1988;81:1209-1216.

154. Adragna NC, Fonseca P, Lauf PK. Hydroxyurea affects cell morphology, cation transport, and red blood cell adhesion in cultured vascular endothelial cells. *Blood.* 1994;83:533-560.

155. Maiocchi SL, Morris JC, Thomas SR. Regulation of the nitric oxide oxidase activity of myeloperoxidase by pharmacological agents. *Biochem Pharmacol.* 2017;135:90-115.

156. Kinney TR, Helms RW, O'Branski EE, et al. Safety of hydroxyurea in children with sickle cell anemia: results of the HUG-KIDS study, a phase I/II trial. *Blood.* 1999;94:1550-1554.

157. Kosaryan M, Zafari M, Alipur A, et al. The effect and side effect of hydroxyurea therapy on Patients with β-thalassemia: a systematic review to December 2012. *Hemoglobin.* 2014;38:262-271.

158. Voskaridou E, Kalotychou V, Loukopoulos D. Clinical and laboratory effects of long-term administration of hydroxyurea to patients with sickle cell/b-thalassemia. *Br J Haematol.* 1995;89:479-484.

159. Thelander L, Reichard P. Reduction of ribonucleotides. *Annu Rev Biochem.* 1979;48:133-158.

160. Elford HL. Effect of hydroxyurea on ribonucleotide reductase. *Biochem Biophys Res Commun.* 1968;33:129-135.

161. Nicander B, Reichard P. Relations between synthesis of deoxyribonucleotides and DNA replication in 3T6 fibroblasts. *J Biol Chem.* 1986;260:5376-5381.

162. Thelander L, Erikson S, Akerman M. Ribonucleotide reductase from calf thymus. *J Biol Chem.* 1980;255:7426-7432.

163. Eriksson S, Thelander L, Akerman M. Allosteric regulation of calf thymus ribonucleotide diphosphate reductase. *Biochemistry.* 1979;18:2948-2952.

164. Cory JG, Fleischer AE, Munro JB III. Reconstitution of the ribonucleotide reductase in mammalian cells. *J Biol Chem.* 1978;253:2898-2901.

165. Mann GJ, Musgrove EA, Fox RM, et al. Ribonucleotide reductase M1 subunit in cellular proliferation, quiescence, and differentiation. *Cancer Res.* 1988;48:5151-5156.

166. Thelander M, Graslund A, Thelander L. Subunit M2 of mammalian ribonucleotide reductase. *J Biol Chem.* 1985;260:2737-2741.

167. Engstrom Y, Eriksson S, Jildevik I, et al. Cell cycle-dependent expression of mammalian ribonucleotide reductase. *J Biol Chem.* 1985;260:9114-9116.

168. Nyholm S, Thelander L, Graslund A. Reduction and loss of the iron center in the reaction of the small subunit of mouse ribonucleotide reductase with hydroxyurea. *Biochemistry.* 1993;32:11569-11574.

169. Satyamoorthy K, Chitnis M, Basrur V. Sensitization of P388 murine leukemia cells to hydroxyurea cytotoxicity by hydrophobic iron-chelating agents. *Anticancer Res.* 1986;6:329-333.

170. Moran RE, Straus MJ. Cytokinetic analysis of L1210 leukemia after continuous infusion of hydroxyurea in vivo. *Cancer Res.* 1979;39:1616-1622.

171. Cress AE, Gerner EW. Hydroxyurea inhibits ODC induction, but not the G1 to S-phase transition. *Biochem Biophys Res Commun.* 1979;87:773-780.

172. Cokic VP, Smith RD, Beleslin-Cokic BB, et al. Hydroxyurea induces fetal hemoglobin by the nitric oxide-dependent activation of soluble guanylyl cyclase. *J Clin Invest.* 2003;111(2):231-239.

173. Plucinski TM, Fager RS, Reddy GP. Allosteric interaction of components of the replitase complex is responsible for enzyme cross-inhibition. *Mol Pharmacol.* 1990;38:86-88.

174. Ying S, Chen Z, Medhurst A, et al. DNA-PKcs and PARP1 bind to unresected stalled DNA replication forks where they recruit XRCC1 to mediate repair. *Cancer Res.* 2018;76:1078-1088.

175. Kim TM, Son MIY, Dodds S, et al. Deletion of BRCA2 exon 27 causes defects in response to both stalled and collapsed replication forks. *Mutat Res.* 2014;766-767:66-72.

176. Von Hoff DD, Waddelow T, Forseth B, et al. Hydroxyurea accelerates loss of extrachromosomally amplified genes from tumor cells. *Cancer Res.* 1991;51:6273-6279.

177. Nevaldine BH, Rizwana R, Hahn PJ. Differential sensitivity of double minute chromosomes to hydroxyurea treatment in cultured methotrexate-resistant mouse cells. *Mutat Res.* 1999;406:55-62.

178. McClarty GA, Tonin PN, Srinivasan PR, et al. Relationships between reversion of hydroxyurea resistance in hamster cells and the coamplification of ribonucleotide reductase M2 component, ornithine decarboxylase and P5-8 genes. *Biochem Biophys Res Commun.* 1988;154:975-981.

179. Zhou BS, Hsu NY, Pan BC, et al. Overexpression of ribonucleotide reductase in transfected human KB cells increases their resistance to hydroxyurea: M2 but not M1 is sufficient to increase resistance to hydroxyurea in transfected cells. *Cancer Res.* 1995;55:1328-1333.

180. Choy BK, McClarty GA, Chan AK, et al. Molecular mechanisms of drug resistance involving ribonucleotide reductase: hydroxyurea resistance in a series of clonally related mouse cell lines selected in the presence of increasing drug concentrations. *Cancer Res.* 1988;48:7524-7531.

181. Abid MR, Li Y, Anthony C, et al. Translational regulation of ribonucleotide reductase by eukaryotic initiation factor 4E protein synthesis to the control of DNA replication. *J Biol Chem.* 1999;274:35991-35998.

182. Wong SJ, Myette M, Wereley JP, et al. Increased sensitivity of hydroxyurea-resistant leukemic cells to gemcitabine. *Clin Cancer Res.* 1999;5:439-453.

183. Yen Y, Grill SP, Dutschman GE, et al. Characterization of a hydroxyurea-resistant human KB cell line with supersensitivity to 6-thioguanine. *Cancer Res.* 1994;54:3689-3691.

184. Kubota M, Takimoto T, Tanizawa A, et al. Differential modulation of 1-β-D-arabinofuranosylcytosine metabolism by hydroxyurea in human leukemic cell lines. *Biochem Pharmacol.* 1988;37:1745-1749.

185. Robichaud NJ, Fram RJ. Potentiation of ara-C induced cytotoxicity by hydroxyurea in LoVo colon carcinoma cells. *Biochem Pharmacol.* 1987;36:1673-1677.

186. Schilsky RL, Ratain MJ, Vokes EE, et al. Laboratory and clinical studies of biochemical modulation by hydroxyurea. *Semin Oncol.* 1992;19:84-89.

187. Creasey WA, Capizzi RL, DeConti RC. Clinical and biochemical studies of high-dose intermittent therapy of solid tumors with hydroxyurea. *Cancer Chemother Rep.* 1970;54:191-194.

188. Tracewell WG, Trump DL, Vaughan WP, et al. Population pharmacokinetics of hydroxyurea in cancer patients. *Cancer Chemother Pharmacol.* 1995;35:417-422.

189. Dong M, McGann PT, Mizuno T, et al. Development of a pharmacokinetic-guided dose individualization strategy for hydroxyurea treatment in children with sickle cell anemia. *Br J Clin Pharmacol.* 2016;81:742-752.

190. Estepp JH, Melloni C, Thornburg CD, et al. Pharmacokinetics and bioequivalence of a liquid formulation of hydroxyurea in children with sickle cell anemia. *J Clin Pharmacol.* 2016;56:298-306.

191. Veale D, Cantwell BM, Kerr N, et al. Phase I study of high-dose hydroxy-urea in lung cancer. *Cancer Chemother Pharmacol.* 1988;1:53-56.

192. Rodriguez GI, Kuhn JG, Weiss GR, et al. A bioavailability and pharmacoki-netic study of oral and intravenous hydroxyurea. *Blood.* 1998;91:1533-1541.

193. Blumenreich MS, Kellihan MJ, Joseph UG, et al. Long-term intravenous hydroxyurea infusions in patients with advanced cancer: a phase I trial. *Cancer.* 1993;71:2828-2832.

194. Fishbein WN, Carbone PP. Hydroxyurea: mechanism of action. *Science.* 1963;142:1069-1070.

195. Adamson RH, Ague SL, Hess SM, et al. The distribution, excretion, and metabolism of hydroxyurea-14C. *J Pharmacol Exp Ther.* 1965;150:322-334.

196. Colvin M, Bono VH Jr. The enzymatic reduction of hydroxyurea to urea by mouse liver. *Cancer Res.* 1970;30:1516-1519.

197. Beckloff GL, Lerner HJ, Frost D, et al. Hydroxyurea in biological fluids: dose concentration relationship. *Cancer Chemother Rep.* 1963;48:57-58.

198. Kennedy BJ, Smith LR, Goltz RW. Skin changes secondary to hydroxyurea. *Arch Dermatol.* 1975;111:183-187.

199. Worley B, Glassman SJ. Acral ketatosis and leucocytoclastic vasculitis occurring during treatment of essential thrombocythaemia with hydroxy-urea. *Clin Exp Dermatol.* 2016;41:166-169.

200. Renfro L, Kamino H, Raphael B, et al. Ulcerative lichen planus-like der-matitis associated with hydroxyurea. *J Am Acad Dermatol.* 1991;24:143-145.

201. Sirieix ME, Debure C, Baudot N, et al. Leg ulcers and hydroxyurea: forty-one cases. *Arch Dermatol.* 1999;135:818-820.

202. Sears ME. Erythema in areas of previous irradiation in patients treated with hydroxyurea. *Cancer Chemother Rep.* 1965;40:31-32.

203. Heddle R, Calvert AF. Hydroxyurea-induced hepatitis. *Med J Aust.* 1980;1:121.

204. Kavuru MS, Gadsden T, Lichtin A, et al. Hydroxyurea-induced acute inter-stitial lung disease. *South Med J.* 1994;87:767-769.

205. Cheung AYC, Browne B, Capen C. Hydroxyurea-induced fever in cervical carcinoma: case report and review of the literature. *Cancer Invest.* 1999;17:245-248.

206. Rana S, Houston PE, Wang WC, et al. Hydroxyurea and growth in young children with sickle cell disease. *Pediatrics.* 2014;134:465-472.

207. Lederman HM, Connolly MA, Kalpathi R, et al. Immunologic effects of hydroxyurea in sickle cell anemia. *Pediatrics.* 2014;134:686-695.

208. Diav-Citrin O, Hunnisett L, Sher G, et al. Hydroxyurea use during preg-nancy: a case report in sickle cell disease and review of the literature. *Am J Hematol.* 1999;60:148-150.

Antimitotic Drugs

Cindy H. Chau, William D. Figg, and Bruce A. Chabner

Because of the central role of mictrotubules in cell division, antimicrotubule agents are highly effective constituents of most standard regimens for cancers.[1] Following the discovery of the antitumor activity of vinca alkaloids in the 1950s, the subsequent search for antimitotic drugs among natural sources yielded compounds displaying unique structure, and unique biochemical and clinical properties. Drugs such as the vinca alkaloids, taxanes, and eribulin were isolated from a variety of plant and animal sources, reflecting the importance of antimitotic strategies for self-defense. Adding to the success of antimitotic research, new formulations of antitubulin drugs have won marketing approval, including a nanoparticle form of vincristine for childhood leukemia[2] and antibody-antimitotic conjugates for lymphomas[3] and breast cancer.[4] Notwithstanding the success of microtubule inhibitors, attempts to target mitotic kinases and other cellular constituents that play critical roles in mitosis have not yet met with success.

Microtubule Structure

Microtubules are composed of two closely related peptides, which form a heterodimer of tightly linked α and β subunits.[1] The α- and β-tubulins contain approximately 450 amino acids with a molecular weight of 50 kDa and are encoded by a family of closely related genes.[5] When tubulin molecules assemble into microtubules, they form linear "protofilaments," which align side by side around a hollow central core. The β-subunit of one dimer lies head to tail in contact with the α-tubulin subunit of the next, as shown in Figure 11.1. Each microtubule is composed of 13 protofilaments, wound together in an imperfect helix. One turn of the helix contains 13 tubulin dimers, each from a different protofilament. These microtubules can grow and shrink by the addition or removal of subunits from their ends, a process governed by the hydrolysis of GTP and known as "dynamic instability." Because microtubules are composed of heterodimers, they are polarized, with α-tubulin exposed at the slow-growing *minus* end and β-tubulin at the *plus* end. A GTP cap at the plus end stabilizes the microtubule and prevents its disassembly. The addition and removal of subunits occurs most rapidly at the plus end, while net shortening occurs at the minus end.[6]

Microtubules are nucleated through attachment to centrioles at microtubule-organizing centers (MTOCs). Contained within the MTOC is another distinct subunit, γ-tubulin.[7] γ-Tubulin combines with several other associated proteins to form a circular structure known as the γ-tubulin ring complex. This complex serves as a scaffold for the polymerization of α/β-tubulin heterodimers into microtubules. The complex essentially *caps* the minus end, while microtubule growth continues away from MTOC in the plus direction.

Functional diversity of microtubules is achieved through their association with various regulatory proteins, particularly the microtubule-associated proteins (MAPs), through variations in tubulin isotype composition, and through posttranslational tubulin modifications, such as phosphorylation and acetylation.[8] The intrinsic dynamicity of microtubules is also influenced by the tubulin isotype composition, and the sensitivity of microtubules to both depolymerizing and polymerizing agents is also a function of the tubulin isotypes, their posttranslational modifications, and MAPs. There are multiple isotypes of α- and β-tubulins, each distinguished by different C-terminal amino acid sequences. Isotypes are encoded by a multigene family.

Modified regions of polymerized tubulin provide sites for the binding of MAPs, which regulate the dynamic behavior of cytoplasmic microtubules, generally by modifying GTP hydrolysis.[9] MAPs have two binding domains, one of which binds to microtubules and also to free tubulin molecules, facilitating the initial nucleation step of tubulin polymerization. The other domain links the microtubule to other cellular components, promoting movement. MAPs, such as the end-binding proteins, destabilize microtubules by promoting hydrolysis of GTP (Fig. 11.2). Other MAPs, the dyneins (GTPases) and kinesins (ATPases), transform chemical energy into mechanical sliding force and move solutes and subcellular organelles along microtubules. Dyneins move intracellular organelles away from the plus end, while kinesins move chromosomes, vesicles, and organelles in the opposite direction. Motor proteins, which play critical roles in mitosis, premeiotic events, and organelle transport, have become strategic targets for anticancer therapeutic development.[10]

Microtubule Function

The microtubules are principal components of the mitotic spindle that correctly separates, or segregates, the duplicate set of chromosomes into two daughter cells during cell division. The integrity of the mitotic spindle is required for cells to pass through various cell cycle checkpoints. Errors in chromosome segregation are recognized, activating checkpoint proteins that trigger programmed cell death or apoptosis.[11] The microtubules also play critical roles in many interphase functions such as maintaining cellular shape and serving as a scaffold for attachment and movement of cellular organelles, secretion, neurotransmission, and intracellular signaling.[12]

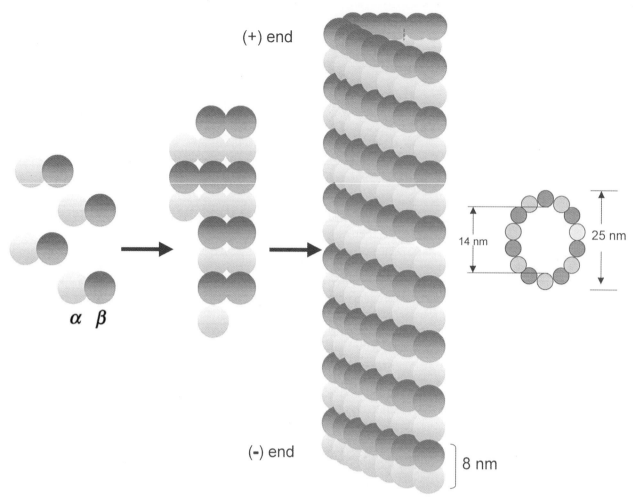

FIGURE **11.1** Microtubular structure. Heterodimers of α-tubulin and β-tubulin assemble to form a short microtubule nucleus. Nucleation is followed by elongation of the microtubule at both ends to form a cylinder that is composed of tubulin heterodimers arranged head to tail in 13 protofilaments. Net addition of heterodimers takes place at the plus (+) end, with β-tubulin facing the solvent, and a loss of dimers happens predominantly at the minus end (−).

FIGURE **11.2** Model for the effects of GTP hydrolysis on microtubular structure. The protofilaments that join to form a dynamically unstable microtubule (MT) are shown at the left, structure I. The highly stable MT-GTP (as mimicked experimentally by the analog GMPCPP) is shown in structure II. End-binding proteins (EBs) promote the hydrolysis of GTP and the release of Pi, destabilizing the microtubules. With the binding of end proteins and release of Mg^2, it enters a transition state, mimicked by the MT-GTPγS structure III, in which Pi is hydrolyzed, and the lattice undergoes compaction. In the next step, structure IV, Pi is released to leave MT-GDP, resulting in a twisted, strained, and unstable state. Taxane binding to β tubulin stabilizes the MT-GDP state. (From Zhang R, Alushin GM, Brown A, Nogales E. Mechanistic Origin of Microtubule Dynamic Instability and Its Modulation by EB Proteins. *Cell*. 2015;162:849-859, with permission.)

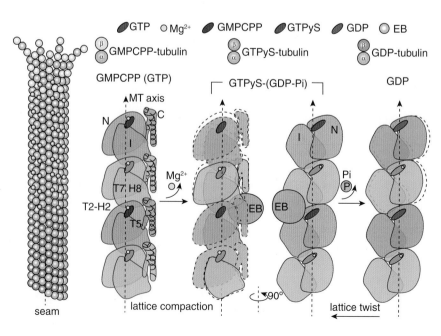

The unique functions of microtubules depend on their polymerization dynamics, created by a constantly shifting equilibrium between α-β-tubulin heterodimer subunits and microtubule polymers.[13] Tubulin polymerization occurs by a rapid elongation of the microtubule through the reversible, noncovalent addition of α-β-tubulin heterodimers, primarily at its plus end (Fig. 11.1). Microtubule assembly and disassembly are governed not only by the concentration of free tubulin but also by chemical mediators that promote assembly (e.g., Mg^{2+}, GTP) or disassembly (Ca^{2+}) and by the relative concentrations of GTP and GDP at critical points along the microtubule. Two processes are principally responsible for the unique functionality and dynamics of microtubules in the living cell. The first, known as *treadmilling*, is the continuous process of growth at one end of the microtubule and the shortening at the opposite end.[14] Treadmilling plays a role in many microtubule functions, most notably in the formation of the mitotic spindle and the polar movement and segregation of the chromosomes during the anaphase stage of mitosis. In the second dynamic process, known as *dynamic instability*, the plus ends of microtubules alternate between states of slow sustained growth and rapid shortening.[13] The minus end is bound tightly to the MTOC, which slows both assembly and disassembly of the subunits. The rate of dynamic instability accelerates during mitosis, enabling the mitotic spindle to grow, find and attach to chromosomes, and align chromosomes for proper cell division. These mechanisms are altered by MAPs, ion concentrations, tubulin isotypes, and posttranslational modifications.

The essential property of microtubules is their "dynamic instability," or the rapid switching between phases of growth and shrinkage.[6] Each tubulin dimer associates with two molecules of GTP; GTP bound to α-tubulin at N-site is nonexchangeable, whereas the other bound to β-tubulin at the E or exchangeable site can be hydrolyzed to GDP, which in turn can be replaced by a new GTP molecule. Free dimers readily exchange GDP for GTP, rendering them available for incorporation into protofilaments. At the plus end of the microtubule, the newly incorporated α-tubulin contacts the GTP of the terminal β tubulin and forms a pocket that promotes hydrolysis. Taxanes stabilize the microtubule in its GDP-bound state and prevent its exchange and microtubule disassembly.

Hydrolysis of GTP at the β-tubulin site is promoted by end-binding proteins and leads to compaction and twisting of the polymer, introducing tension to the microtubule and fueling the kinetic functions of the microtubule and its associated proteins[15] (Fig. 11.2). During elongation of the microtubule, GTP hydrolysis lags behind subunit addition, thus forming a "GTP cap" that stabilizes the plus end and promotes further extension of the polymer. However, when the rate of subunit addition decreases, hydrolysis catches up and the GTP cap is lost, promoting rapid depolymerization of the microtubule. The switch from growth to shrinkage is known as *catastrophe*, and the switch from shrinkage to growth is known as *rescue*. Although tubulin polymerization and dissociation occur simultaneously at each end, the net changes in length at the more kinetically dynamic plus end are much larger over time than those at the minus end.

As the cell enters mitosis and as the nuclear envelop breaks down and releases the now condensed chromosomes, the cell enters a phase of rapid reorganization of the microtubular apparatus. The microtubules of the interphase array disassemble and are replaced by a new population of mitotic spindle microtubules, which are much more dynamic and whose MTOCs are the newly duplicated centrosomes at each of the two poles of the cell.[16]

Dynamic instability and treadmilling are vital to the assembly and function of the newly formed mitotic spindle, in that they create significant energy for the precise alignment of the chromosomes and their attachment to the spindle during metaphase, as well as chromosome separation during anaphase. Although mitotic spindles can form in the presence of low concentrations of antimicrotubule agents, in some cells, mitosis cannot progress beyond the mitotic cell cycle checkpoint at the metaphase/anaphase transition, triggering apoptosis.[17] In others, "slippage" of multinucleated cells into the postmitotic interphase of the cell cycle occurs, with incompletely and inaccurately segregated chromosomes, leading to apoptosis.[17] "Slippage" may explain the activity of the taxanes and vinca alkaloids in slowly cycling solid tumors.

Vinca Alkaloids

The vinca alkaloids were originally discovered as products of the pink periwinkle plant *Catharanthus roseus* G. Don (formerly *Vinca rosea* Linn). The early folk medicinal uses of extracts of *C. roseus* for controlling hemorrhage, scurvy, toothache, and diabetes, and for the healing of chronic wounds led to the screening of these compounds for their hypoglycemic activity and then for anticancer properties.[18] The clinical efficacy of the naturally occurring vinca alkaloids vincristine (VCR) and vinblastine (VBL) led to the subsequent development of various semisynthetic analogs including vinorelbine (VRL, 5′-norhydro-VBL), vindesine (VDS), and the bifluorinated vinflunine (VFL).

The vinca alkaloids have in common a large dimeric asymmetric structure composed of a dihydroindole nucleus (vindoline), the major alkaloid in the periwinkle, linked by a carbon-carbon bridge to an indole nucleus (catharanthine), which is found in much lower quantities in the plant (Fig. 11.3). VCR and VBL differ in the substituent (R_1) attached to the nitrogen of the vindoline nucleus, where VCR possesses a formyl group and VBL has a methyl group.

Despite the minor structural differences between VCR and VBL, they differ in their antitumor activity and toxicity. Because of its virtual absence of myelosuppressive effects, VCR is valuable as a part of curative therapy for childhood acute lymphocytic leukemia and lymphomas, as well as pediatric Ewing's and other soft tissue sarcomas. In adults with cancer, VCR is an essential part of the combination chemotherapeutic regimens for acute lymphocytic leukemia and non-Hodgkin's lymphoma. VBL has been an integral component of combination therapeutic regimens for germ cell malignancies (with cisplatin and bleomycin, PVB) and Hodgkin's disease (with doxorubicin, bleomycin, and DTIC, ABVD). VCR, VBL, and VRL are approved for use in the United States. VRL is approved in the United States either as a single agent or in combination with cisplatin to treat non–small cell lung cancer and has also been registered for advanced breast cancer in other countries. VRL has the additional advantage of being administered orally,[19] in contrast to other available vinca alkaloids. Other analogs (VDS and VFL) are approved outside the United States but have limited utility in practice. Vinflunine is approved in Europe for second-line treatment of

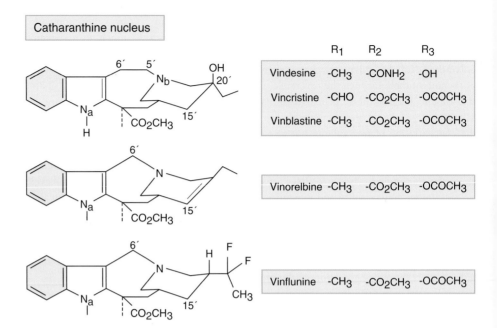

	R₁	R₂	R₃
Vindesine	-CH₃	-CONH₂	-OH
Vincristine	-CHO	-CO₂CH₃	-OCOCH₃
Vinblastine	-CH₃	-CO₂CH₃	-OCOCH₃

| Vinorelbine | -CH₃ | -CO₂CH₃ | -OCOCH₃ |

| Vinflunine | -CH₃ | -CO₂CH₃ | -OCOCH₃ |

FIGURE 11.3 Structures of the vindoline nucleus and catharanthine nucleus in various vinca alkaloids. Modifications for each analogue are indicated.

metastatic urothelial cancer after failure of platinum-based therapy, based on a 2.6-month survival advantage compared to best supportive care. The key features of these vinca alkaloids are listed in Table 11.1.

Mechanism of Action

The vinca alkaloids induce cytotoxicity by inhibiting microtubule polymerization. Nanomolar concentrations, which are readily achieved in plasma during clinical administration, induce typical inhibition of mitosis. Although the vinca alkaloids preferentially disrupt proliferating cells and tissues, they also affect nonproliferating tissues that are rich in tubulin, such as neurons and platelets.

The vinca alkaloids bind to microtubules at two binding sites, each with different affinities including high-affinity sites (K_d, 1 to 2 µmol) located at the ends of microtubules and low-affinity sites (K_d, 0.25 to 0.3 mmol) located along the sides of microtubule surfaces. The binding of the vinca alkaloids to high-affinity sites suppresses tubulin polymerization. This engagement disrupts treadmilling and dynamic instability but has less effect on the microtubule mass. Low concentrations of the vinca alkaloids enhance dynamic instability at the minus end of microtubules, but suppress dynamic instability at the plus end. The result is attenuated activity, neither growing nor shortening, of the microtubular apparatus and a potent block at the metaphase/anaphase boundary in mitosis.[13]

The cytotoxic actions of the vinca alkaloids are principally ascribed to their effects on formation of the mitotic spindle and disruption of orderly chromosome segregation. Mitotic checkpoints detect the abnormal segregation of chromosomes and promote apoptosis. Following vinca alkaloid treatment, mitotic progress is delayed in a metaphase-like state with chromosomes "stuck" at the spindle poles, unable to move to the spindle equator. The cell-cycle signal to the anaphase-promoting complex, which is required for the cell to transition from metaphase to anaphase, is blocked, mitotic figures accumulate, and the cells eventually undergo apoptosis. For surviving cells, cytokinesis may not occur, allowing cells to progress into interphase, resulting in multinucleation.

Other explanations have been offered for the vinca effects on slowly dividing cells; the drugs, through their interaction with microtubules, disrupt an array of cell functions, including neurotransmission and secretory functions, cell migration, and angiogenesis. The vinca alkaloids and other antimicrotubule agents disrupt malignant angiogenesis with surprising potency.[20] In vitro, 0.1 to 1.0 pmol/L VBL blocks endothelial proliferation, chemotaxis, and spreading on fibronectin, all essential steps in angiogenesis. Vinca treatment causes an inhibition of signaling by c-Jun N-terminal kinase and cell surface tyrosine kinases and activates apoptotic pathways. These actions by microtubule disrupting agents perturb both malignant and nonmalignant cells in the nonmitotic cell-cycle phases.[20] Altered signaling

<table>
TABLE

11.1   *Key features of the vinca alkaloids*
</table>

	Vincristine	Vinblastine	Vindesine	Vinorelbine	Vinflunine
Mechanism of action	Low concentrations inhibit microtubule dynamic instability and treadmilling. High concentrations inhibit polymerization of tubulin				
Standard adult dosage	1.4 mg/m² weekly	First dose: 3.7 mg/m², dose range: 5.5–7.4 mg/m² weekly	3–4 mg/m² every 1–2 wk	25–30 mg/m² weekly	280–320 mg/m² every 3 wk
Pharmacokinetics (terminal half-life)	85 h	25 h	24 h	27–43 h	~40 h
Metabolism	Hepatic, cytochrome P-450 CYP3A5 (major); CYP3A4 (minor)	CYP3A4	CYP3A subfamily	CYP3A4	CYP3A4
Principal toxicity	Peripheral neuropathy	Neutropenia	Neutropenia	Neutropenia	Neutropenia
Other toxicities	Constipation, abdominal pain, SIADH, alopecia, extravasation injury	Thrombocytopenia, anemia, alopecia, peripheral neuropathy (mild), SIADH, constipation, N/V, extravasation injury, mucositis	Peripheral neuropathy (mild), alopecia, N/V, SIADH, mucositis, alopecia, extravasation injury	Peripheral neuropathy (mild), anemia, thrombocytopenia, constipation, N/V, fatigue, SIADH, mucositis, alopecia, extravasation injury	Thrombocytopenia, anemia, fatigue, constipation, N/V, mucositis, peripheral neuropathy (mild), alopecia, extravasation injury

N/V, nausea and vomiting; SIADH, syndrome of inappropriate antidiuretic hormone secretion.

inhibits BCL-2 and other antiapoptotic proteins and may explain the synergistic interaction of the vincas with other cancer drugs in curative combinations for leukemias and lymphomas.

In summary, the relationships between the antiproliferative actions of the vinca alkaloids and various relevant subcellular effects, such as microtubule stabilization and microtubule depolymerization, result in mitotic arrest. These effects occur even at the lowest effective drug concentrations with little or no microtubule depolymerization or disorganization of the mitotic spindle apparatus. With increasing drug concentrations, the organization of microtubules and chromosomes in arrested mitotic spindles deteriorates in a manner that is common to all vinca derivatives. Current evidence, as related to knowledge of pharmacokinetics in humans (prolonged retention in tissues), suggests that the antiproliferative effects of the vinca alkaloids result as much from loss of dynamic instability as from actual depolymerization of the microtubules.

Mechanistic and Functional Differences

With regard to the disruptive effects of the vinca alkaloids on microtubule dynamics, the naturally occurring vinca alkaloids VCR and VBL, the semisynthetic analog VRL, and the bifluorinated analog VFL impart similar actions but differ in their affinities for a common binding site on tubulin: VCR > VBL > VRL > VFL.[21] They also differ in their spectrum of antitumor activity in experimental tumor systems and in their effects on microtubular dynamics.[22]

The explanation for the differential effects of the various vinca alkaloids on normal tissues and tumors is not clear. Peripheral neurotoxicity, possibly due to drug-induced microtubule loss or altered microtubule dynamics in axonal processes, is a common adverse effect of first-generation vinca alkaloids. VCR, the most potent of the analogs in humans and the most neurotoxic, has the greatest affinity for tubulin.[22] In contrast, VFL's lower affinity for tubulin binding may contribute to its reduced incidence of peripheral neuropathy. One possible factor determining patterns of toxicity to normal tissues versus tumor may be tubulin isotype composition, which is highly variable among tissues and which may determine relative binding affinities in different tissues. Intracellular drug accumulation and tubulin binding vary according to tubulin isotype composition.[23] Neurons are enriched in α-β-tubulin classes II and III, and the relatively high drug binding affinities for these isotypes may explain, in part, why the vinca alkaloids produce neurotoxicity. Other factors that determine neurotoxicity of analogues may be differences in transport, interaction with MAPs, or disruption of neurosecretory function.

Cellular Pharmacology

The vinca alkaloids are rapidly taken up into cells, steady-state intracellular/extracellular concentration ratios ranging from 5- to 500-fold greater than plasma depending on the cell type and culture conditions.[24] Retention varies considerably among cells and tissues, but in general, these drugs are lipophilic, bind avidly to tubulin, and remain in cells long after extracellular drug disappears. Although the binding affinity for tubulin appears to be less for VFL than for the other vinca alkaloids, its intracellular accumulation is highest among the analogues.[25]

An energy-requiring uptake mechanism, as well as temperature-independent, nonsaturable mechanisms, analogous to simple diffusion, may both contribute to uptake of these lipophilic compounds.[24] Although both drug concentration and treatment duration are important determinants of drug accumulation and cytotoxicity, the duration of exposure above a critical threshold concentration is perhaps the most important determinant of vinca alkaloid cytotoxicity.[26] Cytotoxicity is directly related to the extracellular concentration of drug when the duration of treatment is kept constant; for prolonged exposure to VCR, the concentration yielding 50% inhibition of cell growth ranges from 1 to 5 nmol/L.

Mechanisms of Resistance

Resistance to the vinca alkaloids develops rapidly in vitro with continuous exposure to these agents. Two types of mechanisms of resistance to the vinca alkaloids have been well characterized. The first mechanism is pleiotropic or multidrug resistance (MDR), which can be either innate (primary) or acquired. The ATP-binding cassette (ABC) transporters export a variety of natural products and lipophilic substrates across cellular compartments. These membrane-spanning proteins mediate resistance to the natural products such as vinca alkaloids, taxanes, and anthracyclines, and many other synthetic compounds, including targeted molecules. The most extensively studied ABC transporters conferring resistance to the vinca alkaloids and taxanes are the permeability glycoprotein (Pgp), or the *MDR1*-encoded gene product MDR1 (ABC subfamily B1; ABCB1), and the multidrug resistance protein (MRP1) (ABC subfamily C1; ABCC1).[27,28]

MDR1 is a 170-kDa energy-dependent transmembrane transport pump that regulates the efflux of a large range of amphipathic hydrophobic substances, resulting in decreased drug accumulation. The specific Pgp associated with resistance to the vinca alkaloids shows structural diversity from the exporter that confers taxane resistance, due to posttranslational modification or other membrane-associated proteins. The composition of membrane gangliosides in cancer cells resistant to the vinca alkaloids has also been shown to differ from that of wild-type cells.[29] VCR resistance, as assessed ex vivo, correlates with Pgp overexpression, particularly in childhood acute lymphoblastic leukemia (ALL).[30] Resistance to the vinca alkaloids is also conferred by MRP1, which is a 190-kDa membrane-spanning protein that shares 15% amino acid homology with MDR1.[27,31] MRP1 transports vincas, taxanes, etoposide, and doxorubicin, and its increased expression confers resistance to the latter two agents, but vinca alkaloids and taxanes are only modestly affected. Moreover, both transporters do not confer a significant resistance to vinflunine.[32] The reversal of drug resistance of MDR1 and MRP1 is easily demonstrated in vitro by compounds that compete directly to blocking the efflux of the cytotoxic drugs and increase intracellular drug retentions. However, the interpretation of clinical studies of resistance modulation has been confounded by the fact that MDR modulators affect drug retention in normal tissues and decrease drug clearance, thereby enhancing toxicity.[33] Strategies aimed at reversing resistance to vincas in the clinic with inhibitors of both MDR1 and MRP1 have been uninterpretable due to these pharmacokinetic alterations.

The second less well-characterized mechanism of vinca alkaloid resistance relates to the diversity of tubulin isotypes.[34] Mammalian cells have six α- and seven β-tubulin isotypes, whose expression may influence microtubule dynamics. Structural alterations in α- or β-tubulin due to either genetic mutations and consequential amino acid substitutions or posttranslational modifications have been identified in cancer cells with acquired resistance to the antimicrotubule drugs. Tubulin isotype expression is altered in resistance cells and may influence the response to vinca alkaloids. Decreased expression of class III β-tubulin, which increases the rate of microtubule assembly, is associated with vinca alkaloid resistance, while knockdown of either class II or IVb β-tubulin with siRNA hypersensitizes lung cancer cell lines to the effects of the vinca alkaloids.[34] The expression of class II β-tubulin, which may be linked to suppression of p53 function, may also confer vinca alkaloid resistance.[35]

Increased expression of MAPs, particularly MAP4, which promote microtubule assembly and hyperstability, perhaps by mechanisms similar to those linked with alterations in α- and β-tubulins, has also been associated with vinca alkaloid resistance.[34] Various alterations in the principal components of the apoptotic pathway may confer resistance to the vinca alkaloids. Experimental evidence suggests that VBL and other antimicrotubule agents induce proapoptotic effects by phosphorylating the antiapoptotic factor Bcl-xL, whereas some VBL-resistance mutants that undergo reduced apoptosis have defects in BcL-xL phosphorylation.[36]

Clinical Pharmacology

The clinical pharmacology of the vinca alkaloids were incompletely understood until technical advances in extraction and chromatographic detection (electrochemical and fluorescence), which have made HPLC-mass spectrometry the most feasible means of separating and quantifying the minute concentrations of the vinca alkaloids and their metabolites.[37]

The vinca alkaloids are most commonly administered intravenously as a bolus injection or brief infusion. The vinca alkaloids exhibit large volumes of distribution, high clearance rates followed by long terminal half-lives ($t_{1/2}$), extensive hepatic metabolism, and biliary/fecal elimination of metabolites. Interindividual variability in their pharmacologic behavior has been attributed to many factors, including differences in protein and tissue binding, hepatic metabolism, and biliary clearance. In comparative studies of the vincas, VBL has the shortest terminal $t_{1/2}$ and the highest clearance rate; and VCR, VFL, and VDS have slower clearance and longer terminal half-lives.[38] The longest terminal $t_{1/2}$ and lowest clearance rate of VCR may account, in part, for its greater propensity to induce neurotoxicity.

Although prolonged infusion schedules may avoid excessively toxic peak concentrations and may increase the duration of drug exposure in plasma above biologically relevant threshold concentrations for any given tumor, there is little evidence to support the notion that prolonged infusion schedules are more effective than bolus schedules. Rapid distribution of drug and high avidity of binding of the vinca alkaloids to tubulin are likely responsible for the efficacy of intermittent administration schedules.

Vincristine

After conventional doses of VCR (1.4 mg/m^2) given as brief infusions, peak plasma concentrations (C_{peak}) approach 400 nmol/L.[39] VCR binds extensively to both plasma proteins (reported values in the range of 48% to 75%) and formed blood elements, particularly platelets, which contain high concentrations of tubulin. The platelet count has been inversely related to drug exposure.[38] Poor drug penetration across the blood-brain barrier has been documented in most studies. The low penetration of VCR across the blood-brain barrier and other tumor sanctuary sites can be attributed to its large size and the fact that it is an avid substrate for the ABC transporters, which maintain the integrity of these blood-tissue barriers. Inadvertent administration of vincristine into the subarachnoid space leads to convulsions and death. In humans receiving intravenous drug, VCR concentrations in cerebrospinal fluid are 20- to 30-fold lower than in plasma and do not exceed 1.1 nmol/L.[40] After intravenous injection, VCR is rapidly distributed to body tissues followed by triphasic elimination, with a high volume of distribution and terminal half-life about 85 hours, suggesting slow clearance from tissue compartments.[41]

Protracted VCR administration schedules has attracted interest as their pharmacokinetics closely simulate the optimal in vitro conditions for cytotoxicity.[42] For example, VCR concentrations of 100 to 400 nmol/L are achieved only briefly after bolus injection, and levels generally decline to less than 10 nmol/L in 2 to 4 hours. Exposure to 100 nM VCR for 3 hours is required to kill 50% of L1210 murine or CEM human lymphoblastic leukemia cells, whereas longer treatment durations of 6 to 12 hours achieve this degree of cytotoxicity at much lower drug concentrations (10 nM), while no lethal effects occur at VCR concentrations below 2 nM. A 0.5-mg intravenous bolus injection of VCR followed by a continuous infusion at dosages of 0.5 to 1.0 mg/m^2/d for 5 days results in steady-state VCR concentrations ranging from 1 to 10 nmol/L. Prolonged infusions of the vinca alkaloids are employed in several widely used chemotherapy regimens that have been associated with robust activity, such as EPOCH, which is comprised of etoposide, doxorubicin, and VCR given by continuous infusion on days 1 to 4, oral prednisone on days 1 to 5, and cyclophosphamide IV on day 5 of courses repeated every 3 week.[43]

VCR is metabolized and excreted primarily by the hepatobiliary system.[41] Within 72 hours after the administration of radiolabeled VCR, approximately 12% of the radioactivity is excreted in the urine (consisting mainly of metabolites), and approximately 70% to 80% is excreted in the feces (40% of which consists of metabolites).[39,40] VCR metabolites are rapidly excreted into bile.[44] VCR metabolism is mediated by hepatic cytochrome P-450 CYP3A subfamily. VCR is preferentially metabolized by CYP3A4 and CYP3A5 to form the major metabolite M1 (a secondary amine), with CYP3A5 being more efficient in catalyzing the M1 formation.[45] Thus, genetically polymorphic expression of CYP3A5 may contribute to the observed interindividual variability in vincristine exposure and response.

Because the drug clearance occurs primarily by hepatic metabolism, the vinca alkaloids, as a group, must be used with caution in patients with hepatic dysfunction. A 50% reduction in the dose is recommended if direct bilirubin is above 3 mg/dL. With VCR the risk of ileus and with VLB the risk of severe and prolonged myelosuppression are high in the presence of liver failure.

Vinblastine

The clinical pharmacology of VBL is similar to that of VCR, with rapid tissue uptake and extensive binding to plasma proteins and formed blood elements. Plasma disappearance fits a triexponential pharmacokinetic model with a rapid distribution phase ($t_{1/2\alpha} < 5$ minutes) and terminal half-life of approximately 25 hours.[46] The principal mode of VBL disposition is hepatic metabolism and biliary excretion, with small amounts of metabolite recovered in urine. Fecal excretion of the parent compound is low, which indicates that hepatic metabolism is extensive with CYP3A isoforms primarily responsible for drug biotransformation.[47] At least one metabolite, desacetylvinblastine, which may be as active as the parent compound, has been identified in both urine and feces.

Vindesine, Vinorelbine, and Vinflunine

Pharmacokinetic parameters for these three analogs are given in Table 11.1. All behave similarly to VCR and VBL, with plasma disposition characterized by a triphasic model, large volume of distribution, and long terminal half-lives. They are tightly protein bound and extensively metabolized by CYP3A isoforms. Their 4-O-deacetyl metabolites have antitumor activity, but other metabolites are inactive. These drugs should also be used with caution in patients with hepatic dysfunction.

Vinorelbine was the first vinca alkaloid to display oral activity,[19] exhibiting similar pharmacokinetics to IV-administered drug. The oral formulation of VRL, which is approved in some European countries, is rapidly absorbed after oral ingestion with bioavailability of approximately 40% and is not affected by food intake.

Drug Interactions

There are few meaningful drug interactions between vinca compounds and other cancer drugs, the most important being to restrict their use with other neurotoxic drugs, such as the platinum analogues, taxanes, and brentuximab vedotin (an antibody conjugate with an antimitotic, auristatin E derivative), as the neurotoxicity will be additive. Treatment with the vinca alkaloids lowers drug levels of phenytoin and has precipitated seizures, an interaction most likely due to induction of CYP3A metabolism.[48] The same drugs as well as H$_2$ blockers induce CYP isoenzymes and accelerate vinca clearance. Administration of the vinca alkaloids with erythromycin, clarithromycin, antifungal azoles, and other inhibitors of CYP3A may also lead to severe toxicity. The vinca alkaloids inhibit glucuronidation of AZT to its 5'-O-glucuronide metabolite.[49] Lastly, corticosteroids may induce CYP metabolism and alter vinca pharmacokinetics and response.[50]

Dosage and Administration

The vinca alkaloids are most commonly administered by direct intravenous injection or through the side-arm tubing of a running intravenous infusion. Experienced oncology personnel should administer these agents because drug extravasation can cause severe soft tissue injury.

Vincristine

For adults, the conventional weekly dose is 1.4 mg/m². A restriction of the absolute single dose of VCR to 2.0 mg/m², which is often referred to as *capping*, has at times been adopted, based on early reports of substantial neurotoxicity at higher doses. However, this restriction is largely empirical; some authorities have blamed capping for less than optimal results of combination therapy of Hodgkin's disease.[51] VCR dosage modifications should be based on toxicity, particularly peripheral and autonomic neuropathy. However, dosage should not be reduced for mild peripheral neurotoxicity (tingling of fingers or toes), particularly if the agent is being used in a potentially curative setting. Instead, doses should be modified for serious neurotoxicity, including severe symptomatic sensory changes, motor (foot drop) and cranial nerve deficits, and ileus. In clearly palliative situations, dose reduction, lengthened dosing interval, or selection of alternative agents may be justified in the event of moderate neurotoxicity. A prophylactic regimen, consisting of stool softeners, dietary bulk, and laxatives, to prevent the consequences of constipation, is also recommended for patients receiving VCR.

VCR is a potent vesicant and should only be given IV. Inadvertent intrathecal injection of VCR or other vinca alkaloids induces a severe myeloencephalopathy characterized by ascending motor and sensory neuropathies, encephalopathy, and rapid death.[52] Although the issue has not been evaluated carefully, the major role of the liver in the disposition of VCR implies that dose modifications should be considered for patients with hepatic dysfunction, as indicated above. Dosage reductions for renal dysfunction are not indicated.

Vinblastine

For VBL administration, initiate weekly dosing regimens at 2.5 and 3.7 mg/m² for children and adults, respectively, followed by gradual dose escalation based on hematologic tolerance. Because the severity of the leukopenia that may occur with identical VBL doses varies widely among individuals, VBL dosing as a single agent may require significant adjustment, based on white blood cell nadirs. For most adult patients, however, the weekly dosage is 5.5 to 7.4 mg/m². The most commonly used schedule is a bolus injection of 6 to 8 mg/m² in cyclic combination chemotherapy regimens every 3 to 4 weeks. Five-day continuous infusions of VBL, 1.5 to 2.0 mg/m²/d, have been used and achieved plasma steady state levels of 2 nmol/L,[38] but no evidence exists to favor prolonged infusion versus standard bolus administration. Although specific guidelines have not been established, VBL dosages should be modified for patients with hepatic dysfunction, especially biliary obstruction, as indicated above.

Vindesine, Vinorelbine, and Vinflunine

Standard schedules for these three analogs are given in Table 11.1. Dose adjustment, as indicated above, should be employed in the presence of hepatic dysfunction but is not indicated for compromised renal function.

Toxicity of Vinca alkaloids

The principal toxicities of the vinca alkaloids differ despite their structural and pharmacologic similarities. Peripheral neurotoxicity is the predominant toxicity of VCR, whereas myelosuppression predominates with VBL, VDS, VRL, and VFL. Nevertheless, peripheral neurotoxicity is often noted following multiple cycles of treatment with all of the vinca alkaloids and may become apparent after inadvertent high-dose treatment or in settings involving patients with underlying neuropathy. VCR can cause myelosuppression in heavily pretreated patients.

Neurologic

The vinca alkaloids, particularly VCR, can induce neurotoxicity characterized by a peripheral, symmetric mixed sensorimotor, and autonomic polyneuropathy.[53] The primary neuropathologic effects are axonal degeneration and decreased axonal transport as a result of interference with axonal microtubule function. Initially, only symmetric sensory impairment and paresthesia in distal extremities are noticed. Neuritic pain and loss of deep tendon reflexes may develop with continued treatment, followed by disabling foot drop, wrist drop, wide spread motor loss, ataxia, and generalized paresis. Back, bone, and limb pain, possibly of neuritic origin, can occasionally occur. Nerve conduction studies confirm axonal degeneration. Cranial nerve palsies may be associated with hoarseness, diplopia, jaw pain, and facial palsies. These symptoms may require evaluation for brain or spinal cord metastases as an alternative explanation. Auditory loss has also been reported, and caution is warranted when used in combination with other ototoxic agents. Acute, severe autonomic neurotoxicity is uncommon, but ileus, urinary retention, or hypotension may arise as a consequence of high-dose therapy (>2 mg/m²) or in patients with altered hepatic function or with predisposing hereditary neurological disorders such as Charcot-Marie-Tooth disease, Guillain-Barré syndrome, or familial neuropathies. In adults, the neurotoxic effects of VCR may begin with cumulative doses as little as 5 to 6 mg, and manifestations may be profound after cumulative doses of 15 to 20 mg. Children are less sensitive than adults, but older persons are particularly prone. Hepatic dysfunction or obstructive liver disease increases the risk of developing severe neuropathy because of impaired drug metabolism and delayed biliary excretion.[54]

The only known effective intervention for vinca alkaloid neurotoxicity is discontinuation of the drug or reduction of the dose or frequency of drug administration. Antidotes, including thiamine, vitamin B_{12}, folinic acid, pyridoxine, and neuroactive agents (e.g., sedatives, tranquilizers, and anticonvulsants) have no value.

The manifestations of neurotoxicity are similar but less severe and less frequent for the other vinca alkaloids. Neurotoxicity is usually mild and not dose limiting for VBL and VDS, while VRL and VFL are infrequently responsible for neurotoxic events.

The inadvertent intrathecal administration of the vinca alkaloids causes an ascending myeloencephalopathy that is usually fatal. Reports of immediate cerebrospinal fluid withdrawal and lavage with Ringer's lactate solution supplemented with fresh frozen plasma (15 mL/L) at a rate of 55 mL/h for 24 hours have provided encouraging results, in that two affected patients survived with significant paraplegia, but intact cerebral function.[52,55] To prevent this mistake, pharmacy, nursing, and physicians should be trained not to administer intrathecal methotrexate and intravenous VCR in a single setting, and the drugs should not be delivered together.

Hematologic

Neutropenia is the principal dose-limiting toxicity of VBL, VDS, VRL, and VFL. Thrombocytopenia and anemia are usually less common and less severe. The onset of neutropenia is usually 7 to 11 days after treatment, and recovery is generally by days 14 to 21. Myelosuppression is not typically cumulative. Hematologic toxicity of clinical relevance is uncommon after VCR treatment but may be a major manifestation following inadvertent administration of high dosages.

Gastrointestinal

Gastrointestinal autonomic dysfunction, as manifested by bloating, constipation, ileus, and abdominal pain, occurs most commonly with VCR and less frequently, albeit more readily apparent at high doses, with the other vinca alkaloids. Paralytic ileus (particularly in pediatric patients), intestinal necrosis, and perforation have been reported.[56] Poor intestinal transit may result in the impaction of stool in the upper colon. An empty rectum may be noted on digital examination, and an abdominal radiograph may be useful in diagnosing this condition. This condition may be responsive to high enemas and laxatives. A routine prophylactic regimen to prevent constipation is therefore recommended for all patients receiving VCR. The ileus, which may mimic a "surgical abdomen," usually resolves with conservative therapy alone after termination of treatment. Patients who receive high dosages of VCR and less frequent with other vinca alkaloids or have hepatic dysfunction may be especially prone to develop severe ileus. Mucositis, stomatitis, and pharyngitis occur more frequently with VBL than with VRL or VDS and are uncommon with VCR. Nausea, vomiting, and diarrhea may also occur to a lesser extent. Asymptomatic and transient elevations in liver function test results, particularly alkaline phosphatase levels, have been noted. Pancreatitis has also been reported with VRL.[57]

Extravasation

All vinca alkaloids are potent vesicants and may cause severe tissue damage if extravasation occurs. Injection site reactions, including erythema, pain, and venous discoloration, are common. Discomfort and signs of phlebitis may also occur along the course of an injected vein, with resultant sclerosis. The risk of phlebitis increases if veins are not adequately flushed after treatment. If extravasation is suspected, treatment should be discontinued, and aspiration of any residual drug remaining in the tissues should be attempted. The treatment of choice for minimizing both discomfort and cellulitis consists of the application of local heat immediately for 1 hour four times daily for 3 to 5 days and the injection of hyaluronidase (150 to 1,500 total units) subcutaneously, through six clockwise injections in a circumferential manner using a 25-gauge needle (changing the needle with each injection) into surrounding tissues.[58] Surgical debridement of necrotic tissue may be necessary.

Miscellaneous

All the vinca alkaloids, except VFL, possibly due to insufficient clinical experience, have been implicated as a cause of syndrome of inappropriate antidiuretic hormone secretion (SIADH) by directly affecting the hypothalamus, neurohypophyseal tract, or posterior pituitary. Patients who are receiving intensive hydration are particularly prone to severe hyponatremia secondary to SIADH, which may result in generalized seizures.[59] This entity has been associated with elevated plasma levels of antidiuretic hormone and usual remits in 2 to 3 days. Hyponatremia generally responds to

fluid restriction. Alopecia occurs in a small proportion of patients, particularly those receiving cumulative treatment with VBL, VRL, VDS, and VFL. Hand-foot syndrome is a rare toxicity of VRL. VBL may cause photosensitivity reactions, possibly as a result of corneal irritation. Myalgia and arthralgia have been reported with all vinca alkaloids, including VFL.

The primary cardiovascular toxicities (e.g., hypotension, cardiac arrhythmias) result from autonomic dysfunction. While chest pain has been noted in association with the vincas, there is no clear association of these drugs with coronary occlusive events, strokes, or peripheral vascular toxicities. Vinca drugs, especially VFL, may rarely cause acute dyspnea and pneumonitis; these reactions were particularly noticed when the drugs were combined with mitomycin C. Reactions take the form of acute bronchospasm during infusion, or a subacute cough and dyspnea, occasionally with interstitial infiltrates, beginning within 1 hour after treatment. The use of corticosteroids may be beneficial in severe cases, and patients have been retreated without sequelae. VCR-induced autonomic neurotoxicity may produce bladder atony, thereby causing polyuria, dysuria, incontinence, and urinary retention.[60]

Pharmacogenetics

The human cytochrome P450 3A (CYP3A) isozymes are involved in the metabolism of the vinca alkaloids. The hepatic clearances of vincristine were fivefold higher for CYP3A5 high expressers than low expressers, indicating that polymorphic expression of CYP3A5 may be a determinant in the CYP-mediated clearance of vincristine.[61,62] CYP3A5 polymorphism may account for lower rates of neurotoxicity and dosage reductions among African American patients with ALL who are receiving treatment with VCR compared with Caucasian patients.[63,64] CYP3A4 polymorphisms have been associated with differential clinical outcomes in patients with Hodgkin's lymphoma who undergo treatment with vinca alkaloids.[65] P450 CYP isoform polymorphisms have also been related to clinical outcome in patients with non–small cell lung cancer undergoing treatment with VRL.[66]

In a study of children with ALL, an inherited polymorphism (T allele at rs924607) in the promoter region of *CEP72* was associated with increased risk and severity of VCR-related peripheral neuropathy, with the cumulative incidence of neuropathy significantly higher and the average grade of neuropathy significantly greater in patients homozygous for the *CEP72* risk allele (TT) compared to all other patients.[67] The *CEP72* gene encodes a centrosomal protein that is essential for microtubule formation, and the variant allele creates a binding site for a transcriptional repressor, leading to lower *CEP72* mRNA expression. These data were further confirmed in another study of adults with ALL where the CEP72 polymorphism identified adults at increased risk of VCR-induced peripheral neuropathy.[50]

Since ABCB1 is implicated in the resistance and pharmacokinetics of vinca alkaloids, in vitro studies suggest that *ABCB1* polymorphisms at the 1236, 2677, and/or 3435 positions significantly minimize protein functionality. Several clinical studies have tested the hypothesis that genetic variations in the above genes (*CYP3A4/5*, *CEP72*, *ABCB1*) and other genes may contribute to interpatient variation in VCR pharmacokinetics, treatment response, and toxicity (reviewed in Ref.[68]). However, results of these studies remain inconclusive. When SNPs of the *ABCB1* gene were retrospectively analyzed in children with ALL treated with VCR, no association was found between the SNPs C3435T or G2677T and VCR pharmacokinetics or toxicity. A recent study suggests that focusing on haplotype analysis rather than individual polymorphisms to determine the effects of *ABCB1* SNPs in terms of drug response and clinical outcome may be helpful.[54]

Taxanes

The taxanes are the most important new class of chemotherapeutic drugs in the past two decades. The prototypical taxane, paclitaxel, and docetaxel have demonstrated antitumor activity in a broad array of solid tumors. Paclitaxel was discovered by Wall, Wani, and colleagues at Research Triangle Institute as part of a National Cancer Institute plant screening program.[69] In 1964, a crude extract with antitumor activity was isolated from the bark of the Pacific yew, *Taxus brevifolia*, a slowly growing evergreen found in the old-growth forests of the Pacific Northwest. Paclitaxel was identified as the active chemical constituent of the extract in 1971. Interest in the agent accelerated in 1979 after Horwitz and colleagues described its unique mechanism of stabilizing microtubules,[69] as compared to the destabilizing effect of vincas.

Paclitaxel is produced by *Taxomyces andreanae*, a fungal endophyte isolated from the inner bark of the Pacific yew. Commercial production now depends on semisynthesis, using, a precursor, 10-deacetylbaccatin III. The precursor is isolated from the needles of more abundant yew species such as the European yew, *Taxus baccata*. Docetaxel, derived semisynthetically from 10-deacetylbaccatin III, is slightly more water soluble than paclitaxel and is a more potent antimicrotubule agent in vitro.[70] Cabazitaxel, a synthetically modified taxane, which closely resembles the earlier products, was approved in 2014 for treatment of endocrine-resistant prostate cancer.[71] A fourth taxane, albumin microparticulate formulation (also known as protein-bound paclitaxel particles for injection or nanoparticle albumin-bound paclitaxel or nab-paclitaxel [Nab-T]) has received regulatory approval for treatment of breast and pancreatic cancer in the United States and elsewhere.[72] The key clinical and pharmacological features of the taxanes are displayed in Table 11.2.

The taxanes are important components for treating ovarian, breast, pancreatic, prostate, and lung cancers. Paclitaxel is now used in both adjuvant therapy, in combination with doxorubicin or carboplatin, and as a single agent in metastatic breast cancer, as well as treatment of ovarian cancer in combination with carboplatin, and with a platinum analogue in metastatic non–small cell lung cancer. Docetaxel has the same spectrum of activity but is used primarily for second line for lung cancer and for adjuvant and metastatic breast cancer, gastroesophageal cancer, and metastatic prostate cancer with antiandrogens or in hormone refractory disease.

The antitumor spectra for paclitaxel and docetaxel are nearly identical. Differences in clinical efficacy end points and the regulatory indications between paclitaxel and docetaxel largely reflect different drug development paths, study designs, and dose schedules and not necessarily inherent superiority of one taxane over the other.

Nab-T received its first approval in the United States for the treatment of breast cancer after failure of anthracycline-based chemotherapy for metastatic disease or relapse within 6 months of adjuvant therapy. It is a formulation of paclitaxel within particles of human serum albumin, in contrast to earlier formulations of paclitaxel in polyoxyethylated castor oil (Cremophor EL). Nab-T is associated with fewer hypersensitivity reactions, does not require a complex pretreatment regimen, and has a similar spectrum of activity and toxicity when used against breast cancer and non–small cell lung cancer, and unique activity with gemcitabine against pancreatic cancer.

The most recent addition to the taxane group is cabazitaxel, which is approved for docetaxel-resistant prostate cancer. It closely resembles docetaxel and paclitaxel in its pharmacological properties but is a poor substrate for the MDR transporter that confers resistance to docetaxel. Taxane activity in prostate cancer may be related to their ability to block androgen receptor transit to the nucleus, an action circumvented by androgen receptor splice variants that activate androgen response pathways in the absence of ligand.[73]

Structures

The structures of paclitaxel, docetaxel, and cabazitaxel are shown in Figure 11.4. The taxanes are complex alkaloid esters, consisting of a 15-member taxane ring system linked to an unusual four-member oxetane ring at positions C-4 and C-5.[74] The taxane rings of both paclitaxel and docetaxel, but not 10-deacetylbaccatin III, are linked to an ester at the C-13 position, which is essential to its interaction with microtubules. Substitutions at the C-2′ and C-3′ positions are also required for the unique antimicrotubule action of the taxanes. Acetyl substitution at C-2′ results in a substantial loss of activity. The structures of paclitaxel and docetaxel differ in substitutions at the C-10 taxane ring position and on the ester side chain attached at C-13, which renders docetaxel slightly more water soluble and more potent than paclitaxel. Neither the acetyl group at C-10 nor the phenyl group at C-5′ is required for in vitro activity, and the structures of paclitaxel and docetaxel differ at these positions.

Mechanism of Action

The taxanes bind with high affinity to the β-tubulin component of protofilaments along the length of the microtubule.[75] The binding sites are distinct from those of exchangeable GTP, colchicine, podophyllotoxin, and the vinca alkaloids. Photoaffinity labeling found paclitaxel binding to the N-terminal 1 to 31 amino acids and to residues 217 to 233 of the β-tubulin subunit.[76] X-ray crystallographic models of the β-tubulin N-terminus indicate that His 227 and Asp 224 are critical to binding the C-2 benzoyl side chain of paclitaxel, and modeling data also indicate that both paclitaxel and docetaxel bind to the interior surface of the microtubule lumen.[77] Other antimicrotubule natural products that stabilize microtubules, such as the epothilones and eleutherobins, occupy the same binding sites. Paclitaxel binds to microtubules with high affinity (K_d, 10 nmol), although the binding affinities of docetaxel and cabazitaxel are several fold higher.[78] Cabazitaxel, docetaxel, and paclitaxel promote microtubule assembly in vitro in the absence of Ca^{2+}, GTP, MAPs, and in cold solutions, conditions that inhibit assembly in the absence of drug.

TABLE

11.2 *Key features of the taxanes, eribulin, and epothilones*

	Paclitaxel	Docetaxel	Nab-paclitaxel	Ixabepilone	Eribulin
Mechanism of action	Low concentrations inhibit microtubule dynamics (dynamic instability and treadmilling). High concentrations inhibit depolymerization of tubulin.				Unique tubulin-binding site, otherwise same
Standard dosage (mg/m^2)	135–175 mg/m^2 over 3 h every 3 wk; 135 mg/m^2 over 24 h every 3 wk; 100 mg/m^2 over 3 h every 2 wk; or 80 mg/m^2 over 1 h weekly	60–100 mg/m^2 over 1 h every 3 wk (75 mg/m^2 is the most common dose used)	260 mg/m^2 over 30 min every 3 wk; or 100–120 over 30 min weekly	40 mg/m^2 over 3 h every 3 wk; dose capped at 2.2 mg/m^2 for body surface areas exceeding this value	1.4 mg/m^2 on day 1 and day 8, every 3 wk
Principal toxicity	Neutropenia	Neutropenia	Neutropenia	Neutropenia	Neutropenia
Other toxicities	Peripheral neuropathy, HSR, anemia, thrombocytopenia, myalgia, arthralgia, asthenia, alopecia	Peripheral neuropathy, HSR (mild to moderate), fluid retention, anemia, thrombocytopenia, myalgia, arthralgia, alopecia, cutaneous	Peripheral neuropathy, anemia, thrombocytopenia, asthenia, alopecia	Peripheral neuropathy, HSRs, anemia, thrombocytopenia, asthenia, alopecia	Sensory neuropathy, anemia, asthenia, alopecia
Premedication (to prevent HSR)	Corticosteroid plus H$_1$- and H$_2$-histamine antagonists before each treatment	Corticosteroids with each treatment to prevent fluid retention; H$_1$-histamine antagonists	None	H$_1$- and H$_2$-histamine antagonists before each treatment; for patients who experience an HSR, corticosteroid plus H$_1$- and H$_2$-histamine antagonists	None
Pharmacokinetic behavior	Nonlinear for short infusions (3 h); linear for longer infusions (24 h)	Dose proportional up to 115 mg/m^2	Dose proportional	Dose proportional	Dose proportional
Terminal half-life ($T_{1/2}$)	13–20 h	~11 h	13–27 h	~52 h	~40 h
Primary route of elimination	CYP3A4 and CYP2B8	CYP 3A4/5	Same as paclitaxel	CYP3A4	Fecal elimination of unchanged drug

HSR, hypersensitivity reaction; Nab-paclitaxel, protein-bound paclitaxel particles for injection.

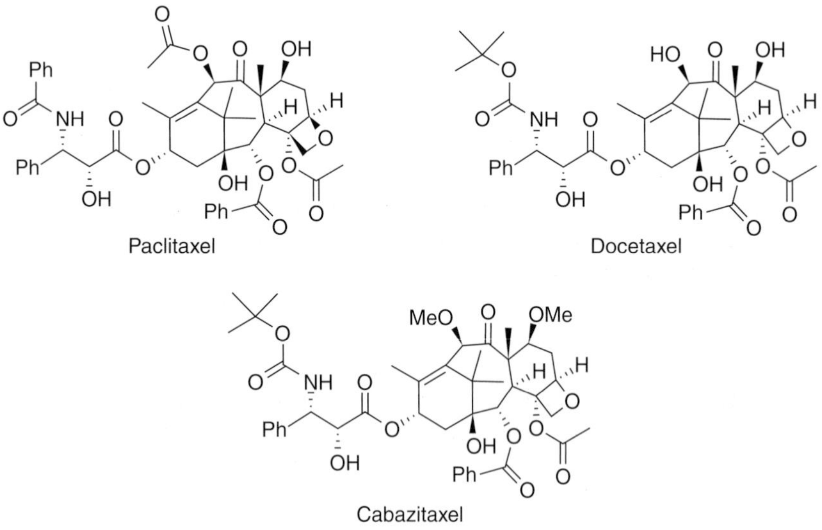

FIGURE 11.4 Structures of taxane analogues: paclitaxel **(A)**, docetaxel **(B)**, and cabazitaxel **(C)**.

In contrast to the vincas, the taxanes disrupt microtubule dynamics by stabilizing the microtubule against depolymerization, mimicking the GTP bound state, and preventing the essential dynamic instability and treadmilling of the mitotic spindle.[6] Binding of the taxanes enhances tubulin polymerization, induces a conformation change in tubulin, and increases tubulin affinity for neighboring tubulin molecules. There is one paclitaxel-binding site on each tubulin dimer of the microtubule, and the ability of paclitaxel to enhance polymerization is associated with nearly 1:1 stoichiometric binding of paclitaxel to β tubulin in microtubules. At submicromolar concentrations that are readily achieved in the clinic, binding is stoichiometric, and tubulin polymerization is enhanced. However, substoichiometric concentrations suppress microtubule dynamics without increasing the amount of polymerized tubulin.[79]

The taxanes inhibit tubulin dissociation at both microtubule ends, but the ends remain free for tubulin addition. Most studies with docetaxel indicate that it suppresses tubulin dynamics similar to paclitaxel, but the structural aspects of abnormal microtubule confirmation induced by paclitaxel, docetaxel, and cabazitaxel may differ.[80] Paclitaxel induced the formation of microtubules with predominantly 12 protofilaments, whereas 13 or 14 protofilaments are usually evident in docetaxel-induced microtubules. A detailed comparison of the binding properties of the taxane analogues by Churchill has disclosed significant differences in their molecular interactions with dimers and their allosteric effects, despite their common binding site, and their functional impacts.[78]

The antitumor effects of paclitaxel occur due to its ability to arrest cells in metaphase on bipolar spindles. Taxanes induce the formation of abnormal spindles, with failure of chromatids to attach to microtubules at their kinetochores. This failure to pair chromosomes on the mitotic spindle activates the mitotic checkpoint, arrests cell in mitosis, and induces apoptosis. Currently, there is a debate on whether paclitaxel induces tumor cell death by a mechanism other than mitotic arrest. While paclitaxel has long been recognized to induce mitotic arrest, concentrations that have been used in cell culture to characterize the mechanism of action may be much higher than intratumoral concentrations. Recent evidence in breast cancer demonstrates that intratumoral concentrations of paclitaxel are too low to cause mitotic arrest and that

clinically relevant doses of paclitaxel actually induce chromosome missegregation in highly abnormal, multipolar spindles.[81,82] This results into daughter cells with abnormal number of chromosomes that will undergo cell death in the subsequent interphase. Mitotic arrest was not necessary for paclitaxel response in patients with breast cancer.[82]

Taxanes can elicit other anticancer effects, mediating cellular events that can activate subsequent downstream apoptotic pathways. The tumor suppressor gene *p53* participates in cell death signaling and restrains cell-cycle progression following exit from a prolonged mitotic block. Microtubule disruption induces *p53*, inhibits cyclin-dependent kinases (CDK; e.g., p21/Waf-1), and activates signaling pathways related to apoptosis (e.g., Jun N-terminal kinase, BCL-2 family members).[83] Caspase-dependent and -independent mechanisms of cell death result. The taxanes enhance the effects of ionizing radiation in vitro at clinically achievable concentrations (<50 nmol/L) and in vivo, perhaps by inhibition of cell-cycle progression into mitosis, retaining cell in the most radiosensitive G-2 phase of the cell cycle.[84] The taxanes inhibit angiogenesis at concentrations below those that induce cytotoxicity (0.1 to 5 nM),[85] explaining efficacy in vascular stents.

Paclitaxel enclosed in albumin nanoparticles slowly releases into the circulation and likely has the same basic functions as the unencapsulated drug. However, the albumin coat may result in increased accumulation of paclitaxel microparticles in tumor tissue by transmembrane uptake of the nanoparticle through an albumin-specific glycoprotein 60–mediated mechanism, *secreted protein acidic and rich in cysteine* (SPARC),[86] followed by incorporation into intracellular acidic vesicles, and then digestion of the particle and intracellular release of the drug.

Mechanisms of Resistance

The MDR phenotype, which is mediated by the ABC transporter family and confers cross-resistance to a wide range of natural product drugs, is the best characterized mechanism of resistance to the taxanes. The most important ABC transporters implicated in taxane resistance is the *MDR1*-encoded gene product MDR1 or Pgp (ABC subfamily B1; *ABCB1*) and MDR3 (ABC subfamily *ABCB4*).[27,84] In contrast to the vinca alkaloids, ABCC1 (MRP1) and ABCC2

(MRP2) confer a lower level of resistance to the taxanes.[87] The clinical relevance of MDR1 and MRP overexpression to taxane resistance remains unclear, although cabazitaxel development was undertaken in part because of its lower susceptibility to MDR1. Early clinical observations of the antitumor profile of the taxanes, particularly in women with breast cancer who respond to the taxanes following the development of progressive disease while receiving treatment with the anthracyclines, suggest that cross-resistance to the taxanes and anthracycline is incomplete, but the role of MDR as a major cause of anthracycline resistance in this setting is not certain. Similar to the vinca alkaloid resistance, taxane resistance associated with the MDR phenotype can be reversed by many classes of drugs, including the calcium channel blockers, tamoxifen, and cyclosporine A.[33] Plasma concentrations of the principal component of the vehicles used to formulate paclitaxel (Cremophor EL) and docetaxel/cabazitaxel (polysorbate-80) (Tween 80) can also reverse MDR-mediated resistance.[88] However, clinical attempts to reverse taxane resistance with various transport inhibitors have yielded inconclusive results.[33]

Alterations in cytoskeletal components, tubulin-binding sites, and microtubule dynamics, as well as tubulin gene amplifications and isotype switching, have also been implicated in drug resistance to the taxanes (reviewed in Ref.[34]). Cancers grown in vitro and those sampled from patients resistant to tubulin-binding agents, including the taxanes, may exhibit alterations in MAP proteins, tubulin content, tubulin isotype profiles, and tubulin polymerization dynamics. Significantly higher levels of class I, III, and IV isotypes of β-tubulin have been associated with taxane resistance in both preclinical and clinical studies. High cellular levels of β-III tubulin increase the dynamic instability of microtubules and impede microtubule assembly, whereas low levels are associated with rapid microtubule assembly. High expression of the β-III tubulin isotype appears to independently predict a poor response and reduced survival in patients with non–small cell lung and breast cancer following treatment with taxanes.[34,89,90] Overexpression of both class III and IVa β-tubulin appears to be most germane to conferring resistance to the taxanes and other microtubule-stabilizing agents. Moreover, a loss of wild-type γ-actin, with concomitant expression of mutant isoforms, was identified in tumor samples from ALL patients at relapse, associating γ-actin to drug resistance.[91]

In addition to transport and tubulin factors, taxane cytotoxicity is also dependent on a host of signaling and DNA repair factors, including impairment of apoptosis, DNA repair, and survival pathways such as AKT and survivin.[92] Transfection of cells with HER-2, a member of the epidermal growth factor receptor, which is amplified and overexpressed in approximately 30% of breast cancers, confers taxane resistance.[93] Consistent with these observations, inactivation of HER-2 by the antibody trastuzumab sensitizes breast cancer cells to the taxanes, and the treatment of women with HER-2–overexpressing breast cancer with trastuzumab combined with paclitaxel increases survival in both the adjuvant and metastatic setting, compared to paclitaxel alone.[94] Various other factors have been implicated in taxane resistance. In prostate cancer cell lines, resistance to docetaxel was mediated by increased expression of miR-141,[95] which decreases the translation of apoptotic genes, while low levels of miR-200c up-regulated CYP1B1 and induced resistance in renal carcinomas.[96] Loss of KDM5D, which demethylates histone H3K4, leads to androgen receptor activation

and docetaxel resistance in prostate cancer cells[97] and correlated with poorer survival in patients. Finally, the exocrine subset of pancreatic ductal carcinoma, highly resistant to taxanes, became sensitive to paclitaxel when CYP3A5, a paclitaxel-metabolizing CYP, was inhibited.[98]

Clinical Pharmacology

Sensitive HPLC assays, particularly those using tandem mass spectroscopy and solid-phase extraction, detect paclitaxel and docetaxel concentrations in the low nanomolar range in minute quantities of plasma (0.05 mL) and simultaneously measure metabolites.[99] The taxanes are administered by intravenous infusion. Rapid drug distribution to all tissues except for central nervous system and avid intracellular concentration result in large volumes of distribution and long terminal $t_{1/2}$ values.

Paclitaxel

Paclitaxel has been studied at doses of 15 to 825 mg/m^2 and infused over 0.5 to 96 hours at both weekly and every 3-weeks dosing cycles. The pharmacokinetics of paclitaxel are nonlinear following short (<6 hours, mainly 3 hours) but not long (>24 hours) infusions.[100] For prolonged infusion schedules, paclitaxel plasma concentrations declined in a biphasic manner with an initial rapid decline representing distribution to the peripheral compartment and a slower drug elimination phase. With improvements in analytical assays, a three compartment model seems to be more accurate to depict the elimination of paclitaxel. The pharmacokinetics become nonlinear for shorter infusion durations because the elimination clearance varies with the dose administered.[101] With increasing plasma concentration of paclitaxel, there is a disproportionately larger increase in drug exposure accompanied by decrease in proportional drug elimination from body tissues. The clinical implications of this nonlinear pattern are that dose escalation may result in a disproportionate increase in drug exposure and hence toxicity, whereas dose reduction may result in a disproportionate decrease in drug exposure and affect its efficacy. The use of shorter infusion schedules also results in higher plasma concentrations of paclitaxel's Cremophor vehicle, which may be responsible for an appearance of nonlinearity (or pseudo-nonlinearity).[102] Key pharmacokinetic parameters of paclitaxel are presented in Table 11.2.

Paclitaxel clearance depends on metabolism by hepatic cytochrome P-450 oxidases, followed by biliary excretion.[103] It is metabolized primarily by CYP2C8 to the largely inactive metabolite 6-hydroxypaclitaxel and by CYP3A4 to 3′-phenylhydroxypaclitaxel (minor), as well as dihydroxylated metabolites.[104,105] In humans, 71% of an administered dose of paclitaxel is excreted in the feces within 5 days as either parent compound or metabolites, 6α-hydroxypaclitaxel accounting for 26% of the dose; only 5% is unchanged paclitaxel. Renal clearance of paclitaxel and metabolites is minimal.

Docetaxel

The pharmacokinetics of docetaxel on a 1-hour infusion schedule are linear at doses of 115 mg/m^2 or less and optimally fit a three-compartment model.[106] As with paclitaxel, plasma protein binding is high (>85% to 95%), binding in plasma primarily to α_1-acid glycoprotein, albumin, and lipoproteins. Because of its lipophilic properties, docetaxel has a large volume of distribution and avidly accumulates in all tissues except brain and testes. Terminal $t_{1/2}$ values range from 11.1 to 18.5 hours. Studies have focused on determining factors that may influence the large interindividual variability of docetaxel pharmacokinetics; however, precise factors are not yet completely understood.[107] The principal determinants of docetaxel clearance are body surface area, hepatic function, and plasma α_1-acid glycoprotein concentrations.[107,108] The main pharmacokinetic determinants of toxicity, particularly neutropenia, are total drug exposure and the time in which plasma levels exceed biologically relevant concentrations. Free drug concentrations are also predictive of neutropenia.[109]

Docetaxel is metabolized by the hepatic cytochrome P-450 mixed-function oxidase, specifically, CYP3A4 and CYP3A5 are the primary contributors, oxidizing and cyclizing the C-13 side chain and not the taxane ring.[105] These metabolites seem to be much less active than docetaxel. Both parent and metabolites are predominantly eliminated into the bile and excreted mainly in feces as metabolites. In patients with moderate impairment of hepatic function, clearances are reduced by 50%.

Nab-Paclitaxel

Nab-T doses of 80 to 360 mg/m^2 yielded dose linear paclitaxel pharmacokinetics. Approximately 89% to 98% of paclitaxel is protein bound in plasma. Plasma concentration data fit a two-compartment model. At the recommended dose of 260 mg/m^2, given as a 1-hour infusion every 3 weeks, the C_{max} in plasma was 7.7 µg/mL, and the primary elimination half life was 9 hours.[110] Subsequent studies found a terminal half-life of 13 to 27 hours and clearance of 13 to 15 L/h/m^2.[111-114] In humans, the clearance for nab-paclitaxel (13.2 L/h/m^2) was significantly greater than those for paclitaxel in Cremophor (8.9 L/h/m^2).[113] The greater clearance of nab-paclitaxel may be due to the binding of paclitaxel to albumin, which results in increased uptake of nab-paclitaxel in tumor and normal tissue via the SPARC receptor. Renal impairment has no impact on the clearance of the drug, while the maximal elimination rate decreased by about 22% to 25% in patients with moderate and severe hepatic impairment.[111] A 50% decrease in neutrophils correlated with the duration of a drug concentration above 720 ng/mL.

Kurzrock and colleagues have evaluated hepatic arterial infusion of nab-paclitaxel at doses up to 300 mg/m^2 given over 4 hours.[115] Clearance was dose independent at 22 to 24 L/h/m^2, and the plasma $t_{1/2}$ varied from 10 hours at 180 mg/m^2 over a 1-hour infusion to 2.6 hours for 300 mg/m^2 over 4 hours. C_{max} varied in the range from about 2 to 4.8 mg/L depending on the duration of infusion, markedly lower than the value for intravenous infusion and reflecting about a 40% extraction of drug in its first pass through the liver (Fig. 11.5). The drug was well tolerated and gave a 30% response rate and 60% disease control rate in patients with predominant hepatic metastases, without dose limiting toxicity.

Cabazitaxel

Following a 1-hour intravenous infusion, plasma concentrations of cabazitaxel can be described by a three-compartment model with a terminal half-life of 95 hours.[116] The pharmacokinetics of cabazitaxel is similar to docetaxel, except cabazitaxel has a larger volume of distribution, a longer terminal $t_{1/2}$, and a clearance of 30 to 45 L/h/m^2. Cabazitaxel is mainly bound to human serum albumin (82%) and lipoproteins. It is extensively metabolized in the liver (>95%), mainly by the CYP3A4/5 isoenzyme (80% to 90%), and to a lesser extent by CYP2C8. Cabazitaxel is the main circulating moiety in human plasma with seven metabolites detected in plasma. Cabazitaxel is mainly excreted in the feces as numerous metabolites (76% of the dose), while renal excretion of cabazitaxel and metabolites account for 3.7% of the dose (2.3% as unchanged drug in urine).

Drug Interactions

Both sequence-dependent pharmacokinetic and toxicologic interactions between paclitaxel and several other chemotherapy agents have been noted, but the number of clinically significant drug-drug interactions has been surprisingly low in light of the importance of cytochrome P-450 metabolism in drug disposition. In multi-drug regimens for breast cancer, paclitaxel or docetaxel are usually sequenced prior or after to either cisplatin or carboplatin. Cisplatin followed by paclitaxel (24-hour schedule) induces more profound neutropenia than the reverse sequence, due to a 33% reduction in the clearance of paclitaxel after cisplatin.[117] The least toxic sequence—paclitaxel before cisplatin—induced more cytotoxicity in vitro and was selected for clinical development for patients with ovarian and non–small cell lung cancer. Treatment with paclitaxel on either a 3- or 24-hour schedule followed by carboplatin results in equivalent neutropenia and less thrombocytopenia as compared with carboplatin as a single agent, which is not explained by pharmacokinetic interactions.[118] Sequencing paclitaxel by 24-hour infusion immediately before anthracyclines reduces the clearance rates of both doxorubicin and doxorubicinol.[119] Although neither sequence-dependent pharmacologic interactions nor exacerbation of acute toxicity occurs between when doxorubicin and a 3-hour infusion of paclitaxel are combined, this regimen leads to a higher incidence of cardiotoxicity than an equivalent cumulative doxorubicin dose given without paclitaxel. The precise etiology for these interactions is unclear. Experimental data indicate that paclitaxel enhances the metabolism of doxorubicin to cardiotoxic metabolites, such as doxorubicinol, in cardiomyocytes.[120] Clinically relevant drug-drug interactions for docetaxel (reviewed in Nieuweboer et al.[107]) are challenging to identify given its large interindividual variability; however, decreased docetaxel clearance or enhanced toxicity have been described when docetaxel was given concomitantly with topotecan or doxorubicin, respectively.[107] In addition, drug interactions may also result from inducers/inhibitors of CYP isoenzymes that are involved in the metabolism of paclitaxel (CYP3A4 and CYP2C8) and docetaxel (CYP3A). For example, potent inhibitors of CYP3A4 (e.g., ketoconazole and protease inhibitors) may increase drug exposure.

Dosage and Administration

Paclitaxel

Effective premedication regimens have decreased the incidence of major adverse reactions and have led to evaluations of paclitaxel in a broad range of schedules. Although the paclitaxel dose schedule consisting of 135 mg/m^2 over 24 hours was initially approved for patients with ovarian cancer, further approval was subsequently

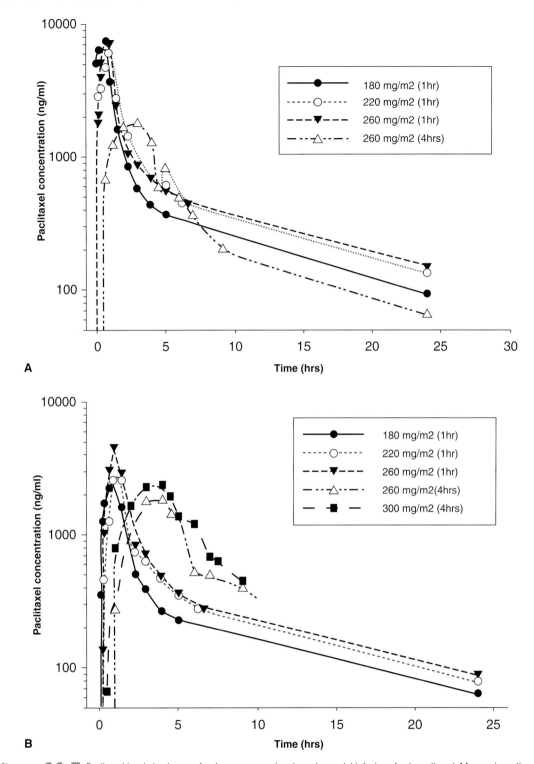

FIGURE 11.5 Paclitaxel levels in plasma after intravenous or intrahepatic arterial infusion of nab-paclitaxel. Mean nab-paclitaxel concentrations in plasma after intravenous (A) or intrahepatic arterial infusion (B) over 1 or 4 hours at the indicated doses. (From Siqing F, Culotta KS, Falchook GS, et al. Pharmacokinetic evaluation of nanoparticle albumin-bound paclitaxel delivered via hepatic arterial infusion in patients with predominantly hepatic metastases. *Cancer Chemother Pharmacol.* 2016;77:357-364, with permission.)

obtained for paclitaxel, 175 mg/m^2 on a 3-hour schedule in ovarian and other malignancies. In patients with advanced breast and ovarian cancers, the schedules are equivalent, particularly with regard to event-free and overall survival, and the shorter infusion is more convenient for patients. Based on in vitro studies, which indicated that the duration of exposure above a biologically relevant threshold is one of the most important determinants of cytotoxicity, more protracted infusion schedules were evaluated; however, there is no clear evidence that protracted schedules are superior with regard to efficacy or toxicities.[121] There has also been considerable interest in a 1-hour infusion weekly, which results in substantially less myelosuppression than every 3-week schedules. Weekly paclitaxel has yielded superior response rates compared with every 3-week schedules, particularly in breast cancer treatment, but not for ovarian cancer.[122,123] Standard dosages are listed on Table 11.2. Premedication with dexamethasone, antihistamine, and an H_2-receptor antagonist before treatment is recommended to prevent major HSRs.

Following intracavitary administration, paclitaxel concentrations in the peritoneal and pleural cavities are several orders of magnitude greater than plasma concentrations, which remain biologically relevant, and the results of a single randomized trial indicate that the administration of intraperitoneal paclitaxel in conjunction with carboplatin administered intravenously confers a modest survival advantage in previously untreated women with optimally debulked advanced ovarian cancer.[124] However, inconvenience and catheter-related complications have prevented its widespread adoption.

Patients with moderate-to-severe elevations in serum concentrations of hepatocellular enzymes or bilirubin (or both) are more likely to develop severe toxicity than patients without hepatic dysfunction.[125] Therefore, it is prudent to reduce paclitaxel doses by at least 50% in patients with abnormal serum bilirubin or significant (five to ten times) elevations in hepatic transaminases.

Contact of paclitaxel with plasticized polyvinyl chloride equipment or devices must be avoided because of the risk of patient exposures to plasticizers that may be leached from polyvinyl chloride infusion bags or sets. Paclitaxel solutions should be diluted and stored in glass or polypropylene bottles or suitable plastic bags (polypropylene or polyolefin) and administered through polyethylene-lined administration sets that include an in-line filter with a microporous membrane not greater than 0.22 μm.

Docetaxel

Regulatory approval was granted in the United States for docetaxel as a 1-hour infusion in a dose range of 60 to 100 mg/m² once every 3 weeks in patients with breast, non–small cell lung, prostate, gastric, or head and neck cancers. Like paclitaxel, docetaxel is also administered on a weekly schedule of 40 mg/m², but the weekly schedule actually appears less effective in adjuvant breast cancer therapy, although hematologic toxicity is much less than with conventional every 3-week schedules.[126] However, weekly administration schedules have been associated with a higher incidence of cumulative asthenia and neurotoxicity, particularly with docetaxel doses exceeding 36 mg/m²/wk.[127]

Patients with hepatic dysfunction (bilirubin > ULN, AST, and/or ALT >1.5 × ULN concomitant with alkaline phosphatase >2.5 × ULN) should not receive docetaxel due to increased risk of toxicity. The polysorbate 80 formulation of docetaxel was associated with an unacceptably high rate of hypersensitivity reactions and profound fluid retention in patients who did not receive premedication; thus, premedication with a dexamethasone regimen is recommended before treatment similar to paclitaxel. Glass bottles or polypropylene or polyolefin plastic products should be used for preparation and storage, and docetaxel should be administered through polyethylene-lined administration sets.

Nab-Paclitaxel

The recommended dosage schedule Nab-T for the treatment of patients with metastatic breast cancer is 260 mg/m² as a 30-minute IV infusion every 3 weeks. Nab-T, 125 to 150 mg/m², given on days 1, 8, and 15 in a 3-week cycle is an alternative schedule that appeared more effective than either every 3-week nab-paclitaxel or weekly Cremophor-based paclitaxel in achieving pathological complete remission in a neoadjuvant regimen for breast cancer.[128] The two paclitaxel formulations cause equal hematological toxicity, but nab-paclitaxel produced higher rates of grades 3 to 4 peripheral sensory neuropathy (8% to 15% versus 3%). No premedication to prevent HSRs or edema is indicated prior to administration.

Dose adjustments is recommended for hepatic impairment. It is also recommended that patients who experience severe neutropenia (neutrophil < 500/μL for at least 7 days) or severe sensory neuropathy should have the dosage reduced to 220 mg/m² for subsequent courses. Additional dose reduction or discontinuation of Nab-T may be necessary if the neuropathy worsens with continued treatment. The use of PVC-free containers and administration sets, as well as in-line filters, is not necessary.

Cabazitaxel

Cabazitaxel is approved for docetaxel-resistant prostate cancer based on a phase III trial of men with metastatic castrate-resistant prostate cancer demonstrating improved overall median survival on cabazitaxel compared to mitoxantrone.[129] It is given in a standard dose of 25 mg/m² every 3 weeks as a 1-hour infusion with daily oral prednisone and premedication prior to infusion to prevent hypersensitivity reactions. It is provided in a Tween 80 formulation, which requires further dissolution in ethanol and saline prior to administration. Dose adjustment for hepatic dysfunction aligns with guidelines for paclitaxel, dose reductions in patients with mild to moderate hepatic dysfunction and contraindicated in severe impairment.[130] No dose adjustment is necessary to renal dysfunction.[131] Dose adjustments are also recommended for severe neutropenia, febrile neutropenia, and severe diarrhea or neuropathy.

Toxicity of Taxanes

Despite having similar structural features, the toxicity spectra of paclitaxel, docetaxel, and Nab-T do not completely overlap (see Table 11.2). Myelosuppression, primarily neutropenia, is the principal toxicity of all three agents, but neurotoxicity is more frequent and severe with multiple doses of Nab-T.

Paclitaxel

Hematologic

Neutropenia is the principal toxicity of paclitaxel. The onset is usually on days 8 to 10, and recovery is generally complete by days 15 to 21 on every 3-week dosing regimens. A critical pharmacologic determinant of the severity of neutropenia is the duration that plasma drug concentrations are maintained above biologically relevant levels (0.05 to 0.1 μmol/L), which may explain why neutropenia is more severe with more protracted infusions.[103] The main determinant of the severity of neutropenia, aside from pharmacokinetics and dose, is the extent of prior myelotoxic therapy. Neutropenia is noncumulative, and the duration of severe neutropenia is usually brief. At paclitaxel doses exceeding 175 mg/m² on a 24-hour schedule and 225 mg/m² on a 3-hour schedule, nadir neutrophil counts are typically less than 500/μL for fewer than 5 days. Patients who have received extensive prior therapy can usually tolerate paclitaxel doses of 175 to 200 mg/m² over 3 or 24 hours. More frequent administration schedules, particularly weekly treatment schedules with doses of 80 to 100 mg/m², are associated with less severe neutropenia. Platelet and red blood cell counts are less affected by taxanes, except in heavily pretreated patients.

Hypersensitivity

The incidence of major HSRs in early trials was approximately 30% but declined to 1% to 3% following development of effective premedication.[132] Major HSRs, which are characterized by dyspnea with bronchospasm, urticaria, hypotension, and chest, abdominal, and back pain, usually occur within the first 10 minutes after the first (and less frequently after the second) treatment and resolve completely after stopping treatment. They occur infrequently (1% to 2% of infusions) after pretreatment with antihistamines and dexamethasone. Although the incidence of minor HSRs, such as isolated flushing and rash, is about 40%, major reactions do not generally occur after minor HSRs. Mechanisms of HSR to taxanes may involve complement activation induced by the solvent (Cremophor EL for paclitaxel and polysorbate 80 for docetaxel) or an immunologically mediated release of histamine or other vasoactive substances directed against the taxane moiety or the vehicle.[132] A management approach for HSRs based on skin testing and rapid drug desensitization has been shown to be effective and safe method for taxane rechallenge.[132]

Peripheral Neurotoxicity

Peripheral neuropathy, another dose-limiting toxicity of paclitaxel, is characterized by sensory symptoms, such as numbness in a symmetric glove-and-stocking distribution,[133] and a loss of deep tendon reflexes. Axonal degeneration and demyelination neuronopathy is particularly severe at higher doses or when combined with other neurotoxic agents such as cisplatin. Severe neurotoxicity is uncommon when paclitaxel is given alone at doses of 135 to 175 mg/m² on a 3- or 24-hour schedule every 3 weeks or below 100 mg/m² on a weekly schedule, but most "low-risk" patients experience only mild or moderate effects. Patients with preexisting neuropathy caused by other drugs or comorbidities (diabetes, alcoholism) are prone to paclitaxel-induced neuropathy, as are patients over age 70. Symptoms may begin as soon as 24 to 72 hours after treatment with higher doses (≥250 mg/m²) but usually occur only after multiple courses at 135 to 250 mg/m² every 3 weeks. Neurotoxicity is generally more pronounced when paclitaxel is administered on short infusion schedules, indicating that peak plasma concentration may be a principal pharmacologic determinant. The combination of paclitaxel on a 3-hour schedule or a weekly schedule and cisplatin is particularly neurotoxic for non–small cell lung cancer patients, while paclitaxel with carboplatin produces less neurotoxicity. There are no antidotes of proven value to prevent or treat the neuropathy.[134] Transient myalgia and arthralgia of uncertain etiology, usually noted 24 to 48 hours after therapy and apparently dose-related, are also common, and a myopathy has been described in patients receiving high doses with cisplatin.[135]

Cardiac

Paclitaxel treatment has been associated with cardiac rhythm disturbances, most of which were subclinical and only discovered with cardiac monitoring during infusion of drug.[136] The most common disturbance, a transient, asymptomatic bradycardia, was noted in 29% of patients in one trial and, in the absence of hemodynamic effects, is not an indication for discontinuing paclitaxel. These bradyarrhythmias are likely true adverse effects of paclitaxel as related taxanes affect cardiac automaticity and conduction and occur in humans and animals after ingesting of yew plants. There is also no evidence that chronic, long-term treatment with paclitaxel causes progressive cardiac dysfunction. Routine cardiac monitoring during paclitaxel therapy is not necessary but is advisable for patients who may not be able to tolerate bradyarrhythmias, such as those with atrioventricular conduction disturbances or ventricular dysfunction. The combination of paclitaxel and doxorubicin is associated with a higher frequency of congestive cardiotoxicity than with the same cumulative doxorubicin dose given alone, especially when the dose of doxorubicin exceeds 360 mg/m². Paclitaxel may increase the incidence of congestive heart failure when given with trastuzumab, a known cadiotoxin.[137]

Other Toxicities

The taxanes as a class often cause dermatological adverse events.[138] Paclitaxel and the other taxanes induces reversible alopecia of the scalp in a dose-related fashion and loss of all facial and body hair in heavily pretreated patients. In a small fraction of patients, the alopecia is permanent. Rash, especially in the intertriginous areas, is common, as is photosensitivity and in 5% to 10% of taxane-treated patients, a desquamation and erythema of the dorsum of the hands and, less commonly, feet. Pain and erythema associated with the hand-foot syndrome may require steroid cream or oral corticosteroids. Scleroderma-like skin changes and even subacute cutaneous lupus erythematosus, especially in photoexposed areas, are noted with taxane treatment. Nail disorders, most prominently onycholysis, may be associated with rash, particularly in patients treated on weekly schedules. Drug-related gastrointestinal effects, such as vomiting and diarrhea, are uncommon. Higher paclitaxel doses or protracted (96-hour) infusional administration can cause mucositis. Rarely neutropenic enterocolitis and gastrointestinal necrosis have been noted in patients given high doses of paclitaxel in combination with doxorubicin or cyclophosphamide.[139] Severe hepatotoxicity, pancreatitis, and pulmonary toxicity (e.g., acute bilateral pneumonitis) have also been noted rarely. In contrast to the vinca alkaloids, the agent is not a potent vesicant, but extravasations of large volumes can cause moderate soft tissue injury.

Docetaxel

Hematologic

Neutropenia is the principal toxicity of docetaxel.[140] Following treatment with docetaxel administered over 1 hour every 3 weeks, neutropenia was noted within 1 week, and resolution typically occurs by day 15. At a dose of 100 mg/m² administered over 1 hour, neutrophil counts fall below 500/μL, and the incidence of neutropenic complications is high. Severe neutropenia at 75 mg/m² is common, but the duration is brief, and febrile neutropenia is much less common. Neutropenia is significantly less when lower doses are administered on a weekly schedule. The most important determinant of neutropenia is the extent of prior treatment. Thrombocytopenia and anemia are usually modest.

Hypersensitivity

HSRs have been reported in approximately 31% of patients receiving docetaxel without premedication in early phase II studies.[132] Major reactions characterized by dyspnea, bronchospasm, and hypotension typically occur during the first or second course and within minutes after the start of treatment. Symptoms generally resolve within 15 minutes after cessation of treatment, and docetaxel infusion can be resumed without sequelae after treatment with an H2-receptor antagonist. Fortunately, however, most events are minor and rarely result in discontinuation of treatment. Both the incidence and severity of HSRs appear to be reduced by premedication with corticosteroids and H1-receptor and H2-receptor antagonists, but the corticosteroid premedication regimen is principally administered to prevent fluid retention. Patients with severe HSRs to paclitaxel may be at increased risk of similar reactions to docetaxel.[132]

Fluid Retention

Docetaxel induces a unique fluid retention syndrome characterized by edema, weight gain, and pleural or peritoneal collections. Fluid retention is cumulative and unrelated to hypoalbuminemia or cardiac, renal, or hepatic dysfunction. Instead, increased capillary permeability and insufficient lymphatic drainage appear to be responsible.[141] Premedication with corticosteroids largely remedies this side effect and increases the number of courses and cumulative docetaxel dose before the onset of this toxicity.[142] Aggressive use of diuretics may accelerate fluid loss in cases of ascites or pleural effusion.

Neurotoxicity

Docetaxel neurotoxicity is similar to that of paclitaxel, but less frequent and less severe. Patients typically complain of paresthesia and numbness, but peripheral motor effects may also occur. Docetaxel can be considered as a substitute for paclitaxel in high-risk patients with underlying neuropathy.[143] Nevertheless, mild-to-moderate peripheral neurotoxicity occurs in approximately 40% of previously untreated patients. Severe toxicity has been unusual with every 3-week docetaxel doses less than 100 mg/m^2, except in patients with antecedent neurotoxicity and relevant disorders, such as alcohol abuse and diabetes mellitus. Malaise, myalgia, and arthralgia have been prominent complaints in patients who have been treated with large cumulative doses, particularly when docetaxel is administered on a weekly schedule.[135]

Other Toxicities

Skin toxicity, manifested as the dorsal hand-foot syndrome or rash, may occur in approximately 50% of patients; corticosteroid premedication reduces the incidence.[138] Other toxicities are as described above for paclitaxel that are deemed to be a class effect of the taxanes. Stomatitis is more common with docetaxel than paclitaxel, but still infrequent.

Nab-Paclitaxel

The toxicity profile of Nab-T is similar to the other taxanes: neutropenia is dose-limiting toxicity, neuropathy as a later complication.[133] The rate of HSRs, particularly major reactions, is about the same as that of Cremophor-based paclitaxel. Premedication regimen to prevent HSRs is not necessary. Nab-T caused a greater degree of severe sensory neuropathic symptoms (10% versus 2%), severe arthralgia/myalgia (8% versus 2%), and asthenia (8% versus 3%) as compared to Cremophor-based paclitaxel, possibly the function of higher doses of Nab-T tolerated. Additional toxicities, most of which are noted with other taxane formulations, include increased lacrimation, conjunctivitis, radiation recall, rash, and uncommonly Stevens-Johnson syndrome, toxic epidermal necrolysis, photosensitivity reactions, and, in patients previously treated with capecitabine, palmar-plantar erythrodysesthesia.

Cabazitaxel

Most common toxicities associated with cabazitaxel were hematologic with the rates (all grade) of neutropenia, leukopenia, and anemia being greater than 90%. Diarrhea, fatigue, and asthenia were the most common grade 3 or higher nonhematologic adverse events. Cabazitaxel is associated with less peripheral neuropathy, nail disorders, alopecia, and dysgeusia than is docetaxel; however, it induces a high rate of grade ≥3 neutropenia, which needs to be proactively managed to avoid febrile neutropenia.[144]

Pharmacogenetics

Genetic variants in drug-metabolizing enzymes, transporters (that taxanes are substrates for), and other proteins have been shown to influence the pharmacology of the taxanes. Several allelic variants of these genes alter functional activity, thereby contributing to interindividual differences in taxane metabolism and predisposing patients to variable toxicities. Pharmacogenetics studies have been conducted on genes encoding: (a) efflux transporters of the ATP-binding cassette family (*ABCB1, ABCG2, ABCC1, ABCC10,* and *ABCC2*); (b) influx transporters of the solute carrier (SLC) family (*SLCO1B1* and *SLCO1B3*); (c) CYP-metabolizing isoenzymes of taxanes (*CYP3A4, CYP3A5,* and, for paclitaxel, *CYP2C8*); and more recently (d) targets of taxanes such as the *β*-tubulin gene encoding the *β*-subunit of tubulin dimers (*TUBB2A*) and microtubule-associated genes (*MAP4* and *MAPT*).

A systematic review was conducted for pharmacogenetics studies on paclitaxel- and docetaxel-induced toxicities and revealed inconclusive results.[145] Some studies have suggested that polymorphisms in *CYP2C8* or *ABCB1* cause pharmacokinetic variation, while others show no effect. The *CYP2C8*3* had lower clearance of paclitaxel, while *ABCB1* (2677G>T/A) variant allele had a significantly higher clearance of paclitaxel.[146] A study of docetaxel clearance found greater clearance with patients with the *CYP3A4*1B* and *CYP3A5*1A* variants.[147] Inconclusive data for risk of toxicity and effects on drug exposure were reported on variants in *CYP3A4, CYP3A5, ABCB1,* and, for paclitaxel, *CYP2C8*. The genetic variants *CYP2C8*3*[148-150] for paclitaxel and *CYP3A4*1B/CYP3A5*3* for taxanes[151,152] have shown predictive potential for hematological toxicity and neurotoxicity. Two variants in *ABCB1* (3435C>T and 2677G>T/A) have frequently been identified for their association with neurological, GI, and hematological adverse events.[153-155]

Recent genome-wide association studies have found several genetic variants associated with risk of peripheral neuropathy during treatment with paclitaxel[156-159] and with docetaxel.[160]

One study found that the *CYP1B1*3* (4326 C>G) allele was significantly associated with progression-free survival, independent of paclitaxel clearance[161] and with survival in prostate cancer patients receiving docetaxel.[162] In a study of patients with metastatic breast cancer, the *ABCB1* (3435 C>T) variant allele showed a significantly lower disease control rate and lower overall survival rate.[163] Other studies associated *ABCB1* (2677G>T/A) with response to paclitaxel.[164,165] Variations in methodological approach, sample size, study design, treatment schedule, and toxicity end point affect consistency of results. Substantial validation in multiple cohorts and prospective studies is required to fully understand their relevance and potential translation into clinical practice.

Other Natural Products that Enhance Tubulin Polymerization

Tubulin is a major strategic target for plant and animal defense mechanisms. In addition to taxanes and vincas, numerous other natural toxins that modify tubulin polymerization and function include: the **epothilones** (isolated from myxobacterium *Sorangium cellulosum*), **discodermolide** (from the Caribbean sponge *Discodermia dissoluta*), **eleutherobin** (from the soft coral *Eleutherobia* sp.), the **taccalonolides** (from *Tacca chantrieri*), **peloruside A** (from the New Zealand marine sponge *Mycale hentscheli*), **laulimalide** (from the marine sponge *Cacospongia mycofijiensis*), and the **sarcodictyins** (from the Mediterranean stoloniferan coral *Sarcodictyon roseum*). Epothilones, discodermolide, eleutherobins, and the sarcodictyins bind to microtubules at or near the taxane-binding site, and possess a common pharmacophore that may enable the development of synthetic or semisynthetic compounds with improved pharmaceutical properties.[166] Laulimalide binds to a unique site on microtubules.

Epothilones

Of the above candidates, only epothilones and the semisynthetic, eribulin, have been approved for clinical use. Ixabepilone (IX) (Fig. 11.6), a semisynthetic analog of epothilone B with a modified lactam substitution as compared to the naturally occurring molecule, has received approval in the United States and elsewhere alone or in combination with capecitabine for the treatment of patients with metastatic or locally advanced breast cancer resistant to anthracyclines and taxanes.[167] Because of its toxicity and modest activity, IX is rarely used in clinical practice. Epothilone D (KOS-862), which lacks a potentially toxic epoxide, showed anticancer activity and less neurotoxicity in patients with breast and ovarian cancers in early trials, but its development has been discontinued as have other analogues of IX.[168]

Mechanism of Action

Epothilones competitively inhibit binding of paclitaxel to tubulin polymers in vitro, suggesting a common binding site and mechanism.[169] Epothilone B promotes tubulin polymerization in the absence of GTP and MAPs, and do so more avidly than paclitaxel. The features of their antitumor action closely resemble those of the taxanes: mitotic arrest, p53-mediated apoptosis, and in cells progressing to interphase, multinucleation and cell death.

Mechanisms of Resistance

A critical difference between the epothilones, taxanes, and vinca alkaloids is that overexpression of the ABC transporters Pgp and MRP1 minimally affects the cytotoxicity of the epothilones.[170] Epothilones have strong antiproliferative activity in paclitaxel-resistant human cancer cells with high expression of Pgp, while tumor samples from patients with IX-responsive malignancies may show significant expression of MDR1 and MRP1 mRNA.[168]

β-III-tubulin overexpressing tumors, which are resistant to taxanes, remain sensitive to epothilones.[171] In preclinical systems, cancer cells with point mutations involving βI and various other β-tubulins at sites that are critical for microtubule stabilization are resistant to the IX.[172] Additionally, the transporter, MRP-7 (ABCC10), appears to confer resistance to epothilone B, other natural products, and nucleoside analogues that are not substrates for Pgp.[173]

Ixabepilone

Clinical Pharmacology

In cancer patients, IX exhibits dose-proportional pharmacokinetics in the dose range of 15 to 57 mg/m^2.[174] Following administration of a standard 40 mg/m^2 dose, C_{max} and terminal phase $t_{1/2}$ values average 252 ng/mL and 52 hours, respectively. Like the taxanes and vincas, IX's volume of distribution at steady state is large, with mean values exceeding 1,000 L, reflecting rapid tissue uptake and binding. Protein binding is modest (67% to 77%) compared to taxanes.

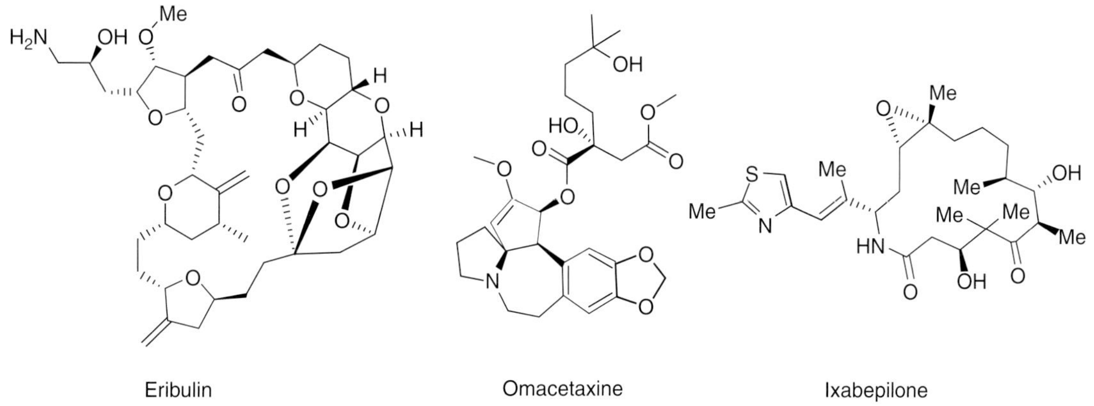

Eribulin   Omacetaxine   Ixabepilone

FIGURE **11.6** Structures of eribulin and ixabepilone.

The principal mode of clearance of IX is hepatic metabolism by CYP3A4.[175] Little parent compound is excreted (1.6% and 5.6% of the dose in feces and urine, respectively). More than 30 inactive metabolites are excreted into human urine and feces, but no single metabolite accounts for more than 6% of the administered dose.

Drug Interactions

IX does not induce CYP isoenzymes and would not be expected to affect disposition of other substrates for these enzymes. However, coadministration of IX with ketoconazole, a potent CYP3A4 inhibitor, increases IX AUC values by 79%, on average, compared to IX given alone.[175] Therefore, strong inhibitors or inducers of CYP3A4 should be used with caution in patients receiving of IX. IX has no known metabolic interaction with capecitabine.

Dosage and Administration

The recommended dosage of IX is 40 mg/m^2 intravenously over 3 hours every 3 weeks. Doses for patients with body surface areas greater than 2.2 m^2 should be calculated based on 2.2 m^2. To minimize major HSRs, all patients should be premedicated 1 hour before treatment with both an H$_1$-histamine and H$_2$-histamine antagonist. For patients who experience an HSR, a corticosteroid is added to the above pretreatment regimen. Dose modification and/or treatment delay are recommended for patients who develop clinically relevant grades of neuropathy and/or myelosuppression.

As IX clearance primarily depends on CYP3A4 metabolism, dose reductions are necessary for patients with altered hepatic function. Dose reduction to 32 mg/m^2 in patients with AST or ALT elevations from 2.5 to 10 times the upper limit of normal (ULN) and bilirubin up to 1.5 times the ULN is recommended. For patients with AST or ALT elevations up to 10 times the ULN and bilirubin ranging from 1.5 to 3 times the ULN of normal, doses should be reduced to 20 mg/m^2. If well tolerated, the dose can be increased up to, but should not exceed, 30 mg/m^2 in subsequent cycles. IX monotherapy should not be administered to patients with ALT and/or AST above 10 times the ULN and/or bilirubin above 3.0 mg/dL. Ixabepilone combined with capecitabine is not recommended for patients who have AST, ALT levels, and/or bilirubin levels exceeding the ULN. In a population pharmacokinetic study of ixabepilone as monotherapy, there was no meaningful effect of mild and moderate renal insufficiency (creatinine clearance >30 mL/min) on the pharmacokinetics of ixabepilone. Ixabepilone in combination with capecitabine has not been evaluated in patients with calculated creatinine clearance less than 50 mL/min.

Based on pharmacokinetic studies, if a strong CYP3A4 inhibitor must be coadministered, dose reduction to 20 mg/m^2, which should adjust the IX AUC to that observed without inhibitors, should be considered.[175]

Toxicity

Neurotoxicity

Peripheral neurotoxicity is the most common serious toxicity observed with ixabepilone both as monotherapy and when combined with capecitabine.[176] Symptoms, including a burning sensation, hyperesthesia, hypoesthesia, paresthesia, discomfort, and neuropathic pain, are reported by 60% to 70% of breast cancer patients who had previously received a taxane after treatment with ixabepilone alone or in combination with capecitabine. Disabling

toxicity (grades 3 and 4) was noted in 14% on monotherapy and 23% with capecitabine, respectively. In heavily pretreated patients, neuropathy is first noticed during the first three cycles and becomes progressively more serious thereafter, and may require dose reduction, treatment delay, and discontinuation of IX. Following treatment discontinuation and/or dose reduction, manifestations usually resolve in 4 to 6 weeks, as compared to neuropathy due to the taxanes and vinca alkaloids, which resolves more slowly and incompletely. Patients who have hepatic insufficiency and/or diabetes mellitus are at an increased risk of developing severe neuropathy.

Myelosuppression

Dose-dependent myelosuppression, principally neutropenia, is common following IX treatment.[177] Effects on platelets and red blood cells are not dose limiting. Grade 4 neutropenia (<500 cells/μL) has occurred in 36% of patients treated with ixabepilone in combination with capecitabine and in 23% of patients treated with monotherapy; however, febrile neutropenia and infection with neutropenia have been reported in 5% or fewer patients on monotherapy or with capecitabine. Myelosuppression does not generally worsen with successive treatment but may necessitate dose reduction if severe.

Hypersensitivity

Since IX is formulated in polyoxyethylated castor oil, severe HSRs, largely secondary to this diluent, do occur. All patients should receive premedication with H$_1$- and H$_2$-histamine antagonists approximately 1 hour before treatment. In the case of severe HSRs, treatment should be stopped and aggressive supportive measures (e.g., epinephrine, corticosteroids) started. Corticosteroid pretreatment and prolonging the infusion time may allow successful retreatment of patients who had experienced prior reactions.[177]

Other Toxicities

Patients treated with ixabepilone have developed cognitive dysfunction, lethargy, and discoordination in the peritreatment period, possibly due to the effects of ethanol in the diluent. Myalgia and arthralgia in the peritreatment period have also been noted. Various cardiac disturbances, including myocardial infarction, arrhythmia, left ventricular dysfunction, and congestive heart failure, have also been observed but may have been incidental. Ileus, colitis, gastritis, gastrointestinal hemorrhage, hepatic injury, erythema multiforme, various rashes, and muscle spasm have all been reported as uncommon side effects. Nail disorders, including onycholysis and subungual hemorrhagic bullae, occur after treatment courses.

Natural Products that Disrupt Tubulin Dynamics

Other natural and semisynthetic agents under evaluation bind to the vinca or colchicine-binding domains of tubulin. The dolastatins, which constitute a series of oligopeptides isolated from the sea hare, *Dolabella auricularia*, were evaluated clinically but failed to show advantage over other therapeutics that target tubulin.[178] Auristatin and related analogs, which are among the most potent derivatives of dolastatin-10, have proven activity when linked to anti-CD30 antibody for treatment of Hodgkin's lymphoma (see Chapter 29, Monoclonal Antibodies).

Eribulin

Eribulin mesylate (Fig. 11.6), a synthetic macrocyclic ketone analogue of the marine natural product halichondrin B, which was originally isolated from the marine sponge *Halichondria okadai*, is approved for treatment of metastatic breast cancer and for soft tissue sarcomas.[179,180] Halichondrin analogues bind to tubulin at a unique site at the positive end of the microtubule, inhibit tubulin polymerization, induce mitotic arrest and apoptosis, as well as possess marked growth-inhibitory properties very similar to the vincas, but in some cell lines, it is not cross-resistant with other tubulin binders and is active in the subnanomolar range.[181] Eribulin also exhibits effects on peripheral nerves, angiogenesis, vascular remodeling, and reversal of epithelial-to-mesenchymal transition.[181]

The pharmacokinetics of eribulin is linear with a terminal half-life of approximately 40 hours and a large volume of distribution. No accumulation of eribulin is observed with weekly administration. Metabolite concentrations represented less than 0.6% of parent compound, confirming that there are no major human metabolites of eribulin. Cytochrome P-450 3A4 (CYP3A4) negligibly metabolizes eribulin *in vitro*. Unchanged eribulin accounted for approximately 91% and less than 10% of total eribulin in feces and urine, respectively.[182] There is minimal risk of drug-drug interactions in the clinical setting.[183]

Approval of eribulin for breast cancer patients progressing after two lines of therapy was granted based on the results of the weekly schedule of eribulin, as compared to physician's choice (a variety of drugs, including capecitabine), in which the drug produced no improvement in progression-free survival, but a 3-month advantage in overall survival.[184,185] In 2017, eribulin received approval for treatment of patients with unresectable or metastatic liposarcoma who have received a prior anthracycline-containing regimen.[180] The recommended treatment dose is 1.4 mg/m^2 administered intravenously over 2 to 5 minutes on days 1 and 8 of a 21-day cycle. Dose reduction to 1.1 mg/m^2 is recommended for mild hepatic impairment and for moderate to severe renal impairment and 0.7 mg/m^2 for moderate hepatic impairment.[186,187] Eribulin does not require a vehicle for formulation and has a much reduced propensity for causing HSRs. The primary toxicities were neutropenia (grades 3 to 4 in 50% of patients) at about day 15 on the weekly schedule, and in a shorter duration on the 3-week schedule, and peripheral (mainly sensory) neuropathy, which in phase II to III studies developed in 30% to 50% of patients with breast cancer, including 10% to 20% with grades 3 to 4 toxicity.[179] The neuropathy tended to develop later (at 11 weeks) and led to treatment discontinuation less frequently (3%) than it did for patients on ixabepilone. Prior treatment with a taxane may increase the incidence of neuropathy.

References

1. Jordan MA, Kamath K. How do microtubule-targeted drugs work? An overview. *Curr Cancer Drug Targets.* 2007;7:730-742.
2. Douer D. Efficacy and Safety of Vincristine Sulfate Liposome Injection in the Treatment of Adult Acute Lymphocytic Leukemia. *Oncologist.* 2016;21:840-847.
3. Bighin C, Pronzato P, Del Mastro L. Trastuzumab emtansine in the treatment of HER-2-positive metastatic breast cancer patients. *Future Oncol.* 2013;9:955-957.
4. Gravanis I, Tzogani K, van Hennik P, et al. The European Medicines Agency Review of Brentuximab Vedotin (Adcetris) for the Treatment of Adult Patients With Relapsed or Refractory CD30+ Hodgkin Lymphoma or Systemic Anaplastic Large Cell Lymphoma: Summary of the Scientific Assessment of the Committee for Medicinal Products for Human Use. *Oncologist.* 2016;21:102-109.
5. Li H, DeRosier DJ, Nicholson WV, Nogales E, Downing KH. Microtubule structure at 8 A resolution. *Structure.* 2002;10:1317-1328.
6. Alushin GM, Lander GC, Kellogg EH, Zhang R, Baker D, Nogales E. High-resolution microtubule structures reveal the structural transitions in alpha-beta-tubulin upon GTP hydrolysis. *Cell.* 2014;157:1117-1129.
7. Zheng Y, Jung MK, Oakley BR. Gamma-tubulin is present in Drosophila melanogaster and Homo sapiens and is associated with the centrosome. *Cell.* 1991;65:817-823.
8. Luduena RF. Multiple forms of tubulin: different gene products and covalent modifications. *Int Rev Cytol.* 1998;178:207-275.
9. Vale RD. Microtubule motors: many new models off the assembly line. *Trends Biochem Sci.* 1992;17:300-304.
10. Verhey KJ, Gaertig J. The tubulin code. *Cell Cycle.* 2007;6:2152-2160.
11. Bhalla KN. Microtubule-targeted anticancer agents and apoptosis. *Oncogene.* 2003;22:9075-9086.
12. Wilson L, Jordan MA. *Pharmacological Probes of Microtubule Function.* New York: Wiley-Liss; 1994.
13. Mitchison T, Kirschner M. Dynamic instability of microtubule growth. *Nature.* 1984;312:237-242.
14. Margolis RL, Wilson L. Microtubule treadmilling: what goes around comes around. *Bioessays.* 1998;20:830-836.
15. Zhang R, Alushin GM, Brown A, Nogales E. Mechanistic Origin of Microtubule Dynamic Instability and Its Modulation by EB Proteins. *Cell.* 2015;162:849-859.
16. Zhai Y, Kronebusch PJ, Simon PM, Borisy GG. Microtubule dynamics at the G2/M transition: abrupt breakdown of cytoplasmic microtubules at nuclear envelope breakdown and implications for spindle morphogenesis. *J Cell Biol.* 1996;135:201-214.
17. Zhu Y, Zhou Y, Shi J. Post-slippage multinucleation renders cytotoxic variation in anti-mitotic drugs that target the microtubules or mitotic spindle. *Cell Cycle.* 2014;13:1756-1764.
18. Johnson IS. Historical background of Vinca alkaloid research and areas of future interest. *Cancer Chemother Rep.* 1968;52:455-461.
19. Rowinsky EK, Noe DA, Trump DL, et al. Pharmacokinetic, bioavailability, and feasibility study of oral vinorelbine in patients with solid tumors. *J Clin Oncol.* 1994;12:1754-1763.
20. Bates D, Eastman A. Microtubule destabilising agents: far more than just antimitotic anticancer drugs. *Br J Clin Pharmacol.* 2017;83:255-268.
21. Kruczynski A, Barret JM, Etievant C, Colpaert F, Fahy J, Hill BT. Antimitotic and tubulin-interacting properties of vinflunine, a novel fluorinated Vinca alkaloid. *Biochem Pharmacol.* 1998;55:635-648.
22. Jordan MA, Himes RH, Wilson L. Comparison of the effects of vinblastine, vincristine, vindesine, and vinepidine on microtubule dynamics and cell proliferation in vitro. *Cancer Res.* 1985;45:2741-2747.
23. Sullivan KF. Structure and utilization of tubulin isotypes. *Annu Rev Cell Biol.* 1988;4:687-716.
24. Zhou XJ, Placidi M, Rahmani R. Uptake and metabolism of vinca alkaloids by freshly isolated human hepatocytes in suspension. *Anticancer Res.* 1994;14:1017-1022.
25. Simoens C, Lardon F, Pauwels B, et al. Comparative study of the radiosensitizing and cell cycle effects of vinflunine and vinorelbine, in vitro. *BMC Cancer.* 2008;8:65.
26. Jackson DV Jr, Bender RA. Cytotoxic thresholds of vincristine in a murine and a human leukemia cell line in vitro. *Cancer Res.* 1979;39:4346-4349.
27. Kavallaris M, Annereau JP, Barret JM. Potential mechanisms of resistance to microtubule inhibitors. *Semin Oncol.* 2008;35:S22-S27.
28. Li W, Zhang H, Assaraf YG, et al. Overcoming ABC transporter-mediated multidrug resistance: molecular mechanisms and novel therapeutic drug strategies. *Drug Resist Updat.* 2016;27:14-29.
29. Peterson RH, Meyers MB, Spengler BA, Biedler JL. Alteration of plasma membrane glycopeptides and gangliosides of Chinese hamster cells accompanying development of resistance to daunorubicin and vincristine. *Cancer Res.* 1983;43:222-228.

30. Pieters R, Hongo T, Loonen AH, et al. Different types of non-P-glycoprotein mediated multiple drug resistance in children with relapsed acute lymphoblastic leukaemia. *Br J Cancer.* 1992;65:691-697.

31. Hipfner DR, Deeley RG, Cole SP. Structural, mechanistic and clinical aspects of MRP1. *Biochim Biophys Acta.* 1999;1461:359-376.

32. Etievant C, Kruczynski A, Barret JM, Tait AS, Kavallaris M, Hill BT. Markedly diminished drug resistance-inducing properties of vinflunine (20′,20′-difluoro-3′,4′-dihydrovinorelbine) relative to vinorelbine, identified in murine and human tumour cells in vivo and in vitro. *Cancer Chemother Pharmacol.* 2001;48:62-70.

33. Callaghan R, Luk F, Bebawy M. Inhibition of the multidrug resistance P-glycoprotein: time for a change of strategy? *Drug Metab Dispos.* 2014;42:623-631.

34. Kavallaris M. Microtubules and resistance to tubulin-binding agents. *Nat Rev Cancer.* 2010;10:194-204.

35. Arai K, Matsumoto Y, Nagashima Y, Yagasaki K. Regulation of class II beta-tubulin expression by tumor suppressor p53 protein in mouse melanoma cells in response to Vinca alkaloid. *Mol Cancer Res.* 2006;4:247-255.

36. Upreti M, Galitovskaya EN, Chu R, et al. Identification of the major phosphorylation site in Bcl-xL induced by microtubule inhibitors and analysis of its functional significance. *J Biol Chem.* 2008;283:35517-35525.

37. Damen CW, Rosing H, Schellens JH, Beijnen JH. High-performance liquid chromatography coupled with mass spectrometry for the quantitative analysis of vinca-alkaloids in biological matrices: a concise survey from the literature. *Biomed Chromatogr.* 2010;24:83-90.

38. Nelson RL. The comparative clinical pharmacology and pharmacokinetics of vindesine, vincristine, and vinblastine in human patients with cancer. *Med Pediatr Oncol.* 1982;10:115-127.

39. Gidding CE, Kellie SJ, Kamps WA, de Graaf SS. Vincristine revisited. *Crit Rev Oncol Hematol.* 1999;29:267-287.

40. Jackson DV Jr, Sethi VS, Spurr CL, McWhorter JM. Pharmacokinetics of vincristine in the cerebrospinal fluid of humans. *Cancer Res.* 1981;41:1466-1468.

41. Rahmani R, Zhou XJ. Pharmacokinetics and metabolism of vinca alkaloids. *Cancer Surv.* 1993;17:269-281.

42. Jackson DV. The periwinkle alkaloids. In: Lokich JJ, ed. *Cancer Chemotherapy by Infusion.* Chicago, IL: Precept Press; 1990:155-185.

43. Sparano JA, Lee JY, Kaplan LD, et al. Rituximab plus concurrent infusional EPOCH chemotherapy is highly effective in HIV-associated B-cell non-Hodgkin lymphoma. *Blood.* 2010;115:3008-3016.

44. Jackson DV Jr, Castle MC, Bender RA. Biliary excretion of vincristine. *Clin Pharmacol Ther.* 1978;24:101-107.

45. Dennison JB, Kulanthaivel P, Barbuch RJ, Renbarger JL, Ehlhardt WJ, Hall SD. Selective metabolism of vincristine in vitro by CYP3A5. *Drug Metab Dispos.* 2006;34:1317-1327.

46. Owellen RJ, Hartke CA, Hains FO. Pharmacokinetics and metabolism of vinblastine in humans. *Cancer Res.* 1977;37:2597-2602.

47. Zhou-Pan XR, Seree E, Zhou XJ, et al. Involvement of human liver cytochrome P450 3A in vinblastine metabolism: drug interactions. *Cancer Res.* 1993;53:5121-5126.

48. Jarosinski PF, Moscow JA, Alexander MS, Lesko LJ, Balis FM, Poplack DG. Altered phenytoin clearance during intensive chemotherapy for acute lymphoblastic leukemia. *J Pediatr.* 1988;112:996-999.

49. Rajaonarison JF, Lacarelle B, Catalin J, Durand A, Cano JP. Effect of anticancer drugs on the glucuronidation of 3′-azido-3′-deoxythymidine in human liver microsomes. *Drug Metab Dispos.* 1993;21:823-829.

50. Stock W, Diouf B, Crews KR, et al. An Inherited Genetic Variant in CEP72 Promoter Predisposes to Vincristine-Induced Peripheral Neuropathy in Adults With Acute Lymphoblastic Leukemia. *Clin Pharmacol Ther.* 2017;101:391-395.

51. Sulkes A, Collins JM. Reappraisal of some dosage adjustment guidelines. *Cancer Treat Rep.* 1987;71:229-233.

52. Dyke RW. Treatment of inadvertent intrathecal injection of vincristine. *N Engl J Med.* 1989;321:1270-1271.

53. Swain SM, Arezzo JC. Neuropathy associated with microtubule inhibitors: diagnosis, incidence, and management. *Clin Adv Hematol Oncol.* 2008;6:455-467.

54. Maggini V, Buda G, Martino A, et al. MDR1 diplotypes as prognostic markers in multiple myeloma. *Pharmacogenet Genomics.* 2008;18:383-389.

55. Slyter H, Liwnicz B, Herrick MK, Mason R. Fatal myeloencephalopathy caused by intrathecal vincristine. *Neurology.* 1980;30:867-871.

56. Sharma RK. Vincristine and gastrointestinal transit. *Gastroenterology.* 1988;95:1435-1436.

57. Tester W, Forbes W, Leighton J. Vinorelbine-induced pancreatitis: a case report. *J Natl Cancer Inst.* 1997;89:1631.

58. Goolsby TV, Lombardo FA. Extravasation of chemotherapeutic agents: prevention and treatment. *Semin Oncol.* 2006;33:139-143.

59. Hoang M, Varughese J, Ratner E. Syndrome of Inappropriate Antidiuretic Hormone after vinorelbine treatment. *J Oncol Pharm Pract.* 2013;19:380-383.

60. Gottlieb RJ, Cuttner J. Vincristine-induced bladder atony. *Cancer.* 1971;28:674-675.

61. Dennison JB, Jones DR, Renbarger JL, Hall SD. Effect of CYP3A5 expression on vincristine metabolism with human liver microsomes. *J Pharmacol Exp Ther.* 2007;321:553-563.

62. Dennison JB, Mohutsky MA, Barbuch RJ, Wrighton SA, Hall SD. Apparent high CYP3A5 expression is required for significant metabolism of vincristine by human cryopreserved hepatocytes. *J Pharmacol Exp Ther.* 2008;327:248-257.

63. Renbarger JL, McCammack KC, Rouse CE, Hall SD. Effect of race on vincristine-associated neurotoxicity in pediatric acute lymphoblastic leukemia patients. *Pediatr Blood Cancer.* 2008;50:769-771.

64. Sims RP. The effect of race on the CYP3A-mediated metabolism of vincristine in pediatric patients with acute lymphoblastic leukemia. *J Oncol Pharm Pract.* 2016;22:76-81.

65. Ribrag V, Koscielny S, Casasnovas O, et al. Pharmacogenetic study in Hodgkin lymphomas reveals the impact of UGT1A1 polymorphisms on patient prognosis. *Blood.* 2009;113:3307-3313.

66. Pan JH, Han JX, Wu JM, Sheng LJ, Huang HN. CYP450 polymorphisms predict clinic outcomes to vinorelbine-based chemotherapy in patients with non-small-cell lung cancer. *Acta Oncol.* 2007;46:361-366.

67. Diouf B, Crews KR, Lew G, et al. Association of an inherited genetic variant with vincristine-related peripheral neuropathy in children with acute lymphoblastic leukemia. *JAMA.* 2015;313:815-823.

68. van de Velde ME, Kaspers GL, Abbink FCH, Wilhelm AJ, Ket JCF, van den Berg MH. Vincristine-induced peripheral neuropathy in children with cancer: a systematic review. *Crit Rev Oncol Hematol.* 2017;114:114-130.

69. Wani MC, Horwitz SB. Nature as a remarkable chemist: a personal story of the discovery and development of Taxol. *Anticancer Drugs.* 2014;25:482-487.

70. Cortes JE, Pazdur R. Docetaxel. *J Clin Oncol.* 1995;13:2643-2655.

71. Cassinello J, Carballido Rodriguez J, Anton Aparicio L. Role of taxanes in advanced prostate cancer. *Clin Transl Oncol.* 2016;18:972-980.

72. Gradishar WJ. Albumin-bound paclitaxel: a next-generation taxane. *Expert Opin Pharmacother.* 2006;7:1041-1053.

73. Martin SK, Pu H, Penticuff JC, Cao Z, Horbinski C, Kyprianou N. Multinucleation and Mesenchymal-to-Epithelial Transition Alleviate Resistance to Combined Cabazitaxel and Antiandrogen Therapy in Advanced Prostate Cancer. *Cancer Res.* 2016;76:912-926.

74. Gueritte-Voegelein F, Guenard D, Lavelle F, Le Goff MT, Mangatal L, Potier P. Relationships between the structure of taxol analogues and their antimitotic activity. *J Med Chem.* 1991;34:992-998.

75. Schiff PB, Fant J, Horwitz SB. Promotion of microtubule assembly in vitro by taxol. *Nature.* 1979;277:665-667.

76. Ojima I, Chakravarty S, Inoue T, et al. A common pharmacophore for cytotoxic natural products that stabilize microtubules. *Proc Natl Acad Sci U S A.* 1999;96:4256-4261.

77. Nogales E, Wolf SG, Downing KH. Structure of the alpha beta tubulin dimer by electron crystallography. *Nature.* 1998;391:199-203.

78. Churchill CD, Klobukowski M, Tuszynski JA. Elucidating the mechanism of action of the clinically approved taxanes: a comprehensive comparison of local and allosteric effects. *Chem Biol Drug Des.* 2015;86:1253-1266.

79. Jordan MA, Toso RJ, Thrower D, Wilson L. Mechanism of mitotic block and inhibition of cell proliferation by taxol at low concentrations. *Proc Natl Acad Sci U S A.* 1993;90:9552-9556.

80. Prota AE, Bargsten K, Zurwerra D, et al. Molecular mechanism of action of microtubule-stabilizing anticancer agents. *Science.* 2013;339:587-590.

81. Weaver BA. How Taxol/paclitaxel kills cancer cells. *Mol Biol Cell.* 2014;25:2677-2681.

82. Zasadil LM, Andersen KA, Yeum D, et al. Cytotoxicity of paclitaxel in breast cancer is due to chromosome missegregation on multipolar spindles. *Sci Transl Med.* 2014;6:229ra43.

83. Mielgo A, Torres VA, Clair K, Barbero S, Stupack DG. Paclitaxel promotes a caspase 8-mediated apoptosis through death effector domain association with microtubules. *Oncogene.* 2009;28:3551-3562.

84. Barbuti AM, Chen ZS. Paclitaxel Through the Ages of Anticancer Therapy: Exploring Its Role in Chemoresistance and Radiation Therapy. *Cancers (Basel).* 2015;7:2360-2371.

85. Bocci G, Di Paolo A, Danesi R. The pharmacological bases of the antiangiogenic activity of paclitaxel. *Angiogenesis.* 2013;16:481-492.

86. Desai NP, Trieu V, Hwang LY, Wu R, Soon-Shiong P, Gradishar WJ. Improved effectiveness of nanoparticle albumin-bound (nab) paclitaxel versus polysorbate-based docetaxel in multiple xenografts as a function of HER2 and SPARC status. *Anticancer Drugs.* 2008;19:899-909.

87. Cole SP, Sparks KE, Fraser K, et al. Pharmacological characterization of multidrug resistant MRP-transfected human tumor cells. *Cancer Res.* 1994;54:5902-5910.

88. Webster LK, Cosson EJ, Stokes KH, Millward MJ. Effect of the paclitaxel vehicle, Cremophor EL, on the pharmacokinetics of doxorubicin and doxorubicinol in mice. *Br J Cancer.* 1996;73:522-524.

89. Seve P, Dumontet C. Is class III beta-tubulin a predictive factor in patients receiving tubulin-binding agents? *Lancet Oncol.* 2008;9:168-175.

90. Seve P, Mackey J, Isaac S, et al. Class III beta-tubulin expression in tumor cells predicts response and outcome in patients with non-small cell lung cancer receiving paclitaxel. *Mol Cancer Ther.* 2005;4:2001-2007.

91. Verrills NM, Po'uha ST, Liu ML, et al. Alterations in gamma-actin and tubulin-targeted drug resistance in childhood leukemia. *J Natl Cancer Inst.* 2006;98:1363-1374.

92. Li W, Fan J, Banerjee D, Bertino JR. Overexpression of p21(waf1) decreases G2-M arrest and apoptosis induced by paclitaxel in human sarcoma cells lacking both p53 and functional Rb protein. *Mol Pharmacol.* 1999;55:1088-1093.

93. Yu D, Liu B, Tan M, Li J, Wang SS, Hung MC. Overexpression of c-erbB-2/neu in breast cancer cells confers increased resistance to Taxol via mdr-1-independent mechanisms. *Oncogene.* 1996;13:1359-1365.

94. Slamon DJ, Leyland-Jones B, Shak S, et al. Use of chemotherapy plus a monoclonal antibody against HER2 for metastatic breast cancer that overexpresses HER2. *N Engl J Med.* 2001;344:783-792.

95. Yao YS, Qiu WS, Yao RY, et al. miR-141 confers docetaxel chemoresistance of breast cancer cells via regulation of EIF4E expression. *Oncol Rep.* 2015;33:2504-2512.

96. Chang I, Mitsui Y, Fukuhara S, et al. Loss of miR-200c up-regulates CYP1B1 and confers docetaxel resistance in renal cell carcinoma. *Oncotarget.* 2015;6:7774-7787.

97. Komura K, Jeong SH, Hinohara K, et al. Resistance to docetaxel in prostate cancer is associated with androgen receptor activation and loss of KDM5D expression. *Proc Natl Acad Sci U S A.* 2016;113:6259-6264.

98. Noll EM, Eisen C, Stenzinger A, et al. CYP3A5 mediates basal and acquired therapy resistance in different subtypes of pancreatic ductal adenocarcinoma. *Nat Med.* 2016;22:278-287.

99. Zhang SQ, Chen GH. Determination of Paclitaxel in Human Plasma by UPLC-MS-MS. *J Chromatogr Sci.* 2008;46:220-224.

100. Stage TB, Bergmann TK, Kroetz DL. Clinical pharmacokinetics of paclitaxel monotherapy: an updated literature review. *Clin Pharmacokinet.* 2018;57:7-19.

101. Gianni L, Kearns CM, Giani A, et al. Nonlinear pharmacokinetics and metabolism of paclitaxel and its pharmacokinetic/pharmacodynamic relationships in humans. *J Clin Oncol.* 1995;13:180-190.

102. Sparreboom A, van Zuylen L, Brouwer E, et al. Cremophor EL-mediated alteration of paclitaxel distribution in human blood: clinical pharmacokinetic implications. *Cancer Res.* 1999;59:1454-1457.

103. Kearns CM, Gianni L, Egorin MJ. Paclitaxel pharmacokinetics and pharmacodynamics. *Semin Oncol.* 1995;22:16-23.

104. Cresteil T, Monsarrat B, Dubois J, Sonnier M, Alvinerie P, Gueritte F. Regioselective metabolism of taxoids by human CYP3A4 and 2C8: structure-activity relationship. *Drug Metab Dispos.* 2002;30:438-445.

105. Shou M, Martinet M, Korzekwa KR, Krausz KW, Gonzalez FJ, Gelboin HV. Role of human cytochrome P450 3A4 and 3A5 in the metabolism of taxotere and its derivatives: enzyme specificity, interindividual distribution and metabolic contribution in human liver. *Pharmacogenetics.* 1998;8:391-401.

106. Baker SD, Zhao M, Lee CK, et al. Comparative pharmacokinetics of weekly and every-three-weeks docetaxel. *Clin Cancer Res.* 2004;10:1976-1983.

107. Nieuweboer AJ, de Morree ES, de Graan AJ, Sparreboom A, de Wit R, Mathijssen RH. Inter-patient variability in docetaxel pharmacokinetics: a review. *Cancer Treat Rev.* 2015;41:605-613.

108. Hirth J, Watkins PB, Strawderman M, Schott A, Bruno R, Baker LH. The effect of an individual's cytochrome CYP3A4 activity on docetaxel clearance. *Clin Cancer Res.* 2000;6:1255-1258.

109. Minami H, Kawada K, Sasaki Y, et al. Pharmacokinetics and pharmacodynamics of protein-unbound docetaxel in cancer patients. *Cancer Sci.* 2006;97:235-241.

110. Ibrahim NK, Desai N, Legha S, et al. Phase I and pharmacokinetic study of ABI-007, a Cremophor-free, protein-stabilized, nanoparticle formulation of paclitaxel. *Clin Cancer Res.* 2002;8:1038-1044.

111. Biakhov MY, Kononova GV, Iglesias J, et al. Nab-paclitaxel in patients with advanced solid tumors and hepatic dysfunction: a pilot study. *Expert Opin Drug Saf.* 2010;9:515-523.

112. Chen N, Li Y, Ye Y, Palmisano M, Chopra R, Zhou S. Pharmacokinetics and pharmacodynamics of nab-paclitaxel in patients with solid tumors: disposition kinetics and pharmacology distinct from solvent-based paclitaxel. *J Clin Pharmacol.* 2014;54:1097-1107.

113. Gardner ER, Dahut WL, Scripture CD, et al. Randomized crossover pharmacokinetic study of solvent-based paclitaxel and nab-paclitaxel. *Clin Cancer Res.* 2008;14:4200-4205.

114. Sparreboom A, Scripture CD, Trieu V, et al. Comparative preclinical and clinical pharmacokinetics of a Cremophor-free, nanoparticle albumin-bound paclitaxel (ABI-007) and paclitaxel formulated in Cremophor (Taxol). *Clin Cancer Res.* 2005;11:4136-4143.

115. Siqing F, Culotta KS, Falchook GS, et al. Pharmacokinetic evaluation of nanoparticle albumin-bound paclitaxel delivered via hepatic arterial infusion in patients with predominantly hepatic metastases. *Cancer Chemother Pharmacol.* 2016;77:357-364.

116. Yap TA, Pezaro CJ, de Bono JS. Cabazitaxel in metastatic castration-resistant prostate cancer. *Expert Rev Anticancer Ther.* 2012;12:1129-1136.

117. Rowinsky EK, Citardi MJ, Noe DA, Donehower RC. Sequence-dependent cytotoxic effects due to combinations of cisplatin and the antimicrotubule agents taxol and vincristine. *J Cancer Res Clin Oncol.* 1993;119:727-733.

118. Belani CP, Kearns CM, Zuhowski EG, et al. Phase I trial, including pharmacokinetic and pharmacodynamic correlations, of combination paclitaxel and carboplatin in patients with metastatic non-small-cell lung cancer. *J Clin Oncol.* 1999;17:676-684.

119. Holmes FA, Madden T, Newman RA, et al. Sequence-dependent alteration of doxorubicin pharmacokinetics by paclitaxel in a phase I study of paclitaxel and doxorubicin in patients with metastatic breast cancer. *J Clin Oncol.* 1996;14:2713-2721.

120. Perotti A, Cresta S, Grasselli G, Capri G, Minotti G, Gianni L. Cardiotoxic effects of anthracycline-taxane combinations. *Expert Opin Drug Saf.* 2003;2:59-71.

121. Wilson WH, Berg SL, Bryant G, et al. Paclitaxel in doxorubicin-refractory or mitoxantrone-refractory breast cancer: a phase I/II trial of 96-hour infusion. *J Clin Oncol.* 1994;12:1621-1629.

122. Chan JK, Brady MF, Penson RT, et al. Weekly vs. Every-3-Week Paclitaxel and Carboplatin for Ovarian Cancer. *N Engl J Med.* 2016;374:738-748.

123. Green MC, Buzdar AU, Smith T, et al. Weekly paclitaxel improves pathologic complete remission in operable breast cancer when compared with paclitaxel once every 3 weeks. *J Clin Oncol.* 2005;23:5983-5992.

124. Armstrong DK, Bundy B, Wenzel L, et al. Intraperitoneal cisplatin and paclitaxel in ovarian cancer. *N Engl J Med.* 2006;354:34-43.

125. Joerger M, Huitema AD, Huizing MT, et al. Safety and pharmacology of paclitaxel in patients with impaired liver function: a population pharmacokinetic-pharmacodynamic study. *Br J Clin Pharmacol.* 2007;64:622-633.

126. Kudlowitz D, Muggia F. Defining risks of taxane neuropathy: insights from randomized clinical trials. *Clin Cancer Res.* 2013;19:4570-4577.

127. Hainsworth JD, Burris HA III, Greco FA. Weekly administration of docetaxel (Taxotere): summary of clinical data. *Semin Oncol.* 1999;26:19-24.

128. Untch M, Jackisch C, Schneeweiss A, et al. Nab-paclitaxel versus solvent-based paclitaxel in neoadjuvant chemotherapy for early breast cancer (GeparSepto-GBG 69): a randomised, phase 3 trial. *Lancet Oncol.* 2016;17:345-356.

129. de Bono JS, Oudard S, Ozguroglu M, et al. Prednisone plus cabazitaxel or mitoxantrone for metastatic castration-resistant prostate cancer progressing after docetaxel treatment: a randomised open-label trial. *Lancet.* 2010;376:1147-1154.

130. Sarantopoulos J, Mita AC, He A, et al. Safety and pharmacokinetics of cabazitaxel in patients with hepatic impairment: a phase I dose-escalation study. *Cancer Chemother Pharmacol.* 2017;79:339-351.

131. Azaro A, Rodon J, Machiels JP, et al. A phase I pharmacokinetic and safety study of cabazitaxel in adult cancer patients with normal and impaired renal function. *Cancer Chemother Pharmacol.* 2016;78:1185-1197.

132. Picard M, Castells MC. Re-visiting Hypersensitivity Reactions to Taxanes: A Comprehensive Review. *Clin Rev Allergy Immunol.* 2015;49:177-191.

133. Kudlowitz D, Muggia F. Clinical features of taxane neuropathy. *Anticancer Drugs.* 2014;25:495-501.

134. Hershman DL, Lacchetti C, Dworkin RH, et al. Prevention and management of chemotherapy-induced peripheral neuropathy in survivors of adult cancers: American Society of Clinical Oncology clinical practice guideline. *J Clin Oncol.* 2014;32:1941-1967.

135. Chiu N, Chiu L, Chow R, et al. Taxane-induced arthralgia and myalgia: a literature review. *J Oncol Pharm Pract.* 2017;23:56-67.

136. Arbuck SG, Strauss H, Rowinsky E, et al. A reassessment of cardiac toxicity associated with Taxol. *J Natl Cancer Inst Monogr.* 1993;117-130.

137. Jerian S, Keegan P. Cardiotoxicity associated with paclitaxel/trastuzumab combination therapy. *J Clin Oncol.* 1999;17:1647-1648.

138. Sibaud V, Leboeuf NR, Roche H, et al. Dermatological adverse events with taxane chemotherapy. *Eur J Dermatol.* 2016;26:427-443.

139. Seewaldt VL, Cain JM, Goff BA, Tamimi H, Greer B, Figge D. A retrospective review of paclitaxel-associated gastrointestinal necrosis in patients with epithelial ovarian cancer. *Gynecol Oncol.* 1997;67:137-140.

140. Markman M. Management of toxicities associated with the administration of taxanes. *Expert Opin Drug Saf* 2003;2:141-146.

141. Semb KA, Aamdal S, Oian P. Capillary protein leak syndrome appears to explain fluid retention in cancer patients who receive docetaxel treatment. *J Clin Oncol.* 1998;16:3426-3432.

142. Piccart MJ, Klijn J, Paridaens R, et al. Corticosteroids significantly delay the onset of docetaxel-induced fluid retention: final results of a randomized study of the European Organization for Research and Treatment of Cancer Investigational Drug Branch for Breast Cancer. *J Clin Oncol.* 1997;15:3149-3155.

143. Rose PG, Smrekar M. Improvement of paclitaxel-induced neuropathy by substitution of docetaxel for paclitaxel. *Gynecol Oncol.* 2003;91:423-425.

144. Meisel A, von Felten S, Vogt DR, et al. Severe neutropenia during cabazitaxel treatment is associated with survival benefit in men with metastatic castration-resistant prostate cancer (mCRPC): a post-hoc analysis of the TROPIC phase III trial. *Eur J Cancer.* 2016;56:93-100.

145. Frederiks CN, Lam SW, Guchelaar HJ, Boven E. Genetic polymorphisms and paclitaxel- or docetaxel-induced toxicities: a systematic review. *Cancer Treat Rev.* 2015;41:935-950.

146. Green H, Soderkvist P, Rosenberg P, et al. Pharmacogenetic studies of Paclitaxel in the treatment of ovarian cancer. *Basic Clin Pharmacol Toxicol.* 2009;104:130-137.

147. Baker SD, Verweij J, Cusatis GA, et al. Pharmacogenetic pathway analysis of docetaxel elimination. *Clin Pharmacol Ther.* 2009;85:155-163.

148. Angelini S, Botticelli A, Onesti CE, et al. Pharmacogenetic Approach to Toxicity in Breast Cancer Patients Treated with Taxanes. *Anticancer Res.* 2017;37:2633-2639.

149. Hertz DL, Motsinger-Reif AA, Drobish A, et al. CYP2C8*3 predicts benefit/risk profile in breast cancer patients receiving neoadjuvant paclitaxel. *Breast Cancer Res Treat.* 2012;134:401-410.

150. Hertz DL, Roy S, Motsinger-Reif AA, et al. CYP2C8*3 increases risk of neuropathy in breast cancer patients treated with paclitaxel. *Ann Oncol.* 2013;24:1472-1478.

151. Kus T, Aktas G, Kalender ME, et al. Polymorphism of CYP3A4 and ABCB1 genes increase the risk of neuropathy in breast cancer patients treated with paclitaxel and docetaxel. *Onco Targets Ther.* 2016;9:5073-5080.

152. Leskela S, Jara C, Leandro-Garcia LJ, et al. Polymorphisms in cytochromes P450 2C8 and 3A5 are associated with paclitaxel neurotoxicity. *Pharmacogenomics J.* 2011;11:121-129.

153. Kim HS, Kim MK, Chung HH, et al. Genetic polymorphisms affecting clinical outcomes in epithelial ovarian cancer patients treated with taxanes and platinum compounds: a Korean population-based study. *Gynecol Oncol.* 2009;113:264-269.

154. Sissung TM, Baum CE, Deeken J, et al. ABCB1 genetic variation influences the toxicity and clinical outcome of patients with androgen-independent prostate cancer treated with docetaxel. *Clin Cancer Res.* 2008;14:4543-4549.

155. Sissung TM, Mross K, Steinberg SM, et al. Association of ABCB1 genotypes with paclitaxel-mediated peripheral neuropathy and neutropenia. *Eur J Cancer.* 2006;42:2893-2896.

156. Apellaniz-Ruiz M, Lee MY, Sanchez-Barroso L, et al. Whole-exome sequencing reveals defective CYP3A4 variants predictive of paclitaxel dose-limiting neuropathy. *Clin Cancer Res.* 2015;21:322-328.

157. Baldwin RM, Owzar K, Zembutsu H, et al. A genome-wide association study identifies novel loci for paclitaxel-induced sensory peripheral neuropathy in CALGB 40101. *Clin Cancer Res.* 2012;18:5099-5109.

158. Leandro-Garcia LJ, Inglada-Perez L, Pita G, et al. Genome-wide association study identifies ephrin type A receptors implicated in paclitaxel induced peripheral sensory neuropathy. *J Med Genet.* 2013;50:599-605.

159. Schneider BP, Li L, Radovich M, et al. Genome-Wide Association Studies for Taxane-Induced Peripheral Neuropathy in ECOG-5103 and ECOG-1199. *Clin Cancer Res.* 2015;21:5082-5091.

160. Hertz DL, Owzar K, Lessans S, et al. Pharmacogenetic Discovery in CALGB (Alliance) 90401 and Mechanistic Validation of a VAC14 Polymorphism that Increases Risk of Docetaxel-Induced Neuropathy. *Clin Cancer Res.* 2016;22:4890-4900.

161. Marsh S, Somlo G, Li X, et al. Pharmacogenetic analysis of paclitaxel transport and metabolism genes in breast cancer. *Pharmacogenomics J.* 2007;7:362-365.

162. Sissung TM, Danesi R, Price DK, et al. Association of the CYP1B1*3 allele with survival in patients with prostate cancer receiving docetaxel. *Mol Cancer Ther.* 2008;7:19-26.

163. Chang H, Rha SY, Jeung HC, et al. Association of the ABCB1 gene polymorphisms 2677G>T/A and 3435C>T with clinical outcomes of paclitaxel monotherapy in metastatic breast cancer patients. *Ann Oncol.* 2009;20:272-277.

164. Green H, Soderkvist P, Rosenberg P, Horvath G, Peterson C. mdr-1 single nucleotide polymorphisms in ovarian cancer tissue: G2677T/A correlates with response to paclitaxel chemotherapy. *Clin Cancer Res.* 2006;12:854-859.

165. Johnatty SE, Beesley J, Paul J, et al. ABCB1 (MDR 1) polymorphisms and progression-free survival among women with ovarian cancer following paclitaxel/carboplatin chemotherapy. *Clin Cancer Res.* 2008;14:5594-5601.

166. Risinger AL, Giles FJ, Mooberry SL. Microtubule dynamics as a target in oncology. *Cancer Treat Rev.* 2009;35:255-261.

167. Thomas ES, Gomez HL, Li RK, et al. Ixabepilone plus capecitabine for metastatic breast cancer progressing after anthracycline and taxane treatment. *J Clin Oncol.* 2007;25:5210-5217.

168. Lee JJ, Swain SM. The epothilones: translating from the laboratory to the clinic. *Clin Cancer Res.* 2008;14:1618-1624.

169. Giannakakou P, Gussio R, Nogales E, et al. A common pharmacophore for epothilone and taxanes: molecular basis for drug resistance conferred by tubulin mutations in human cancer cells. *Proc Natl Acad Sci U S A.* 2000;97:2904-2909.

170. Lee JJ, Kelly WK. Epothilones: tubulin polymerization as a novel target for prostate cancer therapy. *Nat Clin Pract Oncol.* 2009;6:85-92.

171. Dumontet C, Jordan MA, Lee FF. Ixabepilone: targeting betaIII-tubulin expression in taxane-resistant malignancies. *Mol Cancer Ther.* 2009;8:17-25.

172. Wang Y, O'Brate A, Zhou W, Giannakakou P. Resistance to microtubule-stabilizing drugs involves two events: beta-tubulin mutation in one allele followed by loss of the second allele. *Cell Cycle.* 2005;4:1847-1853.

173. Hopper-Borge E, Xu X, Shen T, Shi Z, Chen ZS, Kruh GD. Human multidrug resistance protein 7 (ABCC10) is a resistance factor for nucleoside analogues and epothilone B. *Cancer Res.* 2009;69:178-184.

174. Lee FY, Smykla R, Johnston K, et al. Preclinical efficacy spectrum and pharmacokinetics of ixabepilone. *Cancer Chemother Pharmacol.* 2009;63:201-212.

175. Goel S, Cohen M, Comezoglu SN, et al. The effect of ketoconazole on the pharmacokinetics and pharmacodynamics of ixabepilone: a first in class epothilone B analogue in late-phase clinical development. *Clin Cancer Res.* 2008;14:2701-2709.

176. Vahdat LT, Thomas ES, Roche HH, et al. Ixabepilone-associated peripheral neuropathy: data from across the phase II and III clinical trials. *Support Care Cancer.* 2012;20:2661-2668.

177. Yardley DA. Proactive management of adverse events maintains the clinical benefit of ixabepilone. *Oncologist.* 2009;14:448-455.

178. Poncet J. The dolastatins, a family of promising antineoplastic agents. *Curr Pharm Des.* 1999;5:139-162.

179. Doherty MK, Morris PG. Eribulin for the treatment of metastatic breast cancer: an update on its safety and efficacy. *Int J Womens Health.* 2015;7:47-58.

180. Osgood CL, Chuk MK, Theoret MR, et al. FDA Approval Summary: Eribulin for Patients with Unresectable or Metastatic Liposarcoma who have Received a Prior Anthracycline-Containing Regimen. *Clin Cancer Res.* 2017;23:6384-6389.

181. Dybdal-Hargreaves NF, Risinger AL, Mooberry SL. Eribulin mesylate: mechanism of action of a unique microtubule-targeting agent. *Clin Cancer Res.* 2015;21:2445-2452.

182. Swami U, Chaudhary I, Ghalib MH, Goel S. Eribulin—a review of preclinical and clinical studies. *Crit Rev Oncol Hematol.* 2012;81:163-184.

183. Zhang ZY, King BM, Pelletier RD, Wong YN. Delineation of the interactions between the chemotherapeutic agent eribulin mesylate (E7389) and human CYP3A4. *Cancer Chemother Pharmacol.* 2008;62:707-716.

184. Cortes J, O'Shaughnessy J, Loesch D, et al. Eribulin monotherapy versus treatment of physician's choice in patients with metastatic breast cancer (EMBRACE): a phase 3 open-label randomised study. *Lancet.* 2011;377:914-923.

185. Kaufman PA, Awada A, Twelves C, et al. Phase III open-label randomized study of eribulin mesylate versus capecitabine in patients with locally advanced or metastatic breast cancer previously treated with an anthracycline and a taxane. *J Clin Oncol.* 2015;33:594-601.

186. Devriese LA, Witteveen PO, Marchetti S, et al. Pharmacokinetics of eribulin mesylate in patients with solid tumors and hepatic impairment. *Cancer Chemother Pharmacol.* 2012;70:823-832.

187. Tan AR, Sarantopoulos J, Lee L, et al. Pharmacokinetics of eribulin mesylate in cancer patients with normal and impaired renal function. *Cancer Chemother Pharmacol.* 2015;76:1051-1061.

Alkylating and Methylating Agents

Stanton L. Gerson, Lachelle D. Weeks, and Bruce A. Chabner

Alkylating agents are antitumor drugs that act through the covalent binding of alkyl groups to cellular molecules. This binding is mediated by reactive intermediates formed from a parent alkylating compound. Historically, alkylating agents have played an important role in the development of cancer chemotherapy. The nitrogen mustards mechlorethamine (HN_2, "nitrogen mustard") and tris(β-chloroethyl) amine (HN_3) were the first nonhormonal agents to show significant antitumor activity in humans.[1,2] Clinical trials of nitrogen mustards in lymphoma evolved from the observation that lymphoid atrophy, in addition to lung and mucous membrane irritation, was produced by sulfur mustard during the First and Second World Wars. Antitumor evaluation, based on the pioneering laboratory work of Goodman and Gilman,[3] showed that related but less reactive nitrogen mustards, the bischloroethylamines (Fig. 12.1), were less toxic and caused regression of lymphoid tumors in mice. The first clinical studies produced dramatic lymphoma regression in some patients, and the antitumor effects were confirmed by an organized multi-institution study.[1,2] This demonstration of efficacy encouraged efforts to find additional chemical agents with antitumor activity, leading to the wide variety of antitumor agents in use today. The nonclassical alkylating agents including methylating agents such as procarbazine and temozolomide will be discussed later in this chapter. A long known property of alkylating agents to induce DNA damage has taken on renewed interest as these sites of DNA damage lead to altered gene expression, neoantigen induction, and novel immunotherapy targets. Despite the enthusiastic development of targeted agents, classical alkylating agents continue to occupy a central position in cancer chemotherapy, both in conventional combination regimens and in high-dose protocols with hematopoietic cell transplantation (HCT). Improved understanding of resistance mechanisms has led to the development of targeted agents that block these resistance pathways to enhance the efficacy of alkylating agents.

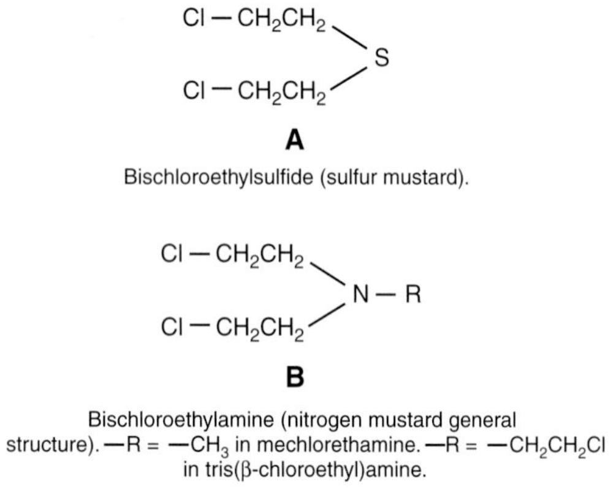

Alkylating Reactions

Alkylation reactions occur by two mechanisms: S_N1 and S_N2. In S_N1 reactions, the rate-limiting step is the formation of a carbonium ion that can react rapidly with a nucleophile. This reaction follows first-order kinetics with a rate that depends solely on the concentration of the alkylating agent. In contrast, S_N2 reactions follow second-order kinetics and depend on the concentrations of both the alkylating agent and the nucleophile. Such reactions involve a transition-state entity formed by both reactants that decomposes to form the alkylated cellular constituent. Agents such as chloroethylnitrosoureas, through a S_N1 type of mechanism, form covalent adducts with oxygen and nitrogen atoms in DNA. Compounds with S_N2 predominant mechanisms, such as busulfan, tend to react more slowly, with little alkylation of oxygen sites. Because alkylating agents are designed to produce reactive intermediates, the parent compounds typically have short elimination half-lives of less than 5 hours.

As a class, the alkylating agents share a common target (DNA) and are cytotoxic, mutagenic, and carcinogenic. The activity of most alkylating agents is enhanced by radiation, hyperthermia, nitroimidazoles, glutathione depletion, immune checkpoint inhibition, and inhibition of DNA repair. They differ greatly, however, in their toxicity profiles and antitumor activity. These differences are undoubtedly the result of differences in pharmacokinetic features, lipid solubility, ability to penetrate the central nervous system (CNS), membrane transport properties, detoxification reactions, and specific enzymatic reactions capable of repairing alkylation sites on DNA.[4-6] Application of techniques such as magnetic resonance imaging and mass spectrometry to the study of the alkylation mechanism and the chemical nature of the intermediates involved have led to a detailed understanding of these reactions.[7,8] Such approaches, coupled with improved techniques for studying cellular damage[9,10] and for determining mechanisms of detoxification,[11] make it possible to predict sites of alkylation and allow scientists to understand and modify the biologic consequences of such alkylations. The induction of DNA damage by alkylating agents and the resulting neoantigens create new targets for immunotherapy and immune check point inhibitors that recognize new peptides from damaged tumor cells, as displayed on MHC class 2 by antigen-presenting macrophages and recognized by activated T cells.

Alkylating Agents Used Clinically

The important pharmacologic properties of the clinically useful alkylating agents are summarized in Table 12.1.

A

Bischloroethylsulfide (sulfur mustard).

B

Bischloroethylamine (nitrogen mustard general structure). —R = —CH₃ in mechlorethamine. —R = —CH₂CH₂Cl in tris(β-chloroethyl)amine.

FIGURE **12.1** Structures of bischloroethylsulfide and bischloroethylamine. **A.** Bischloroethylsulfide (sulfur mustard). **B.** Bischloroethylamine (nitrogen mustard general structure).

TABLE
12-1 *Key features of selected alkylating agents*

	Cyclophosphamide	Ifosfamide	Melphalan	BCNU	Busulfan	Bendamustine
Mechanism of action	All agents produce alkylation of DNA through the formation of reactive intermediates that attack nucleophilic sites.					
Mechanisms of resistance	Increased capacity to repair alkylated lesions, for example, guanine O^6-alkyl transferase (nitrosoureas, busulfan) Increased expression of glutathione-associated enzymes, including γ-glutamyl cysteine synthetase, γ-glutamyl transpeptidase, and glutathione-S-transferases Increased ALDH (cyclophosphamide) Decreased expression or mutation of p53					
Dose/schedule (mg/m²)	400 to 2,000 IV 100 PO qd	1,000 to 4,000 IV	8 PO qd × 5 d	200 IV	2 to 4 mg qd	70 to 100 mg daily, on day 1 and 2 of a 28-day cycle
Oral bioavailability	100%	Unavailable	30% (variable)	Not known	50% or greater	?
Pharmacokinetics Primary elimination $t_{1/2}$ (h)	3 to 10 (parent) 1.6 (aldophosphamide) 8.7 (phosphoramide mustard)	7 to 15 (parent)	1 (parent)	0.25 to 0.75[a] (nonlinear increase with dose from 170 to 720 mg/m²)	2 to 3 h	0.5 (parent)
Metabolism and excretion	Microsomal hydroxylation activates, then chemical decomposition Hydrolysis to phosphoramide mustard (active) and acrolein Excretion as inactive oxidation products	Microsomal hydroxylation activates, then chemical decomposition Hydrolysis to phosphoramide mustard and acrolein Excretion as inactive oxidation and dechloroethylated products	Spontaneously decomposes 20% to 35% excreted unchanged in urine	Decomposes to active and inert products; also P-450–mediated inactivation	Enzymatic conjugation with glutathione	Chemical decomposition Excretion primarily in feces
Toxicity						
Bone marrow	Acute, platelets spared	Acute but mild	Delayed, nadir at 4 wk	Delayed, nadir 4 to 6 wk	Acute and delayed marrow aplasia	Acute but mild
Other	Hemorrhagic cystitis, cardiac toxicity, IADH	Hemorrhagic cystitis, encephalopathy	—	Pulmonary fibrosis, renal failure, hypotension	Addisonian syndrome, seizures, pulmonary fibrosis, venoocclusive disease	Mucositis, infections, tumor lysis syndrome
Precautions	Use MESNA with high-dose therapy	Always coadminister MESNA	Decomposes if administered over <1 h	—	Monitor AUC with high-dose therapy induces phenytoin metabolism	

[a]Jones RB, Matthes SM, Dufton C, et al. Nitrosoureas. In: Grochow LB, Ames MM, eds. *A Clinician's Guide to Chemotherapy Pharmacokinetics and Pharmacodynamics.* Baltimore, MD: Williams & Williams; 1998:331. See Reference[12].
AUC, area under the concentration–time curve; BCNU, bischloroethylnitrosourea; IADH, inappropriate antidiuretic hormone syndrome; IV, intravenously; MESNA, 2-mercaptoethane sulfonate; PO, per os; $t_{1/2}$, plasma half-life.

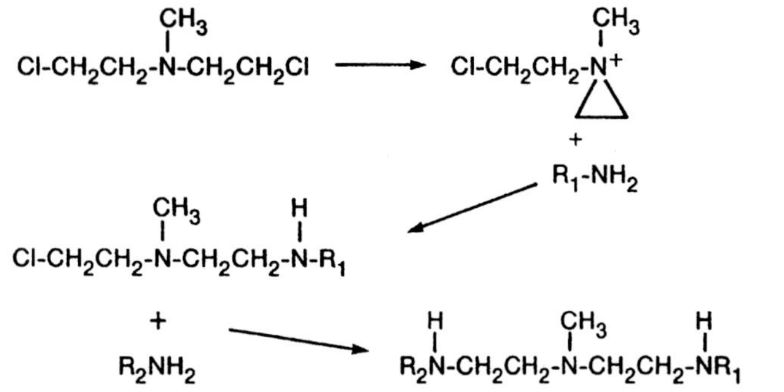

FIGURE **12.2** Alkylation mechanism of nitrogen mustards. (Reprinted from Colvin M. Molecular pharmacology of alkylating agents. In: Cooke ST, Prestayko AW. eds. *Cancer and Chemotherapy: Antineoplastic Agents*, vol 3. 1st ed. New York: Academic Press;1981:291. Copyright © 1981 Academic Press, Inc. With permission.)

Nitrogen Mustards

The prototypic alkylating agents have been the bischloroethylamines or nitrogen mustards. The first nitrogen mustard to be used extensively in the clinic was *mechlorethamine (mustine)* (Fig. 12.1), sometimes referred to by its original code name HN_2 or by the term *nitrogen mustard*. The mechanism of nitrogen mustard alkylation is shown in Figure 12.2. In the initial step, chlorine is lost and the *β*-carbon reacts with the nucleophilic nitrogen atom to form the cyclic, positively charged, and very reactive aziridinium moiety. Reaction of the aziridinium ring with a nucleophile (electron-rich atom) yields the initial alkylated product. Formation of a second aziridinium by the remaining chloroethyl group allows for a second alkylation, which produces a cross-link between the two alkylated nucleophiles.

Numerous analogs of mechlorethamine were synthesized in which the methyl group was replaced by a variety of chemical groups that stabilized the molecule. Most of these compounds proved to have less antitumor activity than mechlorethamine, but many other derivatives have a higher therapeutic index, a broader range of clinical activity, and can be administered both orally and intravenously. These drugs, which for the most part have replaced mechlorethamine in clinical use are *melphalan* (L-phenylalanine mustard), *chlorambucil, bendamustine, cyclophosphamide,* and *ifosfamide* (Fig. 12.3). The latter two agents are unique in that they require

metabolic activation and undergo a complex series of activation and degradation reactions (to be described in detail later in this chapter).

These derivatives have electron-rich groups substituted on the nitrogen atom. This alteration reduces the electrophilicity of the nitrogen and renders the molecules less reactive. Melphalan and chlorambucil retain alkylating activities and seem to be more tumor selective than nitrogen mustard. Cyclophosphamide and ifosfamide, on the other hand, possess no intrinsic alkylating activity and must be metabolized to produce alkylating compounds.

Cyclophosphamide remains the most widely used alkylating agent.[13] It is an essential component of drug regimens for non-Hodgkin's lymphoma (NHL) (CHOP—cyclophosphamide, doxorubicin, vincristine [Oncovin], prednisone), other lymphoid malignancies, and solid tumors in children. Cyclophosphamide is also used in combination treatments for breast cancer and in high-dose chemotherapy with bone marrow restoration. More than other alkylating agents, its properties as an immunomodulator has led to its use post stem cell infusion to block the function of recipient as well as donor T cells responding to host antigens improving engraftment, especially in haplotransplant settings and reducing acute graft versus host disease (GVHD).

- Ifosfamide, an isomeric analog of cyclophosphamide, was introduced into clinical use in 1972. It is currently approved for the treatment of relapsed testicular germ cell tumors[14] and for the treatment of both pediatric and adult soft tissue sarcomas.[15,16] It is used in combination with etoposide and carboplatin for relapsed lymphomas.

- Melphalan is primarily employed in multiple myeloma,[17] occasionally in malignant melanoma, and in high-dose chemotherapy with marrow transplantation.

- *Chlorambucil,* an oral medication, has single-agent activity against chronic lymphocytic leukemia (CLL) and small B-cell lymphomas.[18]

- Originally described in 1963, *bendamustine* (Fig. 12.3) has emerged as an effective treatment for patients with CLL and indolent NHL.[19–22]

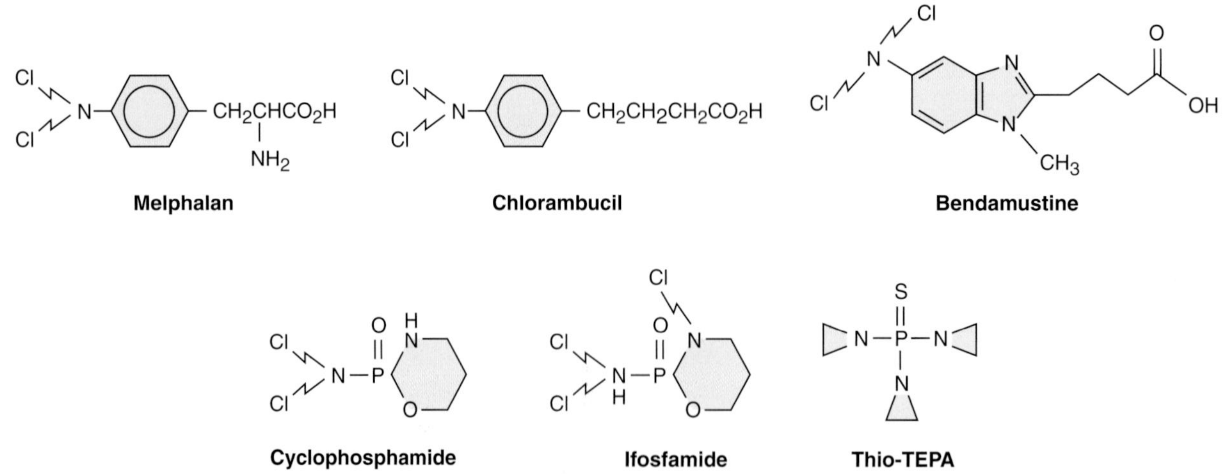

FIGURE **12.3** Alkylating agent structures.

Aziridines

The stable aziridines are analogs of the reactive ring-closed intermediates of the nitrogen mustards. Compounds bearing two or more aziridine groups, such as *thiotepa* (Fig. 12.3 [thiotepa, triethylenethiophosphoramide]), have clinical activity against breast and ovarian cancer,[23] but thiotepa is currently used as an occasional component of high-dose regimens.[24] It was originally tested for antitumor activity because the nitrogen mustards alkylate through an aziridine intermediate. Both thiotepa and its primary desulfurated metabolite *TEPA* (triethylenephosphoramide) have cytotoxic activity in vitro.

Alkyl Alkane Sulfonates

The major clinical representative of the alkyl alkane sulfonates is *busulfan*, which is widely used in high-dose regimens in preparation for stem cell transplantation for the treatment of acute myelogenous leukemia (AML).[25] Of the alkyl alkane sulfonates, compounds with one to eight methylene units between the sulfonate groups have antitumor activity, but maximal cross-linking and activity are achieved by compounds with four units.[26] The mechanism of action of the alkyl alkane sulfonates is shown in Figure 12.4.

Busulfan exhibits second-order alkylation kinetics. The compound reacts more extensively with thiol groups of amino acids and proteins[27] than do the nitrogen mustards. These reactions along with interactions with DNA may contribute to cytotoxicity. Brookes and Lawley[28,29] were able to demonstrate the reaction of busulfan with the N-7 position of guanine.[30,31] The cytotoxic potential of busulfan correlates with adenine-to-guanine cross-linking.[30] Busulfan is markedly cytotoxic to hematopoietic stem cells. This effect is seen clinically in the prolonged aplasia that may follow busulfan administration and can be shown experimentally in stem cell cloning systems.[32] The pharmacologic basis for this property of busulfan is not well understood but may involve damage to the mesenchymal stem cells in the microenvironment. In recent years, an intravenous formulation has simplified the dose appropriate administration of busulfan to achieve optimal blood levels during high-dose myeloablative treatments.

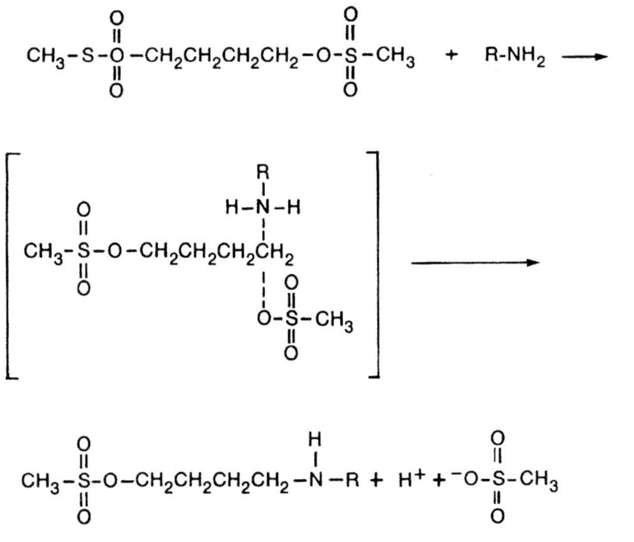

Nitrosoureas

The nitrosourea antitumor agents were discovered in a drug screening effort that focused on analogues of methylnitrosoguanidine and methylnitrosourea.[33] Chloroethyl derivatives such as *chloroethylnitrosourea* and *BCNU (carmustine)* (Fig. 12.5) possess marked antitumor activity and had activity against tumor in the CNS.[34] In addition to chloroethyl alkylating activity, the available nitrosoureas can also carbamoylate nucleophiles.[35] Closely related methylating agents, *procarbazine*, *temozolomide*, and *dacarbazine (DTIC)*, are lipophilic and penetrate the CNS (see nonclassical alkylating agents, this chapter).

The nitrosoureas exhibit only partial cross-resistance with other alkylating agents, and a number of studies established unique aspects of the mechanism of the alkylation reaction for these compounds (Fig. 12.6). BCNU cross-links DNA after the formation of initial monoadducts, particularly at the N-7 position of guanine. As shown in Figure 12.6, the diazonium hydroxide intermediate formed during BCNU hydrolysis decomposes to form a 2-chloroethyl carbonium ion (or equivalent), a strong electrophile, capable of alkylation of guanine, cytidine, and adenine bases.[36] In a subsequent step occurring over hours, the chloride is displaced by electron-rich nitrogen on the complementary DNA strand base to form a cross-link. DNA-protein cross-links are also possible by initiating chloroethylation at the amino or sulfhydryl group of protein.[37]

Isocyanates resulting from the spontaneous breakdown of many of the methyl- and chloroethylnitrosoureas are also shown in Figure 12.6. The role of isocyanate-mediated carbamoylation in antitumor effects is incompletely understood, but this activity may be responsible for some toxicities associated with nitrosourea therapy.[38]

High-dose BCNU, etoposide, and cisplatin comprise the BEP regimen used for autologous stem cell transplantation in patients with refractory or relapsed lymphoma.[30] Another high-dose BCNU-containing regimen, BEAM (BCNU, etoposide, cytarabine, melphalan), has also been used with success with autologous hematopoietic stem cell transplant in patients with NHL.[31] BCNU had attracted interest as an adjuvant to radiation therapy in the treatment of

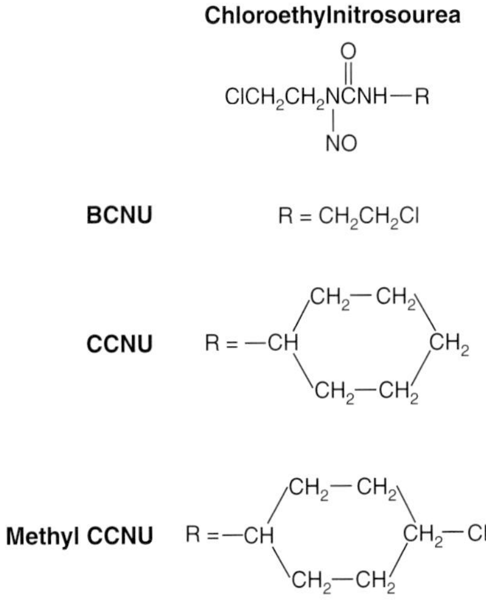

FIGURE **12.4** Structure and alkylating mechanism of busulfan, an alkane sulfonate. (Reprinted from Colvin M. Molecular pharmacology of alkylating agents. In: Cooke ST, Prestayko AW. eds. *Cancer and Chemotherapy: Antineoplastic Agents*, vol 3. 1st ed. New York: Academic Press;1981:291. Copyright © 1981 Academic Press, Inc. With permission.)

FIGURE **12.5** Structures of nitrosoureas. BCNU, bischloroethylnitrosourea; CCNU, cyclohexylchloroethylnitrosourea.

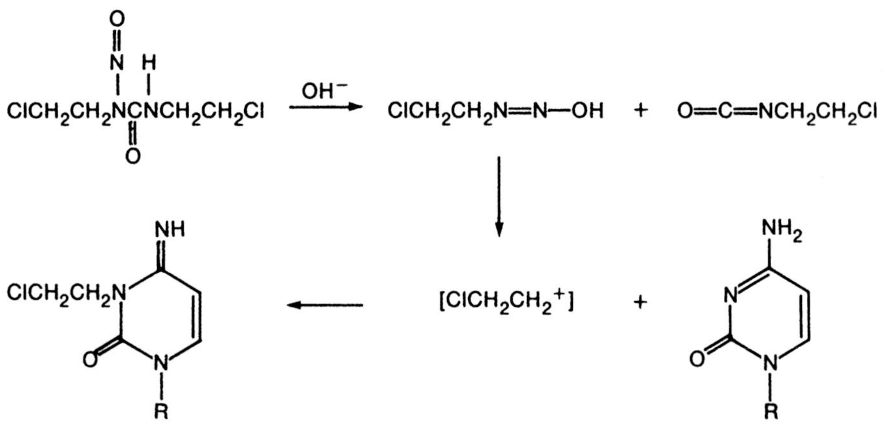

FIGURE **12.6** Alkylation of nucleoside by bischloroethylnitrosourea (BCNU).

patients with grade III and IV astrocytoma but has been replaced by temozolomide.[39] BCNU-impregnated polymer wafers implanted in the tumor bed at the time of surgical resection provide a controlled release form of local chemotherapy.[40]

Streptozotocin is a unique methylnitrosourea with methylating activity that lacks carbamoylating activity, and this class of agents is discussed in depth in the second part of this chapter. It is used exclusively in the treatment of metastatic islet cell carcinoma of the pancreas and malignant carcinoid tumors.[41] The dose-limiting toxicities in humans have been gastrointestinal and renal but not hematopoietic.

Prodrugs of Alkylating Agents

Therapy with alkylating agents is compromised by a high level of toxicity to normal tissues and a lack of tumor selectivity. Cyclophosphamide and ifosfamide were prodrugs synthesized in the hope that high levels of phosphamidases in epithelial tumors would selectively activate the drugs.[42] Strategies for more selective delivery of alkylating agent to tumor have been explored including cleavable tumor-directed antibody-alkylating agent conjugates,[43] alkylating agent-glutathione conjugates (which might be selectively cleaved by glutathione transferase [GST] P1 expressed in high levels in tumor cells)[44], or viral vectors delivering activating enzymes to tumor cells.[45]

Cellular Pharmacology

Cellular Uptake

The uptake of alkylating agents into cells is an important determinant of cellular specificity. Many are highly lipid soluble (including the active metabolites of the methylating agents, cyclophosphamide, and ifosfamide, as well as chlorambucil) and readily enter cells by passive diffusion. Mechlorethamine uptake depends upon the choline transport system.[46] Melphalan is transported into several cell types by at least two active transport systems, which also carry leucine and other neutral amino acids across the cell membrane.[47] High levels of leucine in the medium protect cells from the cytotoxic effects of melphalan by competing with melphalan for transport.[48] In contrast to mechlorethamine and melphalan, the highly lipid-soluble nitrosoureas BCNU and CCNU enter cells by passive diffusion.[49] Chlorambucil uptake also occurs through simple passive diffusion.

Studies of cellular uptake of alkylating agents that require metabolic activation (such as cyclophosphamide or ifosfamide) are hampered by uncertainty about which metabolite, or even parent drug, is the most critical moiety for transport.

Sites of Alkylation

Any alkylating agent producing reactive intermediates binds to a variety of cellular constituents[50] including nucleic acids, proteins, amino acids, and nucleotides. As an example, the active alkylating species from a bis-chloroethyl nitrogen mustard demonstrates selectivity for nucleophiles in the following order: (a) oxygens of phosphates, (b) oxygen substituents on DNA bases, (c) amino groups of purines, (d) amino groups of proteins, (e) sulfur atoms of methionine, and (f) thiol groups of cysteinyl residues of glutathione.[51] DNA is generally favored as the primary target. Proof of this hypothesis may be emerging from three areas of research where cytotoxicity correlates with (a) activity of DNA repair enzymes, perhaps best shown for BCNU and repair by alkyl guanine alkyltransferase (AGT)[52]; (b) changes in a matrix of genetic and epigenetic events measured and analyzed by gene expression arrays[53]; and (c) specific DNA adducts shown by mass spectrometric analysis.[54] The stringency of such analyses requires that alternative toxic pathways not involving DNA must be excluded, a difficult requirement to meet.

In the DNA molecule, the phosphoryl oxygens of the sugar phosphate backbone are obvious electron-rich targets for alkylation. Alkylation of the phosphate groups occurs[55] and can result in strand breakage from hydrolysis of the resulting phosphotriesters. Although the biologic significance of the strand breakage caused by phosphate alkylation remains uncertain, the process is so slow that it seems unlikely to be a major determinant of cytotoxicity, even for monofunctional agents.[56] Alkylation of the O-6 atom and of the extracyclic nitrogen of guanine appears to be particularly important for carcinogenesis.[57]

Studies of the base specificity of alkylation by the chemotherapeutic alkylating agents have been much less extensive. Busulfan and mechlorethamine alkylate the N-7 position of guanine. Guanine cross-links (two guanine molecules abridged at the N-7 position by an alkylating agent) have been isolated from acid hydrolysates of the reaction mixtures.[28]

Reaction of the nitrogen mustard with native DNA, however, produces alkylation of the N-1 position of adenine in addition to N-7–alkylated guanine. The enhanced alkylation of the N-7 position of guanine may result from base stacking and charge transfer that enhance the nucleophilic character of the N-7 position. Melphalan preferentially alkylates guanine N-7 or adenine N-3.[58]

Base sequence influences the alkylating reaction. The N-7 position of guanine is most electronegative and, therefore, most vulnerable to attack by the aziridinium cation intermediate of the nitrogen mustards when the base is flanked by guanines on its 3' and 5' sides. The key site of DNA attack for the nitrosoureas as well as nonclassic methylating agents such as procarbazine and dacarbazine seems to be the O-6 methyl group of guanine (about 9% of alkylation).[6] Enhanced repair of this site is associated with drug resistance.[59] Thus, the preferred sites for alkylation vary by alkylating agent and chemical environment around the DNA base in question. Recent studies have identified that the relatively innocuous N^7-alkylation can become a site of toxic damage if its normal and efficient repair by base excision repair (BER) is interrupted.

DNA Cross-linking

On the basis of their isolation of the guanines linked at N-7 by alkylating agents, Brookes and Lawley[58] postulated that the bifunctional alkylating agents such as the nitrogen mustards produced interstrand and intrastrand DNA-DNA cross-links and that these cross-links were responsible for the inactivation of the DNA and cytotoxicity. On the basis of the Watson-Crick DNA model, these authors suggested that appropriate spatial relationships for cross-linking by nitrogen mustards or sulfur mustard occurred between the N-7 positions of guanine residues in complementary DNA strands (Fig. 12.7).

The importance of cross-linking is supported by the fact that the bifunctional alkylating agents, with few exceptions, are much more effective antitumor agents than the analogous monofunctional agents. Furthermore, increasing the number of alkylating units on the molecule beyond two does not usually increase the antitumor activity of the compound.

Direct evidence that DNA cross-linking occurs as the result of treatment of DNA or cells with bifunctional alkylating agents was provided initially by relatively insensitive physical techniques. The alkaline elution method[48] detects DNA cross-linking in cells and tumor-bearing animals exposed to minimal cytotoxic levels of alkylating agents.[60] DNA cross-linking by bifunctional alkylating agents correlates with cytotoxicity and that DNA in

drug-resistant cells has lower levels of cross-linkage.[61] The alkaline elution technique also detects DNA-protein as well as DNA-DNA cross-links.[62] DNA-protein cross-links likely do not play a major role in cytotoxicity and may be overcome by replication bypass mechanisms.[63]

In addition to these target effect-response studies, silencing of the AGT promoter in gliomas correlates with improved antitumor activity and survival in patients treated with BCNU.[64] Because AGT repairs guanine alkylation products produced by BCNU, decreased enzyme activity would be expected to increase DNA alkylation, implying that DNA is a critical target for BCNU effects. It is now standard of care to test for MGMT promoter methylation in clinical decisions of whether to add temozolomide to the treatment of gliomas.

Thus, evidence increasingly supports the hypothesis that DNA adduct formation is the major mechanism of alkylating agent cytotoxicity.

Chloroethylnitrosoureas cross-link via a unique mechanism.[37] The spontaneous decomposition of the chloroethylnitrosoureas generates a chloroethyldiazonium hydroxide entity that can alkylate DNA bases to produce an alkylating chloroethylamine group on the nucleotide in the DNA strand (Fig. 12.2). This group could then alkylate an adjacent nucleotide on the complementary DNA strand in a slower step, producing an interstrand cross-link.

The mechanism of alkylation by thiophosphates such as thiotepa likely begins with protonation of the aziridine N, which leads to ring opening. Cross-linking can proceed by one of several mechanisms, either activation of the free chloroethyl carbon or activation of a second aziridine ring on the original molecule. Monofunctional DNA alkylations exceed cross-links in number and are potentially cytotoxic. This hypothesis is supported by the fact that certain clinically effective agents, such as procarbazine and dacarbazine, are monofunctional alkylating compounds and do not produce cross-links in experimental systems. The basis of the cytotoxic effects of monofunctional alkylation appears to be through mismatch repair (MMR)-mediated processes, since cells lacking MMR are often methylating agent tolerant. The futile cycling of repair reactions through MMR efficiently removes bases opposite O^6-methylguanine and reinserts a thymine, with repeated attempt to repair the O^6-mG:T mismatch and further futile repair. This produces single-strand break and double-strand break (DSB) that are cytotoxic, especially in the second round of DNA synthesis, after formation of the O^6-mG:T mismatch.

Data suggest that alkylation is nonuniform along the DNA strand and may be concentrated in specific regions. One determinant of regional specificity of DNA alkylations may be chromatin structure[10]; areas of active transcription seem to be most vulnerable. Additionally, evidence shows that nitrogen mustards such as mechlorethamine preferentially cross-link at 5'-GNC sequence.[65]

Tumor Resistance

The emergence of alkylating agent–resistant tumor cells is a major problem that limits the clinical effectiveness of these drugs. Cellular resistance mechanisms identified in preclinical experimental settings include drug uptake, enhanced antiapoptosis pathways, activation of survival pathways, enhanced intratumoral drug inactivation, and changes in DNA repair.

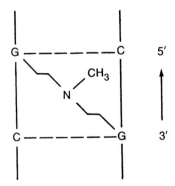

FIGURE 12.7 Cross-linking of DNA by nitrogen mustard. (Modified and reproduced from Brookes P, Lawley PD. The reaction of monofunctional and difunctional alkylating agents with nucleic acids. *Biochem J.* 1961;80:486, with permission.)

Decreased Cellular Uptake of Selected Alkylating Agents

Several of the drugs (melphalan, nitrogen mustard) of this class require active transport into cells. One mechanism for drug resistance is decreased drug entry into the cell. This mechanism was best demonstrated in L5178Y lymphoblast cells resistant to mechlorethamine.[46] The extracellular domain of the leucine-melphalan transporter expresses CD98. Reduced expression of CD98 on human myeloma cells is associated with melphalan resistance.[66] The glutathione-dependent efflux transporters MRP1 and MRP2 can confer resistance to chlorambucil.[67]

Resistance Due to Inactivation by Glutathione or GSTs

Intracellular inactivation of alkylating agents has been implicated in human tumor resistance. Early studies showed increased levels of sulfhydryls associated with resistance in experimental tumors and increased nonprotein sulfhydryl content, particularly in the form of glutathione, in resistant tumor cell lines. While increased intracellular glutathione content may be found in resistant cells, elevated GST activity may also play a role,[68] and increased aldehyde dehydrogenase (ALDH) activity, which converts

aldophosphamide to the inactive carboxyphosphamide, was present in cells resistant to cyclophosphamide.[69–71]

DNA Repair and Alkylating Agent Resistance

Enhanced repair of DNA lesions generated by alkylation plays a clearly established role in resistance of experimental and human tumor cells to alkylating agents. Because DNA appears to be the most critical target for the alkylating agents, its repair has been a major focus of study, and several mechanisms involved in repairing alkylation and strand breaks are summarized in Figure 12.8.

Enhanced excision of alkylated nucleotides from DNA as a mechanism of resistance to alkylating agents was first demonstrated in bacteria and later in mammalian cells. Bacterial, fungal, and mammalian cells are capable of excising and repairing sites of alkylation, as well as removing cross-links and repairing single-strand break and DSBs.[59]

Alkylguanine DNA Alkyltransferase Mediated Repair

Repair of DNA alkylation products and cross-links involves multiple systems, each composed of one or several distinct enzymes (see Fig. 12.8). The simplest of these catalyzes the transfer of

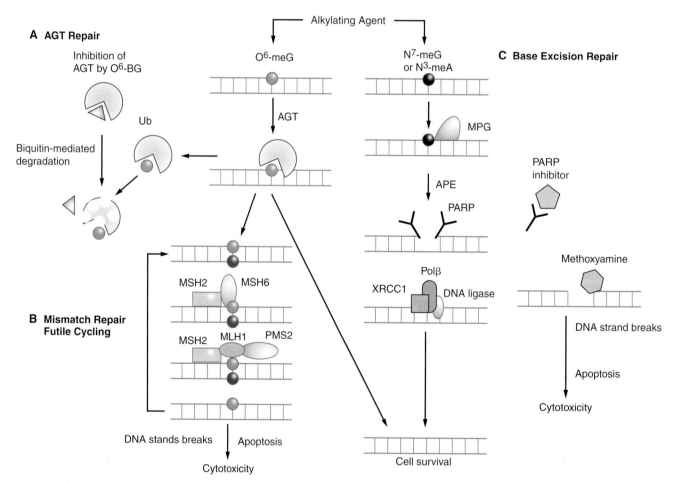

FIGURE **12.8** DNA repair pathways that play an important role in resistance to alkylating agents. **A.** AGT. **B.** Mismatch repair. **C.** Base excision repair. Targeted therapies to improve tumor sensitivity including O^6-benzylguanine, PARP inhibition, and methoxyamine are indicated. AGT, alkylguanine transferase; O^6-meG, O^6-methylguanine; N^7-meG, N^7-methylguanine; N^3-meA, N^3-methyladenine; O^6-BG, O^6-benzylguanine; Ub, ubiquitin; PARP, poly-ADP-ribose polymerase; Polβ, DNA polymerase β; MPG, methylpurine glycosylase. Not shown are components of the double-strand break repair complexes. (Adapted from Sarkaria JN, Kitange GJ, James CD, et al. Mechanisms of chemoresistance to alkylating agents in malignant glioma. *Clin Cancer Res.* 2008;14(10):2900-2908. Copyright © 2008 American Association for Cancer Research. With permission from AACR.)

alkyl substituents (methyl-, ethyl-, benzyl-, 2-chloroethyl-, and pyridyloxobutyl-) from the O^6-position of guanine to an active cysteine acceptor site within the protein in a single enzyme repair process. This enzyme, alkylguanine-O^6-alkyl transferase (AGT), is encoded by the MGMT (O^6-methylguanine methyltransferase) gene in humans and is homologous to the bacterial alkyltransferase gene, ada.

Several clinical trials have established an inverse correlation between AGT content in brain tumors and the response to treatment of brain tumor patients receiving BCNU, temozolomide, and other alkylating agents.[72,73] Lower levels of AGT activity result from epigenetic silencing due to MGMT promoter methylation. Tumors with methylated MGMT are highly responsive to these agents, while those with fully expressed AGT tend to be resistant. The availability of 5′ cytosine methylation–specific PCR (MSP) provides a facile assessment of MGMT promoter methylation and has value as a predictive assay for response to alkylating agent–based chemotherapy. MGMT promoter methylation has been correlated with survival in patients with glioma treated with nitrosoureas and temozolomide[64,74] and prolonged progression-free survival (PFS) in patients treated with temozolomide.[75] Together, these data illustrate a role for MGMT gene function in glioma chemoresistance to alkylating agents.[76,77]

Mismatch Repair

A second DNA repair system, MMR, recognizes the mismatch created by alkylation of DNA bases, and, after unsuccessful attempts at repair, triggers cell cycle arrest and apoptosis. For example, O^6-alkylation of guanine leads to mispairing of the damaged base with thymine, creating a distortion in the DNA double helix, which is recognized by components of the MMR complex. MMR deficiency has been associated with resistance to alkylating agents owing to the inability to recognize the mismatch and initiate the cycle of futile repair attempts, cell cycle arrest, and apoptosis.[78] Several proteins comprise the MMR pathway (hMLH1, hPMS2, hMSH2, hMSH3, and hMSH6), which is programmed to correct erroneous DNA base pairing.

In MMR competent cells during DNA replication, DNA polymerase mispairs unresolved O^6-methylguanine with thymine. The mismatch triggers attempts to remove the mispaired thymine. If repair is successful, subsequent rounds of replication continue to mispair O^6-methylguanine with thymine, resulting in repetitive futile cycles of MMR. This futile cycle may induce DSBs, which in turn, trigger p53-dependent cell cycle arrest and apoptosis.[79] Loss of MMR competence creates tolerance to the mispaired bases and allows cell replication and survival, provided the DNA lesions are compatible with viability. The loss of MLH6 may occur in glioma cells selected by resistance to temozolomide.[80]

Interactions of MMR proteins with cell cycle checkpoint proteins have been implicated in apoptosis. hMLH1 has been associated with signaling ATR-dependent G2 cell cycle arrest in response to DNA methylation,[81] and MMR proteins may initiate degradation of cyclin D1 following alkylation to promote cell cycle arrest in response to alkylation.[62] Functional MSH2 and hMLH1 activate p73-dependent apoptosis pathways via c-Abl.[82]

Resistance to alkylating agents conferred by MMR deficiency is further illustrated by hereditary nonpolyposis colon cancer, which is caused by mutations in hMLH1 or hMSH2 genes. Colon cancer cells harboring these mutations are resistant to alkylating agents,[83] as are other cell lines deficient in hMLH1.[84]

DNA Excision Repair

DNA excision repair pathways provide a comprehensive mechanism for recognizing and removing damaged bases or nucleotide segments from a single DNA strand and then resynthesizing the new DNA segment, using the opposing undamaged strand as a template. Excision repair complexes includes BER and nucleotide excision repair (NER).

Base Excision Repair

In response to DNA alkylation, BER is initiated by the action of damage-specific DNA glycosylases that recognize and excise single-base lesions such as N^3-methyladenine and N^7-methylguanine formed by temozolomide. This pathway is also important for essing 5-FU nucleotide incorporated into DNA or deoxyuridylate incorporated into DNA during treatment with pemetrexed. Related thymidylate synthase inhibitors also initiate incorporation of uracil into DNA.[85] Release of the damaged base produces an apurinic/apyrimidinic (AP) site, which is excised by the APE endonuclease (Fig. 12.9). The missing segment is then resynthesized by DNA

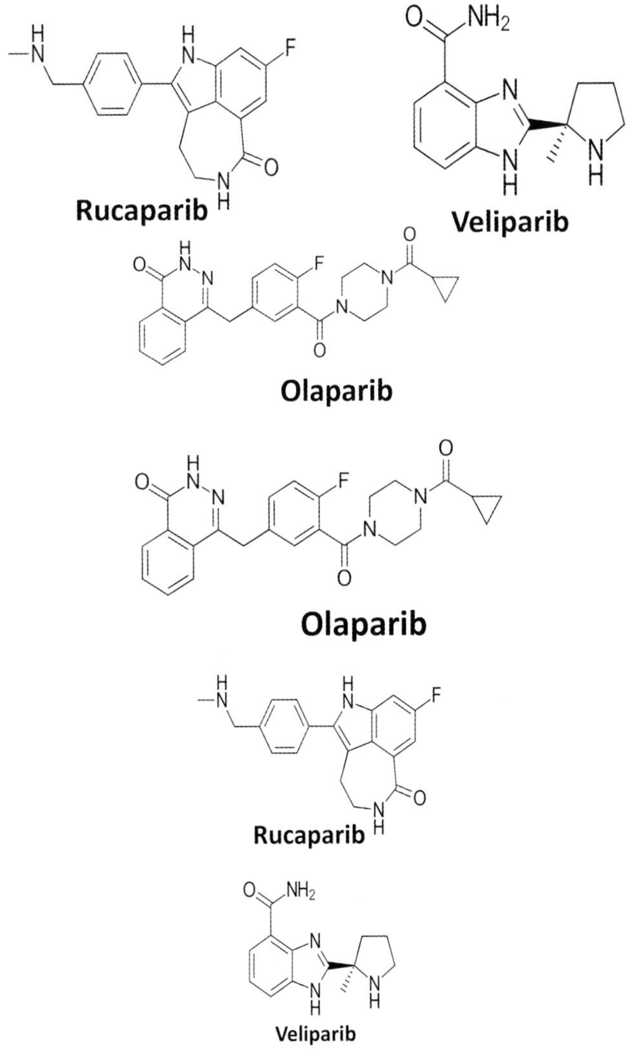

FIGURE **12.9** Structure of PARP inhibitors

polymerase and sealed by DNA ligase. Persistent AP sites are recognized by topoisomerase I and II, and these may form cleavable complexes that induce apoptotic signals. The enzyme PARP plays a pivotal role in the recognition of strand breaks and in the formation of DNA strand break intermediates that attract repair complexes. The N^3-methyladenine and N^7-methylguanine are the most common adducts created by alkylation and account for greater than 80% of all methylation events. However, these lesions contribute modestly to the cytotoxicity of alkylating agents due to the efficiency of the BER pathway. Perturbation of BER capacity through alterations of glycosylase expression or through pathway inhibition greatly decreases the efficiency of N^3- and N^7-methyl adduct repair.[86] Targeting of BER, as described below, is particularly effective in enhancing the sensitivity to platinating agents in various cell line tumors, especially breast cancers deficient in BRCA 1 and BRCA 2, and to alkylating agents in MMR-deficient tumors.[87]

Nucleotide Excision Repair

NER is an additional mechanism for excising bulky alkylation products and DNA intrastrand cross-links. The pathway includes multiple proteins that recognize DNA adducts, such as those produced by alkyl lesions and incise 3′ and 5′ to the damaged base(s), causing release of the damaged nucleotides and surrounding segments of DNA. Excision is followed by resynthesis of the missing segment, using the opposing strand as a template. Components of the NER complex also have a role in repair of DSBs. NER-deficient mammalian cells, such as those derived from patients with xeroderma pigmentosum (XP), are hypersensitive to alkylating and cross-linking agents.[88] Studies of the effects of NER deficiency on the toxicity of alkylating agents are most extensive in rodent models, but there is evidence that polymorphic variants of ERCC1 confer increased alkylating agent sensitivity for both normal and malignant tissues, influence response to treatment, and greater toxicity.[89] The role of NER in alkylating agent sensitivity and resistance in clinical cancer treatment is under active investigation, and recent evidence from the D'Andrea laboratory implicates increased ERCC2 expression as a factor in bladder cancer resistance to platinum therapies.[90]

Cross-link Repair

Interstrand cross-links covalently tether strands of DNA, preventing unwinding of duplex DNA and prohibiting polymerase access. Both strands of DNA are involved in this lesion, precluding straightforward excision repair and gap-filling pathways. Consequently, the repair of interstrand DNA cross-links is complex, integrating elements of the NER pathway, a variety of less well-understood activities to form a DSB, insertion of new bases, and homologous recombination (HR). Polymerase zeta can also mediate bypass DNA synthesis past a cross-link. Though mechanisms are incompletely understood, several mammalian cell types have extreme sensitivity to cross-linking agents. Fanconi's anemia (FA)[91] and Bloom's (BLM) syndrome cells[92] are both hypersensitive to alkylating agents that cause interstrand cross-links. FA pathway and the BLM helicase are believed to be activated in response to replication stalling due to cross-linked DNA; their dysfunction in the inherited disorders accounts for alkylating agent sensitivity.[93] Furthermore, mutations in excision repair genes ERCC1 and ERCC4 (XPF) also render cells sensitive to cross-linking by alkylating agents, suggesting these genes play a role in the repair of cross-links in addition to their role in NER.[94]

Akt and Mitochondrial-Linked Apoptosis

The Akt family in humans is comprised of three genes (Akt1, Akt2, and Akt3) encoding for serine/threonine protein kinases (PKB). Akt activation occurs downstream of various receptor tyrosine kinases and phosphatidylinositol 3-kinase (PI3K). The PI3K/Akt pathway is frequently activated in human cancer and has been implicated in tumor cell proliferation, cellular survival, and chemotherapy resistance. In response to alkylation, Akt is induced in cancer cells in an MMR-dependent manner.[95]

PI3K/Akt-mediated chemotherapy resistance is conferred via antiapoptotic effects. Activated Akt is thought to inhibit apoptosis by phosphorylating molecules upstream and downstream of the mitochondrial apoptotic pathway. Akt-dependent phosphorylation of proapoptotic BH3 family members such as Bad, Bax, and Bim-EL decreases the ability of these proteins to hold mitochondria in an open configuration, resulting in a reduction in cytochrome c release. Akt can phosphorylate caspase-9 to inhibit its ability to activate executioner caspase 3.[96] Akt reduces cytochrome c release through modification of the antiapoptotic Bcl-2 homologous Mcl-1.[97] Akt exerts indirect inhibition of apoptosis through effects on p53, the most important regulator of apoptosis.[98]

Akt also drives chemoresistance by promoting cell growth. Akt is involved in the survival pathway of mammalian target of rapamycin (mTOR), a serine/threonine kinase that is implicated in protein synthesis control.[99] Akt activates mTOR complex 1 (mTORC1, or mTOR-raptor complex) indirectly by inhibiting phosphorylation of tuberous sclerosis complex 2, thereby allowing Ras-related small G protein (Rheb)-GTP to activate mTORC1 signaling.[100]

Defects in Cell Cycle Arrest and Apoptosis

In cells that experience genotoxic stress during replication, activation of cell cycle arrest (checkpoint) factors triggers the signaling cascades, leading to delayed progression through S phase in order to allow time for DNA repair.[101] In the presence of DNA damage, an S-phase cell cycle checkpoint is activated by the checkpoint kinases ataxia-telangiectasia mutated (ATM) and ATM- and Rad3-related (ATR). Activation depends on the type of DNA damage: ATM is recruited to DNA DSBs induced by agents such as ionizing radiation (IR), whereas ATR is recruited to sites of replication protein A (RPA)-coated single-stranded DNA (ssDNA). These sites accumulate at stalled replication forks or at sites of single-strand damage.[102,103] The involvement of ATM and ATR in the response to carcinogen-induced DNA damage has been established,[104] which can be measured by accumulation of H2AX and by showing an enhanced sensitivity of ATM- and ATR-defective cells to methylating agents.

Two parallel branches of the DNA damage–dependent S-phase checkpoint are thought to cooperate by inhibiting distinct steps of DNA replication. One branch is activated by the phosphorylation of structural maintenance of chromosomes 1 (SMC1), a cohesin that is activated by ATM or ATR.[105] The second branch, consisting of the ATR-Chk1 or ATM-Chk2 complexes, regulates turnover of CDC25A, a phosphatase that regulates Cdk2 and consequently blocks the initiation of replication.[106]

Defects in damage recognition or apoptotic signaling may lead to relative resistance.[107] For example, loss of normal p53 function, up-regulation of the antiapoptotic proteins, Bcl-2 or Bcl-X$_L$, or overexpression of the epidermal growth factor receptor (EGFR) can disrupt the normal apoptotic response to DNA damage caused by alkylating agents.[108] Apoptotic cell death after DNA damage is mediated through p53, which blocks cell cycle progression, initiates attempts to repair damage, and ultimately activates apoptotic pathways. Loss of p53 has recently been noted to be associated with increased DNA replication starts, and replication start collapse in early S phase may lead to increased sensitivity in cancer cells after unrepaired incorporation of U, 5-FU, or N^7-mG after chemotherapy exposure.[109,110]

Reversal of Resistance

Exposure to alkylating agents leads to induction of a series of compensatory defensive responses in cell cycle drug-activating and drug-inactivating enzymes and induction of DNA repair capacity. Efforts to prevent or reverse tumor cell resistance have involved modulation of glutathione detoxification, as well as inhibition of DNA repair. Because of differences in repair mechanisms, combinations of alkylating agents in high doses have also been tested in breast cancer and other tumors, to no clear benefit.[111,112]

Glutathione Inhibition

Because of the pivotal importance of GSH in alkylating agent detoxification, three pharmacological approaches to modulation have been adopted: (a) precursors of GSH or other sulfhydryls replete sulfhydryls content in normal tissues, thus reducing the host toxicity; (b) specific inhibitors of GSH biosynthetic enzymes selectively decrease intracellular GSH in tumors; (c) inhibitors of detoxifying enzymes (GSTs) decrease the tumor cell's ability to protect itself against alkylating metabolites.

1. Because GSH cannot readily cross cell membranes, early efforts to increase intracellular GSH relied on administration of a precursor, L-2-oxothiazolidine-4-carboxylate, that must be enzymatically metabolized to L-cysteine, one of the three constituents of GSH.

2. A number of agents, including diethyl maleate, phorone, and dimethyl fumarate, have been used to deplete GSH by chemical interaction but proved too toxic clinically. By far, the most effective approach in reducing the GSH biosynthetic capacity of a tumor cell has been achieved by administering amino acid sulfoximines,[113] which inhibit γ-glutamylcysteine synthetase. The lead compound to emerge from these studies was L-buthionine (SR)-sulfoximine (BSO), the R-stereoisomer of which inhibits γ-glutamylcysteine synthetase.[114] GSH levels are low in unperturbed tumor cells adding to the rationale for BSO to improve the therapeutic index of alkylating agents. Although BSO caused differential sensitization of tumors in animal models, trials in humans failed to clearly demonstrate therapeutic index improvement,[115,116] and enthusiasm for clinical use of BSO has waned.

3. An alternative approach to decreasing GSH effects is to inhibit the enzymes that use GSH as a cofactor. GST overexpression was determined to be at least one contributing mechanism to the alkylating agent–resistant phenotype, providing a rationale for the use of GST inhibitors as modulating agents.

Specific inhibitors of GST P1 have now been developed and are being studied clinically but with inconclusive clinical results.[117,118]

4. A very different approach to modulation of alkylator toxicity was suggested in studies by the U.S. army, which examined over 4,000 synthetic thiol derivatives as radioprotectors.[119] One of these compounds, WR2721, 5-2-(3-aminopropylamino)-[$H_2N(CH_2)_3NH(CH_2)_2$-S-PO_3H_2], has been shown to dephosphorylate selectively in normal tissues through catalysis by alkaline phosphatase.[120] This agent, with the generic name of amifostine, is approved for ameliorating renal toxicity in patients receiving cisplatin and for reducing xerostomia in patients receiving head and neck irradiation. In experimental tumors, it enhanced the antitumor activity of many alkylating agents,[121] and in clinical trials, it showed some modest effect on the neutropenia caused by cyclophosphamide but failed to produce measurable benefit in patients receiving combined radiochemotherapy (with cisplatin and cyclophosphamide) and those with head and neck cancer.[122] Similarly, its ability to reduce toxicity of high-dose chemotherapy with HCT remains unproven.[123]

Inhibition of DNA Alkyl Adduct Repair

As discussed previously, silencing of MGMT by methylation of its promoter ablates expression of AGT, a key repair enzyme for alkylation adducts of O^6-guanine, and correlates with sensitivity of human gliomas to treatment with various drugs, including BCNU and temozolomide.[83,124] Preclinical data support the concept that inhibition of AGT sensitizes human glioma xenograft to the same drugs and that resistance can be restored by mutations in AGT that decrease binding of inhibitors to the enzyme. AGT binds irreversibly to the guanine cross-link (or removes the mono-methyl adduct by covalent transfer resulting in its inactivation) and is permanently inactivated in the process. Small molecular weight analogs of O^6-methyl guanine can inactivate AGT and sensitize tumor cells. The most potent of these inhibitors is O^6-benzyl guanine (BG), a compound that has reached clinical development. Its evaluation has been slowed by uncertainty regarding the optimal dose in combination with chemotherapy drugs. A trial with BCNU and OBG (120 mg/m^2) in patients with multiple myeloma depleted AGT by 94% in bone marrow tumor cells but produced responses in only 4 of 17 patients.[125] BG clearly enhances BCNU hematotoxicity, leading to a clinical study using a mutant P140K MGMT delivered by lentiviral vector to hematopoietic stem cells with clinical efficacy in patients with glioma treated with the combination of temozolomide and BG.[126]

Inhibition of BER

BER is one of the fundamental mechanisms for removing nonbulky DNA adducts, as created by oxidative stress and reactive molecules. This multistep pathway begins when alkylated bases are excised by lesion-specific glycosylases to create apurinic/apyrimidinic (AP) sites. These sites are then substrates for endonuclease cleavage of the phosphodiester backbone, creating single-strand breaks. The single-strand break is identified by poly-adenosine diphosphate-ribose polymerase (PARP), an essential component of BER. Binding of

PARP to strand breaks promotes poly(ADP) ribosylation of nuclear accessory proteins, forming negatively charged branch polymers that recruit enzymes that accomplish repair of the gap. The gap is filled by reading off the complementary DNA strand before the single strand is resealed. If the BER system is blocked by inhibitors of one of the important components in the pathway, single-strand breaks accumulate and may be converted into DSBs by an encounter with a replication fork.

Inhibitors of various steps in BER have been identified. The first of these was methoxyamine, an orally available compound that binds to the aldehydic oxygen of the AP site and prevents access of BER enzymes.[127] In model systems, methoxyamine leads to accumulation of DNA breaks and potentiates the cytotoxicity of alkylating agents. It has entered clinical trials, with temozolomide, pemetrexed, and fludarabine.

Potent inhibitors of PARP have been developed and approved for clinical use in ovarian cancer.[128–130] Three are now FDA approved: olaparib, veliparib, and rucaparib (Fig. 12.10). By inactivating BER, these compounds create a flurry of single-strand breaks and ultimately DSB in cells deficient in DSB repair. In preclinical experiments, PARP inhibitors enhance the activity of methylating agents and sensitize cells to DNA damage, even in the presence of high levels of expression of AGT[131] and are particularly effective against cells defective in DSB repair. Research is ongoing into the use of PARP inhibition in other malignancies as single-agent therapy and as sensitizers of known chemotherapeutics. Preclinical models find evidence of synergy of PARP inhibitors and temozolomide, although clinical trials have not confirmed improved outcomes.[132] PARP inhibitors have been approved for relapsed, platinum-sensitive ovarian cancer in BRCA-mutated disease and for maintenance therapy after platinum-based induction in both BRCA-mutated and wild-type ovarian tumors and for BRCA-mutated Her-2-negative metastatic breast cancers.

Clinical Pharmacology

The primary pharmacokinetics properties of standard alkylating agents are given in Table 12.1. Although some agents are too reactive chemically to provide more than momentary exposure of tumor cells to parent drug (the best examples are mechlorethamine and BCNU), others are stable in their parent form and even others require metabolic activation, as in the case of cyclophosphamide and ifosfamide. Doses of some alkylating agents may need to be adjusted for organ dysfunction and may require pharmacokinetic monitoring in individual patients, as with high-dose busulfan, to execute rational treatment regimens.

Activation, Decomposition, and Metabolism

Decomposition Versus Metabolism

A principal route of degradation of most of the reactive alkylating agents is spontaneous hydrolysis of the alkylating entity (i.e., alkylation by water). For example, mechlorethamine rapidly undergoes reaction to produce 2-hydroxyethyl-2-chloroethylmethylamine and bis-2-hydroxyethylmethylamine (Fig. 12.11). Likewise, both melphalan and chlorambucil undergo similar hydrolysis to form the mono-hydroxyethyl and bishydroxyethyl products, although less rapidly than the aliphatic nitrogen mustards.[132,133] The mono-hydroxylated products are less active alkylators than their chloro-alkyl precursors.

Most alkylating agents also undergo some degree of enzymatic metabolism. For example, if mechlorethamine radiolabeled in the methyl group is administered to mice, approximately 15% of the radioactivity can be recovered as exhaled carbon dioxide, which indicates that enzymatic demethylation is occurring. For the phosphoramide mustards and nitrosoureas, enzymatic metabolism plays a significant role in determining their pharmacokinetic profile.

Cyclophosphamide and Ifosfamide

Cyclophosphamide is activated to alkylating and cytotoxic metabolites by cytochrome P-450 isozymes 2B6, 2C9, and 3A4.[134,135] The

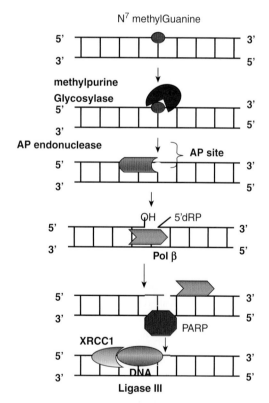

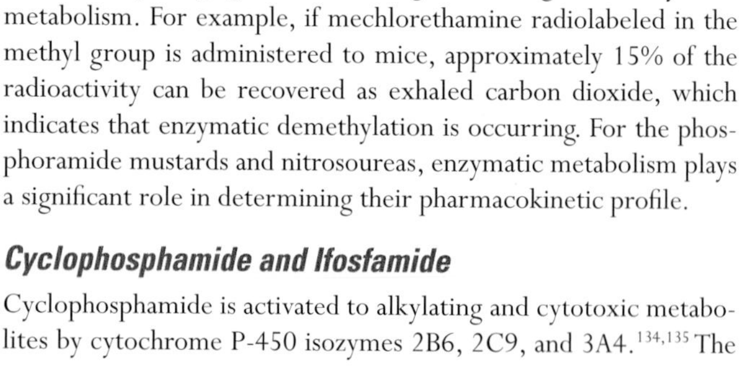

FIGURE 12.10 Endonuclease repair of mis-incorporation of uracil and uracil analogs into DNA. Base excision repair: Temozolomide methylation of DNA results in N^7-methylguanine and N^3-methyladenine. Both are repaired by base excision repair. Initiating with the removal of the base by methylpurine glycosylase, the AP endonuclease (AP endo) recognizes the abasic (AP) site, and clips the backbone. The remaining sugar deoxyribose is removed by polymerase beta (pol beta), which then fills in the correct base (in the example shown, a guanine-G), while the backbone is stabilized by PARP and XRCC1, and the lesion ligated by DNA ligase III.

FIGURE 12.11 Hydrolysis products of mechlorethamine

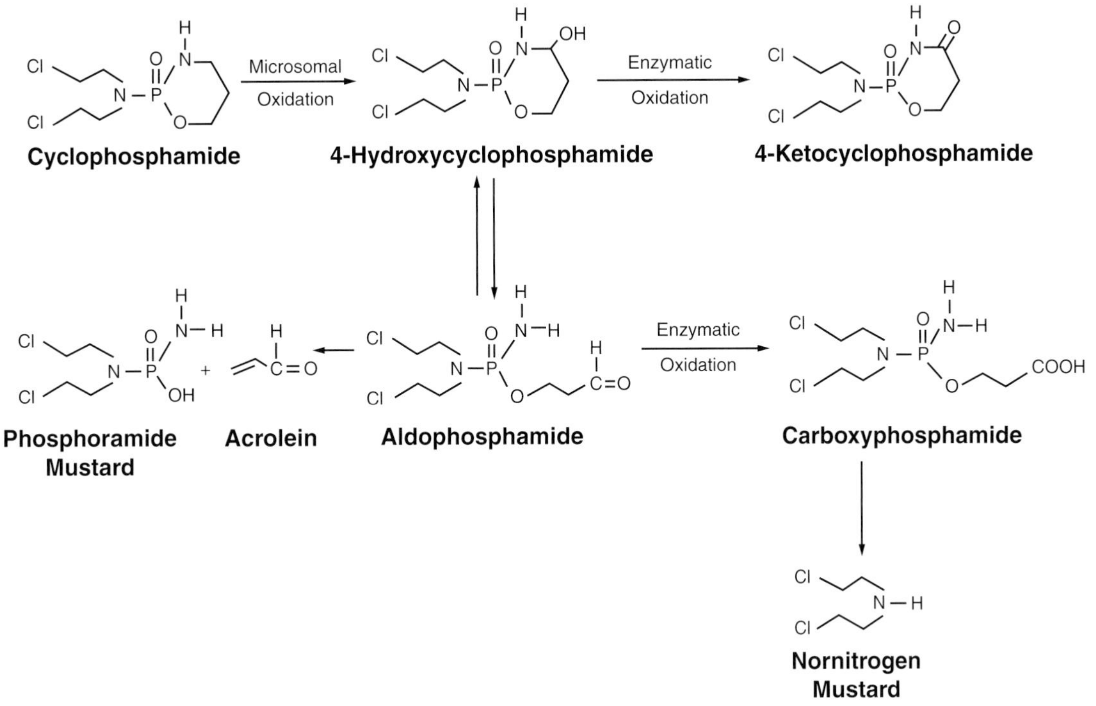

FIGURE **12.12** Metabolism of cyclophosphamide.

complex metabolic transformations are illustrated in Figure 12.12. The initial metabolic step is the oxidation of the ring carbon adjacent to the nitrogen to produce 4-hydroxycyclophosphamide, which establishes equilibrium with aldophosphamide. Aldophosphamide undergoes a spontaneous (nonenzymatic) elimination reaction to form phosphoramide mustard and acrolein. Phosphoramide mustard, which is generally believed to be the DNA cross-linking agent of clinical significance, is a circulating metabolite that does not enter cells easily due to its anionic form. Thus, the intracellular generation of phosphoramide mustard from aldophosphamide is believed to be important to a therapeutic result. A major detoxification route is the oxidation of aldophosphamide to the inactive carboxyphosphamide by ALDH1A1 and, to a much lesser extent, by ALDH3A1 and ALDH5A1 in the liver and in red blood cells. The concentration of ALDH in a variety of cell types appears inversely proportional to cytotoxicity, supporting its crucial role in determining cytotoxicity.[93] The high enzyme concentration in hematopoietic progenitor cells may explain the ability of cyclophosphamide to produce major myelosuppression without myeloablation in patients receiving high doses without transplantation. Likewise, cancer stem cells expressing ALDH may also be drug resistant.

Multiple metabolites can react with glutathione (GSH). Some of these reactions with GSH may be reversible while others are irreversible; the latter are associated with detoxification pathways. Several-fold differences in the extent of metabolite formation have been observed among patients, and these interindividual differences may be due to polymorphisms in cytochrome P-450 enzymes. CYP3A4 and 3A5 genotypes may influence response or survival in patients treated with cyclophosphamide. A minor (approximately 10%) alternative oxidative pathway leads to N-dechloroethylation and the formation of the neurotoxic chloroacetaldehyde. Cytochrome

P-450 3A4 is the main enzyme responsible for this undesirable secondary oxidation with a minor contribution from cytochrome P-450 2B6.

The metabolism of ifosfamide (Fig. 12.13) parallels that of cyclophosphamide but with some differences in isozyme specificities and reaction kinetics. Activation of ifosfamide to 4-hydroxyifosfamide is catalyzed by the hepatic cytochrome P-450 isoform 3A4. Aldo-ifosfamide partitions between ALDH1A1-mediated detoxification to carboxy-ifosfamide and a spontaneous (nonenzymatic) elimination reaction to yield isophosphoramide mustard and acrolein. Isophosphoramide is the DNA cross-linking agent of clinical significance. Hydroxylation proceeds at a slower rate for ifosfamide than for cyclophosphamide, which results in a longer plasma half-life for the parent compound. Dechloroethylation of ifosfamide produces inactive metabolites (primarily mediated by cytochrome P-450 isozyme 2B6 and 3A4) and competes with the activation step as a major pathway of elimination.[135,136]

Both cyclophosphamide (above doses of 4 g/m²) and ifosfamide (above doses of 5 g/m²) exhibit dose-dependent nonlinear pharmacokinetics, with significant delays in elimination at higher doses.[137] Interestingly, both drugs also induce their own metabolism, resulting in significant shortening of the elimination half-life for the parent compound when the drugs are administered on multiple consecutive days.[138,139] Both agents can undergo further chemical reaction to form acrolein, which is toxic to bladder. This compound may also form O^6G adducts, and these may be recognized and removed by AGT.

Nitrosoureas

The decomposition of nitrosoureas to generate the alkylating chloroethyldiazonium hydroxide entity has been mentioned, and the

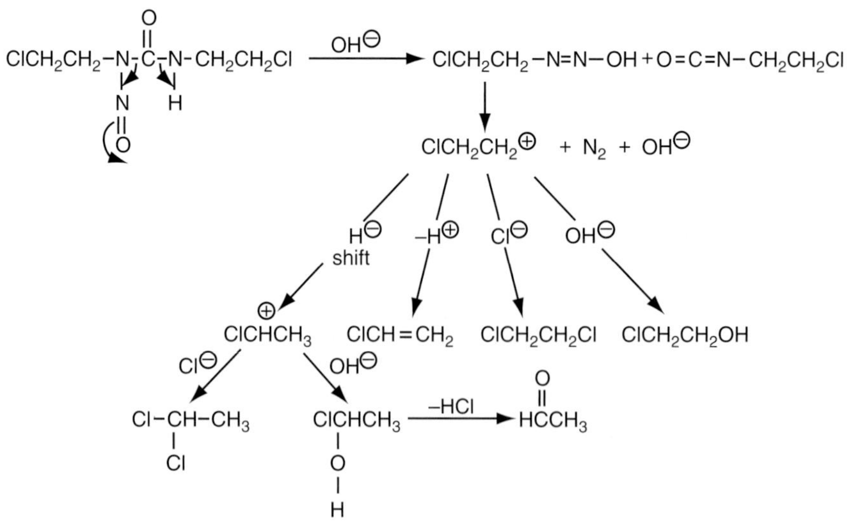

FIGURE **12.13** Metabolic activation of ifosfamide to its active form, 4-hydroxyifosfamide, and further metabolic transformation to chloroacetaldehyde and other end products. NADPH, reduced form of nicotinamide adenine dinucleotide phosphate.

products generated by this decomposition in aqueous solution are illustrated in Figure 12.14.

The nitrosoureas also undergo metabolic transformation. BCNU can be inactivated through denitrosation reactions catalyzed by both cytosolic and microsomal enzymes. Class μ glutathione S-transferase is a major catalyst of the cytosolic denitrosation reaction. Enhancement of P-450 activity in vivo by phenobarbital abolished the therapeutic effect of BCNU against the 9L intracerebral rat tumor and decreased the therapeutic activity of CCNU and BCNU against this tumor.[140] The phenobarbital-treated rats had increased plasma clearance of BCNU. The plasma clearance of parent BCNU decreases and the plasma half-life increases as doses escalate from standard-dose (150 to 200 mg/m[2]) to high-dose regimens (600 mg/m[2]) (Table 12.1).

CCNU and methyl-CCNU undergo hydroxylation of their cyclohexyl ring to produce a series of metabolites that represent the major circulating species after treatment with these drugs. These metabolites have increased alkylating activity but diminished carbamoylating effects.[140]

Clinical Pharmacokinetics

Gas chromatography-mass spectrometry and high-pressure liquid chromatography (HPLC) have generated pharmacokinetic information (Table 12.1) for alkylating agents and their metabolites.

Melphalan

In patients who received 0.6 mg/kg of the drug intravenously, the peak levels of melphalan, as measured by HPLC, were 4.5 to 13 μmol/L (1.4 to 4.1 μg/mL), and the mean terminal-phase half-life ($t_{1/2\beta}$) of the drug in the plasma was 1 hour.[133] Dose adjustment is not indicated at conventional doses, but in high-dose regimens, there are conflicting data regarding adjustment for renal function.[141] The 24-hour urinary excretion of the parent drug averaged 13% of the administered dose. Inactive monohydroxy and dihydroxy metabolites appear in plasma within minutes of drug administration.

Other studies have demonstrated low and variable systemic availability of the drug after oral dosing.[121,133] Food slows its absorption. After oral administration of melphalan, 0.6 mg/kg, much lower peak levels of drug of approximately 1 μmol/L (0.3 μg/mL) were seen. The time to achieve peak plasma levels varied considerably and occurred as late as 6 hours after dosing. The low bioavailability was caused by incomplete absorption of the drug from the gastrointestinal tract because 20% to 50% of an oral dose could be recovered in the feces. Regional administration of melphalan is possible by both intracavitary[142] and limb perfusion methods.[143]

Chlorambucil

After the oral administration of 0.6 mg/kg of chlorambucil,[133,144] peak levels of 2.0 to 6.3 μmol/L (0.6 to 1.9 μg/mL) occur within 1 hour. Peak plasma levels of phenylacetic acid mustard, an oxidation product of chlorambucil with alkylating activity, range from 1.8 to 4.3 μmol/L (0.5 to 1.18 μg/mL), and the peak levels of this metabolite are achieved 2 to 4 hours after dosing. The terminal-phase half-lives for chlorambucil and phenylacetic acid mustard are 92 and 145 minutes, respectively. Less than 1% of the administered dose of chlorambucil is excreted in the urine as either chlorambucil (0.54%) or phenylacetic acid mustard (0.25%). Approximately 50% of the radioactivity from carbon-14–labeled chlorambucil administered orally is excreted in the urine in 24 hours. Of this material, over 90% appears to be the monohydroxy and dihydroxy hydrolysis products of chlorambucil and phenylacetic acid mustard.

Cyclophosphamide

Cyclophosphamide is well absorbed after oral administration to humans.[145] The systemic availability of the unchanged drug after oral administration of 100-mg doses (1 to 2 mg/kg) was 97% of that after intravenous injection of the same dose. A comparison of oral versus intravenous cyclophosphamide in the same patient revealed no difference in the area under the curve (AUC) for the primary cytotoxic metabolites, hydroxycyclophosphamide, and phosphoramide mustard.[146] After intravenous administration, the peak plasma levels of the parent compound are dose dependent. Peak levels are 4, 50, and 500 nmol/mL after the administration of 1 to 2 mg/kg,[147] 6 to 15 mg/kg,[148] and 60 mg/kg,[149] respectively. The terminal-phase half-life of cyclophosphamide varies considerably among patients (3 to 10 hours). In patients less than 19 years of

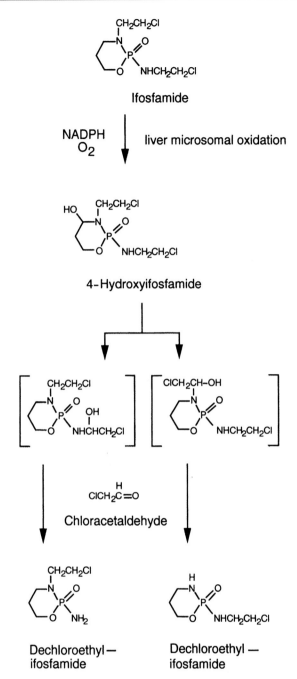

FIGURE 12.14 Decomposition of bischloroethylnitrosourea (BCNU) in buffered aqueous solution.

age, the plasma half-life of parent drug is 1.5 hours.[150] Peak alkylating levels are achieved 2 to 3 hours after drug administration, and the terminal half-life of plasma alkylating activity is 7.7 hours with a plateau-like level of plasma alkylating activity maintained for at least 6 hours.

The predominant metabolites found in plasma are nor-nitrogen mustard and phosphoramide mustard, with lesser concentrations of the putative transport forms aldophosphamide and 4-hydroxycyclophosphamide. The peak plasma levels of the major metabolites of cyclophosphamide, 4-hydroxycyclophosphamide/aldophosphamide, were 1.4 and 2.6 nmol/mL after injection of doses of 10 and 20 mg of radiolabeled cyclophosphamide per kilogram, respectively. Subsequent studies have determined that

4-hydroxycyclophosphamide/aldophosphamide has a half-life of approximately 1.5 hours in children and 1 to 5 hours in adults receiving conventional[146] or high-dose[151] cyclophosphamide. The AUC for 4-hydroxycyclophosphamide and aldophosphamide at conventional doses of drug ranged from 3 to 19 nmol/mL × hours and seems independent of either peak plasma levels or the plasma half-life of the parent drug or hydroxycyclophosphamide.

Because the initial metabolism of cyclophosphamide is hepatic, modulation of the activity of P-450 in vivo might be expected to alter the pharmacokinetics of the drug. Pretreatment with phenobarbital, a known P-450 inducer, reduces the plasma half-life of the parent compound in both humans and experimental animals.[152] Also, with repeated doses of cyclophosphamide, the plasma half-life of parent compound becomes progressively shorter[153] and that of 4-hydroxycyclophosphamide increases, which indicates that cyclophosphamide can induce the P-450 enzymes responsible for its metabolism.

The pharmacokinetics of cyclophosphamide and its metabolites has been incompletely studied in patients with renal failure. Because both parent drug and active metabolites are excreted, albeit to a limited extent, by the kidneys, caution should be used when cyclophosphamide is administered to such patients.[154]

Ifosfamide

After single doses of 3.8 to 5.0 g/m², the terminal half-life of ifosfamide was 6.3 hours, on day 1 decreasing to 3.8 hours on day 5. Also, the alkylating activity excreted in the urine is about 21%.[155,156] As with cyclophosphamide, ifosfamide clearance increases during continuous infusion or with multiple daily doses, reaching a steady state 2 to 3 days after drug administration is begun.[157] Whereas less than 10% of a dose of cyclophosphamide is dechlorethylated, as much as 50% of a dose of ifosfamide may be excreted in the urine as dechlorethylated products. Because the slower activation rate of ifosfamide results in more prolonged exposure to the bladder-toxic metabolite acrolein, the disulfide detoxifier MESNA is routinely administered in association with ifosfamide.

Thiotepa

Thiotepa is rapidly desulfurated to TEPA and other alkylating species.[158-161] The conversion of thiotepa to TEPA is mediated by P-450 isoenzymes. Both thiotepa and TEPA have cytotoxic activity. Aside from individual variability, the plasma terminal half-life of intact thiotepa is a relatively consistent 1.2 to 2 hours. TEPA appears in plasma within 5 minutes of thiotepa administration. In 120 minutes, its plasma concentration reaches that of thiotepa, but it persists longer, with a half-life of 3 to 21 hours, so that after 24 hours TEPA concentration × time exceeds that of the parent drug. In 24 hours, only 1.5% of the administered thiotepa is excreted in the urine unchanged, together with 4.2% as TEPA and 23.5% as other alkylating species.[162] The pharmacokinetics in children resembles that in adults.[159,160]

Bendamustine

Bendamustine has a similar mechanism of action to the other chloroethylating agents. It has three distinct structural elements: a mechlorethamine group, which acts as the chloroethylating agent; a benzimidazole ring, which may interfere with nucleotide metabolism; and a butyric acid side chain, which may react with proteins and membranes (Fig. 12.4).[19] Clinically, bendamustine acts as an alkylating agent and not an antimetabolite. Bendamustine produces strand breaks at a number far greater than equimolar concentrations of cyclophosphamide or melphalan. Furthermore, bendamustine-induced strand breaks are repaired slowly compared to those produced by other alkylating agents perhaps because of the bulk of the adduct. Furthermore, bendamustine shows only partial cross-resistance with other alkylating agents. This improved activity in resistant populations has been attributed to both extensive strand break formation and failed repair.

Current use of bendamustine is in lymphoid malignancies. It is indicated for fludarabine-refractory CLL[20] often in combination with rituximab,[22] where response rates in excess of 50% are noted, including patients with complete responses, and its superior activity has been confirmed in a phase III trial comparing chlorambucil with bendamustine, where 68% of bendamustine-treated patients compared to only 31% in chlorambucil-treated patients had a complete or partial response rate ($P < 0.0001$).[21] Bendamustine is also active against refractory indolent B-cell lymphomas with a more favorable therapeutic index than CHOP-rituximab (α-CD20) treatment. Additionally, a clinical trial evaluating the efficacy of bendamustine-rituximab combination therapy found that the combination is well tolerated and active against follicular lymphomas and Waldenstrom's macroglobulinemia.[22]

Bendamustine is tightly bound to human serum plasma proteins (94% to 96%) and is mainly found in extracellular spaces. Bendamustine is primarily metabolized via spontaneous hydrolysis of either of the chloroethyl arms to hydroxyethyl metabolites, which are significantly less active than parent drug. Two active minor metabolites, M3 (a hydroxy metabolite) and M4 (an N-desmethyl product), are formed via cytochrome P-450 1A2. Bendamustine clearance in humans is approximately 700 mL/min. After a single dose of 120 mg/m² bendamustine IV over 1 hour, the intermediate $t_{1/2}$'s of the parent compound is approximately 40 minutes. The mean apparent terminal elimination $t_{1/2}$ of M3 and M4 is approximately 3 hours and 30 minutes, respectively.[163]

Nitrosoureas

In humans after short-term infusion (15 to 75 minutes) of 60 to 170 mg/m², initial peak levels of up to 5 μmol/L of BCNU are achieved. The plasma concentration decay curves were biexponential, with a distribution-phase half-life of 6 minutes and a second-phase half-life of 68 minutes. With high-dose BCNU, longer elimination half-lives of 22 to 45 minutes have been reported.[164]

Busulfan

Busulfan is primary employed in high-dose regimens associated with bone marrow reconstitution. It is routinely administered over 3 to 4 consecutive days, with dosing every 6 hours or once daily. The daily dose is usually in the range of 3.2 mg/kg, or approximately 120 mg/m². The drug bioavailability by the oral route is variable among patients.[165] The drug exhibits circadian rhythmicity in its pharmacokinetics, particularly in children, with higher drug levels and slower elimination in the evening. The primary elimination half-life is approximately 2.5 hours in both children and adults, although interpatient variability is considerable at both low and high doses. It is the preferred agent for HST of genetic disorders.

The relationship between intravenous dose and AUC within the same patient appears to be predictable over multiple days of administration during high-dose therapy. Because of variable bioavailability, there is less consistency with the oral formulation. A range of threefold AUC in plasma levels after oral dosing is found among individuals in various cohorts studied.[166] Thus, intravenous administration is the preferred route. Clearance declines with age and with increases in body weight, which leads to potential underdosing of children in high-dose regimens.[167] Busulfan clearance for patients older than 18 years averages 2.64 to 2.9 mL/min/kg, whereas for children aged 2 to 14, clearance averages 4.4 to 4.5 mL/min/kg, and for children aged 3 or younger, it is 6.8 to 8.4 mL/min/kg.[168] Mean volume of distribution at steady state was larger in children less than 1 year of age (0.77 ± 0.24 versus 0.64 ± 0.11 L/kg; $P = 0.040$) and children less than 4 year of age (0.73 ± 0.18 versus 0.64 ± 0.11 L/kg; $P = 0.001$) than in older children.[169] Thus, larger doses must be used in the younger age groups to achieve the desired cytotoxic exposure.

Because of its high lipid solubility and low level of protein binding, busulfan penetrates readily into the brain and cerebrospinal fluid. The ratio of drug concentration in cerebrospinal fluid to plasma approximates 1.[170] Positron-labeled busulfan has been used to track uptake into the brain, revealing that approximately 20% of a standard dose rapidly enters the CNS.[171] This access to the brain may enhance the activity of this drug against leukemia and lymphoma cells in the CNS, but it also may explain its propensity to cause seizures. Prophylaxis with anticonvulsants is required in patients receiving high-dose busulfan. Busulfan enhances the clearance of phenytoin (Dilantin) and, in some patients, lowers the drug's plasma concentration below the therapeutic range, which increases the risk of seizures.[172] Phenytoin levels should be monitored in the setting of busulfan therapy or an alternative, non–P-450 metabolized anticonvulsant should be used.

Monitoring of drug levels and adjustment of doses to reach desired levels of drug exposure (AUC) have become an accepted aspect of high-dose intravenous busulfan with stem cell transplantation.

A mean steady-state plasma busulfan concentration of 200 to 600 ng/mL (0.8 to 3.2 μM) is associated with an optimal outcome: a low rate of graft rejection or relapse and a low incidence of serious or fatal toxicity (venoocclusive disease and neurotoxicity).[173] The clearance rate fell almost fourfold, from 20 mL/min/kg in the youngest patients (<age 2) to 5 mL/min/kg in patients over age 20. These findings argued for flexible dosing adjusted for patient age. Later studies established the efficacy of drug level monitoring in allowing dose adjustment in individual patients to achieve optimal results.[124,174–176]

Exposures below 900 μM × min are associated with a high risk of relapse, while AUC levels above 1,500 μM × min increase the risk of venous occlusive disease of the liver and other potentially fatal adverse events.[173] A target AUC of 1,200 μM × min seems to be a reasonable and safe target. An approach is to administer a small, test dose (0.8 mg/kg) of busulfan, from which an AUC parameter is calculated and used to make an extrapolation to the desired AUC.[124] The test dose method produced a highly accurate estimate of the actual high-dose AUC in two trials[176]; fewer than 5% of patients had AUC values that fell out of the desired range.

Toxicity

Nausea and Vomiting

Although nausea and vomiting are not life-threatening toxic reactions, they are a frequent side effect of alkylating agent therapy and require antiemetics. The marked effectiveness of the newer centrally acting antiemetics (H_3 antagonists) suggests that the emetic effect of these drugs is at most only partially mediated by direct gastrointestinal toxicity.

Hematopoietic Suppression

The usual dose-limiting toxicity of the alkylating agents is suppression of hematopoiesis. Characteristically, this suppression involves all formed elements of the blood: leukocytes, platelets, and red cells. However, the degree, time course, and cellular pattern of the hematopoietic suppression produced by the various alkylating agents differ. Many alkylating agents also cause lymphopenia, which can result in immunosuppression that outlasts the myelosuppression. Clinically significant platelet suppression may be seen when the dose of cyclophosphamide exceeds 30 mg/kg, but relative platelet sparing is characteristic of the drug. Even at the high doses (200 mg/kg or greater) of cyclophosphamide used in preparation for bone marrow transplantation, recovery of endogenous hematopoietic elements occurs within 21 to 28 days and has allowed these high doses to be used without transplantation in patients with aplastic anemia. This stem cell–sparing property of cyclophosphamide is related to stem cell possession of high concentrations of ALDH, an enzyme required for conversion of the phosphoramide mustard into the inactive metabolite carboxycyclophosphamide. As such, cumulative damage to the bone marrow is uncommonly seen when cyclophosphamide is given as a single agent, and repeated high doses of the drug can be given without progressive lowering of leukocyte and platelet counts. This has allowed cyclophosphamide to be successfully employed posttransplant to block lymphocyte activation and reduce acute GVHD, particularly in the setting of haploidentical transplantation.

The hematopoietic depression produced by the nitrosoureas is characteristically delayed. The onset of leukocyte and platelet depression occurs 3 to 4 weeks after drug administration and may last an additional 2 to 3 weeks. Thrombocytopenia appears earlier and usually is more severe than leukopenia. Even if the nitrosourea is given at 6-week intervals, hematopoietic recovery may not occur between courses, and dose reduction is often necessary for repeat courses.

Immunosuppression

Alkylating agents suppress both humoral and cellular immunities. Cyclophosphamide is a particularly potent immunosuppressive alkylating agent affecting both basal B- and T-cell functions. Appropriate low doses of cyclophosphamide in vivo may enhance immunologic responses by selective inhibition of the function of regulatory T cells.[177] Much of this inhibition of T-cell function comes from apoptosis and increased activation-induced cell death through Fas (CD95) up-regulation.[178] However, some immunosuppressive effects of cyclophosphamide may involve mechanisms other than lethal damage to lymphocytes. Induction of B-cell tolerance by cyclophosphamide occurs in vivo (or by activated cyclophosphamide

in vitro). It is reversible and is associated with failure of the cyclophosphamide-treated B cell to regenerate a surface immunoglobulin receptor after capping with anti-immunoglobulin serum.[179] Also, 4-hydroperoxycyclophosphamide, an activated analog of cyclophosphamide, blocks the differentiation of regulatory T-cell precursors at drug levels that are not cytotoxic and do not produce measurable DNA cross-linking in drug-sensitive cell lines.[180]

Clinically, there is significant interest in the immunomodulatory effects of the alkylating agents in the setting of cancer therapy, particularly cyclophosphamide. Suppression of the recipient immune response before allogeneic transplantation with cyclophosphamide has been in clinical application since Santos et al.[181] showed that matched sibling bone marrow can be successfully transplanted into recipients who have been pretreated with large doses of cyclophosphamide. Alkylating agents are also used in lymphodepleting regimens prior to administration of chimeric antigen receptor (CAR) T cell and genetically engineered T-cell administration for treatment of variety of malignancies. More recently, cyclophosphamide given at 50 mg/kg/d after stem cell transplant has been shown to enhance allograft tolerance and reduce the incidence of GVHD.[182] Since cyclophosphamide is minimally toxic to hematopoietic stem cells due to their high levels of aldehyde dehydrogenase, the transient immunosuppression of high dose cyclophosphamide is followed by predictable immune reconstitution. High-dose cyclophosphamide therapy is followed by predictable patterns of immune system reconstitution.

Interstitial Pneumonitis, Lung Injury, and Fibrosis

Both BCNU[183] and busulfan[184,185] produce pulmonary fibrosis when administered in lower doses over prolonged periods. Virtually all alkylating agents have been associated with similar patterns of acute lung injury or fibrosis, though much less frequently than with busulfan or BCNU. Busulfan is infrequently used in this dosing pattern, but BCNU is still used in this manner to treat brain tumors. Both drugs are primarily given in short (1 to 4 day) courses of high-dose therapy with HCT. With this dosing pattern, busulfan produces less frequent lung toxicity. BCNU causes a dose-dependent pattern of acute lung injury in marrow transplant regimens, with a frequency variation of 5% to 60%, depending on the regimen and dose of BCNU.[186] This acute injury is manifested by cough, dyspnea, with or without fever, and hypoxemia, frequently with minimal radiographic findings. It can occur in an acute form or subacutely in the months after treatment. Although these problems can become life threatening or progress to fibrosis, the acute injury responds well to treatment with prednisone, which is most often administered routinely or at the first signs of cough or fever.

Renal and Bladder Toxicity

A toxicity that is relatively unique to the oxazaphosphorines (cyclophosphamide and ifosfamide) is hemorrhagic cystitis, which may range from a mild cystitis to severe bladder damage with massive hemorrhage.[187,188] Hemorrhagic cystitis is often a devastating, life-threatening, or extremely debilitating treatment complication, so great emphasis should always be placed on prevention. This toxicity is caused by the excretion of acrolein, a metabolite of both cyclophosphamide and ifosfamide in the urine, with subsequent direct irritation of the bladder mucosa.[187] This toxicity is usually seen within weeks of the administration of high-dose cyclophosphamide but can occur at any time after repeated doses of ifosfamide or lower-dose cyclophosphamide. Chronic cystitis caused by cyclophosphamide has been associated with the later development of malignant transitional cell tumors of the bladder.[188] The most effective agent for preventing oxazaphosphorine-induced cystitis is 2-mercaptoethane sulfonate (MESNA), which dimerizes to an inactive metabolite in plasma but hydrolyzes in urine to yield the active parent that conjugates with alkylating species and prevents cystitis. MESNA should be administered routinely to all patients receiving ifosfamide and to any patient receiving high-dose cyclophosphamide, or any patient on standard doses who has a history of drug-induced cystitis.[189] MESNA is usually given in divided doses every 4 hours in dosages of 60% of those of the alkylating agent. Experiments in animals and clinical evaluation indicate that the systemic administration of sulfhydryl compounds does not impair the antitumor or immunosuppressive effect of cyclophosphamide.[190]

At high doses of ifosfamide, severe renal tubular damage with elevation of serum urea and creatinine has been seen, along with a Fanconi-like tubular acidosis and salt-wasting syndrome.[191,192] High-dose cyclophosphamide can also produce the syndrome of inappropriate antidiuretic hormone excretion, resulting in transient water retention.[193] Chronic administration of nitrosoureas can infrequently produce renal damage.[194,195] High-dose melphalan has been associated with renal tubular injury and proteinuria.[147]

Gonadal Atrophy

Alkylating agents have profound toxic effects on reproductive tissue. A depletion of testicular germ cells but preservation of Sertoli's cells was described by Spitz[196] in the first extensive review of the histologic effects of mechlorethamine in patients. This toxic effect and its functional counterpart of aspermia have subsequently been well documented in both animals[197] and humans.[198,199] The probability of aspermia or amenorrhea increases with increasing dose and cumulative dose of alkylating agents. Because of the widespread availability of sperm banking, patients who will undergo treatment with alkylating agents and who wish to father children should be counseled to be evaluated for sperm banking prior to treatment. (Egg harvesting and storage of embryos as well as newer successful experiments with egg storage and storage and reimplantation of pretreatment harvested ovarian tissue have yielded successful pregnancies.) Oligospermia or anovulation may be associated with advanced malignancy in the absence of treatment. Ovulation and sperm counts may return in uncommon cases after tumor remission induced by either conventional or high-dose alkylating agents.[200,201] The risk of amenorrhea and infertility after alkylating agents increases with increasing age, as well as dose and cumulative dose of alkylating agents used.

Teratogenesis

All alkylating agents are teratogenic. Studies have been carried out in a number of systems, both in vivo and in embryo culture in vitro.[148] The teratogenic action seems to be the result of direct cytotoxicity to the developing embryo.[202]

Because of the demonstrated teratogenicity of the alkylating agents in animals, appropriate concern has existed about the potential effects of their administration to patients during pregnancy.

In 1968, Nicholson[203] reviewed literature reports of women treated with cytotoxic agents during pregnancy. In the 25 instances in which the alkylating agents were given during the first trimester of pregnancy and the status of the fetus was recorded, four cases of fetal malformation occurred. No instances of malformed fetuses were reported when alkylating agents or other cytotoxic drugs were administered during the second or third trimester. Thus, administration of alkylating agents during the first trimester presents a definite risk of a malformed viable infant, but the risk is lower beyond that point. Other reports confirm the risk of malformation in children born to mothers who had received chlorambucil,[204] cyclophosphamide,[205] or nitrogen mustard and procarbazine[206] during the first trimester and the birth of normal infants to mothers receiving alkylating agents during the second or third trimester.[207,208]

Treatment-Related Leukemias

Treatment-related or secondary leukemia, usually AML, often preceded by myelodysplastic syndrome (MDS), arises in patients who have a history of exposure to alkylating agents. Cases of secondary leukemia have been described in patients treated with all commonly used alkylating agents (see Chapter 42). Alkylating agent–associated AML is often preceded by MDS with deletions in chromosomes 5 or 7.[209,210] The risk of AML is greatest 4 to 7 years after therapy but later as well, likely due to the requirement for subsequent genetic events following the initial chromosomal deletions.[162] The routine use of sequential chemotherapy and radiation for treatment of Hodgkin's disease is best avoided except in cases of advanced disease, and if used together, combined in the lowest possible dose.[211] Underlying genetic deficits, such as neurofibromatosis type 1 (NF1)[212] or defects in DNA repair related to FA,[210] may lead to increased susceptibility to treatment-related leukemia. Recently, clonal hematopoiesis of indeterminate potential (CHIP) has been identified to evolve as a function of age and is linked to a finite number of acquired mutations in genes associated with AML and MDS. It is possible that older individuals with a solid tumors who undergo treatment with alkylating agents in the setting of CHIP are more likely to develop a treatment-related myeloid malignancy.[213] These leukemias are characterized by a low response rate to conventional treatment, although they may respond to demethylating epigenetic treatments such as decitabine; despite initial responses in some patients, most patients relapse, and there is a poor long-term survival rate.

Other malignancies, including solid tumors may develop up to 20 years after treatment with alkylating agents.[211]

Organ Toxicity in High-Dose Chemotherapy

Alkylating agents have become a logical tool, either alone or in combination with other drugs or irradiation, for high-dose chemotherapy regimens.[214–216] Cross-resistance among alkylating agents and the closely related platinum analogues is incomplete, so patients treated with conventional doses of cyclophosphamide or melphalan may have complete responses to high-dose regimens containing other alkylators. A second important consideration is that for many alkylating agents, there is a linear increase in tumor killing as the dose increases. In this high-dose setting, multiple new toxicities become apparent, including acute fluid imbalance; a syndrome of inappropriate antidiuretic hormone secretion after cyclophosphamide (SIADH); hemorrhagic myocarditis; nephrogenic diabetes insipidus after cyclophosphamide therapy[217]; hypertension with combinations of alkylating agents[218]; venoocclusive disease of the liver; metabolic abnormalities such as idiopathic hyperammonemia[219]; interstitial pneumonitis[220,221]; and late vasculitis with pulmonary hemorrhage.[222] Additionally, lack of adequate bladder irrigation or failure to administer protective compounds such as MESNA may lead to hemorrhagic cystitis. The dose-limiting extramedullary toxicities of the alkylating agents encountered in common high-dose regimens are listed in Table 12.2.

Among these toxicities, melphalan produces severe gastrointestinal toxicity. Venoocclusive disease (VOD) of the liver, reflecting endothelial damage and subsequent clot formation in the small hepatic venules, occurs in as many as 20% of patients who undergo high-dose chemotherapy with nitrosoureas, busulfan, thiotepa, or carboplatin, treatable with defibrotide.[232] Drug level monitoring, as described earlier, can largely prevent this complication in patients receiving high-dose busulfan. Mucositis and enterocolitis are major side effects of many regimens such as etoposide, melphalan, thiotepa.

Cutaneous toxicity is frequently noted during high-dose chemotherapy, including a variety of rashes,[233] most often a macular erythematous eruption.

Pulmonary drug toxicity occurs frequently with all high-dose regimens, both as an acute manifestation of pulmonary injury, and in the months following transplantation, when pulmonary fibrosis may develop.[234] Pulmonary drug toxicity is commonly associated with carmustine when the acute or chronic dose exceeds 1,200 mg/m^2 of body surface.

TABLE 12.2   Alkylating agents in high-dose chemotherapy

Dose-Limiting Extramedullary Toxicities of Single Agents

Drug	MTD[a] (mg/m^2)	Fold Increase Over Standard Dose	Major Organ Toxicities
Cyclophosphamide	7,000	7.0	Cardiac
Ifosfamide	16,000	2.7	Renal, CNS
Thiotepa	1,000	18.0	GI, CNS
Melphalan	180	5.6	GI
Busulfan	640	9.0	GI, hepatic
BCNU	1,050	5.3	Lung, hepatic
Cisplatin	200	2.0	PN, renal
Carboplatin	2,000	5.0	Renal, PN, hepatic
Etoposide	3,000	6.0	GI

Combination High-Dose Chemotherapy Regimens

Regimen	Dose	Major Toxicities	Regimen MTD[b]	References
Cyclophosphamide	6,000			
BCNU	300	Lung, GI	0.47	[223]
Etoposide	750			
Busulfan	640	Lung, GI, hepatic	1.0	[224]
Cyclophosphamide	8,000			
Ifosfamide	16,000			
Carboplatin	1,800	Renal, hepatic, GI	0.8	[225]
Etoposide	1,500			
Cyclophosphamide	5,250			
Etoposide	1,200			[226]
Cisplatin	180			
Cyclophosphamide	6,000			
Thiotepa	500	GI, cardiac	0.59	[227]
Carboplatin	800			
Cyclophosphamide	5,625			
BCNU	600	Lung, hepatic, renal	0.57	[228]
Cisplatin	165			

[a]See references.[12,229–231]
[b]See Eder et al.[227] for calculation of regimen MTD.
BCNU, bischloroethylnitrosourea; CNS, central nervous system; GI, gastrointestinal; MTD, maximum tolerated dose; PN, peripheral neuropathy.

Hemorrhagic myocarditis is an infrequent but serious cardiac complication associated with cyclophosphamide in total does of 200 mg/kg or greater. Other reported cardiac complications include nonbacterial thrombotic endocarditis and catheter-associated right-sided endocarditis during marrow infusion and after chemotherapy.[235]

The highly lipid-soluble alkylators, especially busulfan, the nitrosoureas, and thiotepa, cause CNS dysfunction, including seizures, altered mental status, cerebellar dysfunction, cranial nerve palsies, and coma.[236] High-dose ifosfamide produces neurotoxicity at least in part due to a metabolite chloroacetaldehyde (Fig. 12.11).[237] Patients with hypoalbuminemia, renal insufficiency, and those treated with higher doses of ifosfamide are at increased risk for neurotoxicity.[238] Concomitant use of aggressive intravenous fluids appears to increase the renal excretion of CNS-toxic metabolites and reduce the risk of CNS injury.

Methylating Agents

Classic alkylating agents, such as the prototype nitrogen-mustard compounds, typically contain a chloroethyl group, and their biologic activity results from polyfunctional alkylation of biologic macromolecules (see earlier in the chapter). Compounds with diverse chemical structures are also capable of covalent binding to biologic macromolecules and have important clinical activity.

These compounds, referred to here as the *nonclassic alkylating agents*, include procarbazine (PCB), dacarbazine (DTIC), and temozolomide (TMZ).

Although these agents lack bifunctionality, they share a common structural feature, an *N*-methyl group, which mediates their activity.[239] These agents are essentially prodrugs, which undergo metabolic transformation to active intermediates, and become potent methyl donors, most importantly to specific sites in DNA. They are effective in unique settings and regimens, and indeed, DTIC is part of curative regimens for lymphomas. Additionally, TMZ is the primary agent for treating glioblastoma multiforme.

Procarbazine

PCB was synthesized as part of an effort to develop new monoamine oxidase inhibitors at the Hoffman-La Roche Laboratories[239,240] and had antitumor activity in preclinical testing.[240] Early clinical trials demonstrated significant efficacy against Hodgkin's disease, for which it remains a component of some multidrug regimens for Hodgkin's lymphoma and NHLs.[241,242] It is also a part of multidrug regimens for high-grade glioma[243] but has been largely replaced by TMZ.

Mechanism of Action and Cellular Pharmacology

The most compelling evidence to date suggests that the cytotoxicity of PCB is mediated by its role as a methylating agent (Fig. 12.15).

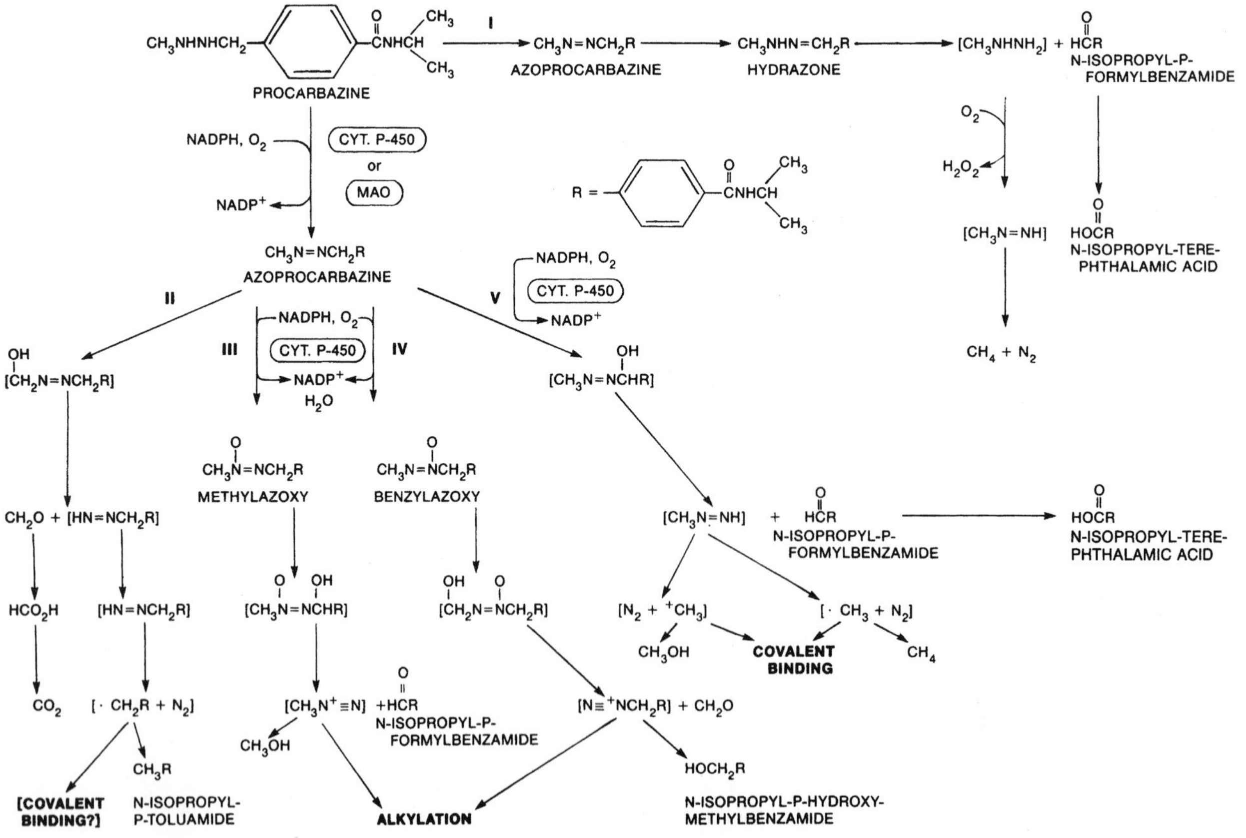

FIGURE **12.15** Chemical and metabolic reactions of procarbazine, leading to the generation of reactive intermediates. I, Chemical breakdown of procarbazine in aqueous solution; II, III, IV, and V, proposed metabolic activation pathways in vivo. Intermediates not identified in vivo or in vitro are indicated by brackets. See text for detailed description. CYT, cytochrome; MAO, monoamine oxidase; NADP, nicotinamide adenine dinucleotide; NADPH, nicotinamide adenine dinucleotide phosphate.

Adult Fisher rats treated with carbon radiolabeled PCB displayed O^6-[^{14}C]methylguanine, a known mutagenic and carcinogenic adduct[244-246] that is also thought to contribute to cytotoxicity,[247] as well as lesser amounts of 7-[^{14}C]methylguanine. Further evidence for alkylation as its primary mechanism came from the observation that PCB given to athymic nude mice bearing human malignant gliomas and medulloblastoma xenografts resulted in greater growth delays in tumors lacking O^6-alkylguanine-DNA alkyl transferase (AGT),[248] the enzyme mediating repair of O^6-methylguanine.

Mechanisms of Resistance

Resistance develops rapidly in tumor cells after exposure to PCB. The inverse correlation between CNS xenograft response to PCB and AGT activity, and the finding that O^6-methylguanine was found in significantly higher levels in two sensitive lines with low-AGT levels as compared with O^6-methylguanine levels in a resistant line with a high-AGT content, suggests that resistance to this methylating agent is secondary to AGT-mediated repair of O^6-methylguanine, similar to nitrosourea resistance mediated by this enzyme.[249] As noted below, loss of MMR can also mediate potent resistance to this class of agents.

Drug Interactions

PCB undergoes extensive hepatic microsomal metabolism as part of its activation pathway. A variety of potentially toxic metabolites are generated by microsomal metabolism, as shown in Figure 12.16, but have not been extensively studied in human subjects, and their contribution to cytotoxicity is largely inferred by the DNA adducts generated. A second pathway of importance is inhibition monoamine oxidase, which is widespread in tissues and plasma, and responsible for drug-drug and drug-food interactions. The activity of other drugs that are substrates for microsomal metabolism may be enhanced in the presence of PCB, as shown by a prolonged pentobarbital-induced sleep time in animals.[250,251] Therefore, patients taking hypnotics or sedative metabolized by CYP enzymes may experience potentiated effects of this drug interaction. Conversely, cimetidine, antifungal imidazoles, and antibiotics that affect microsomal metabolism may increase or decrease PCB metabolism and thereby alter PCB activity and toxicity (Fig 12.16).

Pretreatment of rats with phenobarbital before PCB administration resulted in increased PCB clearance and a slight decrease in concentrations of the azometabolite. In as much as phenobarbital or phenytoin pretreatment increased the survival of tumor-bearing mice treated with PCB, it may be presumed that microsomal enzyme induction resulted in increased production of active PCB metabolites.[252] It is not known whether this drug interaction may be useful clinically to achieve therapeutic advantage through biochemical modulation of PCB activity.

Monoamine oxidase inhibition[253] and pyridoxal phosphate depletion[254] by PCB cause CNS depression. This also may potentiate the sedative effects of other CNS depressants. This inhibition of monoamine oxidase also predisposes patients to acute hypertensive reactions after concomitant therapy with tricyclic antidepressants and sympathomimetic drugs, as well as after ingestion of tyramine-rich foods, such as red wine, bananas, ripe cheese, and yogurt. Finally, a disulfiram-like reaction manifested by sweating, facial flushing, and headache may occur in patients who ingest alcohol while taking PCB (Table 12.3).

Toxicity

PCB, which is administered orally, causes anorexia and mild nausea and vomiting, which is probably of central origin and often abates with continued use.[255] In some patients, it is often helpful to escalate the dosage in a stepwise fashion over the first several days of drug administration to minimize these gastrointestinal side effects. Mild-to-moderate reversible leukopenia and thrombocytopenia are the most common dose-limiting toxicity of PCB. Depression of peripheral leukocyte and platelet counts becomes apparent after 1 week of therapy and may persist for 2 weeks or longer after discontinuation of the drug. PCB also may cause hemolysis in patients with glucose-6-phosphate dehydrogenase deficiency.[256] PCB generally does not cause mucosal injury.

Patients receiving PCB orally may occasionally experience neurotoxicity manifest by drowsiness, depression, agitation, and paresthesias of the extremities.[257] These effects are probably a result of central monoamine oxidase inhibition or may be related to drug-induced depletion of pyridoxal phosphate.[253,258,259]

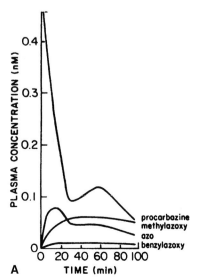

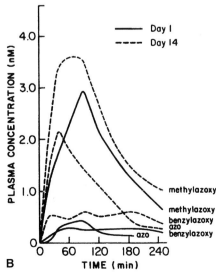

FIGURE **12.16** **A.** Procarbazine (PCB) disappearance and azo and azoxy metabolite kinetics in rat plasma after administration of PCB, 150 mg/kg, intraperitoneally. **B.** Plasma concentrations of azo and azoxyprocarbasine metabolites in a patient after the administration of PCB, 250 mg/kg/d, orally, on days 1 and 14 of a 14-day treatment schedule. (Reprinted from Shiba DA, Weinkam RJ. Quantitative analysis of procarbazine, procarbazine metabolites and chemical degradation products with application to pharmacokinetic studies. *J Chromatogr.* 1982;229(2):397-407. Copyright © 1982 Elsevier. With permission.)

TABLE

12.3 *Key features of procarbazine*

Factor	Result
Mechanism of action	Metabolic activation required: methylation of nucleic acids; inhibition of DNA, RNA, and protein synthesis
Metabolism	Converted to azo-PCB by erythrocyte and liver microsomes
	Subsequent metabolism to *N*-isopropyl-*p*-formylbenzamide, *N*-isopropyl-*p*-hydroxymethyl benzamide, *N*-isopropyl-*p*-toluamide, *N*-isopropyl-*N*-isopropylterephthalamic acid (inactive), methane, and carbon dioxide
	Possible formation of methyldiazene free radical "active intermediate"
Pharmacokinetics	Half-life = 7 min
	Approximately 100% bioavailability from oral route, peak plasma concentration reached within 60 min
	Equilibration between plasma and cerebrospinal fluid in 15 to 30 min
Elimination	Renal elimination of ≥75% in 24 h
Drug and food interactions	PCB may inhibit hepatic microsomal drug metabolism and therefore potentiate activity of barbiturates, antihistamines, narcotics, and phenothiazines
	Alcohol use may cause "disulfiram-like" reaction
	Sympathomimetics, tricyclic antidepressants, or tyramine-rich foods may cause severe hypertension from PCB inhibition of monoamine oxidase
Toxicity	Myelosuppression
	Gastrointestinal (nausea and vomiting); rare, hepatic dysfunction
	Neurotoxicity (drowsiness, depression, agitation, paresthesias)
	Cutaneous or pulmonary hypersensitivity (rare)
	Azoospermia; anovulation
	Carcinogenesis (associated with secondary malignancy in treated patients)
	Teratogenesis
Precautions	Dose modification may be necessary in hepatic and/or renal dysfunction
	Avoid alcohol
	Avoid tyramine-rich foods, sympathomimetics, tricyclic antidepressants, hypnotics, antihistamines, narcotics, phenothiazines

When PCB is administered intravenously, neurotoxic effects become more pronounced and are dose limiting. After a single high-dose intravenous bolus (2 g/m²) or a 5-day continuous infusion of PCB, patients experienced severe nausea and vomiting, confusion, and even coma lasting several days.[258,259] Myelosuppression does not occur when PCB is administered in this way. However, there is also a parallel lack of clinical antitumor effect, which emphasizes the importance of first-pass hepatic metabolism for activation of PCB to antiproliferative intermediates. The pattern of toxicity after small, intermittent intravenous doses is more like that seen after oral administration,[239,245] although it is unlikely that this schedule offers any clinical benefit over that of conventional oral dosing.

PCB also may cause hypersensitivity reactions, including maculopapular skin rash, eosinophilia, pulmonary infiltrates, or, rarely, transient hepatic dysfunction.[260–262] The skin rash usually responds to concomitant glucocorticosteroid treatment, and the PCB may be continued without further sequelae. In contrast, PCB-induced interstitial pneumonitis usually necessitates drug discontinuation.

PCB has potent immunosuppressive properties including lymphopenia.[263] These immunosuppressive properties have led to trials for treatment of lupus erythematosus and suppression of GVHD after bone marrow transplantation, although neither use is common, particularly in light of its leukemogenic potential. The successful use of PCB in curative regimens has directed increasing

attention and concern to the chronic and late toxicities of this agent. PCB causes profound azoospermic[264] and has teratogenic,[247] mutagenic,[265] and carcinogenic[266] properties in experimental animals, and some of these effects are associated with PCB use in humans.

PCB is highly toxic to reproductive organs, causing azoospermia and anovulation.[267,268] More than 90% of men receiving PCB in combination with classic alkylating agents, such as in MOPP combination chemotherapy for Hodgkin's disease, have irreversible azoospermia. Approximately 50% of women thus treated have permanent drug-induced ovarian failure. In pregnant animals, administration of PCB causes congenital skeletal and CNS abnormalities.[247,265–269] Although evidence for direct causation of lethal and nonlethal mutations in human fetuses is lacking, women of childbearing potential should be advised against pregnancy during chemotherapy. In women treated with MOPP chemotherapy and who regain normal ovarian function, there seems to be no impairment of fertility nor any increased birth defects in offspring.[268,270]

PCB is highly leukemogenic.[266] The increased incidence of secondary leukemias and solid malignancies in patients after treatment with MOPP, combination chemotherapy exacerbated by the use of radiation therapy, pointed to PCB as the responsible carcinogen.[271] Because this regimen also contains an alkylating agent with carcinogenic properties, it is difficult to implicate PCB alone.[271] Indeed, studies in experimental systems suggest that additive or interactive effects of classic alkylating agents with PCB may account for the observed mutagenesis.[272]

The mechanisms of PCB gonadal toxicity and somatic genotoxicity are mostly the result of DNA alkylation of and cytotoxicity to proliferative tissues, although some authors have invoked separate pathways for anticancer and antigonadal effects (78,79).

Dacarbazine

History

DTIC was chemically synthesized as a purine antagonist. As reviewed by Montgomery,[273] a compounds designed as analogs of aminoimidazole carboxamide (AIC), an intermediate in purine ring synthesis, were synthesized in the late 1950s and had significant antitumor activity in experimental testing. The addition of nitrous acid to form a 5-diazoimidazole derivative seemed to responsible for this antitumor activity, and the further addition of a third nitrogen group to form the 5-triazene resulted in a light-sensitive compound that spontaneously converted back to the diazo analog. Dimethyl substitution of the triazine resulted in a more stable but still light-sensitive derivative, DTIC, which was highly active and was developed for clinical use.[274] Subsequent research revealed the alkylating potential of this compound.

DTIC is an modestly active single agent in the treatment of metastatic malignant melanoma,[275] but its primary value is found in the combination therapy of Hodgkin's disease.[276] It is most commonly used as part of the doxorubicin, bleomycin, vinblastine, and DTIC (ABVD) and actinomycin D, bleomycin, and vincristine (ABV) regimens for Hodgkin's disease.[277] In addition, DTIC has modest activity in the treatment of sarcomas,[278] neuroblastoma,[279] and primary and neuroendocrine brain tumors. The key features of DTIC are summarized in Table 12.4.

Mechanism of Action and Cellular Pharmacology

There is convincing evidence that, similar to PCB, the production of O^6-methylguanine is the primary cytotoxic event after administration of DTIC.[280] Xenografts, or cell lines with negligible levels of AGT, are more sensitive to DTIC than are xenografts or cell lines with high levels of AGT.[281,282] Furthermore, DTIC depletes AGT levels in human colon cancer HT 29 xenografts in athymic mice[283] and in human peripheral blood cells in patients treated for metastatic melanoma.[284] The active methylating metabolite is produced by first a cytochrome P-450 oxidation of the side chain 3-methyl group, followed by rearrangement of thee triazene side chain to yield a highly reaction N=NCH$_3$ moiety, as shown in Figure 12.16, and yielding 5-aminoimidazole-4-carboxamide, the major metabolite found is plasma within minutes of drug administration.

Preclinical and clinical studies suggest that elevated levels of AGT may be responsible for resistance to this agent.[282,285] Furthermore, resistance to all methylators, including DTIC, is seen in the setting of a deficiency of DNA mismatch repair.[286]

Drug Interactions

At present, there are no known drug or food interactions with DTIC that are of clinical importance. Although the initial step for metabolic activation of DTIC is catalyzed by microsomal metabolism, the interaction of phenobarbital, or other commonly used cytochrome P-450–inducing agents, with DTIC has not been reported.

DTIC activity against L1210 murine leukemia is potentiated by alkylating agents, such as melphalan, and by doxorubicin.[273] Activity is also enhanced when DTIC is combined with the nitrosoureas

TABLE 12.4	Key features of dacarbazine [5-(3,3-dimethyl-1-triazeno) imidazole-4-carboxamide, DTIC, DIC, NSC-45388]
Factor	**Result**
Mechanism of action	Metabolic activation probably required; methylation of nucleic acids; direct DNA damage; inhibition of purine synthesis
Metabolism	Oxidative *N*-methylation to 5-aminoimidazole-4-carboxamide via formation of 5(3-hydroxymethyl-3-methyltriazen-1-yl) imidazole-4-carboxamide and 5-(3-methyltriazen-2-yl) imidazole-4-carboxamide
	$t_{1/2}\alpha = 3$ min; $t_{1/2}\beta = 41$ min
	$V_d = 0.6$ L/kg; Cl = 15 mL/kg/min
	20% protein bound
	Variable oral absorption
	Poor CSF penetration (plasma/CSF ratio = 7:1 at equilibrium)
Elimination	Renal excretion: 50% as unchanged dacarbazine and 9% to 18% as 5-aminoimidazole-4-carboxamide
	Minor hepatobiliary and pulmonary excretion
Toxicity	Myelosuppression
	Gastrointestinal (nausea and vomiting)
	Influenza-like syndrome (fever, myalgia, and malaise)
	Infrequent alopecia, cutaneous hypersensitivity, or photosensitivity
	Rare hepatic vein thrombosis and hepatic necrosis
	Possible carcinogenesis and teratogenesis
Precautions	Dose modification may be necessary in hepatic and/or renal dysfunction

Cl, clearance; CSF, cerebrospinal fluid; $t_{1/2}$, half-life; V_d, apparent volume of distribution.

bischloromethyl-nitrosourea (BCNU) and chloroethylcyclo-hexylnitrosourea (CCNU). The mechanism(s) for the potentiation observed using these combinations may be related to the ability of nitrosoureas to deplete AGT and thereby sensitize cells to methylating agents.

Clinical Pharmacology

DTIC is supplied in sterile vials containing 100 or 200 mg DTIC for intravenous administration. As a single agent of the usual dose is 250 mg/m² daily for 5 days every 3 to 4 weeks.[287] The latter schedule was developed in an attempt to minimize the gastrointestinal toxicity from DTIC, which tends to lessen with repeated administration of small doses. HPLC and mass spectroscopy have been used to study triazine pharmacology, but our understanding of DTIC pharmacology in humans is incomplete. After oral administration, the drug is absorbed slowly and variably; therefore, intravenous administration is the preferred route. Intravenous boluses of 2.65 to 6.85 mg/kg (approximately 120 to 300 mg/m²) produced peak plasma concentrations of 10 to 30 µg/mL. After intravenous administration, a biphasic plasma disappearance is found, consistent with a two-compartment model with an initial half-life of 3 minutes and a terminal half-life of 41 minutes. Approximately 20% of DTIC is loosely bound to plasma protein.[288] In humans, the mean volume of distribution for DTIC was 0.6 L/kg, and the total body clearance was 15.4 mL/kg/min. In one study, approximately 50% of an intravenous dose of DTIC was recovered in the urine as parent drug, and the renal clearance was calculated to be between 5 and 10 mL/kg/min, exceeding the glomerular filtration rate, and suggesting that tubular secretion may be involved in the renal excretion of DTIC. Altered schedules of intravenous drug administration did not change the AUC (concentration × time), confirming a lack of schedule dependence for DTIC pharmacokinetics.[289]

DTIC penetrates poorly into the CSF. At equilibrium, the ratio between plasma and spinal fluid was 7:1.[288] However, DTIC has activity against transplantable murine ependymoblastoma, and there are reports of activity against primary and metastatic brain tumors in humans.[275]

The major metabolite of DTIC found in plasma and urine is AIC (Fig. 12.16) with cumulative excretion in the urine accounting for 9% to 20% of parent compound.[288,289] AIC is also formed in vitro from DTIC in the presence of liver microsomes and by some tumor cells. After the intraperitoneal administration of [^{14}CO-methyl] DTIC to rats or mice, 4% of the dose is recovered as respiratory $^{14}CO_2$ in 6 hours, and 9% of the dose is recovered as $^{14}CO_2$ in 24 hours. Presumably, the expired radiolabeled $^{14}CO_2$ is derived from the formaldehyde produced after N-demethylation of DTIC. These findings, as well as the identification of 5-(3-hydroxymethyl-3-methyltriazen-1-yl) imidazole-4-carboxamide (HMTIC) as a urinary metabolite of DTIC in rats, are consistent with a metabolic pathway for DTIC, as shown in Figure 12.16, in which MTIC is the primary active metabolite, responsible for transferring its methyl group to DNA.

Toxicity

The most frequent toxic reaction to DTIC treatment is moderately severe nausea and vomiting, and this occurs in 90% of patients.[290] These symptoms may persist for up to 12 hours after infusion.

The severity of gastrointestinal toxicity decreases with successive doses when the drug is given on a 5-day schedule. Above 1,200 mg/m² as a rapid intravenous bolus, DTIC frequently causes severe, but short-lived, watery diarrhea. After rapid infusion of a high dose (>1,380 mg/m²) of DTIC, hypotension may occur.

Myelosuppression is a common dose-related toxicity of DTIC, although the degree of leukopenia and thrombocytopenia is variably mild to moderate. Significant myelosuppression occurs when more than 1,380 mg/m² is given as a single intravenous bolus or above a total of 1,000 mg/m² on the 5-day schedule.[290] Usually, there is sufficient recovery so that DTIC may be administered every 21 to 28 days on the 5-day schedule.

Less frequent toxic reactions include a flu-like syndrome with fever up to 39°C, myalgias, and malaise lasting several days after DTIC treatment. Headache, facial flushing, facial paresthesias, pain along the injection vein, alopecia, and abnormal hepatic and renal function tests are less common. Photosensitivity to DTIC has been reported in several patients, especially after high-dose therapy.[291] Therefore, patients should be advised to avoid sunlight exposure for several days after DTIC therapy. Hepatic vein occlusion associated with fever, eosinophilia, and hepatic necrosis and resulting in death have been attributed to DTIC as a distinct clinical pathologic syndrome.[292] The mechanism for this toxicity is unknown.

DTIC markedly depresses antibody responses and allograft rejection in mice for up to 60 days after a single injection. Drug-resistant lymphomas in mice were found to be highly immunogenic, perhaps as a result of mutations in the MMR system and mutations arising from the O^6-methylguanine:T mispairing (see below), such that large inoculum of the DTIC-resistant tumors were rejected by immunocompetent animals. Consistent with its alkylating potential, DTIC has mutagenic, carcinogenic, and teratogenic properties in experimental systems.[293] In rodents, DTIC causes lymphoma and tumors of the thymus, lung, uterus, or mammary glands when given orally or by single or multiple injections.[294] The monomethyl triazeno derivative also caused similar tumors but in a lower frequency compared with DTIC.[295] It is not firmly established whether DTIC is carcinogenic for humans. In a retrospective analysis of patients receiving either MOPP or ABVD (plus or minus radiation therapy) for Hodgkin's disease, Valagussa et al.[296] reported no treatment-associated secondary malignancies in patients receiving ABVD. Subsequently, isolated cases of acute leukemia occurring after DTIC therapy have been reported,[297] but these remain rare. Finally, DTIC causes dose-dependent fetal malformations and fetal resorptions when administered to pregnant rats and rabbits.[298] Teratogenic effects were observed in the urogenital system, skeleton, eye, and cardiovascular system.

Temozolomide

History

Several series of 1,2,4-triazines and 1,2,4-triazinones were synthesized in England in the 1960s and 1970s, and selected compounds proved to have activity against murine tumors.[299] Selection of the next generation of imidazotetrazinones focused on TMZ (Figs. 12.17 and 12.18). This compound, with a different spectrum of activity against murine tumors,[300] was less active and considerably

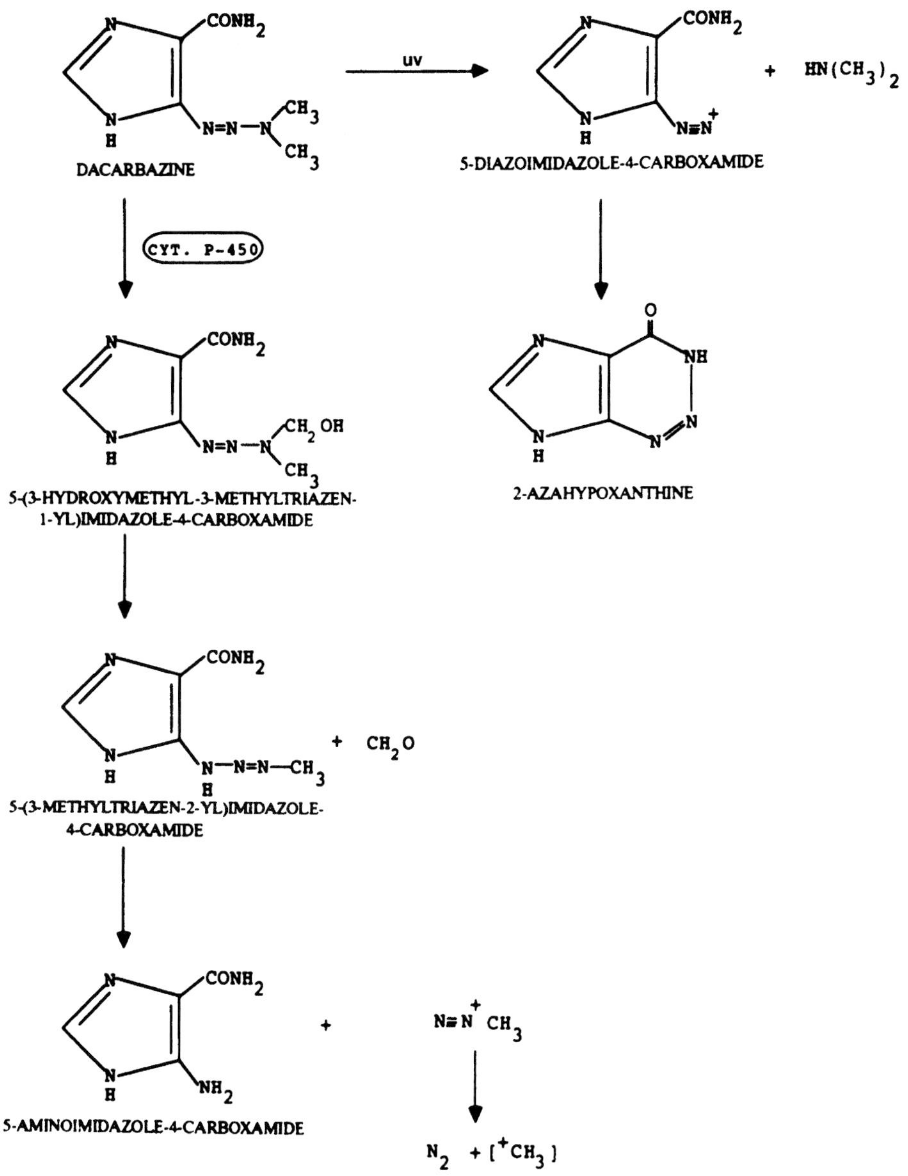

FIGURE **12.17** Light-activated and metabolic reactions of dacarbazine, leading to the generation of reactive intermediates. CYT, cytochrome; UV, ultraviolet.

less toxic than the parent mitozolomide and displayed remarkable capacity to penetrate all body tissues, including the brain[301]; TMZ had the favorable property of spontaneously undergoing ring opening in aqueous solution with resulting generation of the monomethyl triazine MTIC, the same metabolite formed by metabolic

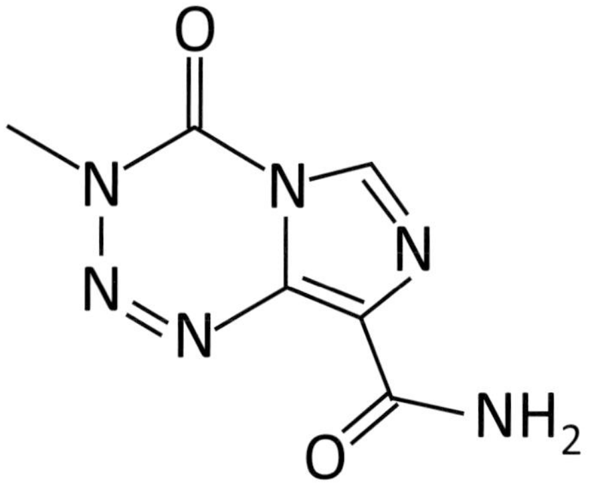

FIGURE **12.18** Structure of temozolomide.

dealkylation of DTIC.[302] The inefficient demethylation of DTIC in humans (despite rapid demethylation in mice) coupled with the nonenzymatic conversion of TMZ to MTIC suggested a potential benefit for the use of TMZ. Table 12.4 lists the key features of TMZ.

Phase I trials of oral TMZ on a single-dose schedule demonstrated the dose-limiting toxicity to be myelosuppression with trivial clinical benefits.[303] However, based on preclinical data supporting a multiple-dose regimen, another phase I trial using a 5-day schedule was conducted, with myelosuppression again the dose-limiting toxicity. Greater clinical activity was noted: four responses (two partial and two complete) in 23 patients with metastatic melanoma and two partial responses in four patients with high-grade glioma.[303] The promising results in gliomas were confirmed in subsequent trials,[304] and TMZ is now established as the primary agent, with radiation therapy, for treatment of high-grade gliomas, with superior activity to PCB,[305] and notable single-agent activity either prior to or concurrent with radiotherapy.[75,306,307] Furthermore, TMZ has been shown to be active in the treatment of other primary brain tumors, including low-grade glioma,[308] oligodendroglioma,[309,310] and meningioma.[310]

General Mechanism of Action and Cellular Pharmacology

The spontaneous conversion of TMZ is initiated by the effect of water at the highly electropositive C^4 position of TMZ. This activity opens the ring, releases CO_2, and generates the reactive methylating agent MTIC. The initial proposal was that this effect of water was catalyzed in the close environment of the major groove of DNA,[311] but confirming this mechanism has been difficult, and it is known that TMZ converts readily to MTIC in free solution in the absence of DNA.[312] MTIC degrades to the methyldiazonium cation, $N=NCH_3$, which transfers the methyl group to DNA and to the final degradation product AIC, which is excreted via the kidneys.[313] The methylation of DNA appears to be the principal mechanism responsible for the cytotoxicity of TMZ to malignant cells (see following discussion). The methyldiazonium cation can also react with RNA and with soluble and cellular proteins.[314] However, the methylation of RNA and the methylation or carbamoylation of protein do not appear to have any known significant role in the antitumor activity of TMZ.[314] Further studies are required to clarify the role of these targets in the biochemical mechanism of action of TMZ.

The spontaneous conversion of TMZ and MTIC depends on pH. Under acidic conditions, TMZ is stable; however, its chemical stability decreases at a pH of greater than 7.0 and is converted rapidly to MTIC in that environment.[313] In contrast, MTIC is more stable under basic conditions and rapidly degrades to the methyldiazonium cation and AIC at a pH of less than 7.0.[313] A comparison of the half-life of TMZ in phosphate buffer (pH, 7.4; $t_{1/2} = 1.83$ hours)[313] indicates that the conversion of TMZ to MTIC is a chemically controlled reaction with little or no enzymatic component. The spontaneous conversion of TMZ may contribute to its highly reproducible pharmacokinetics in comparison with other alkylating agents such as DTIC and PCB, which must undergo metabolic conversion in the liver and are thus subject to interpatient variation in metabolic rates of conversion.

Among the lesions produced in DNA after treatment of cells with TMZ, the most common is methylation at the N^7-position of guanine, followed by methylation at the O^3 position of adenine (3%) and the O^6-position of guanine (7%).[313] Although the N^7-methylguanine and O^3-methyladenine adducts probably contribute to the antitumor activity of TMZ in some, if not all, sensitive cells, their role is modest.[87] The critical role of the O^6-methylguanine adduct, which accounts for 5% of the total adducts formed by TMZ,[313] in the agent's antitumor activity is supported by the correlation between the sensitivity of tumor cell lines to TMZ and the activity of the DNA repair protein AGT, which specifically removes alkyl groups at the O^6-position of guanine. Cell lines that have low levels of AGT are sensitive to the cytotoxicity of TMZ, whereas cell lines that have high levels of this repair protein are much more resistant to it.[315] This correlation also has been observed in human glioblastoma xenograft models.[316] The preferential alkylation of guanine and adenine and the correlation of sensitivity to the drug with the ability to repair the O^6-alkylguanine lesion are also features of the pharmacology of DTIC and the nitrosourea alkylating agents BCNU and CCNU.[317,318]

The cytotoxic mechanism of TMZ appears to be related to the failure of the DNA mismatch repair system to find a complementary base for methylated guanine. This system involves the formation of a complex of proteins that recognize the O^6-methylguanine: thymidine mismatch, which is preferentially incorporated by DNA polymerases and repeatedly recognized by the MMR complex. In a process termed aberrant repair, the repair process is targeted to the DNA strand opposite the O^6-methylguanine, removes the T, only to have the polymerase reinsert a T, resulting in long-lived nicks in the DNA.[319] These nicks are converted into DSBs during DNA replication, blocking the cell cycle at the G_2M boundary.[320] In murine (and human) leukemia cells, sensitivity to TMZ correlates with increased fragmentation of DNA and apoptotic cell death. More recent work has shown that TMZ induces G_2-M arrest through activation of Chk1 kinase with subsequent phosphorylation of cdc 25 phosphatase and cdc2.[321] This has been shown to be p53 independent, although p53 also has impacts on G_2-M arrest duration and outcome. Specifically, p53 wild-type cells undergo prolonged G_2-M arrest and senescence, whereas p53-deficient cells bypass cell cycle arrest and die by mitotic catastrophe. Additionally, O^6-methylguanine–induced apoptosis is executed by the mitochondrial damage pathway, requires DNA replication, and is mediated by p53 and Fas/CD95/Apo-1.[322]

DNA adducts formed by TMZ and the subsequent DNA damage or alteration of specific genes may cause cell death or reduce the metastatic potential of tumor cells. For example, mutations caused by adduct formation may result in altered surface antigens on tumor cells that contribute enhanced immunogenicity in the host.[323] The effects of enhanced immunologic response range from complete tumor rejection to reduced growth rates and reduced metastatic potential.[324] Additional evidence suggests that TMZ can reduce the metastatic potential of Lewis lung carcinoma cells[325] and induce differentiation in the K562 erythroleukemia cell line.[326] It has been postulated that TMZ-induced DNA damage and subsequent cell cycle arrest may reduce the metastatic properties of some tumor cells.[326]

Mechanism of Resistance

AGT DNA Repair Protein

AGT repair of guanine alkylation is the primary mechanism of resistance to TMZ and other methylating agents.[327] AGT functions as the first line of defense against TMZ by removing the alkyl groups from the O^6-position of guanine, in effect reversing the cytotoxic lesion of TMZ. AGT levels can be correlated with the sensitivity of tumor cell lines to TMZ and the alkylating agents BCNU and DTIC.[317,328,329] The role of AGT in resistance to TMZ is also evidenced by the ability of the virally transfected human AGT gene to confer a high level of resistance to TMZ and other methylating and chloroethylating agents on cells that are devoid of endogenous AGT activity and sensitive to alkylation.[330]

AGT levels in human tumor tissues and normal tissue specimens derived from the brain, lung, and ovary vary widely over a 100-fold range, with some human tumors having no detectable activity.[331,332] While constitutively expressed, MGMT promoter methylation is responsible for gene silencing in tumors, leading to loss of expression. Some specimens from all tumor types examined in these studies have demonstrated a complete absence of AGT activity: as many as 22% of primary brain tumor specimens have no detectable AGT activity.[331] Similar findings with respect to AGT levels in brain tumor cells have been observed in in vitro models.[333] AGT activity has been localized to both the cytoplasm and the nucleus of the cell, although the function of cytoplasmic AGT and its mechanism of transport to the nucleus are unknown. AGT transfers the methyl group to an internal cysteine residue, acting as methyltransferase and methyl acceptor protein. In the process, AGT becomes irreversibly inactivated, and new AGT must be synthesized to restore AGT activity.[249] Therefore, the number of O^6-methylguanine adducts that can be repaired is limited by the number of AGT molecules of the protein available. Elevated AGT levels (measured by immunohistochemistry or implied by methylation of the promoter of the gene) in newly diagnosed glioblastoma multiforme directly correlated with lack of response to TMZ[305] or survival.[74]

Deficiency in Mismatch Repair Pathway

Although AGT is clearly important in the resistance of cells to TMZ, some cell lines that express low levels of AGT are nevertheless resistant, indicating that other resistance mechanisms may be involved.[334,335] A deficiency in the MMR pathway as a result of mutations in any one of the proteins that recognize and repair DNA (i.e., including GTBP, hMSH2, hPMS2, hMLH1, and MSH6) can render cells tolerant to methylation and the cytotoxic effects of TMZ. This deficiency in the MMR pathway results in a failure to recognize and repair the O^6-methylguanine adducts produced by TMZ and other methylating agents.[83,286,315] The DNA damage that results from failure to repair the O^6-methylguanine adducts produces a particular type of genomic instability, microsatellite instability, that is associated with some familial and sporadic cancers, such as hereditary nonpolyposis colorectal cancer,[336] and in colon cancers, sensitivity to immune checkpoint inhibitors. The high level of TMZ resistance in tumor cells that are deficient in MMR is unrelated to the level of AGT and is, therefore, unaffected by AGT inhibitors. Recent studies suggest that while MSH6 mutations do not occur commonly in newly diagnosed glioblastoma, they are seen in approximately 26% of glioblastoma that have recurred after treatment with alkylating agents, notably temozolomide.[80,337,338] A methylator-resistant human glioblastoma multiforme xenograft, D-245 MG (PR), in athymic nude mice by serially treating the parent xenograft, D-245 MG, with PCBD-245 MG xenografts expressed the human mismatch repair proteins hMSH2 and hMLH1, whereas the resistant xenografts, D-245 MG (PR), expressed hMLH1 but not hMSH2, thus defects in MMR, as found in TMZ-resistant human gliomas, also confer resistance to PCB.[286,339,340]

Base Excision Repair and Temozolomide Resistance

O^6-methylguanine adducts are sensitive to AGT repair, while TMZ-initiated adducts, N^7-methylguanine and N^3-methyladenine, are not susceptible to AGT and produce cytotoxicity (particularly N^3-methyladenine), independently of DNA mismatch repair activity.[87,335,341,342] These lesions are promptly repaired by a series of enzymatic steps including N-methylpurine-DNA glycosylase, AP endonuclease, poly (ADP-ribose) polymerase (PARP) DNA polymerase β, x-ray repair cross complementing 1, and ligase III. Tumor cells resistant to TMZ because of DNA mismatch repair deficiency have been rendered susceptible to this methylator by inhibition of BER. Strategies have included inhibition of PARP[343–345] and use of methoxyamine.[346] Intriguingly, moderate enhancement of TMZ activity following BER disruption was also

seen in DNA mismatch repair–proficient cells.[87,335,341,342] While interruption of BER can sensitize cells to temozolomide, it does not appear that BER mediates TMZ resistance. Early phase clinical trials with methoxyamine[347] and PARP inhibitors combined with TMZ are in progress.

Drug Interactions

There are no known adverse reactions with other drugs. However, compounds that deplete AGT such as O^6-benzylguanine,[318] will increase TMZ toxicity.

Clinical Pharmacology and Toxicity

TMZ is supplied in capsules containing 5, 25, 100, or 250 mg for oral use, although an intravenous formulation has recently been approved for commercial use. In the initial phase I trial in the United Kingdom, TMZ was administered as a single intravenous dose at doses of 50 to 200 mg/m² and subsequently was given orally to fasted patients as a single dose, up to a total dose of 200 to 1,000 mg/m². Additionally, oral doses of 750 to 1,000 mg/m² were divided into five equal doses and administered daily for 5 days at 4-week intervals.

The pharmacokinetics of TMZ were evaluated in the United Kingdom phase I trials.[303] After intravenous administration, plasma TMZ concentrations declined biexponentially consistent with a two-compartment open model and a terminal elimination half-life of 1.8 hours. After oral administration, plasma TMZ concentrations were consistent with a one-compartment oral model, with rapid absorption and maximum plasma concentrations occurring 0.7 hour after treatment. The clearance of TMZ was 11.8 L/h, and the pharmacokinetics were independent of the dosage (with a linear relationship between dose and area under the time × concentration curve). Oral bioavailability was considered to be complete.

In 1993, Schering-Plough began the worldwide development of TMZ. Data from these studies confirmed the safety, tolerability, and pharmacokinetics of TMZ reported in the CRC phase I study (Table 12.5).[348–352] Food has a minor effect on absorption of oral TMZ.

TABLE 12.5 *Key features of temozolomide {8-carbamoyl-3-methylimidazo [5,1-d]-1,2,3,5-tetrazin-4(3H)-one}*

Factor	Result
Mechanism of action	Methylation of nucleic acids
Metabolism	Chemical conversion of 5(3-methyltriazeno) imidazole-4-carboxamide in aqueous solution
Pharmacokinetics (IV or PO)	Volume of distribution: 28.3 L Elimination half-life: 1.8 h Distribution half-life: 0.26 h Clearance: 11.76 L/h[253]
Drug and food interactions	Unknown
Toxicity	Myelosuppression Nausea and vomiting Elevated hepatic transaminases

IV, intravenously; PO, per os.

Phase I studies of TMZ also were expanded to include pediatric cancer patients. A phase I study was conducted to define the multiple-dose pharmacokinetics of TMZ in this population. In this study, 19 patients between 3 and 17 years old were given TMZ over a dosage range of 100 to 240 mg/m^2/d. TMZ was absorbed rapidly, had an AUC that increased in a dosage-related manner, and showed no evidence of accumulation. The plasma half-life, whole-body clearance, and volume of distribution were independent of dosage (Table 12.6).[350] Compared with adult patients treated with 200 mg/m^2/d, children appeared to have a higher AUC (48.7 versus 34.5 mg/h/mL), most likely because children have a larger ratio of body surface area to volume. Despite higher concentrations at dosages equivalent to those used in adult patients, the bone marrow function in pediatric patients appears to allow greater exposure to the drug before dose-limiting bone marrow toxicity develops.[350]

Subsequent phase I trials sponsored by Schering-Plough in adult[348,351–353] and pediatric patients[350] with advanced cancer also have confirmed that hematologic toxicity, specifically lymphopenia, thrombocytopenia, and neutropenia, is dose limiting. Neutropenia or thrombocytopenia appeared 21 to 28 days after the first dose of each cycle and recovered to grade 1 myelosuppression within 7 to 14 days. Grade 4 toxicity occurred at cumulative oral dosages of more than 1,000 mg/m^2 over 5 days, but little other toxicity was seen.[353] Grade 3 or 4 myelosuppression occurred in less than 10% of patients studied but can be prolonged upon repeated or continuous dosing, particularly in brain tumor patients. Few other toxicities are noted even at higher and cumulative doses.

A dosage of 200 mg/m^2 of TMZ given on a 5-day schedule and repeated every 28 days is appropriate for patients who have not received prior chemotherapy or radiation therapy. Patients who are pretreated with chemotherapy receive a lower starting dose of TMZ (i.e., 150 mg/m^2), which can be escalated to 200 mg/m^2 in subsequent courses in the absence of grade 3 or 4 myelosuppression.[353] The effect of prior treatment with chemotherapy, radiation, or both, on the maximum tolerated dose (MTD) of TMZ has been evaluated.[353] Clearance from the plasma was significantly less in patients with prior exposure to nitrosourea,[353] possibly contributing to the decreased tolerance to TMZ in these patients.[353] Other schedules including 21 days out of 28 and 7 days on/7 days off, and fixed doses of 75 mg a day and 200 mg a day for 5 days have also been evaluated, though they have not yet produced convincing changes in activity.[354]

References

1. Goodman LS, Maxwell MW, Dameshek W, et al. Nitrogen mustard therapy: use of methyl-bis(beta-chloroethyl)amine hydrochloride and tris(beta-chloroethyl)amine hydrochloride for Hodgkin's disease, lymphosarcoma, leukemia and certain allied and miscellaneous disorders. *J Am Med Assoc.* 1946;132:26-132.
2. Jacobson LO, Spurr CL, Barron ESG, et al. Nitrogen mustard therapy: studies on the effect of methyl-bis (beta-chloroethyl) amine hydrochloride on neoplastic diseases and allied disorders of the hematopoietic system. *J Am Med Assoc.* 1946;132:263-271.
3. Goodman LS, Wintrobe MM, Dameschek W, et al. Use of methyl-bis (beta-chloroethyl) amine hydrochloride for Hodgkin's disease, lymphosarcoma, leukemia. *JAMA.* 1946;132:126.
4. Harris AL. DNA repair and resistance to chemotherapy. *Cancer Surv.* 1985;4:601-624.
5. Russo JE, Hilton J, Colvin OM. The role of aldehyde dehydrogenase isoenzymes in cellular resistance to the alkylating agent cyclophosphamide. In: Weiner, H, Flynn TG, eds. *Enzymology and Molecular Biology of Carbonyl Metabolism.* New York: Alan R. Liss; 1989.
6. Brent, TP, Houghton PJ, Houghton JA. O6-Alkylguanine-DNA alkyltransferase activity correlates with the therapeutic response of human rhabdomyosarcoma xenografts to 1-(2-chloroethyl)-3-(trans-4-methylcyclohexyl)-1-nitrosourea. *Proc Natl Acad Sci U S A.* 1985;82:2985-2989.
7. Colvin M, Brundrett RB, Kan MN. Alkylating properties of phosphoramide mustard. *Cancer Res.* 1976;36:1121-1126.
8. Brundrett RB, Cowens JW, Colvin M. Chemistry of nitrosoureas. Decomposition of deuterated 1,3-bis(2-chloroethyl)-1-nitrosourea. *J Med Chem.* 1976;19:958-961.
9. Ewig RA, Kohn KW. DNA damage and repair in mouse leukemia L1210 cells treated with nitrogen mustard, 1,3-bis(2-chloroethyl)-1-nitrosourea, and other nitrosoureas. *Cancer Res.* 1977;37:2114-2122.
10. Sudhakar S, Tew KD, Schein PS, et al. Nitrosourea interaction with chromatin and effect on poly(adenosine diphosphate ribose) polymerase activity. *Cancer Res.* 1979;39:1411-1417.
11. Bolton MG, Colvin OM, Hilton J. Specificity of isozymes of murine hepatic glutathione S-transferase for the conjugation of glutathione with L-phenylalanine mustard. *Cancer Res.* 1991;51:2410-2415.
12. Jones RB, Matthes SM, Dufton C, et al. Nitrosoureas. In: Grochow LB, Ames MM, eds. *A Clinician's Guide to Chemotherapy Pharmacokinetics and Pharmacodynamics.* Baltimore, MD: Williams & Williams; 1998:331.
13. Friedman OM, Myles A, Colvin M. Cyclophosphamide and certain structurally related phosphoramide mustard. In: *Advances in Cancer Chemotherapy*, vol. 1. New York: Marcel Dekker; 1979.
14. Niederle N, Scheulen ME, Cremer M, et al. Ifosfamide in combination chemotherapy for sarcomas and testicular carcinomas. *Cancer Treat Rev.* 1983;10(suppl A):129-135.
15. Nielsen OS, Judson I, van Hoesel Q, et al. Effect of high-dose ifosfamide in advanced soft tissue sarcomas. A multicentre phase II study of the EORTC Soft Tissue and Bone Sarcoma Group. *Eur J Cancer.* 2000;36:61-67.
16. van Oosterom AT, Mouridsen HT, Nielsen OS, et al. Results of randomised studies of the EORTC Soft Tissue and Bone Sarcoma Group (STBSG) with two different ifosfamide regimens in first- and second-line chemotherapy in advanced soft tissue sarcoma patients. *Eur J Cancer.* 2002;38:2397-2406.
17. Venon MD, Roccaro AM, Gay J, et al. Front line treatment of elderly multiple myeloma in the era of novel agents. *Biologics.* 2009;3:99-109.
18. Galton DAG, Israels LG, Nabarro JDN, et al. Clinical trials of p-(di-2-chloroethylamino)-phenylbutyric acid (CB 1348) in malignant lymphoma. *Br Med J.* 1955;2:1172-1176.
19. Leoni LM, Bailey B, Reifert J, et al. Bendamustine (Treanda) displays a distinct pattern of cytotoxicity and unique mechanistic features compared with other alkylating agents. *Clin Cancer Res.* 2008;14:309-317.
20. Bergmann MA, Goebeler ME, Herold M, et al. Efficacy of bendamustine in patients with relapsed or refractory chronic lymphocytic leukemia: results of a phase I/II study of the German CLL Study Group. *Haematologica.* 2005;90:1357-1364.
21. Knauf WU, Lissichkov T, Aldaoud A, et al. Phase III randomized study of bendamustine compared with chlorambucil in previously untreated patients with chronic lymphocytic leukemia. *J Clin Oncol.* 2009;27:4378-4384.
22. Robinson KS, Williams ME, van der Jagt RH, et al. Phase II multicenter study of bendamustine plus rituximab in patients with relapsed indolent B-cell and mantle cell non-Hodgkin's lymphoma. *J Clin Oncol.* 2008;26:4473-4479.
23. Gordinier ME, Kudelka AP, Kavanagh JJ, et al. Thiotepa in combination with cisplatin for primary epithelial ovarian cancer: a phase II study. *Int J Gynecol Cancer.* 2002;12:710-714.
24. van der Wall E, Beijnen JH, Rodenhuis S. High-dose chemotherapy regimens for solid tumors. *Cancer Treat Rev.* 1995;21:105-132.
25. Santos GW, Tutschka PJ, Brookmeyer R, et al. Marrow transplantation for acute nonlymphocytic leukemia after treatment with busulfan and cyclophosphamide. *N Engl J Med.* 1983;309:1347-1353.

26. Haddow A, Timmis GM. Myleran in chronic myeloid leukaemia; chemical constitution and biological action. *Lancet.* 1953;264:207-208.

27. Roberts JJ, Warwick GP. Metabolic and chemical studies of 'myleran': formation of 3-hydroxytetrahydrothiophene-1,1-dioxide in vivo, and reactions with thiols in vitro. *Nature.* 1959;184:1288-1289.

28. Lawley PD, Brookes P. Methylation of adenine in deoxyadenylic acid or deoxyribonucleic acid at N-7. *Biochem J.* 1964;92:19C-20C.

29. Iwamoto T, Hiraku Y, Oikawa S, et al. DNA intrastrand cross-link at the 5′-GA-3′ sequence formed by busulfan and its role in the cytotoxic effect. *Cancer Sci.* 2004;95:454-458.

30. Wadhwa PD, Fu P, Koc ON, et al. High-dose carmustine, etoposide, and cisplatin for autologous stem cell transplantation with or without involved-field radiation for relapsed/refractory lymphoma: an effective regimen with low morbidity and mortality. *Biol Blood Marrow Transplant.* 2005;11:13-22.

31. Zaucha R, Gooley T, Holmberg L, et al. High-dose chemotherapy with BEAM or Busulphan/Melphalan and Thiotepa followed by hematopoietic cell transplantation in malignant lymphoma. *Leuk Lymphoma.* 2008;49:1899-1906.

32. Fried W, Kedo A, Barone J. Effects of cyclophosphamide and of busulfan on spleen colony-forming units and on hematopoietic stroma. *Cancer Res.* 1977;37:1205-1209.

33. Skinner WA, Gram HF, Greene MO, et al. Potential anticancer agents. XXXI. The relationship of chemical structure to antileukaemic activity with analogues of 1-methyl-3-nitro-1-nitrosoguanidine (NSC-9369). *J Med Pharm Chem.* 1960;2:299-333.

34. Schabel FM Jr, Johnson TP, McCaleb GS, et al. Experimental evaluation of potential anticancer agents VIII. Effects of certain nitrosoureas on intracerebral L1210 leukemia. *Cancer Res.* 1963;23:725-733.

35. Carter SK, Newman JW. Nitrosoureas: 1,3-bis(2-chloroethyl)-1-nitrosourea (NSC-409962; BCNU) and 1-(2-chloroethyl)-3-cyclohexyl-1-nitrosourea (NSC-79037; CCNU)—clinical brochure. *Cancer Chemother Rep 3.* 1968;1:115-151.

36. Penketh PG, Shyam K, Sartorelli AC. Comparison of DNA lesions produced by tumor-inhibitory 1,2-bis(sulfonyl)hydrazines and chloroethylnitrosoureas. *Biochem Pharmacol.* 2000;59:283-291.

37. Ludlum DB, Kramer BS, Wang J, et al. Reaction of 1,3-bis(2-chloroethyl)-1-nitrosourea with synthetic polynucleotides. *Biochemistry.* 1975;14:5480-5485.

38. Panasci LC, Green D, Nagourney R, et al. A structure-activity analysis of chemical and biological parameters of chloroethylnitrosoureas in mice. *Cancer Res.* 1977;37:2615-2618.

39. Prados MD, Yung WK, Fine HA, et al. Phase 2 study of BCNU and temozolomide for recurrent glioblastoma multiforme: North American Brain Tumor Consortium study. *Neuro Oncol.* 2004;6:33-37.

40. Perry J, Chambers A, Spithoff K, et al. Gliadel wafers in the treatment of malignant glioma: a systematic review. *Curr Oncol.* 2007;14:189-194.

41. Rougier P, Mitry E. Chemotherapy in the treatment of neuroendocrine malignant tumors. *Digestion.* 2000;62(suppl 1):73-78.

42. Gomori G. Histochemical demonstration of sites of phosphamidase activity. *Proc Soc Exp Biol Med.* 1948;69:407-409.

43. Deonarain MP, Epenetos AA. Targeting enzymes for cancer therapy: old enzymes in new roles. *Br J Cancer.* 1994;70:786-794.

44. Tew KD. TLK-286: a novel glutathione *S*-transferase-activated prodrug. *Expert Opin Investig Drugs.* 2005;14:1047-1054.

45. Chase M, Chung RY, Chiocca EA. An oncolytic viral mutant that delivers the CYP2B1 transgene and augments cyclophosphamide chemotherapy. *Nat Biotechnol.* 1998;16:444-448.

46. Wolpert MK, Ruddon RW. A study on the mechanism of resistance to nitrogen mustard (HN2) in Ehrlich ascites tumor cells: comparison of uptake of HN2–14-C into sensitive and resistant cells. *Cancer Res.* 1969;29: 873-879.

47. Begleiter A, Lam HY, Grover J, et al. Evidence for active transport of melphalan by two amino acid carriers in L5178Y lymphoblasts in vitro. *Cancer Res.* 1979;39:353-359.

48. Kohn KW, Erickson LC, Ewig RA, et al. Fractionation of DNA from mammalian cells by alkaline elution. *Biochemistry.* 1976;15:4629-4637.

49. Begleiter A, Lam HP, Goldenberg GJ. Mechanism of uptake of nitrosoureas by L5178Y lymphoblasts in vitro. *Cancer Res.* 1977;37:1022-1027.

50. Skipper HE, Bennett LL Jr, Langham WH. Over-all tracer studies with C14 labeled nitrogen mustard in normal and leukemic mice. *Cancer.* 1951;4:1025-1027.

51. Coles B. Effects of modifying structure on electrophilic reactions with biological nucleophiles. *Drug Metab Rev.* 1984;15:1307-1334.

52. Magull-Seltenreich A, Zeller WJ. Inhibition of O6-alkylguanine-DNA alkyltransferase in animal and human ovarian tumor cell lines by O6-benzylguanine and sensitization to BCNU. *Cancer Chemother Pharmacol.* 1995;35:262-266.

53. Shipp MA, Ross KN, Tamayo P, et al. Diffuse large B-cell lymphoma outcome prediction by gene-expression profiling and supervised machine learning. *Nat Med.* 2002;8:68-74.

54. Osborne MR, Lawley PD. Alkylation of DNA by melphalan with special reference to adenine derivatives and adenine-guanine cross-linking. *Chem Biol Interact.* 1993;89:49-60.

55. Bannon P, Verly W. Alkylation of phosphates and stability of phosphate triesters in DNA. *Eur J Biochem.* 1972;31:103-111.

56. Verly WG. Commentary. Monofunctional alkylating agents and apurinic sites in DNA. *Biochem Pharmacol.* 1974;23:3-8.

57. Dunn WC, Tano K, Horesovsky GJ, et al. The role of O6-alkylguanine in cell killing and mutagenesis in Chinese hamster ovary cells. *Carcinogenesis.* 1991;12:83-89.

58. Brookes P, Lawley PD. The reaction of mono- and di-functional alkylating agents with nucleic acids. *Biochem J.* 1961;80:496-503.

59. Silber JR, Blank A, Bobola MS, et al. O6-methylguanine-DNA methyltransferase-deficient phenotype in human gliomas: frequency and time to tumor progression after alkylating agent-based chemotherapy. *Clin Cancer Res.* 1999;5:807-814.

60. Thomas CB, Osieka R, Kohn KW. DNA cross-linking by in vivo treatment with 1-(2-chloroethyl)-3-(4-methylcyclohexyl)-1-nitrosourea of sensitive and resistant human colon carcinoma xenograms in nude mice. *Cancer Res.* 1978;38:2448-2454.

61. Erickson LC, Bradley MO, Ducore JM, et al. DNA crosslinking and cytotoxicity in normal and transformed human cells treated with antitumor nitrosoureas. *Proc Natl Acad Sci U S A.* 1980;77:467-471.

62. Lan Z, Sever-Chroneos Z, Strobeck MW, et al. DNA damage invokes mismatch repair-dependent cyclin D1 attenuation and retinoblastoma signaling pathways to inhibit CDK2. *J Biol Chem.* 2002;277:8372-8381.

63. Ewig RA, Kohn KW. DNA-protein cross-linking and DNA interstrand cross-linking by haloethylnitrosoureas in L1210 cells. *Cancer Res.* 1978;38:3197-3203.

64. Esteller M, Garcia-Foncillas J, Andion E, et al. Inactivation of the DNA-repair gene MGMT and the clinical response of gliomas to alkylating agents. *N Engl J Med.* 2000;343:1350-1354.

65. Sawyer GA, Frederick ED, Millard JT. Flanking sequences modulate diepoxide and mustard cross-linking efficiencies at the 5′-GNC site. *Chem Res Toxicol.* 2004;17:1057-1063.

66. Harada N, Nagasaki A, Hata H, et al. Down-regulation of CD98 in melphalan-resistant myeloma cells with reduced drug uptake. *Acta Haematol.* 2000;103:144-151.

67. Calcutt G, Connors TA. Tumour sulphydryl levels and sensitivity to the nitrogen mustard merophan. *Biochem Pharmacol.* 1963;12:839-845.

68. Robson CN, Lewis AD, Wolf CR, et al. Reduced levels of drug-induced DNA cross-linking in nitrogen mustard-resistant Chinese hamster ovary cells expressing elevated glutathione *S*-transferase activity. *Cancer Res.* 1987;47:6022-6027.

69. Hilton J. Role of aldehyde dehydrogenase in cyclophosphamide-resistant L1210 leukemia. *Cancer Res.* 1984;44:5156-5160.

70. Chute JP, Muramoto GG, Whitesides J, et al. Inhibition of aldehyde dehydrogenase and retinoid signaling induces the expansion of human hematopoietic stem cells. *Proc Natl Acad Sci U S A.* 2006;103:11707-11712.

71. Hess DA, Wirthlin L, Craft TP, et al. Selection based on CD133 and high aldehyde dehydrogenase activity isolates long-term reconstituting human hematopoietic stem cells. *Blood.* 2006;107:2162-2169.

72. Gerson SL. Clinical relevance of MGMT in the treatment of cancer. *J Clin Oncol.* 2002;20:2388-2399.

73. Rabik CA, Njoku MC, Dolan ME. Inactivation of O6-alkylguanine DNA alkyltransferase as a means to enhance chemotherapy. *Cancer Treat Rev.* 2006;32:261-276.

74. Hegi ME, Diserens AC, Gorlia T, et al. MGMT gene silencing and benefit from temozolomide in glioblastoma. *N Engl J Med.* 2005;352:997-1003.

75. Stupp R, Mason WP, van den Bent MJ, et al. Radiotherapy plus concomitant and adjuvant temozolomide for glioblastoma. *N Engl J Med.* 2005;352:987-996.

76. Liu L, Gerson SL. Targeted modulation of MGMT: clinical implications. *Clin Cancer Res.* 2006;12:328-331.

77. Gerson SL. MGMT: its role in cancer aetiology and cancer therapeutics. *Nat Rev Cancer.* 2004;4:296-307.

78. Servitzoglou M, De Vathaire F, Oberlin O, Patte C, Thomas-Teinturier C. Dose-effect relationship of alkylating agents on testicular function in male survivors of childhood lymphoma. *Pediatr Hematol Oncol.* 2015;32(8):613-623.

79. Alp BF, Kesik V, Malkoç E, et al. The effect of melatonin on procarbazine induced testicular toxicity on rats. *Syst Biol Reprod Med.* 2014.

80. Cahill DP, Codd PJ, Batchelor TT, et al. MSH6 inactivation and emergent temozolomide resistance in human glioblastomas. *Clin Neurosurg.* 2008;55:165-171.

81. Wang Y, Qin J. MSH2 and ATR form a signaling module and regulate two branches of the damage response to DNA methylation. *Proc Natl Acad Sci U SA.* 2003;100:15387-15392.

82. Sun G, Jin S, Baskaran R. MMR/c-Abl-dependent activation of ING2/p73alpha signaling regulates the cell death response to *N*-methyl-*N'*-nitro-*N*-nitrosoguanidine. *Exp Cell Res.* 2009;315:3163-3175.

83. Liu L, Markowitz S, Gerson SL. Mismatch repair mutations override alkyltransferase in conferring resistance to temozolomide but not to 1,3-bis (2-chloroethyl)nitrosourea. *Cancer Res.* 1996;56:5375-5379.

84. Taverna P, Liu L, Hanson AJ, et al. Characterization of MLH1 and MSH2 DNA mismatch repair proteins in cell lines of the NCI anticancer drug screen. *Cancer Chemother Pharmacol.* 2000;46:507-516.

85. Yan Y, Han X, Qing Y, et al. Inhibition of uracil DNA glycosylase sensitizes cancer cells to 5-fluorodeoxyuridine through replication fork collapse-induced DNA damage. *Oncotarget.* 2016;7(37):59299-59313. doi:10.18632/oncotarget.11151.

86. Trivedi RN, Almeida KH, Fornsaglio JL, et al. The role of base excision repair in the sensitivity and resistance to temozolomide-mediated cell death. *Cancer Res.* 2005;65:6394-6400.

87. Liu L, Taverna P, Whitacre CM, et al. Pharmacologic disruption of base excision repair sensitizes mismatch repair-deficient and -proficient colon cancer cells to methylating agents. *Clin Cancer Res.* 1999;5:2908-2917.

88. Murray D, Vallee-Lucie L, Rosenberg E, et al. Sensitivity of nucleotide excision repair-deficient cells to ionizing radiation and cyclophosphamide. *Anticancer Res.* 2002;22:21-26

89. Vilmar A, Sørensen JB. Excision repair cross-complementation group 1 (ERCC1) in platinum-based treatment of non-small cell lunch cancer with special emphasis on carboplatin: a review of current literature. *Lung Cancer.* 2009;64:131-139.

90. Van Allen EM, Mouw KW, Kim P, et al. Somatic ERCC2 mutations correlate with cisplatin sensitivity in muscle-invasive urothelial carcinoma. *Cancer Discov.* 2014;4(10):1140–1153. doi:10.1158/2159-8290.

91. Chen CC, Taniguchi T, D'Andrea A. The Fanconi anemia (FA) pathway confers glioma resistance to DNA alkylating agents. *J Mol Med.* 2007;85:497-509.

92. Kurihara T, Inoue M, Tatsumi D. Hypersensitivity of Bloom's syndrome fibroblasts to *N*-ethyl-*N*-nitrosourea. *Mutat Res.* 1987;184:147-151.

93. Pichierri P, Franchitto A, Rosselli F. BLM and the FANC proteins collaborate in a common pathway in response to stalled replication forks. *EMBO J.* 2004;23:3154-3163.

94. Hoy CA, Thompson LH, Mooney CL, et al. Defective DNA cross-link removal in Chinese hamster cell mutants hypersensitive to bifunctional alkylating agents. *Cancer Res.* 1985;45:1737-1743.

95. Caporali S, Levati L, Starace G, et al. AKT is activated in an ataxia-telangiectasia and Rad3-related-dependent manner in response to temozolomide and confers protection against drug-induced cell growth inhibition. *Mol Pharmacol.* 2008;74:173-183.

96. Gardai SJ, Hildeman DA, Frankel SK, et al. Phosphorylation of Bax Ser184 by Akt regulates its activity and apoptosis in neutrophils. *J Biol Chem.* 2004;279:21085-21095.

97. Qi XJ, Wildey GM, Howe PH. Evidence that Ser87 of BimEL is phosphorylated by Akt and regulates BimEL apoptotic function. *J Biol Chem.* 2006;281:813-823.

98. Levine AJ. p53, the cellular gatekeeper for growth and division. *Cell.* 1997;88:323-331.

99. Easton JB, Houghton PJ. mTOR and cancer therapy. *Oncogene.* 2006;25:6436-6446.

100. Manning BD, Cantley LC. AKT/PKB signaling: navigating downstream. *Cell.* 2007;129:1261-1274.

101. Abraham RT. Cell cycle checkpoint signaling through the ATM and ATR kinases. *Genes Dev* 2001;15:2177-2196.

102. Cortez D, Guntuku S, Qin J, et al. ATR and ATRIP: partners in checkpoint signaling. *Science.* 2001;294:1713-1716.

103. Lee JH, Paull TT. ATM activation by DNA double-strand breaks through the Mre11-Rad50-Nbs1 complex. *Science.* 2005;308:551-554.

104. Cliby WA, Roberts CJ, Cimprich KA, et al. Overexpression of a kinase-inactive ATR protein causes sensitivity to DNA-damaging agents and defects in cell cycle checkpoints. *EMBO J.* 1998;17:159-169.

105. Musio A, Montagna C, Mariani T, et al. SMC1 involvement in fragile site expression. *Hum Mol Genet.* 2005;14:525-533.

106. Bartek J, Lukas C, Lukas J. Checking on DNA damage in S phase. *Nat Rev Mol Cell Biol.* 2004;5:792-804.

107. Kirsch DG, Kastan MB. Tumor-suppressor p53: implications for tumor development and prognosis. *J Clin Oncol.* 1998;16:3158-3168.

108. Sarkaria JN, Kitange GJ, James CD, et al. Mechanisms of chemoresistance to alkylating agents in malignant glioma. *Clin Cancer Res.* 2008;14:2900-2908.

109. Singh S, Vaughan CA, Frum RA, Grossman SR, Deb S, Palit Deb S. Mutant p53 establishes targetable tumor dependency by promoting unscheduled replication. *J Clin Invest.* 2017;127(5):1839–1855.

110. Pappas K, Xu J, Zairis S, et al. p53 Maintains Baseline Expression of Multiple Tumor Suppressor Genes. *Mol Cancer Res.* 2017;15(8):1051-1062. doi:10.1158/1541-7786.

111. Teicher BA, Crawford JM, Holden SA, et al. Glutathione monoethyl ester can selectively protect liver from high dose BCNU or cyclophosphamide. *Cancer.* 1988;62:1275-1281

112. Antman K, Eder JP, Elias A, et al. High-dose combination alkylating agent preparative regimen with autologous bone marrow support: the Dana-Farber Cancer Institute/Beth Israel Hospital experience. *Cancer Treat Rep.* 1987;71:119-125.

113. Griffith OW, Meister A. Differential inhibition of glutamine and gamma-glutamylcysteine synthetases by alpha-alkyl analogs of methionine sulfoximine that induce convulsions. *J Biol Chem.* 1978;253:2333-2338.

114. Campbell EB, Hayward ML, Griffith OW. Analytical and preparative separation of the diastereomers of L-buthionine (SR)-sulfoximine, a potent inhibitor of glutathione biosynthesis. *Anal Biochem.* 1991;194:268-277.

115. Bailey HH, Mulcahy RT, Tutsch KD, et al. Phase I clinical trial of intravenous L-buthionine sulfoximine and melphalan: an attempt at modulation of glutathione. *J Clin Oncol.* 1994;12:194-205.

116. O'Dwyer PJ, Hamilton TC, LaCreta FP, et al. Phase I trial of buthionine sulfoximine in combination with melphalan in patients with cancer. *J Clin Oncol.* 1996;14:249-256.

117. Johansson AS, Ridderstrom M, Mannervik B. The human glutathione transferase P1-1 specific inhibitor TER 117 designed for overcoming cytostatic-drug resistance is also a strong inhibitor of glyoxalase I. *Mol Pharmacol.* 2000;57:619-624.

118. Vergote I, Finkler N, del Campo J, et al. Phase 3 randomised study of canfosfamide (Telcyta, TLK286) versus pegylated liposomal doxorubicin or topotecan as third-line therapy in patients with platinum-refractory or -resistant ovarian cancer. *Eur J Cancer.* 2009;45:2324-2332.

119. Yuhas JM, Spellman JM, Culo F. The role of WR-2721 in radiotherapy and/or chemotherapy. *Cancer Clin Trials.* 1980;3:211-216.

120. Capizzi RL, Scheffler BJ, Schein PS. Amifostine-mediated protection of normal bone marrow from cytotoxic chemotherapy. *Cancer.* 1993;72:3495-3501.

121. Alberts DS, Chang SY, Chen HS, et al. Kinetics of intravenous melphalan. *Clin Pharmacol Ther.* 1979;26:73-80.

122. Haddad R, Sonis S, Posner M, et al. Randomized phase 2 study of concomitant chemoradiotherapy using weekly carboplatin/paclitaxel with or without daily subcutaneous amifostine in patients with locally advanced head and neck cancer. *Cancer.* 2009;115:4514-4523.

123. Phillips GL II. The potential of amifostine in high-dose chemotherapy and autologous hematopoietic stem cell transplantation. *Semin Oncol.* 2002;29:53-56.

124. Kletzel M, Jacobsohn D, Duerst R. Pharmacokinetics of a test dose of intravenous busulfan guide dose modifications to achieve an optimal area under the curve of a single daily dose of intravenous conditioning regimen with hematopoietic stem cell transplantation. *Biol Blood Marrow Transplant.* 2006;12:472-479.

125. Batts ED, Maisel C, Kane D, et al. O6-benzylguanine and BCNU in multiple myeloma: a phase II trial. *Cancer Chemother Pharmacol.* 2007;60:415-421.

126. Adair JE, Johnston SK, Mrugala MM, et al. Gene therapy enhances chemotherapy tolerance and efficacy in Glioblastoma patients. *J Clin Invest.* 2014;124:4082-4092.

127. Armi PF, Cooper BW, Williams BM, et al. Phase I clinical trial of methoxyamine in combination with fludarabine for patients with advanced hematologic malignancies. *Oncotarget.* 2017;8:79864-79875.

128. Pujade-Lauraine E, Ledermann JA, Selle F, et al. Olaparib tablets as maintenance therapy in patients with platinum-sensitive, relapsed ovarian cancer and a BRCA ½ mutation (SOLO2/ENGOT-Ov21): a double-blind, randomized, placebo-controlled, phase 3 trial. *Lancet Oncol.* 2017;18:1274-1284

129. Coleman RL, Oza AM, Larusso D, et al. Rucaparib maintenance treatment for recurrent ovarian carcinoma after response to platinum therapy (ARIEL3): a randomized, double-blind, placebo-controlled, phase 3 trial. *Lancet.* 2017; 390:1949-1961.

130. Mirza MR, Monk BJ, Herrstedt J, et al. Niraparib maintenance therapy in platinum sensitive, recurrent ovarian cancer. *N Engl J Med.* 2016;375:2154-2164

131. Plummer R, Jones C, Middleton M, et al. Phase I study of the poly(ADP-ribose) polymerase inhibitor, AG014699, in combination with temozolomide in patients with advanced solid tumors. *Clin Cancer Res.* 2008;14:7917-7923.

132. Erice O, Smith MP, White R, et al. MGMT expression predicts PARP-mediated resistance to temozolomide. *Mol Cancer Ther.* 2015;14:1236-1246.

133. Alberts DS, Chang SY, Chen HS, et al. Comparative pharmacokinetics of chlorambucil and melphalan in man. *Recent Results Cancer Res.* 1980; 74:124-131.

134. Chang TK, Weber GF, Crespi CL, et al. Differential activation of cyclophosphamide and ifosfamide by cytochromes P-450 2B and 3A in human liver microsomes. *Cancer Res.* 1993;53:5629-5637.

135. Colvin M. The comparative pharmacology of cyclophosphamide and ifosfamide. *Semin Oncol.* 1982;9:2-7.

136. Allen LM, Creaven PJ. In vitro activation of isophosphamide (NSC-109724), a new oxazaphosphorine, by rat liver microsomes. *Cancer Chemother Rep.* 1972;56:603-610.

137. Kerbusch T, de Kraker J, Keizer HJ, et al. Clinical pharmacokinetics and pharmacodynamics of ifosfamide and its metabolites. *Clin Pharmacokinet.* 2001;40:41-62.

138. Chen TL, Kennedy MJ, Anderson LW, et al. Nonlinear pharmacokinetics of cyclophosphamide and 4-hydroxycyclophosphamide/aldophosphamide in patients with metastatic breast cancer receiving high-dose chemotherapy followed by autologous bone marrow transplantation. *Drug Metab Dispos.* 1997;25:544-551.

139. D'Incalci M, Bolis G, Facchinetti T, et al. Decreased half life of cyclophosphamide in patients under continual treatment. *Eur J Cancer.* 1979;15: 7-10.

140. Nieto Y, Vaughan WP. Pharmacokinetics of high-dose chemotherapy. *Bone Marrow Transplant.* 2004;33:259-269.

141. Tattersall MH, Jarman M, Newlands ES, et al. Pharmacokinetics of melphalan following oral or intravenous administration in patients with malignant disease. *Eur J Cancer.* 1978;14:507-513

142. Markman M. Melphalan and cytarabine administered intraperitoneally as single agents and combination intraperitoneal chemotherapy with cisplatin and cytarabine. *Semin Oncol.* 1985;12:33-37.

143. Roberts MS, Wu ZY, Siebert GA, et al. Pharmacokinetics and pharmacodynamics of melphalan in isolated limb infusion for recurrent localized limb malignancy. *Melanoma Res.* 2001;11:423-431.

144. Chang SY, Alberts DS, Farguhar D, et al. Hydrolysis and protein binding of melphalan. *J Pharm Sci.* 1978: 67: 682-684.

145. Juma FD, Rogers HJ, Trounce JR. Pharmacokinetics of cyclophosphamide and alkylating activity in man after intravenous and oral administration. *Br J Clin Pharmacol.* 1979;8:209-217.

146. Struck RF, Alberts DS, Horne K, et al. Plasma pharmacokinetics of cyclophosphamide and its cytotoxic metabolites after intravenous versus oral administration in a randomized, crossover trial. *Cancer Res.* 1987;47: 2723-2726.

147. Peters WP, Stuart A, Klotman M, et al. High-dose combination cyclophosphamide, cisplatin, and melphalan with autologous bone marrow support. A clinical and pharmacologic study. *Cancer Chemother Pharmacol.* 1989;23:377-383.

148. Klein NW, Vogler MA, Chatot CL, et al. The use of cultured rat embryos to evaluate the teratogenic activity of serum: cadmium and cyclophosphamide. *Teratology.* 1980;21:199-208.

149. Jardine I, Fenselau C, Appler M, et al. Quantitation by gas chromatography-chemical ionization mass spectrometry of cyclophosphamide, phosphoramide mustard, and nornitrogen mustard in the plasma and urine of patients receiving cyclophosphamide therapy. *Cancer Res.* 1978;38: 408-415.

150. Sladek NE, Doeden D, Powers JF, et al. Plasma concentrations of 4-hydroxycyclophosphamide and phosphoramide mustard in patients repeatedly given high doses of cyclophosphamide in preparation for bone marrow transplantation. *Cancer Treat Rep.* 1984;68:1247-1254.

151. Graham MI, Shaw IC, Souhami RL, et al. Decreased plasma half-life of cyclophosphamide during repeated high-dose administration. *Cancer Chemother Pharmacol.* 1983;10:192-193.

152. Jao JY, Jusko WJ, Cohen JL. Phenobarbital effects on cyclophosphamide pharmacokinetics in man. *Cancer Res.* 1972;32:2761-2764.

153. Erlichman C, Soldin SJ, Hardy RW, et al. Disposition of cyclophosphamide on two consecutive cycles of treatment in patients with ovarian carcinoma. *Arzneimittelforschung.* 1988;38:839-842.

154. Bagley CM Jr, Bostick FW, DeVita VT Jr. Clinical pharmacology of cyclophosphamide. *Cancer Res.* 1973;33:226-233.

155. Brade WP, Herdrich K, Varini M. Ifosfamide—pharmacology, safety and therapeutic potential. *Cancer Treat Rev.* 1985;12:1-47

156. Singer JM, Hartley JM, Brennan C, Nicholson PW, Souhami RL. The pharmacokinetics and metabolism of ifosfamide during bolus and infusional administration: a randomized cross-over study. *Br J Cancer.* 1998;77(6):978-984.

157. Boddy AV, Cole M, Pearson AD, et al. The kinetics of the auto-induction of ifosfamide metabolism during continuous infusion. *Cancer Chemother Pharmacol.* 1995;36:53-60.

158. Cohen BE, Egorin MJ, Kohlhepp EA, et al. Human plasma pharmacokinetics and urinary excretion of thiotepa and its metabolites. *Cancer Treat Rep.* 1986;70:859-864.

159. Heideman RL, Gillespie A, Ford H, et al. Phase I and pharmacokinetic evaluation of thiotepa in the cerebrospinal fluid and plasma of pediatric patients: evidence for dose-dependent plasma clearance of thiotepa. *Cancer Res.* 1989;49:736-741.

160. Kletzel M, Kearns GL, Wells TG, et al. Pharmacokinetics of high dose thiotepa in children undergoing autologous bone marrow transplantation. *Bone Marrow Transplant.* 1992;10:171-175.

161. O'Dwyer PJ, LaCreta F, Engstrom PF, et al. Phase I/pharmacokinetic reevaluation of thioTEPA. *Cancer Res.* 1991;51:3171-3176.

162. Tucker MA, Coleman CN, Cox RS, et al. Risk of second cancers after treatment for Hodgkin's disease. *N Engl J Med.* 1988;318:76-81.

163. Schoffsky P, Seeland G, Engel H, et al. Weekly administration of bendamustine: a Phase I study in patients with advanced progressive solid tumours. *Ann Oncol.* 2000;11:729-734.

164. Henner WD, Peters WP, Eder JP, et al. Pharmacokinetics and immediate effects of high-dose carmustine in man. *Cancer Treat Rep.* 1986;70:877-880.

165. Peters WP, Henner WD, Grochow LB, et al. Clinical and pharmacologic effects of high dose single agent busulfan with autologous bone marrow support in the treatment of solid tumors. *Cancer Res.* 1987;47:6402-6406.

166. Kashyap A, Wingard J, Cagnoni P, et al. Intravenous versus oral busulfan as part of a busulfan/cyclophosphamide preparative regimen for allogeneic hematopoietic stem cell transplantation: decreased incidence of hepatic venoocclusive disease (HVOD), HVOD-related mortality, and overall 100-day mortality. *Biol Blood Marrow Transplant.* 2002;8:493-500.

167. Grochow LB, Krivit W, Whitley CB, et al. Busulfan disposition in children. *Blood.* 1990;75:1723-1727.

168. Vassal G, Fischer A, Challine D, et al. Busulfan disposition below the age of three: alteration in children with lysosomal storage disease. *Blood.* 1993;82:1030-1034.

169. Bartelink IH, Bredius RG, Ververs TT, et al. Once-daily intravenous busulfan with therapeutic drug monitoring compared to conventional oral busulfan improves survival and engraftment in children undergoing allogeneic stem cell transplantation. *Biol Blood Marrow Transplant.* 2008;14:88-98.

170. Hassan M, Ehrsson H, Smedmyr B, et al. Cerebrospinal fluid and plasma concentrations of busulfan during high-dose therapy. *Bone Marrow Transplant.* 1989;4:113-114.

171. Hassan M, Thorell JO, Warne N, Stone-Elander S. 11C-labeling of busulphan. *Int J Rad Appl Instrum A.* 1991;42:1055-1059.

172. Grigg AP, Shepherd JD, Phillips GL. Busulphan and phenytoin. *Ann Intern Med.* 1989;111:1049-1050.

173. Slattery JT, Sanders JE, Buckner CD, et al. Graft-rejection and toxicity following bone marrow transplantation in relation to busulfan pharmacokinetics. *Bone Marrow Transplant.* 1995;16:31-42.

174. Gaziev J, Nguyen L, Puozzo C, et al. Novel pharmacokinetic behavior of intravenous busulfan in children with thalassemia undergoing hematopoietic stem cell transplantation: a prospective evaluation of pharmacokinetic and pharmacodynamic profile with therapeutic drug monitoring. *Blood.* 2010;115(22):4597-4604.

175. Ciurea SO, Andersson BS. Busulfan in hematopoietic stem cell transplantation. *Biol Blood Marrow Transplant.* 2009;15:523-536.

176. Russell JA, Kangarloo SB. Therapeutic drug monitoring of busulfan in transplantation. *Curr Pharm Des.* 2008;14:1936-1949.

177. Makinodan T, Santos GW, Quinn RP. Immunosuppressive drugs. *Pharmacol Rev.* 1970;22:189-247.

178. Strauss G, Osen W, Debatin KM. Induction of apoptosis and modulation of activation and effector function in T cells by immunosuppressive drugs. *Clin Exp Immunol.* 2002;128(2):255-266

179. Shand FL, Howard JG. Cyclophosphamide inhibited B cell receptor regeneration as a basis for drug-induced tolerance. *Nature.* 1978;271: 255-257.

180. Ozer H, Cowens JW, Colvin M, et al. In vitro effects of 4-hydroperoxycyclophosphamide on human immunoregulatory T subset function. I. Selective effects on lymphocyte function in T-B cell collaboration. *J Exp Med.* 1982;155:276-290.

181. Santos GW, Sensenbrenner LL, Anderson PN, et al. HL-A-identical marrow transplants in aplastic anemia, acute leukemia, and lymphosarcoma employing cyclophosphamide. *Transplant Proc.* 1976;8(4):607-610.

182. Luznik L, Bolanos-Meade J, Zahurak M, et al. High-dose cyclophosphamide as single-agent, short-course prophylaxis of graft-versus-host disease. *Blood.* 2010; 115:3224-3230

183. Aronin PA, Mahaley MS Jr, Rudnick SA, et al. Prediction of BCNU pulmonary toxicity in patients with malignant gliomas: an assessment of risk factors. *N Engl J Med.* 1980;303:183-188.

184. Burns WA, McFarland W, Matthews MJ. Busulfan-induced pulmonary disease. Report of a case and review of the literature. *Am Rev Respir Dis.* 1970;101:408-413.

185. Willson JK. Pulmonary toxicity of antineoplastic drugs. *Cancer Treat Rep.* 1978;62:2003-2008.

186. Cao TM, Negrin RS, Stockerl-Goldstein KE, et al. Pulmonary toxicity syndrome in breast cancer patients undergoing BCNU-containing high-dose chemotherapy and autologous hematopoietic cell transplantation. *Biol Blood Marrow Transplant.* 2000;6:387-394.

187. Philips FS, Sternberg SS, Cronin AP, et al. Cyclophosphamide and urinary bladder toxicity. *Cancer Res.* 1961;21:1577-1589.

188. Forni AM, Koss LG, Geller W. Cytological study of the effect of cyclophosphamide on the epithelium of the urinary bladder in man. *Cancer.* 1964;17:1348-1355.

189. Andriole GL, Sandlund JT, Miser JS, et al. The efficacy of mesna (2-mercaptoethane sodium sulfonate) as a neuroprotectant in patients with hemorrhagic cystitis receiving further oxazaphosphorine chemotherapy. *J Clin Oncol.* 1987;5:799-803.

190. Botta JA Jr, Nelson LW, Weikel JH Jr. Acetylcysteine in the prevention of cyclophosphamide-induced cystitis in rats. *J Natl Cancer Inst.* 1973;51:1051-1058.

191. DeFronzo RA, Abeloff M, Braine H, et al. Renal dysfunction after treatment with isophosphamide (NSC-109724). *Cancer Chemother Rep.* 1974; 58:375-382.

192. Moncrieff M, Foot A. Fanconi syndrome after ifosfamide. *Cancer Chemother Pharmacol.* 1989;23:121-122.

193. DeFronzo RA, Braine H, Colvin M, et al. Water intoxication in man after cyclophosphamide therapy. Time course and relation to drug activation. *Ann Intern Med.* 1973;78:861-869.

194. Silver HK, Morton DL. CCNU nephrotoxicity following sustained remission in oat cell carcinoma. *Cancer Treat Rep.* 1979;63:226-227.

195. Harmon WE, Cohen HJ, Schneeberger EE, et al. Chronic renal failure in children treated with methyl CCNU. *N Engl J Med.* 1979;300:1200-1203.

196. Spitz S. The histological effects of nitrogen mustards on human tumors and tissues. *Cancer.* 1948;1:383-398.

197. Toppari J, Bishop PC, Parker JW, et al. Cytotoxic effects of cyclophosphamide in the mouse seminiferous epithelium: DNA flow cytometric and morphometric analysis. *Fundam Appl Toxicol.* 1990;15:44-52.

198. Richter P, Calamera JC, Morgenfeld MC, et al. Effect of chlorambucil on spermatogenesis in the human with malignant lymphoma. *Cancer.* 1970; 25:1026-1030.

199. Miller DG. Alkylating agents and human spermatogenesis. *JAMA.* 1971;217: 1662-1665.

200. Hinkes E, Plotkin D. Reversible drug-induced sterility in a patient with acute leukemia. *JAMA.* 1973;223:1490-1491.

201. Blake DA, Heller RH, Hsu SH, et al. Return of fertility in a patient with cyclophosphamide-induced azoospermia. *Johns Hopkins Med J.* 1976;139: 20-22.

202. Sadler TW, Kochhar DM. Chlorambucil-induced cell death in embryonic mouse limb buds. *Toxicol Appl Pharmacol.* 1976;37:237-256.

203. Nicholson HO. Cytotoxic drugs in pregnancy. Review of reported cases. *J Obstet Gynaecol Br Commonw.* 1968;75:307-312.

204. Steege JF, Caldwell DS. Renal agenesis after first trimester exposure to chlorambucil. *South Med J.* 1980;73:1414-1415.

205. Toledo TM, Harper RC, Moser RH. Fetal effects during cyclophosphamide and irradiation therapy. *Ann Intern Med.* 1971;74:87-91.

206. Garrett MJ. Letter: teratogenic effects of combination chemotherapy. *Ann Intern Med.* 1974;80:667.

207. Ortega J. Multiple agent chemotherapy including bleomycin of non-Hodgkin's lymphoma during pregnancy. *Cancer.* 1977;40:2829-2835.

208. Lergier JE, Jiménez E, Maldonado N, et al. Normal pregnancy in multiple myeloma treated with cyclophosphamide. *Cancer.* 1974;34:1018-1022.

209. Rowley JD, Golomb HM, Vardiman JW. Nonrandom chromosome abnormalities in acute leukemia and dysmyelopoietic syndromes in patients with previously treated malignant disease. *Blood.* 1981;58:759-767.

210. Davies SM. Therapy-related leukemia associated with alkylating agents. *Med Pediatr Oncol.* 2001;36:536-540.

211. Schellong G, Riepenhausen M, Creutzig U, et al. Low risk of secondary leukemias after chemotherapy without mechlorethamine in childhood Hodgkin's disease. German-Austrian Pediatric Hodgkin's Disease Group. *J Clin Oncol.* 1997;15:2247-2253.

212. Chao RC, Pyzel U, Fridlyand J, et al. Therapy-induced malignant neoplasms in Nf1 mutant mice. *Cancer Cell.* 2005;8:337-348.

213. Ganguly BB, Banerjee D, Agarwal MB. Impact of chromosomal alterations, genetic mutations, and clonal hematopoiesis of indeterminate potential (CHIP) on the classification and risk stratification of MDS. *Blood Cells Mol Dis.* 2017;69:90-100. doi:10.1016/j.bcmd 2017 10.001.

214. Lazarus HM, Herzig RH, Graham-Pole J, et al. Intensive melphalan chemotherapy and cryopreserved autologous bone marrow transplantation for the treatment of refractory cancer. *J Clin Oncol.* 1983;1:359-367.

215. Leff RS, Thompson JM, Johnson DB, et al. Phase II trial of high-dose melphalan and autologous bone marrow transplantation for metastatic colon carcinoma. *J Clin Oncol.* 1986;4:1586-1591.

216. Takvorian T, Canellos GP, Ritz J, et al. Prolonged disease-free survival after autologous bone marrow transplantation in patients with non-Hodgkin's lymphoma with a poor prognosis. *N Engl J Med.* 1987;316:1499-1505.

217. Finn G, Denning D. Transient nephrogenic diabetes insipidus following high-dose cyclophosphamide chemotherapy and autologous bone marrow transplantation. *Cancer Treat Rep.* 1987;71:220-221.

218. Graves SW, Eder JP, Schryber SM, et al. Endogenous digoxin-like immunoreactive factor and digitalis-like factor associated with the hypertension of patients receiving multiple alkylating agents as part of autologous bone marrow transplantation. *Clin Sci (Lond).* 1989;77:501-507.

219. Mitchell RB, Wagner JE, Karp JE, et al. Syndrome of idiopathic hyperammonemia after high-dose chemotherapy: review of nine cases. *Am J Med.* 1988;85:662-667.

220. Ozsahin M, Belkacémi Y, Pène F, et al. Interstitial pneumonitis following autologous bone-marrow transplantation conditioned with cyclophosphamide and total-body irradiation. *Int J Radiat Oncol Biol Phys.* 1996;34:71-77.

221. Pecego R, Hill R, Appelbaum FR, et al. Interstitial pneumonitis following autologous bone marrow transplantation. *Transplantation.* 1986;42:515-517.

222. Seiden MV, O'Donnell WJ, Weinblatt M, et al. Vasculitis with recurrent pulmonary hemorrhage in a long-term survivor after autologous bone marrow transplantation. *Bone Marrow Transplant.* 1990;6:345-347.

223. Kessinger A, Armiage JO, Smith DM, et al. High-dose therapy and autologous peripheral blood stem cell transplantation for patients with lymphoma. *Blood.* 1989;74:1260-1265.

224. Jones RJ, Piantadosi S, Mann RB, et al. High-dose cytotoxic therapy and bone marrow transplantation for relapsed Hodgkin's disease. *J Clin Oncol.* 1990;8:527-537.

225. Wilson WH, Jain V, Bryant G, et al. Phase I and II study of high-dose ifosfamide, carboplatin and etoposide with autologous bone marrow rescue in lymphomas and solid tumor. *J Clin Oncol.* 1992;10:1712-1722.

226. Dunpy FR, Spitzer G, Buzdar AU, et al. Treatment of estrogen receptor-negative or hormonally refractory breast cancer with double high-dose chemotherapy intensification and bone marrow support. *J Clin Oncol.* 1990;8:1207-1216.

227. Eder JP, Elias A, Shea TC, et al. A phase I-II study of cyclophosphamide, thiotepa, and carboplatin with autologous bone marrow transplantation in solid tumor patients. *J Clin Oncol.* 1990;8:1239-1245.

228. Peters WP, Shpall EJ, Jones RB, et al. High-dose combination alkylating agents with bone marrow support as initial treatment for metastatic breast cancer. *J Clin Oncol.* 1988;6:1368-1376.

229. Phillips GL, Wolff SN, Fay JW, et al. Intensivie 1,3-bis(2-chloroethyl)-1-nitrosourea (BCNU) monochemotherapy and autologous bone marrow transplantation for malignant gliomas. *J Clin Oncol.* 1986;4:639-645.

230. Gianni AM, Bregni M, Siena S, et al. Recombinant human granulocyte-macrophage colong-stimulating factor reduces hematologic toxicity and widens clinical applicability of high-dose cyclophosphamide treatment in breast cancer anc non-Hodgkin's lymphoma. *J Clin Oncol.* 1990;8:768-778.

231. Reid JM, Pendergrass TW, Krailo MD, et al. Plasma pharmacokinetics and cerebrospinal fluid concentration of idarubincin idarubicinol in pediatric leukemia patients: a Children's Cancer Study Group report. *Cancer Res.* 1990;50:6525-6528.

232. Fulgenai A, Ferrero ME. Defibrotide in the treatment of hepatic veno-occlusive disease. *Hepat Med.* 2016; 8:105-113.

233. Linassier C, Colombat P, Reisenleiter M, et al. Cutaneous toxicity of autologous bone marrow transplantation in nonseminomatous germ cell tumors. *Cancer.* 1990;65:1143-1145.

234. Jochelson M, Tarbell NJ, Freedman AS, et al. Acute and chronic pulmonary complications following autologous bone marrow transplantation in non-Hodgkin's lymphoma. *Bone Marrow Transplant.* 1990;6:329-331.

235. Martino P, Micozzi A, Venditti M, et al. Catheter-related right-sided endocarditis in bone marrow transplant recipients. *Rev Infect Dis.* 1990;12:250-257.

236. Phillips GL, Fay JW, Herzig GP, et al. Intensive 1,3-bis(2-chloroethyl)-1-nitrosourea (BCNU) autologous bone marrow transplantation therapy of refractory cancer: a preliminary report. *Exp Hematol.* 1979;7(suppl 5):372-383.

237. Goren MP, Wright RK, Pratt CB, et al. Dechloroethylation of ifosfamide and neurotoxicity. *Lancet.* 1986;2:1219-1220.

238. Thigpen T. Ifosfamide-induced central nervous system toxicity. *Gynecol Oncol.* 1991;42:191-192.

239. Zeller P, Gutmann H, Hegedus B, et al. Methylhydrazine derivatives, a new class of cytotoxic agents. *Experientia.* 1963;19:129.

240. Bollag W. The tumor-inhibitory effects of the methylhydrazine derivative Ro4-6467/1 (NSC 77213). *Cancer Chemother Rep.* 1963;33:1-4.

241. De Vita VT Jr, Hubbard SM, Longo DL. The chemotherapy of lymphomas: looking back, moving forward–the Richard and Hinda Rosenthal Foundation award lecture. *Cancer Res.* 1987;47:5810-5824.

242. DeVita VT Jr, Canellos GP, Chabner B, et al. Advanced diffuse histiocytic lymphoma, a potentially curable disease. *Lancet.* 1975;1:248-250.

243. Newton HB, Junck L, Bromberg J, et al. Procarbazine chemotherapy in the treatment of recurrent malignant astrocytomas after radiation and nitrosourea failure. *Neurology.* 1990;40:1743-1746.

244. Bedell MA, Lewis JG, Billings KC, et al. Cell specificity in hepatocarcinogenesis: preferential accumulation of O6-methylguanine in target cell DNA during continuous exposure to rats to 1,2-dimethylhydrazine. *Cancer Res.* 1982;42:3079-3083.

245. Rossi SC, Conrad M, Voigt JM, et al. Excision repair of O6-methylguanine synthesized at the rat H-ras N-methyl-N-nitrosourea activation site and introduced into *Escherichia coli. Carcinogenesis.* 1989;10:373-377.

246. Swenberg JA, Bedell MA, Billings KC, et al. Cell-specific differences in O6-alkylguanine DNA repair activity during continuous exposure to carcinogen. *Proc Natl Acad Sci U S A.* 1982;79:5499-5502.

247. Chaube S, Murphy ML. Fetal malformations produced in rats by N-isopropyl-alpha-(2-methylhydrazino)-p-toluamide hydrochloride (procarbazine). *Teratology.* 1969;2:23-31.

248. Schold SC Jr, Brent TP, von Hofe E, et al. O6-alkylguanine-DNA alkyltransferase and sensitivity to procarbazine in human brain-tumor xenografts. *J Neurosurg.* 1989;70:573-577.

249. Pegg AE. Mammalian O6-alkylguanine-DNA alkyltransferase: regulation and importance in response to alkylating carcinogenic and therapeutic agents. *Cancer Res.* 1990;50:6119-6129.

250. Lee IP, Lucier GW. The potentiation of barbiturate-induced narcosis by procarbazine. *J Pharmacol Exp Ther.* 1976;196:586-593.

251. Oliverio VT, Denham C, Devita VT, et al. Some pharmacologic properties of a new antitumor agent, N-isopropyl-alpha-(2-methylhydrazino)-p-toluamide, hydrochloride (Nsc-77213). *Cancer Chemother Rep.* 1964;42:1-7.

252. Shiba DA, Weinkam RJ. The in vivo cytotoxic activity of procarbazine and procarbazine metabolites against L1210 ascites leukemia cells in CDF1 mice and the effects of pretreatment with procarbazine, phenobarbital, diphenylhydantoin, and methylprednisolone upon in vivo procarbazine activity. *Cancer Chemother Pharmacol.* 1983;11:124-129.

253. De Vita VT, Hahn MA, Oliverio VT. Monoamine oxidase inhibition by a new carcinostatic agent, N-isopropyl-a92-methylhydrazino)-p-toluamide (MIH). *Proc Soc Exp Biol Med.* 1965;120:561-565.

254. Chabner BA, DeVita VT, Considine N, et al. Plasma pyridoxal phosphate depletion by the carcinostatic procarbazine. *Proc Soc Exp Biol Med.* 1969;132:1119-1122.

255. DeVita VT, Serpick A, Carbone PP. Preliminary clinical studies with ibenzmethyzin. *Clin Pharmacol Ther.* 1966;7:542-546.

256. Sponzo RW, Arseneau JC, Canellos GP. Procabazine induced oxidative haemolysis: relationship in vivo red cell survival. *Br J Haematol.* 1974;27:587-595.

257. Weiss HD, Walker MD, Wiernik PH. Neurotoxicity of commonly used antineoplastic agents (first of two parts). *N Engl J Med.* 1974;291:75-81.

258. Casimir A, Kavanaugh J, Liu F. Phase 1 trial of intravenous PCB administered as a 5 day continuous infusion: correlation with plasma levels of pyridoxal phosphate. *Proc Am Assoc Cancer Res.* 1983;24:144.

259. Chabner BA, Sponzo R, Hubbard S, et al. High-dose intermittent intravenous infusion of procarbazine (NSC-77213). *Cancer Chemother Rep.* 1973;57:361-363.

260. Dunagin WG. Clinical toxicity of chemotherapeutic agents: dermatologic toxicity. *Semin Oncol.* 1982;9:14-22.

261. Garbes ID, Henderson ES, Gomez GA, et al. Procarbazine-induced interstitial pneumonitis with a normal chest x-ray: a case report. *Med Pediatr Oncol.* 1986;14:238-241.

262. Lokich JJ, Moloney WC. Allergic reaction to procarbazine. *Clin Pharmacol Ther.* 1972;13:573-574.

263. Liske R. A comparative study of the action of cyclophosphamide and procarbazine on the antibody production in mice. *Clin Exp Immunol.* 1973;15:271-280.

264. Parvinen LM. Early effects of procarbazine (N-isopropyl-L-(2-methylhydrazino)-p-toluamide hydrochloride) on rat spermatogenesis. *Exp Mol Pathol.* 1979;30:1-11.

265. Pueyo C. Natulan induces forward mutations to L-arabinose-resistance in *Salmonella typhimurium. Mutat Res.* 1979;67:189-192.

266. Sieber SM, Correa P, Dalgard DW, et al. Carcinogenic and other adverse effects of procarbazine in nonhuman primates. *Cancer Res.* 1978;38:2125-2134.

267. Schilsky RL, Lewis BJ, Sherins RJ, et al. Gonadal dysfunction in patients receiving chemotherapy for cancer. *Ann Intern Med.* 1980;93:109-114.

268. Schilsky RL, Sherins RJ, Hubbard SM, et al. Long-term follow up of ovarian function in women treated with MOPP chemotherapy for Hodgkin's disease. *Am J Med.* 1981;71:552-556.

269. Johnson JM, Thompson DJ, Haggerty GC, et al. The effect of prenatal procarbazine treatment on brain development in the rat. *Teratology.* 1985;32:203-212.

270. Andrieu JM, Ochoa-Molina ME. Menstrual cycle, pregnancies and offspring before and after MOPP therapy for Hodgkin's disease. *Cancer.* 1983;52: 435-438.

271. Henry-Amar M. Quantitative risk of second cancer in patients in first complete remission from early stages of Hodgkin's disease. *NCI Monogr.* 1988;(6):65-72.

272. Goldstein LS. Dominant lethal mutations induced in mouse spermatogonia by mechlorethamine, procarbazine and vincristine administered in 2-drug and 3-drug combinations. *Mutat Res.* 1987;191:171-176.

273. Montgomery JA. Experimental studies at Southern Research Institute with DTIC (NSC-45388). *Cancer Treat Rep.* 1976;60:125-134.

274. Shealy YF, Montgomery JA, Laster WR Jr. Antitumor activity of triazeno-imidazoles. *Biochem Pharmacol.* 1962;11:674-676.

275. Comis RL. DTIC (NSC-45388) in malignant melanoma: a perspective. *Cancer Treat Rep.* 1976;60:165-176.

276. Frei E III, Luce JK, Talley RW, et al. 5-(3,3-dimethyl-1-triazeno)imidazole-4-carboxamide (NSC-45388) in the treatment of lymphoma. *Cancer Chemother Rep.* 1972;56:667-670.

277. Bonadonna G, Valagussa P, Santoro A. Alternating non-cross-resistant combination chemotherapy or MOPP in stage IV Hodgkin's disease. A report of 8-year results. *Ann Intern Med.* 1986;104:739-746.

278. Gottlieb JA, Benjamin RS, Baker LH, et al. Role of DTIC (NSC-45388) in the chemotherapy of sarcomas. *Cancer Treat Rep.* 1976;60:199-203.

279. Finklestein JZ, Albo V, Ertel I, et al. 5-(3,3-Dimethyl-1-triazeno)imidazole-4-carboxamide (NSC-45388) in the treatment of solid tumors in children. *Cancer Chemother Rep.* 1975;59:351-357.

280. Clarke DA, Barclay RK, Stock CC, et al. Triazenes as inhibitors of mouse sarcoma 180. *Proc Soc Exp Biol Med.* 1955;90:484-489.

281. D'Incalci M, Citti L, Taverna P, et al. Importance of the DNA repair enzyme O6-alkyl guanine alkyltransferase (AT) in cancer chemotherapy. *Cancer Treat Rev.* 1988;15:279-292.

282. Gibson NW, Hartley J, La France RJ, et al. Differential cytotoxicity and DNA-damaging effects produced in human cells of the Mer+ and Mer- phenotypes by a series of alkyltriazenylimidazoles. *Carcinogenesis.* 1986;7:259-265.

283. Mitchell RB, Dolan ME. Effect of temozolomide and dacarbazine on O6-alkylguanine-DNA alkyltransferase activity and sensitivity of human tumor cells and xenografts to 1,3-bis(2-chloroethyl)-1-nitrosourea. *Cancer Chemother Pharmacol.* 1993;32:59-63.

284. Lee SM, Thatcher N, Dougal M, et al. Dosage and cycle effects of dacarbazine (DTIC) and fotemustine on O6-alkylguanine-DNA alkyltransferase in human peripheral blood mononuclear cells. *Br J Cancer.* 1993;67: 216-221

285. Lunn JM, Harris AL. Cytotoxicity of 5-(3-methyl-1-triazeno)imidazole-4-carboxamide (MTIC) on Mer+, Mer+Rem- and Mer- cell lines: differential potentiation by 3-acetamidobenzamide. *Br J Cancer.* 1988;57:54-58.

286. Friedman HS, Johnson SP, Dong Q, et al. Methylator resistance mediated by mismatch repair deficiency in a glioblastoma multiforme xenograft. *Cancer Res.* 1997;57:2933-2936.

287. Buesa JM, Gracia M, Valle M, et al. Phase I trial of intermittent high-dose dacarbazine. *Cancer Treat Rep.* 1984;68:499-504.

288. Loo TL, Luce JK, Jardine JH, et al. Pharmacologic studies of the antitumor agent 5-(dimethyltriazeno)imidazole-4-carboxamide. *Cancer Res.* 1968;28:2448-2453.

289. Breithaupt H, Dammann A, Aigner K. Pharmacokinetics of dacarbazine (DTIC) and its metabolite 5-aminoimidazole-4-carboxamide (AIC) following different dose schedules. *Cancer Chemother Pharmacol.* 1982;9:103-109

290. Luce JK, Thurman WG, Isaacs BL, et al. Clinical trials with the antitumor agent 5-(3,3-dimethyl-1-triazeno)imidazole-4-carboxamide(NSC-45388). *Cancer Chemother Rep.* 1970;54:119-124.

291. Beck TM, Hart NE, Smith CE. Photosensitivity reaction following DTIC administration: report of two cases. *Cancer Treat Rep.* 1980;64: 725-726.

292. Ceci G, Bella M, Melissari M, et al. Fatal hepatic vascular toxicity of DTIC. Is it really a rare event? *Cancer.* 1988;61:1988-1991.

293. Tamaro M, Dolzani L, Monti-Bragadin C, et al. Mutagenic activity of the dacarbazine analog p-(3,3-dimethyl-1-triazeno)benzoic acid potassium salt in bacterial cells. *Pharmacol Res Commun.* 1986;18:491-501.

294. Schmid FA, Hutchinson DJ, Chemotherapeutic, carcinogenic, and cell-reguloatory effects of triazenes. *Cancer Res.* 1974;34:1671-1675

295. Beal DD, Skibba JL, Croft WA, et al. Carcinogenicity of the antineoplastic agent, 5-(3,3-dimethyl-1-triazeno)-imidazole-4-carboxamide, and its metabolites in rats. *J Natl Cancer Inst.* 1975;54:951-957.

296. Valagussa P, Santoro A, Fossati Bellani F, et al. Absence of treatment-induced second neoplasms after ABVD in Hodgkin's disease. *Blood.* 1982;59: 488-494.

297. Carey RW, Kunz VS. Acute non-lymphocytic leukemia (ANLL) following treatment with dacarbazine for malignant melanoma. *Am J Hematol.* 1987;25:119-121.

298. Thompson DJ, Molello JA, Strebing RJ, et al. Reproduction and teratology studies with oncolytic agents in the rat and rabbit. II. 5-(3,3-dimethyl-1-triazeno) imidazole-4-carboxamide (DTIC). *Toxicol Appl Pharmacol.* 1975;33:281-290.

299. Harrap KA, Connors TA, Stevens MFG. Second-generation azolotetrazi-nones. In: *New Avenues in Developmental Cancer Chemotherapy.* London, UK: Academic Press, 1987:335.

300. Horspool KR, Stevens MF, Newton CG, et al. Antitumor imidazotetrazines. 20. Preparation of the 8-acid derivative of mitozolomide and its utility in the preparation of active antitumor agents. *J Med Chem.* 1990;33:1393-1399.

301. Stevens MF, Hickman JA, Langdon SP, et al. Antitumor activity and pharmacokinetics in mice of 8-carbamoyl-3-methyl-imidazo[5,1-d]-1,2,3,5-tetrazin-4(3H)-one (CCRG 81045; M & B 39831), a novel drug with potential as an alternative to dacarbazine. *Cancer Res.* 1987;47:5846-5852.

302. Tsang LL, Quarterman CP, Gescher A, et al. Comparison of the cytotoxicity in vitro of temozolomide and dacarbazine, prodrugs of 3-methyl-(triazen-1-yl) imidazole-4-carboxamide. *Cancer Chemother Pharmacol.* 1991;27:342-346.

303. Newlands ES, Blackledge GR, Slack JA, et al. Phase I trial of temozolomide (CCRG 81045: M&B 39831: NSC 362856). *Br J Cancer.* 1992;65: 287-291.

304. Vogelbaum MA, Berkey B, Peereboom D, et al. Phase II trial of preirradiation and concurrent temozolomide in patients with newly diagnosed anaplastic oligodendrogliomas and mixed anaplastic oligoastrocytomas: RTOG BR0131. *Neuro Oncol.* 2009;11:167-175.

305. Friedman HS, McLendon RE, Kerby T, et al. DNA mismatch repair and O6-alkylguanine-DNA alkyltransferase analysis and response to Temodal in newly diagnosed malignant glioma. *J Clin Oncol.* 1998;16:3851-3857.

306. Stupp R, Dietrich PY, Ostermann Kraljevic S, et al. Promising survival for patients with newly diagnosed glioblastoma multiforme treated with concomitant radiation plus temozolomide followed by adjuvant temozolomide. *J Clin Oncol.* 2002;20:1375-1382.

307. Stupp R, Hegi ME, Mason WP, et al. Effects of radiotherapy with concomitant and adjuvant temozolomide versus radiotherapy alone on survival in glioblastoma in a randomised phase III study: 5-year analysis of the EORTC-NCIC trial. *Lancet Oncol.* 2009;10:459-466.

308. Ziu M, Kalkanis SN, Gilbert M, Ryken TC, Olson JJ. The role of initial chemotherapy for the treatment of adults with diffuse low grade glioma : a systematic review and evidence-based clinicalpractice guideline. *J Neurooncol.* 2015;125(3):585-607.

309. van den Bent MJ, Taphoorn MJ, Brandes AA, et al. Phase II study of first-line chemotherapy with temozolomide in recurrent oligodendroglial tumors: the European Organization for Research and Treatment of Cancer Brain Tumor Group Study 26971. *J Clin Oncol.* 2003;21:2525-2528.

310. Chamberlain MC, Tsao-Wei DD, Groshen S. Temozolomide for treatment-resistant recurrent meningioma. *Neurology.* 2004;62:1210-1212.

311. Lowe PR, Sansom CE, Schwalbe CH, et al. Antitumor imidazotetrazines. 25. Crystal structure of 8-carbamoyl-3-methylimidazo[5,1-d]-1,2,3,5-tetrazin-4(3H)-one (temozolomide) and structural comparisons with the related drugs mitozolomide and DTIC. *J Med Chem.* 1992;35: 3377-3382.

312. Clark AS, Deans B, Stevens MF, et al. Antitumor imidazotetrazines. 32. Synthesis of novel imidazotetrazinones and related bicyclic heterocycles to probe the mode of action of the antitumor drug temozolomide. *J Med Chem.* 1995;38:1493-1504.

313. Denny BJ, Wheelhouse RT, Stevens MF, et al. NMR and molecular modeling investigation of the mechanism of activation of the antitumor drug temozolomide and its interaction with DNA. *Biochemistry.* 1994;33:9045-9051.

314. Bull VL, Tisdale MJ. Antitumour imidazotetrazines–XVI. Macromolecular alkylation by 3-substituted imidazotetrazinones. *Biochem Pharmacol*. 1987;36: 3215-3220.

315. Wedge SR, Porteous JK, Newlands ES. 3-aminobenzamide and/or O6-benzylguanine evaluated as an adjuvant to temozolomide or BCNU treatment in cell lines of variable mismatch repair status and O6-alkylguanine-DNA alkyltransferase activity. *Br J Cancer*. 1996;74:1030-1036.

316. Friedman HS, Dolan ME, Pegg AE, et al. Activity of temozolomide in the treatment of central nervous system tumor xenografts. *Cancer Res*. 1995;55:2853-2857.

317. D'Atri S, Piccioni D, Castellano A, et al. Chemosensitivity to triazene compounds and O6-alkylguanine-DNA alkyltransferase levels: studies with blasts of leukaemic patients. *Ann Oncol*. 1995;6:389-393.

318. Dolan ME, Moschel RC, Pegg AE. Depletion of mammalian O6-alkylguanine-DNA alkyltransferase activity by O6-benzylguanine provides a means to evaluate the role of this protein in protection against carcinogenic and therapeutic alkylating agents. *Proc Natl Acad Sci U S A*. 1990;87:5368-5372.

319. Karran P, Macpherson P, Ceccotti S, et al. O6-methylguanine residues elicit DNA repair synthesis by human cell extracts. *J Biol Chem*. 1993;268:15878-15886.

320. Karran P, Hampson R. Genomic instability and tolerance to alkylating agents. *Cancer Surv*. 1996;28:69-85.

321. Hirose Y, Berger MS, Pieper RO. Abrogation of the Chk1-mediated G(2) checkpoint pathway potentiates temozolomide-induced toxicity in a p53-independent manner in human glioblastoma cells. *Cancer Res*. 2001;61:5843-5849.

322. Roos W, Baumgartner M, Kaina B. Apoptosis triggered by DNA damage O6-methylguanine in human lymphocytes requires DNA replication and is mediated by p53 and Fas/CD95/Apo-1. *Oncogene*. 2004;23: 359-367.

323. Bianchi R, Citti L, Beghetti R, et al. O6-methylguanine-DNA methyltransferase activity and induction of novel immunogenicity in murine tumor cells treated with methylating agents. *Cancer Chemother Pharmacol*. 1992;29:277-282.

324. Allegrucci M, Fuschiotti P, Puccetti P, et al. Changes in the tumorigenic and metastatic properties of murine melanoma cells treated with a triazene derivative. *Clin Exp Metastasis*. 1989;7:329-341.

325. Tentori L, Leonetti C, Aquino A. Temozolomide reduces the metastatic potential of Lewis lung carcinoma (3LL) in mice: role of alpha-6 integrin phosphorylation. *Eur J Cancer*. 1995;31A:746-754.

326. Tisdale MJ. Antitumour imidazotetrazines-X. Effect of 8-carbamoyl-3-methylimidazo[5,1-d]-1,2,3,5-tetrazin-4-(3H)-one (CCRG 81045; M & B 39831; NSC 362856) on DNA methylation during induction of haemoglobin synthesis in human leukaemia cell line K562. *Biochem Pharmacol*. 1986;35:311-316.

327. Pegg AE, Dolan ME, Moschel RC. Structure, function, and inhibition of O6-alkylguanine-DNA alkyltransferase. *Prog Nucleic Acid Res Mol Biol*. 1995;51:167-223

328. Baer JC, Freeman AA, Newlands ES, et al. Depletion of O6-alkylguanine-DNA alkyltransferase correlates with potentiation of temozolomide and CCNU toxicity in human tumour cells. *Br J Cancer*. 1993;67: 1299-1302.

329. Redmond SM, Joncourt F, Buser K, et al. Assessment of P-glycoprotein, glutathione-based detoxifying enzymes and O6-alkylguanine-DNA alkyltransferase as potential indicators of constitutive drug resistance in human colorectal tumors. *Cancer Res*. 1991;51:2092-2097.

330. Wang G, Weiss C, Sheng P, et al. Retrovirus-mediated transfer of the human O6-methylguanine-DNA methyltransferase gene into a murine hematopoietic stem cell line and resistance to the toxic effects of certain alkylating agents. *Biochem Pharmacol*. 1996;51:1221-1228.

331. Citron M, Decker R, Chen S, et al. O6-methylguanine-DNA methyltransferase in human normal and tumor tissue from brain, lung, and ovary. *Cancer Res*. 1991;51:4131-4134.

332. Frosina G, Rossi O, Arena G, et al. O6-alkylguanine-DNA alkyltransferase activity in human brain tumors. *Cancer Lett*. 1990;55:153-158.

333. Yarosh DB. The role of O6-methylguanine-DNA methyltransferase in cell survival, mutagenesis and carcinogenesis. *Mutat Res*. 1985;145:1-16.

334. Bobola MS, Tseng SH, Blank A, et al. Role of O6-methylguanine-DNA methyltransferase in resistance of human brain tumor cell lines to the clinically relevant methylating agents temozolomide and streptozotocin. *Clin Cancer Res*. 1996;2:735-741.

335. Tentori L, Leonetti C, Scarsella M, et al. Combined treatment with temozolomide and poly(ADP-ribose) polymerase inhibitor enhances survival of mice bearing hematologic malignancy at the central nervous system site. *Blood*. 2002;99:2241-2244.

336. Ionov Y, Peinado MA, Malkhosyan S, et al. Ubiquitous somatic mutations in simple repeated sequences reveal a new mechanism for colonic carcinogenesis. *Nature*. 1993;363:558-561.

337. Cancer Genome Atlas Research Network. Comprehensive genomic characterization defines human glioblastoma genes and core pathways. *Nature*. 2008;455:1061-1068.

338. Yip S, Miao J, Cahill DP, et al. MSH6 mutations arise in glioblastomas during temozolomide therapy and mediate temozolomide resistance. *Clin Cancer Res*. 2009;15:4622-4629.

339. Kat A, Thilly WG, Fang WH, et al. An alkylation-tolerant, mutator human cell line is deficient in strand-specific mismatch repair. *Proc Natl Acad Sci U S A*. 1993;90:6424-6428.

340. Koi M, Umar A, Chauhan DP, et al. Human chromosome 3 corrects mismatch repair deficiency and microsatellite instability and reduces N-methyl-N'-nitro-N-nitrosoguanidine tolerance in colon tumor cells with homozygous hMLH1 mutation. *Cancer Res*. 1994;54:4308-4312.

341. Tentori L, Leonetti C, Scarsella M. Systemic administration of the PARP inhibitor GPI 15427 increases the anti-tumor activity of temozolomide in melanoma, glioma and lymphoma preclinical models in vivo. *Proc Am Assoc Cancer Res*. 2003;44:1253.

342. Tentori L, Portarena I, Torino F, et al. Poly(ADP-ribose) polymerase inhibitor increases growth inhibition and reduces G(2)/M cell accumulation induced by temozolomide in malignant glioma cells. *Glia*. 2002;40:44-54.

343. Bowman KJ, White A, Golding BT, Griffin RJ, Curtin NJ. Potentiation of anti-cancer agent cytotoxicity by the potent poly(ADP-ribose) polymerase inhibitors NU1025 and NU1064. *Br J Cancer*. 1998;78:1269-1277.

344. Calabrese CR, Batey MA, Thomas HD, et al. Identification of potent nontoxic poly(ADP-Ribose) polymerase-1 inhibitors: chemopotentiation and pharmacological studies. *Clin Cancer Res*. 2003;9:2711-2718.

345. Curtin NJ, Wang LZ, Yiakouvaki A, et al. Novel poly(ADP-ribose) polymerase-1 inhibitor, AG14361, restores sensitivity to temozolomide in mismatch repair-deficient cells. *Clin Cancer Res*. 2004;10:881-889.

346. Yan L, Bulgar A, Miao Y, et al. Combined treatment with temozolomide and methoxyamine: blocking apurininc/pyrimidinic site repair coupled with targeting topoisomerase II{alpha}. *Clin Cancer Res*. 13:1532-1539, 2007

347. Caimi PF, Cooper BW, William BM, Dowlati A, Barr PM, Fu P, Pink J, Xu Y, Lazarus HM, de Lima M, Gerson SL. Phase I clinical trial of the base excision repair inhibitor methoxyamine in combination with fludarabine for patients with advanced hematologic malignancies. *Oncotarget*. 2017 8(45):79864-79875. doi:10.18632/oncotarget.20094.

348. Brada M, Judson I, Beale P, et al. Phase I dose-escalation and pharmacokinetic study of temozolomide (SCH 52365) for refractory or relapsing malignancies. *Br J Cancer*. 1999;81:1022-1030.

349. Dhodapkar M, Rubin J, Reid JM, et al. Phase I trial of temozolomide (NSC 362856) in patients with advanced cancer. *Clin Cancer Res*. 1997;3: 1093-1100.

350. Estlin EJ, Lashford L, Ablett S, et al. Phase I study of temozolomide in paediatric patients with advanced cancer. United Kingdom Children's Cancer Study Group. *Br J Cancer*. 1998;78:652-661.

351. Hammond LA, Eckardt JR, Baker SD, et al. Phase I and pharmacokinetic study of temozolomide on a daily-for-5-days schedule in patients with advanced solid malignancies. *J Clin Oncol*. 1999;17:2604-2613.

352. Reidenberg P, Statkevich P, Judson I. Effect of food on the oral bioavailability of temozolomide, a new chemotherapeutic agent. *Proc Am Soc Clin Pharmacol Ther*. 1996;59:70.

353. Reidenberg P, Willalona M, Eckhardt G. Phase 1 clinical and pharmacokinetic study of temozolomide in advanced cancer patients stratified by extent of prior therapy. *Proc Eur Soc Med Oncol*. 1996;7:99.

354. Perry JR, Rizek P, Cashman R, Morrison M, Morrison T. Temozolomide rechallenge in recurrent malignant glioma by using a continuous temozolomide schedule: the "rescue" approach. *Cancer*. 2008;113: 2152-2157.

Platinum Analogues

Lauren Amable, Eddie Reed, and Bruce A. Chabner

Collectively, cisplatin, carboplatin, and oxaliplatin are major contributors to systemic therapy, for a very broad range of malignancies—with the exception of taxanes, the most active class of anticancer agents. Cisplatin was discovered when Rosenberg and colleagues[1,2] in a set of experiments involving *Escherichia coli* observed the dramatic inhibition of bacterial replication caused by an electric current passed through platinum electrodes on cellular replication. The current released cis-platinum chloride complex into solution. Following those seminal experiments, a rapid series of basic, preclinical, and clinical studies yielded evidence of similar activity against many human tumors and resulted in Food and Drug Administration (FDA) approval for the treatment of testicular cancer. Within 15 years, cisplatin's effectiveness in testicular, ovarian, lung, head and neck, and bladder cancer was established; new analogues (oxaliplatin) and more recent studies have established the value of this class of drugs in treatment of a broad range of the most common human cancers and numerous rarer cancers as well.

Because of the particularly troublesome toxicities of renal damage, nausea and vomiting, deafness, and peripheral neuropathy, major efforts were undertaken to identify analogues of cisplatin that have equivalent clinical effectiveness but without the toxicities of the parent compound. Carboplatin, the first such analogue to achieve widespread clinical use (Fig. 13.1), proved to be equally effective as cisplatin in ovarian cancer, lung cancer, and several other malignancies, but for unclear reasons, less effective than cisplatin in the treatment of germ cell malignancy. Carboplatin is less neurotoxic, emetogenic, and nephrotoxic than cisplatin but more myelosuppressive.

Among newer platinum analogs, only oxaliplatin (Fig. 13.1) has received FDA approval. For unclear reasons, oxaliplatin is particularly effective in colorectal cancer, in combination with 5-fluorouracil (Chapter 8). Colon cancer is a disease for which neither cisplatin nor carboplatin shows meaningful benefit. Understanding the molecular basis for these peculiarities for these three compounds could potentially unlock new insights as to how cancer cells escape the effects of DNA-damaging agents.

Chemistry

Cisplatin and carboplatin are divalent inorganic complexes and are highly water soluble and readily activated by water displacement of the chloride or carboxylate groups, respectively. Oxaliplatin is a divalent oxalate salt and not entirely cross-resistant with carboplatin and cisplatin in model tumor systems. The more complex leaving groups of carboplatin and oxaliplatin tend to reduce reactivity in aqueous solution, decrease renal toxicity and hearing loss, and the bulky cyclohexyl substitution on oxaliplatin may alter susceptibility to repair of DNA adducts, as will be explained below. The structures of the three FDA-approved analogues are shown in Figure 13.1, and important aspects of their chemistry are summarized in Table 13.1 and in previous reviews.[3] Three other platinum analogues, nedaplatin (Japan) with a glycolate leaving group, heptaplatin (Korea) with a nonleaving seven member chelate attached to the metal, and lobaplatin (China) with a complex chelate and a lactate leaving group, are marketed in single countries.[4]

The most exciting of new developments in the chemistry of platinum analogues is the utilization of nanoparticle (NP) drug delivery systems. A variety of nanoparticle carriers have been adapted to deliver platinum-based drugs to tumors with promising results including: polymeric NPs, polymeric micelles, dendrimers,

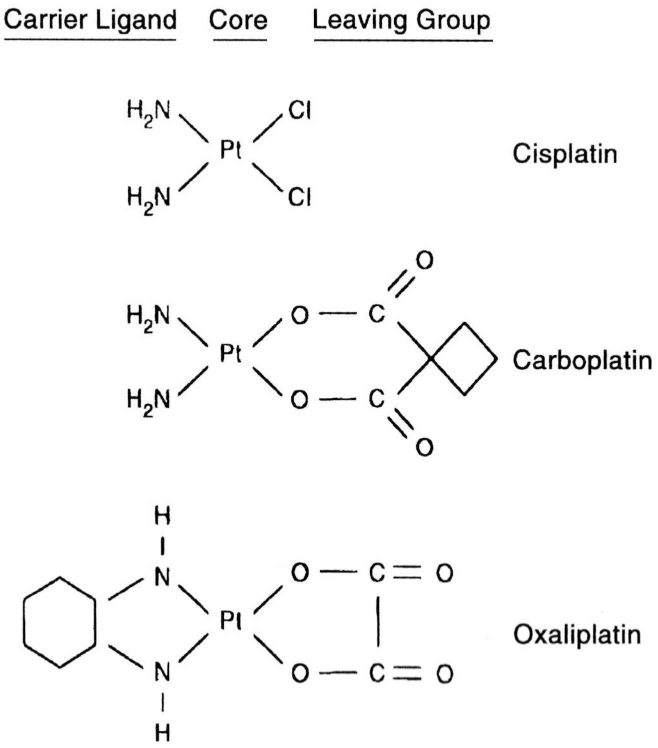

FIGURE 13.1 Two-dimensional structures are shown for cisplatin, carboplatin, and oxaliplatin. The core structures are the same based on the cis configuration of Pt(II). The leaving groups are different for the three compounds. The carrier ligand is different for oxaliplatin

TABLE

13.1 *Important issues regarding platinum chemistry*

1. Analogs in the *cis* configuration are clinically active. Analogs in the *trans* configuration are not.
2. The bond angles for the platinum core of these drugs are fixed; therefore, DNA bends to accommodate the structure of the drug.
3. The leaving group is important in platinum pharmacology, and the specific carrier ligand is important as well.
4. The aquation chemistry of the cisplatin compound suggests that either the parent or the hydroxylated form can passively penetrate cells. However, current data suggest that cisplatin, carboplatin, and oxaliplatin are actively transported into and out of the cell.
5. The aquation chemistry for oxaliplatin is similar to that of cisplatin. For carboplatin, esterase activity for the carboxylato-leaving group is necessary to generate the reactive species of the compound.
6. All clinically active platinum compounds that have been studied form bifunctional DNA adducts. This type of DNA damage appears to be responsible for the cell-killing effect of these analogs.

liposomes, nanocapsules, ferromagnetic NPs, gold NPs, carbon nanotubes, and many others.[5] The usage of nanoparticle delivery systems promotes drug accumulation in tumor while reducing toxic side effects. The accumulation is due to the enhanced permeability and retention (EPR) effect.[6] Nanoparticles and liposomes accumulate due to tumor tissue having leaky vasculature and poor lymphatic clearance.

Two cisplatin NP formulations, Lipoplatin and Nanoplatin (NC-6004), have evoked particular interest. Lipoplatin is a PEGylated liposomal cisplatin nanoparticle composed of soy phosphatidylcholine, cholesterol, dipalmitoyl phosphatidylglycerol, and methoxy-PEG-distearoyl phosphatidylethanolamine. The drug contains 9% cisplatin and 91% lipid.[7] In clinical trials, Lipoplatin accumulated more in tumor tissues compared to normal tissues, and side effects such as nephrotoxicity, neuropathy, ototoxicity, and hair loss were not observed.[8] It failed to show convincing clinical activity.

Nanoplatin, or NC-6004, is a polymeric micelle containing platinum loaded onto poly(ethylene glycol)-poly(aspartic acid) (PEG-P(Glu)).[9] Polymeric micelles contain a hydrophobic core, which provides a space to load therapeutic agents, surrounded by a hydrophilic shell to stabilize the micelle in aqueous solution. Cisplatin and the polymer are mixed at a molar ratio of 1:1, and the particle has an average diameter of 16 nm. Compared to drug alone, micelles delivered increased cisplatin to tumors and provided comparable antitumor activity.[10] Preclinical data of Nanoplatin suggested prolonged circulation in blood increased tumor accumulation resulting in tumor growth inhibition coupled with reduced nephrotoxicity and neurotoxicity.[11] Like lipoplatin, it has not shown significant clinical activity.[12]

Cellular Pharmacology

Cisplatin is able to cross cell membranes because of its simple chemistry. It is a small, rigid planar molecule. At physiologic pH of 7.4, either as the dichloride salt or with dissociation of its chlorides and their replacement by -OH molecules, the uncharged molecule diffuses into the cell (Fig. 13.2). However, work by a number of laboratories strongly suggests that simple diffusion of cisplatin across cell membranes does not fully explain transmembrane trafficking of platinum drugs.[13–17] Specific membrane transport proteins may promote influx and efflux of the drug, such as the CTR1, ATP7A, and ATP7B transporters.

Copper transporter 1, CTR1, is a significant contributor to the active uptake of platinum drugs by cells, including cisplatin, carboplatin, and oxaliplatin.[13,15] In addition, the human organic cation transporters (OCT) 1, 2, and 3 have been implicated in modulating the cellular uptake of platinum compounds, specifically as it may relate to human renal toxicity.[16,17] Cisplatin is primarily imported by OCT2, while OCT1 transports carboplatin and oxaliplatin, and OCT3 transports primarily oxaliplatin. ATPase copper transporters, ATP7A and ATP7B, are the major contributors to platinum drug efflux in cancer cells.[14]

Once inside the cell, three different fates await the platinum compound. First, it may be exported from the cell by active transport proteins. A second fate is to become reactive by displacement of the chloride groups of cisplatin, or carboxylato groups of carboplatin (Fig. 13.2). These entities rapidly bind covalently to sulfhydryl groups, such as glutathione or metallothioneins, or to methionine or cysteine amino acids on proteins. A third fate is for the activated platinum complex to react nonspecifically with several intracellular nucleophiles, including electron-rich sites on RNAs, and DNA.

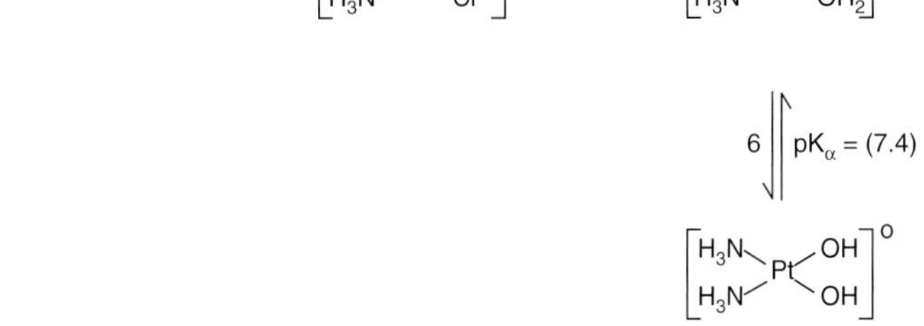

FIGURE **13.2** Aquation and hydrolysis equilibria of cisplatin. Note that reactions 3 and 6 are favored at physiologic pH and yield products that have a neutral charge and that theoretically could readily cross cell membranes. (Reprinted from Lim MC, Martin RB. Nature of cis amine Pd(II) and antitumor cis amine Pt(II) complexes in aqueous-solutions. *Inorg Nucl Chem.* 1976;38(10):1911-1914. Copyright © 1976 Elsevier. With permission.)

Through this relatively nonspecific interaction of the highly reactive platinum moiety with a range of subcellular molecules, cisplatin damages the cell. The measured affinity for RNA is greater than that for DNA, which, in turn, is greater than that for proteins. Because of transit time from the cellular membrane into the nucleus, the sum total of reactions with DNA is lower than that with intracellular protein.

Table 13.2 summarizes the relative proportions of the cellular DNA lesions formed after exposure to cisplatin, carboplatin, or oxaliplatin. The reactions with cellular DNA determine the bulk of cisplatin-related antiproliferative effects. The N7 nitrogen of deoxyguanosine is the favored site for mono-adduct formation on DNA, and this reaction leads to intrastrand cross-links. N7-d(GpG) and the N7-d(ApG) intrastrand adducts account for more than 80% of total platinum-DNA damage that forms after cisplatin exposure to isolated DNA,[18] tissue culture cells,[19,20] or isolated cells from patients in clinical settings.[21–23] In subsequent, more detailed studies, the intrastrand N7-d(GpG) and the N7-d(ApG) adducts were most clearly correlated with cell killing (Fig. 13.3).[3] These two adducts are associated with severe kinking of the DNA double helix.[24] One exceptional study found that in a Burkitt's lymphoma cell line, adduct formation with protein was correlated with cell death in a time frame that could not be explained by DNA damage.[25]

Kinking of the DNA is caused by rigid bond angles within the cisplatin molecule.[24] The DNA double helix thereby bends to accommodate the platinum adduct. This kinking is recognized and repaired by the nucleotide excision repair pathway, which involves the genes ERCC1, XPA, and others.[26–28] In contrast, most bifunctional alkylating agents have bond angles that allow the drug to bend and thereby to accommodate to the structure of the DNA. HMGBox proteins are abundant in the nucleus, have a high affinity for 1,2-d(GpG) intrastrand cross-links, and protect the adduct against repair. This finding is of particular relevance for testicular cancer treatment, as these cells express the HMGB4 isoform, perhaps accounting for the high cure rate of this malignancy.[28]

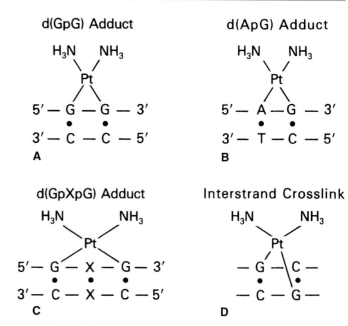

FIGURE 13.3 Bifunctional adducts of cisplatin with DNA. Lesions indicated in panels **A**, **B**, and **C** represent different intrastrand adducts, which together account for more than 90% of total platinum binding to DNA. The lesion indicated in panel **D** is the interstrand cross-link measured by alkaline elution and accounts for less than 5% of total platinum binding to DNA. See text for discussion.

Carboplatin is similar to cisplatin in most respects and is active as a clinical agent in many of the same malignancies. The major subcellular differences between these two drugs include the need for an esterase activity to release the carboxylato-leaving group of the carboplatin molecule and thereby to expose the reactive aquated arms for covalent binding to target sites. Thus, there is a delayed time frame for the formation of the specific DNA lesions, such as the N7-d(GpG) and N7-d(GpG) adducts, as compared with cisplatin.[29] For almost all matters, the subcellular behaviors of cisplatin and carboplatin appear to be the same.

Oxaliplatin is FDA approved for the treatment of colorectal cancer. The major subcellular differences between cisplatin and oxaliplatin include the carrier ligand effects involving the less reactive leaving groups of the oxaliplatin compound,[30,31] the bulkier non-leaving group, which is difficult for DNA polymerase to bypass, and differences in the rates of formation and repair of oxaliplatin-DNA damage, as compared with cisplatin.[30,32,33] One study has raised the possibility that oxaliplatin, unlike the other platinum analogues, may kills cells by inducing ribosomal stress rather than its formation of DNA adducts, although further evidence is needed to support this interesting possibility.[34] Differences in clinical pharmacology and in clinical toxicity are also discussed later in this chapter.

Mechanism(s) of Cytotoxicity

The consensus is that cisplatin and its analogs exert their cytotoxic effects by covalently binding to purine DNA bases and disrupting the normal functions of cellular DNA, blocking cell progression at the G_2M checkpoint, and inducing attempts to repair. Accumulation of strand breaks leads to apoptosis. Platinum analogs that have therapeutic activity form a preponderance of DNA intrastrand adducts as

TABLE 13.2	*Types of DNA lesions caused by cisplatin, carboplatin, and oxaliplatin*	
DNA lesion	**% of total DNA damage**	**Comment**
N7-d(GpG)-intrastrand adduct	~60	Possibly lethal to cells
N7-d(ApG)-intrastrand adduct	~30	Possibly lethal to cells
N7-d(GpXpG)-intrastrand adduct	~10	Potential lethality unclear
N7-d(X)-d(X)-interstrand cross-link	<2	Biologic importance unclear
		Levels correlate with cellular toxicity

opposed to DNA interstrand cross-links or DNA-platinum-protein cross-links, although encounter of adducts by a replication fork can convert single-strand damage to double-strand breaks.

Early studies of cisplatin and transplatin compared the relative importance of DNA damage versus protein binding in terms of causing tumor cell kill in tissue culture.[3] Some laboratories have sought to correlate tumor cell kill with one or more of the different intrastrand lesions, the N7-d(GpG) adduct or the N7-d(ApG) adduct or the N7-d(GpXpG) adduct.[30] There are conflicting reports over which lesion(s) may be more associated with the cytotoxic effects of these drugs and which lesion(s) may be more associated with the mutagenic effects of these drugs. These studies have not been definitive because of the complexity of the mix of DNA adducts after cisplatin exposure, as shown in Table 13.2. When platinum agents are allowed to react with isolated DNA or cells, or are given to animals, the proportions of the various DNA adducts are relatively constant.

Cells deficient in double-strand break repair, such as BRCA1 or BRCA2 mutant cells, and basal-type breast cancer cells (which tend to express low levels of BRCA1 RNA and are often p53 mutant), are highly sensitive to cisplatin, raising the possibility that accumulation of double-strand breaks (DSBs), as a result of attempts to repair either single-strand or double-strand cross-links, is ultimately responsible for cell death.[35] BRCA1 and BRCA2 function in the repair of double-strand breaks via the homologous recombination (HR) repair pathway. BRCA1 and BRCA2 facilitate the recruitment of the complex of proteins, such as CtIP, RAD51, ATR, and BRCA2, to the DSBs to repair the damage.[36,37] BRCA1 additionally plays several roles such as regulating BRCA2, checkpoint function, transcriptional regulation, chromatin remodeling, and ubiquitination,[38] all of which may explain the increased sensitivity to cisplatin in BRCA-deficient cells.

Cell death may occur through apoptotic or nonapoptotic pathways. The apoptotic pathways may be mediated through mismatch repair (MMR) genes,[39–42] p53,[43] and/or decreased bcl2/bax/bclX$_L$.[44,45] Overwhelming DNA damage is associated with acute, nonapoptotic cell death. Reports of experimental and clinical studies over the past three decades show that cisplatin enhances immune-mediated killing of tumor cells[3] as will be discussed below. The advent of oxaliplatin has raised questions about the effects of different carrier ligands on platinum's ability to induce cellular damage and evade DNA repair processes. Saris and colleagues[32] found that a ligand bound to the platinum core, when opposite the *cis* configuration of the reactive bonds, can exert tremendous influence on subcellular pharmacology of the drug. The carrier cyclohexyl ligand reduces DNA repair efficiency and increases cell killing.[30–33,41]

Recognition of platinum adducts by high mobility group (HMG) proteins were initially thought to promote DNA repair; however, recent studies suggest that the presence of HMG proteins delayed DNA repair by shielding the repair machinery from access to DNA lesions.[46] Alteration of HMG protein expression results in changes of cisplatin efficacy, further supporting the model of repair machinery shielding.[47] HMGB4 proteins are highly expressed in the testis and contribute to the increased responsiveness to cisplatin in testicular tumors.[47]

A difference between oxaliplatin and cisplatin or carboplatin is the relative inability of DNA polymerase alpha to perform replicative bypass over an oxaliplatin-DNA lesion as compared with a cisplatin or carboplatin-DNA lesion. DNA polymerase beta is a key protein involved in repair of the 1,2GG adduct formed by oxaliplatin; cells deficient in this enzyme are hypersensitive to oxaliplatin but not to cisplatin.[48] Thus, cells that depend on replicative bypass as a major mechanism of platinum resistance may be comparatively more sensitive to oxaliplatin than the other platinum compounds. Others have shown that the carrier ligand has substantial effects on the clinical pharmacology of platinum analogs, as will be discussed later.

Cisplatin affects the mitochondria on multiple levels. Reactive oxygen species (ROS) produced via the mitochondria are induced by cisplatin treatment, resulting in the enhancement of cytotoxicity.[49] Changes in mitochondria function[50,51] and dynamics of mitochondria fusion and fission have been implicated in cisplatin resistance. In chemoresistant cells, a higher level of mitochondria fusion was observed, and it was suggested that this change promotes cell survival.[52] Cisplatin preferentially binds mitochondrial DNA in comparison to nuclear DNA with a fourfold higher DNA-platinum adduct concentration.[53,54] The mitochondria lack NER to repair the mitochondria DNA-pt adduct damage[55] further contributing to mitochondria dysfunction. Mitochondrial damage may thus contribute to the cytotoxic action of cisplatin and repair of that damage may play a role in resistance to cisplatin- and platinum-based compounds.[56]

Platinum agents give additive or synergistic activity with a range of other anticancer agents. Cisplatin is thought to be relatively non–cell cycle-specific in terms of its cell-killing effects, although cross-links form with greatest efficiency during S-phase. It tends to synergize with agents that reduce the intracellular levels of purine and pyrimidine precursors needed for DNA replication or repair, including 5-fluorouracil[57] and gemcitabine.[58] Oxaliplatin down-regulates thymidylate synthase, perhaps adding to its beneficial interaction with fluoropyrimidines (see Chapter 8). Platinums also show additive or supraadditive cell killing with agents that alter mitosis (paclitaxel),[59] with inhibitors of DNA repair activity (PARP),[60,61] and with down-regulation or inhibition of ERCC1.[62–66] Positive interactions with interleukins,[64] inhibitors of AP-1,[66] proteasome inhibitors,[65] and topoisomerase inhibitors have been described,[67] as well as with agents from virtually every class of chemotherapy.[3]

Cisplatin is widely used as a radiation sensitizer for head and neck cancer, locally advanced lung cancers, and cervical cancer. For maximum synergy, cisplatin is usually given prior to or with radiation.[68] The mechanism of sensitization is dependent on the nonhomologous end-joining (NHEJ) repair pathway.[69,70] Exposure to radiation results in both single-strand DNA (SSB) and double-strand DNA (DSB) breaks. While cisplatin does not increase the number of DSBs, having a DNA-pt adduct near a DSB results in the complete abrogation of NHEJ repair.[71] The presence of an unrepaired DSB is catastrophic and results in cell death. Alterations in the DNA damage response (DDR) pathway additionally delay repair of DSBs induced by irradiation.[72]

In summary, the primary mechanism of cell killing for this class of compounds is covalent binding to purine bases of cellular DNA. This covalent binding leads to bending of the DNA helix at a fixed angle, with local denaturing of the DNA strand. This DNA damage is detected by components of the repair complex and is converted into a strand break. Adducts are removed and breaks are repaired primarily by the NER and double-strand break repair process. When not effectively repaired, cell killing may occur through apoptotic or nonapoptotic pathways. In clinical use, platinum compounds are highly synergistic with irradiation and with other DNA-damaging agents, perhaps as a result of their ability to overwhelm mechanisms that protect and repair DNA. The possible contribution of drug-induced, immune-mediated cell killing, which may occur in the intact host, is discussed next.

Immune Effects of Platinum Agents

The interactions of platinum derivatives with the immune system are poorly understood. In the first human clinical studies of positive immune modulation by cisplatin,[3,73,74] monocyte function in mice and in patients with epithelial ovarian cancer improved posttreatment.[73] Preclinical studies in FAS-knockout mice suggested that the ability of intraperitoneal cisplatin to effect Lewis lung tumor cell kill depending on the presence of Fas-Fas ligand interaction.[75] Cisplatin induced up-regulation of Jun/JNK, which in turn may lead to up-regulation of Fas in Fas-competent cells,[76-78] and to greater immunogenicity and greater immune-mediated cell killing. An obligatory role for CD8+ T cells, and the need for costimulatory up-regulation in cisplatin treatment of murine papillomavirus–induced tumors was suggested by interesting studies of the TC-1 and C3 tumors in mice. Checkpoint inhibitors PD-1 and PDl-1 have clear antitumor activity in a number of human tumors.

Platinum based chemotherapy enhances response to various immune therapies in experimental settings,[79-83] and impressively improved progression free survival and over-all survival when used in combination with a PD-1 checkpoint inhibitor (pembrolizumab) in non-small cell lung cancer, as compared to PD-1 alone, demonstrating that such combinations are feasible, safe, and effective, despite fears of the immunosuppressive effects of chemotherapy.[81]

Mechanisms of Resistance

The mechanisms of resistance to platinum agents have been studied most extensively for cisplatin. These are summarized in Table 13.3. Four types of pathways or mechanisms confer intrinsic or acquired resistance to platinum compounds: altered cellular accumulation of drug, cytosolic inactivation of drug, altered DNA repair/physiology, or an altered apoptotic process that results in increased tolerance to DNA damage.[84] In early studies of cisplatin resistance in cell culture models,[3,19,29] DNA repair, cytosolic inactivation, and cellular accumulation of drug contributed to the overall pattern of resistance.

Altered Cellular Accumulation

Chemically, the pH of the blood compartment is such that the redox state of cisplatin in the bloodstream favors the uptake of a neutral species of drug, from the blood into the cell. This uptake is mediated across the drug concentration gradient, from high levels in the blood to the lower levels within the cells.[3] Even though cisplatin chemistry suggests the possibility that passive forces may play a dominant role in transmembrane cellular uptake, other studies suggest a more active process. Holzer and colleagues[15] have shown that when the copper transporter CTR1 is inactivated within cells, cellular accumulation of drug is dramatically reduced. Under these conditions, cells became more resistant to platinum exposures, including cisplatin, carboplatin, and oxaliplatin in his experimental model.

TABLE 13.3	Mechanisms of cellular resistance to platinum compounds

Alterations in transmembrane cellular accumulation of drug:
- Three transmembrane carriers for cisplatin have been identified. OCT-1 (CTR1), the carnitine transporter, and copper transporters, while ATP7A and ATP7B, and certain ABC transporters contribute to drug efflux.
- Altered cellular accumulation has been associated with inhibition of a variety of membrane proteins, including Na, K-adenosine triphosphatase.

Cytosolic inactivation of drug:
- Glutathione transferase conjugation of activated platinum occurs with possible active transport out of the cell. This may occur for drug conjugated to reduced glutathione, by the multidrug resistance protein (MRP) class of adenosine triphosphate–dependent transporters.
- Metallothioneins and glutathione inactivate platinum-based drugs.
- Other sulfhydryl-containing groups, such as cysteines and methionines on proteins, inactivate drug.

DNA damage repair:
- Expression of nucleotide excision repair increases the level of drug resistance (NER; this pathway is responsible for the repair of cisplatin-DNA damage).
- Enhanced mRNA and protein expression of ERCC1, ERCC2, and other NER genes in platinum-resistant tumors.
- Defective mismatch repair (MMR) may be responsible for failure to link unrepaired DNA damage to apoptotic pathways.
- Polymerase bypass or translesional DNA synthesis is observed to occur preferentially in cisplatin-resistant cells.
- Expression of HMG proteins may shield cells from cisplatin or carboplatin adduct repair, conferring sensitivity

Resistance to apoptosis:
- Loss of p53, increased expression of EZH2, increased expression of antiapoptotic genes.

Reduced drug accumulation appears to be a consistent observation in cisplatin-resistant tumor cell lines. Active efflux of cisplatin has been described in vitro, particularly as medicated by the copper transporters, ATP7A and ATP7B,[14] as well as other proteins.[85] Overexpression of either ATP7A or ATP7B in vitro results in increased resistance to cisplatin. In several studies, increased expression of either transporter is associated with a poor response to cisplatin therapy. The role of transporters has not been confirmed in studies of clinical chemotherapy.

Cytosolic Inactivation of Drug

Proteins or peptides with increased levels of sulfhydryl groups may confer cellular resistance to cisplatin through covalent binding to the active moieties of the compound. Such molecules include glutathione[86,87] and metallothionein.[88,89] Up-regulation of either results in inactivation of cisplatin in the cytoplasm, reducing DNA damage. Binding of cisplatin to glutathione (GSH) leads to the excretion of the drug from the cell, primarily by the MRP transporters. Cytosolic inactivation of drug appears to be particularly important at high levels of platinum resistance.[3] Metallothioneins (MTs) are low molecular weight proteins that regulate the homeostasis of cellular metals. MTs bind other reactive metals, including iron, cadmium, copper, and zinc as well as cisplatin to detoxify the cell from excess metal. Several cell lines resistant to cisplatin display increased overexpression of MTs, but clinical confirmation is lacking.

DNA Repair and Drug Sensitivity/Resistance

Platinum compounds form bulky lesions with cellular DNA, which are repaired by the NER complex.[28,62] This is the same pathway that repairs DNA damage from polycyclic aromatic hydrocarbons and from ultraviolet light. There are 17 proteins involved in the DNA repairosome that repairs cisplatin-DNA adduct including ERCC1, XPA, XPF, XPB, XPD, and others.[3,28,62] Cells deficient in NER, as in cell lines established from patients with the xeroderma pigmentosa disorder, show extreme sensitivity to platinum damage, as do a subset of human ovarian cancers with inactivating mutations in the NER pathway and extreme sensitivity to cisplatin.[90,92] Of great interest is the finding that these ovarian cancers were resistant to PARP inhibitors, which are uniquely effective against tumors with defects in a different pathway, homologous recombination.

In sequence, the platinum-DNA lesion is recognized by the repairosome, the 3′ cut into the DNA strand is made 15 to 23 bases from the site of the lesion, a helicase function is implemented, and then the 5′ cut is made.[26,27] The 5′ cut is implemented by the ERCC1-XPF heterodimer, which is the last substep in the excision of cisplatin-DNA damage. Gap-filling and ligase activities follow.

ERCC1 is a useful biomarker for the activity of nucleotide excision repair. NER is the DNA repair pathway that is primarily responsible for the repair of platinum-DNA lesions. ERCC1 is up-regulated and/or down-regulated in concert with other genes involved in the NER repairosome, which include XPA, XPB, XPD, XPF, and select other NER genes. Thus, ERCC1 is highly up-regulated when the NER process is activated and is down when the NER process is relatively inactive.

The possible relationships between platinum-DNA adduct levels in tissues from cancer patients and clinical end points in those patients have been explored.[91–93] In some studies, adduct was measured with the use of an enzyme-linked immunosorbent assay that detected only a fraction of the total amount of DNA damage. In other studies, including the Amable and Reed laboratory, adduct was assayed by atomic absorbance spectrometry with Zeeman background correction and now by inductively coupled plasma-mass spectrometry (ICP-MS), which measures total DNA-bound platinum.[93,94] Measurement of DNA-platinum adducts by ICP-MS is the most sensitive method as it is able to capture platinum levels as low as part per trillion (ppt) levels. ICP-MS is very attractive when analyzing DNA-pt adduct levels in patient samples, where quantities might be limited.

Generally, platinum-DNA adduct levels in peripheral blood cell DNA parallel the adduct levels formed in tumor tissues taken from the same patients, a finding that suggest a shared competency in cellular pharmacology (transport, inactivation, DSB repair) between normal and tumor tissue. Consistent with this observation, platinum-DNA adduct levels in peripheral blood cell DNA correlated well with independent assessments of tumor response or the duration of progression-free survival: the higher the adduct level, the greater the likelihood of response. The correlation between platinum-DNA adduct levels and disease response was consistently seen using treatment programs that were totally or predominantly platinum based. As previously discussed, NER is responsible for the repair of cisplatin-DNA adduct, and ERCC1 is an essential gene in the NER pathway. The mRNA expression of ERCC1 in tumor tissues directly correlates with clinical resistance to platinum therapy in ovarian cancer,[95,96] gastric cancer,[97] colorectal cancer,[98] and lung cancer.[99,100] Up-regulation of ERCC1 and other genes in the NER process suggests increased levels of DNA repair activity, which has been clearly demonstrated in vitro,[101–103] and loss of components of the NER complex is associated with cisplatin sensitivity of ovarian cancer cells in vitro.[66,103,104]

Several studies show that other genes critical to the NER process, such as XPA, XPD (ERCC2), and others, show up-regulation of mRNA expression concurrent with clinical resistance to platinum-based therapy.[95,96,105] Among the more definitive studies, ERCC2 was clearly implicated in cisplatin resistance in bladder cancer.[105] These studies are fully consistent with a large number of in vitro studies showing a similar direct relationship between expression of components of the NER pathway and cellular resistance.

Platinum-DNA adduct repair occurs in two phases in vitro.[28] The first phase occurs over the first 6 to 8 hours after the drug exposure, during which 60% to 80% of all DNA damage is removed from the cells. The second phase occurs more slowly and may last for many hours. It is not complete after 24 hours. A similar pattern was observed in a study of the in vitro removal of platinum from the DNA of peripheral blood cells,[21] indicating that what happens in vitro parallels what happens in human patients.

The first phase of cisplatin-DNA adduct repair is predominated by transcription-coupled, or gene-specific, repair.[106–108] In this process, transcriptionally active genes are repaired first, before the rest of the genome. The quiescent parts of cellular DNA are repaired in a more leisurely fashion by the cell, taking many hours. This is a function of the three-dimensional state of DNA structure in which transcriptionally active genes are more open and can be readily accessed by the DNA repair protein machinery. Epigenetic approaches to relax and unwind chromatin structure resulted in increased adduct formation and cisplatin sensitivity.[109,110] The gene-specific repair of cisplatin-DNA damage occurs over the first 6 to 8 hours after the cisplatin exposure and is most prominent in cisplatin-resistant cells.

The importance of DNA repair to cellular and clinical resistance to platinum compounds has been confirmed by many laboratory and clinical studies. In one such clinical study, Olaussen et al.[111] showed that in patients with early-stage lung cancer, ERCC1 was useful in determining which patients would benefit from adjuvant platinum-based chemotherapy. In another important clinical study, Viguier et al.[112] showed that a specific ERCC1 codon 118 polymorphism was predictive for response to oxaliplatin-based chemotherapy in advanced colon cancer. This polymorphism is associated with reduced expression of ERCC1 mRNA and protein. These are but two of a large number of recent studies confirming the potential usefulness of ERCC1 as a clinically important biomarker for successful treatment with cisplatin, carboplatin, or oxaliplatin.[84] Such use of ERCC1 may become more important as efforts are made to avoid the toxicities of platinum-based compounds and when assessment of ERCC1 can predict the likelihood of therapeutic response. Other mechanisms of evading DNA damage may affect the outcomes of treatment with this class of drugs. Enhanced replicative bypass of platinum-DNA lesions has been suggested to be a mechanism of tumor cell resistance to platinum compounds. The presence of a DNA-pt adduct causes replication DNA polymerases to stall, requiring replacement with a translesion polymerase to continue DNA synthesis. Replication bypass of adducts involves three translation polymerases: Pol η, REV1, and Pol ζ.[113] REV1 and Pol ζ are major determinants to resistance to cisplatin, oxaliplatin, satraplatin, and picoplatin, whereas Pol η contributes to the tolerance of only cisplatin. Instability of replication forks that encounter DNA breaks may lead to apoptosis. The loss of the PTIP protein, which has the function of recruiting a nuclease to stalled forks, stabilizes damaged DNA and leads to resistance to cisplatin and other DNA-damaging agents.[114] Another mechanism of resistance arises from loss of SLFN11, a factor that suppresses DNA damage repair; silencing of SLFN11 in a patient derived xenograft model resulted from up-regulation of EZH2 and increased methylation of its target histone marker, K3K27me3.[115] Neither of these mechanisms have been demonstrated in clinical specimens.

Altered Apoptosis/Increased Tolerance to DNA Damage

Apoptosis in response to cisplatin is mediated through the MMR complex,[39–45] bcl2, MAPK pathway, p53, and NF-κB pathways[116] as previously discussed. Sensitivity to drug-induced apoptosis may be altered in cells that have inherited or acquired defects in MMR (loss of hMLH1, hMLH2, or MSH6). This altered sensitivity to apoptosis results in enhanced tumor cell survival and, therefore, greater resistance to chemotherapy. In cell lines deficient in MMR, the activity of NER may be increased, thus clouding the relationship of MSH to platinum sensitivity.

Clinical Pharmacology: Pharmacokinetics and Toxicity

The clinical pharmacology profiles of cisplatin, carboplatin, and oxaliplatin are summarized in Tables 13.4 to 13.6.[35,117,118] All three drugs are given by slow intravenous infusion, with hydration.

TABLE 13.4	Key features of cisplatin
Dosage	50 to 75 mg/m² IV every 3 to 4 wk.
	Other dosing regimens may be used in selected situations.
	Usually administered in normal saline with vigorous IV prehydration (at least 0.5 L of saline with 12.5 g of mannitol).
Mechanism of action	Covalently binds to DNA bases and disrupts DNA function.
	Toxicity may be related to DNA damage and/or protein damage.
Metabolism	Inactivated intracellularly and in the bloodstream by conjugation to sulfhydryl groups.
	Drug covalently binds to glutathione, metallothionein, and sulfhydryls on proteins.
Pharmacokinetics	After IV bolus, primary plasma $t_{1/2}$ of parent compound = 60 min.
Elimination	Approximately 25% of an IV dose is excreted from the body during the first 24 h.
	Of that portion eliminated, excretion is renal >90% and bile <10%.
	Extensive long-term protein binding has been observed in many tissues.
Drug interactions	Thiosulfates administered IV may inactivate drug systemically.
	Amifostine (WR2721) may also act to inactivate drug but preferentially in healthy tissues.
	May show enhanced efficacy, and increased toxicity, with a range of other cytotoxic agents.
Toxicity	Renal insufficiency with cation wasting.
	Nausea and vomiting.
	Peripheral neuropathy.
	Auditory impairment (high tone loss).
	Myelosuppression (thrombocytopenia > WBC > RBC).
	Visual impairment (rare).
	Hypersensitivity.
	Seizures (rare).
	Leukemia.
Precautions	Use with caution in the presence of other nephrotoxic drugs (such as aminoglycosides).
	Monitor serum electrolytes and cations (especially Mg^{2+} and Ca^{2+}) and creatinine.
	Maintain high urine flow during cisplatin administration.
	Aggressive premedication with antiemetics is recommended.
	Caution should be used if the 24-h creatinine clearance is <60 mL/min. Consideration should be given to using alternative agents such as carboplatin in this setting.

RBC, red blood cell count; $t_{1/2}$, half-life; WBC, white blood cell count.

TABLE

13.5   *Key features of carboplatin*

Dosage	Generally dosed by AUC, in mg/mL × min. Usual dosing range is 4 to 6 mg/m^2 × min.
	Calvert formula is generally used for calculating the AUC. A measured creatinine clearance is recommended.
	Calvert formula is AUC (carboplatin) = dose/(creatinine clearance + 25).
	The older dosing method is 1 mg cisplatin = 4 mg carboplatin. This approach is not recommended. AUC dosing is associated with greater patient safety, particularly with respect to myelosuppression.
Mechanism of action	Covalent binding to DNA.
Metabolism	Conversion to a DNA-reactive species occurs more quickly in cells than in IV solutions, which suggests the activity of esterases in cleavage of the dicarboxylate side group.
Pharmacokinetics	After IV bolus, $t_{1/2}$ = 1.3 to 1.7 h.
Elimination	Approximately 90% is excreted in the urine in 24 h.
Drug interactions	See cisplatin (Table 13.4).
Toxicity	Myelosuppression is more prominent than with cisplatin.
	Nausea and vomiting may occur but are much less prominent than with cisplatin.
	Nephrotoxicity can occur, particularly at higher dosages and in patients with prior renal dysfunction.
Precautions	AUC dosing is very important in the setting of preexistent renal dysfunction.

AUC, area under the concentration × time curve; $t_{1/2}$, half-life.

Both cisplatin and oxaliplatin rapidly disappear from plasma after administration, entering tissues and binding covalently to nucleophilic groups on macromolecules. Carboplatin, a more stable complex, disappears with a $t^{1/2}$ from plasma of 2 hours, the majority of a dose undergoing renal excretion.

For oxaliplatin, the volume of distribution is 50-fold greater than for cisplatin. Oxaliplatin undergoes extensive nonenzymatic conversion to reactive species. Maximum plasma concentrations reach 1 to 1.5 µg/mL for patients receiving 80 to 130 mg/m^2 doses and fall with a plasma $t^{1/2}$ of 0.288 hours. Oxaliplatin is excreted as

TABLE

13.6   *Key features of oxaliplatin*

Dosage	Up to 85 mg/m^2 every 2 wk; or up to 130 mg/m^2 every 3 wk.
	Given as a 2-, 4-, or 6-h infusion; 6-h infusions are used most commonly.
	Administer in a 5% dextrose IV solution (different from cisplatin or carboplatin)
Mechanism of action	DNA damage. May have unique properties based on unique carrier ligand. 1,2-Diaminocyclohexane carrier ligand is the nonleaving group.
Metabolism	Not fully characterized. Drug accumulates in red blood cells of humans and rats but does not accumulate in plasma (cisplatin accumulates in plasma with repeated dosing).
Pharmacokinetics	With a 4-h infusion:
	Free platinum levels decrease in a triphasic fashion.
	Terminal $t_{1/2}$ = 14 min
	Volume of distribution = 349 L
	Total clearance = 222 mL/min; renal clearance = 121 mL/min
Elimination	Renal elimination is important. Characterization in humans is not complete.
Drug interactions	Most effective in gastrointestinal malignancies, given in combination with fluorouracil analogs.
	Synergizes with antimetabolites; additional studies warranted.
Toxicity	When given with 5-fluorouracil, major toxicities include:
	Myelosuppression (neutropenia primarily).
	Diarrhea ± stomatitis.
	Peripheral neuropathy (sensory much greater than motor).
	Nausea and vomiting, mild to moderate.
	Rare toxicities: anaphylaxis, hemolytic anemia, laryngopharyngeal dysesthesias.
Precautions	Similar to those for cisplatin and carboplatin (Tables 13.4 and 13.5).

$t_{1/2}$, half-life.

low molecular weight metabolites in the urine, and less than 2% is excreted in the feces. In patients with renal dysfunction, dose reduction is not necessary if the creatinine clearance is greater than 20 mL/min.[118]

Administration

The primary consideration in administering cisplatin is the prevention of its renal toxicity. While doses vary from 20 mg/m^2 per day for 5 days to a single dose of 100 mg/m^2, the usual single doses in combination regimens are in the range of 50 to 70 mg/m^2. In the absence of saline pretreatment, the incidence of nephrotoxicity exceeds 50% for any of these doses. In the low chloride environment of the urine, the drug undergoes aquation and, in the nephron, attacks the renal epithelium. Therefore, urine volume and chloride content must be maximized to prevent renal damage. A review of hydration schemes emphasizes that a number of different strategies have been employed.[119] The key ingredient is saline prehydration, usually 1 to 2 L given 2 to 4 hours prior to drug administration, to increase chloride content in the urine and prevent drug activation, followed by saline hydration in conjunction with the drug. Diuretics, such as furosemide, and mannitol infusion have been employed to increase urine volume. Magnesium supplementation in the intravenous fluid (8 to 16 mEq) is employed in the pretreatment fluid, particularly in patients with hypomagnesemia, and with doses of cisplatin greater than 50 mg/m^2. The duration of drug infusion is usually 2 to 4 hours depending on dose. Current recommendations are summarized in Table 13.7.

While adequate pretreatment hydration must also be assured prior to carboplatin and oxaliplatin, these agents have much reduced capacity to produce renal damage. Therefore, pretreatment with 500 to 1,000 mL saline is usually sufficient for these agents. Since carboplatin is eliminated primarily by renal excretion,

its dosing is dependent on the Calvert formula: Dose (mg) = target AUC (usually 5 mg/mL × minutes) × (creatinine clearance + 25). Oxaliplatin can safely be given at full doses to patients with a creatinine clearance greater than 20 mL/min. The acute neurotoxicity of oxaliplatin is directly related to dose and to the duration of drug infusion. The more severe toxicities are seen at higher doses and with shorter infusion times. Therefore, oxaliplatin doses should not exceed 85 mg/m^2 every 2 weeks or 130 mg/m^2 every 3 weeks. The oxaliplatin infusion should always be at least over 2 hours in duration. Oxaliplatin dosing guidelines are provided in Table 13.6. When given in combination with other agents, as in the treatment of colorectal cancer, these doses should never be exceeded. A number of oxaliplatin-based combination therapy regimens are under investigation in a range of diseases.

Kidney Toxicity

Renal toxicity is common with all clinically utilized platinum analogs, and particularly so with cisplatin.[120] Although the bulk of cisplatin is eliminated by covalent binding to macromolecules, a portion of drug is filtered through the glomerulus and interacts with renal tubules. The problem is greatest with cisplatin, a more reactive molecule than the analogs. Kidney damage from carboplatin and from oxaliplatin tends to be less severe and may be subclinical in many cases. Preclinical models suggest that the proximal renal tubule is less sensitive to platinum damage than the distal tubule, although both are affected.

Renal excretory dysfunction may become evident after several cycles of therapy with cisplatin or carboplatin, even in the face of a normal serum creatinine, likely the result of tubular damage.[120] This phenomenon has been observed with a number of heavy metals, such as lead. This finding is important because drugs of other classes (such as antibiotics) may be needed by cancer patients and require adequate renal clearance.

Loss of Mg^{2+} and Ca^{2+} in the urine is a common result of platinum-related renal toxicity. The treating physician should monitor serum levels of these cations and consider their replacement during the course of treatment as needed; zinc and selenium may also become deficient. Symptomatic hypomagnesemia and hypocalcemia may result, with muscle weakness and tetany as common complaints.[121]

Because of the key role of kidney function in cisplatin administration, questions have arisen as to whether patients with only a solitary kidney can be safely treated postnephrectomy. In the presence of a normal serum creatinine, this does appear to be safe.[122]

Nausea and Vomiting

Cisplatin is clearly the most emetogenic of the platinum analogs, although severe nausea may be seen with carboplatin and with oxaliplatin.[4,118,119] Emesis was severe and persistent during the early clinical trials of cisplatin and led to drug discontinuation in many patients. Fortunately, modern antiemetic regimens have greatly decreased this toxicity. It is not clear whether this emetogenic effect is mediated primarily through the CNS or through peripheral mechanisms. However, for cisplatin in particular, the most aggressive antiemetic regimens are necessary to ensure patient comfort and patient compliance with future treatment. Premedication for nausea and vomiting should be aggressive and

TABLE 13.7	*Hydration for administration of cisplatin*
Cisplatin dose	**Hydration and administration**
<50 mg/m^2	Outpatient
	Short duration (2 to 6 h)
	2 to 4 L normal saline
	Consider potassium supplementation, per electrolyte monitoring
>50 mg/m^2	Outpatient
	Short duration (2 to 6 h)
	2 to 4 L normal saline
	Consider potassium and/or magnesium supplementation
>100 mg/m^2	As above, consider addition of mannitol

From Crona DJ, Faso A, Nishijima TF, McGraw KA, Galsky MD, Milowsky MI. A systematic review of strategies to prevent cisplatin-induced nephrotoxicity. *Oncologist.* 2017;22(5):609-19. doi:10.1634/theoncologist.2016-0319

focused on preventing the development of symptoms. Aggressive prevention can also prevent delayed nausea and vomiting.

Adequate prevention of nausea and vomiting can be ensured by following the guidelines of the 2004 Perugia International Antiemesis Consensus Conference.[123] Generally, level 4 antiemesis regimens should always be used for cisplatin-based regimens. Level 4 antiemesis regimens consist of a defined combination before and after chemotherapy. Before chemotherapy, one should administer a 5-HT3 receptor antagonist on day 1, dexamethasone (20 mg IV on day 1, with repeated doses orally on days 2 to 4, as necessary), and aprepitant (125 mg 1 hour before cisplatin on day 1, plus 80 mg once daily on the mornings of days 2 and 3). Newer regimens incorporating NK-1 antagonists such as netupitant, with palonsetron and dexamethoasone may further improve control of emesis.

For carboplatin or for oxaliplatin, level 3 antiemesis, consisting of a 5-HT3 receptor antagonist and dexamethasone prior to and after chemotherapy, is indicated.[117] However, for some patients, level 4 antiemesis therapy will be needed, even for carboplatin and for oxaliplatin.

Neurotoxicity

Neurotoxicity is a major side effect of cisplatin and is a frequent problem with carboplatin and oxaliplatin.[117,118] Platinum drugs primarily affect the dorsal root ganglia, and adducts can be identified in this tissue.[124,125] Clinical neurotoxicity can be manifested primarily as a peripheral sensory neuropathy with auditory impairment, and, much less commonly, spinal cord degeneration (Lhermitte's syndrome), visual disturbances and cortical blindness, seizures, papilledema, and retrobulbar neuritis. The presentation of neurotoxicity varies among the agents. While cisplatin and carboplatin ordinarily cause a progressive sensory neuropathy, with numbness and tingling of extremities, paresthesia of digits, and loss of ankle reflexes, oxaliplatin may lead to acute transient paresthesia in the distal extremities and throat pain (laryngopharyngeal dysesthesia) associated with swallowing of cold liquids, and a chronic, progressive sensory neuropathy. Symptoms of neurotoxicity are associated with conduction defects upon peripheral nerve testing. The majority of patients receiving these drugs for multiple cycles will report neuropathic symptoms. Oxaliplatin generates a chronic sensory peripheral neurotoxicity that is associated with cumulative platinum dose. Unlike the neurotoxicity of carboplatin and cisplatin, oxaliplatin-induced neurotoxicity is usually fully reversible over 3 to 4 months after stopping the drug. Attempts to reverse or prevent platinum analogue neuropathy have been largely unsuccessful. Several exhaustive reviews have concluded that there is no convincing evidence for the myriad of drugs, including nerve growth factor, sulfhydryls, Mg^{2+}, antioxidants, vitamins, or ion channel modulators.[125–127] Neither has a pharmacogenomic study revealed a relationship between variants in ion channels, DNA repair pathways, and drug transporters with neurotoxicity.[125] Perhaps, the greatest interest is in amifostine, a sulfhydryl known to modify renal toxicity by conjugation with activated cisplatin, but concerns linger as to the potential reversal of the drugs' antitumor effect. For example, one study assessed the effect of vitamin B_6 on preventing peripheral neuropathy in patients with ovarian cancer who received platinum-based combination chemotherapy.[128] The group randomized to receive vitamin B_6 had significantly less toxicity than the similarly treated group that did not receive vitamin B_6. However, the

group receiving vitamin B_6 also had a significantly reduced response rate and a significantly reduced survival. Thus, neurotoxicity, when severe, is usually managed by dose reductions and/or dose delays.

Myelosuppression

Trilineage cumulative myelosuppression is commonly seen with cisplatin and with carboplatin but less so with oxaliplatin. Cisplatin causes more thrombocytopenia than leukopenia, while both thrombocytopenia and leukopenia are common after carboplatin. Leukopenia can be ameliorated by granulocyte colony–stimulating factor, and anemia responds to erythropoietin. Platinum-based therapy of ovarian cancer is associated with a fourfold increase in the risk of developing acute myelogenous leukemia.[129] Carboplatin and cisplatin have been associated with secondary AML.

Ototoxicity

Auditory impairment can be overt, with clinically dramatic reductions in auditory acuity after several cycles of cisplatin-based therapy, or they can be more subtle. Some patients may complain of the loss of the ability to filter out extraneous noises during a conversation, for example, in a restaurant. High-frequency tones (4,000 to 8,000 Hz) are most affected.[130] Severe ototoxicity appears to occur less frequently with carboplatin or with oxaliplatin. A clinical trial evaluating the protective effects of sodium thiosulfate against hearing loss in children treated with cisplatin has yielded initial positive results, and awaits confirmatory studies.[131]

Acute Hypersensitivity

Acute hypersensitivity reactions, including IgE-mediated anaphylaxis (facial edema, bronchospasm, tachycardia, hypotension), occur in 10% to 15% of patients who are treated with any of the three platinum compounds, usually after the seventh or eighth exposure to the drug. If treatment with platinum-based therapy is of crucial importance, desensitization may be attempted using slow infusions of dilutions of the clinical formulation (1:1,000, then 1:100, and lower dilutions as tolerated until the infusion is completed). This approach is successful in up to 50% of patients.[61] Rarely, hemolytic anemia can be seen with drugs in this class. Life-threatening acute hypersensitivity may be problematic with carboplatin or with cisplatin. One should be alert to this possibility for any patient who is being retreated with a new round of 6 monthly treatments. It is not clear to what extent this risk may exist with oxaliplatin.

Mild forms of hypersensitivity may be treated with corticosteroid and antihistamine pretreatment and with a longer period of drug infusion.[61]

Clinical Concepts of Platinum Resistance

In the treatment of gynecologic malignancies, specifically in ovarian cancer, recurrent disease after carboplatin treatment, usually with paclitaxel, may be either platinum sensitive or platinum resistant.[132,133] If a patient with ovarian cancer is more than 2 years out from the most recent dose of platinum (having responded to that therapy), there is a greater than 70% likelihood that the disease will respond to retreatment with cisplatin- or carboplatin-based therapy.

The percentage of patients who will respond decreases with the shortening of the disease-free period. Patients who have disease recurrence within the first 6 months after the most recent dose of platinum have a low likelihood of response to retreatment with cisplatin or carboplatin and are considered to have platinum-resistant disease. This concept is firmly established for cases of epithelial ovarian cancer. The applicability of this concept to other diseases commonly treated with platinum-based therapy is uncertain.

As discussed above, some clinicians are convinced that clinical treatment decisions can be made based on whether a tumor specimen expresses detectable levels of ERCC1/ERCC2 protein or not.[111] If ERCC1/2 protein is not detected in the lung cancer specimen, these tumors are likely platinum sensitive. If ERCC1/2 protein is easily detected, a nonplatinum regimen is utilized instead. These tumors are likely to be platinum resistant.

Common Clinical Uses

The platinum compounds constitute the mainstay of therapy for a wide range of malignancies. This includes potentially curative therapies for advanced-stage testicular and ovarian germ cell tumors, and epithelial ovarian cancer; platinum-based regimens are commonly employed for upper aerodigestive tumors, urinary bladder cancers, and small cell and non–small cell lung cancer. Effective oxaliplatin-based therapies also are in place for advanced stages and for adjuvant therapy of colorectal cancer. Cisplatin, in conjunction with radiation, is curative for a significant subset of locally advanced head and neck malignancies and cervical cancer. There is a rapidly growing interest in cisplatin as an effective agent in BRCA1 and BRCA2 mutant breast cancer and in triple negative (HER2/neu, estrogen receptor, and progesterone receptor-negative) breast cancers, which share similar gene expression profiles and exhibit striking clinical sensitivity to cisplatin as neoadjuvant chemotherapy.[134,135] Eighteen of twenty-eight (64%) of triple-negative patients responded partially or completely to single-agent cisplatin, including 2 of 2 complete responses in BRCA1 mutant tumors,[134] while 10 of 12 BRCA1 mutant tumors responded completely to cisplatin in a second neoadjuvant trial.[135] Whether the basis for this sensitivity is a common underlying defect in double-strand break repair has not been established, but the hypothesis is intriguing. Cisplatin-based regimens are now a frequently used alternative in neoadjuvant therapy of triple-negative breast cancer and in metastatic triple-negative disease.[136]

Table 13.8 is a summary of the current use of platinum analogs in several major malignancies. An extensive review of the data is beyond the scope of this text but is easily obtained in major texts, or online. Generally, in most circumstances where the cisplatin and carboplatin have been tested in phase III trials, cisplatin is clearly the more toxic agent. Cisplatin commonly causes renal toxicity, neurotoxicity, auditory toxicity, and a range of other side effects. That said, there are several diseases where cisplatin remains the mainstay of therapy because of the strong advantage in clinical efficacy. Those diseases include testicular, bladder, small cell lung, esophageal, gastric, basal-type breast, and cervical cancer. In several of these malignancies (cervix, head and neck), cisplatin's utility is due in part to its role as a radiation sensitizer. In non–small cell lung cancer and in head and neck cancers, cisplatin and carboplatin are both highly effective.

In ovarian cancer, cisplatin and carboplatin are viewed as having equivalent clinical efficacy, with carboplatin associated with a much lower rate of observed toxicities. For this reason, carboplatin has supplanted cisplatin in this disease. In colorectal cancer, the level of efficacy seen for oxaliplatin in phase II clinical trials far exceeded the historical phase II data for cisplatin and carboplatin. Its lack of dependence on MMR may account for this difference. Oxaliplatin is, therefore, considered much more efficacious in this disease than the other two compounds, even though direct comparisons are mostly lacking. Oxaliplatin-fluorouracil-leucovorin (FOLFOX) combinations are increasingly used in upper gastro-intestinal malignancy, often with irinotecan (FOLFIRINOX).

A better understanding of the molecular processes that underlie the clinical differences between cisplatin, carboplatin, and oxaliplatin and mechanisms of resistance to these agents may open the door for the development of more effective regimens in this class, with an even better therapeutic index and broader efficacy.

TABLE

13.8   *Disease comparisons of platinum analogues*

Ovarian cancer	Prospective randomized trials showed clinical equivalency for cisplatin and carboplatin. Cisplatin was more toxic.
Testicular cancer	Prospective randomized trials showed clinical superiority for cisplatin combinations over carboplatin combinations.
Non–small cell lung cancer	Meta-analyses suggest that cisplatin-based regimens MAY offer improved efficacy over carboplatin-based regimens.
Small cell lung cancer	Recent randomized trials suggest that carboplatin-based regimens may have equal efficacy and less toxicity.
Colorectal cancer	Phase II data for oxaliplatin are strongly superior over historical phase II data for cisplatin or carboplatin.
Bladder cancer	Prospective randomized trials showed clinical superiority for cisplatin combinations over carboplatin combinations.
Cervix cancer	Cisplatin is optimal radiosensitizer. Carboplatin is active. Oxaliplatin is much less active than cisplatin or carboplatin.
Gastric cancer	Cisplatin-based regimens appear superior. Oxaliplatin-based regimens may be equivalent to cisplatin-based regimens. Carboplatin less active.
Esophageal cancer	Cisplatin is optimal radiosensitizer. Carboplatin is active. Generally, cisplatin/5-FU is used concurrent with radiation.
Head and neck cancers	Cisplatin is optimal radiosensitizer. Carboplatin is active.

References

1. Rosenberg B, Van Camp L, Krigas T. Inhibition of cell division in Escherichia coli by electrolysis products from a platinum electrode. *Nature.* 1965;205:698-699.

2. Rosenberg B, Van Camp L, Trosko JE, Mansour VH. Platinum compounds: a new class of potent antitumour agents. *Nature.* 1969;222(5191):385-386.

3. Reed E. Cisplatin and analogs. In: Chabner B, Longo D, eds. *Cancer Chemotherapy and Biotherapy: Principles and Practice.* 3rd ed. Philadelphia, PA: Lippincott Williams & Wilkins; 2001:447-465.

4. Johnstone TC, Suntharalingam K, Lippard SJ. The next generation of platinum drugs: targeted Pt(II) agents, nanoparticle delivery, and Pt(IV) prodrugs. *Chem Rev.* 2016;116(5):3436-3486. doi:10.1021/acs.chemrev.5b00597.

5. Duan X, He C, Kron SJ, Lin W. Nanoparticle formulations of cisplatin for cancer therapy. *Wiley Interdiscip Rev Nanomed Nanobiotechnol.* 2016;8(5):776-791. doi:10.1002/wnan.1390.

6. Maeda H, Bharate GY, Daruwalla J. Polymeric drugs for efficient tumor-targeted drug delivery based on EPR-effect. *Eur J Pharm Biopharm.* 2009;71(3):409-419. doi:10.1016/j.ejpb.2008.11.010.

7. Boulikas T. Clinical overview on Lipoplatin: a successful liposomal formulation of cisplatin. *Expert Opin Investig Drugs.* 2009;18(8):1197-1218. doi:10.1517/13543780903114168.

8. Jehn CF, Boulikas T, Kourvetaris A, Kofla G, Possinger K, Luftner D. First safety and response results of a randomized phase III study with liposomal platin in the treatment of advanced squamous cell carcinoma of the head and neck (SCCHN). *Anticancer Res.* 2008;28(6B):3961-3964.

9. Yue Z, Cao Z. Current strategy for cisplatin delivery. *Curr Cancer Drug Targets.* 2016;16(6):480-488.

10. Nishiyama N, Kato Y, Sugiyama Y, Kataoka K. Cisplatin-loaded polymer-metal complex micelle with time-modulated decaying property as a novel drug delivery system. *Pharm Res.* 2001;18(7):1035-1041.

11. Uchino H, Matsumura Y, Negishi T, et al. Cisplatin-incorporating polymeric micelles (NC-6004) can reduce nephrotoxicity and neurotoxicity of cisplatin in rats. *Br J Cancer.* 2005;93(6):678-687. doi:10.1038/sj.bjc.6602772.

12. Plummer R, Wilson RH, Calvert H, et al. A Phase I clinical study of cisplatin-incorporated polymeric micelles (NC-6004) in patients with solid tumours. *Br J Cancer.* 2011;104(4):593-598. doi:10.1038/bjc.2011.6.

13. Kruh GD. Lustrous insights into cisplatin accumulation: copper transporters. *Clin Cancer Res.* 2003;9(16 Pt 1):5807-5809.

14. Samimi G, Katano K, Holzer AK, Safaei R, Howell SB. Modulation of the cellular pharmacology of cisplatin and its analogs by the copper exporters ATP7A and ATP7B. *Mol Pharmacol.* 2004;66(1):25-32. doi:10.1124/mol.66.1.25.

15. Holzer AK, Manorek GH, Howell SB. Contribution of the major copper influx transporter CTR1 to the cellular accumulation of cisplatin, carboplatin, and oxaliplatin. *Mol Pharmacol.* 2006;70(4):1390-1394. doi:10.1124/mol.106.022624.

16. Zhang S, Lovejoy KS, Shima JE, et al. Organic cation transporters are determinants of oxaliplatin cytotoxicity. *Cancer Res.* 2006;66(17):8847-8857. doi:10.1158/0008-5472.CAN-06-0769.

17. Ciarimboli G, Ludwig T, Lang D, et al. Cisplatin nephrotoxicity is critically mediated via the human organic cation transporter 2. *Am J Pathol.* 2005;167(6):1477-1484. doi:10.1016/S0002-9440(10)61234-5.

18. Eastman A. Reevaluation of interaction of cis-dichloro(ethylenediamine)platinum(II) with DNA. *Biochemistry.* 1986;25(13):3912-3915.

19. Eastman A, Schulte N, Sheibani N, Sorenson C. Mechanisms of resistance to platinum drugs. In: Nicolini M, ed. *Platinum and Other Metal Coordination Compounds in Cancer Chemotherapy.* Boston, MA: Springer; 1988:178-196.

20. Fichtinger-Schepman AM, van der Veer JL, den Hartog JH, Lohman PH, Reedijk J. Adducts of the antitumor drug cis-diamminedichloroplatinum(II) with DNA: formation, identification, and quantitation. *Biochemistry.* 1985; 24(3):707-713.

21. Fichtinger-Schepman AM, van Oosterom AT, Lohman PH, Berends F. cis-Diamminedichloroplatinum(II)-induced DNA adducts in peripheral leukocytes from seven cancer patients: quantitative immunochemical detection of the adduct induction and removal after a single dose of cis-diamminedichloroplatinum(II). *Cancer Res.* 1987;47(11):3000-3004.

22. Fichtinger-Schepman AM, van Oosterom AT, Lohman PH, Berends F. Interindividual human variation in cisplatinum sensitivity, predictable in an in vitro assay? *Mutat Res.* 1987;190(1):59-62.

23. Fichtinger-Schepman AM, van Dijk-Knijnenburg HC, van der Velde-Visser SD, Berends F, Baan RA. Cisplatin- and carboplatin-DNA adducts: is PT-AG the cytotoxic lesion? *Carcinogenesis.* 1995;16(10):2447-2453.

24. Gelasco A, Lippard SJ. NMR solution structure of a DNA dodecamer duplex containing a cis-diammineplatinum(II) d(GpG) intrastrand cross-link, the major adduct of the anticancer drug cisplatin. *Biochemistry.* 1998;37(26): 9230-9239. doi:10.1021/bi973176v.

25. Ducore JM, Erickson LC, Zwelling LA, Laurent G, Kohn KW. Comparative studies of DNA cross-linking and cytotoxicity in Burkitt's lymphoma cell lines treated with cis-diamminedichloroplatinum(II) and L-phenylalanine mustard. *Cancer Res.* 1982;42(3):897-902.

26. Sancar A. Mechanisms of DNA excision repair. *Science.* 1994;266(5193):1954-1956.

27. de Laat WL, Jaspers NG, Hoeijmakers JH. Molecular mechanism of nucleotide excision repair. *Genes Dev.* 1999;13(7):768-785.

28. Reed E. Platinum-DNA adduct, nucleotide excision repair and platinum based anti-cancer chemotherapy. *Cancer Treat Rev.* 1998;24(5):331-344.

29. Micetich KC, Barnes D, Erickson LC. A comparative study of the cytotoxicity and DNA-damaging effects of cis-(diammino)(1,1-cyclobutanedicarboxylato)-platinum(II) and cis-diamminedichloroplatinum(II) on L1210 cells. *Cancer Res.* 1985;45(9):4043-4047.

30. Reardon JT, Vaisman A, Chaney SG, Sancar A. Efficient nucleotide excision repair of cisplatin, oxaliplatin, and Bis-aceto-ammine-dichloro-cyclohexylamine-platinum(IV) (JM216) platinum intrastrand DNA diadducts. *Cancer Res.* 1999;59(16):3968-3971.

31. Luo FR, Wyrick SD, Chaney SG. Cytotoxicity, cellular uptake, and cellular biotransformations of oxaliplatin in human colon carcinoma cells. *Oncol Res.* 1998;10(11-12):595-603.

32. Saris CP, van de Vaart PJ, Rietbroek RC, Blommaert FA. In vitro formation of DNA adducts by cisplatin, lobaplatin and oxaliplatin in calf thymus DNA in solution and in cultured human cells. *Carcinogenesis.* 1996; 17(12):2763-2769.

33. Raymond E, Faivre S, Chaney S, Woynarowski J, Cvitkovic E. Cellular and molecular pharmacology of oxaliplatin. *Mol Cancer Ther.* 2002;1(3):227-235.

34. Bruno PM, Liu Y, Park GY, et al. A subset of platinum-containing chemotherapeutic agents kills cells by inducing ribosome biogenesis stress. *Nat Med.* 2017;23(4):461-471. doi:10.1038/nm.4291.

35. Rottenberg S, Jaspers JE, Kersbergen A, et al. High sensitivity of BRCA1-deficient mammary tumors to the PARP inhibitor AZD2281 alone and in combination with platinum drugs. *Proc Natl Acad Sci U S A.* 2008;105(44):17079-17084. doi:10.1073/pnas.0806092105.

36. Chen L, Nievera CJ, Lee AY, Wu X. Cell cycle-dependent complex formation of BRCA1.CtIP.MRN is important for DNA double-strand break repair. *J Biol Chem.* 2008;283(12):7713-7720. doi:10.1074/jbc.M710245200.

37. Jensen RB, Carreira A, Kowalczykowski SC. Purified human BRCA2 stimulates RAD51-mediated recombination. *Nature.* 2010;467(7316):678-683. doi:10.1038/nature09399.

38. Murphy CG, Moynahan ME. BRCA gene structure and function in tumor suppression: a repair-centric perspective. *Cancer J.* 2010;16(1):39-47. doi:10.1097/PPO.0b013e3181cf0204.

39. Aebi S, Fink D, Gordon R, et al. Resistance to cytotoxic drugs in DNA mismatch repair-deficient cells. *Clin Cancer Res.* 1997;3(10):1763-1767.

40. Drummond JT, Anthoney A, Brown R, Modrich P. Cisplatin and adriamycin resistance are associated with MutLalpha and mismatch repair deficiency in an ovarian tumor cell line. *J Biol Chem.* 1996;271(33):19645-19648.

41. Nehme A, Baskaran R, Nebel S, et al. Induction of JNK and c-Abl signalling by cisplatin and oxaliplatin in mismatch repair-proficient and -deficient cells. *Br J Cancer.* 1999;79(7-8):1104-1110. doi:10.1038/sj.bjc.6690176.

42. Vaisman A, Varchenko M, Umar A, et al. The role of hMLH1, hMSH3, and hMSH6 defects in cisplatin and oxaliplatin resistance: correlation with replicative bypass of platinum-DNA adducts. *Cancer Res.* 1998;58(16):3579-3585.

43. Siemer S, Ornskov D, Guerra B, Boldyreff B, Issinger OG. Determination of mRNA, and protein levels of p53, MDM2 and protein kinase CK2 subunits in F9 cells after treatment with the apoptosis-inducing drugs cisplatin and carboplatin. *Int J Biochem Cell Biol.* 1999;31(6):661-670.

44. Arriola EL, Rodriguez-Lopez AM, Hickman JA, Chresta CM. Bcl-2 over-expression results in reciprocal downregulation of Bcl-X(L) and sensitizes human testicular germ cell tumours to chemotherapy-induced apoptosis. *Oncogene.* 1999;18(7):1457-1464. doi:10.1038/sj.onc.1202420.

45. Henkels KM, Turchi JJ. Cisplatin-induced apoptosis proceeds by caspase-3-dependent and -independent pathways in cisplatin-resistant and -sensitive human ovarian cancer cell lines. *Cancer Res.* 1999;59(13):3077-3083.

46. Huang JC, Zamble DB, Reardon JT, Lippard SJ, Sancar A. HMG-domain proteins specifically inhibit the repair of the major DNA adduct of the anti-cancer drug cisplatin by human excision nuclease. *Proc Natl Acad Sci U S A.* 1994;91(22):10394-10398.

47. Park S, Lippard SJ. Binding interaction of HMGB4 with cisplatin-modified DNA. *Biochemistry.* 2012;51(34):6728-6737. doi:10.1021/bi300649v.

48. Yang J, Parsons J, Nicolay NH, et al. Cells deficient in the base excision repair protein, DNA polymerase beta, are hypersensitive to oxaliplatin che-motherapy. *Oncogene.* 2010;29(3):463-468. doi:10.1038/onc.2009.327.

49. Marullo R, Werner E, Degtyareva N, et al. Cisplatin induces a mitochondrial-ROS response that contributes to cytotoxicity depending on mitochondrial redox status and bioenergetic functions. *PLoS One.* 2013;8(11):e81162. doi:10.1371/journal.pone.0081162.

50. Yadav N, Chandra D. Mitochondrial and postmitochondrial survival signaling in cancer. *Mitochondrion.* 2014;16:18-25. doi:10.1016/j.mito.2013.11.005

51. Shin DH, Choi YJ, Park JW. SIRT1 and AMPK mediate hypoxia-induced resistance of non-small cell lung cancers to cisplatin and doxorubicin. *Cancer Res.* 2014;74(1):298-308. doi:10.1158/0008-5472.CAN-13-2620.

52. Kong B, Tsuyoshi H, Orisaka M, Shieh DB, Yoshida Y, Tsang BK. Mitochondrial dynamics regulating chemoresistance in gynecological can-cers. *Ann NY Acad Sci.* 2015;1350:1-16. doi:10.1111/nyas.12883.

53. Olivero OA, Semino C, Kassim A, Lopez-Larraza DM, Poirier MC. Preferential binding of cisplatin to mitochondrial DNA of Chinese hamster ovary cells. *Mutat Res.* 1995;346(4):221-230.

54. Giurgiovich AJ, Diwan BA, Olivero OA, Anderson LM, Rice JM, Poirier MC. Elevated mitochondrial cisplatin-DNA adduct levels in rat tissues after transplacental cisplatin exposure. *Carcinogenesis.* 1997;18(1):93-96.

55. Olivero OA, Chang PK, Lopez-Larraza DM, Semino-Mora MC, Poirier MC. Preferential formation and decreased removal of cisplatin-DNA adducts in Chinese hamster ovary cell mitochondrial DNA as compared to nuclear DNA. *Mutat Res.* 1997;391(1-2):79-86.

56. Marrache S, Pathak RK, Dhar S. Detouring of cisplatin to access mito-chondrial genome for overcoming resistance. *Proc Natl Acad Sci U S A.* 2014;111(29):10444-10449. doi:10.1073/pnas.1405244111.

57. Rothenberg ML, Oza AM, Bigelow RH, et al. Superiority of oxaliplatin and fluorouracil-leucovorin compared with either therapy alone in patients with progressive colorectal cancer after irinotecan and fluorouracil-leucovorin: interim results of a phase III trial. *J Clin Oncol.* 2003;21(11):2059-2069. doi:10.1200/JCO.2003.11.126.

58. Villella J, Marchetti D, Odunsi K, Rodabaugh K, Driscoll DL, Lele S. Response of combination platinum and gemcitabine chemotherapy for recurrent epithelial ovarian carcinoma. *Gynecol Oncol.* 2004;95(3):539-545. doi:10.1016/j.ygyno.2004.07.056.

59. Engblom P, Rantanen V, Kulmala J, Helenius H, Grenman S. Additive and supra-additive cytotoxicity of cisplatin-taxane combinations in ovarian carcinoma cell lines. *Br J Cancer.* 1999;79(2):286-292. doi:10.1038/sj.bjc.6690046.

60. Donawho CK, Luo Y, Luo Y, et al. ABT-888, an orally active poly(ADP-ribose) polymerase inhibitor that potentiates DNA-damaging agents in preclinical tumor models. *Clin Cancer Res.* 2007;13(9):2728-2737. doi:10.1158/1078-0432.CCR-06-3039.

61. Lenz HJ. Management and preparedness for infusion and hypersensitivity reac-tions. *Oncologist.* 2007;12(5):601-609. doi:10.1634/theoncologist.12-5-601.

62. Altaha R, Liang X, Yu JJ, Reed E. Excision repair cross complement-ing-group 1: gene expression and platinum resistance. *Int J Mol Med.* 2004;14(6):959-970.

63. Li Q, Tsang B, Bostick-Bruton F, Reed E. Modulation of excision repair cross complementation group 1 (ERCC-1) mRNA expression by phar-macological agents in human ovarian carcinoma cells. *Biochem Pharmacol.* 1999;57(4):347-353.

64. Li Q, Bostick-Bruton F, Reed E. Effect of interleukin-1 alpha and tumour necrosis factor-alpha on cisplatin-induced ERCC-1 mRNA expression

in a human ovarian carcinoma cell line. *Anticancer Res.* 1998;18(4A):2283-2287.

65. Mimnaugh EG, Yunbam MK, Li Q, et al. Prevention of cisplatin-DNA adduct repair and potentiation of cisplatin-induced apoptosis in ovarian carcinoma cells by proteasome inhibitors. *Biochem Pharmacol.* 2000;60(9):1343-1354.

66. Bonovich M, Olive M, Reed E, O'Connell B, Vinson C. Adenoviral deliv-ery of A-FOS, an AP-1 dominant negative, selectively inhibits drug resis-tance in two human cancer cell lines. *Cancer Gene Ther.* 2002;9(1):62-70. doi:10.1038/sj.cgt.7700409.

67. von Knethen A, Lotero A, Brune B. Etoposide and cisplatin induced apoptosis in activated RAW 264.7 macrophages is attenuated by cAMP-induced gene expression. *Oncogene.* 1998;17(3):387-394. doi:10.1038/sj.onc.1201926.

68. Gorodetsky R, Levy-Agababa F, Mou X, Vexler AM. Combination of cispla-tin and radiation in cell culture: effect of duration of exposure to drug and timing of irradiation. *Int J Cancer.* 1998;75(4):635-42.

69. Myint WK, Ng C, Raaphorst GP. Examining the non-homologous repair process following cisplatin and radiation treatments. *Int J Radiat Biol.* 2002;78(5):417-24. doi:10.1080/09553000110113047.

70. Dolling JA, Boreham DR, Brown DL, Mitchel RE, Raaphorst GP. Modulation of radiation-induced strand break repair by cisplatin in mammalian cells. *Int J Radiat Biol.* 1998;74(1):61-9.

71. Boeckman HJ, Trego KS, Turchi JJ. Cisplatin sensitizes cancer cells to ion-izing radiation via inhibition of nonhomologous end joining. *Mol Cancer Res.* 2005;3(5):277-285. doi:10.1158/1541-7786.MCR-04-0032.

72. Sears CR, Cooney SA, Chin-Sinex H, Mendonca MS, Turchi JJ. DNA damage response (DDR) pathway engagement in cisplatin radiosensitization of non-small cell lung cancer. *DNA Repair (Amst).* 2016;40:35-46. doi:10.1016/j.dnarep.2016.02.004.

73. Kleinerman ES, Zwelling LA, Howser D, et al. Defective monocyte killing in patients with malignancies and restoration of function during chemother-apy. *Lancet.* 1980;2(8204):1102-1105.

74. Kleinerman ES, Zwelling LA, Muchmore AV. Enhancement of naturally occurring human spontaneous monocyte-mediated cytotoxicity by cis-diamminedichloroplatinum(II). *Cancer Res.* 1980;40(9):3099-3102.

75. Merritt RE, Mahtabifard A, Yamada RE, Crystal RG, Korst RJ. Cisplatin augments cytotoxic T-lymphocyte-mediated antitumor immunity in poorly immunogenic murine lung cancer. *J Thorac Cardiovasc Surg.* 2003;126(5):1609-1617. doi:10.1016/S0022.

76. Gupta S, Natarajan R, Payne SG, et al. Deoxycholic acid activates the c-Jun N-terminal kinase pathway via FAS receptor activation in primary hepato-cytes. Role of acidic sphingomyelinase-mediated ceramide generation in FAS receptor activation. *J Biol Chem.* 2004;279(7):5821-5828. doi:10.1074/jbc.M310979200.

77. Schwabe RF, Uchinami H, Qian T, Bennett BL, Lemasters JJ, Brenner DA. Differential requirement for c-Jun NH2-terminal kinase in TNFalpha- and Fas-mediated apoptosis in hepatocytes. *FASEB J.* 2004;18(6):720-722. doi:10.1096/fj.03-0771fje.

78. Shangary S, Lerner EC, Zhan Q, Corey SJ, Smithgall TE, Baskaran R. Lyn regulates the cell death response to ultraviolet radiation through c-Jun N terminal kinase-dependent Fas ligand activation. *Exp Cell Res.* 2003;289(1):67-76.

79. Wilailak S, Dangprasert S, Srisupundit S. Phase I clinical trial of chemoim-munotherapy in combination with radiotherapy in stage IIIB cervical cancer patients. *Int J Gynecol Cancer.* 2003;13(5):652-656.

80. Beyranvand Nejad E, van der Sluis TC, van Duikeren S, et al. Tumor eradica-tion by cisplatin is sustained by CD80/86-mediated costimulation of CD8+ T Cells. *Cancer Res.* 2016;76(20):6017-6029. doi:10.1158/0008-5472.CAN-16-0881.

81. Gandhi L, Rodriquez-Abreu D, Gadgeel S, et al. Pembrolizumab plus che-motherapy in metastatic non-small-cell lung cancer. *New Engl J Med.* 2018; doi:10.1056/NEJMoa1801005.

82. Lens MB, Eisen TG. Systemic chemotherapy in the treatment of malig-nant melanoma. *Expert Opin Pharmacother.* 2003;4(12):2205-2211. doi:10.1517/14656566.4.12.2205.

83. Ohtsukasa S, Okabe S, Yamashita H, Iwai T, Sugihara K. Increased expression of CEA and MHC class I in colorectal cancer cell lines exposed to chemo-therapy drugs. *J Cancer Res Clin Oncol.* 2003;129(12):719-726. doi:10.1007/s00432-003-0492-0.

84. Amable L. Cisplatin resistance and opportunities for precision medicine. *Pharmacol Res.* 2016;106:27-36. doi:10.1016/j.phrs.2016.01.001.

85. Burger H, Loos WJ, Eechoute K, Verweij J, Mathijssen RH, Wiemer EA. Drug transporters of platinum-based anticancer agents and their clinical significance. *Drug Resist Updat.* 2011;14(1):22-34. doi:10.1016/j.drup.2010.12.002.

86. Godwin AK, Meister A, O'Dwyer PJ, Huang CS, Hamilton TC, Anderson ME. High resistance to cisplatin in human ovarian cancer cell lines is associated with marked increase of glutathione synthesis. *Proc Natl Acad Sci U S A.* 1992;89(7):3070-3074.

87. Hosking LK, Whelan RD, Shellard SA, Bedford P, Hill BT. An evaluation of the role of glutathione and its associated enzymes in the expression of differential sensitivities to antitumour agents shown by a range of human tumour cell lines. *Biochem Pharmacol.* 1990;40(8):1833-1842.

88. Pattanaik A, Bachowski G, Laib J, et al. Properties of the reaction of cis-dichlorodiammineplatinum(II) with metallothionein. *J Biol Chem.* 1992; 267(23):16121-16128.

89. Kelley SL, Basu A, Teicher BA, Hacker MP, Hamer DH, Lazo JS. Overexpression of metallothionein confers resistance to anticancer drugs. *Science.* 1988;241(4874):1813-1815.

90. Ceccaldi R, O'Connor KW, Mouw KW, et al. A unique subset of epithelial ovarian cancers with platinum sensitivity and PARP inhibitor resistance. *Cancer Res.* 2015;75(4):628-634. doi:10.1158/0008-5472.CAN-14-2593.

91. Reed E, Ozols RF, Tarone R, Yuspa SH, Poirier MC. Platinum-DNA adducts in leukocyte DNA correlate with disease response in ovarian cancer patients receiving platinum-based chemotherapy. *Proc Natl Acad Sci U S A.* 1987; 84(14):5024-5028.

92. Reed E, Ostchega Y, Steinberg SM, et al. Evaluation of platinum-DNA adduct levels relative to known prognostic variables in a cohort of ovarian cancer patients. *Cancer Res.* 1990;50(8):2256-2260.

93. Darcy KM, Tian C, Reed E. A Gynecologic Oncology Group study of platinum-DNA adducts and excision repair cross-complementation group 1 expression in optimal, stage III epithelial ovarian cancer treated with platinum-taxane chemotherapy. *Cancer Res.* 2007;67(9):4474-4481. doi:10.1158/0008-5472.CAN-06-4076.

94. Lee JM, Peer CJ, Yu M, et al. Sequence-specific pharmacokinetic and pharmacodynamic phase I/Ib study of olaparib tablets and carboplatin in women's cancer. *Clin Cancer Res.* 2017;23(6):1397-1406. doi:10.1158/1078-0432.CCR-16-1546.

95. Dabholkar M, Bostick-Bruton F, Weber C, Bohr VA, Egwuagu C, Reed E. ERCC1 and ERCC2 expression in malignant tissues from ovarian cancer patients. *J Natl Cancer Inst.* 1992;84(19):1512-1517.

96. Dabholkar M, Vionnet J, Bostick-Bruton F, Yu JJ, Reed E. Messenger RNA levels of XPAC and ERCC1 in ovarian cancer tissue correlate with response to platinum-based chemotherapy. *J Clin Invest.* 1994;94(2):703-708. doi:10.1172/JCI117388.

97. Metzger R, Leichman CG, Danenberg KD, et al. ERCC1 mRNA levels complement thymidylate synthase mRNA levels in predicting response and survival for gastric cancer patients receiving combination cisplatin and fluorouracil chemotherapy. *J Clin Oncol.* 1998;16(1):309-316. doi:10.1200/JCO.1998.16.1.309.

98. Shirota Y, Stoehlmacher J, Brabender J, et al. ERCC1 and thymidylate synthase mRNA levels predict survival for colorectal cancer patients receiving combination oxaliplatin and fluorouracil chemotherapy. *J Clin Oncol.* 2001;19(23):4298-4304. doi:10.1200/JCO.2001.19.23.4298.

99. Lord RV, Brabender J, Gandara D, et al. Low ERCC1 expression correlates with prolonged survival after cisplatin plus gemcitabine chemotherapy in non-small cell lung cancer. *Clin Cancer Res.* 2002;8(7):2286-2291.

100. Rosell R, Taron M, Barnadas A, Scagliotti G, Sarries C, Roig B. Nucleotide excision repair pathways involved in Cisplatin resistance in non-small-cell lung cancer. *Cancer Control.* 2003;10(4):297-305.

101. Li Q, Yu JJ, Mu C, et al. Association between the level of ERCC-1 expression and the repair of cisplatin-induced DNA damage in human ovarian cancer cells. *Anticancer Res.* 2000;20(2A):645-652.

102. Wang G, Reed E, Li QQ. Molecular basis of cellular response to cisplatin chemotherapy in non-small cell lung cancer (Review). *Oncol Rep.* 2004;12(5):955-965.

103. Ferry KV, Hamilton TC, Johnson SW. Increased nucleotide excision repair in cisplatin-resistant ovarian cancer cells: role of ERCC1-XPF. *Biochem Pharmacol.* 2000;60(9):1305-13.

104. Lee KB, Parker RJ, Bohr V, Cornelison T, Reed E. Cisplatin sensitivity/resistance in UV repair-deficient Chinese hamster ovary cells of complementation groups 1 and 3. *Carcinogenesis.* 1993;14(10):2177-2180.

105. Van Allen EM, Mouw KW, Kim P, et al. Somatic ERCC2 mutations correlate with cisplatin sensitivity in muscle-invasive urothelial carcinoma. *Cancer Discov.* 2014;4(10):1140-1153. doi:10.1158/2159-8290.CD-14-0623.

106. Furuta T, Ueda T, Aune G, Sarasin A, Kraemer KH, Pommier Y. Transcription-coupled nucleotide excision repair as a determinant of cisplatin sensitivity of human cells. *Cancer Res.* 2002;62(17):4899-4902.

107. Zhen W, Link CJ Jr, O'Connor PM, et al. Increased gene-specific repair of cisplatin interstrand cross-links in cisplatin-resistant human ovarian cancer cell lines. *Mol Cell Biol.* 1992;12(9):3689-3698.

108. Jones JC, Zhen WP, Reed E, Parker RJ, Sancar A, Bohr VA. Gene-specific formation and repair of cisplatin intrastrand adducts and interstrand cross-links in Chinese hamster ovary cells. *J Biol Chem.* 1991;266(11):7101-7107.

109. Stronach EA, Alfraidi A, Rama N, et al. HDAC4-regulated STAT1 activation mediates platinum resistance in ovarian cancer. *Cancer Res.* 2011;71(13):4412-4422. doi:10.1158/0008-5472.CAN-10-4111.

110. Bai T, Tanaka T, Yukawa K, Umesaki N. A novel mechanism for acquired cisplatin-resistance: suppressed translation of death-associated protein kinase mRNA is insensitive to 5-aza-2′-deoxycitidine and trichostatin in cisplatin-resistant cervical squamous cancer cells. *Int J Oncol.* 2006;28(2):497-508.

111. Olaussen KA, Dunant A, Fouret P, et al. DNA repair by ERCC1 in non-small-cell lung cancer and cisplatin-based adjuvant chemotherapy. *N Engl J Med.* 2006;355(10):983-991. doi:10.1056/NEJMoa060570.

112. Viguier J, Boige V, Miquel C, et al. ERCC1 codon 118 polymorphism is a predictive factor for the tumor response to oxaliplatin/5-fluorouracil combination chemotherapy in patients with advanced colorectal cancer. *Clin Cancer Res.* 2005;11(17):6212-6217. doi:10.1158/1078-0432.CCR-04-2216.

113. Sharma S, Shah NA, Joiner AM, Roberts KH, Canman CE. DNA polymerase zeta is a major determinant of resistance to platinum-based chemotherapeutic agents. *Mol Pharmacol.* 2012;81(6):778-787. doi:10.1124/mol.111.076828.

114. Ray Chaudhuri A, Callen E, Ding X, et al. Replication fork stability confers chemoresistance in BRCA-deficient cells. *Nature.* 2016;535(7612):382-387. doi:10.1038/nature18325.

115. Gardner EE, Lok BH, Schneeberger VE, et al. Chemosensitive relapse in small cell lung cancer proceeds through an EZH2-SLFN11 axis. *Cancer Cell.* 2017;31(2):286-99. doi:10.1016/j.ccell.2017.01.006.

116. Zhu H, Luo H, Zhang W, Shen Z, Hu X, Zhu X. Molecular mechanisms of cisplatin resistance in cervical cancer. *Drug Des Devel Ther.* 2016;10:1885-1895. doi:10.2147/DDDT.S106412.

117. Takimoto CH, Graham MA, Lockwood G, et al. Oxaliplatin pharmacokinetics and pharmacodynamics in adult cancer patients with impaired renal function. *Clin Cancer Res.* 2007;13(16):4832-4839. doi:10.1158/1078-0432.CCR-07-0475.

118. Extra JM, Espie M, Calvo F, Ferme C, Mignot L, Marty M. Phase I study of oxaliplatin in patients with advanced cancer. *Cancer Chemother Pharmacol.* 1990;25(4):299-303.

119. Crona DJ, Faso A, Nishijima TF, McGraw KA, Galsky MD, Milowsky MI. A systematic review of strategies to prevent cisplatin-induced nephrotoxicity. *Oncologist.* 2017;22(5):609-619. doi:10.1634/theoncologist.2016-0319.

120. Reed E, Jacob J. Carboplatin and renal dysfunction. *Ann Intern Med.* 1989;110(5):409.

121. Schilsky RL, Anderson T. Hypomagnesemia and renal magnesium wasting in patients receiving cisplatin. *Ann Intern Med.* 1979;90(6):929-931.

122. Kondo M, Hotta Y, Ando R, Yasui T, Kimura K. The impact of a solitary kidney on tolerability to gemcitabine plus cisplatin chemotherapy in urothelial carcinoma patients: a retrospective study. *Cancer Chemother Pharmacol.* 2017;79(5):995-1001. doi:10.1007/s00280-017-3277-x.

123. Hesketh PJ. Chemotherapy-induced nausea and vomiting. *N Engl J Med.* 2008;358(23):2482-2494. doi:10.1056/NEJMra0706547.

124. Dzagnidze A, Katsarava Z, Makhalova J, et al. Repair capacity for platinum-DNA adducts determines the severity of cisplatin-induced peripheral neuropathy. *J Neurosci.* 2007;27(35):9451-7. doi:10.1523/JNEUROSCI.0523-07.2007.

125. Avan A, Postma TJ, Ceresa C, et al. Platinum-induced neurotoxicity and preventive strategies: past, present, and future. *Oncologist.* 2015;20(4):411-432. doi:10.1634/theoncologist.2014-0044.

126. Albers JW, Chaudhry V, Cavaletti G, Donehower RC. Interventions for preventing neuropathy caused by cisplatin and related compounds. *Cochrane Database Syst Rev.* 2014(3):CD005228. doi:10.1002/14651858.CD005228.pub4.

127. Hershman DL, Lacchetti C, Dworkin RH, et al. Prevention and management of chemotherapy-induced peripheral neuropathy in survivors of adult cancers: American Society of Clinical Oncology clinical practice guideline. *J Clin Oncol.* 2014;32(18):1941-1967. doi:10.1200/JCO.2013.54.0914.

128. Wiernik PH, Yeap B, Vogl SE, et al. Hexamethylmelamine and low or moderate dose cisplatin with or without pyridoxine for treatment of advanced ovarian carcinoma: a study of the Eastern Cooperative Oncology Group. *Cancer Invest.* 1992;10(1):1-9.

129. Travis LB, Holowaty EJ, Bergfeldt K, et al. Risk of leukemia after platinum-based chemotherapy for ovarian cancer. *N Engl J Med.* 1999;340(5):351-357. doi:10.1056/NEJM199902043400504.

130. Burkard R, Trautwein P, Salvi R. The effects of click level, click rate, and level of background masking noise on the inferior colliculus potential (ICP) in the normal and carboplatin-treated chinchilla. *J Acoust Soc Am.* 1997;102(6):3620-3627.

131. Freyer Dr, Chen L, Krailo MD, et al. Effects of sodium thiosulfate versus observations on development of cisplatin-induced hearing loss inj children with cancer (ACCL0431), a multi-centre, randomized controlled, open-label, Phase 3 trial. *Lancet Oncol.* 2017;18:63-74.

132. Markman M, Rothman R, Hakes T, et al. Second-line platinum therapy in patients with ovarian cancer previously treated with cisplatin. *J Clin Oncol.* 1991;9(3):389-393. doi:10.1200/JCO.1991.9.3.389.

133. Reed E, Jacob J, Ozols RF, Young RC, Allegra C. 5-Fluorouracil (5-FU) and leucovorin in platinum-refractory advanced stage ovarian carcinoma. *Gynecol Oncol.* 1992;46(3):326-329.

134. Silver DP, Richardson AL, Eklund AC, et al. Efficacy of neoadjuvant Cisplatin in triple-negative breast cancer. *J Clin Oncol.* 2010;28(7):1145-1153. doi:10.1200/JCO.2009.22.4725.

135. Byrski T, Gronwald J, Huzarski T, et al. Pathologic complete response rates in young women with BRCA1-positive breast cancers after neoadjuvant chemotherapy. *J Clin Oncol.* 2010;28(3):375-379. doi:10.1200/JCO.2008.20.7019.

136. Petrelli F, Barni S, Bregni G, de Braud F, Di Cosimo S. Platinum salts in advanced breast cancer: a systematic review and meta-analysis of randomized clinical trials. *Breast Cancer Res Treat.* 2016;160(3):425-437. doi:10.1007/s10549-016-4025-3.

Topoisomerase Inhibitors

Anish Thomas and Yves Pommier

Topoisomerase Biology

The human genome consists of long polymers of nucleic acids, several feet long packed in the nucleus and mitochondria. In addition, DNA molecules consist of two continuous strands that wind around each other in a right-handed duplex helical structure (the "double helix") and need to be separated as single strands to serve as substrates for the synthesis of RNAs during transcription and DNA during replication. These characteristics explain the absolute need for topoisomerases, which act as the "magicians of the genome" to remove DNA and RNA topological problems and enable the function and stability of both the nuclear and mitochondrial genomes.

Nucleic Acid Topological Problems and Their Resolution by Topoisomerases

Figure 14.1 summarizes various topological problems inevitably associated with nucleic acids and how they are resolved by topoisomerases. As mentioned above, transcription and replication require "unzipping" of the two strands of the DNA duplex to serve as templates for new RNA transcripts or daughter DNA strands (Fig. 14.1A). As a result, the DNA duplex becomes overwound (positively supercoiled [Sc+]) ahead of the polymerases and underwound (negatively supercoiled [Sc−]) in the wake of the polymerases. Sc+ DNA, which tightens the helix, antagonizes further unzipping by helicases, while Sc− promotes the formation of alternative DNA structures such as R-loops, guanosine and cytosine quartets (G- and I-motifs, respectively) and Z-DNA (left-handed DNA segments). All topoisomerases remove supercoils, but TOP3 enzymes are only effective toward Sc− as they cleave only single-stranded segments of duplex DNA. Two activities (catenation/decatenation and unknotting/knotting; Figure 14.1B and C) are specific to the type II topoisomerases because of the unique ability of type II enzymes to make DNA double-strand breaks (DSBs) that enable the transport of another DNA duplex through the DSB. Such reactions are critical to unlink catenated daughter DNA molecules at the end of replication (by TOP2α especially; Fig. 14.1B) and to remove DNA knots (Fig. 14.1C). At the end of replication and during DNA repair, hemicatenated molecules are resolved by TOP3α (Fig. 14.1D) in a heterotrimeric "dissolvasome" complex including TOP3α, the Bloom syndrome helicase (BLM), and RMI1 (RecQ-mediated genomic instability 1). The functions of topoisomerases have recently been extended to RNA topological problems with the specific activity of TOP3β as the eukaryotic RNA topoisomerase (Fig. 14.1E).[1]

Classification and Distinctive Features of the Six Human Topoisomerases

The human genome encodes six topoisomerases (Fig. 14.2A): two type IB (TOP1 and TOP1MT encoded by the *TOP1* and *TOP1MT* genes on chromosomes 20q12 and 8q24.3, respectively), two type IA (TOP3α and TOP3β encoded by the *TOP3A* and *TOP3B* genes on chromosomes 17p11.2 and 22q11.22, respectively), and two type IIA (TOP2α and TOP2β encoded by *TOP2A* and *TOP2B* on chromosomes 17q21.22 and 3p24.2, respectively). Notably, two topoisomerase genes associated with cellular proliferation, *TOP1* and *TOP2A*, are frequently amplified in cancers. *TOP2A* is commonly coamplified with proliferation genes including ERBB2 (target of EGFR inhibitors in breast cancers and lung adenocarcinomas), the chromatin-remodeling factor SMARCE1, and the glucose-linked metabolic gene *IGFBP4*. *TOP1* is commonly coamplified with SRC (oncogene protein kinase: https://discover.nci.nih.gov/cellminercdb).

All topoisomerases act by forming covalent and reversible breaks in the DNA backbone, referred to as topoisomerase cleavage complexes (TOPcc), via phosphotyrosyl residues (Fig. 14.2). The breaks (TOPcc) are the catalytic intermediates that support all DNA transactions (swiveling of the helix around its axis or passage of another strand or duplex through the break). TOPcc exhibit limited base-sequence specificity/requirement, which allows topoisomerases to act wherever they are needed.

Type I topoisomerases (TOP1, TOP1MT, TOP3α, and TOP3β) remove DNA supercoils (resolve overwound and underwound DNA duplex; see above) by cleaving on strand of the DNA duplex (Fig. 14.2A). Type IA and type IB enzymes differ in their catalytic mechanisms. Type IA topoisomerases (TOP3α and TOP3β) cleave the DNA by forming a covalent tyrosyl at the 5′-end of a nucleotidic bond and require a divalent metal (Mg^{2+}) as cofactor (Fig. 14.2A and C). Type IA enzymes process DNA (remove negative supercoiling and resolve double-Holiday junctions) by a strand-passing mechanism, in which the TOPcc allows the passage of another strand. By contrast, type IB enzymes (TOP1 and TOP1MT) act by letting the DNA swivel around its axis at the break site. Type IB enzymes (TOP1 and TOP1MT) do not require metal cofactor for catalysis and cleave DNA by covalent linkage of their catalytic tyrosine with the 3′-end of the DNA break (Fig. 14.2B). Type IB enzymes are therefore simpler molecular machines and are closely related to lambda integrase and Cre recombinase, but without the strict DNA sequence requirement of lambda integrase and Cre recombinase.

Type II topoisomerases (TOP2α and TOP2β) exhibit a broader range of activities than type I enzymes (see Fig. 14.1). In addition to supercoiling removal, they can decatenate (and catenate) and unknot

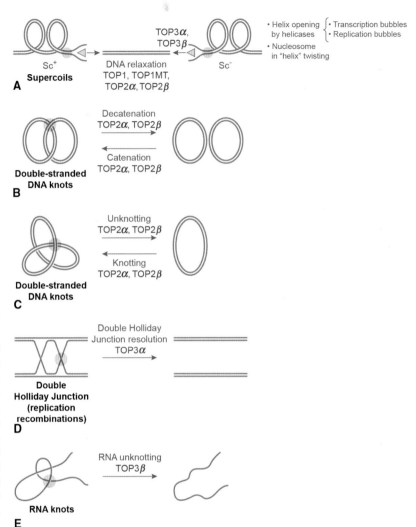

FIGURE **14.1** Topological problems resolved by topoisomerases. **A.** Transcription and replication generate positive supercoiling (Sc+) ahead and negative supercoiling (Sc–) behind transcription and replication complexes. While TOP1, TOP1MT, TOP2α, and TOP2β topoisomerases are able to remove Sc–, TOP3 enzymes (TOP3α and TOP3β) are not able to remove Sc+ and can only dissipate Sc–. **B.** TOP2 enzymes specifically decatenate intertwined duplex DNA circles (post replicatixon) by making double-strand break at crossover point (*yellow circle*). **C.** In addition, TOP2 enzymes allow the crossover of duplex DNA within single molecules, thereby unknotting and knotting duplex DNA circles. **D.** TOP3α can decatenate double-Holiday junctions by strand passage in association with RMI1 and RMI2 (heterotrimeric TRR complex) and the Bloom syndrome helicase BLM. Such structures are generated during replication and recombinations. **E.** TOP3β in association with TDRD3 acts also as the vertebrate RNA helicase, which can unknot RNA molecules.

(and knot) DNA. This is due to the fact that TOP2 enzymes cleave both strands of duplex in concert with a canonical 4 base pair stager (with a 5′-overhang) (Fig. 14.2A). TOP2cc DNA DSB act a 2-gate device for passing another DNA duplex (from the same DNA molecule for supercoiling relaxation and unknotting/knotting) or passing another DNA molecule (decatenation/catenation) (see Fig. 14.1). Like type IA enzymes, TOP2s break the DNA by covalent linkage of their catalytic tyrosine to the 5′-end of the break (Fig. 14.2A and C) and require Mg^{2+} as cofactor (coordinated by the TOPRIM motif). They also require ATP for the remodeling (and regeneration) of the overall enzyme structure during each breakage-relegation cycle.

Genetic analyses have established the essentiality of topoisomerases for development, cellular survival, and proliferation. TOP2A and TOP3A in metazoans (including humans and TOP2 and Top3 in yeast) are essential. TOP1 is essential in metazoans but not in yeast, where inactivation of TOP1 leads to genomic instability (especially in the ribosomal repeats). *TOP2B* knockout mice develop in utero but die at birth from neuromuscular synapse dysfunction. *TOP3B* knockout mice are viable, but suffer from global organ dysfunctions as they age. Genetic inactivation of *TOP3B* causes mental disorders (schizophrenia and mental retardation).[7,8] TOP1MT knockout mice have the mildest phenotype but suffer from defective organ regeneration under stress conditions (enhanced cardiotoxicity of doxorubicin and delayed liver regeneration).[9,10]

Topoisomerase Cleavage Complexes (TOPcc) and Their DNA Damaging Effects

Anticancer topoisomerase inhibitors all act by trapping TOPcc and poisoning topoisomerases as they break DNA. The molecular mechanism of poisoning is common to all inhibitors. The drugs act as "interfacial inhibitors"[4]; they intercalate into the DNA break sites of the TOPcc (Fig. 14.2A, bottom schemes) and prevent the reversal of the cleavage complex (curved arrows in Fig. 14.2B and C). The sequestration of topoisomerases in the TOPcc results in an overall reduction of topoisomerase enzymatic activity. Yet, the anticancer activity of the anticancer topoisomerase inhibitors is not due to the reduction of enzymatic activity, but to the trapping of the TOPcc. This concept is important, as anticancer drug responses to both TOP1 and TOP2 inhibitors is positively correlated with high topoisomerase levels in cancer cells, and a common mechanism of drug resistance is down-regulation of topoisomerases.

Topoisomerases can also be trapped by DNA lesions generated by anticancer drugs that alter DNA bases (such as adducts produced by platinum derivatives and base substitution by cytarabine). The drugs alter the DNA structure, which in turn prevents the proper resealing of the DNA breaks associated with the TOPcc (reviewed in Ref. [3]).

Drug-trapped TOPcc kill cells primarily by interfering with DNA replication and transcription. Both processes are coupled with

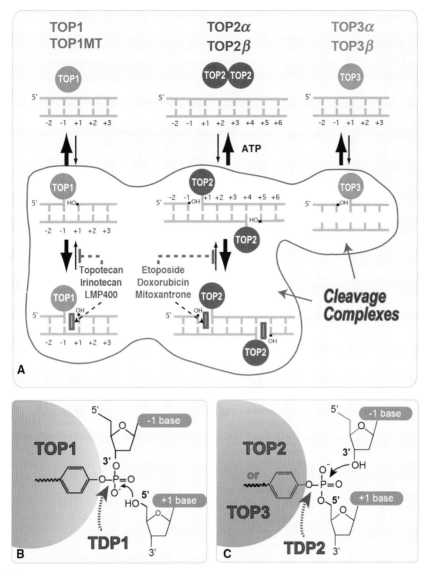

FIGURE **14.2** **A.** The human nuclear genome encodes 6 topoisomerases: two type IB enzymes, TOP1 and TOP1MT; two type IIA, TOP2α and TOP2β; and two type IA, TOP3α and TOP3β. Type I enzymes (TOP1, TOP1MT, TOP3α, and TOP3β) change DNA topology by making transient DNA single-strand breaks through the covalent linkage of their enzyme catalytic tyrosine to one end of the DNA break. These catalytic intermediates are commonly referred to *cleavage complexes*. The cleavage complexes for TOP2α and TOP2β are DNA double-strand breaks covalently linked to enzyme homodimers. TOP1, TOP2α, and TOP2β topoisomerases are the targets of widely used anticancer drugs,[2,3] which act as *interfacial inhibitors* by binding at the topoisomerase-DNA interfaces and blocking the reversal of the cleavage complexes.[4] Consequently, topoisomerase inhibitors block the catalytic cycle of their topoisomerase target enzymes. TOP1 is the unique target of topotecan and irinotecan. Both drugs are water-soluble derivatives of the alkaloid camptothecin.[5] In addition to camptothecins, TOP1 can be targeted by a different chemical class, the indenoisoquinolines.[6] TOP2α and TOP2β are both the targets of several chemical classes including the epipodophyllotoxin derivatives (etoposide and teniposide), the anthracyclines (doxorubicin, daunorubicin, idarubicin, and epirubicin), and mitoxantrone. **B.** TOP1 cleaves the DNA by transesterification reaction and reversible covalent linkage to the DNA 3'-end. If the 5'-hydroxyl-end of the DNA fails to reverse the reaction (curved arrow), tyrosyl DNA phosphodiesterase 1 (TDP1) excises the TOP1 covalent complex. **C.** TOP2 and TOP3 enzymes cleave the DNA with opposite polarity (covalent linkage to the DNA 5'-end) and rescue by TDP2.

the topoisomerases that remove the supercoiling associated with DNA tracking by RNA and DNA polymerases and enable initiation and termination of transcription and replication. Trapping of TOP1 ahead of replication forks is toxic to cells as replication forks collide into the trapped TOP1cc, which generate "replication runoff" lesions with DNA double-stranded ends (DSE) comprising the broken template strand and the aborted daughter strand (Fig. 14.3A). TOPcc also cause steric blocks that interfere with the dynamics of

chromatin during chromatin remodeling associated with transcription, replication, and DNA repair. In addition, the DNA DSBs generated by TOP2cc are at the origin of chromosome breaks, which are highly toxic but also can give rise to translocations and chromosome rearrangements. This is the molecular basis for the secondary leukemia induced by TOP2 inhibitors (discussed in Ref.[11]) (Fig. 14.3B).

To end this section, we wish to add two remarks regarding TOPcc. First, the trapping of TOPcc in bacteria by antibiotics is

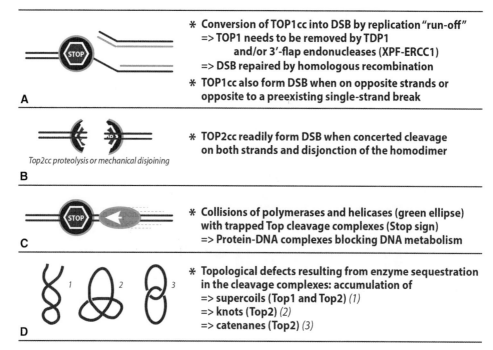

FIGURE **14.3** Schematic representation of the cytotoxic mechanisms of topoisomerase inhibitors. The anticancer activity of clinical topoisomerase inhibitors is due to the trapping of the cleavage complexes (**A–C**) rather than catalytic inhibition (**D**).

the mechanism of action of the widely used antibacterial quinolone derivatives such as norfloxacin or ciprofloxacin. The structural differences between the bacterial type II enzymes (gyrase and TOPOIV) and the human TOP2 (TOP2α and TOP2β) are the basis for the selectivity of the antibiotics, as they do not trap the host TOP2 enzymes. Second, TOPcc form readily under physiological conditions as the genome is exposed to a variety of common alterations (oxidized bases, mismatches, abasic sites, nick, misincorporated ribonucleotides, carcinogenic and oxidative adducts) (reviewed in Ref.[11]). The TOPcc generated by alterations embedded in the human genome are particularly prone to the generation of abortive TOPcc, which, in turn, are source of genomic instability, chromosome rearrangements, and cancer initiation.

Repair of TOPcc

Because of the prevalence of TOPcc under physiological conditions, all cells (from humans to yeasts) encode specific enzymes dedicated to the excision of irreversible (aborted) TOPcc. The two main pathways for removing TOPcc are the phosphodiesterase and the endonuclease pathways. Two tyrosyl DNA phosphodiesterases (TDPs) remove TOPcc: TDP1 and TDP2. Schematically, TDP1 excises TOP1cc and TDP2 TOP2cc (Fig. 14.4). Yet, both enzymes can serve as backup for each other, and TDP1 can excise TOP2cc and TDP2 can excise TOP1cc with much reduced efficiency compared their preferred substrates (for details, see Refs.[11,12]). The process of recruitment of the TDPs to the aborted TOPcc is not fully elucidated. Nevertheless, recent studies revealed that TDP1 is recruited to TOP1cc by PARP1 and that PARP inhibitors inhibit the TDP1 repair pathway for TOP1 inhibitors.

Aborted TOPcc are also processed by endonucleases. Instead of just clipping the topoisomerase-DNA bond, endonucleases excise a segment of the DNA covalently attached to the trapped topoisomerase (Fig. 14.4). Recent studies[13] have established that MRE11

(meiotic recombination endonuclease 11–like protein) is a key endonuclease for the excision of TOP2cc as part of the MRN complex comprising MRE11, NBN (nibrin; also called Nbs1 for Nijmegen breakage syndrome protein 1), and RAD50. The activity of MRE11 on aborted TOP2cc is consistent with the known role of MRE11 in processing the meiotic DSB produced by SPO11 (a type II topoisomerase from the topoisomerase 6 family) during meiotic recombination. It is notable that MRE11 is susceptible to genomic inactivation in mismatch repair (MMR)-deficient cells, such as colon cancers.[14] Further studies are warranted to explore whether such MRE11-deficient cancers would be selectively sensitive to TOP2 inhibitors.

In case of TOP1cc, XPF (xeroderma pigmentosum group F, which is annotated under ERCC4 in HUGO nomenclature) may act as an endonuclease for the excision of TOP1-DNA complex as an alternative for the TDP1-PARP1 pathway.[15] The translational implication is that tumors with deficient XPF-ERCC1 rely solely on TDP1 for repair, and should be selectively sensitive to the combination of TOP1 inhibitors with TDP1 or PARP1 inhibitors, thereby creating a novel synthetic lethal paradigm.[15]

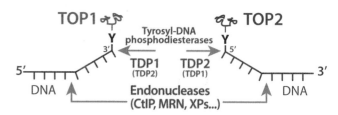

FIGURE **14.4** Repair pathways for the excision of topoisomerase cleavage complexes. The redundancy of these pathways (endonuclease versus phosphodiesterase pathways) creates potential synthetic lethal scenarios, for instance, inhibition of the TDP1-PARP1 pathways by PARP inhibitors in XPF-ERCC1–deficient tumors or inhibition of the TDP2 pathway in MRE11-deficient mismatch repair-deficient tumors.

FDA-Approved TOP1 Warheads

The two camptothecin TOP1 inhibitors topotecan (Hycamtin) and irinotecan (Camptosar) (Fig. 14.5) are widely used.

Topotecan

Topotecan is a water-soluble camptothecin derivative containing a stable basic side chain at position 9 of the A ring of 10-hydroxycamptothecin. Clinical trials of topotecan were initiated in 1989; topotecan was approved for use as second-line chemotherapy in patients with advanced ovarian cancer in 1996, for the treatment of small cell lung cancer (SCLC) after failure of initial or subsequent chemotherapy in 1998, and for treatment of stage IVB recurrent or persistent cervical cancer that is not amenable to curative treatment with surgery and/or radiation therapy in combination with cisplatin in 2006. Key features of topotecan are listed in Table 14.1.

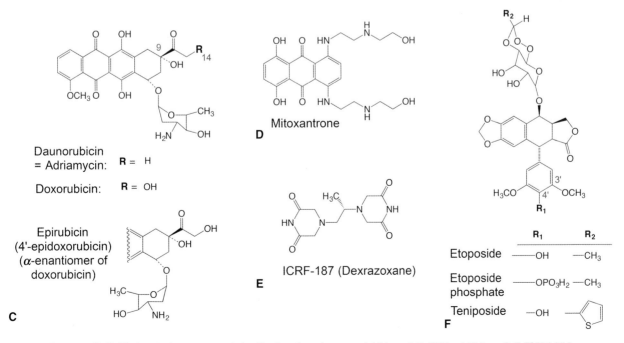

FIGURE **14.5** Chemical structures and classification of topoisomerase inhibitors. **A,B.** TOP1cc inhibitors. **C–F.** TOP2 inhibitors. Anthracyclines **(C)** and anthracenediones **(D)** are DNA intercalator TOP2cc poisons, whereas dexrazoxane **(E)** is a TOP2 catalytic inhibitor. Demethylepipodophyllotoxins **(F)** are nonintercalator TOP2cc poisons without the off-target effects (DNA intercalation, oxygen radical production) of anthracyclines and anthracenediones.

TABLE	
14.1 *Key features of topotecan*	

Mechanism of action	Topoisomerase I poison. Stabilizes the cleavable complex in which TOP1 is covalently bound to DNA at a single-stranded break site.
Metabolism	Nonenzymatic hydrolysis of the lactone ring generates the less active open-ring hydroxy carboxylic acid. *N*-desmethyl is a minor metabolite.
Elimination	About 26% to 41% excreted unchanged in urine over 24 h. Concentrated in the bile at levels that are 1.5 times higher than the simultaneous plasma levels.
Pharmacokinetics	Terminal half-life of topotecan lactone is 3 h; approximate clearance of 62 L/h/m^2 (range, 14 to 155 L/h/m^2) reported for 30-min topotecan infusions.
Toxicity	Myelosuppression, predominantly neutropenia with thrombocytopenia
	Nausea and vomiting (mild)
	Diarrhea (mild)
	Fatigue
	Alopecia
	Skin rash
	Elevated liver function test results
	Mucositis
Modifications for organ dysfunction	In minimally pretreated patients, no dosage adjustments appear to be necessary for patients with mild renal impairment (creatinine clearance 40 to 60 mL/min), but dosage adjustment to 0.75 mg/m^2/d is recommended for patients with moderate renal impairment (20 to 39 mL/min). Further dosage adjustments may be necessary for patients with extensive prior chemotherapy or radiation therapy. Dosage adjustments are not required for hyperbilirubinemia up to 10 mg/dL.
Precautions	For febrile or severe grade 4 neutropenia lasting >3 d, the dosage for subsequent courses should be reduced by 0.25 mg/m^2/d. Monitoring of blood counts is essential.

Clinical Pharmacology

The most common dose and schedule of topotecan administration is a 30-minute IV infusion of 1.5 mg/m^2 daily for 5 days every 3 weeks.[16] This regimen has been tested widely and is used in ovarian and lung cancer. Five-day continuous infusions of topotecan at 2.0 mg/m^2/d have been tested in patients with hematologic malignancies, although in these studies gastrointestinal toxicities such as mucositis and diarrhea became more problematic. Prolonged 21-day infusion schedules at 0.5 to 0.6 mg/m^2/d have been disappointing in phase II studies. Other schedules tested in phase I or phase II studies include a single 30-minute infusion, 24-hour infusions, and 3-, 5-, and 14-day continuous infusions. Oral administration has also been tested clinically and has been found comparable with IV administration in randomized studies.[17-19]

General Pharmacokinetics

After IV topotecan administration, the lactone ring undergoes rapid hydrolysis to generate the inactive carboxylate species. Less than 1 hour after the start of an infusion, most of the circulating drug in plasma is in the carboxylate form, and this species predominates for the duration of the monitoring period. In most studies, the ratio of the lactone to total topotecan area under the concentration versus time curve (AUC) ranges from 20% to 35%. Interindividual variation in the AUC and the total body clearance is quite large for both lactone and total topotecan (lactone plus carboxylate). In general, plasma concentrations and AUC levels tend to increase with increasing doses, consistent with linear pharmacokinetics, although, in some studies, nonlinearity in drug clearance at higher-dose levels was seen.[20]

For topotecan lactone, the terminal half-life ranges from 2.0 to 3.5 hours, which is relatively short compared with that of other chemotherapeutic agents. Consequently, no accumulation is observed when topotecan is administered daily for 5 consecutive days. Population pharmacokinetic studies in patients treated with IV or orally administered topotecan revealed that patient characteristics (i.e., gender, height, weight) and laboratory values (i.e., serum creatinine concentration) give a moderate ability to predict the clearance of topotecan in an individual patient.[21,22]

Absorption

The most common route for topotecan administration is IV; however, oral formulations using prolonged administration schedules have undergone preclinical and clinical testing. In humans, the reported oral bioavailability ranges from 30% to 42%[23] and is influenced by multiple factors. First, the relatively high pH in the small bowel leads to conversion to the carboxylate form, which is poorly absorbed by the intestinal walls. Second, the bioavailability is reduced by protein-mediated, outward-directed transport of topotecan by ABCG2.[24,25] Third, the bioavailability is partly influenced by the binding of topotecan to food, proteins, and intestinal fluids and/or by decomposition in the gastrointestinal fluid.

Metabolism

Topotecan undergoes a reversible pH-dependent hydrolysis of its lactone moiety; it is the lactone form that is pharmacologically active. At pH ≤ 4, the lactone is exclusively present, whereas the ring-opened hydroxy acid form predominates at physiologic pH.

In vitro studies in human liver microsomes indicate that metabolism of topotecan to an *N*-demethylated metabolite represents a minor metabolic pathway.

Because topotecan is metabolized in the liver only to a minor extent, the pharmacokinetics in patients with impaired liver function does not significantly differ from those in patients with normal hepatic function.[26,27] About 30% of the dose is excreted in the urine, and renal clearance is an important determinant of topotecan elimination.[26,27] Therefore, dose modifications are recommended for patients with impaired renal function and are not required for patients with liver dysfunction.

Adverse Reactions

Dose-related, reversible, and noncumulative myelosuppression is the most important side effect of topotecan.[28] Neutropenia occurs more frequently and is often more severe than thrombocytopenia, and it is more severe in heavily pretreated patients. Besides myelosuppression, stomatitis (24% to 28% of patients) and late-onset diarrhea (40%) can occur at higher doses. Other nonhematological toxicities include alopecia, nausea, vomiting, fatigue, and asthenia.

Hematologic toxicity is more pronounced with the shorter oral regimens but is still mostly mild and noncumulative, whereas diarrhea is a severe and intractable side effect of more prolonged daily administration.[29] An analysis of the pharmacokinetic-pharmacodynamic relationships revealed that the total area under the curve per course did not differ between the various regimens and that the daily-times-five schedule provided the best systemic exposure and toxicity profile.[30]

Antitumor Activity

The antitumor activity of topotecan, given as a single agent using various schedules of administration, was established in a variety of phase II studies, including ovarian cancer, SCLC, NSCLC, breast cancer, myelodysplastic syndrome, and chronic myelomonocytic leukemia. Marginal activity was seen in head and neck cancer, prostate cancer, pancreatic cancer, gastric cancer, esophageal carcinoma, hepatocellular carcinoma, and recurrent malignant glioma, as well as when topotecan was used as consolidation treatment after first-line standard chemotherapy for ovarian cancer.[31]

In a phase III study, the daily-times-five IV topotecan was compared with paclitaxel (3-hour infusion of 175 mg/m^2/d every 3 weeks) in ovarian cancer. Topotecan and paclitaxel were equally effective with regard to response rates, progression-free survival, and overall survival.[32] In an open-label, multicenter study comparing the activity and tolerability of oral versus IV topotecan in patients with relapsed epithelial ovarian cancer after failure of one platinum-based regimen,[18] oral doses of topotecan were administered as 2.3 mg/m^2/d and IV doses as 1.5 mg/m^2/d for 5 consecutive days every 3 weeks. No difference in response rates between the two treatment arms was reported. Although a small, statistically significant difference in survival favored the IV formulation, in the context of second-line palliative treatment for ovarian cancer, this difference in outcome has only limited clinical significance. For this reason, oral topotecan could be an alternative treatment modality in this setting because of its convenience and good tolerability.

Another phase III study compared single-agent topotecan with combination chemotherapy consisting of cyclophosphamide, doxorubicin, and vincristine (CAV) in patients with SCLC which relapsed after first-line platinum-based chemotherapy.[33] Although the response rate, time to disease progression, and overall survival were similar, the palliation of disease-related symptoms was better with topotecan. In a randomized trial performed by the Eastern Cooperative Oncology Group (ECOG), topotecan was compared with best support of care in patients with extensive-stage SCLC.[34] In this trial, topotecan was administered as consolidation therapy after response induction with cisplatin and etoposide. Although topotecan produced a moderate increase in the time to disease progression, it did not improve survival. Finally, similar to the study of ovarian cancer, oral topotecan was compared to IV administration in patients with relapsed and chemosensitive SCLC. The oral formulation was similar in efficacy, resulted in less severe neutropenia, and was more convenient.[19] Topotecan has also shown some activity against hematological malignancies and advanced cervical cancer[35]; it is approved in combination with cisplatin for recurrent or resistant (stage IVB) cervical cancer.

Irinotecan

Irinotecan (CPT-11) was the first camptothecin derivative with increased aqueous solubility to enter clinical trials and became commercially available in Japan for treatment of lung cancer, cervical cancer, and ovarian cancer in 1994. In the United States, irinotecan was approved in 1996 for use in patients with advanced colorectal cancer refractory to 5-FU, and in 2000, it was approved as a component of first-line therapy in combination with 5-FU/LV for the treatment of metastatic colorectal cancer or for patients who have progressed following initial 5-FU–based chemotherapy. Key features of irinotecan are listed in Table 14.2.

Clinical Pharmacology

Systemic exposure to irinotecan can vary up to 10-fold among patients receiving standard doses.[36] Pharmacokinetic and pharmacodynamic properties of irinotecan can be affected by a variety of factors, including inherited genetic variability, age, sex, malnutrition, polypharmacy, complex physiological changes due to concomitant disease, organ dysfunction, and tumor invasion.

Pharmacodynamics

Irinotecan is unique among camptothecin analogues in that it must first be converted by a carboxylesterase-converting enzyme to the active metabolite SN-38.[37] SN-38 is the major metabolite responsible for irinotecan's biologic effects, including efficacy and toxicity. SN-38 is approximately 1,000 times as potent as irinotecan as an inhibitor of TOP1 purified from human and rodent tumor cell lines.[5]

Pharmacokinetics

After intravenous infusion of irinotecan in humans, irinotecan plasma concentrations decline in a multiexponential manner, with a mean terminal elimination half-life of about 6 to 12 hours. The plasma half-life of SN-38 is relatively long compared with that of the other camptothecins, approximately 10 to 20 hours. The prolonged duration of exposure to SN-38 is probably a function of its sustained production from irinotecan in tissues by carboxylesterase (CES) 2 because direct injection of SN-38 into rats resulted in extremely rapid plasma clearance, with a half-life of only 7 minutes.[38]

TABLE

14.2   *Key features of irinotecan*

Mechanism of action	After metabolic activation to SN-38, the mechanism of action is the same as for topotecan.
Metabolism	Irinotecan is a prodrug that requires enzymatic cleavage of the C-10 side chain by an irinotecan carboxylesterase–converting enzyme to generate the biologically active metabolite SN-38. Irinotecan can also undergo hepatic oxidation of its dipiperidine side chain to form the inactive metabolite 7-ethyl-10-[4-*N*-(5-aminopentanoic acid)-1-piperidino] carbonyloxycamptothecin (APC). Like topotecan non-enzymatic hydrolysis of the lactone E-ring generate the inactive carboxylate derivative.
Elimination	Elimination of irinotecan occurs by urinary excretion, biliary excretion, and hepatic metabolism. About 16% (range, 11.1% to 20.9%) of an administered dose of irinotecan is excreted unchanged in the urine. SN-38 is glucuronidated, and both the conjugated and unconjugated forms are excreted in the bile. Glucurono conjugated SN-38 can be converted back to SN-38 by bacteria in the gut, leading to diarrhea.
Pharmacokinetics	Approximate terminal half-life of irinotecan lactone is 6.8 h (range, 5.0 to 9.6 h) and approximate clearance is 46.9 L/h/m^2 (range, 39.0 to 53.5 L/h/m^2). Approximate terminal half-life of SN-38 lactone is 11 h (range, 9.1 to 13.0 h).
Toxicity	Early-onset diarrhea within hours or during the infusion is associated with cramping, vomiting, flushing, and diaphoresis. Consider atropine 0.25 to 1.0 mg SC or IV in patients experiencing cholinergic symptoms. Late-onset diarrhea can occur later than 12 h after drug administration.
	Myelosuppression, predominantly neutropenia
	Alopecia
	Nausea and vomiting
	Mucositis
	Fatigue
	Elevated hepatic transaminases
	Pulmonary toxicity (uncommon) associated with a reticulonodular infiltrate, fever, dyspnea, and eosinophilia
Modifications for organ dysfunction	No definite recommendations are available for patients with impaired renal or hepatic dysfunction. Caution is warranted in patients with Gilbert's disease.
Precautions	Severe delayed-onset diarrhea may be controlled by high-dose loperamide given in an initial oral dose of 4 mg followed by 2 mg every 2 h during the day and 4 mg every 4 h during the night. High-dose loperamide should be started at the first sign of any loose stool and continued until no bowel movements occur for a 12-h period. Particular caution is also warranted in monitoring and managing toxicities in elderly patients (>64 y) or those who have previously received pelvic/abdominal irradiation.

Metabolism

Irinotecan is subject to extensive metabolic conversion by various enzyme systems, including esterases to form the active metabolite SN-38. The main CES responsible for the clinical activation of irinotecan in humans is CES2.[39] CES activity in human liver is found in the microsomal fractions, and this enzyme has been cloned and characterized.[40]

SN-38 is predominantly detoxified by a drug-metabolizing UDP-glucuronosyltransferase (UGT) 1A1 to form SN-38 glucuronide (SN-38G), which is present in the plasma and bile of patients receiving irinotecan chemotherapy.[37] The relative AUC value of the active metabolite SN-38 to irinotecan varies from 0.9% to 11%. Irinotecan can also undergo CYP3A4-mediated oxidative metabolism to several inactive oxidation products, one of which can be hydrolyzed by CES to release SN-38.

The decrease in plasma concentrations of SN-38G tends to parallel the decrease in SN-38 over time, suggesting that UGT is the rate-limiting step for the elimination of SN-38.

The UGT1A isoforms UGT1A1, UGT1A3, UGT1A6, UGT1A7, and UGT1A9 have all been implicated in the glucuronidation of SN-38,[41] although UGT1A1 is believed to be predominantly responsible for SN-38 metabolism in humans.[42,43] UGT1A1 is known to

be a highly polymorphic enzyme. UGT1A1 activity is reduced in individuals with genetic polymorphisms that lead to reduced enzyme activity such as the UGT1A1*28 polymorphism. Approximately 10% of the North American population is homozygous for the UGT1A1*28 allele (also referred to as UGT1A1 7/7 genotype). In a prospective study, in which irinotecan was administered as a single agent (350 mg/m^2) on a once-every-3-week schedule, patients with the UGT1A1 7/7 genotype had a higher exposure to SN-38 than patients with the wild-type UGT1A1 allele (UGT1A1 6/6 genotype).

In addition to hepatic metabolism, elimination of irinotecan also occurs by urinary and fecal excretion. Up to 37% of the administered irinotecan dose is excreted unchanged in the urine over 48 hours after a short 90-minute infusion, with only less than 0.3% being excreted as SN-38.[44] Biliary secretion of irinotecan, SN-38, and SN-38G also contributes substantially to drug elimination. The canalicular multispecific organic anion transporter ABCC2 (cMOAT; MRP2) is believed to be responsible for the biliary secretion of irinotecan carboxylate, SN-38 carboxylate, and the carboxylate and lactone forms of SN-38G.[45] SN-38 is also a substrate for other transport systems in the bile canaliculi such as ABCC1 (MRP1) and ABCG2 (BCRP; MXR), but not ABCB1.[24,37] OATP1B1 (OATP-C), which transports a variety of drugs and their metabolites from blood into hepatocytes, showed transport activity for SN-38 but not for irinotecan and SN-38G.[46]

Adverse Reactions

The principal DLT for all irinotecan schedules is delayed diarrhea and neutropenia. Severe, occasionally life-threatening toxicity occurs sporadically, even in relatively low-risk patients enrolled in well-controlled clinical trials. The co-occurrence of diarrhea and neutropenia places patients at greatest risk.[47] The frequency of severe diarrhea (grade 3 or 4) can be reduced by more than 50% if an intensive treatment with loperamide is used. Neutropenia is typically dose related, generally of brief duration and noncumulative, and occurs in 14% to 47% of patients treated once every 3 weeks, and less frequently using the weekly schedule (12% to 19%). In approximately 3% of patients, the neutropenia is associated with fever. In one phase I study, where irinotecan was given as a 96-hour continuous infusion for 2 weeks every 3 weeks, thrombocytopenia was also dose limiting.[48] Due to inhibition of acetylcholinesterase activity by irinotecan within the first 24 hours after dosing of the drug, an acute cholinergic reaction can be observed. Interindividual variability in the pharmacokinetics of irinotecan is at least one of the major causes of irinotecan-induced severe toxicity.[49-51]

Antitumor Activity

The most commonly used schedules of irinotecan administration are 30- or 90-minute IV infusions of 125 mg/m² given weekly for 4 of every 6 weeks or 350 mg/m² given every 3 weeks. In Japan, regimens of 100 mg/m² every week or 150 mg/m² every other week also have been used. The weekly times four schedule is more popular in North America, and the every-3-week schedule was developed predominantly in Europe. None of these regimens show clear superiority with regard to antitumor efficacy in comparative clinical studies.[37] Remarkably, the dose intensity of all applied dosage regimens of irinotecan is approximately 100 mg/m²/wk, which suggests a schedule independency.

Phase II studies consistently revealed response rates of 10% to 35% to single-agent irinotecan in advanced or metastatic colorectal cancer independent of the applied schedules. There was no apparent difference between the various schedules with respect to the median remission duration and median survival time.[52] In a randomized phase III study comparing treatment with irinotecan given as an IV infusion at a dose of 300 to 350 mg/m² every 3 weeks to best supportive care in patients refractory to previous treatment with 5-FU–based chemotherapy, the 1-year survival rate was significantly greater for the irinotecan-treated group than for the control group, 36% and 14% ($P < 0.01$), respectively.[53] Another randomized phase III study comparing treatment with irinotecan to three different continuous IV infusion schedules of 5-FU in patients with previously treated advanced colorectal cancer revealed a survival advantage for the irinotecan-treated group in comparison to the 5-FU–treated group.[54] Apart from colorectal cancer antitumor activity, single-agent irinotecan has also shown activity in phase II studies in several other solid malignancies, including breast cancer, relapsed or refractory non-Hodgkin's lymphomas, and SCLC.

FDA-Approved TOP2 Warheads

TOP2-targeting drugs used in clinic can be divided into intercalating and nonintercalating TOP2 poisons (Fig. 14.5). The intercalators include doxorubicin and other anthracyclines and anthracenediones. Nonintercalating TOP2 poisons include the epipodophyllotoxins, etoposide and teniposide. We refer to the drugs covered in this section as "warheads" because they are effective as free drugs and because several of them are also used as warheads for "targeted delivery" to tumors.

Daunorubicin (Daunomycin) and Doxorubicin

The anthracycline antibiotics doxorubicin and daunorubicin (Fig. 14.5), initially discovered in the 1960s, are used widely in current oncologic practice. Their key features are summarized in Table 14.3. Doxorubicin is widely used for the treatment of solid tumors, especially breast cancer and lymphoma, while daunorubicin is routinely included as part of chemotherapeutic induction programs for AML and ALL. The doxorubicin analogue epirubicin is like the parent compound with respect to its acute toxicity profile and spectrum of antitumor efficacy but is significantly less potent and only slightly less cardiotoxic. The modestly decreased cardiac toxicity of epirubicin is only a marginal advantage since other means are currently available to lessen the risk of anthracycline-induced heart damage. Idarubicin, a daunorubicin analogue, has significant activity in AML but is less active against solid tumors and, thus, is an appropriate alternate anthracycline only in the setting of acute leukemia.

Clinical Pharmacology

Doxorubicin has been successfully administered in a wide range of schedules. There is little evidence that changes in the schedule make a measurable difference in antitumor activity. The most common schedule of doxorubicin is 45 to 60 mg/m² every 21 days. The antitumor activity of doxorubicin and its myelosuppressive effect are proportional to the AUC, not to peak drug levels. Cardiac toxicity correlates with the peak drug level in plasma; weekly dosing at 20 to 30 mg/m² seems to be less cardiotoxic and approximately as effective as bolus dosing. A 96-hour infusion is convincingly less cardiotoxic while preserving antitumor activity.[55] As an added benefit, prolonged infusions dramatically lessen the nausea and vomiting associated with bolus administration of doxorubicin. The only major negative aspect of infusional doxorubicin is a tendency for mucositis, which increases in intensity as the infusion is prolonged. Daunorubicin is usually administered as a brief intravenous infusion in doses of 30 to 45 mg/m² daily for 3 days as induction therapy for AML.

Pharmacokinetics and Metabolism

The pharmacokinetics of anthracyclines is dominated by tissue binding. During the early distributive phase, drug levels fall rapidly as the drug gains ready access to all tissues except the brain. During this phase, the bulk of the drug binds to DNA throughout the body, and, in general, tissue levels of the drug are proportional to their DNA content.[56] In addition, plasma protein binding accounts for approximately 75% of the drug in the plasma.[57] Despite this plasma protein binding, tissue/plasma ratios range from 10:1 to 500:1 by virtue of the higher affinity of the drugs for DNA compared to plasma.

After bolus administration, or after the conclusion of a constant IV infusion, an initial doxorubicin half-life of 10 minutes is followed

TABLE

14.3   *Key features of daunorubicin and doxorubicin*

Mechanism of action	Pleiotropic effects including (a) stabilization of the TOP2 cleavage complexes, in which TOP2 is covalently bound to the ends of a DNA double-strand break, (b) inhibition of TOP2 catalytic activity at concentration above µM, (c) generation of reactive oxygen intermediates, and (d) stimulation of apoptosis.
Metabolism	Reduction of side-chain carbonyl to alcohol, resulting in some loss of cytotoxicity
	One-electron reduction to semiquinone free radical intermediate by flavoproteins, leading to aerobic production of superoxide anion, hydrogen peroxide, and hydroxyl radical
	Two-electron reduction, resulting in formation of aglycone species that can be conjugated for export in the bile
Pharmacokinetics	*Doxorubicin:* V_d = 25 L; protein binding = 60% to 70%; CSF/plasma ratio, very low; $t_{1/2\alpha}$ = 10 min; $t_{1/2\beta}$ = 1 to 3 h; $t_{1/2\gamma}$ = 30 h. Circulates predominantly as parent drug; doxorubicinol is the most common metabolite, although a substantial fraction of patients form doxorubicin 7-deoxyaglycone and doxorubicinol 7-deoxyaglycone; substantial interpatient variation in biotransformation; no apparent dose-related change in clearance; clearance in men > women.
	Daunomycin: V_d, protein binding, and CSF/plasma ratio similar to doxorubicin; $t_{1/2\alpha}$ = 40 min; $t_{1/2\beta}$ = 20 to 50 h. Metabolism to daunomycin faster than for equivalent doxorubicin metabolism, although interpatient variation remains high.
Elimination	Only 50% to 60% of parent drug accounted for known routes of elimination, which include reduction of the side-chain carbonyl by hepatic aldo-keto-reductases, aglycone formation, and excretion of biliary conjugates and metabolites. A substantial fraction of the parent compound is bound to DNA and cardiolipin in tissues and is slowly dissociated, contributing to prolonged disappearance. While changes in anthracycline pharmacokinetics may be difficult to demonstrate in patients with mild alterations in liver function, drug clearance is definitely decreased in the presence of significant hyperbilirubinemia or patients with a marked burden of metastatic tumor in the liver.
Drug interactions	Heparin binds to doxorubicin, causing aggregation; coadministration of both drugs leads to increased doxorubicin clearance. In rodents, phenobarbital has been shown to increase, and morphine decrease, doxorubicin disappearance; drugs that diminish hepatic reduced glutathione pools (acetaminophen and BCNU) sensitize the liver to anthracycline toxicity.
Toxicity	Myelosuppression
	Mucositis
	Alopecia
	Cardiac toxicity
	Severe local tissue damage after drug extravasation
Precautions	Acute and chronic cardiac decompensation can occur. Most common is cumulative dose-related congestive cardiomyopathy, which is more frequent in patients with underlying hypertensive heart disease or those who have received mediastinal radiation with a cardiac dose >2,000 cGy.
	Radiation sensitization of normal tissues, including chest wall and esophagus, is common and may occur many years after radiation exposure.
	Extravasation damage to extremities has resulted in loss of limb function.

by a secondary half-life of 1 to 3 hours. The terminal half-life of 30 to 50 hours accounts for over 70% of the total drug AUC of doxorubicin. As a result of this prolonged terminal phase, plasma levels of drug remain above 10 nM for the greater part of a week after a single dose of 60 mg/m² of doxorubicin.[57] Doxorubicinol is the primary active metabolite of doxorubicin in human plasma but is present in concentrations far smaller than those of the parent compound.[58]

Daunorubicin is cleared rapidly from plasma, with a primary half-life of 40 minutes; the loss of parent drug from plasma correlates with the rapid appearance of C(4)-O-demethyl daunorubicin, daunorubicin, their aglycones, and various sulfate and glucuronide metabolites in the bile. Within hours after a bolus dose of

daunorubicin, the predominant circulating form of the drug is the alcohol metabolite,[59] which has a somewhat longer (23 to 40 hours) half-life than its parent (15 to 30 hours). Unlike doxorubicin, the metabolism of daunorubicin is a major determinant of the plasma pharmacology of daunorubicin.

Men with normal hepatic function have approximately twice the clearance rate of doxorubicin (administered as an IV bolus) as compared to clearance in women[60]; higher drug clearance has been associated with an increased conversion rate of doxorubicin to its major alcohol metabolite. The pharmacodynamic implications of these findings are uncertain.

Approximately 50% of the drug is excreted in the bile, both as parent drug and as various metabolites, including glucuronides, aglycones, and sulfates. Less than 10% of administered drug appears in the urine but is sufficient to cause a reddish-orange discoloration of the urine in many patients.

Adverse Reactions

Bone Marrow Suppression and Mucositis

Bone marrow suppression, mucositis, and related gastrointestinal mucosal injury are common after anthracycline administration. Both myelosuppression and mucositis follow an acute course, with maximal toxicity within 7 to 10 days of drug administration and rapid recovery thereafter. For daunorubicin, bone marrow suppression is more common than mucositis and is the usual dose-limiting toxicity, while doxorubicin causes equally severe toxicity to marrow and mucosa after bolus dose administration. With weekly dosing or continuous infusion, mucositis frequently becomes the dose-limiting toxicity of doxorubicin.

Extravasation Injury

Extravasation of most anthracyclines leads to severe local injury that can continue to progress over weeks to months. These drugs should not be given by intramuscular or subcutaneous routes. Extravasation may occur with or without accompanying stinging or burning sensation, even if blood return was well on aspiration of the infusion needle. If any signs or symptoms of extravasation have occurred, the infusion should be stopped immediately. If extravasation is suspected, application of ice 15 minutes intermittently to the site may be helpful. Because of the progressive nature of extravasation, close observation and consultation with surgery are recommended. Blistering, ulceration, and persistent pain are indications for wide excision followed by split-thickness skin grafting.

Dexrazoxane has been approved for the treatment of anthracycline extravasation injury based on two prospective, nonrandomized, multicenter studies involving 80 patients with presumed anthracycline extravasations.[61] In this study, patients with fluorescence-positive tissue biopsies were treated with a 3-day schedule of IV dexrazoxane (1,000, 1,000, and 500 mg/m^2) through a different venous access location. The first dose was administered as soon as possible and within 6 hours following extravasation. Patients were assessed for efficacy (the possible need for surgical resection) and toxicity during the treatment period and regularly for the next 3 months. In 53 of 54 (98.2%) patients assessable for efficacy, dexrazoxane prevented surgery-requiring necrosis. One patient (1.8%) required surgical debridement. Toxic effects included transient elevation of alanine aminotransferases, nausea, and local pain at the dexrazoxane injection site.

Cardiac Toxicity

The cardiac toxicity of doxorubicin and the other anthracyclines is unique in terms of its pathology and mechanism.[62] Although the major limiting factors in the clinical use of anthracyclines in adults are bone marrow suppression, mucositis, and drug resistance, cardiac toxicity can develop while the tumor is still responsive to the drug. This complication develops during or after the use of the anthracyclines alone or in combination with other chemotherapeutic agents but also with the cardiotoxic monoclonal antibody, trastuzumab.[63] The observed potentiation of anthracycline-induced heart damage by trastuzumab serves as a contraindication to the concurrent use of trastuzumab and doxorubicin in patients whose tumors exhibit high levels of HER2/neu expression, a group that could benefit most from this combination. In addition, children are more sensitive to the cardiac toxicity of this drug, and this has become a significant problem in the use of doxorubicin in pediatric oncology.[64]

The anthracyclines manifest both acute and chronic cardiac toxicities. The acute toxicity is detected most commonly as a range of arrhythmias, including heart block. In its more extreme form, acute injury can include a pericarditis-myocarditis syndrome with onset of fever, pericarditis, and congestive heart failure.[65] This syndrome can occur at low cumulative doses of doxorubicin and can have a fatal outcome. There has been no clear correlation between the manifestation of arrhythmias and the development of the chronic cardiomyopathy.

Chronic cardiac toxicity develops as a result of cumulative injury to the myocardium, the pathology of which has been documented by endomyocardial biopsy.[66,67] With each dose of doxorubicin, there is progressive injury to the myocardium, so that the grade increases steadily with total dose of drug administered. The major changes observed in myocytes are dilation of the sarcoplasmic reticulum and disruption of myofibrils. Early in the development of this toxicity, these changes appear focally in scattered myocytes surrounded by normal-appearing cells. As the toxicity progresses, the frequency of altered cells increases until a significant proportion of the myocardium is involved. Later, the picture is complicated by the development of diffuse myocardial fibrosis. The pathology is unique to the anthracyclines and allows the pathologist to distinguish this from other processes such as viral cardiomyopathy or ischemic heart injury.

The clinical presentation of anthracycline-induced cardiotoxicity is typical of congestive heart failure (CHF): ankle edema, cough, weight gain, and, in extreme cases, pulmonary edema. While "safe" dose limits can be specified for patient populations, individual subjects may develop CHF early in their course of treatment. There is no safe "lifetime" dose of these agents for any individual patient. Risk factors include female gender, concurrent or prior exposure to chest irradiation, cardiac comorbidity, and age. The clinical risk of CHF is low at total doses of doxorubicin below 250 to 300 mg/m^2 or 600 to 700 mg/m^2 of daunorubicin,[68,69] although cases of fatal congestive cardiomyopathy have been observed after a single dose of doxorubicin. Above these doses, the risk steadily accelerates. The total dose limit at which the risk becomes unacceptable is largely arbitrary, and the risk may in part be dependent upon the treatment schedule used. For doxorubicin, the most commonly used total dose limit applied in the past has been 450 to 500 mg/m^2, at which the risk of clinically evident cardiac toxicity has generally been estimated to be 1% to 10%, rising to 7% to 20% at total doses of 550 mg/m^2. The corresponding limit applied for safe levels of daunorubicin is 900 to 1,000 mg/m^2. However, large trials that have prospectively evaluated heart function with radionuclide-gated cardiac blood pool scans strongly suggest that subclinical, but not inconsequential, reductions in ejection fraction can be detected routinely after 250 to 300 mg/m^2 doxorubicin.[70–72] Furthermore, changes in ejection fraction may or may not predict the development of heart failure in a specific patient.

While doxorubicin-induced congestive heart failure may have a fatal outcome, it is eminently treatable with standard measures, and many patients (probably well over half) recover or stabilize at a lower, but clinically acceptable, level of cardiac function.[73-75] Congestive heart failure may however occur many months after the discontinuation of doxorubicin, and patients who appear stabilized with adequate medical management are at increased risk during subsequent intercurrent illnesses.[75,76] Children are at risk of developing congestive heart failure many years after discontinuing doxorubicin even if treated long term with an angiotensin-converting enzyme inhibitor.[77] Ejection fraction measurement by radionuclide scan or echocardiography accurately reflects the status of cardiac contractility and is the standard for early detection of cardiotoxicity of anthracyclines.[78,79] Cardiac MRI may be used when the above imaging modalities are inconclusive and avoids radiation exposure. A significant drop in contractility (below 40% or >15% from baseline) is usually seen before the onset of congestive heart failure; however, this may not be the case in an individual patient.[80] Other approaches that are being investigated to monitor and predict anthracycline cardiac toxicity include strain and straining rate imaging, troponins, and assessment of genetic variants.[81,82] With appropriate monitoring during therapy and observing close limits, clinically significant cardiac toxicity can be avoided in most patients and can be detected before overt failure in the few who develop this complication. The importance of routine monitoring during cancer treatment and posttreatment surveillance has been emphasized in professional society guidelines.[83,84]

Medical management of congestive heart failure employs standard measures: diuresis and afterload reduction. With conservative treatment, many patients experience improvement. This improvement may be gradual and recovery can take more than 1 year. Cardiac transplantation may be indicated in younger patients cured of their malignancy.

Lessening the Risk of Cardiac Toxicity

The overall risk of cardiotoxicity from doxorubicin use in an adult population is 2%, or less, depending on patient age, total dose, and other risk factors. Fortunately, much can now be done to lessen the risk of cardiac toxicity. First, patient characteristics associated with increased risk have been identified. Hypertension and pre-existing cardiac disease predisposing to diastolic dysfunction significantly increase the risk that a patient will develop clinically cardiac abnormalities at a lower cumulative drug dose.[74] Cardiac irradiation clearly increases the sensitivity of the heart to anthracyclines; at a radiation dose of 20 Gy, the slope of the cardiac biopsy score versus the cumulative doxorubicin dose doubles so that a dose of 250 mg/m^2 becomes equal to 500 mg/m^2 in the absence of radiation.[85,86] Computer-based radiation treatment planning should be used to minimize cardiac radiation exposure in patients with breast cancer and lymphoma who will receive an anthracycline.

It is now clear that peak drug concentration is a major contributor to the risk of cardiac toxicity from doxorubicin.[55] In contrast, both in vitro and in patients, the antitumor activity of doxorubicin is a function of AUC not peak drug level. Thus, shifting from bolus drug administration to weekly dosing or prolonged infusion results in a significant reduction in the incidence of cardiac toxicity.[87] In clinical settings where cardiac toxicity has proved to be a serious problem, such as in the pediatric malignancies, the incidence of adverse cardiac effects reaches 25% in those receiving up to 300 mg/m^2, and the late incidence of adverse cardiac events, such

as failure, decreased ventricular dimension, and myocardial infarction in adulthood, increases 3- to 10-fold as compared to normal controls.[88]

Dexrazoxane (Fig. 14.5), a catalytic inhibitor of TOP2[2,89] is the only agent that has shown consistent ability to block the development of anthracycline-induced cardiac toxicity in a wide range of animal models.[90] Randomized, controlled clinical trials have proven that this agent dramatically reduces the incidence of cardiac toxicity in patients with breast cancer.[91-94] Dexrazoxane-treated patients had significantly smaller decreases in left ventricular ejection fraction at each dose level of doxorubicin, and their cardiac biopsies reflected less histologic change. However, the effect of dexrazoxane on antitumor activity remains controversial.[92,93,95] There is some evidence that the use of dexrazoxane concurrently with the initiation of fluorouracil, doxorubicin, and cyclophosphamide therapy interferes with the antitumor efficacy of the regimen, and this use is not recommended.[92,93] Dexrazoxane is approved by the U.S. Food and Drug Administration for reducing the incidence and severity of cardiomyopathy associated with doxorubicin administration in women with metastatic breast cancer who have received a cumulative doxorubicin dose of 300 mg/m^2 and are continuing to receive doxorubicin therapy to maintain tumor control. It is not recommended for use with the initiation of doxorubicin therapy.

The recommended dose ratio of dexrazoxane to doxorubicin is 10:1 (e.g., 500 mg/m^2 of dexrazoxane: 50 mg/m^2 of doxorubicin). Dexrazoxane is administered as an infusion up to 15 minutes in duration with a 30-minute fixed interval from the completion of dexrazoxane infusion to the initiation of doxorubicin.

Biochemical Mechanism of Anthracycline Cardiac Toxicity

The major site of anatomical damage after drug exposure is the sarcoplasmic reticulum, a major site of calcium regulation. Doxorubicin injury to the sarcoplasmic reticulum leads to calcium release.[96,97] Calcium is then taken up by the mitochondria, which do that in preference to ATP generation. This sequence would account for the lower ATP levels and accumulation of calcium within the mitochondria.

Cardiac toxicity from anthracyclines has also been related to doxorubicin-induced free radical formation.[98,99] Within the heart muscle, there are several sites where enzyme activity can reduce doxorubicin to the corresponding semiquinone; doxorubicin-stimulated oxygen radical formation by cardiac sarcoplasmic reticulum, cytosol, and mitochondria has been conclusively demonstrated.[100,101]

Recent studies have implicated Top2$\boldsymbol{\beta}$,[102] which is expressed by cardiomyocytes and nonreplicating cells.[103,104] Top2$\boldsymbol{\beta}$-doxorubicin-DNA ternary cleavage complex can induce DNA DSBs both in the nuclear and mitochondrial genomes leading to cell death in cardiomyocytes. TOP2$\boldsymbol{\beta}$-deleted mouse embryonic fibroblasts have been shown to be resistant to doxorubicin-induced cell death,[105] and mice without the mitochondrial topoisomerase TOP1MT die of cardiac failure due to lack of regeneration of intact mitochondrial DNA (mtDNA), which needs to replace the mtDNA damaged by anthracyclines.[10]

Secondary Leukemia

A second important late toxicity of anthracyclines, and particularly doxorubicin, is secondary leukemia, which have been linked to chromosome translocations following TOP2 poisoning.[106]

Indeed, TOP2 inhibitors are mutagenic as they produce DSBs in DNA through inhibition of TOP2.[11] In addition, anthracyclines oxidize DNA bases through generation of free radicals, which poison TOP2.[11] The risk of secondary AML is 2% or less in most clinical settings but presents a significant issue for adjuvant therapy of breast cancer, and for pediatric uses, where the expectation of cure is high.

Anthracenediones

Anthracenediones were synthesized in the late 1970s and were found to have potent antitumor activity against the P388 and L1210 murine leukemias. The most active of this series is mitoxantrone (Fig. 14.5). Subsequent preclinical and clinical evaluation has demonstrated significant differences between mitoxantrone and the anthracyclines in terms of mechanism of action, lesser cardiac toxicity, diminished potential for extravasation injury, and reduced nausea and vomiting or alopecia. The narrow spectrum of antitumor activity of mitoxantrone has confined it to breast and prostate cancer, leukemias, and lymphomas and has limited the opportunity to replace doxorubicin with mitoxantrone in clinical practice. Its key features are given in Table 14.4.

Clinical Pharmacology

The recommended dosage for bolus intravenous administration of mitoxantrone is 12 mg/m^2/d for 3 days for treatment of AML and 12 to 14 mg/m^2/d once every 3 weeks for patients with solid tumors. The drug has activity against breast cancer,[107] ovarian cancer,[108] non-Hodgkin's lymphoma,[109] and prostate cancer[110] in addition to acute leukemia. It is however rarely used in clinical practice in place of anthracyclines.[111] Mitoxantrone is administered as a 30-minute infusion and rarely causes extravasation injury if infiltrated. It should not be administered in solutions containing heparin.

Pharmacokinetics

The plasma disappearance of mitoxantrone is characterized by a rapid preliminary phase distribution and cellular uptake followed by a long terminal half-life of 23 to 42 hours.[112,113] During this final phase of drug disappearance, drug concentrations in plasma

approximate 1 ng/mL or 2 nM, a level at the margin of cytotoxicity. The pharmacokinetics of mitoxantrone is linear over the dose range from 8 to 14 mg/m^2 administered as a short infusion.[114] Less than 30% of the drug can be accounted for by the fraction of drug that appears in the urine (<10%) or the stool (<20%). Like doxorubicin, mitoxantrone distributes with high concentrations into tissues (liver > bone marrow > heart > lung > kidney) and remains in these sites for weeks after therapy.[112] Although specific guidelines are not available for dose adjustment in patients with hepatic dysfunction, the terminal half-life may be prolonged to greater than 60 hours in patients with liver impairment.[113,115]

Toxicity

The primary advantages of mitoxantrone, in comparison to doxorubicin, are its much-reduced incidence of cardiac toxicity, the mild nausea and vomiting that follow intravenous administration, and minimal alopecia. A small percentage (1% to 5%) of patients will develop congestive heart failure after treatment with mitoxantrone in the absence of prior anthracycline exposure.[116–118] The risk of cardiac toxicity is greatest in cancer patients who have received prior anthracyclines or chest irradiation[116,119] and in those with underlying cardiac disease. Other toxicities include a reversible leukopenia, with recovery within 14 days of drug administration; mild thrombocytopenia; nausea and vomiting; secondary leukemia[120]; and rarely abnormal liver enzymes in patients receiving dose levels appropriate for solid tumors.[121] One minor, and at times alarming, side effect of mitoxantrone is a bluish discoloration of the sclera, fingernails, and urine.

Epipodophyllotoxins

Extracts from the mayapple or mandrake plant have long been used as a source of folk medicine. The active principle, podophyllotoxin, acts as an antimitotic agent that binds to tubulin at a site distinct from that occupied by the vinca alkaloids. A number of semisynthetic derivatives of podophyllotoxin have been made. Two demethylepipodophyllotoxin derivatives, which target TOP2 instead of tubulin, are used in cancer chemotherapy, etoposide (VP-16) and teniposide (VM-26) (Table 14.5; Fig. 14.5).[2,11,89]

Pharmacokinetics

Following a single IV dose, etoposide elimination from plasma follows a two-compartment pharmacokinetic model with a terminal half-life of 6 to 8 hours in patients with normal renal function. For both epipodophyllotoxins, there is a large interpatient variability in pharmacokinetic parameters, around ±35%.[122,123] The volume of distribution averages 4 to 10 L/m^2. The peak plasma concentration and the AUC are proportional to the administered dose[124] up to 800 mg/m^2. Protein binding averages 96% but is nonlinear and influenced by the individual concentration of drug and albumin,[125] resulting in elevated free drug concentrations in patients with low serum albumin. Other conditions, including elevated serum bilirubin, which competes for albumin binding, also increase the concentration of the free drug, or biologically active drug, resulting in greater toxicity.[126,127] Two direct consequences of the high protein binding are (a) the correlation between the unbound fraction of etoposide and acute toxicity and (b) poor diffusion in the central nervous system, as well as in pleural and ascitic fluids. Etoposide

TABLE 14.4	*Key features of mitoxantrone*
Mechanism of action	Inhibition of TOP2; DNA intercalation (like anthracyclines)
Pharmacokinetics	Plasma $t_{1/2}$ = 23 to 42 h
Elimination	Hepatic metabolism (side-chain oxidation)
Toxicity	Acute myelosuppression
	Cardiac dysfunction (especially after doxorubicin)
	Blue tint to fingernails, sclerae
Precautions	Prior doxorubicin
	Hepatic dysfunction (reduce doses 50% for bilirubin elevation)
	Pre-existing cardiac disease

TABLE 14.5	*Key features of epipodophyllotoxin derivatives*	
	Etoposide (VP-16)	**Teniposide (VM-26)**
Mechanism of action	Inhibition of both TOP2α and β Nonintercalator	Same but ≈10-fold more potent
Pharmacokinetics	Terminal half-life = 6 to 8 h	Terminal half-life = 9.5 to 21 h
Elimination	Hepatic metabolism Renal excretion 35% to 40%	Probable hepatic metabolism
Toxicities	Neutropenia Thrombocytopenia (mild) Alopecia Hypersensitivity Mucositis (high doses)	Same as etoposide
Precautions	Reduced dose proportionate to creatinine clearance	Possible increased toxicity in hepatic failure

cerebrospinal fluid (CSF) concentrations are less than 5% of simultaneously measured plasma levels.[122,127]

The elimination half-life is independent of the dose. Etoposide is eliminated by both renal and nonrenal mechanisms, whereas teniposide is mostly eliminated through nonrenal mechanisms.[128] Approximately, 40% of etoposide is cleared through the kidney unchanged.[126,129] Thus, etoposide doses should be reduced in proportion to reductions in creatinine clearance.

Several metabolites of etoposide have been identified in humans.[122,130,131] The main metabolite etoposide-glucuronide is eliminated in the urine. O-demethylation by cytochrome P450 3A (CYP3A4) metabolizes etoposide (and teniposide) to a catechol metabolite, which is further oxidized to a quinone.[128,132] The etoposide-o-dihydroxy also can be converted to the o-quinone derivative. Both these, as well as the 4-demethylepipodophyllotoxin, remain active against TOP2. Moreover, the orthoquinone and semiquinone free radicals of etoposide may covalently bind to DNA and induce DNA strand breakage by TOP2-independent mechanisms.[133,134]

Biliary excretion is a minor route of elimination. Minor alterations in liver function, such as transaminase elevations, do not require dose reduction if renal function remains normal. Elevated bilirubin decreases the clearance of unbound etoposide,[135] leading to a greater hematologic toxicity. Therefore, etoposide dose should be reduced by 50% in patients with total bilirubin levels of 1.5 to 3.0 mg/dL, and no etoposide should be given to patients with more than 5.0 mg/dL bilirubin.[131] Anticonvulsant therapy, when given concomitantly with etoposide, may induce hepatic enzyme induction, resulting in a higher etoposide clearance.[136]

Oral Etoposide

Prolonged administration of etoposide aims for extended TOP2 inhibition, thus preventing tumor cells from repairing the TOP2-associated DNA breaks. Oral administration of etoposide represents the most feasible and convenient strategy to maintain effective concentrations of drug for extended times. Nevertheless, the efficacy of oral etoposide therapy is contingent on circumventing pharmacokinetic limitations, mainly low and variable bioavailability.[137] Pharmacokinetic-pharmacodynamic relationships indicate that severe toxicity is avoided when peak plasma concentrations do not exceed 3 to 5 mg/L and the trough concentration of drug at 24 hours is under 0.3 mg/L.

Oral etoposide is formulated in hydrophilic gelatin capsules. Peak plasma levels are obtained 0.5 to 4 hours after administration.[138] The mean bioavailability is 50%[138,139] with substantial interpatient and intrapatient variability (range 19% to 100%).[140] Bioavailability is not linear and decreases with doses greater than 200 mg, possibly implying a saturable absorptive mechanism in the GI tract. In addition to saturation of uptake, the very low aqueous solubility and the low stability at acid pH likely contribute to the erratic etoposide bioavailability.[140] The intestinal P-glycoprotein mediates the efflux of etoposide, and oral bioavailability of etoposide is not affected by food. The 50 mg/m^2 dose has the highest bioavailability (91% to 96%). By contrast, the bioavailability of doses lower than 100 mg (50 mg/m^2) approaches 75%,[139] while above doses of 100 mg/m^2, bioavailability decreases below 50%. Etoposide has been given orally over a prolonged 21-day schedule at a dose of 50 mg/m^2/d with dose-limiting myelosuppression. A pharmacodynamic model was prospectively tested for the therapeutic monitoring of 21-day oral etoposide.[141]

Etoposide Phosphate

Etoposide phosphate (Etopophos) has been designed as a prodrug of etoposide to obtain a water-soluble compound almost immediately converted to etoposide in plasma by host endogenous phosphatase(s). Thus, etoposide phosphate simplifies the formulation of etoposide by being water soluble and readily converted to etoposide.[142-144] Etoposide phosphate can be administered IV in saline solution over 5-minute infusions without signs of hypotension or acute effects.[142] As it is not formulated with polyethylene glycol (PEG), polysorbate 80, or ethanol, etoposide phosphate does not cause acidosis. Given as a continuous infusion, etoposide phosphate is stable in pumps for at least 7 days. Etoposide phosphate is better suited for bolus administration, high-dose treatment, and continuous infusions, provided equivalent antitumor activity to etoposide is demonstrated.

The molecular weights of etoposide and etoposide phosphate are close (558.57 and 568.55, respectively). To avoid confusion, doses of etoposide phosphate may be expressed as molar equivalent doses of etoposide. The toxicity of etoposide phosphate is similar to that of etoposide.[145] The maximum tolerated dose has been reported at 100 mg/m^2/d of etoposide equivalent for 5 days or 150 mg/m^2/d for dosing on days 1, 3, and 5. Etoposide phosphate may exhibit better intestinal absorption than etoposide with a mean bioavailability of 68% and has been proposed to overcome the intersubject and intrasubject variability in absorption observed with oral etoposide.[146] However, the same large interindividual variability of etoposide phosphate and etoposide AUC has been reported with 42.3% and 48.4%, as coefficients of variation.[147]

Teniposide (VM-26)

Similar to etoposide, teniposide exhibits biexponential disposition following intravenous administration. Only 10% to 20% of administered teniposide is found in the urine as metabolites. The large volume of distribution is consistent with the high degree of protein binding (>99%). Nonrenal clearance is similar to etoposide, as is the volume of distribution. An inverse relationship between serum γ-glutamyl-transpeptidase and teniposide plasma clearance has been reported, suggesting an important hepatic component to clearance. A linear relationship exists between dose and AUC. In humans, CSF levels of teniposide are barely detectable, although teniposide is considered clinically more effective than etoposide in the treatment of primary or secondary brain tumors.[148] Teniposide slowly diffuses into and is then slowly eliminated from third-space compartments such as ascites. Teniposide is available only for intravenous administration, but the IV formulation of teniposide can be used orally. The bioavailability of oral teniposide appears similar to that of oral etoposide in that absorption is decreased at higher doses and is increased with smaller consecutive daily doses. The mean bioavailability is 41%.[149,150] The MTD for oral teniposide given over 21 days is 100 mg/d, and the dose-limiting toxicity is myelosuppression.

Pharmacodynamics

Etoposide activity shows marked schedule dependency, which is both concentration- and time-dependent.[127] Etoposide clearance is not correlated with body surface area.[151] Dosing according to body surface area is a poor predictor of the peak or steady-state etoposide concentration or AUC.[152] Hematologic toxicity correlates better to the AUC of unbound etoposide than to the AUC of total etoposide.[153] Steady-state etoposide plasma levels of more than 1 μg/mL are tumoricidal but are associated with severe myelosuppression when the etoposide plasma levels are continuously higher than 3 μg/mL. The maintenance of a minimum plasma concentration between 2 and 3 μg/mL appears critical for efficacy. Intrapatient pharmacokinetic variability is small (12% to 15%).[127] Various limited sampling methods have been proposed to estimate etoposide AUC from one or two plasma concentration measurements.[154,155] In patients receiving 21-day oral VP-16, etoposide plasma concentrations are correlated with neutrophil count at the nadir.[141]

In the absence of measured plasma concentrations, it has been suggested to simplify VP-16 dosing to a fixed dose independent of body surface area, 260 mg instead of 150 mg/m^2.[127] Interestingly, a study in 52 patients with SCLC found independent prognostic factors regarding overall survival were LDH, etoposide clearance, and etoposide AUC.[156]

Acute Toxicity: Hematologic and Nonhematologic Toxicities

Myelosuppression is the dose-limiting acute toxicity of etoposide and is not cumulative. While the single daily MTD is 300 mg/m^2, intravenous doses of 150 mg/m^2 for 3 days and orally 50 mg/m^2/d over 21 days can be used. In this latter schedule, leukocyte nadirs occur between day 22 and 29. Nonhematological toxicities include nausea and vomiting in 10% to 20% of patients and alopecia in 10% to 30% of patients depending on dose and schedule.

Rare anaphylaxis and chemical phlebitis have been reported. Hypotension was noted in 5% to 8% of patients receiving etoposide but is rare when the drug is given over 1 hour and was probably related to the vehicle (polysorbate 80 plus PEG).[157]

Delayed Toxicity: Etoposide-Induced Secondary Leukemia

The increased frequency of illegitimate recombination events induced by TOP2-reactive agents may account for their leukemogenicity.[11,106,158] Etoposide was demonstrated to be mutagenic in patients.[159] The Childhood Cancer Survivor Study (CCSS) has assembled the largest cohort to date for assessment of late mortality experience of 20,483 survivors. Specific treatment-related risk factors for late mortality were identified including increased risk of death due to subsequent malignancy in patients treated with epipodophyllotoxins (RR = 2.3; 95% CI, 1.2–4.5).[160] Epipodophyllotoxin-associated secondary AML is the best-documented and most frequent secondary malignancy.[161] The follow-up by the National Cancer Institute Cancer Therapy Evaluation Program (CTEP) of patients treated with epipodophyllotoxins did not show evidence of significant variations in the incidence of secondary leukemias in patients who had received low (<1.5 g/m^2), moderate (between 1.5 and 2.99 g/m^2), or high cumulative doses (more than 3 g/m^2).[162] The calculated 6-year rate for development of leukemia was between 0.7% and 3.2%, and the highest rate was observed in the group of patients who received the lowest doses. Most other studies found a correlation between the cumulative dose of etoposide and the risk of secondary leukemias. In a case-control study of the French society of pediatric oncology, 61 patients with secondary leukemia were matched with 196 controls. In multivariate analysis, the risk of leukemia correlated with the type of primary tumor (excess risk in case of Hodgkin's disease and osteosarcoma) and with the cumulative dose of etoposide.[163] The risk of leukemia in patients who received more than 6 g/m^2 was 200-fold higher. The risk of leukemia was not increased by exposure to alkylating agents or radiotherapy. The administration of l-asparaginase prior to etoposide might also increase the risk of leukemia.[164]

The etoposide-induced leukemias frequently involve the long arm of chromosome 11, with translocation of the *MLL* gene at chromosome band 11q23, but other less common abnormalities involve chromosomes 3, 8, 15, 16, 17, 21, or 22.[165-167] The *MLL* (myeloid-lymphoid leukemia or mixed-lineage leukemia) gene resides at 11q23 and participates in the regulation of the differentiation of hematopoietic stem cells. Most of the breakpoints occur in a 9-kb region that includes exons 5 to 11 of the *MLL* gene. This genomic region includes DNA sequences, potentially involved for illegitimate recombinations, such as Alu sequences, VDJ recombinase recognition sites, and TOP2 consensus-binding sequences. Its overall sequence composition is AT rich. AT-rich sequences often correspond to nuclear MARs, where TOP2 cleavage complexes are preferentially formed.[168] More than 20 different translocations involving chromosome 11q23 have been described. TOP2 cleavage assays have shown a correspondence between TOP2 cleavage sites and the translocation breakpoints.[169] The mechanism of the translocation might be a chromosomal breakage by TOP2 followed by the recombination of DNA free ends during DNA repair. Top2*β* rather than Top2*α* has been implicated as the cause of the translocations and leukemia.[170]

In contrast to alkylating agent–associated secondary AML, epipodophyllotoxin-associated AML exhibits a shorter latency period with a median of 24 to 30 months.[161] Their phenotype is most often monocytic (FAB M4 or M5). The outcome of secondary AML is not necessarily worse than that of de novo AML when adjusted for cytogenetic features.[171]

Antitumor Activity

As one of the mainstays of chemotherapy for testicular cancer,[172] SCLC,[173] and bone sarcomas, and in refractory lymphomas, etoposide is widely used.[174] With bleomycin and cisplatin, it effects a nearly 95% cure rate in germ cell tumors of the testis[175] and is a first-line agent in combination therapy of AIDS-related Burkitt's lymphoma and in dose-intense regimens such as ICE, as mentioned previously. A standard regimen for limited stage SCLC combines etoposide, cisplatin, and chest irradiation. A typical regimen combines etoposide 100 mg/m^2 on days 1 to 3 with cisplatin 80 mg/m^2 on day 1, and these drugs are repeated every 3 weeks. Oral etoposide, while feasible, has yet to make a significant impact in clinical chemotherapy but may become useful as palliative treatment, particularly in elderly patients or in patients who are not candidates for intensive combination therapy regimens. Teniposide has very limited use in the clinical practice of medical oncology. Its primary role is to join anthracyclines and antimetabolites in neuroblastoma,[176] pediatric acute myelogenous leukemia,[177-179] and salvage therapy of childhood ALL and lymphomas.[180]

Tumor-Targeted Delivery

Topoisomerase inhibitors have been a mainstay of cancer therapy for many decades. However, conventional topoisomerase inhibitors have several well-established limitations including quick reversal of the trapped DNA-topoisomerase cleavage complex following drug removal and drug resistance mediated by various mechanisms. Further, their effectiveness is often limited by their lack of discrimination between normal tissue and tumor, which leads to systemic toxicities due to adverse effects on normal tissues and limits the achievable doses. Moreover, narrow therapeutic windows necessitate further dose reductions to maintain acceptable tolerability in multidrug combinations that represent the standard-of-care treatment modality for a variety of cancer types. Targeted delivery to tumor cells could overcome some of these limitations of conventional topoisomerase inhibitors. To address these limitations, a variety of site-selective drug delivery strategies have been designed to deliver topoisomerase inhibitors more specifically to tumors including liposomal or nanoparticle formulations to increase plasma half-life and tumor localization and coupling to monoclonal antibodies and other tumor-targeting agents.

Liposomes that are nanosized are also referred to as nanosomes and can be subdivided into stabilized and nonstabilized (conventional) liposomes. Stabilized liposomes can also be subdivided into those that are stabilized by PEG or a non-PEG substitute such as sphingomyelin. Nanoparticles are subdivided into microspheres, which include polymer micelles, and dendrimers. Conjugate formulations consist of the drug linked to nanosized PEG or non-PEG polymers.[181,182] The theoretical advantages of liposomal and nanoparticle-encapsulated and carrier-mediated drugs are increased solubility, prolonged duration of exposure, selective delivery of entrapped drug to the site of action, improved therapeutic index, and potentially overcoming resistance associated with the non–carrier-mediated anticancer agent. The process by which these agents preferentially accumulate in tumor and tissues is called the enhanced permeation and retention (EPR) effect.[183] The pharmacokinetic disposition of these agents is dependent upon the carrier and not the parent drug until the drug is released from the carrier.[184] Thus, the pharmacology and pharmacokinetics of these agents are complex, and detailed studies must be performed to evaluate the disposition of the encapsulated or conjugated form of the drug and the released active drug. The factors affecting the pharmacokinetic and pharmacodynamic variability of these agents most likely include the reticuloendothelial system, which has also been called the mononuclear phagocyte system.[185]

Onivyde

Onivyde (MM-398) is a highly stable nanoliposomal irinotecan that has advantages of site-specific delivery, in vivo drug retention, and extended release of drug compared with the free form of irinotecan.[186] Intraliposomal stabilization of irinotecan was found to reduce the toxicity of the encapsulated agent to healthy tissue while maintaining or increasing its antitumor potency. Compared with free irinotecan, MM-398 is associated with lower maximum concentration, longer elimination half-life, higher area under the curve for SN-38, smaller volume of distribution, and slower plasma clearance of total irinotecan.[186] In phase I studies, the maximum tolerated dose of MM-398 monotherapy was 120 mg/m^2 every 3 weeks and 80 mg/m^2 in combination with leucovorin and 5-fluorouracil.[187] The phase III NAPOLI-1 trial demonstrated a 1.9-month improvement in overall survival with the addition of MM-398 to leucovorin and 5-fluorouracil in patients with metastatic pancreatic ductal adenocarcinoma previously treated with gemcitabine-based therapies.[188] In the combination arm, the median overall survival was 6.1 months compared with 4.2 months with 5-fluorouracil and leucovorin alone. Based on this data, the FDA approved MM-398 in combination with 5-fluorouracil and leucovorin for patients with metastatic pancreatic cancer and disease progression following gemcitabine-based therapy. Grade 3 or 4 adverse events that occurred most frequently in patients who received the combination were neutropenia (27%), diarrhea (13%), vomiting (11%), and fatigue (14%).

DS-8201a

DS-8201a is a HER2-targeting ADC structurally composed of a humanized anti-HER2 antibody, enzymatically cleavable peptide linker and exatecan mesylate (DX-8951f), a novel TOP1 inhibitor, which is more potent in vivo than irinotecan against various tumor xenograft models, including irinotecan-resistant tumors.[189] The DS-8201a linker-payload system allows an enhanced drug-to-antibody ratio of 8 that could reduce plasma exposure and associated off-target toxicities. In preclinical studies, DS-8201a was effective in tumors with low HER2 expression and those that were resistant to ado-trastuzumab emtansine (T-DM1), an ADC composed of HER2 antibody trastuzumab and a tubulin polymerization inhibitor, DM1. In a phase I study, no dose-limiting toxicities were observed, and the maximum tolerated dose was not reached.[190] Consistent with preclinical observations, tumor responses were seen in patients with prior T-DM1 and in low HER2-expressing tumors. Based on these results, the FDA awarded the breakthrough designation for DS-8201a in HER2-positive metastatic breast cancer. DS-8201a is being evaluated in HER2-positive, unresectable, and/or metastatic breast cancer patients who are resistant or refractory to T-DM1.

Sacituzumab Govitecan

Sacituzumab govitecan (IMMU-132) is an ADC targeting TROP-2, a transmembrane glycoprotein that is usually expressed in trophoblast cells that can invade uterine decidua during the process of placental implantation, and an SN-38 payload. The IMMU-132 linker lends intermediate conjugate stability in serum. It is attached to the hydroxyl group on the lactone ring of SN-38 and contains a short PEG moiety to enhance solubility. In the low-pH environment of lysosomes, and in the tumor microenvironment, the carbonate bond between the linker and SN-38 is cleaved, releasing the active form of SN-38, which remains in its active form under such acidic conditions. In a phase I trial, neutropenia was dose limiting, with 12 mg/kg the maximum tolerated dose for cycle 1, but too toxic with repeated cycles; lower doses of 8 and 10 mg/kg were selected for further expansion as patients were most likely to tolerate extended treatment at these doses. Antitumor activity has been observed in patients with triple-negative breast cancer, platinum-resistant urothelial carcinoma, non–small cell and SCLCs.[191,192] Based on responses in previously treated patients with metastatic triple-negative breast cancer, IMMU-132 received a breakthrough therapy designation by the FDA.

PEN-866

PEN-866 (STA-12-8666) employs a novel drug delivery system, HSP90 inhibitor-drug conjugate (HDC) based on the property of small-molecule inhibitors of HSP90 to be preferentially retained in tumor cells in contrast to their rapid clearance from the circulation and normal tissues.[193] HSP90 is highly overexpressed in tumor tissue and is present in an activated configuration that displays greater affinity for selective inhibitors than the resident pool found in normal cells. PEN-866 is comprised of an HSP90-targeting moiety fused via a cleavable carbamate linker to SN-38. CES activity in normal tissue and tumor cleaves the linker region, releasing SN-38 over an extended period.[194] In contrast to ADC, this approach has the theoretical advantage of not requiring a cell surface antigen for binding and active endocytosis. Further, the abundance of HSP90 in tumor cells obviates the requirement for a cytotoxic component active at extremely low concentrations. Preclinical studies have demonstrated activity in pancreatic, breast, sarcoma, and lung cancer models.[195] A phase I study is evaluating PEN-866 in patients with chemotherapy-resistant solid tumors.

Tumor Targeted TOP2 Inhibitors

Liposomal formulations of anthracyclines have shown similar efficacy and less toxicity compared with conventional anthracyclines. Liposomal doxorubicin (Myocet) is approved for the treatment of metastatic breast cancer and pegylated liposomal doxorubicin (Doxil/Caelyx) for the treatment of platinum-resistant ovarian cancer, advanced breast carcinoma, AIDS-related Kaposi's sarcoma,

and multiple myeloma. Several lipid-based nanoformulations of TOP2 inhibitors are in various stages of clinical testing.[196]

Acknowledgments

Anish Thomas and Yves Pommier would like to gratefully acknowledge Alex Sparreboom, Ken-ichi Fujita, William C. Zamboni, James H. Doroshow, and François Goldwasser, contributors to the chapters on topoisomerase inhibitors in the 5th edition of this book. This work was supported by the Center for Cancer Research, the Intramural Program of the NCI (Z01 BC 006150 and ZIA BC 011793).

References

1. Ahmad M, Shen W, Li W, et al. Topoisomerase 3beta is the major topoisomerase for mRNAs and linked to neurodevelopment and mental dysfunction. *Nucleic Acids Res.* 2017;45(5):2704-2713.
2. Pommier Y. Drugging topoisomerases: lessons and challenges. *ACS Chem Biol.* 2013;8(1):82-95.
3. Pommier Y, Leo E, Zhang H, Marchand C. DNA topoisomerases and their poisoning by anticancer and antibacterial drugs. *Chem Biol.* 2010;17(5):421-433.
4. Pommier Y, Marchand C. Interfacial inhibitors: targeting macromolecular complexes. *Nat Rev Drug Discov.* 2012;11(1):25-36.
5. Pommier Y. Topoisomerase I inhibitors: camptothecins and beyond. *Nat Rev Cancer.* 2006;6(10):789-802.
6. Pommier Y, Cushman M. The indenoisoquinoline noncamptothecin topoisomerase I inhibitors: update and perspectives. *Mol Cancer Ther.* 2009;8(5):1008-1014.
7. Stoll G, Pietilainen OP, Linder B, et al. Deletion of TOP3beta, a component of FMRP-containing mRNPs, contributes to neurodevelopmental disorders. *Nat Neurosci.* 2013;16(9):1228-1237.
8. Xu D, Shen W, Guo R, et al. Top3beta is an RNA topoisomerase that works with fragile X syndrome protein to promote synapse formation. *Nat Neurosci.* 2013;16(9):1238-1247.
9. Khiati S, Baechler SA, Factor VM, et al. Lack of mitochondrial topoisomerase I (TOP1mt) impairs liver regeneration. *Proc Natl Acad Sci U S A.* 2015;112(36):11282-11287.
10. Khiati S, Dalla Rosa I, Sourbier C, et al. Mitochondrial topoisomerase I (top1mt) is a novel limiting factor of Doxorubicin cardiotoxicity. *Clin Cancer Res.* 2014;20(18):4873-4881.
11. Pommier Y, Sun Y, Huang SN, Nitiss JL. Roles of eukaryotic topoisomerases in transcription, replication and genomic stability. *Nat Rev Mol Cell Biol.* 2016;17(November 2016):703-721.
12. Pommier Y, Huang SY, Gao R, Das BB, Murai J, Marchand C. Tyrosyl-DNA-phosphodiesterases (TDP1 and TDP2). *DNA Repair (Amst).* 2014;19:114-129.
13. Hoa NN, Shimizu T, Zhou ZW, et al. Mre11 is essential for the removal of lethal topoisomerase 2 covalent cleavage complexes. *Mol Cell.* 2016;64(3):580-592.
14. Takemura H, Rao VA, Sordet O, et al. Defective Mre11-dependent activation of Chk2 by ataxia telangiectasia mutated in colorectal carcinoma cells in response to replication-dependent DNA double strand breaks. *J Biol Chem.* 2006;281(41):30814-30823.
15. Zhang YW, Regairaz M, Seiler JA, Agama KK, Doroshow JH, Pommier Y. Poly(ADP-ribose) polymerase and XPF-ERCC1 participate in distinct pathways for the repair of topoisomerase I-induced DNA damage in mammalian cells. *Nucleic Acids Res.* 2011;39:3607-3620.
16. Saltz L, Sirott M, Young C, et al. Phase-I Clinical and Pharmacology Study of topotecan given daily for 5 consecutive days to patients with advanced solid tumors, with attempt at dose intensification using recombinant granulocyte-colony-stimulating factor. *J Natl Cancer Inst.* 1993;85(18):1499-1507.
17. Eckardt JR, von Pawel J, Pujol JL, et al. Phase III study of oral compared with intravenous topotecan as second-line therapy in small-cell lung cancer. *J Clin Oncol.* 2007;25(15):2086-2092.

18. Gore M, Oza A, Rustin G, et al. A randomised trial of oral versus intravenous topotecan in patients with relapsed epithelial ovarian cancer. *Eur J Cancer.* 2002;38(1):57-63.

19. von Pawel J, Gatzemeier U, Pujol JL, et al. Phase II comparator study of oral versus intravenous topotecan in patients with chemosensitive small-cell lung cancer. *J Clin Oncol.* 2001;19(6):1743-1749.

20. Vanwarmerdam LJC, Huinink WWB, Rodenhuis S, et al. Phase-I clinical and pharmacokinetic study of topotecan administered by a 24-hour continuous-infusion. *J Clin Oncol.* 1995;13(7):1768-1776.

21. Gallo JM, Laub PB, Rowinsky EK, Grochow LB, Baker SD. Population pharmacokinetic model for topotecan derived from phase I clinical trials. *J Clin Oncol.* 2000;18(12):2459-2467.

22. Mould DR, Holford NHG, Schellens JHM, et al. Population pharmacokinetic and adverse event analysis of topotecan in patients with solid tumors. *Clin Pharmacol Ther.* 2002;71(5):334-348.

23. Herben VM, Rosing H, ten Bokkel Huinink WW, et al. Oral topotecan: bioavailability and effect of food co-administration. *Br J Cancer.* 1999;80(9):1380-1386.

24. Brangi M, Litman T, Ciotti M, et al. Camptothecin resistance: role of the ATP-binding cassette (ABC), mitoxantrone-resistance half-transporter (MXR), and potential for glucuronidation in MXR-expressing cells. *Cancer Res.* 1999;59(23):5938-5946.

25. Jonker JW, Smit JW, Brinkhuis RF, et al. Role of breast cancer resistance protein in the bioavailability and fetal penetration of topotecan. *J Natl Cancer Inst.* 2000;92(20):1651-1656.

26. O'Reilly S, Rowinsky E, Slichenmyer W, et al. Phase I and pharmacologic studies of topotecan in patients with impaired hepatic function. *J Natl Cancer Inst.* 1996;88(12):817-824.

27. O'Reilly S, Rowinsky EK, Slichenmyer W, et al. Phase I and pharmacologic study of topotecan in patients with impaired renal function. *J Clin Oncol.* 1996;14(12):3062-3073.

28. Brogden RN, Wiseman LR. Topotecan. A review of its potential in advanced ovarian cancer. *Drugs.* 1998;56(4):709-723.

29. Gelderblom HA, De Jonge MJ, Sparreboom A, Verweij J. Oral topoisomerase 1 inhibitors in adult patients: present and future. *Invest New Drugs.* 1999;17(4):401-415.

30. Gerrits CJ, Schellens JH, Burris H, et al. A comparison of clinical pharmacodynamics of different administration schedules of oral topotecan (Hycamtin). *Clin Cancer Res.* 1999;5(1):69-75.

31. Heron JF. Topotecan: an oncologist's view. *Oncologist.* 1998;3(6):390-402.

32. ten Bokkel Huinink W, Lane SR, Ross GA; International Topotecan Study Group. Long-term survival in a phase III, randomised study of topotecan versus paclitaxel in advanced epithelial ovarian carcinoma. *Ann Oncol.* 2004;15(1):100-103.

33. von Pawel J, Schiller JH, Shepherd FA, et al. Topotecan versus cyclophosphamide, doxorubicin, and vincristine for the treatment of recurrent small-cell lung cancer. *J Clin Oncol.* 1999;17(2):658-667.

34. Schiller JH, Adak S, Cella D, DeVore RF III, Johnson DH. Topotecan versus observation after cisplatin plus etoposide in extensive-stage small-cell lung cancer: E7593—a phase III trial of the Eastern Cooperative Oncology Group. *J Clin Oncol.* 2001;19(8):2114-2122.

35. Long HJ, Bundy BN, Grendys EC, et al. Randomized phase III trial of cisplatin with or without topotecan in carcinoma of the uterine cervix: a gynecologic oncology group study. *J Clin Oncol.* 2005;23(21):4626-4633.

36. Freyer G, Ligneau B, Tranchand B, Ardiet C, Serre Debeauvais F, Trillet Lenoir V. Pharmacokinetic studies in cancer chemotherapy: usefulness in clinical practice. *Cancer Treat Rev.* 1997;23(3):153-169.

37. Mathijssen RH, van Alphen RJ, Verweij J, et al. Clinical pharmacokinetics and metabolism of irinotecan (CPT-11). *Clin Cancer Res.* 2001;7(8):2182-2194.

38. Atsumi R, Okazaki O, Hakusui H. Pharmacokinetics of SN-38 [(+)-(4S)-4,11-diethyl-4,9-dihydroxy-1H- pyrano[3′,4′:6,7]-indolizino[1, 2-b]quinoline-3,14(4H,12H)-dione], an active metabolite of irinotecan, after a single intravenous dosing of 14C-SN-38 to rats. *Biol Pharm Bull.* 1995;18(8):1114-1119.

39. Bencharit S, Morton CL, Howard-Williams EL, Danks MK, Potter PM, Redinbo MR. Structural insights into CPT-11 activation by mammalian carboxylesterases. *Nat Struct Biol.* 2002;9(5):337-342.

40. Danks MK, Morton CL, Krull EJ, et al. Comparison of activation of CPT-11 by rabbit and human carboxylesterases for use in enzyme/prodrug therapy. *Clin Cancer Res.* 1999;5(4):917-924.

41. Hanioka N, Ozawa S, Jinno H, Ando M, Saito Y Sawada J. Human liver UDP-glucuronosyltransferase isoforms involved in the glucuronidation of 7-ethyl-10-hydroxycamptothecin. *Xenobiotica.* 2001;31(10):687-699.

42. Iyer L, Hall D, Das S, et al. Phenotype-genotype correlation of in vitro SN-38 (active metabolite of irinotecan) and bilirubin glucuronidation in human liver tissue with UGT1A1 promoter polymorphism. *Clin Pharmacol Ther.* 1999;65(5):576-582.

43. Iyer L, King CD, Whitington PF, et al. Genetic predisposition to the metabolism of irinotecan (CPT-11). Role of uridine diphosphate glucuronosyltransferase isoform 1A1 in the glucuronidation of its active metabolite (SN-38) in human liver microsomes. *J Clin Invest.* 1998;101(4):847-854.

44. de Jong FA, van der Bol JM, Mathijssen RHJ, et al. Renal function as a predictor of irinotecan-induced neutropenia. *Clin Pharmacol Ther.* 2008;84(2):254-262.

45. de Jong FA, Scott-Horton TJ, Kroetz DL, et al. Irinotecan-induced diarrhea: functional significance of the polymorphic ABCC2 transporter protein. *Clin Pharmacol Ther.* 2007;81(1):42-49.

46. Han JY, Lim HS, Shin ES, et al. Influence of the organic anion-transporting polypeptide 1B1 (OATP1B1) polymorphisms on irinotecan-pharmacokinetics and clinical outcome of patients with advanced non-small cell lung cancer. *Lung Cancer.* 2008;59(1):69-75.

47. Rothenberg ML, Meropol NJ, Poplin EA, Van Cutsem E, Wadler S. Mortality associated with irinotecan plus bolus fluorouracil/leucovorin: summary findings of an independent panel. *J Clin Oncol.* 2001;19(18):3801-3807.

48. Takimoto CH, Morrison G, Harold N, et al. Phase I and pharmacologic study of irinotecan administered as a 96-hour infusion weekly to adult cancer patients. *J Clin Oncol.* 2000;18(3):659-667.

49. Gupta E, Lestingi TM, Mick R, Ramirez J, Vokes EE, Ratain MJ. Metabolic-fate of irinotecan in humans—correlation of glucuronidation with diarrhea. *Cancer Res.* 1994;54(14):3723-3725.

50. Gupta E, Mick R, Ramirez J, et al. Pharmacokinetic and pharmacodynamic evaluation of the topoisomerase inhibitor irinotecan in cancer patients. *J Clin Oncol.* 1997;15(4):1502-1510.

51. Kudoh S, Fukuoka M, Masuda N, et al. Relationship between the pharmacokinetics of irinotecan and diarrhea during combination chemotherapy with cisplatin. *Jpn J Cancer Res.* 1995;86(4):406-413.

52. Vanhoefer U, Harstrick A, Achterrath W, Cao SS, Seeber S Rustum YM. Irinotecan in the treatment of colorectal cancer: clinical overview. *J Clin Oncol.* 2001;19(5):1501-1518.

53. Cunningham D, Glimelius B. A phase III study of irinotecan (CPT-11) versus best supportive care in patients with metastatic colorectal cancer who have failed 5-fluorouracil therapy. *Semin Oncol.* 1999;26(1):6-12.

54. Rougier P, Van Cutsem E, Bajetta E, et al. Randomised trial of irinotecan versus fluorouracil by continuous infusion after fluorouracil failure in patients with metastatic colorectal cancer. *Lancet.* 1998;352(9138):1407-1412.

55. Legha SS, Benjamin RS, Mackay B, et al. Reduction of doxorubicin cardiotoxicity by prolonged continuous intravenous infusion. *Ann Intern Med.* 1982;96(2):133-139.

56. Terasaki T, Iga T, Sugiyama Y, Hanano M. Experimental-evidence of characteristic tissue distribution of adriamycin—tissue DNA concentration as a determinant. *J Pharm Pharmacol.* 1982;34(9):597-600.

57. Greene RF, Collins JM, Jenkins JF, Speyer JL, Myers CE. Plasma pharmacokinetics of adriamycin and adriamycinol: implications for the design of in vitro experiments and treatment protocols. *Cancer Res.* 1983;43(7):3417-3421.

58. Gil P, Favre R, Durand A, Iliadis A, Cano JP Carcassonne Y. Time dependency of adriamycin and adriamycinol kinetics. *Cancer Chemother Pharmacol.* 1983;10(2):120-124.

59. Huffman DH, Bachur NR. Daunorubicin metabolism in acute myelocytic leukemia. *Blood.* 1972;39(5):637-643.

60. Dobbs NA, Twelves CJ, Gillies H, James CA, Harper PG, Rubens RD. Gender affects doxorubicin pharmacokinetics in patients with normal liver biochemistry. *Cancer Chemother Pharmacol.* 1995;36(6):473-476.

61. Mouridsen HT, Langer SW, Buter J, et al. Treatment of anthracycline extravasation with Savene (dexrazoxane): results from two prospective clinical multicentre studies. *Ann Oncol.* 2007;18(3):546-550.

62. Doroshow JH. Doxorubicin-induced cardiac toxicity. *N Engl J Med.* 1991;324(12):843-845.

63. Perez EA, Suman VJ, Davidson NE, et al. Cardiac safety analysis of doxorubicin and cyclophosphamide followed by paclitaxel with or without trastuzumab in the north central cancer treatment group n9831 adjuvant breast cancer trial. *J Clin Oncol.* 2008;26(8):1231-1238.

64. Kremer LCM, Caron HN. Anthracycline cardiotoxicity in children. *N Engl J Med.* 2004;351(2):120-121.

65. Bristow MR, Thompson PD, Martin RP, Mason JW, Billingham ME, Harrison DC. Early anthracycline cardiotoxicity. *Am J Med.* 1978;65(5):823-832.

66. Billingham ME, Mason JW, Bristow MR, Daniels JR. Anthracycline cardiomyopathy monitored by morphologic changes. *Cancer Treat Rep.* 1978;62(6):865-872.

67. Bristow MR, Mason JW, Billingham ME, Daniels JR. Doxorubicin cardiomyopathy—evaluation by phonocardiography, endomyocardial biopsy, and cardiac-catheterization. *Ann Intern Med.* 1978;88(2):168-175.

68. Von Hoff DD, Layard MW, Basa P, et al. Risk factors for doxorubicin-induced congestive heart failure. *Ann Intern Med.* 1979;91(5):710-717.

69. Von Hoff DD, Rozencweig M, Layard M, Slavik M, Muggia FM. Daunomycin-induced cardiotoxicity in children and adults. A review of 110 cases. *Am J Med.* 1977;62(2):200-208.

70. Cottin Y, Touzery C, Dalloz F, et al. Comparison of epirubicin and doxorubicin cardiotoxicity induced by low doses: evolution of the diastolic and systolic parameters studied by radionuclide angiography. *Clin Cardiol.* 1998;21(9):665-670.

71. Perez EA, Suman VJ, Davidson NE, et al. Effect of doxorubicin plus cyclophosphamide on left ventricular ejection fraction in patients with breast cancer in the North Central Cancer Treatment Group N9831 Intergroup Adjuvant Trial. *J Clin Oncol.* 2004;22(18):3700-3704.

72. Swain SM. Adult multicenter trials using dexrazoxane to protect against cardiac toxicity. *Semin Oncol.* 1998;25(4):43-47.

73. Haq MM, Legha SS, Choksi J, et al. Doxorubicin-induced congestive heart-failure in adults. *Cancer.* 1985;56(6):1361-1365.

74. Hershman DL, McBride RB, Eisenberger A, Tsai WY, Grann VR, Jacobson JS. Doxorubicin, cardiac risk factors, and cardiac toxicity in elderly patients with diffuse B-cell non-Hodgkin's lymphoma. *J Clin Oncol.* 2008;26(19):3159-3165.

75. Moreb JS, Oblon DJ. Outcome of clinical congestive-heart-failure induced by anthracycline chemotherapy. *Cancer.* 1992;70(11):2637-2641.

76. Buzdar AU, Marcus C, Smith TL Blumenschein GR. Early and delayed clinical cardiotoxicity of doxorubicin. *Cancer.* 1985;55(12):2761-2765.

77. Lipshultz SE, Lipsitz SR, Sallan SE, et al. Long-term enalapril therapy for left ventricular dysfunction in doxorubicin-treated survivors of childhood cancer. *J Clin Oncol.* 2002;20(23):4517-4522.

78. Alexander J, Dainiak N, Berger HJ, et al. Serial assessment of doxorubicin cardiotoxicity with quantitative radionuclide angiocardiography. *N Engl J Med.* 1979;300(6):278-283.

79. Dresdale A, Bonow RO, Wesley R, et al. Prospective evaluation of doxorubicin-induced cardiomyopathy resulting from postsurgical adjuvant treatment of patients with soft-tissue sarcomas. *Cancer.* 1983;52(1):51-60.

80. Swain SM, Whaley FS, Ewer MS. Congestive heart failure in patients treated with doxorubicin—A retrospective analysis of three trials. *Cancer.* 2003;97(11):2869-2879.

81. Armenian SH, Ding Y, Mills G, et al. Genetic susceptibility to anthracycline-related congestive heart failure in survivors of haematopoietic cell transplantation. *Br J Haematol.* 2013;163(2):205-213.

82. Blanco JG, Sun CL, Landier W, et al. Anthracycline-related cardiomyopathy after childhood cancer: role of polymorphisms in carbonyl reductase genes-a report from the children's oncology group. *J Clin Oncol.* 2012;30(13):1415-1421.

83. Armenian SH, Lacchetti C, Barac A, et al. Prevention and monitoring of cardiac dysfunction in survivors of adult cancers: American society of clinical oncology clinical practice guideline. *J Clin Oncol.* 2017;35(8):893-911.

84. Runowicz CD, Leach CR, Henry NL, et al. American Cancer Society/American Society of clinical oncology breast cancer survivorship care guideline. *J Clin Oncol.* 2016;34(6):611-635.

85. Billingham ME, Bristow MR, Glatstein E, Mason JW, Masek MA, Daniels JR. Adriamycin cardiotoxicity: endomyocardial biopsy evidence of enhancement by irradiation. *Am J Surg Pathol.* 1977;1(1):17-23.

86. Myrehaug S, Pintilie M, Tsang R, et al. Cardiac morbidity following modern treatment for Hodgkin lymphoma: supra-additive cardiotoxicity of doxorubicin and radiation therapy. *Leuk Lymphoma.* 2008;49(8):1486-1493.

87. van Dalen EC, van der Pal HJ, Kremer LC. Different dosage schedules for reducing cardiotoxicity in people with cancer receiving anthracycline chemotherapy. *Cochrane Database Syst Rev* 2016;(3):CD005008.

88. Goorin AM, Chauvenet AR, Perez-Atayde AR, Cruz J, McKone R, Lipshultz SE. Initial congestive heart failure, six to ten years after doxorubicin chemotherapy for childhood cancer. *J Pediatr.* 1990;116(1):144-147.

89. Nitiss JL. Targeting DNA topoisomerase II in cancer chemotherapy. *Nat Rev Cancer.* 2009;9(5):338-350.

90. Ducroq J, Moha ou Maati H, Guilbot S, et al. Dexrazoxane protects the heart from acute doxorubicin-induced QT prolongation: a key role for I(Ks). *Br J Pharmacol.* 2010;159(1):93-101.

91. Lopez M, Vici P, Di Lauro K, et al. Randomized prospective clinical trial of high-dose epirubicin and dexrazoxane in patients with advanced breast cancer and soft tissue sarcomas. *J Clin Oncol.* 1998;16(1):86-92.

92. Swain SM, Whaley FS, Gerber MC, Ewer MS, Bianchine JR, Gams RA. Delayed administration of dexrazoxane provides cardioprotection for patients with advanced breast cancer treated with doxorubicin-containing therapy. *J Clin Oncol.* 1997;15(4):1333-1340.

93. Swain SM, Whaley FS, Gerber MC, et al. Cardioprotection with dexrazoxane for doxorubicin-containing therapy in advanced breast cancer. *J Clin Oncol.* 1997;15(4):1318-1332.

94. Venturini M, Michelotti A, DelMastro L, et al. Multicenter randomized controlled clinical trial to evaluate cardioprotection of dexrazoxane versus no cardioprotection in women receiving epirubicin chemotherapy for advanced breast cancer. *J Clin Oncol.* 1996;14(12):3112-3120.

95. van Dalen E C, Caron HN, Dickinson HO, Kremer LC. Cardioprotective interventions for cancer patients receiving anthracyclines. *Cochrane Database Syst Rev* 2008;(2):CD003917.

96. Emanuelov AK, Shainberg A, Chepurko Y, et al. Adenosine A(3) receptor-mediated cardioprotection against doxorubicin-induced mitochondrial damage. *Biochem Pharmacol.* 2010;79(2):180-187.

97. Keung EC, Toll L, Ellis M, Jensen RA. L-type cardiac calcium channels in doxorubicin cardiomyopathy in rats morphological, biochemical, and functional correlations. *J Clin Invest.* 1991;87(6):2108-2113.

98. Myers C, Bonow R, Palmeri S, et al. A randomized controlled trial assessing the prevention of doxorubicin cardiomyopathy by N-acetylcysteine. *Semin Oncol.* 1983;10(1 suppl 1):53-55.

99. Singal PK, Iliskovic N. Doxorubicin-induced cardiomyopathy. *N Engl J Med.* 1998;339(13):900-905.

100. Davies KJA, Doroshow JH, Hochstein P. Mitochondrial nadh dehydrogenase-catalyzed oxygen radical production by adriamycin, and the relative inactivity of 5-iminodaunorubicin. *FEBS Lett.* 1983;153(1):227-230.

101. Doroshow JH. Effect of anthracycline antibiotics on oxygen radical formation in rat-heart. *Cancer Res.* 1983;43(2):460-472.

102. Zhang S, Liu X, Bawa-Khalfe T, et al. Identification of the molecular basis of doxorubicin-induced cardiotoxicity. *Nat Med.* 2012;18(11):1639-1642.

103. Khiati S, Seol Y, Agama K, et al. Poisoning of mitochondrial topoisomerase I by lamellarin D. *Mol Pharmacol.* 2014;86(2):193-199.

104. Zhang H, Zhang YW, Yasukawa T, Dalla Rosa I, Khiati S, Pommier Y. Increased negative supercoiling of mtDNA in TOP1mt knockout mice and presence of topoisomerases IIalpha and IIbeta in vertebrate mitochondria. *Nucleic Acids Res.* 2014;42(11):7259-7267.

105. Lyu YL, Kerrigan JE, Lin CP, et al. Topoisomerase IIbeta mediated DNA double-strand breaks: implications in doxorubicin cardiotoxicity and prevention by dexrazoxane. *Cancer Res.* 2007;67(18):8839-8846.

106. Cowell IG, Sondka Z, Smith K, et al. Model for MLL translocations in therapy-related leukemia involving topoisomerase IIbeta-mediated DNA strand breaks and gene proximity. *Proc Natl Acad Sci U S A.* 2012;109(23):8989-8994.

107. Neidhart JA, Gochnour D, Roach R, Hoth D, Young D. A comparison of mitoxantrone and doxorubicin in breast-cancer. *J Clin Oncol.* 1986;4(5):672-677.

108. Lawton F, Blackledge G, Mould J, Latief T, Watson R, Chetiyawardana AD. Phase-II study of mitoxantrone in epithelial ovarian-cancer. *Cancer Treat Rep.* 1987;71(6):627-629.

109. Coltman CA Jr, McDaniel TM, Balcerzak SP, Morrison FS, Von Hoff DD. Mitoxantrone hydrochloride (NSC-310739) in lymphoma. A Southwest Oncology Group study. *Invest New Drugs.* 1983;1(1):65-70.

110. Moore MJ, Osoba D, Murphy K, et al. Use of palliative end-points to evaluate the effects of mitoxantrone and low-dose prednisone in patients with hormonally resistant prostate-cancer. *J Clin Oncol.* 1994;12(4):689-694.

111. Britobabapulle F, Catovsky D, Slocombe G, et al. Phase-II study of mitoxantrone and cytarabine in acute myeloid-leukemia. *Cancer Treat Rep* 1987;71(2):161-163.

112. Alberts DS, Peng YM, Leigh S, Davis TP, Woodward DL. Disposition of mitoxantrone in cancer-patients. *Cancer Res.* 1985;45(4):1879-1884.

113. Smyth JF, Macpherson JS, Warrington PS, Leonard RCF, Wolf CR. The clinical-pharmacology of mitoxantrone. *Cancer Chemother Pharmacol.* 1986;17(2):149-152.

114. Repetto L, Vannozzi MO, Balleari E, et al. Mitoxantrone in elderly patients with advanced breast cancer: pharmacokinetics, marrow and peripheral hematopoietic progenitor cells. *Anticancer Res.* 1999;19(1b):879-884.

115. Savaraj N, Lu K, Manuel V, Loo TL. Pharmacology of mitoxantrone in cancer-patients. *Cancer Chemother Pharmacol.* 1982;8(1):113-117.

116. Benjamin RS, Chawla SP, Ewer MS, Carrasco CH, Mackay B, Holmes F. Evaluation of mitoxantrone cardiac toxicity by nuclear angiography and endomyocardial biopsy—an update. *Invest New Drugs.* 1985;3(2):117-121.

117. Shenkenberg TD, Von Hoff DD. Mitoxantrone: a new anticancer drug with significant clinical activity. *Ann Intern Med.* 1986;105(1):67-81.

118. Unverferth DV, Unverferth BJ, Balcerzak SP, Bashore TA, Neidhart JA. Cardiac evaluation of mitoxantrone. *Cancer Treat Rep.* 1983;67(4):343-350.

119. Pai GR, Reed NS, Ruddell WSJ. A case of mitoxantrone-associated cardiomyopathy without prior anthracycline therapy. *Br J Radiol.* 1987;60(719):1125-1126.

120. Kroger N, Damon L, Zander AR, et al.; Solid Tumor Working Party of the European Group for, T. Marrow, G. German Adjuvant Breast Cancer Study and S. F. University of California. Secondary acute leukemia following mitoxantrone-based high-dose chemotherapy for primary breast cancer patients. *Bone Marrow Transplant.* 2003;32(12):1153-1157.

121. Arlin ZA, Silver R, Cassileth P, et al. Phase-I-II trial of mitoxantrone in acute-leukemia. *Cancer Treat Rep.* 1985;69(1):61-64.

122. Hande KR, Wedlund PJ, Noone RM, Wilkinson GR, Greco FA, Wolff SN. Pharmacokinetics of high-dose etoposide (VP-16-213) administered to cancer patients. *Cancer Res.* 1984;44(1):379-382.

123. Rodman JH, Murry DJ, Madden T, Santana VM. Altered etoposide pharmacokinetics and time to engraftment in pediatric patients undergoing autologous bone marrow transplantation. *J Clin Oncol.* 1994;12(11):2390-2397.

124. Allen LM, Creaven PJ. Comparison of the human pharmacokinetics of VM-26 and VP-16, two antineoplastic epipodophyllotoxin glucopyranoside derivatives. *Eur J Cancer.* 1975;11(10):697-707.

125. Stewart CF, Arbuck SG, Fleming RA, Evans WE. Changes in the clearance of total and unbound etoposide in patients with liver dysfunction. *J Clin Oncol.* 1990;8(11):1874-1879.

126. Arbuck SG, Douglass HO, Crom WR, et al. Etoposide pharmacokinetics in patients with normal and abnormal organ function. *J Clin Oncol.* 1986;4(11):1690-1695.

127. D'Incalci M, Rossi C, Zucchetti M, et al. Pharmacokinetics of etoposide in patients with abnormal renal and hepatic function. *Cancer Res.* 1986;46(5):2566-2571.

128. van Schaik RH. CYP450 pharmacogenetics for personalizing cancer therapy. *Drug Resist Updat.* 2008;11(3):77-98.

129. Clark PI, Slevin ML. The clinical pharmacology of etoposide and teniposide. *Clin Pharmacokinet.* 1987;12(4):223-252.

130. D'Incalci M, Farina P, Sessa C, et al. Pharmacokinetics of VP16-213 given by different administration methods. *Cancer Chemother Pharmacol.* 1982;7(2-3):141-145.

131. Hande KR, Wolff SN, Greco FA, Hainsworth JD, Reed G, Johnson DH. Etoposide kinetics in patients with obstructive jaundice. *J Clin Oncol.* 1990;8(6):1101-1107.

132. Stremetzne S, Jaehde U, Schunack W. Determination of the cytotoxic catechol metabolite of etoposide (3'-O-demethyletoposide) in human plasma by high-performance liquid chromatography. *J Chromatogr B.* 1997;703(1-2):209-215.

133. Mans DR, Lafleur MV, Westmijze EJ, et al. Reactions of glutathione with the catechol, the ortho-quinone and the semi-quinone free radical of etoposide. Consequences for DNA inactivation. *Biochem Pharmacol.* 1992;43(8):1761-1768.

134. Mans DR, Lafleur MV, Westmijze EJ, et al. Formation of different reaction products with single- and double-stranded DNA by the ortho-quinone and the semi-quinone free radical of etoposide (VP-16-213). *Biochem Pharmacol.* 1991;42(11):2131-2139.

135. Stewart CF, Fleming RA, Arbuck SG, Evans WE. Prospective evaluation of a model for predicting etoposide plasma protein binding in cancer patients. *Cancer Res.* 1990;50(21):6854-6856.

136. Vecht CJ, Wagner GL, Wilms EB. Interactions between antiepileptic and chemotherapeutic drugs. *Lancet Neurol.* 2003;2(7):404-409.

137. Toffoli G, Corona G, Basso B, Boiocchi M. Pharmacokinetic optimisation of treatment with oral etoposide. *Clin Pharmacokinet.* 2004;43(7):441-466.

138. Stewart DJ, Nundy D, Maroun JA, Tetreault L, Prior J. Bioavailability, pharmacokinetics, and clinical effects of an oral preparation of etoposide. *Cancer Treat Rep.* 1985;69(3):269-273.

139. Hande KR, Krozely MG, Greco FA, Hainsworth JD, Johnson DH. Bioavailability of low-dose oral etoposide. *J Clin Oncol.* 1993;11(2):374-377.

140. Harvey VJ, Slevin ML, Joel SP, Johnston A Wrigley PFM. The effect of food and concurrent chemotherapy on the bioavailability of oral etoposide. *Br J Cancer.* 1985;52(3):363-367.

141. Miller AA, Tolley EA, Niell HB. Therapeutic drug monitoring of 21-day oral etoposide in patients with advanced non-small cell lung cancer. *Clin Cancer Res.* 1998;4(7):1705-1710.

142. Budman DR, Igwemezie LN, Kaul S, et al. Phase-I evaluation of a water-soluble etoposide prodrug, etoposide phosphate, given as a 5-minute infusion on day-1, day-3, and day-5 in patients with solid tumors. *J Clin Oncol.* 1994;12(9):1902-1909.

143. Fields SZ, Igwemezie LN, Kaul S, et al. Phase I study of etoposide phosphate (etopophos) as a 30-minute infusion on day-1, day-3, and day-5. *Clin Cancer Res.* 1995;1(1):105-111.

144. Millward MJ, Newell DR, Mummaneni V, et al. Phase I and pharmacokinetic study of a water-soluble etoposide prodrug, etoposide phosphate (BMY-40481). *Eur J Cancer.* 1995;31a(13-14):2409-2411.

145. Kaul S, Igwemezie LN, Stewart DJ, et al. Pharmacokinetics and bioequivalence of etoposide following intravenous administration of etoposide phosphate and etoposide in patients with solid tumors. *J Clin Oncol.* 1995;13(11):2835-2841.

146. Sessa C, Zucchetti M, Cerny T, et al. Phase-I clinical and pharmacokinetic study of oral etoposide phosphate. *J Clin Oncol.* 1995;13(1):200-209.

147. deJong RS, Mulder NH, Uges DRA, et al. Randomized comparison of etoposide pharmacokinetics after oral etoposide phosphate and oral etoposide. *Br J Cancer.* 1997;75(11):1660-1666.

148. Postmus PE, Haaxma-Reiche H, Smit EF, et al. Treatment of brain metastases of small-cell lung cancer: comparing teniposide and teniposide with whole-brain radiotherapy—A phase III study of the European Organization for the Research and Treatment of Cancer Lung Cancer Cooperative Group. *J Clin Oncol.* 2000;18(19):3400-3408.

149. Smit EF, Ousterhuis BE, Berendsen HH, Sleijfer DT, Postmus PE. Phase I study of oral teniposide (VM-26). *Semin Oncol.* 1992;19(2 suppl 6):35-39.

150. Splinter TA, Holthuis JJ, Kok TC, Post MH. Absolute bioavailability and pharmacokinetics of oral teniposide. *Semin Oncol.* 1992;19(2 suppl 6):28-34.

151. Mick R, Ratain MJ. Modeling interpatient pharmacodynamic variability of etoposide. *J Natl Cancer Inst.* 1991;83(21):1560-1564.

152. Ratain MJ, Mick R, Schilsky RL, Vogelzang NJ, Berezin F. Pharmacologically based dosing of etoposide: a means of safely increasing dose intensity. *J Clin Oncol.* 1991;9(8):1480-1486.

153. Stewart CF, Arbuck SG, Fleming RA, Evans WE. Relation of systemic exposure to unbound etoposide and hematologic toxicity. *Clin Pharmacol Ther.* 1991;50(4):385-393.

154. Gentili D, Zucchetti M, Torri V, et al. A limited sampling model for the pharmacokinetics of etoposide given orally. *Cancer Chemother Pharmacol.* 1993;32(6):482-486.

155. Lum BL, Lane KJ, Synold TW, Goram A, Charnick SB, Sikic BI. Validation of a limited sampling model to determine etoposide area under the curve. *Pharmacotherapy.* 1997;17(5):887-890.

156. You B, Tranchand B, Girard P, et al. Etoposide pharmacokinetics and survival in patients with small cell lung cancer: a multicentre study. *Lung Cancer.* 2008;62(2):261-272.

157. O'Dwyer PJ, Weiss RB. Hypersensitivity reactions induced by etoposide. *Cancer Treat Rep.* 1984;68(7-8):959-961.

158. Pommier Y, Schwartz RE, Zwelling LA, Kohn KW. Effects of DNA intercalating agents on topoisomerase II induced DNA strand cleavage in isolated mammalian cell nuclei. *Biochemistry.* 1985;24(23):6406-6410.

159. Karnaoukhova L, Moffat J, Martins H, Glickman B. Mutation frequency and spectrum in lymphocytes of small cell lung cancer patients receiving etoposide chemotherapy. *Cancer Res.* 1997;57(19):4393-4407.

160. Armstrong GT, Liu Q, Yasui Y, et al. Late mortality among 5-year survivors of childhood cancer: a summary from the childhood cancer survivor study. *J Clin Oncol.* 2009;27(14):2328-2338.

161. Felix CA. Secondary leukemias induced by topoisomerase-targeted drugs. *Biochim Biophys Acta.* 1998;1400(1-3):233-255.

162. Smith MA, Rubinstein L, Anderson JR, et al. Secondary leukemia or myelodysplastic syndrome after treatment with epipodophyllotoxins. *J Clin Oncol.* 1999;17(2):569-577.

163. Le Deley MC, Leblanc T, Shamsaldin A, et al.; P. Societe Francaise d'Oncologie. Risk of secondary leukemia after a solid tumor in childhood according to the dose of epipodophyllotoxins and anthracyclines: a case-control study by the Societe Francaise d'Oncologie Pediatrique. *J Clin Oncol.* 2003;21(6):1074-1081.

164. Pui CH, Relling MV, Behm FG, et al. L-Asparaginase may potentiate the leukemogenic effect of the epipodophyllotoxins. *Leukemia.* 1995;9(10):1680-1684.

165. Pedersen-Bjergaard J, Daugaard G, Hansen SW, Philip P, Larsen SO, Rorth M. Increased risk of myelodysplasia and leukemia after etoposide, cisplatin, and bleomycin for germ-cell tumors. *Lancet.* 1991;338(8763):359-363.

166. Pedersen-Bjergaard J, Pedersen M, Roulston D, Philip P. Different genetic pathways in leukemogenesis for patients presenting with therapy-related myelodysplasia and therapy-related acute myeloid leukemia. *Blood.* 1995;86(9):3542-3552.

167. Pedersen-Bjergaard J, Rowley JD. The balanced and the unbalanced chromosome-aberrations of acute myeloid-leukemia may develop in different ways and may contribute differently to malignant transformation. *Blood.* 1994;83(10):2780-2786.

168. Pommier Y, Cockerill PN, Kohn KW, Garrard WT. Identification within the Simian Virus-40 genome of a chromosomal loop attachment site that contains topoisomerase-II cleavage sites. *J Virol.* 1990;64(1):419-423.

169. Mistry AR, Felix CA, Whitmarsh RJ, et al. DNA topoisomerase II in therapy-related acute promyelocytic leukemia. *N Engl J Med.* 2005;352(15):1529-1538.

170. Azarova AM, Lyu YL, Lin CP, et al. Roles of DNA topoisomerase II isozymes in chemotherapy and secondary malignancies. *Proc Natl Acad Sci U S A.* 2007;104(26):11014-11019.

171. Hijiya N, Ness KK, Ribeiro RC, Hudson MM. Acute leukemia as a secondary malignancy in children and adolescents current findings and issues. *Cancer.* 2009;115(1):23-35.

172. Einhorn LH, Williams SD, Chamness A, Brames MJ, Perkins SM, Abonour R. High-dose chemotherapy and stem-cell rescue for metastatic germ-cell tumors. *N Engl J Med.* 2007;357(4):340-348.

173. Albers P, Siener R, Krege S, et al. Randomized phase III trial comparing retroperitoneal lymph node dissection with one course of bleomycin and etoposide plus cisplatin chemotherapy in the adjuvant treatment of clinical stage I nonseminomatous testicular germ cell tumors: AUO trial AH 01/94 by the German testicular cancer study group. *J Clin Oncol.* 2008;26(18):2966-2972.

174. Williams SD, Birch R, Einhorn LH, Irwin L, Greco FA, Loehrer PJ. Treatment of disseminated germ-cell tumors with cisplatin, bleomycin, and either vinblastine or etoposide. *N Engl J Med.* 1987;316(23):1435-1440.

175. Newlands ES, Bagshawe KD. Epipodophylin derivative (VP 16-23) in malignant teratomas and choriocarcinomas. *Lancet.* 1977;2(8028):87.

176. Bowman LC, Castleberry RP, Cantor A, et al. Genetic staging of unresectable or metastatic neuroblastoma in infants: a Pediatric Oncology Group Study. *J Natl Cancer Inst.* 1997;89(5):373-380.

177. Amylon MD, Shuster J, Pullen J, et al. Intensive high-dose asparaginase consolidation improves survival for pediatric patients with T cell acute lymphoblastic leukemia and advanced stage lymphoblastic lymphoma: a Pediatric Oncology Group study. *Leukemia.* 1999;13(3):335-342.

178. Evans WE, Relling MV, Rodman JH, et al. Conventional compared with individualized chemotherapy for childhood acute lymphoblastic leukemia. *N Engl J Med.* 1998;338(8):499-505.

179. Rivera GK, Buchanan G, Boyett JM, et al. Intensive retreatment of childhood acute lymphoblastic leukemia in first bone marrow relapse. A Pediatric Oncology Group Study. *N Engl J Med.* 1986;315(5):273-278.

180. Solal-Celigny P, Lepage E, Brousse N, et al. Doxorubicin-containing regimen with or without interferon alfa-2b for advanced follicular lymphomas: final analysis of survival and toxicity in the Groupe d'Etude des Lymphomes Folliculaires 86 trial. *J Clin Oncol.* 1998;16(7):2332-2338.

181. Drummond DC, Meyer O, Hong K, Kirpotin DB, Papahadjopoulos D. Optimizing liposomes for delivery of chemotherapeutic agents to solid tumors. *Pharmacol Rev.* 1999;51(4):691-743.

182. Papahadjopoulos D, Allen TM, Gabizon A, et al. Sterically stabilized liposomes: improvements in pharmacokinetics and antitumor therapeutic efficacy. *Proc Natl Acad Sci U S A.* 1991;88(24):11460-11464.

183. Maeda H, Wu J, Sawa T, Matsumura Y, Hori K. Tumor vascular permeability and the EPR effect in macromolecular therapeutics: a review. *J Control Release.* 2000;65(1-2):271-284.

184. Laginha K, Mumbengegwi D, Allen T. Liposomes targeted via two different antibodies: assay, B-cell binding and cytotoxicity. *Biochim Biophys Acta.* 2005;1711(1):25-32.

185. Laverman P, Carstens MG, Boerman OC, et al. Factors affecting the accelerated blood clearance of polyethylene glycol-liposomes upon repeated injection. *J Pharmacol Exp Ther.* 2001;298(2):607-612.

186. Drummond DC, Noble CO, Guo ZX, Hong K, Park JW, Kirpotin DB. Development of a highly active nanoliposomal irinotecan using a novel intraliposomal stabilization strategy. *Cancer Res.* 2006;66(6):3271-3277.

187. Chang TC, Shiah HS, Yang CH, et al. Phase I study of nanoliposomal irinotecan (PEP02) in advanced solid tumor patients. *Cancer Chemother Pharmacol.* 2015;75(3):579-586.

188. Wang-Gillam A, Li CP, Bodoky G, et al.; N.-S. Group. Nanoliposomal irinotecan with fluorouracil and folinic acid in metastatic pancreatic cancer after previous gemcitabine-based therapy (NAPOLI-1): a global, randomised, open-label, phase 3 trial. *Lancet.* 2016;387(10018):545-557.

189. Ogitani Y, Aida T, Hagihara K, et al. DS-8201a, a novel HER2-targeting ADC with a novel DNA topoisomerase I inhibitor, demonstrates a promising antitumor efficacy with differentiation from T-DM1. *Clin Cancer Res.* 2016;22(20):5097-5108.

190. Doi T Iwata H, Tsurutani J, et al. Single agent activity of DS-8201a, a HER2-targeting antibody-drug conjugate, in heavily pretreated HER2 expressing solid tumors. *J Clin Oncol.* 2017;35(15 suppl):108-108.

191. Bardia A, Mayer IA, Diamond JR, et al. Efficacy and safety of anti-trop-2 antibody drug conjugate sacituzumab govitecan (IMMU-132) in heavily pretreated patients with metastatic triple-negative breast cancer. *J Clin Oncol.* 2017;35(19):2141-2148.

192. Gray JE, Heist RS, Starodub AN, et al. Therapy of small-cell lung cancer (SCLC) with a topoisomerase-I-inhibiting antibody-drug conjugate (ADC) targeting Trop-2, sacituzumab govitecan. *Clin Cancer Res.* 2017;23(19):5711-5719.

193. Chiosis G, Neckers L. Tumor selectivity of Hsp90 inhibitors: the explanation remains elusive. *ACS Chem Biol.* 2006;1(5):279-284.

194. Proia DA, Smith DL, Zhang J, et al. HSP90 Inhibitor-SN-38 conjugate strategy for targeted delivery of topoisomerase I inhibitor to tumors. *Mol Cancer Ther.* 2015;14(11):2422-2432.

195. Heske CM, Mendoza A, Edessa LD, et al. STA-8666, a novel HSP90 inhibitor/SN-38 drug conjugate, causes complete tumor regression in preclinical mouse models of pediatric sarcoma. *Oncotarget.* 2016;7(40):65540-65552.

196. Alphandery E, Grand-Dewyse P, Lefevre R, Mandawala C, Durand-Dubief M. Cancer therapy using nanoformulated substances: scientific, regulatory and financial aspects. *Expert Rev Anticancer Ther* 2015;15(10):1233-1255.

Bleomycin, Yondelis, MMC

Bruce A. Chabner

In a search for new antimicrobial and antineoplastic agents, natural products from plants, fungal cultures, and marine organisms have yielded structurally and mechanistically unique products useful for cancer treatment. Collection of raw material, isolation of the active principle and its chemical and mechanistic characterization, and total synthesis of the product represent a series of daunting challenges. Among the successful pioneers in this field, Umezawa et al.[1] isolated a number of bioactive materials for treatment of infectious disease, malaria, and cancer. Among his important contributions were the bleomycins, small glycopeptides from culture broths of the fungus *Streptomyces verticillus*. The most active antitumor agent found was, in fact, a mixture of peptides now known as *bleomycin*, a drug with important activity against Hodgkin's disease, testicular cancer, malignant pleural effusions, and cancers of the cervix and penis. Bleomycin combined with vinblastine, etoposide, and *cis*-platin cures most patients with germ cell tumors of the testis.[2] The drug has attracted great interest because of its unique structure and biochemical action, its virtual lack of toxicity for normal hematopoietic tissue, and its unfortunate ability to cause pulmonary fibrosis. Its primary pharmacologic and pharmacokinetic features are shown in Table 15.1.

Structure and Mechanism of Action

The bleomycins are a family of peptides with a molecular weight of approximately 1,500 (Fig. 15.1). All contain a unique structural component, bleomycinic acid, and differ only in their terminal alkylamine group. Bleomycin A_2, the predominant peptide, has been prepared by total chemical synthesis, as have more than 100 bleomycin analogues, but none has emerged as a superior drug.[3]

The clinical mixture of bleomycin peptides is formulated as a sulfate salt, and its potency is measured in units (U) of antimicrobial activity. Each unit contains between 1.2 and 1.7 mg of polypeptide protein. The powdered clinical mixture is stable for at least 1 year at room temperature and for 4 weeks after reconstitution in aqueous solution at 4°C.

The multiple glycopeptides found in the clinical preparation of bleomycin have been separated and purified by high-performance liquid chromatography (HPLC).[4] The predominant active component, constituting approximately 70% of the commercial preparation, is the A_2 peptide. The native compound isolated from *S. verticillus* is a blue-colored Cu(II) coordinated complex, although the peptide will complex in vitro with other metals including iron, cobalt, zinc, and manganese, in various valence states.[5] The iron and copper complexes are believed to be the active forms in vivo.

The Co(III) complexes have no biologic activity, retain their bound metal tightly, and were formerly used for tumor imaging as the [57]Co complex. Bleomycin has the highest affinity for Cu(II). In initial clinical trials with Cu(II)·bleomycin, patients experienced profound phlebitis. The white apobleomycin, lacking metal, was soon adopted for clinical use. After systemic administration, bleomycin rapidly complexes with Cu(II) derived from plasma proteins.[6] Transport of the Cu(II) bleomycin complex across membranes depends upon the presence of the disaccharide (L-glucose and 3-O-carbamoyl-D-mannose) moiety of bleomycin and its bound metal, Cu(II). Deletion of the disaccharide or the metal markedly impairs uptake and cytotoxicity.[7]

15.1	*Key features of bleomycin pharmacology*
Mechanism of Action	Oxidative Cleavage of DNA Initiated by Hydrogen Abstraction
Metabolism	Activated by microsomal reduction
	Degraded by hydrolase found in multiple tissues
Pharmacokinetics	$t_{1/2}$: 2 to 4 h
Elimination	Renal: 45% to 70% in first 24 h
Drug interactions	None clearly established at a biochemical level
	Oxygen enhances pulmonary toxicity
	cisplatin induces renal failure and increases risk of pulmonary toxicity
Toxicity	Pulmonary interstitial infiltrates and fibrosis
	Desquamation, especially of fingers, elbows
	Raynaud's phenomenon
	Hypersensitivity reactions (fever, anaphylaxis, eosinophilic pulmonary infiltrates)
Precautions	Pulmonary toxicity increased in patients with underlying pulmonary disease
	Age > 70 y
	Renal insufficiency
	Prior chest irradiation
	O_2 during surgery
	Reduce dose if creatinine clearance <80 mL/min

$t_{1/2}$, half-life.

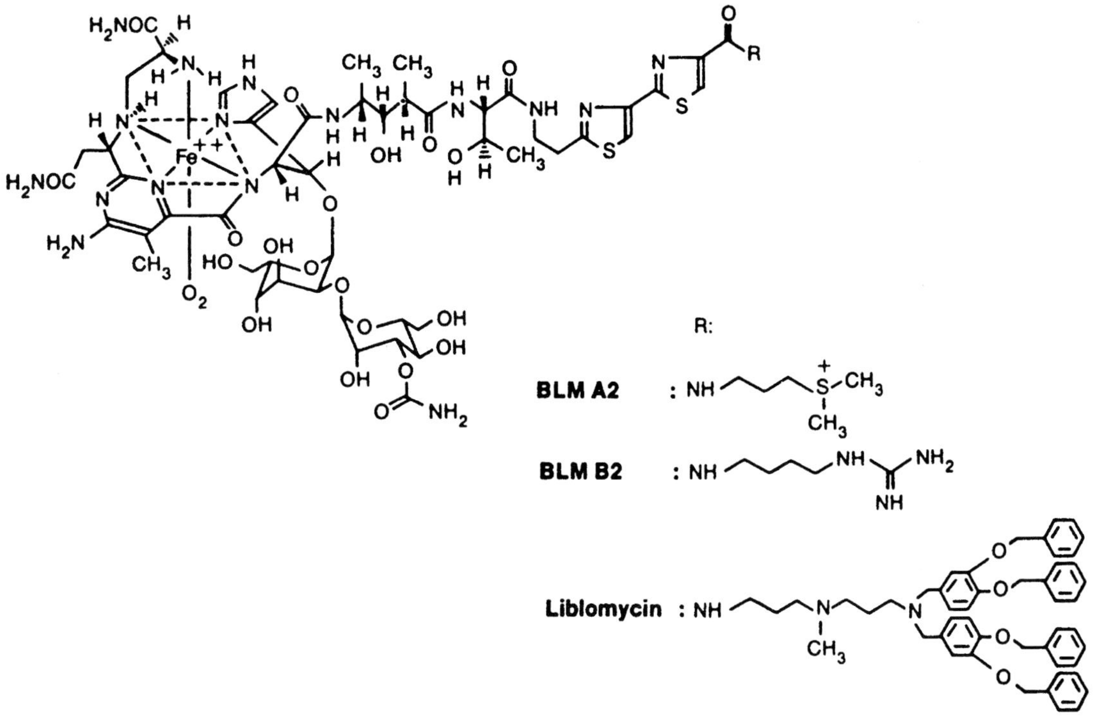

FIGURE **15.1** Structure of bleomycin·Fe(II) complex. The various substitutions on the amino-terminal end of the molecule are shown for bleomycin A₂ (BLM A2) and for bleomycin B₂ (BLM B2; also a component of the clinical preparation).

Intracellularly, Cu(II) complex is converted to reduced Cu(I), which is then replaced by the more abundant Fe(II) metal.[5] Nuclear translocation of the Fe(II)·bleomycin complex proceeds with subsequent DNA damage mediated by the drug's generation of free radicals.

Bleomycin binds Fe(II) by forming a square-pyramidal complex, as indicated in Figure 15.1. Six distinct moieties are required for this metal coordination complex with the pyrimidine, the imidazole, and a secondary amine as undisputed participants.[5] Debate still exists about the arrangement of the remaining ligands.

Mechanism of Antitumor Action

Single- and double-strand DNA breaks are readily observed in cultured cells and in isolated DNA incubated with bleomycin. This breakage is reflected in the chromosomal gaps, deletions, and fragments seen in cytogenetic studies of whole cells incubated with the drug. Other biochemical targets, including RNA and lipid, are attacked by bleomycin and the oxygen radicals it generates, and these interactions may contribute to its action.[8]

The mechanism by which Fe(II)·bleomycin cleaves DNA has been examined using viral, bacterial, mammalian, and synthetic DNAs. Bleomycin is unlike most DNA-damaging agents in that it attacks neither the nucleic acid bases nor the phosphate linkages. In the multistep process, an "activated" Fe(II)·bleomycin·O₂ complex is formed that can directly cleave DNA. Oxygen binding to Fe(II)·bleomycin proceeds most rapidly in the presence of DNA.[9] The proposed sequence of events, producing an activated bleomycin, is outlined in Figure 15.2.

A ternary Fe(II)·bleomycin·O₂ species, which can be trapped with isocyanide, CO, or NO in vitro, is activated by a $1e^-$ reduction.

The e^- can be supplied by a second Fe(II)·bleomycin·O₂ molecule, by H₂O₂, and by microsomal and nuclear reductases, and nicotinamide-adenine dinucleotide phosphate (reduced form) (NADPH), or nicotinamide-adenine dinucleotide (reduced form) (NADH).[10–12] In the absence of DNA, the activated species will self-destruct. The association of O₂Fe(II)·bleomycin with duplex DNA occurs rapidly. The interaction of bleomycin with DNA shows nucleotide sequence selectivity, cleavage occurring preferentially at start sites of active transcription.[13] The guanine-rich telomeric region of chromosome ends is a favored site as well.[14] The binding between bleomycin and DNA proceeds through partial intercalation (insertion between base pairs) of the amino-terminal tripeptide of bleomycin (the *S. tripeptide*).[15] The bithiazole of the S tripeptide binds to guanine groups in the favored sequence of GpT or GpC.[16]

The third step in the action of bleomycin is the generation of single- and double-strand DNA breaks. During the DNA cleavage process, under aerobic conditions, Fe(II)·bleomycin resembles a ferrous oxidase, catalyzing the conversion Fe(II) to Fe(III) and releasing electrons that generate oxygen radicals and other

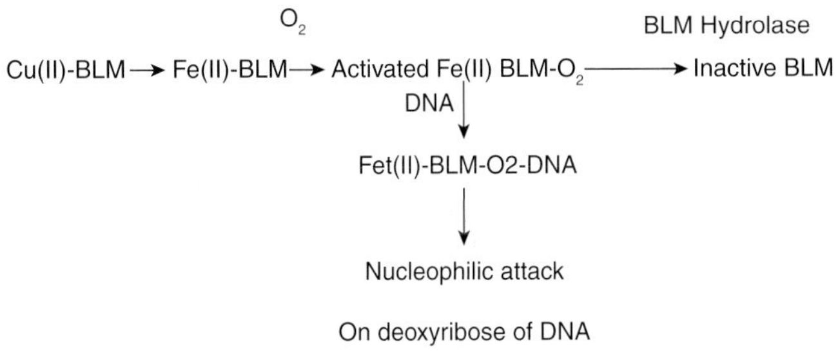

FIGURE **15.2** Model for the activation of cleavage-competent bleomycin (BLM).

reactive species.[17] The active Fe(II) may be regenerated by endogenous reductases, including cytochrome P-450 reductase,[18] an enzyme found in the nucleus and nuclear membrane. Bleomycin bound to DNA consumes oxygen rapidly in vitro, with a maximum velocity of 27 mol oxygen per minute per mole of bleomycin.

The DNA fragments produced after incubation of the substrate with activated bleomycin indicate an attack at the C-3′–C-4′ deoxyribose bond. A proton is extracted at C′-4, leading to a break in the phosphodiester linkage, producing a 5′-oligonucleotide terminating at its 3′ end with a phosphoglycolic acid moiety and a 3′-oligonucleotide containing a 5′-phosphate. In addition, a 3′-(thymin-9′-yl) propenal is released[19] (Fig. 15.3). Under anaerobic conditions, bleomycin (FeIII) is able to cleave DNA, releasing the free base, but the phosphoribose chain remains intact. In cells exposed to bleomycin, free bases and base propenals are detected.

The base propenal compounds have intrinsic cytotoxicity and may contribute to cellular damage.[20]

Bleomycin produces both single- and double-strand DNA breaks in a ratio of approximately 10:1. The highly electronegative 3′-phosphoglycolate and 5′-phosphate groups remaining at the site of DNA single-strand cleavage may promote access of a second bleomycin molecule to the opposing strand, resulting in a double-strand break.

Analysis of the products of DNA cleavage, using either viral or mammalian DNA, has consistently shown a preferential release of thymine or thymine-propenal, with lesser amounts of the other three bases or their propenal derivatives.[8] The propensity for attack at thymine results from the preference for partial intercalation of bleomycin between base pairs in which at least one strand contains the sequence 5′-GpT-3′. The specificity for cleavage of DNA

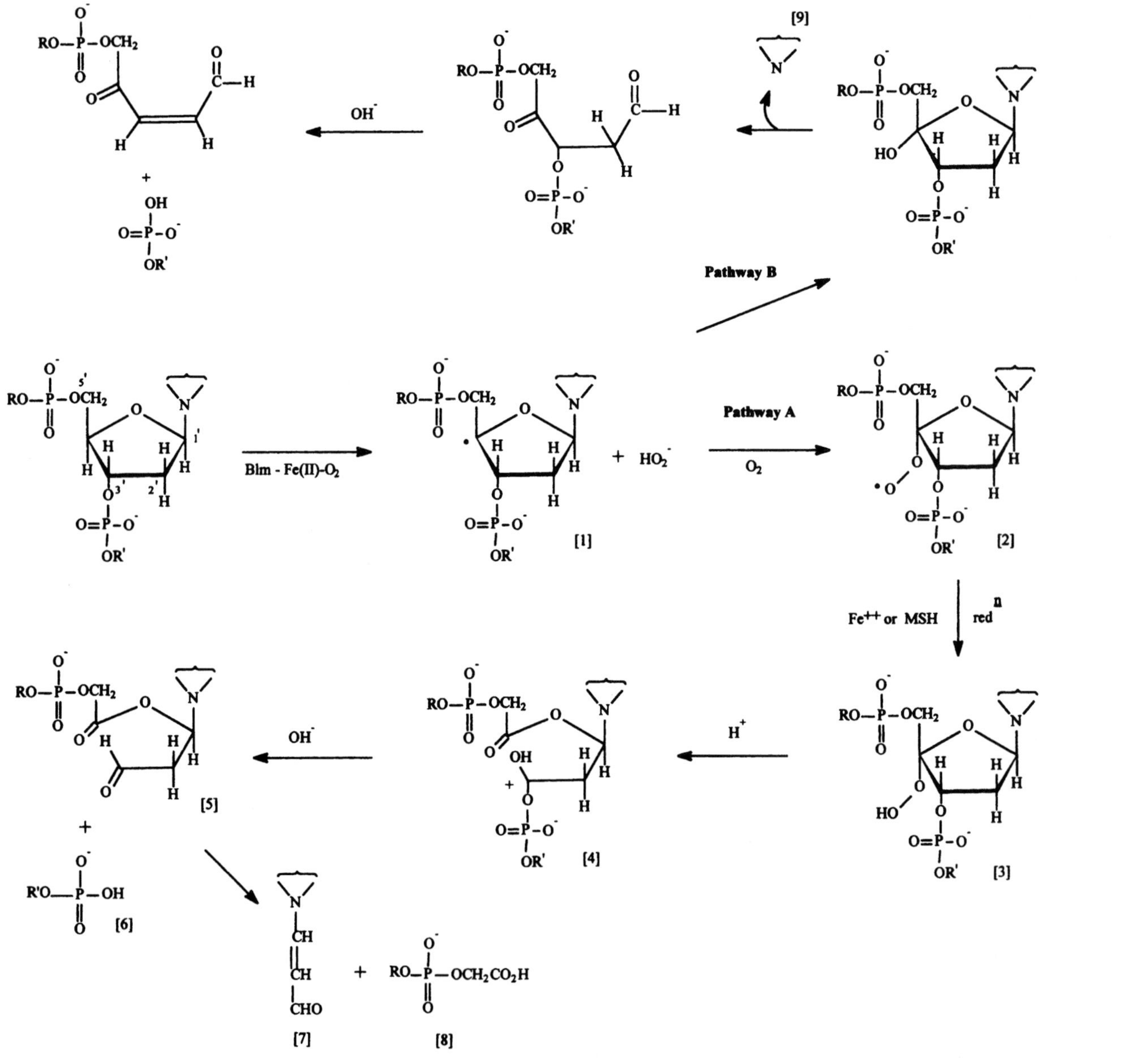

Figure 15.3 Scheme for the cleavage of the 3′–4′ deoxyribose bond by the activated bleomycin·Fe (II)·O_2 complex. In pathway A, the activated drug complex initially abstracts a hydrogen radical from the 4′ position. The unstable intermediate [1] then decomposes in the presence of oxygen [2 and 3], producing the free base propenal [7] and leaving a 3′-phosphoglycolate ester [8] and releasing a 5′-phosphate [6]. Under conditions of limited oxygen, the bleomycin·Fe (II)·O2 complex releases a free base [9] and the DNA strand is susceptible to breakage by alkali.

at a residue located at the 3′ side of G seems to be absolute. A schematic representation of the intercalation and cleavage processes as conceived by Grollman and Takeshita[21] is given in Figure 15.3 and summarizes the structural and sequence specificities discussed above.

Cellular Pharmacology

The cellular uptake of bleomycin is slow and may be mediated by glucose or carotene transporters or endoplasmic vesicles.[7,22] Once bleomycin is internalized, it either translocates to the nucleus to effect DNA damage or can be degraded by bleomycin hydrolase.[23] This enzyme cleaves the carboxamide amine from the β-aminoalaninamide, yielding a weakly cytotoxic deaminobleomycin.[24]

Both the primary amino acid sequence and higher-order structure determined by x-ray crystallography reveal that bleomycin hydrolase is a member of a growing class of self-compartmentalizing or sequestered intracellular proteases.[24] Both yeast and human enzymes are homohexamers with a ring- or barrel-like structure that has the papain-like active sites situated within a central channel in a manner resembling the organization of the active sites in the 20S proteosome.[24] The central channel, which has a strongly positive electrostatic potential in the yeast protein, is slightly negative in human bleomycin hydrolase, perhaps attracting the cationic bleomycin.

Bleomycin hydrolase is found in both normal and malignant cells and is the sole bleomycin-degrading enzyme.[25] This inactivating enzyme is present in relatively low concentrations in the lung and skin, the two normal tissues most susceptible to bleomycin damage.[24,25] Interestingly, pulmonary bleomycin hydrolase levels are highest in animal species or strains resistant to the pulmonary toxicity of bleomycin.[24] Mice that lack the functional gene are more sensitive to the toxic effects of bleomycin.[26] A polymorphism, A1450G, in the coding region is found in 10% of patients with testicular cancer and is associated with a 20% decrease in survival in patients receiving bleomycin, perhaps related to drug toxicity.[27]

DNA is more sensitive to DNA cleavage at the G_2-M and G_1 phases of the cell cycle than at S phase, which may reflect differences in chromatin compaction.[28,29]

The molecular lesions caused by bleomycin include chromosomal breaks and deletions and both single-strand and (less frequently) double-strand breaks. In nonmitotic cells, DNA is organized into nucleosomes, or small beads of heavily transcribed genes, which are joined by long strands, or linker regions. The primary point of attack seems to be in the linker regions of DNA, between nucleosomes.[30] Interestingly, the resulting 180- to 200-base-pair fragments are similar in size to those formed by endonucleases activated during apoptosis.[30,31]

Cells are able to repair bleomycin-induced DNA breaks. Exposure to bleomycin induces p53 phosphorylation and translocation from the cytoplasm to the nucleus, where it initiates DNA repair. The 3′ phosphoglycolate and 5′ deoxyribose ends of DNA strands produced by bleomycin are removed by tyrosyl-DNA phosphodiesterase 1 (TDP 1).[32] TDP 1–deficient cells are hypersensitive to oxidative damage. Both single- and double-strand repair processes are also involved in repair. Homologous recombination (HR) appears to be critical to repair, as HR suppression by Wwox protein, a binding partner of BRCA1, enhances strand breakage, while loss of Wwox induces HR foci, increasing double-strand

break (DSB) repair and promoting bleomycin resistance.[33] The role of other repair pathways in bleomycin damage repair is less clear. Bleomycin exposure rapidly induces base excision repair (BER) and PARP-1 enzyme activity.[34] PARP-1 has an essential role in base excision repair as well as promotes HR and nonhomologous DNA end–joining (NHEJ) repair. However, no specific role of BER in bleomycin toxicity has been defined. Cells from patients with ataxia-telangiectasia, an inherited defect in double-strand repair, are highly sensitivity to bleomycin,[35] as are cells deficient in BRCA1 or in mismatch repair.[36]

Resistance

Several intracellular factors have been identified as contributors to bleomycin tumor resistance: increased drug inactivation by hydrolase,[37] decreased drug accumulation, and increased repair of double-strand DNA breaks.[38] Because Fe(III)·bleomycin requires reduction to Fe(II)·bleomycin, sulfhydryl groups on proteins and peptides are potential factors in binding and inactivating the oxidized bleomycin complex and inducing drug resistance. Tumor lines with elevated levels of glutathione, selected for resistance to doxorubicin, are collaterally sensitive to bleomycin, perhaps due to increased capacity to regenerate bleomycin (FeII).[39] Bleomycin is not affected by P-glycoprotein, the product of the multidrug resistance gene.

Clinical Pharmacokinetics

HPLC is the most specific of several techniques developed for assay of bleomycin in biologic fluids, allowing resolution of the component peptides, but it is more time-consuming than radioimmunoassay.[40,41]

The hallmark of bleomycin pharmacokinetics in patients with normal serum creatinine is a rapid two-phase drug disappearance from plasma; 45% to 70% of the dose is excreted in the urine within 24 hours. For intravenous bolus doses, the primary half-life for plasma disappearance is variously reported to be 2 to 4 hours.[42,43] Peak plasma concentrations reach 1 to 10 mU/mL for intravenous bolus doses of 15 U/m².

Intramuscular injection of bleomycin (2 to 10 U/m²) gave peak plasma levels of 0.13 to 0.6 mU/mL or approximately one tenth the peak level achieved by the intravenous bolus doses[44] (Fig. 15.4). The mean half-life after intramuscular injection was 2.5 hours, or approximately the same as that after intravenous injection. Peak serum concentrations were reached approximately 1 hour after injection. Bleomycin pharmacokinetics also have been studied in patients receiving intrapleural or intraperitoneal injections, routes used in controlling malignant effusions due to breast, lung, and ovarian cancers.[45] Intracavitary bleomycin, in doses of 60 U/m², gives peak plasma levels of 0.4 to 5.0 mU/mL, with a plasma half-life of 3.4 hours after intrapleural doses and 5.3 hours after intraperitoneal injection.[45] Intracavitary levels are 10- to 22-fold higher than simultaneous plasma concentrations.[46] About 45% of an intracavitary dose enters the systemic circulation, and 30% is excreted in the urine.

Bleomycin pharmacokinetics are markedly altered in patients with abnormal renal function, particularly those with creatinine clearance of less than 35 mL/min. Crooke et al.[44] reported a

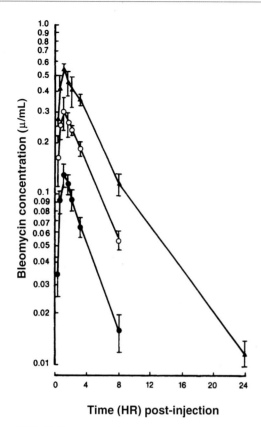

FIGURE **15.4** Pharmacokinetics of bleomycin after intramuscular administration of 2 (●), 5 (○), and 10 (▲) mg of bleomycin per meter square. (From
Oken MM, Crooke ST, Elson MK, et al. Pharmacokinetics of bleomycin after IM
administration in man. *Cancer Treat Rep.* 1981;65:485. With permission.)

patient with a creatinine clearance of 10.7 mL/min and a half-life
of 21 hours. Others have reported a high frequency of pulmonary
toxicity in patients with renal dysfunction secondary to cisplatin
treatment.[47,48] The prudent course is to decrease dosages by 50%
for patients with clearances below 80 mL/min or to give an alternative regimen, substituting ifosfamide for bleomycin for germ cell
tumors.

Clinical Toxicity and Side Effects

The most important toxic actions of bleomycin affect the lungs and
skin; myelosuppression is not usually evident, except in patients
with severely compromised bone marrow function due to extensive
previous chemotherapy[49] and those receiving high-dose therapy.
Fever occurs during the 48 hours after drug administration in one
quarter of patients. Some investigators use a 1-U test dose of bleomycin before an initial dose of drug as rare instances of fatal acute
allergic reactions have been reported.[50]

Pulmonary Toxicity

Pulmonary toxicity is manifest as a subacute or chronic interstitial
pneumonitis complicated in its later stages by progressive interstitial fibrosis, hypoxia, and death.[51] Clinically apparent pulmonary
toxicity, usually manifested with cough, dyspnea, and bibasilar
pulmonary infiltrates on chest radiographs, occurs in 3% to 5%
of patients receiving a total dose of less than 450 U bleomycin;

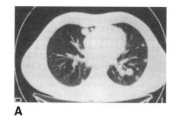 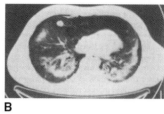

FIGURE **15.5** Computed tomographic scans of the chest before (**A**) and
after (**B**) treatment for testicular cancer. The multiple metastatic pulmonary nodules partially regressed with therapy, but the posttreatment film shows dense bilateral pulmonary fibrosis and a large left pneumothorax and pneumomediastinum.

it increases significantly to a 10% incidence in those treated with
higher cumulative doses (Fig. 15.5). Subclinical evidence of pulmonary toxicity is elicited by spirometry in up to 50% of children
previously receiving bleomycin, findings indicating restrictive function, hyperinflation, and inhomogeneous aeration.[52] Overt toxicity
is also more frequent in patients older than age 70, in those who
have received prior chest irradiation, in those with underlying renal
dysfunction or emphysema, and in patients receiving single doses
greater than 25 U/m².[53] The use of bleomycin in single doses of
more than 30 U should be discouraged because instances of rapid
onset of fatal pulmonary fibrosis as early as 8 weeks after high-dose
bleomycin have been reported.[54] Previous radiotherapy to the chest
predisposes to bleomycin-induced pulmonary toxicity.[55] Although
the risk of lung toxicity increases with cumulative doses greater
than 450 U, severe pulmonary sequelae have been observed at total
doses below 100 U. In the standard regimen for treating testicular
cancer, bleomycin is given in doses of 15 U/m²/wk for 12 doses,
and the incidence of fatal pulmonary toxicity in this low-risk population of young male patients is less than 2%.[56]

While clinically apparent pulmonary toxicity is absent in most
patients receiving bleomycin, serial chest CTs and PET-CT reveal
infiltrates and inflammatory changes during treatment.[57]

Pathogenesis of Pulmonary Toxicity

The potential for bleomycins to cause pulmonary toxicity is easily demonstrated by intravenous infusion or by direct instillation
of the parent molecule into the trachea of a rodent.[58] The terminal
amines of bleomycins are sufficient, by themselves, to cause the toxicity in rodents, and the toxic potency of the bleomycins directly
correlates with the potency of the individual terminal amines, the
A_2 aminopropyl-dimethylsulfonium and the A_5 spermidine having
greater effect than the B_2 agmatine.[59] These findings raise the possibility that modifying the terminal amine might yield a less toxic
analog for clinical use, as yet an unproven hypothesis.

The pathogenesis of bleomycin pulmonary toxicity in rodents
serves as a model for understanding pulmonary fibrosis, an end result
of a broad range of human diseases induced by drugs, autoimmunity,
and infection.[60] Intratracheal instillation of bleomycin in mice or ham-
sters produces rapidly evolving toxicity to alveolar epithelial cells,
epithelial apoptosis, intra-alveolar inflammation, cytokine release by
alveolar macrophages, fibroblast proliferation, and collagen deposition, as well as endothelial cell damage in small pulmonary vessels.
As changes progress from acute inflammation to interstitial fibrosis,
pulmonary function deteriorates, as indicated by a decrease in lung

compliance, a decrease in carbon monoxide diffusion capacity, and terminal hypoxia. Hydroxyproline deposition serves as a quantitative measure of the progression of fibrosis in animal models.

A broad array of cytokines and other mediators, produced by alveolar macrophages and by endothelial cells in response to bleomycin, have been implicated in the molecular pathogenesis of pulmonary fibrosis. These include angiogenic factors including nitrous oxide and vascular endothelial growth factor (VEGF), transforming growth factor-β (TGF-β), tumor necrosis factor-α (TNF-α),[61] interleukins 1β, 2, 3, 4, 5, and 6,[62] and chemokines. TGF-β stimulates the promoter that controls transcription of a collagen precursor.[63] Prostaglandin PGD2 plays a protective role against pulmonary fibrosis in bleomycin models, while PGF2a promotes fibrosis.[64]

Genetic experiments have provided further insight into factors that influence susceptibility to fibrosis and into the central role of cytokines in bleomycin lung toxicity. Bleomycin hydrolase–knockout mice have significantly greater lung and epidermal toxicity than normal controls.[26] Other experiments implicate the central role of TGF-β, which is secreted by alveolar macrophages in response to bleomycin. Mice that lack a necessary TGF-β activation step develop alveolar inflammation but not progressive fibrosis.[65] Mice lacking plasminogen activation are highly susceptible to fibrosis.[66]

The stimulus for cytokine and chemokine release[67] is uncertain, although apoptosis of epithelial cells and the activation of alveolar macrophages, neutrophils, or lymphocytes may play an important role.[60] In mice, genetic deletion of either Fas, which is expressed on pulmonary epithelial cells, or Fas ligand, as expressed on T lymphocytes, does not prevent inflammation but does protect against pulmonary fibrosis.[67] CXCL12, a potent chemokine, is secreted by inflammatory cells in response to lung injury and attracts bone marrow–derived stem cells that establish as fibrocytes in the damaged lung.[68]

In addition to providing important insights regarding the pathogenesis of pulmonary fibrosis, these experiments offer new approaches to prevent or treat bleomycin toxicity. Thus, in various animal models, protection is provided by Fas antigen and anti-Fas ligand antibodies[67]; TNF-α–soluble receptor[61]; TGF-β antibodies[69]; granulocyte-macrophage colony–stimulating factor antibodies[70]; pirfenidone, an inhibitor of platelet-derived growth factor function and procollagen transcription[71]; dehydroproline, an inhibitor of procollagen synthesis[72]; indomethacin[73]; and anti-CXCL12 antibodies. One can add to this list many other drugs and antibodies, including thalidomide, C-KIT inhibitors such as imatinib,[74] and anti-HER 2 antibodies,[75] all of which can ameliorate or prevent bleomycin lung damage in rodents. None of these agents, with the exception of imatinib in a single case report, has yet shown efficacy against bleomycin lung toxicity in a clinical trial.[60,74]

Clinical Syndrome of Pulmonary Toxicity

Clinical symptoms of bleomycin pulmonary injury include a nonproductive cough, dyspnea, and occasionally fever and pleuritic pain. Physical examination usually reveals minimal auscultatory evidence of pulmonary alveolar infiltrates, and initial chest films are often negative or may reveal an increase in interstitial markings, especially in the lower lobes, with a predilection for subpleural areas. Chest radiographs, when positive, reveal patchy reticulonodular infiltrates, which in later stages may coalesce to form areas

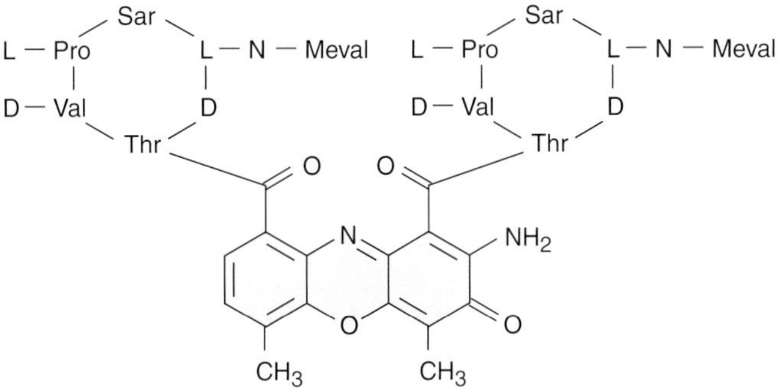

FIGURE 15.6 Structure of actinomycin D. D-Val, D-valine; L-N-Meval, methylvaline; L-Thr, L-threonine; L-Pro, L-proline; Sar, sarcosine.

of apparent consolidation. In occasional patients, the initial radiographic changes may be discrete nodules, with central cavitation, indistinguishable from metastatic tumor or infection[76] (Fig. 15.6). Computed tomographic scans and PET-CT scans[57] show the presence of a diffuse, often bibasilar and subpleural infiltrates at a time of minimal abnormality on plain films of the chest.

Radiologic findings do not differentiate bleomycin lung toxicity from other forms of interstitial lung disease. Arterial oxygen desaturation and a markedly abnormal carbon monoxide diffusion (DLCO) capacity are regular findings in symptomatic patients with bleomycin toxicity, but these findings are common to other causes of diffuse interstitial disease. Open lung biopsy is usually required to distinguish between the primary differential diagnostic alternatives, specifically a drug-induced pulmonary lesion, an infectious interstitial pneumonitis, and neoplastic pulmonary infiltration. The findings on histologic examination of human lung after bleomycin treatment closely resemble those previously described in the experimental animal and include necrosis of type I alveolar cells, an acute inflammatory infiltrate in the alveoli, interstitial and intra-alveolar edema, pulmonary hyaline membrane formation, and intra-alveolar and, later in the course, interstitial fibrosis. In addition, squamous metaplasia of type II alveolar-lining cells has been described as a characteristic finding.[77] In rare cases, a true hypersensitivity pneumonitis may develop, characterized by underlying eosinophilic pulmonary infiltrates and a prompt clinical response to corticosteroids.[78]

Pulmonary function tests, particularly a rapid fall in the carbon monoxide–diffusing capacity, are of possible value in predicting a high risk of pulmonary toxicity. Most patients treated with bleomycin, however, show a progressive (10% to 15%) fall in CO diffusion capacity with increasing total dose and a more marked increase in changes above a 270-U total dose. Whether or not the diffusion capacity test can be used to predict which patients will subsequently develop clinically significant pulmonary toxicity is not clear.[79,80] Some investigators suggest that bleomycin should be halted if the diffusion capacity for carbon dioxide (DCO) falls by 20% to 25% from the initial value, even in the absence of symptoms,[56] although others believe this value may be too restrictive. In toxic patients, and at advanced stages in the evolution of bleomycin pulmonary toxicity, the diffusion capacity as well as arterial oxygen saturation and total lung capacity become markedly abnormal. Long-term assessment of pulmonary function in patients treated with bleomycin for testicular cancer has revealed a return to baseline normal values at a median of 4 years after treatment.[81]

Patients who have received bleomycin seem to be at greater risk of respiratory failure during subsequent surgery,[82] although others have questioned the association of perioperative oxygen supplementation.[83] The sensitivity of bleomycin-treated patients to high concentrations of inspired oxygen is intriguing in view of the molecular action of bleomycin, which is mediated by the formation of oxygen-derived free radicals. Current safeguards for anesthesia in bleomycin-treated patients specify the use of the minimum concentration of supplemental oxygen and modest fluid replacement to prevent pulmonary edema.

No specific therapy is available for patients with bleomycin-induced lung toxicity. Discontinuation of the drug may be followed by a period of continued progression of the pulmonary findings, with partial to complete reversal of the abnormalities in pulmonary function in asymptomatic patients after several months. The inflammatory component of the pathologic process does resolve in experimental models, and interstitial infiltrates regress clinically, but the reversibility of pulmonary fibrosis has not been documented. The value of corticosteroids in promoting recovery from bleomycin-induced lung toxicity remains controversial; beneficial effects have been described in isolated case studies.[84] Long-term follow-up of patients with clinical and radiographic evidence of bleomycin-induced pneumonitis suggests a complete resolution of radiographic, clinical, and pulmonary function abnormalities in most asymptomatic patients 2 years after completion of treatment for testicular cancer.[85] However, in more severe cases, pulmonary fibrosis may be only partially reversible. Bilateral lung transplantation has been employed in one reported case of late respiratory failure.[86] In the absence of symptoms, no specific spirometry or imaging follow-up is indicated once treatment is completed.

Cutaneous Toxicity

A more common but less serious toxicity of bleomycin is its effect on the skin. Approximately, 50% of patients treated with daily or twice-daily doses of this agent develop erythema, induration, and hyperkeratosis and peeling of the skin that may progress to frank ulceration.[87] These changes predominantly affect digits, hands, joints, and areas of previous irradiation. Hyperpigmentation, alopecia, and nail changes also occur during bleomycin therapy. These cutaneous side effects do not necessitate discontinuation of therapy, particularly if clear benefit is being derived from the drug. Rarely, patients may develop Raynaud's phenomenon while receiving bleomycin.[88] Other toxic reactions to bleomycin include hypersensitivity reactions characterized by urticaria, periorbital edema, and bronchospasm. Flagellate dermatitis, with bands of erythematous skin most prominently on the trunk, has been infrequently reported.[89]

Schedules of Administration

Bleomycin has been administered using a number of different schedules and routes, the most common route and schedule are weekly bolus intramuscular injections. A high-dose regimen of continuous intravenous infusion of 25 U/d for 5 days produced the rapid onset of pulmonary toxicity, particularly in patients with previous chest irradiation,[49] but in addition caused hypertensive episodes in 17% of patients and hyperbilirubinemia in 30%. These latter toxicities are rarely seen with conventional intramuscular doses. Continuous intra-arterial infusion also has been used for patients with carcinoma of the cervix,[90] but was modestly effective (a 12% response rate), and 20% of patients developed pulmonary toxicity.

Bleomycin also has been applied topically as a 3.5% ointment in a xipamide (Aquaphor) base. Two-week courses of treatment produced complete regression of Paget's disease of the vulva in four of seven patients with no serious local toxicity.[91]

Bleomycin can be used to sclerose the pleural space in patients with malignant effusions. After thorough evacuation of fluid from the pleural space, 40 U/m^2 is dissolved in 100-mL normal saline and instilled through a thoracostomy tube, which is clamped for 8 hours and then returned to suction. In one third of patients thus treated, the effusion clears completely, about the same response rate as obtained with tetracycline instillation.[92] The only toxic reactions to be expected are fever and pleuritis, both of which resolve in 24 to 48 hours.

The intraperitoneal instillation of bleomycin has been used in patients with ovarian cancer, mesothelioma, and other malignancy confined to the peritoneum[45] but with rare responses. Sixty mg/m^2 of bleomycin per dissolved in 2 L of saline was placed in the peritoneal cavity for a 4- to 8-hour dwell time. Side effects included abdominal pain, fever, rash, and mucositis. A limited pharmacokinetic advantage was observed (the peritoneal area under the concentration × time curve (AUC) was sevenfold greater than the plasma AUC), but the clinical results provide little justification for intraperitoneal therapy.

Bleomycin has been instilled into the urinary bladder in doses of 60 U in 30 mL of sterile water.[93] Seven of twenty-six patients with superficial transitional cell carcinomas had complete disappearance of disease after 7 to 8 weekly treatments. The primary toxic reaction was cystitis. Plasma drug level monitoring revealed little systemic absorption. Bleomycin has occasionally been directly injected into lymphangiomas or cysts,[94] with anecdotal success in ablating the malformations.

Radiation and Drug Interaction

The pharmacologic basis of synergism between bleomycin and radiation therapy has received considerable attention but is poorly understood. Synergistic pulmonary toxicity has been reported in patients receiving bleomycin with or after chest irradiation. Administration of bleomycin within 3 hours of irradiation, either before or after, produces greater than additive effects, possibly owing to the production of free-radical damage to DNA by both agents. This interaction has been tested in a randomized clinical trial of radiation therapy plus or minus bleomycin, 5 mg twice weekly, and methotrexate in patients with head and neck cancer.[95] Those receiving bleomycin and methotrexate had a significantly higher complete response rate and a better 3-year disease-free survival rate. The advent of 5-fluorouracil and the platinum derivatives as radiosensitizers has dampened interest in bleomycin as a radiosensitizer.

TABLE **15.2**	Key features of actinomycin D
Mechanism of Action	Inhibition of RNA Polymerase
Metabolism	Unknown, likely hepatic microsomal metabolism
Pharmacokinetics	$t_{1/2}$: 36 h; clearance 5.3 L/h
Elimination	Renal: 6% to 30%
	Bile: 5% to 11%
Drug interactions	None
Toxicity	Myelosuppression
	Nausea and vomiting
	Mucositis
	Diarrhea
	Necrosis at extravasation site
	Radiation sensitization and recall reactions
Precautions	Avoid extravasation

$t_{1/2}$, half-life.

Actinomycin

In this and the next sections, we consider two fermentation products, actinomycin D and mitomycin C (MMC). Actinomycin D[96] is a valuable drug in treating choriocarcinoma and pediatric sarcomas and has unusual activity in NPM1-mutated acute myeloid leukemia,[97] whereas MMC is effective in treating anal carcinomas.

Actinomycin D (DACT), a product of the *Streptomyces* yeast species, was discovered in 1940.[96] It is a standard agent in combination therapy of Wilms' tumor, neuroblastoma, childhood rhabdomyosarcoma, and Ewing's sarcoma. Key pharmacological features are given in Table 15.2.

Mechanism of Action and Cellular Pharmacology

The structure of DACT, shown in Figure 15.6, consists of a phenoxazinone planar chromophore to which are attached two pentapeptide rings, which vary in structure among the naturally occurring actinomycins. DACT is a strong DNA-binding drug and a potent inhibitor of RNA polymerase and protein synthesis. Actual binding to DNA takes place by intercalation, as the chromophore inserts preferentially between guanine-cytosine base pairs, while the two chains of the pentapeptide rest in the minor groove and form hydrogen bonds with adjoining bases.[98]

DACT enters cells by passive diffusion. High concentrations of DACT inhibit growth and induce cytotoxicity, while at low concentrations and in selected cell lines, it induces differentiation.

Mechanism of Resistance

Resistance to DACT may be related to increased efflux mediated by the P-glycoprotein (Pgp) transporter. Chinese hamster ovary cells exhibiting Pgp amplification were cross-resistant to DACT, vinca alkaloids, anthracyclines, and etoposide.[99] Human tumor cell lines resistant to DACT in vitro amplify the Pgp-encoding MDR gene.

Clinical Pharmacology

The pharmacokinetics of DACT have been analyzed by LC-MS. Studies defined a clearance of 5.3 L/h and a volume of distribution of 7.5 L/70 kg. DACT is eliminated by hepatic metabolism, with less than 20% excreted intact in the urine.[100] It has a long plasma elimination half-life (36 hours).

Toxicity

At the usual clinical dosages of 10 to 15 mcg/kg/d for 5 days, DACT causes nausea, vomiting, diarrhea, mucositis, and hair loss. The major and dose-limiting side effect is myelosuppression, a nadir of white blood cell and platelet counts occurring 8 to 14 days after drug administration.[101] It also causes hepatic enzyme elevations and, less commonly, severe hepatotoxicity with features of venoocclusive disease, as reported in children treated for Wilms' tumor.[102] DACT can act as a radiosensitizer and may cause inflammatory reactions in previously irradiated sites.[103] The clinical consequences of such reactions may be serious, especially when affecting the lung. Corticosteroids may ameliorate these reactions. Extravasation is associated with tissue necrosis.

Mitomycin C

Mitomycin C (Mutamycin; MMC) was isolated from *Streptomyces caespitosus* in 1958.[104] The initial clinical studies used daily low-dose schedules, which resulted in unacceptably severe, cumulative myelosuppression. An intermittent dosing schedule, using bolus injections every 4 to 8 weeks, resulted in more manageable hematological toxicity. With the latter schedule, MMC was active against breast cancer, aerodigestive tract tumors, cervical cancer, and, with bladder instillation, superficial bladder cancer. Its primary current indication is for the treatment of squamous anal cancers with 5-fluorouracil, with or without irradiation.[105] Its key pharmacological features are given in Table 15.3.

Mechanism of Action and Cellular Pharmacology

MMC (Fig. 15.7) has a unique chemical structure in which quinone, aziridine, and carbamate functions are arranged around a pyrrolo[1,2-a]indole nucleus.[106] Mitomycins are the only known naturally occurring compounds containing an aziridine ring, an alkylating entity. MMC is soluble in both aqueous and organic solvents. However, because of its chemical instability in solution, the clinical formulation of MMC is a lyophilized form containing mannitol, an antioxidant (Mitomycin Kyowa). After dissolution in water, MMC is unstable, especially in acidic solutions, in which it spontaneously releases the 9-alpha methoxy group and opens the aziridine ring. It should be administered within several hours of dissolution.

TABLE 15.3	*Key features of mitomycin C*
Mechanism of Action	Alkylation of DNA
Metabolism	Hepatic
Pharmacokinetics	$t_{1/2}\,\alpha$: 2 to 10 min
	$t_{1/2}\,\beta$: 25 to 90 min
Elimination	Renal: 1% to 20%; likely chemical inactivation and hepatic metabolism
Drug interaction	None
Toxicity	Myelosuppression
	Necrosis at extravasation
	Hemolytic uremic syndrome
	Interstitial pneumonitis
	Cardiomyopathy
Precautions	Avoid extravasation

$t_{1/2}$, half-life.

Mechanism of Action: Formation of DNA

MMC induces both single-site alkylation and less frequent but perhaps more biologically important cross-links.[107] DNA cross-linking and alkylation require an initial chemical or enzymatic reduction of the quinone function. The primary mechanism of alkylation is accomplished by activation of the C-1 aziridine and the C-10 carbamate groups (Fig. 15.7), although several additional reactive electrophiles derived from MMC, such as a quinone methide and the oxidized forms of aziridinomitosene and leucoaziridinomitosene, may alkylate DNA as well.[108] Selective removal of the aziridine function of MMC results in a switch from minor to major groove alkylation of DNA, but does not totally eliminate alkylating potential.

MMC is considered the prototypical bioreductive alkylating agent. Two mechanisms exist through which reductive metabolism mediates the cytotoxic effects of MMC.[107–109] First, under anaerobic conditions, one- or two-electron reduction of the quinone groups is followed by spontaneous loss of the carbamate side chain and leads to the formation of reactive unstable intermediates at C-1 and C-10 and the potential for cross-linking. Under aerobic conditions, reduction of the parent molecular leads to formation of semiquinone radicals that react with O_2 to yield superoxide, hydroxyl radicals, or hydrogen peroxide. The reductive activation of MMC

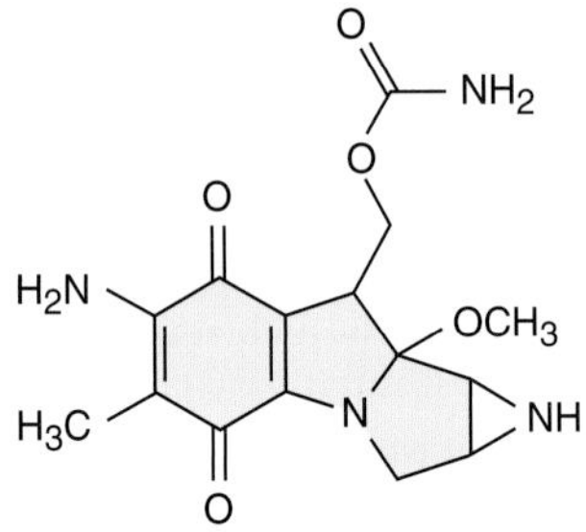

may proceed enzymatically by an NADPH- or NADH-dependent reductase, by DT diaphorase, or by other reductases in cytoplasm or the nucleus.[111–113] The role of these enzymes in determining tumor sensitivity or resistance is suggested by experimental studies, but unproven.

Cumulatively, these various routes to activation imply that the enzymes involved in the reduction of MMC under hypoxic conditions may not be the same as those observed under aerobic conditions and that the products of reduction in various pathways may differ.

Chemical Analysis of DNA Adducts

The preferred covalent interactions between MMC and DNA or DNA fragments occur at the N-2 or N-7 position of guanine.[110,111] Although MMC monoadducts are 10-fold more numerous, interstrand cross-links (Fig. 15.8) are the primary cytotoxic lesion.[111] The primary intracellular metabolite of MMC, 2-7-diaminomitosene, which lacks the 9-alpha methoxy side group, forms monoadducts, but no cross-links, and is noncytotoxic.

Mechanism of Resistance

The mechanisms of resistance to MMC are incompletely understood but likely involve changes in drug accumulation, bioactivation, inactivation of the alkylating species by glutathione and other nucleophiles, or DNA repair. In a series of Chinese hamster ovary cell mutants selected for MMC resistance, a progressive loss of MMC activation capacity and increased capacity for excision repair of DNA were found as cells became more drug resistant.[112] Cells lacking a functional p53 seem insensitive,[110] while cells from subjects with Fanconi anemia, an inherited disease in which the nucleotide excision repair pathway is defective, are supersensitive to MMC.[113] A trial of MMC combined with the PARP inhibitor, veliparib, in solid tumor patients with functional deficiency of the Fanconi pathway gave only five responses of 29 patients treated.[114]

Clinical Pharmacology

MMC has an elimination half-life of 25 to 90 minutes (mean, 54 minutes).[115] MMC is likely cleared from plasma by hepatic metabolism and chemical instability. Impaired renal function does not change the pharmacokinetic behavior of MMC. Urinary recovery of parent drug after intravenous administration ranged from 1% to 20%. An unexplained increase in total body clearance and a decrease in the area under the plasma concentration time curve of MMC were observed in patients receiving combination chemotherapy that included 5-fluorouracil and doxorubicin,[116] an interaction not easily explained in terms of mechanisms of drug elimination or interaction.

MMC is erratically absorbed after oral administration. Intravesical MMC therapy to treat superficial bladder cancer results in extremely low plasma levels, with virtually no systemic side effects.[117] The drug is now used topically or by local injection to prevent fibrosis related to surgery of the conjunctiva, cornea, and other ophthalmologic structures.[118]

FIGURE 15.7 Structure of mitomycin C. Alkylation occurs through reduction of the quinone moieties, with activation of nucleophilic sites at C-1 and C-10.

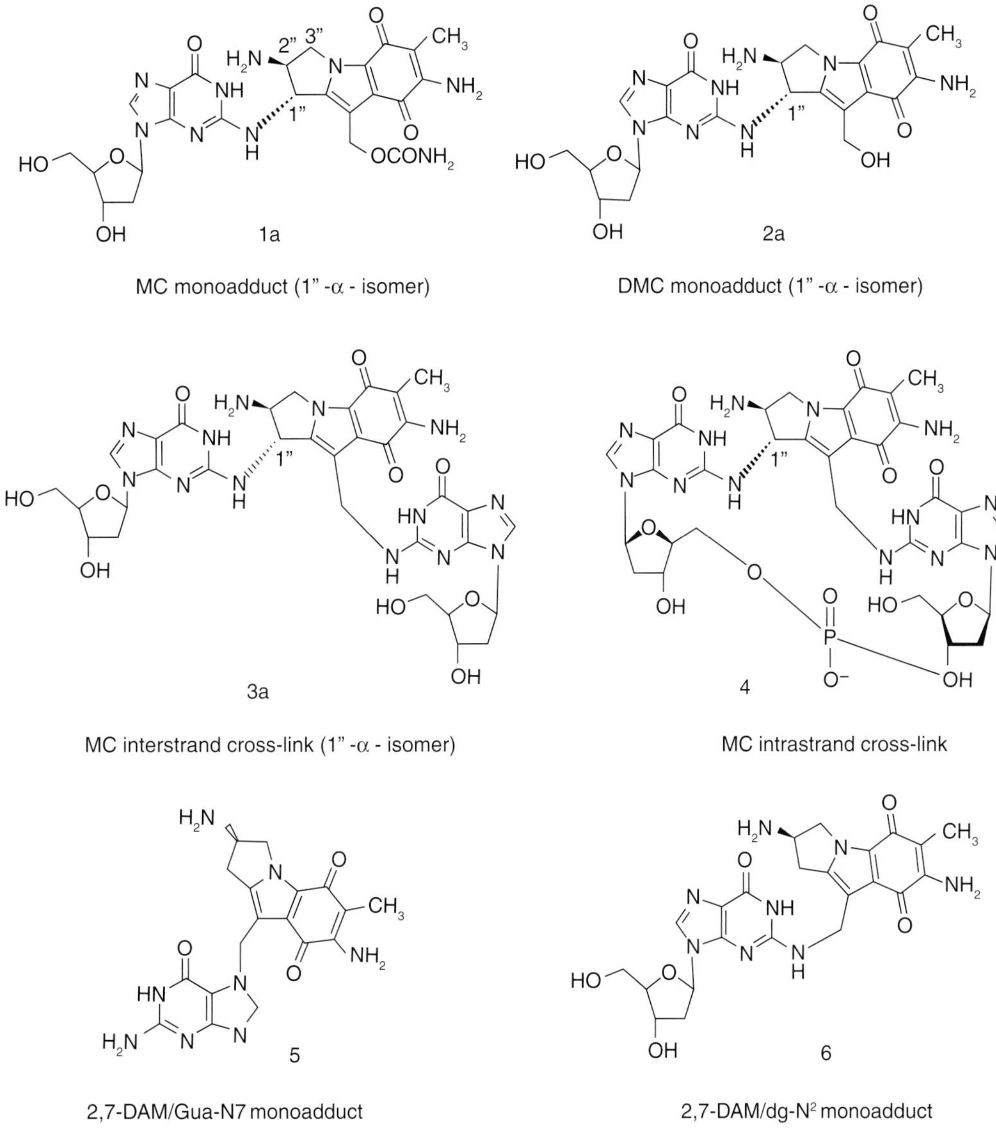

FIGURE **15.8** Six different DNA adducts formed by MMC, by 2,7-diaminomitosene (DAM), and by the 10-decarbamoylated analog (DMC). C-1 and C-10 carbons become sites for alkylation of guanine at the N-2 and N-7 positions. Note the interstrand cross-links produced by MMC. (From Bargonetti J, Champeil E, Tomasz M. Differential toxicity of DNA adducts of mitomycin C. *J Nucl Acids.* 2010. PII: 698960, 6 pages. doi:10.4061/2010/698960, under a Creative Commons 4.0 license.)

Toxicity

The most significant and frequent side effect of MMC is a delayed myelosuppression, which seems to be directly related to schedule and total dose.[119] Below a total dose of 50 mg/m², hematological toxicity is rare. At higher doses, thrombocytopenia is more frequent than leukocytopenia and anemia. High doses of MMC may result in lethal venoocclusive liver disease.[120] Other more frequent and potentially lethal side effects include hemolytic uremic syndrome (HUS), interstitial pneumonitis, and cardiac failure. The incidence of MMC-induced HUS seems to be less than 10% of patients and is primarily seen after single doses of 30 mg/m² and at cumulative doses greater than 50 mg/m².[121] No consistently effective treatment for this syndrome is available, other than drug discontinuation. In these patients, red blood cell transfusion leads to brisk hemolysis and pulmonary edema and should be avoided. Other toxic reactions usually include mild and infrequent anorexia, nausea, vomiting, and diarrhea. Alopecia, stomatitis, and rashes also occur infrequently. Extravasation results in tissue necrosis, with very disabling ulcers that may require plastic surgery.

Pulmonary toxicity of MMC consists of an interstitial pneumonitis. Discontinuation of MMC administration may occasionally lead to recovery, and corticosteroid treatment may be helpful in preventing progression of pulmonary dysfunction. The incidence of pulmonary toxicity is approximately 7% of the treated population.[122] Cardiac failure secondary to MMC occurs 5% to 10% of patients; the incidence rises with cumulative doses greater than 30 mg/m².

Yondelis (Trabectedin)

In the late 1960s, extracts of the Caribbean marine tunicate *Ecteinascidia turbinata*, a sea squirt, were found to inhibit tumor cell

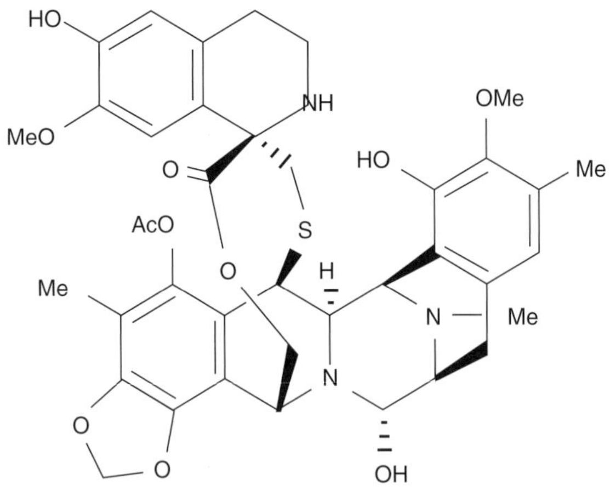

FIGURE **15.9** Structure of trabectedin, which contains three tetrahydroisoquinolone structures, a 10-membered heterocyclic ring, and a cysteine bridge. Lurbinectedin differs only in the substitutions on the third tetrahydroisoloquinolone ring, where a new methoxy group replaces the hydroxyl and the lower methoxy is replaced by a proton.

TABLE 15.4	Key features of trabectedin
Mechanism of Action	Alkylation of DNA, as well as inhibition of RNA polymerase II
Metabolism	Demethylation and CYP3A4-mediated oxidation; metabolism induced by rifampin, blocked by imidazole antifungals (see Machiels et al. *Cancer Chemother Pharmacol.* 2014;74:729-737).
Pharmacokinetics	Terminal $t_{1/2}$: 40 to 50 h
Elimination	Primarily via bile (<2% in urine)
Drug interactions	None (doxorubicin does not affect PK)
Toxicity	Neutropenia
	Thrombocytopenia
	Hepatic toxicity
	Nausea and vomiting
	Fatigue
Precautions	Co-medication with CYP3A4 substrates, inhibitors
	Care should be taken in case of bilirubin increase

$t_{1/2}$, half-life.

proliferation. It is now known that the active molecule is produced by a fungus symbiotic with the sea squirt. In 1984, the active compound, ecteinascidin-743 (now known as trabectedin or Yondelis) was isolated, purified, and synthesized[123] (see Fig. 15.9). Trabectedin belongs to the general class of tetrahydroisoquinolone compounds. A less toxic analogue, lurbinectedin, is undergoing clinical evaluation.[124] As a class, these compounds alkylate DNA and inhibit RNA polymerase II.

Trabectedin is extremely potent, killing tumor cells in vitro at picomolar concentrations. It displayed broad antitumor activity in preclinical testing, and is approved in the United States and many other countries for treatment of soft-tissue sarcomas after doxorubicin failure, and is marketed for platinum-sensitive second-line ovarian cancer in Europe. Its key pharmacological features are given in Table 15.4.

Mechanism of Action

Trabectedin exerts at least two separate actions that may contribute to its cytotoxicity: alkylation of DNA and inhibition of gene transcription.[125,126] It binds to the minor groove of the DNA double helix, showing a preference for GG and GC-rich regions, and forms a covalent bond with the exocyclic N-2 amino group of guanine. This alkylation step depends on the dehydration of the carbinolamine group of the drug, leading to the formation of a reactive iminium intermediate that attacks DNA.[127] Two subunits of trabectedin (A and B) form the primary contacts with DNA, while the C subunit protrudes out of the minor groove and has been implicated as an inhibitor of transcription factors, specifically RNA polymerase II[125] (Fig. 15.9). Alkylation of DNA bends the helix toward its major groove, a structural change that may contribute to inhibition of transcription.[128] The alkylation of DNA triggers induction of proteins involved in both single- and double-stranded DNA repair. Subsequent single-strand breaks are converted to double-strand breaks when encountered by the transcription-coupled nucleotide excision repair (TC-NER) complex.[129]

The status of DNA repair pathways significantly influences tumor response. The drug is most active against cells that have intact TC-NER, in contrast to cisplatin, which is most effective in cells with defective TC-NER.[129] Similarly, the presence of an intact DNA-dependent protein kinase, a component of the nonhomologous end-joining pathway for double-strand break repair, is activated by irradiation or alkylating drugs and paradoxically confers sensitivity. Inhibitors of both base excision repair, such as the PARP inhibitor, olaparib,[130] and inhibitors of ATR and ATM[131] (all implicated in double-strand break recognition and repair) enhance its activity. Deficiency of components of HR repair of double-strand DNA breaks, including BRCA1 and BRCA2, may also sensitize to trabectedin and lurbectedin,[132] as confirmed by early clinical trial results.[133]

A second important action of trabectedin is its ability to inhibit RNA polymerase II and to block transcription.[125] It blocks the tumor-promoting action of the EWSR1-FLI1 fusion transcription factor in Ewing's sarcoma cells.[134] It also inhibits induction of the multidrug resistance gene (MDR1), which is regulated by the transcription factor, NF-Y, although constitutive expression of MDR1 is unaffected.[135] Only at high levels does MDR1 expression confer resistance to trabectedin. These findings suggest its use in combination with other natural products affected by MDR1.

Resistance Mechanisms

Trabectedin is ineffective in cells that constitutively express high levels of the MDR transporter.[136] The cytotoxicity of trabectedin is also significantly influenced by the status of DNA repair pathways. Loss of a key component of TC-NER (the XPG protein) leads to resistance.[137] Conversely, loss of TC-NER leads to enhanced cisplatin sensitivity, thus providing a rationale for combination therapy with these agents, although clinical trials to date have not shown impressive responsiveness to trabectedin in patients refractory to platinum-based regimens.[138] The specific DNA repair changes associated with clinical resistance are not known.

Clinical Pharmacology

Trabectedin is formulated as a lyophilized product. Each vial contains a 250-μg dosage unit in mannitol and 0.05-M phosphate buffer. This formulation, when reconstituted, is light sensitive and stable at room temperature for only a few hours. The usual dose, 1.3 mg/m^2, is administered as a 3- to 24-hour infusion every 3 weeks. Bioanalytical methods utilize HPLC-MS.[139-141]

The predominant mechanism of drug clearance is hepatic metabolism by CYP3A4, as less than 2% of parent compound is excreted in the urine unchanged.[142] Rat or human microsomes convert the drug to N-desmethyl derivative and other oxidative products.

The favored schedule for drug administration is a 24-hour infusion, based on a randomized phase II trial (24-hour versus 3-hour infusion) in soft-tissue sarcoma, demonstrating a significantly improved time to tumor progression for the 24-hour schedule.[143] Shorter infusion schedules produced no apparent advantage in terms of toxicity or response. With the 24-hour infusion, the C_{max} is 1.0 to 10 pg/mL, the drug clearance rate from plasma is 21 to 86 L/h, the terminal half-life in plasma ranges from 26 to 107 hours, and the AUC is 55 to 70 ng × h/mL.[144,145]

Trabectedin has a high volume of distribution (808 to 3,900 L), a slow redistribution from tissues, and a long elimination, with high interpatient variability. Pharmacokinetics are nonlinear with dose for a given infusion regimen, clearance decreasing with drug dose. The drug's clearance decreases with age, but no clear correlation of toxicity with age was observed.[146]

Toxicity

The primary dose-limiting toxicities of trabectedin are myelosuppression, fatigue, and hepatic enzyme elevations.[141,143,145] Myelosuppression (both platelet and neutrophils are affected) correlates with the C_{max} in plasma, while hepatic enzyme elevations are a function of the AUC. Hepatic toxicity consists of acute and rapidly reversible elevations of transaminases, with less notable increases in alkaline phosphatase, and bilirubin. Dexamethasone, 8 mg bid, beginning 24 hours prior to infusion and continuing through days 0 and +1, effectively ameliorates hepatic toxicity.[147]

Drug Interactions

With doxorubicin (60 to 75 mg/m^2), trabectedin in doses of 1.1 mg/m^2 did not improve response or disease progression rates in first-line therapy of soft-tissue sarcoma,[148] but showed outstanding disease control alone in soft-tissue sarcomas,[144,149] and with doxorubicin in uterine and other leiomyosarcomas.[150] In combination with pegylated liposomal doxorubicin (PLD), 30 mg/m^2, trabectedin (1.1 mg/m^2 as a 3-hour infusion) is approved for treatment of platinum-sensitive relapsed ovarian cancer in Europe. Lurbinectedin has yielded promising antitumor response rates alone and combined with doxorubicin or with taxanes in solid tumors. It has the advantage of modest hepatic toxicity.[151]

References

1. Umezawa H, Maeda K, Takeuchi T, et al. New antibiotics, bleomycin A and B. *J Antibiot (Tokyo)*. 1966;19:200-209.
2. Levi JA, Raghavan D, Harvey V, et al. The importance of bleomycin in combination chemotherapy for good-prognosis germ cell carcinoma. *J Clin Oncol*. 1993;11:1300-1305.
3. Takita T, Umezawa Y, Saito S, et al. Total synthesis of bleomycin A$_2$. *Tetrahedron Lett*. 1982;23:521-524.
4. Mistry JS, Sebti SM, Lazo JS. Separation of bleomycins and their deamido metabolites by high-performance cation-exchange chromatography. *J Chromatogr*. 1990;514:86-90.
5. Stubbe J, Kozarich JW. Mechanisms of bleomycin-induced DNA degradation. *Chem Rev*. 1987;87:1107-1136.
6. Umezawa H. Advances in bleomycin studies. In: Hecht SM, ed. *Bleomycin: Chemical, Biochemical, and Biological Aspects*. New York, NY: Springer-Verlag; 1979:24-36.
7. Yu Z, Paul R, Bhattacharya C, et al. Structural features facilitating tumor cell targeting and internalization by bleomycin and its disaccharide. *Biochemistry*. 2015;54:3100-3109.
8. Burger RM. Cleavage of nucleic acids by bleomycin. *Chem Rev*. 1998;98(3):1153-1170.
9. Fulmer P, Pettering DH. Reaction of DNA-bound ferrous bleomycin with dioxygen: activation versus stabilization of dioxygen. *Biochemistry*. 1994;33:5319-5327.
10. Sausville EA, Peisach J, Horwitz SB. A role for ferrous ion and oxygen in the degradation of DNA by bleomycin. *Biochem Biophys Res Commun*. 1976;73:814-822.
11. Mahmutoglu I, Kappus H. Redox cycling of bleomycin-Fe(III) by an NADH-dependent enzyme, and DNA damage in isolated rat liver nuclei. *Biochem Pharmacol*. 1987;36:3677-3681.
12. Burger RM, Kent TA, Horwitz SB, et al. Mossbauer study of iron bleomycin and its activation intermediates. *J Biol Chem*. 1983;258:1559-1564.
13. Chen JK, Yang D, Shen B, Murray V. Bleomycin analogues preferentially cleave at the transcription start sites of actively transcribed genes in human cells. *Int J Biochem Cell Biol*. 2017;85: 56-65.
14. Nyugen TV, Muaary V. Human telomeric DNA sequences are a major target for the antitumour drug bleomycin. *J Biol Inorg Chem*. 2012;17:1-9.
15. Hertzberg RP, Caranfa MJ, Hecht SM. Degradation of structurally modified DNAs by bleomycin group antibiotics. *Biochemistry*. 1988;27:3164-3174.
16. Povirk LF, Hogan M, Dattagupta N. Binding of bleomycin to DNA: intercalation of the bithiazole rings. *Biochemistry*. 1979;18:96-101.
17. Caspary WJ, Niziak C, Lanzo DA, et al. Bleomycin A$_2$: a ferrous oxidase. *Mol Pharmacol*. 1979;16:256-260.
18. Kilkuskie RE, Macdonald TL, Hecht SM. Bleomycin may be activated for DNA cleavage by NADPH–cytochrome P450 reductase. *Biochemistry*. 1984;23:6165-6171.
19. Sausville E, Stein R, Peisach J, et al. Properties and products of the degradation of DNA by bleomycin. *Biochemistry*. 1978;17:2746-2754.
20. Grollman AP, Takeshita M, Pillai KM, et al. Origin and cytotoxic properties of base propenals derived from DNA. *Cancer Res*. 1985;45:1127-1131.
21. Grollman AP, Takeshita M. Interactions of bleomycin with DNA. In: Weber G, ed. *Advances in Enzyme Regulation*. Vol 18. Oxford, UK: Pergamon Press; 1980:67-83.
22. Fugimito J, Higashi H, Kosaki G. Intracellular distribution of [^{14}C]bleomycin and the cytokinetic effects of bleomycin in the mouse tumor. *Cancer Res*. 1976;36:2248-2253.
23. Bršmme D, Rossi AB, Smeekens SP, et al. Human bleomycin hydrolase: molecular cloning, sequencing, functional expression, and enzymatic characterization. *Biochemistry*. 1996;35:6706-6714.
24. Farrell PA, Gonzalez F, Zheng W, et al. Crystal structure of human bleomycin hydrolase, a self compartmentalizing cysteine protease. *Structure*. 1999;7:619-627.
25. Takeda A, Nonaka M, Ishikawa A, et al. Immunohistochemical localization of the neutral cysteine protease bleomycin hydrolase in human skin. *Arch Dermatol Res*. 1999;291:238-240.

26. Schwartz DR, Homanics GE, Hoyt DG. The neutral cysteine protease bleomycin hydrolase is essential for epidermal integrity and bleomycin resistance. *Proc Natl Acad Sci U S A.* 1999;96:4680-4685.

27. de Haas EC, Zwart N, Meijer C, et al. Variation in bleomycin hydrolase gene is associated with reduced survival after chemotherapy for testicular germ cell cancer. *J Clin Oncol.* 2008;26:1817-1823.

28. Olive PL, Banath JP. Detection of DNA double-strand breaks through the cell cycle after exposure to x-rays, bleomycin, etoposide and ^{125}IdUrd. *Int J Radiat Biol.* 1993;64:349-358.

29. Lopez-Larraza DM, Bianchi NO. DNA response to bleomycin in mammalian cells with variable degrees of chromatin condensation. *Environ Mol Mutagen.* 1993;21:258-264.

30. Kuo MT, Hsu TC. Bleomycin causes release of nucleosomes from chromatin and chromosomes. *Nature.* 1978;271:83.

31. Touchekti O, Pron G, Belehradek J Jr, et al. Bleomycin, an apoptosis mimetic drug that induces two types of cell death depending on the number of molecules internalized. *Cancer Res.* 1993;53:5462-5469.

32. Pommier Y, Huang SY, Gao R, et al. Tyrosyl-DNA phosphodiesterases (TDP1 and TDP2). *DNA Repair (Amst).* 2014;19:114-129.

33. Schrock MS, Batar B, Druck T, et al. Wwox-Brca1 interaction: role in DNA repair pathway choice. *Oncogene.* 2016;36(16):2215-2227.

34. Dong F, Soubeyard S, Hache RJG. Activation of PARP-1 in response to bleomycin depends on the Ku antigen and protein phosphatase 5. *Oncogene.* 2010;29:2093-2103.

35. Taylor AMR, Rosney CM, Campbell JB. Unusual sensitivity of ataxia telangiectasia cells to bleomycin. *Cancer Res.* 1979;39:1046-1050.

36. Li HR, Shagisultanova EI, Yamashita K, et al. Hypersensitivity of tumor cell lines with microsatellite instability to DNA double strand break producing chemotherapeutic agent bleomycin. *Cancer Res.* 2004;64:4760-4767.

37. Morris G, Mistry JS, Jani JP, et al. Neutralization of bleomycin hydrolase by an epitope-specific antibody. *Mol Pharmacol.* 1992;42:57-62.

38. Jani JP, Mistry JS, Morris G, et al. In vivo circumvention of human colon carcinoma resistance to bleomycin. *Cancer Res.* 1992;52:2931-2937.

39. Tsuruo T, Hamilton TC, Louie KG, et al. Collateral susceptibility of Adriamycin-, melphalan- and cisplatin-resistant human ovarian tumor cells to bleomycin. *Jpn J Cancer Res.* 1986;77:94194-94195.

40. Shiu GK, Goehl TJ. High-performance liquid chromatographic determination of bleomycin A$_2$ in urine. *J Chromatogr.* 1980;181:127-133.

41. Broughton A, Strong JE. Radioimmunoassay of bleomycin. *Cancer Res.* 1976;36:1418-1421.

42. Crooke ST, Luft F, Broughton A, et al. Bleomycin serum pharmacokinetics as determined by a radioimmunoassay and a microbiologic assay in a patient with compromised renal function. *Cancer.* 1977;39:1430-1434.

43. Alberts DS, Chen HSG, Liu R, et al. Bleomycin pharmacokinetics in man, I: intravenous administration. *Cancer Chemother Pharmacol.* 1978;1:1771-1781.

44. Oken MM, Crooke ST, Elson MK, et al. Pharmacokinetics of bleomycin after IM administration in man. *Cancer Treat Rep.* 1981;65:485-489.

45. Paladine W, Cunningham TJ, Sponzo R, et al. Intracavitary bleomycin in the management of malignant effusions. *Cancer.* 1976;38:1903-1908.

46. Howell SB, Schiefer M, Andrews PA, et al. The pharmacology of intraperitoneally administered bleomycin. *J Clin Oncol.* 1987;5:2009-2016.

47. Dalgleish AG, Woods RL, Levi JA. Bleomycin pulmonary toxicity: its relationship to renal dysfunction. *Med Pediatr Oncol.* 1984;12:313-317.

48. Hinton S, Catalano PJ, Einhorn LH, et al. Cisplatin, etoposide and either bleomycin or ifosfamide in the treatment of disseminated germ cell tumors. *Cancer.* 2003;97:1869-1875.

49. Hubbard SP, Chabner BA, Canellos GP, et al. High-dose intravenous bleomycin in treatment of advanced lymphomas. *Eur J Cancer.* 1975;11:623-626.

50. Levy RL, Chiarillo S. Hyperpyrexia, allergic-type response, and death occurring with bleomycin administration. *Oncology.* 1980;37:316-317.

51. Comis RL. Bleomycin pulmonary toxicity: current status and future directions. *Semin Oncol.* 1992;19(suppl 5):64-70.

52. De A, Guryev I, LaRiviere A, et al. Pulmonary function abnormalities in childhood cancer survivors treated with bleomycin. *Pediatr Blood Cancer.* 2014;61:1679-1684.

53. Parvinen LM, Kikku P, Maekinen E, et al. Factors affecting the pulmonary toxicity of bleomycin. *Acta Radiol Oncol.* 1983;22:417-421.

54. Dee GJ, Austin JH, Mutter GL. Bleomycin-associated pulmonary fibrosis: rapidly fatal progression without chest radiotherapy. *J Surg Oncol.* 1987;35:135-138.

55. Samuels ML, Johnson DE, Holoye PH, et al. Large-dose bleomycin therapy and pulmonary toxicity: a possible role of prior radiotherapy. *JAMA.* 1976;235:1117-1120.

56. Lauritsen J, Kier MG, Bandak, M, et al. Pulmonary function in patients with germ cell cancer treated with bleomycin, etoposide, and cisplatin. *J Clin Oncol.* 2016;34:1492-1499.

57. Falay O, Ozturk E, Bolukbasi Y, et al. Use of fluorodeoxyglucose positron emission tomography for diagnosis of bleomycin-induced pneumonitis in hodgkin lymphoma. *Leuk Lymphoma.* 2017;58:1114-1122.

58. Moeller A, Ask K, Warburton D, et al. The bleomycin animal mode: a useful tool to investigate treatment option for idiopathic pulmonary fibrosis? *Int J Biochem Cell Biol.* 2007;40:362-382.

59. Raisfeld IH. Role of terminal substituents in the pulmonary toxicity of bleomycins. *Toxicol Appl Pharmacol.* 1981;57:355-366.

60. Williamson JD, Sadofsky LR, Hart SP. The pathogenesis of bleomycin-induced lung injury in animals and its applicability to human idiopathic pulmonary fibrosis. *Exp Lung Res.* 2015;41:57-73.

61. Piguet PF, Collart MA, Grau GE, et al. Tumor necrosis factor/cachectin plays a key role in bleomycin induced pneumopathy and fibrosis. *J Exp Med.* 1989;170:6556-6563.

62. Baecher AC, Barth RK. PCR analysis of cytokine induction profiles associated with mouse strain variation in susceptibility to pulmonary fibrosis. *Reg Immunol.* 1993;5:207-217.

63. King SL, Lichter AC, Rowe SW, et al. Bleomycin stimulates pro-alpha (I) collagen promoter through transforming growth factor beta response element by intracellular and extracellular signaling. *J Biol Chem.* 1994;269:13156-13161.

64. Kida T, Ayabe S, Omori K, et al. Prostaglandin D2 attenuates bleomycin-Induced lung inflammation and pulmonary fibrosis. *PLoS One.* 2016;11:e0167729.

65. Coker RK, Laurent GJ, Shahzeidi S, et al. Transforming growth factors-β_1, -β_2, and -β_3 stimulate fibroblast procollagen production in vitro but are differentially expressed during bleomycin-induced lung fibrosis. *Am J Pathol.* 1997;150:981-991.

66. Eitzman DT, McCoy RD, Zheng X, et al. Bleomycin-induced pulmonary fibrosis in transgenic mice that either lack or overexpress the murine plasminogen activator inhibitor-1 gene. *J Clin Invest.* 1996;97:232-237.

67. Kuwano K, Hagimoto N, Kawasaki M, et al. Essential roles of the fas-fas ligand pathway in the development of pulmonary fibrosis. *J Clin Invest.* 1999;104:13-19.

68. Phillips RJ, Burdick MD, Hing K, et al. Circulating fibrocytes traffic to the lungs in response to CXL12 and mediate fibrosis. *J Clin Invest.* 2004;114:438-446.

69. Giri SN, Hyde DM, Hollinger MA. Effect of antibody to transforming growth factor beta on bleomycin-induced accumulation of lung collagen in mice. *Thorax.* 1993;48:959-966.

70. Piguet PF, Grau GE, deKossodo S. Role of granulocyte-macrophage colony stimulating factor in pulmonary fibrosis induced in mice by bleomycin. *Exp Lung Res.* 1993;19:579-587.

71. Gurujeyalakshmi G, Hollinger MA, Giri SN. Pirfenidone inhibits PDGF isoforms in bleomycin hamster model of lung fibrosis at the translational level. *Am J Physiol.* 1999;276:L31131-L31138.

72. Phan SH, Thrall RS, Ward PA. Bleomycin-induced pulmonary fibrosis in rats: biochemical demonstration of increased rates of collagen synthesis. *Am Rev Respir Dis.* 1980;121:5015-5016.

73. Thrau RS, McCormick JR, Jack RM, et al. Bleomycin-induced pulmonary fibrosis in the rat: inhibition by indomethacin. *Am J Pathol.* 1979;95:117-130.

74. Carnevale-Schianca F, Gallo S, Rota-Scalabrini D, et al. Complete resolution of life-threatening bleomycin-induced pneumonitis after treatment with imatinib mesylate in a patient with Hodgkin's lymphoma: hope for severe chemotherapy-induced toxicity. *J Clin Oncol.* 2011;29:e691-e693. doi:10.1200/JCO.2011.35.6733.

75. Faress JA, Nethery DE, Kern EFO, et al. Bleomycin-induced pulmonary fibrosis is attenuated by a monoclonal antibody targeting HER2. *J Appl Physiol.* 2007;103:2077-2083.

76. Talcott JA, Garnick MB, Stomper PC, et al. Cavitary lung nodules associated with combination chemotherapy containing bleomycin. *J Urol.* 1987;138:619-620.

77. Burkhardt A, Gebbers JO, Holtje WJ. Die bleomycin-lunge. *Dtsch Med Wochenschr.* 1977;102:281-289.

78. Holoye PY, Luna MA, MacKay B, et al. Bleomycin hypersensitivity pneumonitis. *Ann Intern Med.* 1978;88:47-49.

79. Comis RL, Kuppinger MS, Ginsberg SJ, et al. Role of single-breath carbon monoxide–diffusing capacity in monitoring the pulmonary effects of bleomycin in germ-free tumor patients. *Cancer Res.* 1979;39:5076-5080.

80. Lucraft HH, Wilkinson PM, Stretton TB., et al. Role of pulmonary function tests in the prevention of bleomycin pulmonary toxicity during chemotherapy for metastatic testicular teratoma. *Eur J Cancer Clin Oncol.* 1982;18:133-139.

81. Osanto S, Bukman A, Van Hoek F, et al. Long-term effects of chemotherapy in patients with testicular cancer. *J Clin Oncol.* 1992;10:574-579.

82. Goldiner PL, Carlon GC, Critkovic E, et al. Factors influencing post-operative morbidity and mortality in patients treated with bleomycin. *Br Med J.* 1978;1:1664-1667.

83. Donat SM, Levy DA. Bleomycin associated pulmonary toxicity: is preoperative oxygen restriction necessary? *J Urol.* 1998;160:1347-1352.

84. Maher J, Daley PA. Severe bleomycin lung toxicity: reversal with high dose corticosteroids. *Thorax.* 1993;48:92–94.

85. Van Barneveld PW, Sleijfer DT, van der Mark TW, et al. Natural course of bleomycin-induced pneumonitis: a follow-up study. *Am Rev Respir Dis.* 1987;135:48-51.

86. Narayan V, Deshpande C, Bermudez CA, et al. Bilateral lung transplantation for bleomycin-associated lung injury. *Oncologist.* 2017;22(5):620-622.

87. Blum RH, Carter SK, Agre K. *Cancer.* 1973;31:903-914.

88. Berger CC, Bokemeyer C, Schneider M, et al. Secondary Raynaud's phenomenon and other late vascular complications following chemotherapy for testicular cancer. *Eur J Cancer.* 1995;31A(13–14):2229-2238.

89. Mowad CM, Mguyen TV, Elenitsas R et al. Bleomycin-induced flagellate dermatitis; a clinical and histopathological review. *Br J Dermatol.* 1994;131:700-702.

90. Morrow CP, DiSaia PJ, Mangan CF, et al. Continuous pelvic arterial infusion with bleomycin for squamous carcinoma of the cervix recurrent after irradiation therapy. *Cancer Treat Rep.* 1977;61:1403-1405.

91. Watring WG, Roberts JA, Lagasse LD, et al. Treatment of recurrent Paget's disease of the vulva with topical bleomycin. *Cancer.* 1978;41:10-11.

92. Kessinger A, Wigton RS. Intracavitary bleomycin and tetracycline in the management of malignant pleural effusions: a randomized study. *J Surg Oncol.* 1987;36:81-83.

93. Bracken RB, Johnson DE, Rodriquez L, et al. Treatment of multiple superficial tumors of bladder with intravesical bleomycin. *Urology.* 1977;9:161-163.

94. Zhang G, Fang Y, Dai BW, et al. Intracystic bleomycin for cystic craniopharyngiomas in children. *Cochrane Database Syst Rev.* 2016;(7):CD008890.

95. Fu K, Phillips TL, Silverberg IJ, et al. Combined radiotherapy and chemotherapy with bleomycin and methotrexate for advanced inoperable head and neck cancer: update of a Northern California Oncology Group randomized trial. *J Clin Oncol.* 1987;5:1410-1418.

96. Waksman SA, Woodruff HB. Bacteriostatic and bactericidal substances produced by soil *Actinomyces. Exp Biol Med.* 1940;45:609–614.

97. Falini B, Brunetti L, Martelli MP. Dactinomycin in NPM1-mutated myeloid Leukemia. *N Engl J Med.* 2015;373:1180-1182.

98. Chen FM, Sha F, Chin K, et al. The nature of actinomycin C binding to d(AACCAXYG) sequence motifs. *Nucleic Acids Res.* 2004;32:271-277.

99. Gupta RS. Podophyllotoxin-resistant mutants of Chinese hamster ovary cells: cross-resistance studies with various microtubule inhibitors and podophyllotoxic analogues. *Cancer Res.* 1983;43:505–512.

100. Hill CR, Cole M, Errington J, et al. Characterization of the clinical pharmacokinetics of actinomycin D and the influence of ABCB1 pharmacogenetic variation on actinomycin D disposition in children with cancer. *Clin Pharmacokinet.* 2014;53:741-751.

101. Frei E. The clinical use of actinomycin. *Cancer Chemother Rep.* 1974;58:49-54.

102. Hazar V, Kutluk T, Akyuz C, et al. Veno-occlusive disease-like hepatotoxicity in two children receiving chemotherapy for Wilms' tumor and clear sarcoma of kidney. *Pediatr Hematol Oncol.* 1998;15:85-89.

103. D'Angio GJ, Farber S, Maddock Cl. Potentiation of x-ray effects by actinomycin D. *Radiology.* 1959;73:175–177.

104. Wakaki S, Marumo H, Tomioka K. Isolations of new fractions of antitumor mitomycins. *Antibiot Chemother.* 1958;8:228-240.

105. Ajani JA, Winter KA, Gunderson LL, et al. Fluorouracil, mitomycin, and radiotherapy vs fluorouracil, cisplatin, and radiotherapy for carcinoma or the anal canal: a randomized controlled trial. *JAMA.* 2008;299: 1914-1921.

106. Stevens CL, Taylor KG, Munk KE, et al. Chemistry and structure of mitomycin C. *J Med Chem.* 1964;8:1–10.

107. Tomasz M, Palom Y. The mitomycin bioreductive antitumor agents: crosslinking and alkylation of DNA as the molecular basis of their activity. *Pharmacol Ther.* 1997;76:73-87.

108. Cummings JS, Spanswick VJ, Smyth JF. Re-evaluation of the molecular pharmacology of mitomycin C. *Eur J Cancer.* 1995;31A:1918-1933.

109. Suresh Kumar G, Lipman R, Cummings J, et al. Mitomycin C-DNA adducts generated by DT-diaphorase: revised mechanism of the enzymatic reductive activation of mitomycin C. *Biochemistry.* 1997;36:14128-14136.

110. Belcourt MF, Hodnick WF, Rockwell S, et al. Differential toxicity of mitomycin C and porfiromycin to aerobic and hypoxic Chinese hamster ovary cells overexpressing human NADPH:cytochrome c (P-450) reductase. *Proc Natl Acad Sci U S A.* 1996;93:456-460.

111. Bargonetti J, Champeil E, Tomasz M. Differential toxicity of DNA adducts of mitomycin C. *J Nucl Acids.* 2010. doi:10.4061/2010/698960.

112. Dulhanty AM, Li M, Whitmore GF. Isolation of Chinese hamster ovary cell mutants deficient in excision repair and mitomycin C bioactivation. *Cancer Res.* 1989;49:117-122.

113. Collins NB, Wilson JB, Bush T, et al. ATR-dependent phosphorylation of FANCA on serine 1449 after DNA damage is important for FA pathway function. *Blood.* 2009;113:2181-2190.

114. Villalona-Calero MA, Duan W, Zhao W, et al. Veliparib alone or in combination with mitomycin C in patients with solid tumors with functional deficiency in homologous recombination repair. *J Natl Cancer Inst.* 2016;108. doi:10.1093/nci/djv437.

115. Den Hartigh J, McVie JG, van Oort WJ, et al. Pharmacokinetics of mitomycin C in humans. *Cancer Res.* 1983;43:5017-5021.

116. Verweij J, Stuurman M, de Vries J, et al. The difference in pharmacokinetics of mitomycin C, given either as a single agent or as part of combination chemotherapy. *J Cancer Res Clin Oncol.* 1986;112:282-284.

117. Dalton JT, Wientjes MG, Pfeffer M. Studies on mitomycin C absorption after intravesical treatment of superficial bladder tumors. *J Urol.* 1991;132:30-33.

118. Panda A, Pe'er J, Aggarwal A, et al. Effect of topical mitomycin C on corneal endothelium. *Am J Ophthalmol.* 2008;145:635-638.

119. Crooke ST, Bradner WT. Mitomycin C: a review. *Cancer Treat Res.* 1976;3:121–139.

120. Lazarus HM, Gottfried MR, Herzig RH. Veno-occlusive disease of the liver after high dose mitomycin C therapy and autologous bone marrow transplantation. *Cancer.* 1982;49:1789–1795.

121. Verweij J, Van der Burg MEL, Pinedo HM. Mitomycin C induced hemolytic uremic syndrome: six case reports and review of the literature on renal, pulmonary and cardiac side effect of the drug. *Radiother Oncol.* 1987;8:33-41.

122. Verweij J, van Zanten T, Souren T. Prospective study of the dose relationship of mitomycin C-induced interstitial pneumonitis. *Cancer.* 1987;60: 756-761.

123. Le VH, Inai M, Williams RM, Kan T. Ecteinascidins. A review of the chemistry, biology, and clinical utility of potent tetrahydroisoquinolone antitumor antibiotics. *Nat Prod Rep.* 2015;32:328-347.

124. Takahashi R, Mabuchi S, Kawano M, et al. Preclinical investigations of PM01183 (Lurbinectedin) as a single agent or in combination with other anticancer agents for clear cell carcinoma of the ovary. *PLoS One.* 2016;11(3):e0151050.

125. Larsen AK, Calmarini CM, D'Incalci M. Unique features of trabectedin mechanism of action. *Cancer Chemother Pharmacol.* 2016;77:663-671.

126. Pommier Y, Kohlhagen G, Bailly C, et al. DNA sequence- and structure-selective alkylation of guanine N2 in the minor groove by ecteinascidin 743, a potent antitumor compound from the Caribbean tunicate *Ecteinascidia turbinata. Biochemistry.* 1996;35:13303-13309.

127. Takebayashi Y, Goldwasser F, Urasaki Y. Ecteinascidin 743 induces protein–linked DNA breaks in human colon carcinoma HCT116 cells and is cytotoxic independently of topoisomerase I expression. *Clin Cancer Res.* 2001;7:185–191.

128. Zewail-Foote M, Hurley LH. Ecteinascidin 743: a minor groove alkylator that bends DNA toward the major groove. *J Med Chem.* 1999;42:2493-2497.

129. Aune GJ, Takagi K, Sordet O, et al. Von Hippel-Lindau—Coupled and transcription-coupled nucleotide excision repair—dependent degradation of RNA polymerase II in response to trabectedin. *Clin Cancer Res.* 2008;14:6449-6455.

130. Ordonez JL, Amaral AT, Carcaboso AM, et al. The PARP inhibitor olaparib enhances the sensitivity of Ewing sarcoma to trabectedin. *Oncotarget.* 2015;5:18875-18890.

131. Lima M, Bouzid H, Soares DG, et al. Dual inhibition of ATR and ATM potentiates the activity of trabectedin and lurbinectedin by perturbing the DNA damage response and homologous recombination repair. *Oncotarget.* 2016;7:25885-25901.

132. Monk BJ, Lorusso D, Italiano A, et al. Trabectedin as a chemotherapy option for patients with BRCA deficiency. *Cancer Treat Rev.* 2016;50:175-182.

133. Delalogue S, Wolp-Diniz R, Bryski T, et al. Activity of trabectedin in germline BRACA 1/20 mutated metastatic breast cancer: results of an international first-in-class phase II study. *Ann Oncol.* 2014;25:1152-1158.

134. Grohar PJ, Griffin LB, Yeung C. et al. Ecteinascidin 743 interferes with the activity of EWS-PL1I1 in Ewing sarcoma cells. *Neoplasia.* 2011;13:145-153.

135. Friedman D, Hu Z, Kolb EA et al. Ecteinascidin-743 inhibits activated but not constitutive transcription. *Cancer Res.* 2002;62:3377-3381.

136. Rinehart KL. Antitumor compounds from tunicates. *Med Res Rev.* 2000;20:1-27.

137. Takebayashi Y, Pourquier P, Zomonjic DB, et al. Antiproliferative activity of ecteinascidin 743 is dependent upon transcription-coupled excision repair. *Nat Med.* 2001;7:961-966.

138. Stevens EV, Nichizula S, Antony S, et al. Predicting cisplatin and trabectedin drug sensitivity in ovarian and colon cancers. *Mol Cancer Ther.* 2008;7:10-18.

139. Rosing H, Hildebrand MJ, Jimeno J, et al. Quantitative determination of ecteinascidin 743 in human plasma by miniaturized high-performance liquid chromatography coupled with electrospray ionization tandem mass spectrometry. *J Mass Spectrom.* 1998;33:1134-1140.

140. Reid JM, Kuffel MJ, Ruben SL, et al. Rat and human liver cytochrome p-450 isoform metabolism of ecteinascidin 743 does not predict gender-dependent toxicity in humans. *Clin Cancer Res.* 2002;8:2952-2962.

141. Ryan DP, Supko JG, Eder JP, et al. Phase I and pharmacokinetic study of ecteinascidin 743 administered as a 762-hour continuous intravenous infusion in patients with solid malignancies. *Clin Cancer Res.* 2001;7:231-242.

142. Sparidans RW, Rosing H, Hildebrand MJ, et al. Search for metabolites of ecteinascidin 743, a novel marine-derived, anticancer agent in man. *Anticancer Drugs.* 2001;12:653-666.

143. Demetri GD, Chawla SP, von Mehren M, et al. Efficacy and safety of trabectedin in patients with advanced or metastatic liposarcoma after failure of prior anthracyclines and ifosfamide: results of a randomized phase II study of two different schedules. *J Clin Oncol.* 2009;27:4188-4196.

144. Kawai A, Araki N, Sugiura H, et al. Trabectedin monotherapy after standard chemotherapy versus best supportive care in patients with advanced translocation-related sarcoma: a randomised, open-label, phase 2 study. *Lancet Oncol.* 2015;16:406-416.

145. von Merhen M, Bookman M, Meropol NJ, et al. Phase I study of the safety and pharmacokinetics of trabectedin with docetaxel in patients with advanced malignancies. *Cancer Chemother Pharmacol.* 2015;75:1047-1055.

146. Garcia-Carbonero R, Supko JG, Maki RG, et al. Ecteinascidin-743 (ET-743) for chemotherapy-naive patients with advanced soft tissue sarcomas: a multicenter phase II and pharmacokinetic study. *J Clin Oncol.* 2005;23:5484-5492.

147. Donald S, Verschoyle RD, Greaves P, et al. Complete protection by high-dose dexamethasone against the hepatotoxicity of the novel antitumor drug yondelis (ET-743) in the rat. *Cancer Res.* 2003;63:5902-5908.

148. Martin-Broto J, Pousa AL, de Las Penas R, et al. Randomized phase II study of trabectedin and doxorubicin compared with doxorubicin alone as first line treatment in patients with advanced soft tissue sarcomas: a Spanish group for research on sarcoma study. *J Clin Oncol.* 2016;34:2294-2302.

149. Demetri GD, von Mehren M, Jones Rl, et al. Efficacy and safety of trabectedin or dacarbazine for metastatic liposarcoma or leiomyosarcoma after failure of conventional chemotherapy: results of a phase III randomized multicenter clinical trial. *J Clin Oncol.* 2016;34:786-793.

150. Paultier P, Floquet A, Chevreau C, et al. Trabectedin in combination with doxorubicin for first-line treatment of advanced uterine or soft-tissue leiomyosarcoma (MS-02): a non-randomised, multi-centre, phase 2 trial. *Lancet Oncol.* 2015;16:457-464.

151. Elez ME, Tabernero J, Geary D, et al. First-in-human phase I study of lurbinectedin (PM01183) in patients with advanced solid tumors. *Clin Cancer Res.* 2014;20:2205-2214.

Epigenetic Agents in Oncology: HDAC Inhibitors, IDH Inhibitors, and EZH2 Inhibitors

Ira Surolia and Susan E. Bates

Histone deacetylase inhibitors (HDACis) are a promising class of anticancer drugs—FDA approved for treatment of certain cancers and undergoing vigorous clinical investigation in oncology as single agents and in drug combinations. They belong to the broader category of drugs that act on the epigenome. Romidepsin (Istodax; Celgene), vorinostat (Zolinza; Merck & Co.), and belinostat (Beleodaq; Spectrum Pharmaceuticals) have all been approved for the treatment of cutaneous or peripheral T-cell lymphomas; and panobinostat (Farydak; Novartis) is approved for the treatment of drug-resistant multiple myeloma. HDACis promote the acetylation of histones.

Chromatin compaction is governed by electrostatic interactions between DNA and histones present as an octamer surrounded by DNA in the nucleosome-chromatin complex. Modification of histone at key sites, through attachment or removal of acetyl, methyl, or phosphate groups, significantly determines the accessibility of DNA to transcription complexes. The enzymes responsible for these modifications (methylases, demethylases, acetyl transferases, and deacetylases, in particular) have been implicated in tumor pathogenesis and have become targets for significant drug development efforts.[1]

HDACs exert a prooncogenic effect, at least in part, by keeping genes involved in differentiation, apoptosis, and cell cycle arrest in a transcriptionally quiescent state. By removing acetyl groups from lysines in the 5′ "tail" of histone proteins, electrostatic interactions with DNA are increased, protranscription acetyl marks are reduced, and gene transcription is inhibited. Histone acetyl transferase (HAT) enzymes function in opposition to the HDACs, increasing acetylation in the epigenetic code, relaxing chromatin, and thereby promoting transcriptional activity (Fig. 16.1).

The mechanisms underlying the ability of the majority of cancers to commandeer the pathways modifying the epigenetic code to manipulate gene expression are incompletely understood. Many cancers display molecular alterations that diminish or dampen HAT activity or shift the balance toward HDAC activity. For example, patients with germline, loss-of-function mutations in CREB-binding protein (CBP), a nuclear protein with intrinsic HAT activity, have a developmental disorder known as Rubinstein-Taybi syndrome.[2] These patients also have an increased incidence of malignant and benign neural and developmental tumors including medulloblastoma, neuroblastoma, pheochromocytoma, nasopharyngeal rhabdomyosarcoma, leiomyosarcoma, seminoma, and embryonal carcinoma. Multiple alterations of HAT proteins are found in cancers; chromosomal translocations

involving HAT proteins are frequent in leukemias; and mutations have been identified in colorectal, breast, and ovarian cancer.[3–5] Table 16.1 lists malignancies characterized by alterations in HDACs and HATs.[6–8,10–12,14,15] HDACis that target these pathways have the potential to reverse mechanisms involved in oncogenesis.

Mechanism of Action

The histone deacetylase (HDAC) enzymes appear to be the major target of the HDACi and are grouped into four different classes based on their similarity to known yeast HDACs.[17,18] The HDACis mainly target class I (HDACs 1, 2, 3, and 8), class IIA (HDACs 4, 5, 7, 9), and IIB (HDACs 6, 10).[1] One classification to consider for HDACis is to divide them based on enzyme specificity: (1) nonselective HDACi, (vorinostat, belinostat, and panobinostat); (2)

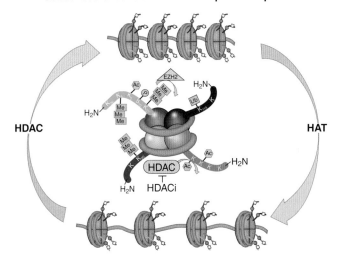

Condensed Chromatin and Transcriptional Repression

Relaxed Chromatin and Transcriptional Activation

FIGURE **16.1** Histone acetyltransferases (HAT) cause decompaction of chromatin and increased chromatin accessiblity, leading to downstream effects stemming from increased transcription. This effect is reversed by histone deacetylases (HDAC). The *inset* shows the structure of a single histone core unit with 146 bp DNA wound around it. Histone tails are rich in lysine residues that may be acetylated (Ac), methylated (Me), or ubiquitinated (Ub). HDAC inhibitors (HDACi) can prevent deacetylation of these lysine residues (K).

TABLE
16.1   *Selected examples of HDAC/HAT abnormalities in malignancy*

HAT/HDAC	Molecular abnormality	Chromosomal Abnormality	Gene Product	Malignancy	Reference
HATs					
CBP (CREB-binding proteins)	Fusion	t(11;16)	MLL/CBP	MDS	6
	Fusion	t(11;16)	MLL/CBP	AML	7
p300	Fusion	t(8;16)	MOZ-CBP	M4/5 AML	8,9
	Fusion	t(11;22)	MLL/p300	t(11;22) AML	10
	Mutations and LOH	22q13		Gastric (intestinal type)	11
	Missense mutation			Colorectal cancer	12,13
HDACs					
HDAC1	Recruitment	t(15;17)	RARa-PML	APL	14
	Recruitment	t(8;21)	AML1-ETO	t(8;21) AML	15,16

selective HDACi, such as class I HDACi (romidepsin and entinostat) and HDAC6 inhibitor (ricolinostat); and (3) multipharmacological HDACi, such as CUDC-101 and CUDC-907.[19]

Table 16.2 lists putative mechanisms of action that have been described for HDACis. It is useful to consider the epigenetic and nonepigenetic effects of HDACi as separate entities. The impact on cell cycle and cell death pathways may not directly follow from epigenetic effects, and as such should be studied separately.[20]

TABLE
16.2   *Putative mechanisms of action of HDACi[a]*

1. Histone acetylation with altered gene expression resulting in cell cycle arrest, growth inhibition, or differentiation
2. Acetylation of nonhistone proteins such as p53, HIF-1s, pRb, STAT-3, Rel A/p65, estrogen receptor impair function and thereby influence cell growth or survival
3. Acetylation of Hsp90 impairs chaperone function resulting in client protein ubiquitination and proteasomal degradation
4. Disruption of aggresome formation through acetylation of tubulin
5. Reduced premitotic phosphorylation of pericentromeric histone H3 and disruption of kinetochore assembly results in prometaphase cell cycle arrest
6. Direct activation of apoptotic pathways—reduction of antiapoptotic proteins such as Bcl-2 and increased expression of proapoptotic proteins such as BAX and BAK
7. Enhanced production of ROS
8. Enhanced antitumor immunity through enhancement of TRAIL or up-regulation of antigen expression that could facilitate cancer cell recognition
9. Disruption of DNA repair through acetylation or down-regulation of proteins such as Ku70, Ku86, BRCA1, and RAD51

[a]Adapted from Piekarz RL, Bates SE. Epigenetic modifiers: basic understanding and clinical development. Clin Cancer Res. 2009;15(12):3918-3926. Copyright © 2009 American Association for Cancer Research. With permission from AACR.

Gene Transcription

The most widely recognized molecular effect of HDACis has been promotion of lysine acetylation in the 5' end of octameric histone proteins in the nucleosome core. HATs and HDACs have opposing roles in the epigenetic modification that controls gene expression. HDACis bind to the HDAC enzyme, thereby inhibiting deacetylation, allowing unregulated acetylation by the HATs. With an increase in the acetyl groups on histones, the positive charge on lysine is neutralized. It is hypothesized that this results in a decrease in the electrostatic forces between the histone octamers and the negative DNA phosphate backbone, opening the chromatin structure and providing increased access. Transcription factors and RNA polymerases can thus more easily reach their respective regions in the now open/accessible chromatin. This leads to transcription of genes such as *CDKN1A*, which encodes p21, and in turn leads to cell cycle arrest and limitation of cell growth.[21–24]

It is certain that the effects on gene transcription are physiologically much more complex, involving multiple transcription factors and alterations in the bromodomain-containing proteins that "read" the acetylation marks. The HAT proteins are part of transcriptional coactivator complexes while HDAC proteins form part of transcriptional corepressor complexes. As such, the activity of transcription factors and nuclear hormone receptors is increasingly recognized as regulated by acetylation. Furthermore, particular lysines are specifically acetylated or methylated as markers for activation of specific genes. This epigenetic code signals transcription of a subset of genes after exposure to the HDACi. Array studies of cancer cell lines have noted that the expression of only 2% to 5% of genes is altered upon exposure to an HDAC inhibitor.[25,26] The number of genes induced approximately equals the number repressed.

Acetylation of Nonhistone Proteins

Acetylation of nonhistone proteins also occurs following HDAC inhibition. Indeed, this may be the principal mechanism of action in some cell types.[27,28] For example, p53 is acetylated at lysines 373 and

382 following exposure to an HDACi, causing decreased proteosomal degradation and inducing expression of p21.[29] One example of nonhistone protein acetylation that has sparked particular interest results from the effects of HDACi on acetylation of Hsp90. Initially demonstrated with vorinostat,[30] acetylation of Hsp90 disrupts the interaction of the chaperone with its client proteins, including cellular molecules associated with tumor development.[31] The long list of Hsp90 client proteins (http://www.picard.ch/downloads/Hsp90interactors) includes many proteins implicated in the onset or maintenance of the malignant phenotype. Cell lines that are addicted to Hsp90 client proteins such as HER-2, the BCR-ABL fusion protein, or mutated and activated EGFR are sensitive not only to Hsp90 inhibitors but also to HDACis.[32] HDACis have also been shown to induce apoptosis in leukemia cell lines with mutations in the FLT-3 gene.[33]

Effects on Cell Cycle

Cell cycle arrest is one of the hallmarks of HDACi activity. HDACi-induced cell cycle arrest commonly occurs at the G1/S cell cycle checkpoint and occasionally at the G2/M boundary.[34,35] G_1/S phase arrest has been ascribed to CDKN1A induction (and its encoded protein p21) and cyclin D and cyclin A gene repression. These events ultimately lead to phosphorylation and decreased activity of retinoblastoma protein (pRb). These effects are primarily mediated by induction of p21 expression. In addition to p21, multiple other genes involved in cell cycle progression have been identified as increased or decreased. Cell cycle arrest may also result from activation of mitotic checkpoints following HDACi-mediated acetylation of pericentromeric chromatin and impairment of kinetochore assembly.[36]

Induction of Apoptosis

Cell death is one of the most well-documented antitumor effects of HDACi and has been directly linked to therapeutic efficacy in preclinical studies. Apoptosis proceeds via one of two pathways: the extrinsic or cell death receptor–mediated pathway, or the intrinsic or mitochondria-mediated pathway. In the extrinsic pathway, death receptors activate caspase 8 and trigger apoptosis via a death-inducing signaling complex. Several HDACis increase expression of TRAIL, DR-5, DR-4, Fas, and Fas-L.[37,38] Death receptor–mediated apoptosis is also facilitated by HDACi-mediated down-regulation of c-FLIP, a protein associated with resistance to TRAIL therapy.[39] In the intrinsic pathway, mitochondrial release of cytochrome c leads to activation of caspase 9 that, in turn, activates caspase 3 and elicits apoptosis.[40] HDACis facilitate the intrinsic apoptosis pathway by down-regulating antiapoptotic proteins such as Bcl-2, Mcl-1, and Bcl-X$_L$ and up-regulating proapoptotic proteins such as Bax and Puma.[41]

Tissue-Type Selectivity

One of the intriguing questions about HDACi efficacy is the basis for their selectivity, and different aspects of mechanism of action have been identified as potential sources. All HDACis approved so far have been in treatment of hematological malignancies. There is emerging evidence of HDACi affecting pathways specific to several hematological malignancies. For instance, diffuse large-cell B-cell lymphomas (DLBCL) harboring mutations in the innate immune system–linked MyD88 gene correlate with sensitivity to the Bruton's tyrosine kinase inhibitor ibrutinib (Imbruvica, Pharmacyclics).[42] The HDACi panobinostat causes STAT3-mediated down-regulation of MyD88 in DLBCL derived cell lines, resulting in an opportunity for a synergistic drug combination between the Bruton's tyrosine kinase inhibitor and the HDACi.[43] As another example, a myeloma cell filled with paraproteins may be more sensitive to the loss of HDAC6-mediated transport to the aggresome than a cell where carcinogenesis does not involve aberrant protein production.[44] Interval dosing with HDACi can increase CD4+ T-cell related HIV expression, useful to reverse HIV latency and clear HIV infection more completely with antiretroviral agents.[45,46] This may also be true of HDACi effect on other latent viral proteins encoded in T cells, and have implications for virus-associated cancers like Kaposi sarcoma and Burkitt lymphoma.[45]

The particular effectiveness of HDACi in T-cell lymphoma is not well understood. HDACi-mediated activation and differentiation of naïve T cells, modulation of the activity of STAT and NFKB pathways all affect lymphocytes in a critical manner.[47] But why cutaneous T-cell lymphoma and peripheral T-cell lymphoma show at times dramatic sensitivity is not understood. Recent observations on the genetics of peripheral T-cell lymphoma have shown that in some subsets, mutation of IDH2, TET2, or DNMT3A promote aberrant methylation. HDACis could in part mitigate this aberrant hypermethylation, and potentially contribute to expression of tumor suppressors that would otherwise be repressed.[48]

Generation of Reactive Oxygen Species

Other mechanistic models include enhanced production of reactive oxygen species (ROS) by certain HDACi as a possible mechanism for cytotoxicity. Treatment of cancer cells with HDACi causes production of ROS followed by ceramide generation, mitochondrial injury, and activation of the caspase cascade that leads to apoptosis.[49–51] Coadministration of a free radical scavenger prevented cellular apoptosis, suggesting a role for ROS in cell death caused by HDAC inhibition.[49] HDACi-induced ROS generation has also been linked to activation of the NFκB pathway.[52]

Inhibition of DNA Repair

HDACis disrupt DNA repair processes through acetylation or down-regulation of proteins such as Ku70, Ku86, BRCA1, and RAD51. The effects of HDACi on DNA repair become apparent when combined with chemotherapy or irradiation. This could be exploited to potentiate the impact of DNA-damaging agents.[53] Enhanced gamma-H2AX foci, associated with double-strand DNA repair, have been reported.[54]

Chemical Structures and Classification of HDACi in Clinical Use

The HDACi family includes a number of structurally unrelated compounds grouped together by their common mechanism of action and classified according to their chemical structures. HDACis generally contain a zinc-binding domain, a capping group, and a straight chain linker connecting the two.[55] A partial list of HDACi

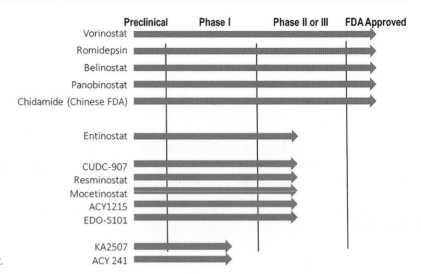

FIGURE 16.2 Graphic display of HDACi in clinical development.

either FDA approved or currently in clinical trials is provided in Figure 16.2 and structures of some of these agents are provided in Figure 16.3.

The first class of agents recognized as HDACis and tested clinically were the short chain and aromatic fatty acids (sodium butyrate,[56] phenylbutyrate,[57] and valproic acid[58]). Sodium butyrate has

been approved for the treatment of urea cycle disorders and valproic acid for seizure disorders. Valproic acid is also used in the treatment of manic depression and in migraine prophylaxis.

Vorinostat or suberoylanilide hydroxamic acid (SAHA), N1-hydroxy-N8-phenyl-octanediamide, belongs to the hydroxamic acid class of HDACi that also includes PCI-24781; givinostat

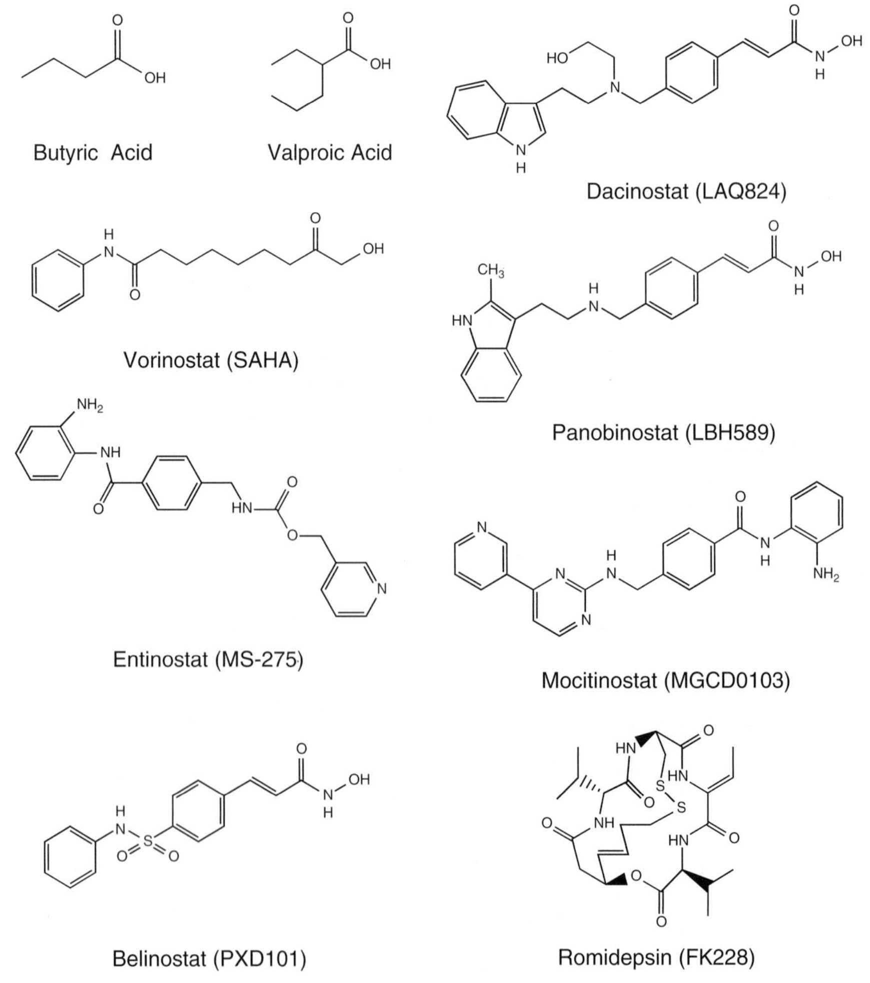

Butyric Acid

Valproic Acid

Dacinostat (LAQ824)

Vorinostat (SAHA)

Panobinostat (LBH589)

Entinostat (MS-275)

Mocitinostat (MGCD0103)

Belinostat (PXD101)

Romidepsin (FK228)

FIGURE 16.3 Chemical structures of selected HDACi.

TABLE

16.3 *Key features of vorinostat/Zolinza® (SAHA)*

Mechanism of action	Inhibition of class I and II HDACs leading to acetylation of histones and nonhistone proteins, altered gene transcription, cell cycle arrest, inhibition of DNA repair, induction of apoptosis
Metabolism	Hydrolysis, β-oxidation followed by glucuronidation by liver enzymes
Pharmacokinetics	$t_{1/2}$ life: 91 to 127 min
Elimination	Liver (99%); remaining 1% is excreted unchanged in urine
Drug interactions	Prolongs PT, INR with concurrent warfarin use
	Concurrent use of other HDACi exacerbates hematological toxicity
Toxicity	Fatigue, nausea, anorexia, vomiting, anemia, thrombocytopenia, EKG changes
Precautions	Do not use in pregnancy
	QTc prolongation: Monitor and correct electrolyte imbalances; monitor QT interval

(ITF2357), {6-[(diethylamino)methyl]naphthalen-2-yl}methyl [4-(hydroxycarbamoyl)phenyl]carbamate; panobinostat (LBH589), (E)-N-hydroxy-3-[4-[[2-(2-methyl-1H-indol-3-yl)ethylamino]methyl]phenyl]prop-2-enamide; dacinostat (LAQ824), 3-[4-[N-(2-Hydroxyethyl)-N-[2-(1H-indol-3-yl)ethyl]aminomethyl]phenyl]-2(E)-propenohydroxamic acid; and belinostat (PXD101), N-hydroxy-3-(phenylsulphamoylphenyl) acrylamide. The path to the discovery of vorinostat began with the observation that dimethylsulfoxide was able to induce synthesis of hemoglobin and differentiation of murine erythroleukemia cells. Synthesis and screening of related polar compounds ultimately led to the selection of vorinostat as the lead compound.[59] It was the structural similarity to trichostatin A that provided the first clue that it was an inhibitor of HDACs.[60] The key features of vorinostat are shown in Table 16.3.

Romidepsin, (1S,4S,7Z,10S,16E,21R)-7-ethylidene-4,21-bis(1-methyletheyl)-2-oxa-12,13-dithia-5,8,20,23-tetraazabicyclo[8.7.6]tricos-16-ene-3,6,9,19,22-pentone, also known as FR901228, FK228, and depsipeptide, is a bicyclic peptide. First

isolated from the fermentation broth of *Chromobacterium violaceum* based on its ability to induce differentiation of H-ras-transformed NIH 3T3 cells,[61] it was later shown to potently inhibit HDACs.[62,63] Subsequent studies revealed it to be a substrate of P-glycoprotein,[64] and clinical development at the National Cancer Institute was initiated based on its unique structure, mechanism, and favorable toxicity profile. The disulfide bond of romidepsin must be reduced inside the cell to yield the drug's active form.[63] The key features of romidepsin are shown in Table 16.4.

The benzamide class of HDACi, including entinostat (MS-275), (pyridylmethyl-N-{4-[(2-aminophenyl)-carbamoyl]-benzyl}-carbamate); tacedinaline (CI-994), 4-(acetylamino)-N-(2-aminophenyl)benzamide; and mocetinostat (MGCD0103), (N-(2-aminophenyl)-4-((4-(pyridin-3-yl)pyrimidin-2-ylamino)methyl)benzamide), are highly potent HDACis now undergoing clinical evaluation. Chidamide also belongs to this class of compounds, is approved by the Chinese FDA for treatment of relapsed/refractory PTCL, and is undergoing clinical trials in the United States and in Japan.[65,66]

TABLE

16.4 *Key features of romidepsin/Istodax® (depsipeptide, FK 228, FR 901228)*

Mechanism of action	Inhibition of class I and II HDAC enzymes leading to acetylation of histones and nonhistone proteins, altered gene transcription, cell cycle arrest, inhibition of DNA repair, induction of apoptosis
Metabolism	Primarily by CYP3A4
Pharmacokinetics	$t_{1/2}$ life: 2.92 h
Elimination	>90% Liver
Drug interactions	With warfarin to prolong PT, INR
	CYP3A4 inducers (barbiturates, carbamazepine, dexamethasone, etc) decrease drug levels. CYP3A4 inhibitors (azole antifungals, some antibiotics, and grapefruit juice) raise drug levels
Toxicity	Fatigue, nausea, anorexia, vomiting, anemia, thrombocytopenia, neutropenia, lymphopenia, infections, and EKG changes
Precautions	Do not use in pregnancy
	ECG changes: Monitor and correct electrolyte imbalances
	Monitor QT interval in patients at risk for QT prolongation
	Can result in failure of estrogen-containing contraceptives

Pharmacokinetics

Pharmacokinetic studies of HDACi have been useful in guiding the route of administration and schedule. They have identified clinical differences among the HDACis, with implications for toxicity and efficacy.

Commonly used as an antiepileptic and not an approved anticancer agent thus far, valproic acid is being studied in combination chemotherapy and radiotherapy trials.[67–69] Extensive pharmacokinetic data are available for valproic acid.[70,71] It has nearly 100% bioavailability, reaching peak plasma concentrations between 50 and 100 mg/L (0.35 to 0.7 mM) between 1 and 4 hours. The half-life in plasma ranges from 7 to 15 hours. It is metabolized primarily in the liver, undergoing beta and omega oxidation via P450 mixed oxidases. Metabolism may be enhanced with concomitant use of agents that induce cytochrome P450 enzymes and may be prolonged with hepatic insufficiency.

While initially tested by the intravenous route, oral administration of vorinostat also produces therapeutic effects. Based on initial studies, the estimated oral bioavailability of vorinostat is 43%; oral administration with a high fat meal resulted in increased absorption.[72] While many dose levels have been studied, the dose used for the FDA registration trial in patients with cutaneous T-cell lymphoma (CTCL) was 400 mg PO qd. At steady state, the area under the concentration versus time curve (AUC) is $6.0 \pm 2.0 \ \mu M \times$ hour, C_{max} $1.2 \pm 0.53 \ \mu M$, and median T_{max} 4 hours. The plasma half-life is estimated to be between 1.5 and 2.0 hours.[72] Vorinostat is 71% bound to human plasma proteins over the range of concentrations of 0.5 to 50 μg/mL. It undergoes biochemical transformation in the liver through phase I hydrolysis and beta-oxidation and phase II conjugation detoxification by glucuronidation to form metabolites such as vorinostat O-glucuronide and 4-anilino-4-oxobutanoic acid.[73] CYP450 enzyme involvement appears not to be significant. Though the mean steady-state concentrations of these metabolites are much higher compared to the parent drug, they are pharmacologically inactive.

Other compounds of the hydroxamic analogue class have been given FDA approval. Belinostat was also tested in both IV and oral formulations. With IV administration, three-compartment pharmacokinetics was demonstrated. Pharmacokinetics is linear for C_{max} and AUC independent of dose.[74] Elimination half-life is independent of dose and ranges from 0.3 to 1.3 hours. The major elimination route is through the bile, and only 0.2% to 2.0% of parent drug is excreted in urine. Oral doses of belinostat up to 1,000 mg daily have been tolerated, but the appropriate oral dose has not been determined in sufficiently large trials.[75] Belinostat is conjugated by UGT1A1 and polymorphic variants that impact protein levels also impact belinostat clearance.[76,77] Table 16.5 lists key features of belinostat. The hydroxamate HDACi, resminostat (formerly 4SC-201, BYK408740), is an oral, pan inhibitor of class I and II HDAC enzymes, and is currently in clinical trials for CTCL, melanoma, and has completed phase 1 drug combination trials in hepatocellular cancer, hematologic malignancies, and colorectal cancer.[78–80]

Panobinostat, approved for multiple myeloma by the intravenous route,[81] has also been studied in oral formulations.[82] With IV administration, maximum plasma concentration and drug exposure increased proportionally with dose. Plasma concentrations peaked close to the end of the 0.5-hour infusion in a phase I trial; the C_{max} range was 120.7 to 565.6 ng/mL with the $t_{1/2}$ in plasma ranging from 7.8 to 17 hours. For oral administration, time to peak concentration ranged from 1 to 1.5 hours, C_{max} 23 to 71 ng/mL, and $AUC_{0–24}$ was 183 to 373 ng h/mL. AUC and C_{max} increased linearly with increasing dose. Its half-life in plasma is about 16 hours.[82] Table 16.6 lists key features of panobinostat.

Approved for CTCL and peripheral T-cell lymphoma (PTCL), romidepsin pharmacokinetics are best described by a first-order, two-compartment model with linear kinetics.[83,84] Pharmacokinetics determined in patients with CTCL treated on the registration trial demonstrated an AUC of 1,549 ng h/mL and C_{max} of 377 ng/mL. The half-life is estimated to be 3 hours. It is greater than 90% protein bound. Metabolism of romidepsin leads to several dozen metabolites without any one being significantly higher in concentration than others.[85] Romidepsin is considered a substrate for CYP3A4 based on in vitro studies. In addition, CYP3A5, CYP2C19, CYP1A1, and CYP2B6 appear to play some role in metabolism of the parent drug.

The benzamide derivatives, which are still in clinical trials, show much longer half-lives than the approved agents. Entinostat half-life is estimated to be 60 to 150 hours. Elimination is biexponential with a fast elimination phase in 4 hours and a slow terminal elimination phase. Interpatient variability is reported. Its long

TABLE

16.5 Key features of belinostat/Beleodaq® (PXD101)

Mechanism of action	Targets class I, II, and IV HDAC
Metabolism	Glucuronidation by UGT1A1
Pharmacokinetics	Elimination $t_{1/2}$ of 1.5 h
Elimination	>90% liver; <2% eliminated by kidneys
Drug interactions	Adalimumab, etanercept, infliximab all increase risk of infection when coadministered
Toxicity	Thrombocytopenia and neutropenia (well tolerated with clinical benefit in patients with platelet count ~100,000/μL)
	Nausea, vomiting, lethargy, fatigue, constipation
Precautions	Do not give to pregnant patients
	Risk for tumor lysis syndrome; hepatotoxicity
	Consider reduced dosing for patients homozygous for the UGT1A1*28 or other allele impairing glucuronidation

TABLE 16.6	Key features of panobinostat/Farydak® (LBH589)
Mechanism of action	Pan-HDAC inhibitor
Metabolism	Reduction, hydrolysis, oxidation, and glucuronidation mediated by the CYP enzymes
Pharmacokinetics	$t_{1/2} = 37$ h
Elimination	>90% liver
Drug interactions	CYP inducers and inhibitors (grapefruit, starfruit) should be avoided
Toxicity	Thrombocytopenia, hematologic toxicities
	Severe diarrhea
	Hypokalemia, hypocalcemia leading to cardiac toxicity
	Nausea, vomiting, decreased intensity of GI side effects when drug taken after high fat meal
Precautions	ECG changes: Monitor and correct electrolyte imbalances
	Avoid concomitant use with QT-prolonging or antiarrhythmic drugs
	Do not give to pregnant patients

half-life may make entinostat a good candidate for combination studies attempting to exploit the unique features of HDACis. For patients treated at the mocetinostat MTD, 45 mg/m² orally three times a week for 2 of every 3 weeks, the observed plasma half-life was 9.9 ± 3.6 hours.[86] Both agents are currently in clinical trials in combination with immunotherapies.[87,88]

Pharmacodynamic Data

To date, only a limited number of pharmacodynamic or biomarker studies have been carried out with HDACi. Perhaps the most direct marker for HDAC inhibition is to measure histone acetylation. This has been readily demonstrated in peripheral blood mononuclear cells by immunoblot or flow cytometric analysis and has also been reported in posttreatment biopsies. Increased acetylation has been observed in PBMCs from patients treated with vorinostat,[72] belinostat,[74] panobinostat,[82] and romidepsin.[89]

Pharmacodynamic studies with vorinostat have suggested that constitutive activation of signaling pathways involving nuclear accumulation of STAT-1 and nuclear localization of phosphorylated STAT-3 may be a marker for resistance in patients with CTCL.[90] Baseline levels of 17 antioxidant genes were lower in RNA obtained from patients with AML with response to vorinostat relative to patients without response, suggesting antioxidant activity might serve as a predictor of clinical efficacy.[91]

A biomarker study was performed in patients with T-cell lymphoma enrolled in a phase II trial with romidepsin.[89] Increased histone acetylation and increased gene expression of *MDR1*, known to be directly up-regulated by HDACi, were observed in PBMC samples within 4 hours of treatment, and, in approximately 40% of patients, lasted from 24 to 48 hours after a single dose. Most patients also had a greater than fourfold increase in hemoglobin F detected in red blood cells. When each surrogate was evaluated for association with either PK parameters or disease response, it was noted that the fold increase in histone acetylation in PBMCs correlated with C_{max} and AUC and inversely correlated with clearance. In addition, the increase in histone

acetylation in PBMCs at the 24-hour time point correlated with response despite the lack of a statistically significant correlation between PK parameters and response. These data suggest that for romidepsin, drug exposure (AUC) may be an important determinant of response.

Gene expression profiling using patient-derived samples has been incorporated in some studies. Genes involved in apoptosis, cell proliferation, immune regulation, and angiogenesis are altered as early as 4 hours after drug administration. More recently, changes in chromatin accessibility seem to reliably correlate with response to romidepsin, though the data need to be validated in a larger patient cohort.[92]

Toxicity

The primary toxicities of HDACi have been hematologic and gastrointestinal, although there are concerns about effects on cardiac conduction.

Gastrointestinal

Anorexia, dysgeusia, nausea, and vomiting are commonly seen in patients receiving HDACi.[72,74,93] As a majority of patients receiving these agents will experience nausea when treated at the MTD, antiemetic prophylaxis is standard. Additional gastrointestinal side effects include constipation or diarrhea, especially for the orally administered agents such as vorinostat or resminostat.[78] Mild elevations in liver function enzymes also occur.[72,81,93]

Constitutional

Fatigue and occasional fever have been observed with HDACi therapy. An increase in serum IL-6 levels has been noted and may play a role in producing the fatigue commonly noted in patients receiving belinostat and potentially other HDACi.[75]

Hematologic

In contrast to classic cytotoxic chemotherapeutic agents, true myelosuppressive effects are minimal. Interestingly, no consistent effect on red blood cell counts has been noted. Leukopenia, granulocytopenia, and thrombocytopenia are usually transient and rapidly reversible, although uncommonly patients may experience significant reductions in platelet count. No cumulative thrombocytopenia has been reported after multiple courses of treatment. Significant bone marrow suppression at 10 to 21 days, as occurs following cytotoxic therapy, has not been observed. Furthermore, treatment with HDACi does not affect colony-forming units from bone marrow cells, and bone marrow biopsies performed in patients treated with HDACi do not demonstrate significant myelosuppression. No bleeding disorders have been reported. However, an increase in the INR was noted in some patients receiving warfarin after the introduction of romidepsin. Physicians need to carefully monitor PT and INR in patients concurrently receiving romidepsin with warfarin or its derivatives (romidepsin package insert).

Cardiac

ECG changes have been reported in clinical trials with the HDACi vorinostat, romidepsin, dacinostat, panobinostat, belinostat, and entinostat and may be considered a class effect,[94] regardless of chemical class. They have been most intensively studied for romidepsin, the most potent of the HDACis. The ECG changes, primarily ST and T wave flattening and ST segment depression, prompted evaluation for myocardial damage or dysfunction following romidepsin; no impact on myocardial wall motion (by echocardiography) was observed, nor was an impact seen on left ventricular ejection fraction, or serum troponin, despite the ECG changes.[95] Notable elevations in troponin were detected only in a patient with a lymphomatous mass involving the myocardium.[96]

The magnitude of HDACi effect on the QT interval has been carefully assessed; increases have been reported in association with HDACi therapy with multiple different agents.[95,97,98] There was increased concern regarding the HDACi after a report of torsades de pointes (polymorphic ventricular tachycardia) in a single patient treated with dacinostat and after several sudden deaths were reported following romidepsin.[99] QT interval prolongation is important as a signal for depolarization delay that could lead to ventricular tachyarrhythmias.[100] The ICH E14 regulatory guidance recommends specific assessment of the potential for QT prolongation as part of the FDA approval process.[101] For romidepsin, an independent cardiology review of 4,910 ECGs in 135 patients determined a relatively minor 5 ± 13.94 ms QT prolongation (including the effect of antiemetics) following infusion.[102]

A thorough study was performed for vorinostat after receiving FDA approval.[103] That study tested a single dose of 800 mg of vorinostat, higher than the dose used for continuous administration and noted that the mean increase of the QTc from baseline was less than 10 ms and that no QTc was noted to be longer than 30 ms from baseline. The QT prolonging effect of the HDACi is in the same range as that of other drugs known to have slight and occasional effects on the QT interval and may reflect an effect on hERG channel trafficking. Vigilance to avoid concomitant use of agents that significantly prolong the QT (e.g., antiarrhythmics such as amiodarone) is therefore prudent and the romidepsin package insert cautions to ensure that patients with history of heart disease, congenital long QT syndrome, and other circumstances that may lead to QT interval prolongation get pretreatment EKG at baseline as well as periodically during treatment. Alternatively,

TABLE 16.7 *Typical cardiac exclusion list from an HDACi clinical trial*

Uncontrolled hypertension
Impaired cardiac function, including any one of the following:
- QTc > 450 ms on screening ECG
- Congenital long QT syndrome
- History or presence of sustained ventricular tachycardia
- History of ventricular fibrillation or torsades de pointes
- Bradycardia, defined as <50 beats/min (patients with a pacemaker and heart rate ≥50 beats/min are eligible)
- New York Heart Association class III to IV congestive heart failure
- Right bundle branch block and left anterior hemiblock (bifascicular block)
- Myocardial infarction or unstable angina within the past 6 mo

HDACi could increase myocardial electrical instability in individual patients with underlying heart disease in a non-QT dependent manner. One possibility is that the ST and T wave changes, along with a median increase in heart rate of ~10 bpm, could indicate altered expression or activity of KATP channels.[104] In addition, many patients having episodes of arrhythmia had uncorrected deficiency of potassium or magnesium, both of which predispose to arrhythmia. We postulated that electrolyte deficiency coupled with the observed ST and T wave changes in the presence of intrinsic cardiac disease was related to the several deaths observed early in development of romidepsin.

Together, these observations led to the recommendation in the FDA-approved package insert for monitoring potassium and magnesium during romidepsin administration. Magnesium and potassium replacement is routine in critical care settings, and monitoring of these electrolytes should be part of good medical management in cancer patients receiving treatment with HDACi.[105] Vorinostat, romidepsin, and panobinostat package inserts recommend monitoring potassium and magnesium; physicians should ensure that potassium and magnesium are within the normal range before administration of these agents. Typical cardiac exclusions in clinical trials of HDACi are included in Table 16.7; and electrolyte administration guidelines are found in Table 16.8.

TABLE 16.8 *Guidelines for electrolyte administration in romidepsin protocols*

Serum K⁺ < 3.5 mmol/L	80 mEq of potassium divided 40 mEq IV and 40 mEq PO
Serum K⁺ < 4.0 mmol/L	40 mEq potassium administered by oral and/or IV routes
Serum Mg⁺⁺ < 0.85 mmol/L	1 g MgSO₄ IV (8.12 mEq) for every 0.05 below 0.85 mmol/L, maximum of 4 g (32.48 mEq)

Other Histone Deacetylase Inhibitor Side Effects

Pulmonary side effects, heralded by a cough and dyspnea, have been noted but are rare.

Renal dysfunction in the form of minor elevations in serum creatinine and/or electrolyte imbalances such as hypocalcemia and hypophosphatemia has occasionally occurred in trials of HDACi. The agents have not been administered to pregnant women because of preclinical evidence of fetal toxicity in rats, such as increased peri-implantation and postimplantation losses and decreased number of live fetuses.[106]

With the FDA approval of four HDACis, it is important to think about using HDACi in the general population. A recent analysis of safety and efficacy in an older population was recently reported, with patients having a median age of 67 to 68 years treated.[107] HDACis must be used with caution in patients with hepatic and renal dysfunction until definitive data are available. With regard to cardiac dysfunction, clinical trials have excluded patients with pre-existing cardiac disorders, long QT syndrome, or other risk factors for arrhythmia or sudden death. Finally, due to the potential reactivation of viral infection by these agents, caution should be used out of concern for reactivating infections or increasing viral loads.

Clinical Uses

Both vorinostat and romidepsin have received FDA approval for the treatment of patients with CTCL. Romidepsin also has significant activity in patients with PTCL, a class of T-cell lymphoma with a poor overall prognosis, and was FDA approved for that indication in 2011. Subsequently, belinostat was also approved for PTCL in the United States, while chidamide was approved for PTCL by the Chinese FDA. While preclinical evidence exists for activity in both solid malignancies and hematological disorders, HDACis have had little success in trials of patients with solid malignancies, but these trials continue in various combinations.

Single-Agent Studies

In general, single-agent HDACi therapy in CTCL and PTCL has shown activity in about one third of patients. This is likely to represent a specific molecular subset in which there is particular activity. However, the defining genetic or epigenetic characteristics in the T-cell lymphomas in this subset have not been determined.

Vorinostat was approved by the FDA in 2006 at a dose of 400 mg once daily for patients with progressive, persistent, or recurrent CTCL on or following two systemic treatments. Objective response rates up to 30% were reported in patients with CTCL, with a response duration over 6 months.[97,108] The pivotal trial in CTCL enrolled 74 patients,[64] stage IIB or higher, and noted both objective response and pruritis relief in 30% of patients.[97]

Romidepsin was approved by the U.S. FDA in 2009 at 14 mg/m^2 on days 1, 8, and 15 of a 28-day cycle for patients with CTCL who previously received at least one prior systemic therapy.[109] Initial phase I trials determined the MTD of 17.8 mg/m^2 administered on days 1 and 5 of a 21-day cycle or 14 mg/m^2 when administered on days 1, 8, and 15 of a 28-day cycle.[93,110] Partial responses (PRs) in T-cell lymphoma in the phase I trial led to two phase II studies.

An overall response rate of 34% in CTCL was noted in the NCI phase 2 trial with a median duration of response of 13.7 months.[111] In an independent international trial, of 96 patients enrolled, 6 patients achieved a CR and 27 patients a PR for an identical overall response rate of 34%.[112] In a PTCL cohort enrolled on the NCI trial, complete responses were observed in 8 and partial responses in 9 of 45 patients, for an overall response rate of 38%.[113] Responses were noted in patients post-stem cell transplant. In the pivotal trial in PTCL, the overall response rate was 25% with a median duration of response of 28 months.[114] Modest responses were seen in trials with patients with AML, and only rare responses were noted in clinical trials where the drug was administered to patients with solid tumors.[115–117]

Belinostat (Beleodaq), an intravenously infused HDACi, received FDA-accelerated approval for the treatment of relapsed or refractory peripheral T-cell lymphoma (PTCL). Approval was based on a single arm phase II, nonrandomized, open-label study of belinostat monotherapy in patients with relapsed/refractory PTCL who had received a median of two lines of prior treatment.[118] Prior therapy with another HDACi was not allowed. The overall response rate among the 120 evaluable patients was 25.8%, with a median duration of response of 8.4 months. The treatment was fairly well tolerated with few patients requiring dose reductions (12.4%). The most common adverse effects reported with belinostat (Beleodaq) included nausea, fatigue, pyrexia, anemia, and vomiting. Incidence of grade 3 to 4 hematologic toxicities was thrombocytopenia, (7%); neutropenia, (6.2%); and anemia, (10.9%). The drug is given in a dose of 1,000 mg/m^2 administered intravenously over 30 min on days 1 through 5 of a 21-day cycle. Other small, early phase trials that studied belinostat in other types of cancer including thymic cancers, ovarian cancer, and hepatocellular carcinoma need more advanced trials to determine clinical benefit.[119–121]

Panobinostat, an orally administered HDACi, received accelerated FDA approval for patients with multiple myeloma who had received at least two prior therapy regimens. It is administered in combination with bortezomib and dexamethasone. A randomized, double-blind, placebo-controlled trial in 768 subjects evaluated the efficacy of the combination of panobinostat (Farydak), bortezomib (Velcade), and dexamethasone relative to bortezomib (Velcade) and dexamethasone alone (control group) in subjects with relapsed or relapsed and refractory multiple myeloma.[122] Median progression-free survival (PFS) reported in the trial was 12 and 8 months in the panobinostat and control arms, respectively. For the subpopulation in which panobinostat received FDA approval, the median progression-free survival (PFS) was 10.6 and 5.8 months in the panobinostat and control arms, respectively. Median overall survival (OS) data from this trial are not mature. Panobinostat labeling contains a boxed warning for severe diarrhea and cardiac ischemic events. Other serious adverse events include bleeding and liver dysfunction. The usual dose of panobinostat is 20 mg (one capsule) orally every other day for three doses per week for 2 consecutive weeks, followed by 1 week off of the medication (a 21-day cycle). Initial treatment with panobinostat is for eight, 21-day cycles. An additional eight cycles (up to a total of 16 cycles) may be given if there is continuing benefit from treatment.

Chidamide (also known as HBI-8000), an HDACi approved by the Chinese FDA (CFDA) in relapsed, refractory PTCL, is being studied in the United States in a clinical trial in combination with immunotherapy in melanoma, renal cell carcinoma, and lung cancer (clinicaltrials.gov accessed in December 2017). The pivotal phase 2 trial in PTCL showed an overall response rate of 28 percent, with a complete response in 14 percent of patients. Median progression-free survival and overall survival were 2.1 and 21.4 months, respectively.[65]

Combination Therapies with Small Molecule Inhibitors, Chemotherapy, Radiation, and Immunotherapy

The promising preclinical activity of HDACis and their consistent efficacy in CTCL and PTCL contrast with the lack of responses to HDACi in solid tumors. Combination therapies have been devised that should exploit the unique activities of HDACi, overcome resistance mechanisms, and provide mechanism-based synergistic activity.

- Synergy based on epigenetic modification is an obvious approach—first, combinations with other drugs that affect gene expression, including the azacytidine analogues, retinoids, or PPAR agonists.[123] Trials combining HDACis with DNA methyltransferase inhibitors are already underway.

- Synergy with cytotoxic chemotherapy has been observed in a number of laboratory investigations and many of these combinations have entered clinical trials. However, many of the laboratory studies utilized long exposures of the HDACi to perform the synergy studies. Exposures of 72 to 96 hours are not likely to be clinically relevant given the short half-life of most HDACis in patients and the ready reversibility of acetylation.

- HDACis impair the function of DNA repair proteins and there is evidence that radiation sensitivity may be enhanced in some settings.[124]

- Since the FDA approval of panobinostat, a pan HDACi, for the treatment of relapsed-refractory multiple myeloma, there is heightened interest in combining proteasome inhibitors with HDACi. One direction for these clinical trials is to use selective HDACi, such as the HDAC6 inhibitor ricolinostat, in combination therapies to target both systems concurrently. An added rationale for these combinations is to minimize the toxicity of the panobinostat-bortezomib combination.[125]

- As discussed, HDACis have effects peculiar to the immune system. One effect of HDACi is to up-regulate components of the immune response that may lead to greater antigen presentation and/or recognition, including tumor-associated antigens; TAP1/2; MHC class I and class II molecules; the CD40, CD80, CD86, and ICAM1 costimulatory/accessory molecules; and death receptors.[126] Other factors supporting the combination of HDACi with immunotherapies include their ability to increase expression of NKG2D ligands on tumors, leading to greater recognition of tumors by NK cells, and decrease the number of MDSC's in the tumor vicinity.[127]

A large number of clinical trials testing these approaches are already underway. Representative examples of trials with immune checkpoint inhibitors are provided in Table 16.9. The

TABLE

16.9 *Clinical trials of combinations of HDACi with immune checkpoint inhibitors*

Clinicaltrials.gov Identifier	Status	Phase	Cancer Type	Epigenetic Drug	Immune Checkpoint Inhibitor	Additional Intervention
NCT02635061	Recruiting	I	Unresectable NSCLC	ACY-241	Nivolumab and ipilimumab	
NCT01686165	Not yet recruiting	II	DLBCL	Belinostat	Rituximab	Yttrium-90
NCT02909452	Recruiting	I	Advanced solid tumors	Entinostat	Pembrolizumab	
NCT02708680	Recruiting	I/II	Triple negative breast cancer	Entinostat	Atezolizumab	
NCT02993991	Not yet recruiting	I	Squamous cell carcinoma of the oral cavity	Mocetinostat	Durvalumab	
NCT02032810	Recruiting	I	Unresectable stage III/IV melanoma	Panobinostat	Ipilimumab	
NCT02512172	Recruiting	I	Advanced colorectal cancer	Romidepsin and/or 5-AZA	Pembrolizumab	
NCT02395627	Recruiting	II	Hormone therapy–resistant breast cancer	Vorinostat	Pembrolizumab	Tamoxifen
NCT02397720	Recruiting	II	AML	5-AZA	Nivolumab	
NCT02508870	Recruiting	I	MDS	5-AZA	Atezolizumab	
NCT02512172	Recruiting	I	MSS advanced CRC	Romidepsin and/or 5-AZA	Pembrolizumab	

combination strategies represent an important and urgent effort to exploit the potential activity of HDACi in solid tumors. It will be very important that these trials determine whether the molecular effect hypothesized to create synergy between two agents has actually occurred. To this end, laboratory correlates will be an essential component of future HDACi clinical trials.

IDH Inhibitors

Isocitrate dehydrogenase (IDH) is an enzyme that catalyzes reactions in the third step of the Krebs citric acid cycle (see Fig. 16.4). In humans, IDH exists in three isoforms: IDH1 and IDH2 use NADP+ as a cofactor and localize to the cytosol as well as to mitochondria. IDH3 utilizes NAD+ and localizes to the mitochondria. The reaction catalyzed by these enzymes is one of only three primary mechanisms of NADPH production in mammalian tissues.[128] Mutant IDH enzymes acquire an altered activity in which the normal product α-KG is converted to 2-hydroxyglutarate (2-HG). Accumulating 2-HG has been found to inhibit alpha-ketoglutarate–dependent dioxygenases, including 5-methylcytosine hydroxylases, needed for reversing DNA methylation, and histone demethylases.[129,130] The net effect is to increase DNA methylation

and histone methylation. Both lead to repression of transcription of genes necessary for progenitor cells to progress to terminally differentiated, lineage committed cells, and inhibition leads to development of a more differentiated phenotype. IDH1/2 mutations can be identified in approximately 20% of AML samples and approximately 5% of MDS samples.[131–133] Additionally, IDH1/2 mutations have been found in solid tumors. Approximately 70% of secondary glioblastomas carry IDH mutations[134,135]; 50% of chondrosarcomas carry IDH1 or IDH2 mutations, with IDH1 mutations predominating; and 23% of intrahepatic cholangiocarcinomas carry primarily IDH1 mutations. IDH1 is responsible for cytosolic IDH production, and IDH2 is the mitochondrial homolog of the gene. Mutant IDH1 appears to need to heterodimerize with WT IDH1 to function, whereas mutant IDH2 does not, and mutant IDH2 produces higher levels of 2-HG accumulation as a result of this difference in its subcellular compartmentalization and enzymatic activity. It is likely because of this difference that IDH2 became the initial drug development target.[136] AG-221, or enasidenib, developed by Agios Pharmaceuticals with Celgene, is an oral selective inhibitor specific for IDH2R140Q and IDH2R172K. As of August 2017, this drug received full FDA approval for relapsed/refractory AML in patients carrying IDH2 mutations. The phase I/II trial that supported approval was based on objective responses in 40.3% of 176 patients and a median overall survival of 9.3 months.[137,138]

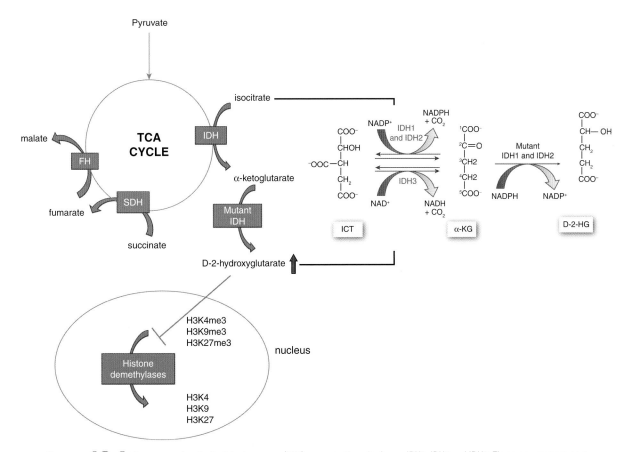

FIGURE 16.4 The enzyme Isocitrate dehydrogenase (IDH) occurs in three isoforms: IDH1, IDH2 and IDH3. These enzymes are part of the TCA/Krebs cycle. The byproduct of the wildtype IDH is alpha-ketoglutarate, a key molecule in many enzymatic activities including DNA and histone demethylation. Mutant IDH generates D-2-hydroxyglutatate from alpha-ketoglutarate. Accumulation of the latter competitively inhibits histone demethylases. The *inset* shows the structure of the metabolites in greater detail: alpha-ketoglutarate and D-2-hydroxyglutarate byproducts of the normal and mutant IDH enzymes, respectfully, differ in the 2-ketone group in the normal pathway being replaced by a hydroxyl group. (Figure adapted from Yang et. al., *Clin. Cancer Res,* 2012 and Cleven et. al., Clin Sarcoma Res. 2017.)

TABLE

16.10   *Key features of enasidenib/IDHIFA® (AG221)*

Mechanism of action	Inhibits isocitrate dehydrogenase 2 enzyme, decreases accumulation of 2-hydroxyglutarate, decreases histone hypermethylation
Metabolism	Primarily by CYP and UGT enzymes
Pharmacokinetics	$t_{1/2}$ = 29 h
Elimination	89% in feces, 11% in urine
Drug interactions	Unknown at this time
Toxicity	Differentiation syndrome may be life threatening. Needs early diagnosis, intervention
	Nausea, vomiting, diarrhea, increased bilirubin, and decreased appetite
Precautions	Inhibits the liver enzyme UGT1A1, involved in bilirubin metabolism. Dosing in patients with liver dysfunction not evaluated
	Preclinical studies show embryo-fetal toxicity

AG-120 is a selective IDH1 inhibitor and has also been tested in AML and is being studied in solid tumors with IDH1 mutations.

Mechanism of Action in Cancer

AG-221 has been shown to allosterically bind to a deep pocket buried in the dimer interface between two IDH2 protein units and exhibits slow-on slow-off binding kinetics. A crystal structure[139] shows that AG-221 stabilizes the open conformation of the IDH2 dimers, thereby inhibiting conversion of alpha-ketoglutarate to 2-HG, and can bind both wild-type–mutant heterodimers and mutant homodimers. Patients with AML treated with this drug on the pivotal phase 1/II trial[138] showed a decrease in 2-HG levels and increased granulocyte count (indicating that leukemic blasts were undergoing differentiation), but did not eradicate IDH mutant clones of leukemic cells. The latter may be because IDH mutant cells may not be exclusively dependent on 2-HG for their survival.[140] The authors of the clinical trial conclude that cell differentiation, and not cell death of myeloblasts, is responsible for efficacy of the drug. Preclinical studies combining IDH inhibitors or 5-Aza with TET2 inhibitors show a more comprehensive decrease in DNA methylation and greater blast differentiation,[141] and clinical trials with these combinations will undoubtedly follow.

One of the important observations from the studies with IDH inhibitors in AML was that, for the first time, there was clinical benefit from partial remission and stable disease. AML has been a disease in which the only treatment response that impacted survival was complete response. The IDH inhibitors are thus a paradigm shift in allowing patients to continue on therapy with control of disease. It will be important to identify the best role for AG221 in the sequence of therapies for AML. A trial combining chemotherapy with AG221 in first-line treatment is expected to start enrolling shortly.

Mechanisms of Resistance

None have been reported at this time.

Pharmacodynamics and Pharmacokinetics

AG221 has a high dose–proportional plasma exposure and an extended half-life (≈137 hours) after multiple doses, reaching steady state by cycle 2 day 1. A 100 mg once per day dose was chosen for the phase 2 cohort. By cycle 2 day 1, AG221 at 100 mg per day reduced plasma 2-HG levels from baseline by a median of 93%.[138] Key features of enasidenib are included in Table 16.10.

Side Effects and Toxicity

The most common adverse events were hyperbilirubinemia, nausea, vomiting, diarrhea, and anorexia.[138] Differentiation syndrome, which can be life-threatening without prompt intervention occurred in 10% of patients. Enasidenib-related grade 3 to 4 adverse events occurred in 99 patients (41%). Most common of these were indirect hyperbilirubinemia, IDH-inhibitor–associated differentiation syndrome (IDH-DS), hematologic adverse events, and infections.

EZH2 Inhibitors

Enhancer of zeste homolog 2 (EZH2) is a histone-lysine N-methyltransferase enzyme. It methylates the lysine 27 residue of histone H3 (H3K27). This histone modification is, in turn, associated with repressed gene transcription when trimethylated (H3K27me3). EZH2 mutations have been observed in a variety of cancers, including lymphoma. No drug in this class currently has FDA approval for any indication. However, tazemetostat (Epizyme, Inc), a first in class oral EZH2 inhibitor, has been granted Fast Track designation by the FDA for relapsed/refractory DLBCL with activating mutations and relapsed/refractory follicular lymphoma with either wild-type EZH2 or EZH2-activating mutations. Once a drug receives *Fast Track* designation, per the FDA, "early and frequent communication between the FDA and a drug company is encouraged throughout the entire drug development and review process. The frequency of communication assures that questions and issues are resolved quickly, often leading to earlier drug approval and access by patients (https://www.fda.gov/ForPatients/Approvals/Fast/ucm405399.htm)."

Mechanism of Action

EZH2 is the enzymatic subunit of polycomb repressive complex 2 (PRC2). As the enzymatic component of the polycomb repressor complex, EZH2 is involved in transcriptional repression through

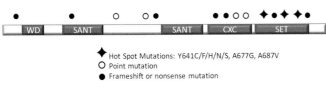

Hot Spot Mutations: Y641C/F/H/N/S, A677G, A687V
○ Point mutation
● Frameshift or nonsense mutation

FIGURE **16.5** Mutation spectrum in EZH2. (Adapted by permission from Nature: Ntziachristos P, Tsirigos A, Van Vlierberghe P, et al. Genetic inactivation of the polycomb repressive complex 2 in T cell acute lymphoblastic leukemia. *Nat Med.* 2012;18(2):298-301. Copyright © 2012 Springer Nature.)

methylation of histone H3 on lysine 27 (H3K27). Thus, EZH2 functions as a histone-lysine methyltransferase. Loss-of-function and activating EZH2 mutations, as well as overexpression have been described and implicated in oncogenesis, depicted in Figure 16.5.[142] Loss-of-function mutations, typically single nucleotide variants or deletions, are found across the gene body, in contrast to hot spot–activating mutations, which are found in the SET methyltransferase domain.[142–145] Aberrant overexpression has been convincingly demonstrated in metastatic prostate cancer, conferring a poor prognosis.[146–148] Recurrent heterozygous point mutations affecting tyrosine 641 (Y641) within the C-terminal catalytic domain of EZH2 occur in 22% of germinal center B cell (GCB), DLBCL, and in 7% to 12% of follicular lymphomas.[149]

Two other hot spot mutations are nearby at A682G, A692V. In vitro biochemical enzymatic assays show that the mutation confers a gain of function of enzyme activity resulting in increased levels of H3K27me3. This mutation shifts the transcriptional balance to repression of target genes, which are largely tumor suppressor genes.[9] Overexpression and activating mutations have been the targets for development of EZH2 inhibitors. Interim reporting from ongoing phase 2 trials show that tazemetostat had an ORR (CR + PR) of 40% in patients with DLBCL with EZH2 mutations and 63% in patients with FL with EZH2 mutations.[13]

In addition, the mammalian switch/sucrose nonfermenting (mSWI/SNF) complex, through its role in chromatin remodeling, has been the focus of interest in several recent seminal studies describing the surprisingly high frequency of mutations in its 10 to 15 biochemically distinct subunits. Some studies suggest the frequency of mutations in mSWI/SNF is similar to the frequency of TP53 mutations associated with cancer, and the SWI/SNF complex is believed to be a tumor suppressor. Mutations in ARID and SMARC subunits are described in a variety of solid tumors and leukemias. Mutations in the BRD7 subunit are described in breast cancer. Many of these mutations destabilize the PRC2 subunit, and depend on the noncatalytic function of EZH2 to stabilize PRC2. There is, therefore, a recognized need for development of EZH2 inhibitors that affect not only EZH2's histone methyltransferase activity but also its nonenzymatic functions.

Clinical Trials

A phase 2 study in patients with synovial sarcoma showed no objective responses, whereas PR was observed in 13% of patients with IN1-negative epithelioid sarcoma in another phase 2 trial leading to expansion of its cohort.[16] Accessing *clinicaltrials.gov* in August 2017 shows ten different phase 1 and phase 2 trials, including NCI-sponsored MATCH trials currently recruiting patients for treatment, primarily with EZH2 inhibitor monotherapy.

Mechanisms of Resistance

In vitro studies in WT and Y641 carrying cell lines show acquisition of mutations under drug selection pressure that may prevent binding of EZH2 inhibitors to their target.[150]

Toxicity and Side Effects

While it is still early in development, some toxicity information can be gleaned from meeting reports. A phase 1 trial with tazemetostat (EPZ-6438, Epizyme) in non-Hodgkin lymphoma reported 20% of patients with grade 3 or 4 drug-related AEs, mainly thrombocytopenia, neutropenia, hypertension, anorexia, and transaminase elevation.[151] The drug was administered at doses ranging between 100 and 800 mg twice daily. Preliminary results from a phase 1 study with GSK2816126 (Glaxo Smith Kline) show similar percentages of drug-related adverse events, though severity of toxicities is not reported from this study that enrolled patients with lymphoma, multiple myeloma, and solid tumors. The most common drug-related adverse events (AEs) reported at >20% incidence were fatigue (53%), nausea (30%), anemia (20%), and vomiting (20%).

References

1. Lane AA, Chabner BA. Histone deacetylase inhibitors in cancer therapy. *J Clin Oncol.* 2009;27(32):5459-5468.
2. Miller RW, Rubinstein JH. Tumors in Rubinstein-Taybi syndrome. *Am J Med Genet.* 1995;56(1):112-115.
3. Ida K, Kitabayashi I, Taki T, et al. Adenoviral E1A-associated protein p300 is involved in acute myeloid leukemia with t(11;22)(q23;q13). *Blood.* 1997;90(12):4699-4704.
4. Sobulo OM, Borrow J, Tomek R, et al. MLL is fused to CBP, a histone acetyltransferase, in therapy-related acute myeloid leukemia with a t(11;16)(q23;p13.3). *Proc Natl Acad Sci U S A.* 1997;94(16):8732-8737.
5. Gayther SA, Batley SJ, Linger L, et al. Mutations truncating the EP300 acetylase in human cancers. *Nat Genet.* 2000;24(3):300-303.
6. Borrow J, Stanton VP, Jr., Andresen JM, et al. The translocation t(8;16)(p11;p13) of acute myeloid leukaemia fuses a putative acetyltransferase to the CREB-binding protein. *Nat Genet.* 1996;14(1):33-41.
7. Taki T, Sako M, Tsuchida M, Hayashi Y. The t(11;16)(q23;p13) translocation in myelodysplastic syndrome fuses the MLL gene to the CBP gene. *Blood.* 1997;89(11):3945-3950.
8. Crowley JA, Wang Y, Rapoport AP, Ning Y. Detection of MOZ-CBP fusion in acute myeloid leukemia with 8;16 translocation. *Leukemia.* 2005;19(12):2344-2345.
9. Souroullas GP, Jeck WR, Parker JS, et al. An oncogenic Ezh2 mutation induces tumors through global redistribution of histone 3 lysine 27 trimethylation. *Nat Med.* 2016;22(6):632-640.
10. Ohnishi H, Taki T, Yoshino H, et al. A complex t(1;22;11)(q44;q13;q23) translocation causing MLL-p300 fusion gene in therapy-related acute myeloid leukemia. *Eur J Haematol.* 2008;81(6):475-480.
11. Koshiishi N, Chong JM, Fukasawa T, et al. p300 gene alterations in intestinal and diffuse types of gastric carcinoma. *Gastric Cancer.* 2004;7(2): 85-90.
12. Ionov Y, Matsui S, Cowell JK. A role for p300/CREB binding protein genes in promoting cancer progression in colon cancer cell lines with microsatellite instability. *Proc Natl Acad Sci U S A.* 2004;101(5):1273-1278.
13. Weigert O, Weinstock DM. The promises and challenges of using gene mutations for patient stratification in follicular lymphoma. *Blood.* 2017;130(13):1491-1498.
14. Grignani F, De Matteis S, Nervi C, et al. Fusion proteins of the retinoic acid receptor-alpha recruit histone deacetylase in promyelocytic leukaemia. *Nature.* 1998;391(6669):815-818.

15. Liu S, Klisovic RB, Vukosavljevic T, et al. Targeting AML1/ETO-histone deacetylase repressor complex: a novel mechanism for valproic acid-mediated gene expression and cellular differentiation in AML1/ETO-positive acute myeloid leukemia cells. *J Pharmacol Exp Ther.* 2007;321(3):953-960.

16. Schoffski P, Agulnik M, Stacchiotti S, et al. Phase 2 multicenter study of the EZH2 inhibitor tazemetostat in adults with synovial sarcoma (NCT02601950). *J Clin Oncol.* 2017;35(15 suppl):11057-11057.

17. Bolden JE, Peart MJ, Johnstone RW. Anticancer activities of histone deacetylase inhibitors. *Nat Rev Drug Discov.* 2006;5(9):769-784.

18. Dokmanovic M, Clarke C, Marks PA. Histone deacetylase inhibitors: overview and perspectives. *Mol Cancer Res.* 2007;5(10):981-989.

19. Li Y, Seto E. HDACs and HDAC inhibitors in cancer development and therapy. *Cold Spring Harbor Perspect Med.* 2016;6(10).

20. Luchenko VL, Litman T, Chakraborty AR, et al. Histone deacetylase inhibitor-mediated cell death is distinct from its global effect on chromatin. *Mol Oncol.* 2014;8(8):1379-1392.

21. Richon VM, Sandhoff TW, Rifkind RA, Marks PA. Histone deacetylase inhibitor selectively induces p21WAF1 expression and gene-associated histone acetylation. *Proc Natl Acad Sci U S A.* 2000;97(18):10014-10019.

22. Sandor V, Senderowicz A, Mertins S, et al. P21-dependent g(1)arrest with downregulation of cyclin D1 and upregulation of cyclin E by the histone deacetylase inhibitor FR901228. *Br J Cancer.* 2000;83(6):817-825.

23. Gui CY, Ngo L, Xu WS, Richon VM, Marks PA. Histone deacetylase (HDAC) inhibitor activation of p21WAF1 involves changes in promoter-associated proteins, including HDAC1. *Proc Natl Acad Sci U S A.* 2004;101(5):1241-1246.

24. Peart MJ, Smyth GK, van Laar RK, et al. Identification and functional significance of genes regulated by structurally different histone deacetylase inhibitors. *Proc Natl Acad Sci U S A.* 2005;102(10):3697-3702.

25. Van Lint C, Emiliani S, Verdin E. The expression of a small fraction of cellular genes is changed in response to histone hyperacetylation. *Gene Expr.* 1996;5(4-5):245-253.

26. Hoshino I, Matsubara H, Akutsu Y, et al. Gene expression profiling induced by histone deacetylase inhibitor, FK228, in human esophageal squamous cancer cells. *Oncol Rep.* 2007;18(3):585-592.

27. Yu X, Guo ZS, Marcu MG, et al. Modulation of p53, ErbB1, ErbB2, and Raf-1 expression in lung cancer cells by depsipeptide FR901228. *J Natl Cancer Inst.* 2002;94(7):504-513.

28. Ray S, Lee C, Hou T, Boldogh I, Brasier AR. Requirement of histone deacetylase1 (HDAC1) in signal transducer and activator of transcription 3 (STAT3) nucleocytoplasmic distribution. *Nucleic Acids Res.* 2008;36(13):4510-4520.

29. Zhao Y, Lu S, Wu L, et al. Acetylation of p53 at lysine 373/382 by the histone deacetylase inhibitor depsipeptide induces expression of p21(Waf1/Cip1). *Mol Cell Biol.* 2006;26(7):2782-2790.

30. Wang Y, Wang SY, Zhang XH, et al. FK228 inhibits Hsp90 chaperone function in K562 cells via hyperacetylation of Hsp70. *Biochem Biophys Res Commun.* 2007;356(4):998-1003.

31. Ding H, Peterson KL, Correia C, et al. Histone deacetylase inhibitors interrupt HSP90*RASGRP1 and HSP90*CRAF interactions to upregulate BIM and circumvent drug resistance in lymphoma cells. *Leukemia.* 2017;31(7):1593-1602.

32. Okabe S, Tauchi T, Nakajima A, et al. Depsipeptide (FK228) preferentially induces apoptosis in BCR/ABL-expressing cell lines and cells from patients with chronic myelogenous leukemia in blast crisis. *Stem Cells Dev.* 2007;16(3):503-514.

33. Li X, Yan X, Guo W, et al. Chidamide in FLT3-ITD positive acute myeloid leukemia and the synergistic effect in combination with cytarabine. *Biomed Pharmacother.* 2017;90:699-704.

34. Gabrielli B, Brown M. Histone deacetylase inhibitors disrupt the mitotic spindle assembly checkpoint by targeting histone and nonhistone proteins. *Adv Cancer Res* 2012;116:1-37.

35. Marson CM. Histone deacetylase inhibitors: design, structure-activity relationships and therapeutic implications for cancer. *Anticancer Agents Med Chem.* 2009;9(6):661-692.

36. Takebayashi S, Nakao M, Fujita N, et al. 5-Aza-2'-deoxycytidine induces histone hyperacetylation of mouse centromeric heterochromatin by a mechanism independent of DNA demethylation. *Biochem Biophys Res Commun.* 2001;288(4):921-926.

37. Kwon SH, Ahn SH, Kim YK, et al. Apicidin, a histone deacetylase inhibitor, induces apoptosis and Fas/Fas ligand expression in human acute promyelocytic leukemia cells. *J Biol Chem.* 2002;277(3):2073-2080.

38. Wang S, El-Deiry WS. TRAIL and apoptosis induction by TNF-family death receptors. *Oncogene.* 2003;22(53):8628-8633.

39. Rippo MR, Moretti S, Vescovi S, et al. FLIP overexpression inhibits death receptor-induced apoptosis in malignant mesothelial cells. *Oncogene.* 2004;23(47):7753-7760.

40. Zhang XD, Gillespie SK, Borrow JM, Hersey P. The histone deacetylase inhibitor suberic bishydroxamate regulates the expression of multiple apoptotic mediators and induces mitochondria-dependent apoptosis of melanoma cells. *Mol Cancer Ther.* 2004;3(4):425-435.

41. Chen S, Dai Y, Pei XY, Grant S. Bim upregulation by histone deacetylase inhibitors mediates interactions with the Bcl-2 antagonist ABT-737: evidence for distinct roles for Bcl-2, Bcl-xL, and Mcl-1. *Mol Cell Biol.* 2009;29(23):6149-6169.

42. Wilson WH, Young RM, Schmitz R, et al. Targeting B cell receptor signaling with ibrutinib in diffuse large B cell lymphoma. *Nat Med.* 2015;21(8):922-926.

43. Mondello P, Brea EJ, De Stanchina E, et al. Panobinostat acts synergistically with ibrutinib in diffuse large B cell lymphoma cells with MyD88 L265 mutations. *JCI Insight.* 2017;2(6):e90196.

44. Hideshima T, Bradner JE, Wong J, et al. Small-molecule inhibition of proteasome and aggresome function induces synergistic antitumor activity in multiple myeloma. *Proc Natl Acad Sci U S A.* 2005;102(24):8567-8572.

45. Archin NM, Kirchherr JL, Sung JA, et al. Interval dosing with the HDAC inhibitor vorinostat effectively reverses HIV latency. *J Clin Invest.* 2017;127(8):3126-3135.

46. Sung JA, Sholtis K, Kirchherr J, et al. Vorinostat renders the replication-competent latent reservoir of human immunodeficiency virus (HIV) vulnerable to clearance by CD8 T cells. *EBioMedicine* 2017;23:52-58.

47. Akimova T, Beier UH, Liu Y, Wang L, Hancock WW. Histone/protein deacetylases and T-cell immune responses. *Blood.* 2012;119(11):2443-2451.

48. Thurn KT, Thomas S, Moore A, Munster PN. Rational therapeutic combinations with histone deacetylase inhibitors for the treatment of cancer. *Future Oncology (London, England).* 2011;7(2):263-283.

49. Bergada L, Yeramian A, Sorolla A, Matias-Guiu X, Dolcet X. Antioxidants impair anti-tumoral effects of Vorinostat, but not anti-neoplastic effects of Vorinostat and caspase-8 downregulation. *PLoS One.* 2014;9(3):e92764.

50. Niu Y, DesMarais TL, Tong Z, Yao Y, Costa M. Oxidative stress alters global histone modification and DNA methylation. *Free Radic Biol Med* 2015;82:22-28.

51. Hegarty SV, Togher KL, O'Leary E, Solger F, Sullivan AM, O'Keeffe GW. Romidepsin induces caspase-dependent cell death in human neuroblastoma cells. *Neurosci Lett* 2017;653:12-18.

52. Bhalla S, Balasubramanian S, David K, et al. PCI-24781 induces caspase and reactive oxygen species-dependent apoptosis through NF-kappaB mechanisms and is synergistic with bortezomib in lymphoma cells. *Clin Cancer Res.* 2009;15(10):3354-3365.

53. Geng L, Cuneo KC, Fu A, Tu T, Atadja PW, Hallahan DE. Histone deacetylase (HDAC) inhibitor LBH589 increases duration of gamma-H2AX foci and confines HDAC4 to the cytoplasm in irradiated non-small cell lung cancer. *Cancer Res.* 2006;66(23):11298-11304.

54. Zhang F, Zhang T, Teng ZH, Zhang R, Wang JB, Mei QB. Sensitization to gamma-irradiation-induced cell cycle arrest and apoptosis by the histone deacetylase inhibitor trichostatin A in non-small cell lung cancer (NSCLC) cells. *Cancer Biol Ther.* 2009;8(9):823-831.

55. Marks PA, Xu WS. Histone deacetylase inhibitors: Potential in cancer therapy. *J Cell Biochem.* 2009;107(4):600-608.

56. Demary K, Wong L, Spanjaard RA. Effects of retinoic acid and sodium butyrate on gene expression, histone acetylation and inhibition of proliferation of melanoma cells. *Cancer Lett.* 2001;163(1):103-107.

57. Davis T, Kennedy C, Chiew YE, Clarke CL, deFazio A. Histone deacetylase inhibitors decrease proliferation and modulate cell cycle gene expression in normal mammary epithelial cells. *Clin Cancer Res.* 2000;6(11):4334-4342.

58. Phiel CJ, Zhang F, Huang EY, Guenther MG, Lazar MA, Klein PS. Histone deacetylase is a direct target of valproic acid, a potent anticonvulsant, mood stabilizer, and teratogen. *J Biol Chem.* 2001;276(39):36734-36741.

59. Marks PA, Breslow R. Dimethyl sulfoxide to vorinostat: development of this histone deacetylase inhibitor as an anticancer drug. *Nat Biotechnol.* 2007;25(1):84-90.

60. Richon VM, Emiliani S, Verdin E, et al. A class of hybrid polar inducers of transformed cell differentiation inhibits histone deacetylases. *Proc Natl Acad Sci U S A.* 1998;95(6):3003-3007.

61. Nakajima H, Kim YB, Terano H, Yoshida M, Horinouchi S. FR901228, a potent antitumor antibiotic, is a novel histone deacetylase inhibitor. *Exp Cell Res.* 1998;241(1):126-133.

62. Ueda H, Nakajima H, Hori Y, Goto T, Okuhara M. Action of FR901228, a novel antitumor bicyclic depsipeptide produced by Chromobacterium violaceum no. 968, on Ha-ras transformed NIH3T3 cells. *Biosci Biotechnol Biochem.* 1994;58(9):1579-1583.

63. Furumai R, Matsuyama A, Kobashi N, et al. FK228 (depsipeptide) as a natural prodrug that inhibits class I histone deacetylases. *Cancer Res.* 2002;62(17):4916-4921.

64. Lee JS, Paull K, Alvarez M, et al. Rhodamine efflux patterns predict P-glycoprotein substrates in the National Cancer Institute drug screen. *Mol Pharmacol.* 1994;46(4):627-638.

65. Shi Y, Jia B, Xu W, et al. Chidamide in relapsed or refractory peripheral T cell lymphoma: a multicenter real-world study in China. *J Hematol Oncol.* 2017;10(1):69.

66. Lu X, Ning Z, Li Z, Cao H, Wang X. Development of chidamide for peripheral T-cell lymphoma, the first orphan drug approved in China. *Intract Rare Dis Res.* 2016;5(3):185-191.

67. Issa JP, Garcia-Manero G, Huang X, et al. Results of phase 2 randomized study of low-dose decitabine with or without valproic acid in patients with myelodysplastic syndrome and acute myelogenous leukemia. *Cancer.* 2015;121(4):556-561.

68. Krauze AV, Myrehaug SD, Chang MG, et al. A phase 2 study of concurrent radiation therapy, temozolomide, and the histone deacetylase inhibitor valproic acid for patients with glioblastoma. *Int J Radiat Oncol Biol Phys* 2015;92(5):986-992.

69. Caponigro F, Di Gennaro E, Ionna F, et al. Phase II clinical study of valproic acid plus cisplatin and cetuximab in recurrent and/or metastatic squamous cell carcinoma of head and neck-V-CHANCE trial. *BMC Cancer.* 2016;16(1):918.

70. Atmaca A, Al-Batran SE, Maurer A, et al. Valproic acid (VPA) in patients with refractory advanced cancer: a dose escalating phase I clinical trial. *Br J Cancer.* 2007;97(2):177-182.

71. Munster P, Marchion D, Bicaku E, et al. Phase I trial of histone deacetylase inhibition by valproic acid followed by the topoisomerase II inhibitor epirubicin in advanced solid tumors: a clinical and translational study. *J Clin Oncol.* 2007;25(15):1979-1985.

72. Kelly WK, O'Connor OA, Krug LM, et al. Phase I study of an oral histone deacetylase inhibitor, suberoylanilide hydroxamic acid, in patients with advanced cancer. *J Clin Oncol.* 2005;23(17):3923-3931.

73. Rubin EH, Agrawal NG, Friedman EJ, et al. A study to determine the effects of food and multiple dosing on the pharmacokinetics of vorinostat given orally to patients with advanced cancer. *Clin Cancer Res.* 2006;12(23):7039-7045.

74. Steele NL, Plumb JA, Vidal L, et al. A phase 1 pharmacokinetic and pharmacodynamic study of the histone deacetylase inhibitor belinostat in patients with advanced solid tumors. *Clin Cancer Res.* 2008;14(3):804-810.

75. Steele NL, Plumb JA, Vidal L, et al. Pharmacokinetic and pharmacodynamic properties of an oral formulation of the histone deacetylase inhibitor Belinostat (PXD101). *Cancer Chemother Pharmacol.* 2011;67(6):1273-1279.

76. Goey AK, Sissung TM, Peer CJ, et al. Effects of UGT1A1 genotype on the pharmacokinetics, pharmacodynamics, and toxicities of belinostat administered by 48-hour continuous infusion in patients with cancer. *J Clin Pharmacol.* 2016;56(4):461-473.

77. Peer CJ, Goey AK, Sissung TM, et al. UGT1A1 genotype-dependent dose adjustment of belinostat in patients with advanced cancers using population pharmacokinetic modeling and simulation. *J Clin Pharmacol.* 2016;56(4):450-460.

78. Brunetto AT, Ang JE, Lal R, et al. First-in-human, pharmacokinetic and pharmacodynamic phase I study of Resminostat, an oral histone deacetylase inhibitor, in patients with advanced solid tumors. *Clin Cancer Res.* 2013;19(19):5494-5504.

79. Kitazono S, Fujiwara Y, Nakamichi S, et al. A phase I study of resminostat in Japanese patients with advanced solid tumors. *Cancer Chemother Pharmacol.* 2015;75(6):1155-1161.

80. Tambo Y, Hosomi Y, Sakai H, et al. Phase I/II study of docetaxel combined with resminostat, an oral hydroxamic acid HDAC inhibitor, for advanced non-small cell lung cancer in patients previously treated with platinum-based chemotherapy. *Invest New Drugs.* 2017;35(2):217-226.

81. Giles F, Fischer T, Cortes J, et al. A phase I study of intravenous LBH589, a novel cinnamic hydroxamic acid analogue histone deacetylase inhibitor, in patients with refractory hematologic malignancies. *Clin Cancer Res.* 2006;12(15):4628-4635.

82. Ellis L, Pan Y, Smyth GK, et al. Histone deacetylase inhibitor panobinostat induces clinical responses with associated alterations in gene expression profiles in cutaneous T-cell lymphoma. *Clin Cancer Res.* 2008;14(14):4500-4510.

83. Woo S, Gardner ER, Chen X, et al. Population pharmacokinetics of romidepsin in patients with cutaneous T-cell lymphoma and relapsed peripheral T-cell lymphoma. *Clin Cancer Res.* 2009;15(4):1496-1503.

84. Fouladi M, Furman WL, Chin T, et al. Phase I study of depsipeptide in pediatric patients with refractory solid tumors: a Children's Oncology Group report. *J Clin Oncol.* 2006;24(22):3678-3685.

85. Shiraga T, Tozuka Z, Ishimura R, Kawamura A, Kagayama A. Identification of cytochrome P450 enzymes involved in the metabolism of FK228, a potent histone deacetylase inhibitor, in human liver microsomes. *Biol Pharm Bull.* 2005;28(1):124-129.

86. Siu LL, Pili R, Duran I, et al. Phase I study of MGCD0103 given as a three-times-per-week oral dose in patients with advanced solid tumors. *J Clin Oncol.* 2008;26(12):1940-1947.

87. Briere D, Sudhakar N, Woods DM, et al. The class I/IV HDAC inhibitor mocetinostat increases tumor antigen presentation, decreases immune suppressive cell types and augments checkpoint inhibitor therapy. *Cancer Immunol Immunother.* 2018;67(3):381-392

88. Pili R, Quinn DI, Hammers HJ, et al. Immunomodulation by entinostat in renal cell carcinoma patients receiving high-dose interleukin 2: A multicenter, single-arm, phase I/II trial (NCI-CTEP#7870). *Clin Cancer Res.* 2017;23(23):7199-7208.

89. Bates SE, Zhan Z, Steadman K, et al. Laboratory correlates for a phase II trial of romidepsin in cutaneous and peripheral T-cell lymphoma. *Br J Haematol.* 2010;148(2):256-267.

90. Fantin VR, Loboda A, Paweletz CP, et al. Constitutive activation of signal transducers and activators of transcription predicts vorinostat resistance in cutaneous T-cell lymphoma. *Cancer Res.* 2008;68(10):3785-3794.

91. Garcia-Manero G, Yang H, Bueso-Ramos C, et al. Phase 1 study of the histone deacetylase inhibitor vorinostat (suberoylanilide hydroxamic acid [SAHA]) in patients with advanced leukemias and myelodysplastic syndromes. *Blood.* 2008;111(3):1060-1066.

92. Qu K, Zaba LC, Satpathy AT, et al. Chromatin accessibility landscape of cutaneous T cell lymphoma and dynamic response to HDAC inhibitors. *Cancer Cell.* 2017;32(1):27-41.

93. Sandor V, Bakke S, Robey RW, et al. Phase I trial of the histone deacetylase inhibitor, depsipeptide (FR901228, NSC 630176), in patients with refractory neoplasms. *Clin Cancer Res.* 2002;8(3):718-728.

94. Molife R, Fong P, Scurr M, Judson I, Kaye S, de Bono J. HDAC inhibitors and cardiac safety. *Clin Cancer Res.* 2007;13(3):1068; author reply 1068-1069.

95. Piekarz RL, Frye AR, Wright JJ, et al. Cardiac studies in patients treated with depsipeptide, FK228, in a phase II trial for T-cell lymphoma. *Clin Cancer Res.* 2006;12(12):3762-3773.

96. O'Mahony D, Peikarz RL, Bandettini WP, Arai AE, Wilson WH, Bates SE. Cardiac involvement with lymphoma: a review of the literature. *Clin Lymphoma Myeloma.* 2008;8(4):249-252.

97. Olsen EA, Kim YH, Kuzel TM, et al. Phase IIb multicenter trial of vorinostat in patients with persistent, progressive, or treatment refractory cutaneous T-cell lymphoma. *J Clin Oncol.* 2007;25(21):3109-3115.

98. Zhang L, Lebwohl D, Masson E, Laird G, Cooper MR, Prince HM. Clinically relevant QTc prolongation is not associated with current dose schedules of LBH589 (panobinostat). *J Clin Oncol.* 2008;26(2):332-333; discussion 333-334.

99. Shah MH, Binkley P, Chan K, et al. Cardiotoxicity of histone deacetylase inhibitor depsipeptide in patients with metastatic neuroendocrine tumors. *Clin Cancer Res.* 2006;12(13):3997-4003.

100. Strevel EL, Siu LL. Cardiovascular toxicity of molecularly targeted agents. *European Journal of Cancer (Oxford, England: 1990).* 2009;45(suppl 1):318-331.

101. Fingert HJ, Varterasian ML. Cardiac safety, risk management, and oncology drug development. *Clin Cancer Res.* 2006;12(12):3646-3647.

102. Turner JR, Karnad DR, Cabell CH, Kothari S. Recent developments in the science of proarrhythmic cardiac safety of new drugs. *Eur Heart J Cardiovasc Pharmacother.* 2017;3(2):118-124.

103. Munster PN, Rubin EH, Van Belle S, et al. A single supratherapeutic dose of vorinostat does not prolong the QTc interval in patients with advanced cancer. *Clin Cancer Res.* 2009;15(22):7077-7084.

104. Noonan AM, Eisch RA, Liewehr DJ, et al. Electrocardiographic studies of romidepsin demonstrate its safety and identify a potential role for K(ATP) channel. *Clin Cancer Res.* 2013;19(11):3095-3104.

105. Morgan M, Maloney D, Duvic M. Hypomagnesemia and hypocalcemia in mycosis fungoides: a retrospective case series. *Leuk Lymphoma.* 2002;43(6):1297-1302.

106. Wise LD, Turner KJ, Kerr JS. Assessment of developmental toxicity of vorinostat, a histone deacetylase inhibitor, in Sprague-Dawley rats and Dutch Belted rabbits. *Birth Defects Res B Dev Reprod Toxicol* 2007;80(1):57-68.

107. Shustov A, Coiffier B, Horwitz S, et al. Romidepsin is effective and well tolerated in older patients with peripheral T-cell lymphoma: analysis of two phase II trials. *Leuk Lymphoma.* 2017;58(10):2335-2341.

108. Mann BS, Johnson JR, He K, et al. Vorinostat for treatment of cutaneous manifestations of advanced primary cutaneous T-cell lymphoma. *Clin Cancer Res.* 2007;13(8):2318-2322.

109. Duvic M, Bates SE, Piekarz R, et al. Responses to romidepsin in patients with cutaneous T-cell lymphoma and prior treatment with systemic chemotherapy. *Leuk Lymphoma* 2017:1-8.

110. Marshall JL, Rizvi N, Kauh J, et al. A phase I trial of depsipeptide (FR901228) in patients with advanced cancer. *J Exp Ther Oncol.* 2002;2(6):325-332.

111. Piekarz RL, Frye R, Turner M, et al. Phase II multi-institutional trial of the histone deacetylase inhibitor romidepsin as monotherapy for patients with cutaneous T-cell lymphoma. *J Clin Oncol.* 2009;27(32):5410-5417.

112. Whittaker SJ, Demierre MF, Kim EJ, et al. Final results from a multicenter, international, pivotal study of romidepsin in refractory cutaneous T-cell lymphoma. *J Clin Oncol.* 2010;28(29):4485-4491.

113. Piekarz RL, Frye R, Prince HM, et al. Phase 2 trial of romidepsin in patients with peripheral T-cell lymphoma. *Blood.* 2011;117(22):5827-5834.

114. Coiffier B, Pro B, Prince HM, et al. Romidepsin for the treatment of relapsed/refractory peripheral T-cell lymphoma: pivotal study update demonstrates durable responses. *J Hematol Oncol* 2014;7:11.

115. Stadler WM, Margolin K, Ferber S, McCulloch W, Thompson JA. A phase II study of depsipeptide in refractory metastatic renal cell cancer. *Clin Genitourin Cancer.* 2006;5(1):57-60.

116. Klimek VM, Fircanis S, Maslak P, et al. Tolerability, pharmacodynamics, and pharmacokinetics studies of depsipeptide (romidepsin) in patients with acute myelogenous leukemia or advanced myelodysplastic syndromes. *Clin Cancer Res.* 2008;14(3):826-832.

117. Whitehead RP, Rankin C, Hoff PM, et al. Phase II trial of romidepsin (NSC-630176) in previously treated colorectal cancer patients with advanced disease: a Southwest Oncology Group study (S0336). *Invest New Drugs.* 2009;27(5):469-475.

118. O'Connor OA, Horwitz S, Masszi T, et al. Belinostat in Patients With Relapsed or Refractory Peripheral T-Cell Lymphoma: Results of the Pivotal Phase II BELIEF (CLN-19) Study. *J Clin Oncol.* 2015;33(23):2492-2499.

119. Giaccone G, Rajan A, Berman A, et al. Phase II study of belinostat in patients with recurrent or refractory advanced thymic epithelial tumors. *J Clin Oncol.* 2011;29(15):2052-2059.

120. Dizon DS, Damstrup L, Finkler NJ, et al. Phase II activity of belinostat (PXD-101), carboplatin, and paclitaxel in women with previously treated ovarian cancer. *Int J Gynecol Cancer.* 2012;22(6):979-986.

121. Yeo W, Chung HC, Chan SL, et al. Epigenetic therapy using belinostat for patients with unresectable hepatocellular carcinoma: a multicenter phase I/II study with biomarker and pharmacokinetic analysis of tumors from patients in the Mayo Phase II Consortium and the Cancer Therapeutics Research Group. *J Clin Oncol.* 2012;30(27):3361-3367.

122. San-Miguel JF, Hungria VT, Yoon SS, et al. Panobinostat plus bortezomib and dexamethasone versus placebo plus bortezomib and dexamethasone in patients with relapsed or relapsed and refractory multiple myeloma: a multicentre, randomised, double-blind phase 3 trial. *Lancet Oncol.* 2014;15(11):1195-1206.

123. Marchi E, Zullo KM, Amengual JE, et al. The combination of hypomethylating agents and histone deacetylase inhibitors produce marked synergy in preclinical models of T-cell lymphoma. *Br J Haematol.* 2015.

124. Akilov OE, Grant C, Frye R, Bates S, Piekarz R, Geskin LJ. Low-dose electron beam radiation and romidepsin therapy for symptomatic cutaneous T-cell lymphoma lesions. *Br J Dermatol.* 2012;167(1):194-197.

125. Vogl DT, Raje N, Jagannath S, et al. Ricolinostat, the first selective histone deacetylase 6 inhibitor, in combination with bortezomib and dexamethasone for relapsed or refractory multiple myeloma. *Clin Cancer Res.* 2017;23(13):3307-3315.

126. Maio M, Covre A, Fratta E, et al. Molecular pathways: At the crossroads of cancer epigenetics and immunotherapy. *Clin Cancer Res.* 2015;21(18): 4040-4047.

127. Kim K, Skora AD, Li Z, et al. Eradication of metastatic mouse cancers resistant to immune checkpoint blockade by suppression of myeloid-derived cells. *Proc Natl Acad Sci U S A.* 2014;111(32):11774-11779.

128. Cairns RA, Mak TW. Oncogenic isocitrate dehydrogenase mutations: mechanisms, models, and clinical opportunities. *Cancer Discov.* 2013;3(7):730-741.

129. Duncan CG, Barwick BG, Jin G, et al. A heterozygous IDH1R132H/WT mutation induces genome-wide alterations in DNA methylation. *Genome Res.* 2012;22(12):2339-2355.

130. Lu C, Ward PS, Kapoor GS, et al. IDH mutation impairs histone demethylation and results in a block to cell differentiation. *Nature.* 2012;483(7390):474-478.

131. Garrett-Bakelman FE, Melnick AM. Mutant IDH: a targetable driver of leukemic phenotypes linking metabolism, epigenetics and transcriptional regulation. *Epigenomics.* 2016;8(7):945-957.

132. Medeiros BC, Fathi AT, DiNardo CD, Pollyea DA, Chan SM, Swords R. Isocitrate dehydrogenase mutations in myeloid malignancies. *Leukemia.* 2017;31(2):272-281.

133. Inoue S, Li WY, Tseng A, et al. Mutant IDH1 downregulates ATM and alters DNA repair and sensitivity to DNA damage independent of TET2. *Cancer Cell.* 2016;30(2):337-348.

134. Nobusawa S, Watanabe T, Kleihues P, Ohgaki H. IDH1 mutations as molecular signature and predictive factor of secondary glioblastomas. *Clin Cancer Res.* 2009;15(19):6002-6007.

135. Ohgaki H, Kleihues P. The definition of primary and secondary glioblastoma. *Clin Cancer Res.* 2013;19(4):764-772.

136. Ward PS, Lu C, Cross JR, et al. The potential for isocitrate dehydrogenase mutations to produce 2-hydroxyglutarate depends on allele specificity and subcellular compartmentalization. *J Biol Chem.* 2013;288(6): 3804-3815.

137. Amatangelo MD, Quek L, Shih A, et al. Enasidenib induces acute myeloid leukemia cell differentiation to promote clinical response. *Blood.* 2017;130(6):732-741.

138. Stein EM, DiNardo CD, Pollyea DA, et al. Enasidenib in mutant IDH2 relapsed or refractory acute myeloid leukemia. *Blood.* 2017;130(6): 722-731.

139. Wang F, Travins J, DeLaBarre B, et al. Targeted inhibition of mutant IDH2 in leukemia cells induces cellular differentiation. *Science (New York, NY).* 2013;340(6132):622-626.

140. Parker SJ, Metallo CM. Metabolic consequences of oncogenic IDH mutations. *Pharmacol Ther* 2015;152:54-62.

141. Thomas D, Majeti R. Optimizing next-generation AML therapy: Activity of mutant IDH2 inhibitor AG-221 in preclinical models. *Cancer Discov.* 2017;7(5):459-461.

142. Ntziachristos P, Tsirigos A, Van Vlierberghe P, et al. Genetic inactivation of the polycomb repressive complex 2 in T cell acute lymphoblastic leukemia. *Nat Med.* 2012;18(2):298-301.

143. Palomo L, Garcia O, Arnan M, et al. Targeted deep sequencing improves outcome stratification in chronic myelomonocytic leukemia with low risk cytogenetic features. *Oncotarget.* 2016;7(35):57021-57035.

144. Shirahata-Adachi M, Iriyama C, Tomita A, Suzuki Y, Shimada K, Kiyoi H. Altered EZH2 splicing and expression is associated with impaired histone H3 lysine 27 tri-Methylation in myelodysplastic syndrome. *Leuk Res* 2017;63:90-97.

145. Grossmann V, Kohlmann A, Eder C, et al. Molecular profiling of chronic myelomonocytic leukemia reveals diverse mutations in >80% of patients with TET2 and EZH2 being of high prognostic relevance. *Leukemia.* 2011;25(5):877-879.

146. Varambally S, Dhanasekaran SM, Zhou M, et al. The polycomb group protein EZH2 is involved in progression of prostate cancer. *Nature.* 2002;419(6907):624-629.

147. Labbe DP, Sweeney CJ, Brown M, et al. TOP2A and EZH2 provide early detection of an aggressive prostate cancer subgroup. *Clin Cancer Res.* 2017;23(22):7072-7083.

148. Lobo J, Rodrigues A, Antunes L, et al. High immunoexpression of Ki67, EZH2, and SMYD3 in diagnostic prostate biopsies independently predicts outcome in patients with prostate cancer. *Urol Oncol.* 2017.

149. Bohers E, Mareschal S, Bouzelfen A, et al. Targetable activating mutations are very frequent in GCB and ABC diffuse large B-cell lymphoma. *Genes Chromosomes Cancer* 2014;53(2):144-153.

150. Gibaja V, Shen F, Harari J, et al. Development of secondary mutations in wild-type and mutant EZH2 alleles cooperates to confer resistance to EZH2 inhibitors. *Oncogene.* 2016;35(5):558-566.

151. Vincent Ribrag J-CS, Jean-Marie M, Anna S, et al. Phase 1 study of tazemetostat (EPZ-6438), an inhibitor of enhancer of Zeste-homolog 2 (EZH2): Preliminary safety and activity in relapsed or refractory non-Hodgkin lymphoma (NHL) patients. 2015.

Differentiating Agents

Bruce A. Chabner

One of the most obvious yet most poorly understood features of malignancy is the failure of cancer cells to differentiate. Malignant cells have the morphologic features of primitive precursors and carry surface markers suggesting that they are blocked at an early step in their maturation. Within this relatively primitive population are cells that preserve the surface antigens (CD38$^+$, CD133$^-$) and properties of stem cells; like their normal counterparts, they may revert to a dormant and drug-resistant state, only later to resume growth.[1] Thus, cancer researchers have turned their attention to understanding the normal process of differentiation, and the signals that block differentiation in tumors. The goal of such work is to speed the development of agents capable of overcoming this hurdle.

From these inquiries have emerged two effective agents, all-trans retinoic acid (ATRA) and arsenic trioxide (ATO) (Fig. 17.1), both of which attack the essential genomic lesion that blocks differentiation in acute promyelocytic leukemia (APL).

The genetic program for myeloid differentiation is controlled by the retinoic acid responsive element (RARE) in DNA, which regulates expression of key transcription factors. Homodimers and heterodimers formed by retinoic acid receptor alpha (RARA) and its partners bind to and regulate the differentiation program controlled by RERE. Dysregulation of the RARE leads to APL, and is caused by a characteristic translocation (t15;17), which fuses RARA to the PML gene. The RARA-PML fusion protein blocks differentiation and leads to leukemic proliferation of promyelocytes. Two small molecules, ATRA and ATO, are able to restore differentiation. They induce differentiation (Fig. 17.2) and ultimately apoptosis of

leukemic cells, thereby restoring normal bone marrow function. The ATO/ATRA combination has become the primary treatment for APL.[2]

We will consider ATO later in this chapter. Cytotoxic agents, including hydroxyurea, 5-azacytidine, decitabine, and cytarabine, may also induce differentiation. The cytidine analogs will be discussed in Chapter 9.

All-trans Retinoic Acid

Sporn and colleagues first reported that retinoids induced differentiation of the human leukemia cell line HL-60 and reversed preneoplastic changes in murine models of epithelial carcinogenesis.[3] However, the first successful clinical trial of a retinoid to treat cancer was reported by Wang, Chen, and colleagues from Shanghai in 1988.[4] They found that ATRA induced complete remission in APL patients refractory to standard chemotherapy. While they were aware of Sporn's earlier work, the mechanism for this effect was unclear; the specific involvement of the retinoic acid receptor in APL had not been elucidated at the time of their report.[5] Subsequent trials showed that ATRA was highly effective in reversing the often fatal coagulopathy (disseminated intravascular coagulation) associated with APL, and, with ATO, induced long-term remission in greater than 90% of APL patients.[2] Key features of ATRA are shown in Table 17.1.

Mechanism of Action

The target of ATRA (Fig. 17.3) is the RAR-α protein (RARA).[6] Under physiological conditions, the three isoforms of RARA homodimerize and form heterodimers with alternative isoforms of RARA, or with the retinoid X receptor alpha (RXRA). The RARA homodimers and heterodimers bind ATRA and function as a chromatin modifier and as a positive transcriptional regulator as the result of their binding to RARE on DNA. In the *absence* of retinoids, these RARA dimers bind corepressors and block differentiation, while in the *presence* of retinoids, the corepressors are expelled from the RARA dimer complex, and replaced by coactivators that initiate transcription and differentiation. They regulate the expression of transcription factors such as RAR-β, C/EBP α, c-Myc, and PU-1,[7] which promote normal myeloid differentiation.

The critical genetic lesion in APL is created by the t(15:17) translocation that merges the retinoid and DNA-binding segment of RARA with PML, a second transcription factor that promotes differentiation. This translocation creates an oncogenic protein, RARA-PML, that has much decreased binding affinity for its physiological ligand, ATRA. The ligand-free RARA-PML fusion protein

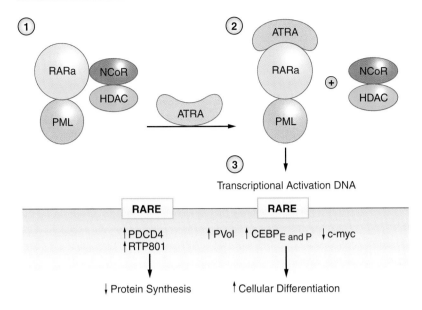

FIGURE **17.2** The RAR-α-PML fusion protein exists in an inhibited state, bound to the nuclear corepressor (NCoR) in complex with histone deacetylase (HDAC) (*1*). In the presence of ATRA (*2*), the NCoR/HDAC complex dissociates, freeing the active RAR-α-PML transcription factor, which binds to RARE (retinoic acid response element) on DNA and regulates expression of multiple genes that inhibit protein synthesis and induce differentiation (*3*).

binds corepressor proteins and blocks the normal differentiation of myeloid cells. The RARA-PML forms heterodimers with other nuclear receptors, particularly (RXRA), and these complexes increase leukemic stem cell renewal and suppress apoptosis.[8] In addition, the fusion protein binds to histone deacetylases and to elements of the polycomb repressive complex, altering histone acetylation and methylation, with a further negative impact on differentiation. In APL cell lines, a key histone acetylase, PCAF (p300/CREB protein associated factor), is critical to ATRA action.[9] This multiplicity of effects is reversed in the presence of high concentrations of ATRA. When ATRA binds to the fusion protein, the resulting complex expels its corepressor proteins, binds activating proteins, and initiates the differentiation program in APL cells; ATRA restores histone acetylation and demethylation, and promotes ubiquitination and degradation of the fusion protein itself.[8]

At least four partner genes other than PML are capable of causing APL when fused to RAR-α but constitute less than 5% of the APL leukemia population. ATRA effectively treats this subset of APL as well. Mutations in isocitrate dehydrogenase (IDH) and FLT3 may contribute to the leukemic proliferation of APL t(15;17). The IDH mutations in acute myeloid leukemia cells produce the oncometabolite 2-hydroxyglutarate, which dysregulates DNA, increases histone methylation, and primes tumor cells for response to ATRA.[10]

Resistance to ATRA therapy in APL patients arises through several different mechanisms. ATRA rapidly induces its own metabolism, "pharmacokinetic resistance." When used as a single agent, remissions last only a few months and, in most patients, are associated with accelerated metabolic clearance of the drug by the CYP26 family of enzymes.[11] Treatment with ATRA induces cytochrome

TABLE 17.1	*Key features of ATRA*
Feature	**ATRA**
Mechanism of action	Binds to RARA-PML fusion protein, activates transcription
Metabolism	CYP26A1. 80% of dose
Dosage and schedule	45 mg/kg/d until remission
Eliminations	Plasma $T_{1/2} < 1$ h
Toxicity	Retinoic acid syndrome (differentiation), dry skin, cheilitis, hepatic enzyme elevation, pseudotumor cerebri, and hypertriglyceridemia
Drug interactions	Imidazoles block metabolism
Precautions	Use with chemotherapy in patients with WBC > 10,000

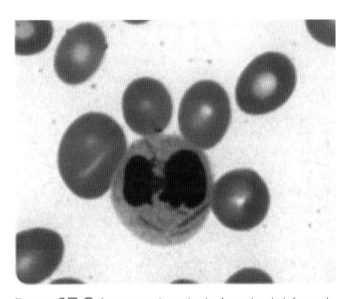

FIGURE **17.3** A mature granulocyte showing Auer rods typical of promyelocytic leukemia cells in the blood smear from a patient on day 16 of ATRA therapy. (Republished with permission of American Society of Hematology from Luu HS, Rahaman PA. Mature neutrophils with Auer rods following treatment with all-trans retinoic acid for acute promyelocytic leukemia. *Blood*. 2015;126(1):121; permission conveyed through Copyright Clearance Center, Inc.)

CYP 26A1 in the tumor as well as the liver, leading to resistance. Mutations in the retinoid-binding site of the fusion protein decrease the affinity of ATRA binding and lead to resistance.[12,13] Even in cells in which the RARA-PML fusion protein is degraded, proliferation may continue, implying that other "drivers" of proliferation may take its place. In these cells, sensitivity to ATRA can be restored by transfection of PML-RARA.[14] Because of the rapid emergence of resistance to ATRA when it is given as a single agent, combination therapy is indicated for remission induction in all PML patients. ATRA is therefore used as standard therapy with ATO in low- and medium-risk patients and with anthracyclines for high-risk patients.[2]

Clinical Pharmacology

ATRA is given orally in doses of 45 mg/d and is continued until remission is achieved. Doses are given in intermittent courses for consolidation. ATRA rapidly abolishes the procoagulant and fibrinolytic activity of the leukemic cells, stops the release of the procoagulant tissue factor, restores fibrinogen levels, and prevents fatal bleeding, and should be initiated even prior to definitive diagnosis in any leukemic patient who presents with bleeding and characteristic myeloid cell histology.[15,16] In patients with hyperleukosis (white blood cell count above 20,000 cells/mm^3), the rapid induction of myeloid differentiation by ATRA leads to expression of integrins on the leukemic cell surface and clogging of small vessels in the lung (the retinoic acid or APL differentiation syndrome).[15,17] Ten to twenty percent of APL patients treated with single-agent ATRA develop pleural or pericardial effusions and experience hypotension, dyspnea, and cardiorespiratory and renal failure. Although controlled trials are lacking, in patients with greater than 10,000 white blood cells/mm^2 in the peripheral blood at the time of diagnosis,

dexamethasone (10 mg intravenously twice daily for 3 days) and anthracyclines should be added to the induction regimen.[15,17]

The above ATRA regimen (45 mg/d) achieves peak concentrations of ATRA of 400 ng/mL. The drug is cleared from plasma with a half-life of less than 1 hour. Its disappearance is hastened by CYP26 inducers, and is inhibited by antifungal imidazoles.[11] Prolonged exposure to high drug concentrations may lead to hypercalcemia and renal failure, a complication treated with bisphosphonates to lower serum calcium and to induce diuresis. Other toxicities of ATRA include dry skin, cheilitis, hepatic enzyme abnormalities, as well as the common retinoid toxicities of pseudotumor cerebri, bone tenderness, hypercalcemia, photosensitivity, and hypertriglyceridemia.[8]

ATRA up-regulates the expression of aquaglyceroporin 9, the ATO transporter, an effect that may account for the excellent 90% 5-year disease-free survival of APL patients treated with these drugs in combination as primary therapy.[1,18]

Arsenic Trioxide

A remarkable addition to the treatment for APL emanated from investigators in Harbin, China, who reported that the majority of patients relapsing and/or refractory to standard ATRA/anthracycline regimens achieved a complete response to a single-agent ATO.[19] Arsenicals have been used in folk medicine for centuries, treating warts, syphilis, ulcers, and leukemia. Several forms of arsenic derivatives have been administered to patients, but a trivalent compound, white arsenic (ATO), which forms arsenous acid (AS(OH)$_3$) in aqueous solution, is easily formulated for intravenous administration, and is well absorbed as an oral solution[20] (see Fig. 17.4). Its key features are shown in Table 17.2.

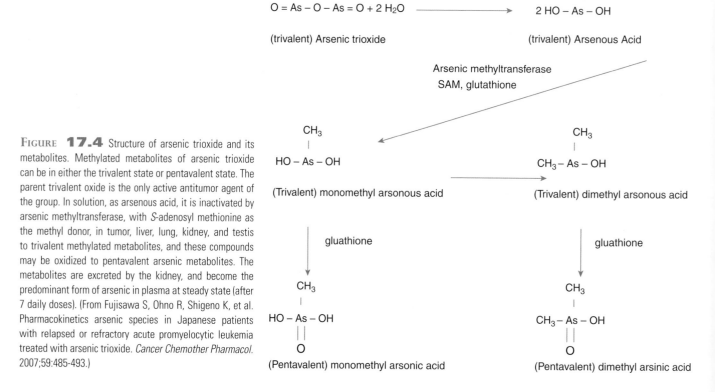

FIGURE **17.4** Structure of arsenic trioxide and its metabolites. Methylated metabolites of arsenic trioxide can be in either the trivalent state or pentavalent state. The parent trivalent oxide is the only active antitumor agent of the group. In solution, as arsenous acid, it is inactivated by arsenic methyltransferase, with *S*-adenosyl methionine as the methyl donor, in tumor, liver, lung, kidney, and testis to trivalent methylated metabolites, and these compounds may be oxidized to pentavalent arsenic metabolites. The metabolites are excreted by the kidney, and become the predominant form of arsenic in plasma at steady state (after 7 daily doses). (From Fujisawa S, Ohno R, Shigeno K, et al. Pharmacokinetics arsenic species in Japanese patients with relapsed or refractory acute promyelocytic leukemia treated with arsenic trioxide. *Cancer Chemother Pharmacol.* 2007;59:485-493.)

17.2   *Key features of ATO*

Features	ATO
Mechanism of action	Induces degradation of fusion protein Increases ROS damage
Metabolism	CYP-mediated methylation inactivates ATO
Dosage and schedule	0.15 mg/kg/d for 28 d (see text for alternative schedule)
Eliminations	Plasma $T_{1/2}$ of 9–11 h
Toxicity	Lengthens QTc, torsade de pointes, leukemic cell maturation syndrome, hyperglycemia, hypertriglyceridemia, hepatic enzyme elevations
Drug interactions	Avoid drugs that prolong QTc (macrolide antibiotics, quinidine, methadone)
Precautions	Monitor and correct serum electrolytes Monitor QTc on EKG during treatment

Mechanism of Action

ATO enters cells via the AQP9 transporter,[18] which is expressed at higher levels in APL and in the M2 AML subtype, as compared to other subtypes of AML. As a general property of arsenicals, ATO attacks sulfhydryl and other reducing molecules.[21] It inactivates the critical enzyme thioredoxin reductase, thereby disabling cellular defenses against reactive oxygen species (ROS).[22] APL cells have a generous intracellular concentration of ROS, probably as the result of their intracellular NADPH oxidase activity,[23] and are particularly susceptible to redox damage. Consistent with the free radical mechanism of toxicity is the observation that the antitumor effects of ATO are antagonized in cell culture by free radical scavengers, such as N-acetylcysteine.[24]

Likely of greater importance is the effect of ATO on RARA-PML stability and function. In the absence of drug, the oncoprotein undergoes sumoylation of the PML segment, which promotes its ability to block differentiation and initiate APL, while phosphorylation of the RARA segment enhances its ability to interact with chromatin remodelers, such as histone deacetylase and the polycomb repressive complexes, 1 and 2, thus exposing new regulatory sites on DNA and altering gene expression. ATO promotes degradation of the protein, covalently binding to cysteine groups in the B domain of the PML segment of RARA-PML.[25] ATO also interacts with and degrades the unrearranged allele of PML in the leukemic cell, an action that seems necessary for antitumor activity of the fusion protein, as mutations in the wild-type allele lead to resistance.[26] ATO interaction with the PML segment of RAR-PML accelerates the formation of nuclear bodies that promote fusion protein ubiquitination, degradation, p53 signaling, and apoptosis.[27]

ATO disrupts the formation of tetramers of the fusion protein with other nuclear receptors, including RXRA, a required partner of RARA-PML, while mutations in RXRA that prevent ATO binding also lead to resistance.[27] Resistance to ATO develops in cells that contain mutation in the B-domain sequence (amino acids 212 to 220), including S214L A216 V, L217F, A216T, L218P, and S220G.[28-30]

The potential for protein degradation by ATO is not confined to PML. It also degrades other oncoproteins, such as EVI-1,[31] BCR-ABL,[32] and NPM-1.[33] ATO has a number of additional biological effects that may contribute to its cytotoxicity. It activates the intrinsic apoptotic pathway that responds to ROS, and downregulates antiapoptotic proteins such as bcl-2. It dampens survival and angiogenic signals.[34] The PI-3 kinase pathway promotes the stem cell features of APL.[27] ATO down-regulates AKT expression, a key component of this pathway.[35] In cell culture, inhibitors of PI-3 kinase and mTOR are synergistic with ATO.[36] Not surprisingly, based on its ability to generate ROS and its proapoptotic effects, ATO enhances the efficacy of irradiation in model systems.[37]

While mutations in RARA-PML, in the wild-type PML allele, and RXRA may explain individual instances of resistance, these explain relapse or lack of response in the minority of patients. A full understanding of resistance has not been achieved.

Clinical Pharmacology

The ATO powder is readily dissolved in saline and yields arsenous acid (Fig. 17.4), and its arsenite anion, which readily forms adducts with nucleophiles such as cysteines in protein and in glutathione. In current clinical use, ATO is given intravenously in doses of 0.15 mg/kg/d for 28 days, followed by 2 weeks of rest, and then resumption of additional courses until remission, but alternative schedules of intermittent administration, such as 0.3 mg/kg/d for 5 days for the first week, followed by 0.25 mg/kg for weeks 2 to 8 are used in combination with ATRA.[38] It is also employed in remission consolidation after a break in therapy. The median plasma maximal total arsenic concentration approaches 0.3 μM,[39] and disappears from plasma with a half-life of 9 to 11 hours. The drug is inactivated by methylation by arsenic methyltransferase, which is found in tumor cells, testes, liver, kidneys, and lung (Fig. 17.4).[40] A minor fraction, about 20%, is excreted as trivalent (active) arsenic in the urine.[41] The major metabolites, monomethylated and dimethylated arsenicals in the trivalent and pentavalent oxidation state, are capable of binding to RARA-PML but do not induce differentiation or degradation of the fusion protein. They are carcinogenic.[40] The methylated metabolites are excreted by the kidneys. Dose modifications for renal or hepatic dysfunction are not necessary.[41] There is no evidence for drug accumulation over the multiple days of treatment for patients with normal renal function. A 40% increase in the area under the plasma concentration curve of trivalent arsenic was found in patients with severe renal impairment, but no increase in side effects was noted in a limited trial.[41] A limited four patient experience with patients in severe renal failure or on dialysis found that 36% to 50% dose reduction (3.6 to 5 mg ATO daily for 28 days, based on monitoring of whole-blood arsenic levels) resulted in long-term complete remission.[42]

Clinical Toxicity

ATO has minimal acute toxic effects. It lengthens the QT interval on EKG, and increases the risk of ventricular arrhythmias. Follow-up of patients treated with the ATO/ATRA combination as primary therapy revealed no significant long-term sequelae, despite fears of carcinogenesis and hepatic and cardiac toxicity, and arsenic or metabolites were undetectable in urine analyzed 2 years after treatment.[43] Patients may acutely experience fatigue, light-headedness, and numbness or tingling of the extremities, and serum chemistries may reveal electrolyte changes, hyperglycemia, and modest hepatic enzyme elevations, all of which are fully reversible with discontinuation of drug. Fewer than 10% of patients with APL develop a leukocyte maturation syndrome similar to that seen with ATRA, with pulmonary distress, effusions, and altered mental status. These symptoms abate with drug discontinuation, corticosteroids, oxygen, and diuretics.[5]

The most serious acute and subacute toxicity relates to prolongation of the QT interval.[44] This toxicity has been ascribed to inhibition of the rapid K^+ efflux channel, a change that slows ventricular repolarization and predisposes to ventricular instability.[45] Drugs that prolong conduction, such as macrolide antibiotics, quinidine, or methadone, should not be used with ATO. It is necessary to confirm a normal QT interval prior to treatment, to monitor the EKG and serum electrolytes at regular intervals (every 3 to 7 days) during therapy, and to correct abnormalities of serum K^+, Ca^+, and Mg^{2+} as necessary. In patients with QTc prolongation of greater than 0.45 seconds, treatment should be suspended until the electrolyte abnormalities are corrected and the QTc returns to normal.

Rarely, patients with prolongation of the QTc develop torsade de pointes, or multifocal ventricular tachycardia, a potentially fatal arrhythmia. This event requires immediate defibrillation, treatment with intravenous magnesium sulfate, and correction of electrolyte abnormalities.[46] Extreme caution should be exercised in resuming ATO treatment in patients who have experienced a ventricular arrhythmia associated with a prolongation of the QTc. Some investigators suggest resuming treatment at a lower dose of 0.10 mg/kg/d, with close monitoring of the EKG and electrolytes.

Alternative formulations of arsenic have entered clinical trials, including an oral formulation of ATO in solution, and a oral tetra-arsenic tetrasulfide,[47] both of which appear to have activity in APL trials.

References

1. Lo-Coco F, Awasati G, Vignetti M, et al. Retinoic acid and arsenic trioxide for acute promyelocytic leukemia. *N Engl J Med.* 2013;369:111-121.
2. Platzbecker U, Awisati G, Cicconi L, et al. Improved outcomes with retinoic acid and arsenic trioxide compared with retinoic acid and chemotherapy in non-high risk acute promyelocytic leukemia: final results of the randomized Italian-German AL0406 trial. *J Clin Oncol.* 2016;35:605-612.
3. Breitman TR, Collins SJ, Keene BR. Terminal differentiation of human promyelocytic leukemia cell line (HL-60) by retinoic acid. *Proc Natl Acad Sci U S A.* 1980;77:2936-2940.
4. Huang ME, Ye YC, Chen SR, et al. Use of all-trans retinoic acid as a differentiation therapy for acute promyelocytic leukemia. *Blood.* 1988;72:567-572.
5. Wang Z-Y, Chen Z. Acute promyelocytic leukemia: from highly fatal to highly curable. *Blood.* 2008;111:2505-2515.
6. Collins SJ. Retinoic acid receptors, hematopoiesis and leukemogenesis. *Curr Opin Hematol.* 2008;15:346-351.
7. Drumea K, Yang ZF, Rosmarin A. Retinoic acid signaling in myelopoiesis. *Curr Opin Hematol.* 2008;15:37-41.
8. Schenk T, Stengel S, Zelent A. Unlocking the potential of retinoic acid in anticancer therapy. *Br J Cancer.* 2014;111:2039-2045.
9. Sunami Y, Araki M, Kan S, et al. Histone acetyltransferase PCAF is required for all-transretinoic acid-induced granulocytic differentiation in leukemia cells. *J Biol Chem.* 2017;292:2815-2829.
10. Boutzen H, Saland E, Larrue C, et al. Isocitrate dehydrogenase 1 mutations prime the all-trans retinoic acid myeloid differentiation pathway in acute myeloid leukemia. *J Exp Med.* 2016;213:483-497.
11. Jing J, Nelson C, Paik J, et al. Physiologically based pharmacokinetic model of All-trans-retinoic acid with applications to cancer populations and drug interactions. *J Pharmacol Exp Ther.* 2017;361:246-258.
12. Rousel MJ, Lanotte M. Maturation sensitive and resistant t(15,17) NB4 cell lines as tools for APL physiopathology, nomenclature of cells and repertory of their known genetic alterations and phenotypes. *Oncogene.* 2001;20:7287-7291.
13. Robertson KA, Emami B, Collins SJ. Retinoic acid-resistant HL-60R cells harbor a point mutation in the retinoic acid receptor ligand binding domain that confers dominant negative activity. *Blood.* 1992;80:1885.
14. Nasr R, Guillemin MC, Ferhi O, et al. Eradication of acute promyelocytic leukemia-initiating cells through PML-RAR degradation. *Nat Med.* 2008;14:1333-1342.
15. Cicconi L, Lo-Cpcp F. Current management of newly diagnosed acute promyelocytic leukemia. *Ann Oncol.* 2016;27:1474-1481.
16. Mantha S, Goldman DA, Devlin SM, et al. Determinants of fatal bleeding during induction therapy for acute promyelocytic leukemia in the ATRA era. *Blood.* 2017;30:1763-1767.
17. Sanz MA, Grimwade D, Tallman MS, et al. Management of acute promyelocytic leukemia: recommendations from an expert panel on behalf of European Leukemianet. *Blood.* 2009;26:1875-1891.
18. Leung J, Pang A, Yuen W-H, et al. Relationship of expression of aquaglyceroporin 9 with arsenic uptake and sensitivity in leukemia cells. *Blood.* 2007;109:740-746.
19. Hu J, Liu Y-F, Wu C-F, et al. Long-term efficacy and safety of all-trans retinoic acid/arsenic trioxide-based therapy in newly diagnosed acute promyelocytic leukemia. *Proc Natl Acad Sci U S A.* 2009;106:3342-3347.
20. Khairul I, Wang QQ, Jiang YH, et al. Metabolism, toxicity and anticancer activities of arsenic compounds. *Oncotarget.* 2017;8:23905-23926.
21. Dilda PJ, Hogg PJ. Arsenical-based cancer drugs. *Cancer Treat Rev.* 2007;33:542-564.
22. Lu J, Chew E-H, Holmgren A. Targeting thioredoxin reductase is a basis for cancer therapy by arsenic trioxide. *Proc Natl Acad Sci U S A.* 2007;104:12288-12293.
23. Wang J, Li L, Cang H, Shi G, et al. NADPH oxidase-derived reactive oxygen species are responsible for the high susceptibility to arsenic cytotoxicity in acute promyelocytic leukemia cells. *Leuk Res.* 2008;32:429-436.
24. Han YH, Kim SZ, Kim SH, et al. Suppression of arsenic trioxide-induced apoptosis in HeLa cells by N-acetylcysteine. *Mol Cells.* 2008;26:18-25.
25. Lallemand-Breitenbach V, Jeanne M, Benhenda S, et al. Arsenic degrades PML or PML-RARalpha through a SUMO-triggered RNF4/ubiquitin-mediated pathway. *Nat Cell Biol.* 2008;10:547-555.
26. Iaccarino L, Ottone T, Divona M, et al. Mutations affecting both the rearranged and the unrearranged *PML* alleles in refractory acute promyelocytic leukaemia. *Br J Haematol.* 2016;172:909-916.
27. De The H, Zhu C. Acute promyelocytic leukaemia: novel insights into the mechanisms of cure. *Nat Rev Cancer.* 2010;16:775-783.
28. Zhu H-H, Qin Y-Z, Huang X-J. Resistance to arsenic therapy in acute promyelocytic leukemia. *N Engl J Med.* 2014;370:1864-1866.
29. Liu J, Zhu HH, Jiang H, et al. Varying responses of PML-RARA with different genetic mutations to arsenic trioxide. *Blood.* 2016;127:243-250.
30. Goto E, Tomita A, Hayakawa F, et al. Missense mutations in PML-RARA are critical for the lack of responsiveness to arsenic trioxide treatment. *Blood.* 2011;119:1600-1609.
31. Verhagen HJMP, Smit MA, Rutten A, et al. Primary acute myeloid leukemia cells with overexpression of EVI-1 are sensitive to all-*trans* retinoic acid. *Blood.* 2016;127:458-463.

32. Gousettis DJ, Gounaris E, Wu EJ, et al. Autophagic degradation of BCR-ABL oncoprotein and generation of antileukemic responses by arsenic trioxide. *Blood.* 2015;125:3455-3465.

33. Hajj HE, Dassouki Z, Berthier C, et al. Retinoic acid and arsenic trioxide trigger degradation of mutated NPM1 resulting in apoptosis of AML cells. *Blood.* 2015;125:3447-3454.

34. Mann KK, Colombo M, Miller WH Jr. Arsenic trioxide decreases AKT protein in a caspase-dependent manner. *Mol Cancer Ther.* 2008;7:1680-1687.

35. Yoon P, Giafis N, Smith J, et al. Activation of mammalian target of rapamycin and the p70 S5 kinase by arsenic trioxide in BCR-ABL-expressing cells. *Mol Cancer Ther.* 2006;5:2815-2823.

36. Billottet C, Banerjee L, Vanhaesebroeck B, et al. Inhibition of class I phosphoinositide 3-kinase activity impairs proliferation and triggers apoptosis in acute promyelocytic leukemia without affecting ATRA-induced differentiation. *Cancer Res.* 2009;69:1027-1036.

37. Kumar P, Gao Q, Ning Y, et al. Arsenic trioxide enhances the therapeutic efficacy of radiation treatment of oral squamous carcinoma while protecting bone. *Mol Cancer Ther.* 2008;7:2060-2069.

38. Burnett AK, Russell NH, Hills RK, et al. Arsenic trioxide and all-*trans* retinoic acid treatment for acute promyelocytic leukaemia in all risk groups (AML17): results of a randomised, controlled, phase 3 trial. *Lancet Oncol.* 2015;16:1295-1305.

39. Fox E, Razzouk BI, Widemann BC, et al. Phase 1 trial and pharmacokinetic study of arsenic trioxide in children and adolescents with refractory or relapsed acute leukemia, including acute promyelocytic leukemia or lymphoma. *Blood.* 2008;111:566-573.

40. Wang QQ, Zhou XY, Zhang YE, et al. Methylated arsenic metabolites bind to PML protein but do not induce cellular differentiation and PML-RARα protein. *Oncotarget.* 2015;28:25646-25659.

41. Sweeney CJ, Takimoto C, Wood L, et al. A pharmacokinetic and safety study of intravenous arsenic trioxide in adult cancer patients with renal impairment. *Cancer Chemother Pharmacol.* 2010;66:345-356.

42. Fitkin F, Roncolato F, Ho WK. Dose-adjusted arsenic trioxide for acute promyelocytic leukaemia in chronic renal failure. *Eur J Haematol.* 2015;95:331-335.

43. Soignet SL, Maslak P, Wang ZG, et al. Complete remission after treatment of acute promyelocytic leukemia with arsenic trioxide. *N Engl J Med.* 1998;339:1341-1348.

44. Drolet B, Simard C, Roden DM. Unusual effects of a QT-prolonging drug, arsenic trioxide, on cardiac potassium currents. *Circulation.* 2004;109:26-29.

45. Gupta A, Lawrence AT, Krishnan K, et al. Current concepts in the mechanisms and management of drug-induced QT prolongation and torsade de pointes. *Am Heart J.* 2007;153:891-899.

46. Alamolhodaei NS, Shirani K, Karimi G. Arsenic cardiotoxicity: an overview. *Environ Toxicol Pharmacol.* 2015;40:1005-1014.

47. Zeidan AM, Gore SD. New strategies in acute promyelocytic leukemia: moving to an entirely oral, chemotherapy-free upfront management approach. *Clin Cancer Res.* 2014;20:4985-4993.

Asparaginase
Bruce A. Chabner

The search for new therapies against cancer has turned recent attention to the altered metabolism of malignant cells. Following the early discovery of the dependence of many tumors on glycolysis,[1] other differences in carbohydrate and lipid metabolism have emerged as essential features of malignant cells. Indeed, mutations in carbohydrate metabolic enzymes, such as isocitrate dehydrogenase,[2] are fundamental to the genesis of subsets of acute myeloid leukemia and cholangiocarcinoma. The first such metabolic dependency to lead to an effective cancer therapy grew out of the observation that guinea pig serum selectively killed acute lymphoid leukemia (ALL) cells, with limited toxicity to normal tissue, an observation that has led to the identification of lymphoid dependence on exogenous asparagine, and the development of bacterial L-asparaginase (L-ASPA) in the treatment of childhood ALL.[3]

L-Asparagine is a nonessential amino acid, which, in most tissues, is synthesized by transamination of L-aspartic acid (Fig. 18.1). The amine group is donated by glutamine, and the reaction is catalyzed by the enzyme L-asparagine synthetase (L-ASPS). This enzyme

is constitutive in many tissues, but the capacity to synthesize asparagine is lacking in human malignancies of lymphocytic derivation, due to epigenetic silencing (gene methylation) or possibly polymorphic variant expression. In tumor cells lacking L-aspS, such as L5178Y murine leukemia cells, the amino acid can be obtained only from a culture medium or, in vivo, from plasma, or from the microenvironment.

The enzyme L-ASPA (L-asparagine aminohydrolase, EC 3.5.1.1), which hydrolyses asparagine to aspartic acid and ammonia as end products, occurs in multiple forms in plants, bacteria, and fungi, and in the plasma of certain animals. In 1953, Kidd reported that guinea pig serum but not rabbit, horse, or human serum inhibited the growth of transplantable lymphomas in rodents.[4] Ten years later, Broome[5] identified the responsible factor in guinea pig plasma, the enzyme L-ASPA. Subsequently, highly purified preparations of L-ASPA from *Escherichia coli*[6] and *Erwinia carotovora* (also known as *Erwinia chrysanthemi*)[7] have become standard components of remission induction, consolidation, and maintenance therapy in childhood and adult ALL.[8] A chemically modified enzyme, pegaspargase (Peg-ASP), with a longer half-life and reduced immunogenicity, was first used in patients hypersensitive to the native *E. coli* enzyme, but has now largely replaced the native enzyme worldwide for first-line therapy of childhood ALL.[9] The key features of L-ASPA are listed in Table 18.1.

Properties and Mechanism of Action

L-ASPA purified from *E. coli*,[10] and now available in recombinant form, was the initial form used in both basic and clinical research. The purified enzyme has a molecular weight of 144,000 Da and is composed of four subunits, which associate as two dimers. The gene coding for the *Erwinia chrysanthemi*[11] enzyme has been cloned and sequenced and expressed in *E. coli*, and its catalytic mechanism has been clarified through crystallographic studies.[12] The dimers in an inactive, open configuration undergo a transition to a catalytically active, or closed form with the binding of substrate. Binding of substrate induces a rotation of threonine 15, and closure of an N-loop against the substrate pocket. Asparagine is much more potent than is glutamine in inducing this active confirmation.

Preparations of enzyme from different bacterial strains show differences in enzyme characteristics such as pH dependence, metal ion dependence, and substrate specificities. For the bacterial class II enzymes, the specific activity of purified enzyme is usually 300 to 400 µmol of substrate cleaved per minute per milligram of protein; the isoelectric point lies between pH 4.6 and 5.5 for

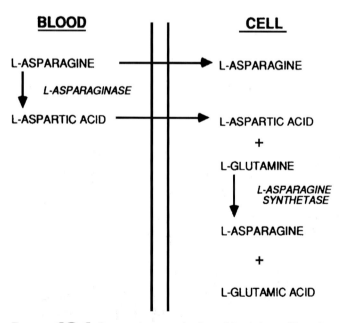

FIGURE 18.1 Sources of L-asparagine for peripheral tissues. The amino acid may be obtained directly from the circulating blood pool of L-asparagine or may be synthesized in the cell by transamination of L-aspartic acid, with L-glutamine acting as the NH₂ donor. The synthetic reaction is catalyzed by L-asparagine synthetase L-ASPS. The liver is a major source of L-asparagine found in plasma. L-ASPA resistance has been ascribed to up-regulation of L-ASPS, but also to increased uptake/retention of L-glutamine and L-asparagine by tumor cells.

TABLE 18.1   *Key features of Escherichia coli L-ASP pharmacology*

	L-Asparaginase (*E. coli*)	Pegaspargase
Mechanism of action	Depletion of the essential amino acid asparagines leads to inhibition of protein synthesis.	Same
Pharmacokinetics	Plasma half-life: 30 h	6 d
	Blood levels proportional to dose	
Dosage	10,000 to 25,000 IU/m^2/dose, interval variable	2,500 IU/m^2 q1–2wk
Elimination	Reticuloendothelial system	Same
Toxicity	Nausea, vomiting, fever, and chills	Same
	Hypersensitivity reactions	
	• Urticaria	
	• Laryngospasm, bronchospasm, dyspnea	
	• Anaphylaxis	
	Decreased protein synthesis:	
	• Albumin	
	• Insulin (with hyperglycemia)	
	• Clotting factors II, V, VII, VIII, IX, and X (with bleeding)	
	• ATIII, protein C and protein S (with thrombosis)	
	• Serum lipoproteins (with hypertriglyceridemia)	
	Pancreatitis	
	Abnormal liver function tests	
	Cerebral dysfunction	
Drug interactions	Asparaginase blocks methotrexate action, "rescues" from methotrexate toxicity.	Same
Precautions	Use with caution in patients with hepatic dysfunction or pancreatitis.	Same
	Hypersensitivity: switch *to Erwinia* preparation	
	Silent inactivation: switch to *Erwinia* preparation	Same

the *E. coli* enzyme and approximates 8.6 for the *Erwinia* protein; and the K_m (Michaelis-Menten constant) for asparagine is 1 to 2 × 10^{-5} mol/L for the *E. coli* enzyme, and 3 to 4 × 10^{-5} for the *Erwinia* protein.[13,14]

The sequence and crystal structure of the *E. coli* enzyme have been solved.[15] The enzyme has only a 46% homology with the *Erwinia chrysanthemi* enzyme; the two enzymes lack antigenic cross-reactivity and differ in biochemical properties. For example, ammonia activates *E. coli* asparaginase, whereas oxygen represses its synthesis; neither affects the *Erwinia* enzyme.[16] The Erwinia enzyme has greater glutaminase activity.

The *E. coli* and *Erwinia* enzymes are highly specific for L-asparagine as substrates and have less relative activity, 3% and 10%, respectively, for glutamine. In contrast, the enzyme from the fungus, *Saccharomyces cerevisiae*, also the subject of pharmaceutical interest, has less affinity and catalytic velocity for asparagine than do the bacterial enzymes, but much reduced glutaminase activity, and reduced antitumor potential.[17] The role of glutamine depletion in enhancing the antitumor activity or contributing to the toxicity of L-ASP preparations is unclear. Cells with high levels of L-ASPS require glutamine as the source of the amino group transferred to aspartate to form asparagine. Glutamine depletion enhances cytotoxicity in cells dependent on L-ASPS activity, but not in cells lacking L-ASPS.[18]

It should be noted that the relevance of cell culture experiments is questionable, as drugs that possess L-ASPA and glutaminase activities produce toxic levels of glutamate, aspartate, and ammonia in the culture medium. These by-products would diffuse into the blood stream in vivo.

While the balance of evidence suggests that glutamine depletion contributes little to the antitumor activity of L-ASPA, it may impair L-ASPA efficacy in vivo. Glutamine allosterically enhances asparaginase activity at low substrate concentrations[12]; therefore, preserving glutamine in plasma may be important in enhancing L-ASPA activity and reaching crucial levels of asparagine depletion. Regarding toxicity, pure glutaminase preparations have been tested clinically and produce high ammonia levels and altered cognitive dysfunction; the hydrolysis of glutamine may contribute to these side effects in the clinical use of bacterial L-ASPA.

The hydrolysis of L-asparagine proceeds according to a reaction mechanism that involves an initial displacement of the amino acid NH$_2$ group during the formation of an enzyme-aspartyl intermediate, followed by hydrolytic cleavage of the latter bond to generate free L-aspartate and active enzyme. The reaction may be summarized as E + Asn ↔ NH$_3$ E • Asp → E + Asp + NH$_3$, where E • Asp represents the enzyme-aspartyl intermediate.[19] A specific threonine in the enzyme catalyzes the nucleophilic attack and displacement of the amide group on the L-asparaginase molecule.

The reaction is irreversibly inhibited by the L-asparagine analog 5-diazo-4-oxo-l-norvaline, which binds covalently to the enzyme's active site.[20]

Cellular Pharmacology

L-ASPA owes its antitumor effects to the rapid and near complete depletion of circulating pools of L-asparagine. Intensive therapy with L-ASPA is critical for the cure of both the common pre-B ALL in children as well as in the effective treatment of the less common T-cell lymphoblastic ALL in adolescents and adults.[21] NK/T-cell lymphoid tumors also display sensitivity to L-ASP.[22] Plasma L-asparagine levels (usually in the range of 4×10^{-5} mol/L) are more than sufficient for L-asparagine–requiring tumor cells, which can grow at a normal rate in tissue culture medium containing 1×10^{-6} mol/L asparagine.[23] Because the K_m of the E. coli enzyme for L-asparagine is 1×10^{-5} mol/L, the hydrolysis of plasma L-asparagine proceeds at less than maximal velocity once levels fall below the K_m, and considerable excess L-ASPA (estimated to be >0.1 IU/mL)[24] is required in plasma to degrade L-asparagine sufficiently to halt tumor growth. *Plasma concentrations of asparagine are not a useful target, as hydrolysis of asparagine continues in the plasma sample after a blood draw, even during refrigeration.*

The cellular effects of L-ASPA result from asparagine depletion and inhibition of protein synthesis. Cytotoxicity correlates well with inhibition of protein synthesis. Inhibition of nucleic acid synthesis is also observed in sensitive cells but is believed to be secondary to the block in protein synthesis. Cells insensitive to asparagine depletion from growth medium in vitro are also insensitive to L-ASPA and show little inhibition of protein synthesis in the presence of the enzyme. These resistant cells tend to have high endogenous activity of L-aspS, although expression levels of this enzyme are an imperfect biomarker for L-ASPA sensitivity (see below).[25] Cell death is dependent upon the activation of programmed cell death, or apoptosis, as suggested by both in vitro and in vivo experiments.[26]

Resistance to L-Asparaginase

Resistance emerges rapidly when L-ASPA is employed as a single agent, both in animal tumor systems and in humans. Cell culture experiments and cells taken from resistant leukemia patients demonstrated elevated levels of L-ASPS, indicating that drug exposure leads to the selection of cells that up-regulate the synthesis of asparagine in the presence of the enzyme.[27] A low or absent expression of L-aspS in ALL cells has been attributed to hypermethylation of the promoter of the L-aspS gene. Up-regulation occurs with hypomethylation of these promoter sequences.[28] However, the role of up-regulation of L-AspS expression (mRNA levels) in clinical resistance is still unclear. The gene is expressed at very low levels in most ALL cells at baseline, but increases modestly and inconsistently during treatment according to prospective trials in human ALL.[29] Adding to further ambiguity, mRNA levels in tumor cells may not accurately reflect enzyme protein levels and enzyme activity in vivo. Further, not all tumors with high L-ASPS activity, such as leukemias with (12:21) TEL/AML1 translocation, are resistant to L-ASPA.[25] While definitive studies on the role of L-ASPS are not yet available, other resistance mechanisms in ALL have been reported,

including up-regulation of glutamine transport and synthesis, variants of L-ASPS with greater activity, and alterations in the apoptotic pathway, and increased provision of asparagine from cells in the tumor microenvironment.[30] In clinical practice, the development of neutralizing antibodies, often in the absence of hypersensitivity symptoms, (so-called silent hypersensitivity),[30] is another common source of resistance.

Chemical Modification and Alternative Sources of Enzyme

Attempts to eliminate the L-glutaminase function have been unsuccessful, as the products lacking this activity have in general had reduced asparaginase activity.[17] In an attempt to reduce the immunogenicity of L-ASPA, eliminate L-glutaminase activity from the molecule, and prolong the enzyme's plasma half-life, the E. coli asparaginase has been chemically modified. The E. coli enzyme conjugated with monomethoxypolyethylene glycol (PEG) displays decreased immunogenicity and a 5-fold increase in plasma half-life (6 days) and retains 50% of its unmodified catalytic activity.[31] Pegaspargase (P-ASPA) is nonimmunogenic in about 70% of patients hypersensitive to the native enzyme. Because of its longer t½, P-ASPA is given in 8- to 10-fold lower doses (2,500 IU/m²), every 2 weeks, and has largely replaced native E. coli enzyme (20,000 IU/m² weekly) for first-line induction treatment of ALL, with equivalent antitumor results.[32] The Erwinia enzyme (20,000 to 25,000 IU/m² weekly) is reserved for use in patients who have hypersensitivity reactions to or silently inactivate the E. coli preparations, but must be used in high doses because of its short t½ of 15 hours. Therapeutic results for patients who are switched midcourse to the Erwinia enzyme are equivalent to the results of patients receiving only P-ASPA.[33]

The in vivo clearance rate of the enzyme and its K_m are two important factors that may play roles in determining the efficacy of asparaginase preparations. Catalytically active L-ASPAs from other bacterial or fungal sources in general have lower substrate affinity and are more rapidly cleared from the circulation in mice, while enzymes from E. coli and Erwinia have high affinity, exhibit longer t½ s, and have greater antitumor activity.[17,34,35]

Clinical Pharmacology

Pharmacokinetics

L-ASPA is readily measured in biologic fluids by a coupled enzymatic assay.[36] The drug is given intramuscularly (IM), or intravenously (IV); IM produces peak plasma levels 50% lower than IV, but IV administration may be less immunogenic, although data are inconclusive on this point.[36] For the native E. coli enzyme, the usual dosages are 25,000 IU/m² once weekly, or 5,000 to 10,000 IU/m² every other day or every 3rd day during induction, with variable dosing and schedules during consolidation. The enzyme level in the plasma required to inhibit tumor cell proliferation is uncertain. L-ASP is detectable in the bloodstream about 11 days after large single doses of the native E. coli enzyme (25,000 IU/m²) and 18 days for P-ASPA.

Most current protocols aim to exceed a nadir of 0.1 IU/mL prior to the next dose. Serum asparagine levels are difficult to measure and interpret due to ongoing enzyme activity in stored blood.

Blood samples collected and stored in the presence of an L-ASPA inhibitor, such as 5-diazo-4-oxo-l-norvaline, may provide more accurate measurements of asparagine.[37]

After intravenous administration, the enzyme distributes primarily within the intravascular space and is degraded in the reticuloendothelial system. The drug penetrates poorly into the cerebrospinal fluid (CSF); concentration of asparagine recovers rapidly, and a weak antileukemic effect is exerted in this sanctuary.[38]

The concentration of native L-ASPA in plasma is proportional to dose in the clinical dose range and has a primary half-life of 30 hours.[39] The *Erwinia* enzyme, although preserving activity in patients hypersensitive to the *E. coli* preparation, has the disadvantage of a shorter half-life in plasma (15 hours).[39] Escalation of the dosage of *Erwinia* enzyme to 20,000 IU/m^2 3 d/wk is recommended to maintain continuous asparagine depletion and equivalent antitumor effects.[40]

Covalent linkage of L-ASPA with PEG, producing P-ASPA, has markedly reduced the clearance of the enzyme, whereas the volume of distribution remains roughly equivalent to the average plasma volume in humans. In plasma, P-ASPA, with a plasma $t\frac{1}{2}$ of 6 days, has a slow total body clearance of 5.3 ± 3.1 mL/h/m^2, and the apparent volume of distribution is 2.1 ± 0.6 L/m^2.[41] The recommended dosage of P-ASPA is 2,500 U/m^2 every 2 weeks, resulting in plasma L-ASPA activity of more than 0.1 IU/mL for 18 days. In patients who develop neutralizing antibodies to the native enzyme, clearance is greatly accelerated, and enzyme may be undetectable in plasma within 4 hours of administration, "silent inactivation."[30,42]

Toxicity

The primary toxicities of L-ASPA fall into two main groups: those related to immunologic sensitization to the foreign protein and those resulting from depletion of asparagine pools and synthesis.

Hypersensitivity and Enzyme Inactivation

Hypersensitivity reactions to L-ASPA are of great concern because they are common, they are associated with L-ASPA inactivation, and they are potentially fatal. Reactions are more frequent when the drug is used as a single agent. Up to 40% of patients receiving single-agent treatment develop evidence of sensitization. Possibly because of the immunosuppressive effect of corticosteroids, 6-mercaptopurine, and other antileukemic agents, the incidence of hypersensitivity reactions falls to less than 20% in patients receiving combination chemotherapy. Other factors that increase the incidence of reactions include doses above 6,000 IU/m^2/d, possibly IV versus IM administration, repeated courses of treatment, and increasing age of patients.[30] Reactions to an initial dose rarely occur; more commonly, hypersensitivity appears during the second week of treatment or later. A gene variant (HSP B*1) in an HLA II allele has been implicated as increasing risk of allergy in about 4% of allergic patients.[43]

Clinical manifestations of hypersensitivity are an important indicator of enzyme inactivation, and include urticaria (approximately two thirds of reported reactions), dyspnea, or full-blown anaphylactic reactions (hypotension, laryngospasm, and cardiac arrest). Rarely, serum sickness–type responses—with arthralgias, proteinuria, and fever—may develop several weeks after treatment.[44] Fatal reactions occur in less than 1% of patients treated, but evidence

of hypersensitivity should prompt a change in treatment to L-ASPA derived from *Erwinia*. Allergic reactions to *Erwinia* L-ASPA may occur in patients who have not previously received *E. coli* enzyme[45] and may ultimately develop in 5% to 20% of patients receiving multiple courses of this enzyme. P-ASPA can also be used in patients hypersensitive to native *E. coli* L-ASPA, but 30% will be hypersensitive to the new drug. Silent enzyme inactivation by neutralizing antibodies occurs in 5% to 10% of patients, and is linked to an increased risk of failure of therapy if undetected.[30,42] Consensus recommendations for monitoring serum L-ASPA are given in Table 18.2.

Because of the frequency and severity of allergic reactions to L-ASPA, routine skin testing was formerly employed for prediction of allergy before the first dose of drug. However, allergic reactions may occur in patients with negative skin tests,[46] and positive skin tests are not invariably predictive of reactions. Hypersensitive patients usually have both Ig E and Ig G antibodies to L-ASPA in serum, but more than half the patients with such antibodies do not display an allergic reaction clinically.[47] Thus, the antibody tests and skin tests have limited value for predicting which patients will have an allergic reaction. Because of concerns about hypersensitivity, personnel administering the drugs should be trained in and prepared to manage anaphylaxis. Patients should be observed for at least 1 hour after administration.

Other toxic effects result from inhibition of protein synthesis; these include hypoalbuminemia, decreased clotting factors, decreased serum insulin with hyperglycemia, and increased serum lipoproteins and triglycerides. Abnormalities in clotting function, either bleeding or more commonly thrombosis, are frequent in association with L-ASPA. Thromboembolic episodes occur in up to 10% to 20% of ALL patients, most frequently during induction therapy and when high-dose glucocorticoids are being administered concurrently.[48] Hemorrhagic events occur less frequently (1% to 2% of ALL patients) and are probably secondary to decreased synthesis of vitamin K–dependent factors, with prolongation of the prothrombin time, partial thromboplastin time, and thrombin time.[49] Platelets from L-ASPA–treated subjects display deficient

---

TABLE

18.2 *Recommendation for monitoring serum L-ASPA level to detect antibody-mediated inactivation[42]*

- All patients should have monitoring of L-ASPA levels in serum during treatment
- Silent inactivation should be identified by to independent samples
- For P-ASPA, measure enzyme level 7 days of first dose:
- "Silent inactivation" is established by day 7 level below 0.1 IU/mL
- For native L-ASPA or *Erwinia* L-ASPA, monitor serum level at nadir prior to next dose:
- Confirm serum levels are acceptable after a gap in L-ASPA treatment, i.e., during consolidation or maintenance therapy
- Switch from P-ASPA or native L-ASPA to *Erwinia* L-ASPA if low or undetectable levels are found

From Van der Sluis IM, Vrooman LM, Pieters R, et. al. Consensus expert recommendations for identification and management of asparaginase hypersensitivity and silent activation. *Hematologica*. 2016;101:279-285. Copyright © 2016 Ferrata Storti Foundation. Reprinted by permission.

aggregation in response to collagen but respond to adenosine diphosphate, arachidonic acid, or epinephrine.[50] Instances of a spontaneous intracranial hemorrhage in children with marked hypofibrinogenemia have been reported.[51]

Thrombotic Complications

Inhibition of the synthesis of anticoagulant proteins is likely responsible for the thrombotic events, which occur in 5% to 35% of ALL patients. The higher rates are found in older, adult patients, and, anecdotally, in higher dose L-ASPA protocols. L-ASPA decreases the synthesis of antithrombin III, a physiologic anticoagulant and protease inhibitor. Circulating levels of this factor fall to 50% or less compared with levels in controls after single large doses of L-ASPA.[44] Also affected is the synthesis of vitamin K–dependent inhibitors of clotting, protein C, and its cofactor, protein S.

Thrombosis in the central nervous system (CNS) is a particularly problematic complication and a diagnostic challenge during therapy with L-ASPA. Clinically diagnosed thrombosis occurred in 1% of patients receiving 30 weeks of continuous native L-ASPA therapy in one pediatric ALL trial, but in prospective studies with careful routine imaging for CNS thrombosis, the rate is consistently higher, approaching 5%.[52] Thrombosis typically involves the transverse or sagittal sinus circulation of the brain, where it causes headache, confusion, seizures, and/or stroke symptoms. Subclinical sinus occlusions can be detected by magnetic resonance imaging in patients who present with modest complaints of headache, and undoubtedly occur more frequently than recognized clinically. Catheter-related venous thrombosis is the most frequent clotting complication and may give rise to superior vena cava or internal jugular vein thrombosis.[53]

Prothrombotic abnormalities (ATIII, factor S or C deficiency) in a Caucasian population are found in patients receiving L-ASPA. Replacement of ATIII in those deficient or prophylactic anticoagulation for patients at high risk may be effective in reducing the incidence, but results with or without heparin or ATIII replacement to date are not definitive.[54–57] Routine low molecular weight heparin prophylaxis has not reduced the rate of symptomatic venous thrombosis.[54] Since heparin effect depends on the level of ATIII, it may be ineffective when used alone in patients receiving L-ASPA and deficient in ATIII. In an attempt to prevent thrombosis, pilot trials have used prophylactic replacement of ATIII in children undergoing L-ASP treatment[55,56] and have reported fewer thrombotic episodes in the small numbers of children thus treated. Combined heparin and ATIII was modestly more effective than ATIII alone (0 versus 12.7%) in an underpowered study in childhood ALL. Larger, more definitive trials of prophylactic anticoagulants, in trials using current high doses of L-ASPA, and examining alternative anticoagulants such as direct thrombin inhibitors, are needed.[55]

For persons who have had a thrombotic event on L-ASPA, prophylactic anticoagulation with low molecular weight heparin and replacement of ATIII if deficient (<60% of normal) are recommended.[55] With this approach, repeated episodes of thrombosis are uncommon.

A careful family history of hypercoagulability should be obtained prior to the initiation of L-ASPA therapy, with consideration given to obtaining laboratory tests to screen for prothrombotic conditions (such as factor V Leiden; ATIII, protein C or S deficiency; elevated factor VIII:c; or prothrombin G20210A mutation).[55]

Other Toxicities

Other toxicities are not as clearly related to the drug's mode of action. Cerebral dysfunction with confusion, stupor, or frank coma occurs as an infrequent complication. Clinically, this syndrome can resemble ammonia toxicity and has, in some cases, been associated with elevated serum ammonia levels and attributed to glutaminase activity.[58] Mental status changes may represent incompletely evaluated cortical sinus thrombosis, which can be visualized by MRI.[59]

Acute pancreatitis is an infrequent, but potentially devastating, complication that occurs in 5% of patients. In most affected individuals, a transient increase in serum amylase concentration may coincide with mild nausea, vomiting, and abdominal pain, and these signs of pancreatitis quickly resolve with discontinuation of the drug. The etiology of pancreatitis is unclear, but in some cases occurs with hypertriglyceridemia, although a causal link has been questioned.[60]

L-ASPA is frequently the cause of abnormal liver function test results (30% to 60% of patients), including increased serum levels of bilirubin, serum transaminases, and alkaline phosphatase. These changes are usually mild and compatible with continued treatment, and fully reverse after therapy. Five percent to eight percent of patients will have grade 3 or 4 toxicity and will not be able to continue L-ASPA until tests normalize.[61] Liver biopsy reveals fatty metamorphosis. Gene variants may predict pancreatitis (variants of CPA2 increase risk[62] and AspS*1 may be protective).[63]

Rarely, patients receiving L-ASPA experience nausea, vomiting, and chills as an immediate reaction, but these side effects can be mitigated by administration of antiemetics, antihistamines, or corticosteroids. Close attention should be given to any symptoms indicative of allergy, as a local allergic reaction frequently heralds a subsequent life-threatening systemic hypersensitivity reaction, and enzyme inactivation. L-ASPA has no known toxicity to gastrointestinal mucosa, and minimal toxicity to bone marrow, and is thus a favorable agent for use in combination chemotherapy. Routine premedications are not recommended because they may mask allergic symptoms

Drug Interactions

The only well-established drug interaction of L-ASPA is its ability to terminate the action of methotrexate.[64] The antagonism of L-asparaginase when given before methotrexate is possibly the result of inhibition of protein synthesis, with consequent prevention of cell entry into the vulnerable S phase of the cell cycle. An alternative explanation for antagonism is derived from the inhibition of methotrexate polyglutamylation by L-asparaginase pretreatment,[65] with decreased retention of methotrexate by tumor cells. L-ASPA may accelerate the clearance of other drugs, including dexamethasone, as a result of its depression of the serum albumin concentration and decreased protein binding of drug.[66]

L-ASPA suppresses immune function in animals and may contribute to higher rates of infection in L-ASPA–treated patients, as reported in ALL trials in which patients were randomized to receive or not receive high doses of E. coli L-ASPA.[67] Hyperglycemia, hypoalbuminemia, and catheter-related thrombosis in patients treated with the drug may also contribute to the risk of infection.

References

1. Vander Heiden MG, Cantley LC, Thompson CB. Understanding the Warburg effect: the metabolic requirements of cell proliferation. *Science.* 2009;324:1029-1033.

2. Medeiros BC, Fathi AT, DiNardo CD, et al. Isocitrate dehydrogenase mutations in myeloid malignancies. *Leukemia.* 2017;31:272-281.

3. Haskell CM, Canellos GP, Leranthal BG, et al. L-asparaginase: therapeutic and toxic effects in patients with neoplastic disease. *N Engl J Med.* 1969;281:1028-1034.

4. Kidd JG. Regression of transplanted lymphomas induced in vivo by means of normal guinea pig serum, I: course of transplanted cancers of various kinds in mice and rats given guinea pig serum, horse serum, or rabbit serum. *J Exp Med.* 1953;98:565-582.

5. Broome JD. Evidence that the L-ASP of guinea pig serum is responsible for its antilymphoma effects, I: properties of the L-ASP of guinea pig serum in relation to those of the antilymphoma substance. *J Exp Med.* 1963;118:99-120.

6. Hill JM, Loeb E, MacLellan P. Response to highly purified L-ASP during therapy of acute leukemia. *Cancer Res.* 1969;29:1574-1580.

7. Ohnuma T, Holland JF, Meyer P. *Erwinia carotovora* asparaginase in patients with prior anaphylaxis to asparaginase from *E. coli. Cancer.* 1972;30:376-381.

8. Rizzari C. Still trying to pick the best asparaginase preparation. *Lancet Oncol.* 2015;16:1580-1581.

9. Dinndorf PA, Gootenberg J, Cohen MH, et al. FDA drug approval summary: pegaspargase (oncaspar) for the first-line treatment of children with acute lymphoblastic leukemia (ALL). *Oncologist.* 2007;12:991-998.

10. Ho PK, Milikin EB, Bobbitt JL, et al. Crystalline L-ASP from *E. coli* B: purification and chemical characterization. *J Biol Chem.* 1970;245:3708-3715.

11. Gilbert HJ, Blazaek R, Bullman HMS, et al. Cloning and expression of the *Erwinia chrysanthemi* asparaginase gene in *Escherichia coli* and *Erwinia carotovora. J Gen Microbiol.* 1986;132(1):151-160.

12. Nyugen HA, Su Y, Lavie A. Structural insights into substrate selectivity of *Erwinia chrysanthemi*-sparaginase. *Biochemistry.* 2016;55:1246-1253.

13. Minton NP, Bullman HMS, Scawen MD, et al. Nucleotide sequence of the *Erwinia chrysanthemi* NCPPB 1066 L-asparaginase gene. *Gene.* 1986;46:25-35.

14. Swain AL, Jaskolski M, Housset D, et al. Crystal structure of *Escherichia coli* L-ASP, an enzyme used in cancer therapy. *Proc Natl Acad Sci U S A.* 1993;90:1474-1478.

15. Michalska K, Jaskolski M. Structural aspects of L-asparaginases, their friends and relations. *Acta Biochim Pol.* 2006;53:627-640.

16. Wade HE, Robinson HK, Phillips BW. L-ASP and glutaminase activities of bacteria. *J Gen Microbiol.* 1971;69:299-312.

17. Costa IM, Schltz L, de Araujo Bianchi Pedra B, et al. Recombinant L-asparaginase 1 from *Saccharomyces cerevisiae*: an allosteric enzyme with antineoplastic activity. *Sci Rep.* 2016;6:36239. doi:10.1038/srep36239.

18. Chan WK, Lorenzi PL, Anishkin A, et al. The glutaminase activity of L-asparaginase is not required for anticancer activity against ASNS-negative cells. *Blood.* 2014;123:3521-2532.

19. Dunlop PC, Meyer GM, Roon RJ. Reactions of asparaginase II of *Saccharomyces cerevisiae*: a mechanistic analysis of hydrolysis and hydroxylaminolysis. *J Biol Chem.* 1980;255:1542-1546.

20. Lachman LB, Handschumacher RE. The active site of L-asparaginase: dimethylsulfoxide effect of 5-diazo-4-oxo-l-norvaline interactions. *Biochem Biophys Res Commun.* 1976;73:1094-1100.

21. Barry E, DeAngelo DJ, Neuberg D, et al. Favorable outcome for adolescents with acute lymphoblastic leukemia treated on Dana-Farber Cancer Institute Acute Lymphoblastic Leukemia Consortium Protocols. *J Clin Oncol.* 2007;25:813-819.

22. Yong W. Clinical study of l-asparaginase in the treatment of L-asparaginase in the treatment of extranodal NK/T-cell lymphoma, nasal type. *Hematol Oncol.* 2016;34:61-68.

23. Amylon MD, Shuster J, Pullen J, et al. Intensive high-dose asparaginase consolidation improves survival for pediatric patients with T cell acute lymphoblastic leukemia and advanced stage lymphoblastic lymphoma: a Pediatric Oncology Group study. *Leukemia.* 1999;13:335-342.

24. Haley EE, Fischer GA, Welch AD. The requirement for L-asparagine of mouse leukemia cells L5178Y in culture. *Cancer Res.* 1961;21:532-536.

25. Stams WAG, Den Boer ML, Beverloo HB, et al. Sensitivity to L-asparaginase is not associated with expression levels of asparagine synthetase in t(12;21) pediatric ALL. *Blood.* 2003;101:2743-2747.

26. Story MD, Voehringer DW, Stephens LC, et al. L-ASP kills lymphoma cells by apoptosis. *Cancer Chemother Pharmacol.* 1993;32:129-133.

27. Haskell CM, Canellos GP. L-ASP resistance in human leukemia-asparagine synthetase. *Biochem Pharmacol.* 1969;18:2578-2580.

28. Ren Y, Roy S, Ding YT, et al. Methylation of the asparagine synthetase promoter in human leukemia cell lines is associated with a specific methyl binding protein. *Oncogene.* 2004;23:3953-3961.

29. Lanvers-Kaminsky C. Asparagine pharmacology: challenges still to be faced. *Cancer Chemother Pharmacol.* 2017;79:439-450.

30. Chien W-W, Beaux C, Rachinel N, et al. Differential mechanisms of asparaginase resistance in B-type acute lymphoblastic leukemia and malignant natural killer cell lines. *Sci Rep.* 2015;5:8068-8076.

31. Holleman A, Den Boer ML, Kazemier KM, et al. Resistance to different classes of drugs is associated with impaired apoptosis in childhood acute lymphoblastic leukemia. *Blood.* 2003;102:4541-4546.

32. Place AD, Stevenson KE, Vrooman LM, et al. Intravenous pegylated asparaginase versus intramuscular native *Escherichia coli* L-asparaginase in newly diagnosed childhood acute lymphoblastic leukemia (DFCI 05-001): a randomized, open-label phase 3 trial. *Lancet Oncol.* 2015;16(16):1677-1690.

33. Ko RH, Jones TL, Radvinsky D, et al. Allergic reactions and antiasparaginase antibodies in children with high-risk acute lymphoblastic leukemia: a children's oncology group report. *Cancer.* 2015;121:4205-4211.

34. Broome JD. Factors which may influence the effectiveness of L-ASPs as tumor inhibitors. *Br J Cancer.* 1968;22:595-602.

35. Asselin BL. The three asparaginases: comparative pharmacology and optimal use in childhood leukemia. *Adv Exp Med Biol.* 1999;456:621-629.

36. Cooney DA, Capizzi RI, Handschumacher RE. Evaluation of L-asparagine metabolism in animals and man. *Cancer Res.* 1970;30:929-935.

37. Asselin BL, Lorenson MY, Whitin JC, et al. Measurement of serum L-asparagine in the presence of L-ASP requires the presence of an L-ASP inhibitor. *Cancer Res.* 1991;51:6568-6573.

38. Hawkins DS, Park JR, Thomson BG, et al. Asparaginase pharmacokinetics after intensive polyethylene glycol-conjugated L-asparaginase therapy for children with relapsed acute lymphoblastic leukemia. *Clin Cancer Res.* 2004;10:5335-5341.

39. Asselin BL, Whitin JC, Coppola DJ, et al. Comparative pharmacokinetic studies of three asparaginase preparations. *J Clin Oncol.* 1993;11:1780-1786.

40. Otten J, Suciu S, Lutz P, et al. The importance of L-ASP (A'ASE) in the treatment of acute lymphoblastic leukemia in children: results of the EORTC 58881 randomized phase trial showing greater efficiency of *Escherichia coli* as compared to *Erwinia* A'ASE (abstract). *Blood.* 1996;88(Suppl 1):669. Abstract 2663.

41. Ho DH, Brown NS, Yen A, et al. Clinical pharmacology of polyethylene glycol-L-ASP. *Drug Metab Dispos.* 1986;14:349-352.

42. Van der Sluis IM, Vrooman LM, Pieters R, et al. Consensus expert recommendations for identification and management of asparaginase hypersensitivity and silent activation. *Hematologica.* 2016;101:279-285.

43. Fernandez CA, Smith C, Yang W, et al. *HLA-DRB!*07.01* is associated with a higher risk of asparaginase allergies. *Blood.* 2014;124:1266-1276.

44. Wacker P, Land VJ, Camitta BM, et al. Allergic reactions to *E. coli* L-asparaginase do not affect outcome in childhood B-precursor acute lymphoblastic leukemia: a Children's Oncology Group Study. *J Pediatr Hematol Oncol.* 2007;29:627-632.

45. Landd VJ, Sutow WW, Fernbach DJ, et al. Toxicity of L-asparaginase in children with advanced leukemia. *Cancer.* 1972;40:339-347.

46. Khan A, Hill JM. Atopic hypersensitivity to L-ASP. *Int Arch Allergy.* 1971;40:463-469.

47. Killander D, Dohlwitz A, Engstedt L, et al. Hypersensitive reactions and antibody formation during L-ASP treatment of children and adults with acute leukemia. *Cancer.* 1976;37:220-228.

48. Nowak-Gottl U, Ahlke E, Fleischhack G, et al. Thromboembolic events in children with acute lymphoblastic leukemia (BFM protocols): prednisone versus dexamethasone administration. *Blood.* 2003;101:2529-2533.

49. Ramsay NKC, Coccia PF, Krivit W, et al. The effect of L-asparaginase on plasma coagulation factors in acute lymphoblastic leukemia. *Cancer.* 1977;40:1398-1401.

50. Shapiro RS, Gerrard JM, Ramsay NK, et al. Selective deficiency in collagen-induced platelet aggregation during L-asparaginase therapy. *Am J Pediatr Hematol Oncol.* 1980;2(3):207-212.

51. Cairo MS, Lazarus K, Gilmore RL, et al. Intracranial hemorrhage and focal seizures secondary to use of L-ASP during induction therapy of acute lymphocytic leukemia. *J Pediatr.* 1980;97:829-833.

52. Payne JH, Vora AJ. Thrombosis and acute lymphoblastic leukemia. *Brit J Haematol.* 2007;138:430-445.

53. Sills RH, Nelson DA, Stockman JA III. L-ASP-induced coagulopathy during therapy of acute lymphocytic leukemia. *Med Pediatr Oncol.* 1978;4:311-313.

54. Sibai H, Seki JT, Wang TQ, et al. Venous thromboembolism prevention during asparaginase-based therapy for acute lymphoblastic leukemia. *Curr Oncol.* 2016;4:355-361.

55. Goyal G, Bhatt VR. L-asparaginase and venous thromboembolism in acute lymphocytic leukemia. *Fuutre Oncol.* 2015;11:2459-2470.

56. Silverman LB, Gelber RD, Dalton VK, et al. Improved outcome for children with acute lymphoblastic leukemia: results of Dana-Farber Consortium Protocol 91-01. *Blood.* 2001;97:1211-1218.

57. Alberts SR, Bretscher M, Wiltsie JC, et al. Thrombosis related to the use of L-ASP in adults with acute lymphoblastic leukemia: a need to consider coagulation monitoring and clotting factor replacement. *Leuk Lymphoma.* 1999;32:489-496.

58. Leonard JV, Kay JDS. Acute encephalopathy and hyperammonaemia complicating treatment of acute lymphoblastic leukemia with asparaginase. *Lancet.* 1986;1:162-163.

59. Bushara KO, Rust RS. Reversible MRI lesions due to pegaspargase treatment of non-Hodgkin's lymphoma. *Pediatr Neurol.* 1997;17:185-187.

60. Raja RA, Schmeigelow K, Sorensen DN, Frndsen TL. Asparaginase-associate pancreatitis is not predicted by hypertriglyceridemia or pancreatic enzyme levels in children with acute lymphoblastic leukemia. *Pediatr Blood Cancer.* 2017;64:32-38.

61. Hijaya N, van der Sluis I. Asparaginase-associated toxicity in children with acute lymphoblastic leukemia. *Leuk Lymphoma.* 2016;57:748-757.

62. Liu C, Yang W, Devidas M, et al. Clinical and genetic risk factors for acute pancreatitis in patients with acute lymphoblastic leukemia. *J Clin Oncol.* 2016;34:2133-2140.

63. Tanfous MB, Sharif-Askari B, Ceppi F, et al. Polymorphisms of asparaginase pathway and asparaginase-related complications in children with acute lymphoblastic leukemia. *Clin Cancer Res.* 2015;21:329-334.

64. Capizzi RL. Schedule-dependent synergism and antagonism between methotrexate and L-ASP. *Biochem Pharmacol.* 1974;23:151-161.

65. Jolivet J, Cole DE, Holcenberg JS, et al. Prevention of methotrexate polyglutamate formation. *Cancer Res.* 1985;45:217-220.

66. Yang L, Panetta JC, Cai X, et al. Asparaginase may influence dexamethasone pharmacokinetics in acute lymphoblastic leukemia. *J Clin Oncol.* 2008;26:1932-1939.

67. Liang DC, Hung IJ, Yang CP, et al. Unexpected mortality from the use of *E. coli* L-ASP during remission induction therapy for childhood acute lymphoblastic leukemia: a report from the Taiwan Pediatric Oncology Group. *Leukemia.* 1999;13:155-160.

Section II
Targeted Agents

Proteasome Inhibitors

Andrew J. Yee, E. Bridget Kim, and Noopur S. Raje

The ubiquitin-proteasome pathway (UPP) is a tightly regulated process involving degradation of intracellular proteins.[1] UPP plays a major role in the cell biology and homeostasis of both normal cells and cancer cells, and alterations in this pathway may lead to cell dysfunction.[2] Enormous efforts have been conducted over the last two decades to obtain a better understanding of this process. Given that intracellular proteolytic mechanisms are ubiquitous in all cells, it is easy to understand why early investigators thought that targeting such a process in tumor cells might be challenging due to the potential for low therapeutic index and lack of tumor specificity. The FDA approval of bortezomib for the treatment of selected hematological malignancies changed this preconception. It validated the proteasome as a therapeutic target and prompted the development of novel proteasome inhibitors (PIs) such as carfilzomib and ixazomib, which are now in clinical use. Proteasome inhibitors have emerged as a landmark development for multiple myeloma, resulting in improvements in overall survival. This chapter summarizes the molecular basis, development, and clinical use of agents targeting the proteasome pathway, with a focus on their use in multiple myeloma.

Ubiquitin-Proteasome Pathway

The UPP has a major role in regulating a broad number of fundamental cellular pathways including apoptosis,[3] cell growth and proliferation,[4] DNA repair,[5] unfolded protein response (UPR),[3,6] and immune response.[7] Alterations in these pathways have been implicated in multiple diseases, particularly cancer.

Broadly speaking, the UPP consists of two major components: the ubiquitinating enzyme complex (UEC) and the degradation system (26S proteasome). Three enzymes make up the UEC, the ubiquitin-activating enzyme (E1), the ubiquitin-conjugating enzyme (E2), and the ubiquitin-conjugating ligase (E3). E1 is a generic enzyme used by the pathways regardless of the protein substrate targeted. By contrast, there are 20 to 30 different ubiquitin-conjugating enzymes (E2) and likely hundreds of E3 ligases. The ligase steps are the points where the specificity of the ubiquitination process is controlled, with most protein substrates having their own distinct ligase.[8,9] Each of these enzymes represents a potential therapeutic target offering unique ways to specifically inhibit the degradation of a very selective protein or groups of proteins. The initial step involves the binding of the UEC to the N-terminus of the target (Fig. 19.1). This enzyme complex catalyzes the covalent linkage of ubiquitin molecules to the ε-amino moieties of internal lysine residues in a processive manner. These ATP-dependent catalytic reactions eventually lead to the generation of a branched polyubiquitinated protein. This ubiquitination process is the primary means by which the cells "tag" or "earmark" specific proteins for degradation at the 26S proteasome.

The second major component of the pathway includes the proteasome (Fig. 19.2), which is composed of two structures, the 20S proteasome and the 19S regulatory subunit. Collectively they form the 26S proteasome complex.[10] The isolated 20S proteasome does not exhibit proteolytic activity in the absence of the 19S regulatory subunit. The 26S proteasome is a large structure with highly processive threonine proteolytic activity, and as a result it cleaves polypeptides at multiple sites, releasing very small peptides ranging in length from 2 to 24 amino acids.[11–13]

The 19S regulatory subunit includes multiple peptidases that disassemble and unfold the polyubiquitin conjugates. It also plays a major role in regulating and facilitating the multiple ATP-dependent processes used by the proteasome including 20S and 19S subunits assembly, protein unfolding, ubiquitination, opening of the regulatory "gate" that allows the protein to enter the 26S lumen, and the action of the isopeptidases leading to the recycling of the ubiquitin molecules.[14]

The 20S proteasome consists of four rings, each containing seven individual globular proteins. As shown in Figure 19.2, the assembly of the rings forms a central lumen through which proteins are funneled. The two outer layers of the 20S proteasome are the α-layers that anchor the 19S regulatory subunit. The two inner rings are the β-layers containing the proteolytic activity of the proteasome. The 19S subunit sits on top and bottom of the 20S subunit, controlling the entry of ubiquitinated proteins into the core of the proteasome.[14] Once the protein enters the lumen of the proteasome, the different proteases digest the protein into smaller peptides fragments. At least three different enzymatic activities have been ascribed to the β-layers, including (1) a caspase-like activity (β1) cleaving proteins near glutamate residues, (2) a trypsin-like function (β2) that cleaves proteins near lysine and arginine residues; and (3) a chymotrypsin-like function (β5) that cleaves proteins near phenylalanine, tyrosine, and tryptophan.[10,15–18]

Chemistry, Structure, and Function of Proteasome Inhibitors

Several classes of synthetic and natural products have the capacity to inhibit proteasomal activity through different mechanisms. Their structures have provided a model upon which many new analogs have been synthesized with better and more specific inhibitory

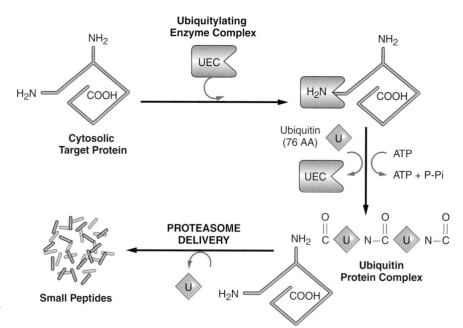

FIGURE 19.1 Schema of the ubiquitin-proteasome pathway.

effects against the 20S proteasome. Based on their inhibitory mechanisms, PIs can be functionally divided into several classes (Fig. 19.3 and Table 19.1).

Peptide Boronates

Sustained efforts to develop novel compounds with high specificity led to the identification of a new class of compounds that are synthetic reversible peptide amides and boronic acid derivatives. The two main members of this class include bortezomib and ixazomib. Bortezomib (previously known as PS-341) preferentially and reversibly inhibits the β5-mediated chymotrypsin-like and β1-mediated caspase-like activities of the proteasome through interaction between the boronic acid on bortezomib and the threonine on β5 or β1 subunits on the proteasome.[22,23] Boronates

are not inactivated by oxidation and are not influenced by the multidrug resistance system.[24] Bortezomib is the first-in-class PI approved by the FDA for the treatment of multiple myeloma (MM) and mantle cell lymphoma (MCL).[25,26] Ixazomib is the first orally active PI approved by the FDA, in combination with lenalidomide and dexamethasone, for the treatment of relapsed MM. Chemically, ixazomib citrate (MLN9708) is a dipeptidyl boronic acid that is rapidly hydrolyzed in water and converts into ixazomib (MLN2238), the active form that potently, reversibly, and selectively inhibits proteasome.[27,28] Another boronate-containing, orally bioavailable small-molecule PI is the investigational drug delanzomib (CEP-18770).[29] Delanzomib induces apoptotic cell death in MM cell lines and in primary purified CD138-positive cells from untreated and bortezomib-treated MM

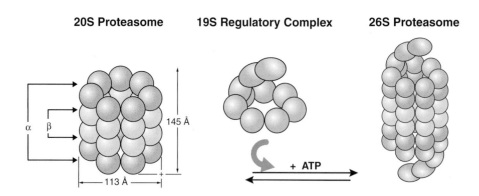

20S Proteasome   **19S Regulatory Complex**   **26S Proteasome**

145 Å

113 Å

- **STACK OF FOUR 7 MEMBERED RINGS; 700 kd; 2,000 kd**
- **700 kDa**
- **14 distinct subunits**
- **Broad substrate specificity**
- **Catalytic nucleophile: Thr of β subunit**

+ ATP

- **2,000 kDa**
- **Degrades ubiquitinated proteins**
- **Proteolysis is ATP-dependent**

FIGURE 19.2 Structure of the 26S proteasome and its assembly.

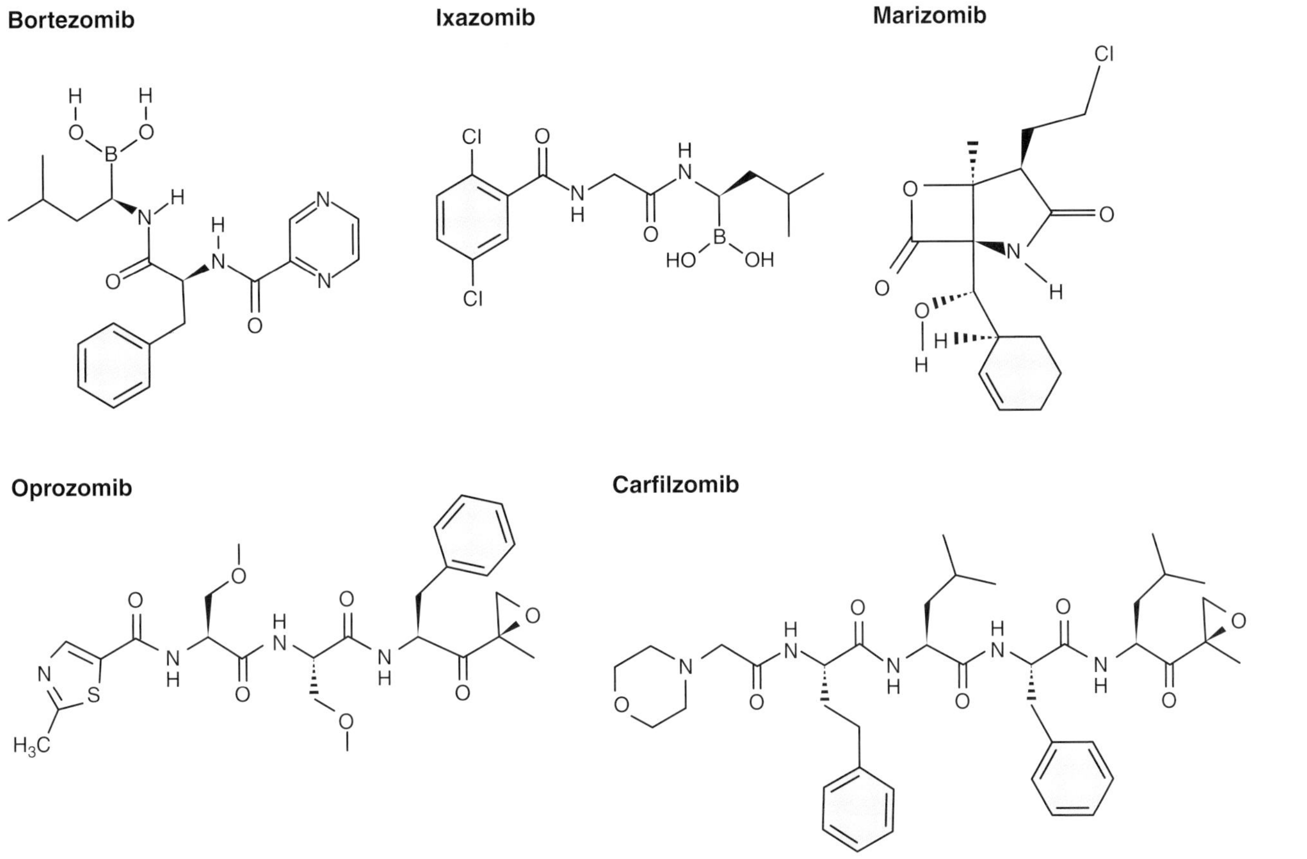

Bortezomib

Ixazomib

Marizomib

Oprozomib

Carfilzomib

FIGURE **19.3** Proteasome inhibitors in clinical use (bortezomib, ixazomib, and carfilzomib) and under development (marizomib and oprozomib).

patients. Compared to bortezomib, delanzomib exhibits a favorable cytotoxicity profile and potently represses osteoclastogenesis. However, delanzomib is no longer under development due to toxicity observed in clinical trials.[30]

β-Lactones

To this class belongs lactacystin, one of the first identified natural PI.[31] Lactacystin and its active component clasto-lactacystin are structurally complex compounds, which makes its synthesis difficult.[31-33] They have potent antitumor activity and induce cell cycle arrest in tumor cell lines.[34,35] However, lactacystin derivatives are not highly selective and inhibit several proteases, limiting their specificity and therapeutic potential. Another class member, marizomib (also known as salinosporamide A or NPI-0052) was isolated from a marine bacterium, *Salinispora tropica*.[36] Its structure is similar to clasto-lactacystin and inhibits the chymotrypsin-like activity of the proteasome more potently than other β-lactones. In contrast with bortezomib, marizomib inhibits all three activities of the proteasome (chymotrypsin-like, trypsin-like, and caspase-like activities)[37] in an irreversible manner.[38-40] Marizomib has strong synergistic activity in preclinical models[41] and is being evaluated in clinical trials.[42,43]

Epoxy Ketones

The first compounds of this class were originally isolated from an unidentified strain of actinomycete. Epoxomicin was identified and characterized as a highly specific inhibitor of the 20S proteasome.[44]

Carfilzomib is structurally related to epoxomicin and has been identified as an irreversible PI.[45] Carfilzomib has a major specificity for the chymotrypsin-like activity of the proteasome and is also more potent than bortezomib, with activity in bortezomib-resistant cells. Carfilzomib has been approved by the FDA as a single agent or as a combination therapy with either dexamethasone or lenalidomide/dexamethasone for the treatment of patients with relapsed or refractory multiple myeloma.[46-48] Oprozomib is an oral epoxyketone currently in development.

Mechanism of Action

One of the first observations suggesting that PIs could be used as anticancer agents was the early discovery that proteasome inhibition leads to inactivation of NF-κB by stabilizing IκB and preventing the translocation of NF-κB to the nucleus.[49,50] NF-κB family is composed of several members including RELA, RELB, REL (cREL), NF-κB1, and NF-κB2. These proteins form heterodimeric and homodimeric complexes, and their activities are regulated by two pathways known as the classical or canonical pathway and the alternative or non-canonical pathway.[51] In both pathways, ubiquitination and degradation of critical components lead to translocation of RELA-p50 dimers (canonical pathway) and REL-p52 and REL-p50 (non-canonical) to the nucleus followed by binding to target gene DNA.[52-55] Abnormal regulation of NF-κB and the signaling pathways that control its activity are involved in cancer development

TABLE
19-1   *Characteristics of proteasome inhibitors*

	Class	IC$_{50}$ Chymotrypsin (β5)	IC$_{50}$ Trypsin (β2)	IC$_{50}$ Caspase (β1)	Binding	Route	Use	Comments
Bortezomib	Boronate	2.4 to 7.9	590 to 4200	24 to 74	Reversible	IV/SC	Approved in MM and mantle cell lymphoma	Widely used in combinations in newly-diagnosed MM and relapsed disease. Peripheral neuropathy is the main adverse event, which is significantly less with weekly and SC dosing. Also used in AL amyloidosis.
Ixazomib	Boronate	3.4	3500	31	Reversible	PO	Approved in MM	First oral PI
Carfilzomib	Epoxyketone	6	3600	2400	Irreversible	IV	Approved in MM	More active than bortezomib in relapsed disease, but associated with increased hypertension and cardiac toxicity. Less risk of peripheral neuropathy than bortezomib.
Oprozomib	Epoxyketone	36 to 82			Irreversible	PO	Under investigation	
Marizomib	β-lactone	3.5	28	430	Irreversible	IV	Under investigation	Can cross blood brain barrier.

Table adapted from several sources.[19-21] IC$_{50}$ values (half-maximal inhibitor concentration) are in nM.

and progression.[56] NF-**κ**B activation affects all hallmarks of cancer through the transcription of genes involved in cell proliferation, angiogenesis, metastasis, inflammation, and suppression of apoptosis.[56-61] Constitutive activation of NF-**κ**B has been described in several solid tumors as well as in a number of hematological malignancies including MM.[62-64] However, further studies in MM established that bortezomib actually triggers NF-**κ**B activation via the canonical pathway but inhibits NF-**κ**B in bone marrow stromal cells.[65] This suggests that bortezomib-induced cytotoxicity in MM cells cannot be fully attributed to inhibition of canonical NF-**κ**B activity.

The endoplasmic reticulum (ER) is an organelle that has an essential role in multiple cellular processes that are required for cell homeostasis and survival. ER stress (ERS), a condition typically associated with accumulation of misfolded or unfolded proteins in the lumen of the ER, triggers an evolutionarily conserved response, the unfolded protein response (UPR).[66] The response of the cell to UPR is first to adapt reestablish homeostasis by increasing the protein folding capacity of the ER.[67,68] The UPR-induced alarm refers to signal transduction events that are commonly associated with cellular stress, including activation of MAPKs, JNK, and p38 MAPK. In addition, kinases responsible for activation of NF-**κ**B may be induced.[67] Finally, when the adaptive mechanisms put in place by the UPR fail to counteract the ERS, then cell death is induced through different mechanisms.[69-72] The important roles of ERS and the UPR in tumor biology make them novel therapeutic targets in cancer. Bortezomib induces ERS-mediated apoptosis and cell cycle arrest across a range of tumors cells, especially MM cells.[73-77]

Interestingly, ERS has also been implicated in the antitumor effects of cisplatin and the heat shock protein 90 inhibitor geldanamycin.[78-80] Bortezomib enhances ERS induced by both compounds, resulting in increased antitumor activity in an orthotopic pancreatic cancer xenograft model.[76] Cells exposed to bortezomib form aggregates of ubiquitin-conjugated proteins, or aggresomes, in vitro and in vivo.[81] Bortezomib-induced aggresome formation may serve a cytoprotective role by allowing cells to dispose of accumulated unfolded proteins that result from proteasome dysfunction[82] and could represent a mechanism of resistance to bortezomib. Notably, bortezomib-induced aggresome formation can be disrupted using histone deacetylase 6 (HDAC6) small interfering RNA or chemical HDAC inhibitors.[76,83-85] These events result in ERS and induction of apoptosis in pancreatic cancer cells, MM, and chronic myeloid leukemia.[86-88] These results provided the rationale for the development of the combination of bortezomib and the HDAC inhibitors vorinostat and later panobinostat in patients with refractory and relapsed MM patients.[89,90]

Bortezomib

Bortezomib reversibly binds to the catalytic site of the 26S proteasome, thereby inhibiting the **β**5/chymotrypsin-like and, to a lesser extent, the **β**2/trypsin-like and **β**1/caspase-like activities.[91,92] Preclinical models have extensively demonstrated that PIs have potent anticancer activities. Lactacystin induces cell death in leukemia cells at concentration of about 5 μM,[93] and bortezomib inhibits tumor growth in a broad variety of tumor models.[94-96]

Normal cells were found to be more resistant to PIs than tumor cells.[97,98] Furthermore, within the dose range of bortezomib that induces tumor growth inhibition in xenograft models, normal hematopoietic cells were not significantly affected by bortezomib. Boronate PIs have been shown to kill tumor cells in culture, as demonstrated by their activity in the tumor cell line screen.[99] Data from the NCI's algorithm COMPARE demonstrated that the mechanism of cytotoxicity of bortezomib was strikingly different from any of the other 60,000 compounds in the library. The average growth inhibition for bortezomib was 7 nM across the entire panel of cells. Cell death was noted at 20 nM for cells incubated for 24 hours with bortezomib.[99] Studies with radiolabeled bortezomib have shown that bortezomib is broadly distributed to all tissues in rats and cynomolgus monkeys, and no detectable drug could be found crossing the blood-brain barrier.[99] In vivo models of drug-resistant human myeloma have shown that a twice weekly schedule of bortezomib administration resulted both in tumor shrinkage and prolonged median survival of treated mice.[100,101]

Clinical Pharmacology

Studies on nonhuman primates have shown that after a single intravenous dose of bortezomib, plasma concentrations decline in a classic biphasic manner with a $t_{1/2}$ **α** of approximately 10 minutes.[102] The terminal elimination phase in humans has been estimated between 5 and 15 hours. Multiple doses of drug appear to result in some decrease in clearance, with a resulting increase in the terminal elimination half-life ($t_{1/2}$) and the area under the curve (AUC), but they have no effect on the estimated maximum plasma concentration (C_{max}) or distribution half-life. Similar pharmacokinetic profiles have also been observed in preclinical studies and do not appear to result in increased toxicity from accumulation of the drug with repeat dosing. The overall disposition of bortezomib is most consistent with a two-compartment pharmacokinetics (PK) model and the principal pathway of elimination is through oxidative deboronation.

Bortezomib is a substrate of cytochrome P450 enzyme 3A4, 2C19, and to a minor extent, 1A2, as demonstrated in the in vitro studies.[103] Co-administration of ketoconazole, a strong CYP3A4 inhibitor, increased bortezomib exposure by 35% in 12 patients with solid tumors, without any reported difference in the occurrence of adverse events between bortezomib plus ketoconazole and the bortezomib alone group.[104] Omeprazole, a strong inhibitor of CYP2C19, has no significant effect on the exposure of bortezomib.[105] Co-administration of a strong CYP3A4 inducer, such as rifampin, is expected to decrease the exposure of bortezomib by at least 45%, potentially reducing efficacy, as with St. John's Wort (*Hypericum perforatum*); therefore, concomitant use of a strong CYP3A4 inducer is not recommended.[105]

Bortezomib in Patients with Renal and Hepatic Dysfunction

A study by the National Cancer Institute Organ Dysfunction Group assessed the PK and pharmacodynamic profiles of bortezomib in patients with advanced malignancies and normal, mild, moderate, or severe renal insufficiency.[106] The study was designed to evaluate safety and tolerability, as well as to determine the maximum tolerated dose (MTD) of bortezomib in this patient population.

Exposure to bortezomib was comparable among all groups and was not affected by the degree of renal impairment. This includes patients with severe renal dysfunction, on dialysis. Bortezomib was also evaluated by the same group in patients with various degree of hepatic impairment who were classified according to the NCI classification of hepatic impairment.[107] Patients received bortezomib doses ranging from 0.5 to 1.3 mg/m². Patients with mild hepatic impairment did not require any dose adjustments. However, patients with moderate or severe hepatic impairment should be started a lower dose, 0.7 mg/m². Moderate and severe impairment were defined as bilirubin >1.5 and 3 × ULN, respectively.

Pharmacodynamics

Proteasome inhibition has been established as a critical pharmacodynamic endpoint for bortezomib. Bortezomib induces inhibition of the 20S proteasome in a dose-dependent manner.[108–110] The majority of the proteasome inhibition occurs within the first hour after administration and proteasome inhibition around 10% to 20% could be detected at 72 hours. This pharmacodynamic endpoint was the rationale for the scheduling of bortezomib once every 72 hours.

Multiple Myeloma

Several phase I studies explored weekly and twice-weekly intravenous bolus schedules in patients with hematological malignancies and solid tumors. Hypotension, syncope, diarrhea, and neurotoxicity were the principal dose limiting toxicities.[109,110] The key phase I study focused on hematological malignancies in 27 heavily pretreated patients.[108] The pivotal finding in this study was that among nine patients with plasma cell dyscrasias (MM and Waldenström's macroglobulinemia), one achieved a complete remission and eight other patients demonstrated a major reduction in paraprotein levels and/or bone marrow plasma cells, suggesting that bortezomib was uniquely effective in MM. In addition, one of three patients with MCL achieved a durable partial remission, as did one patient with follicular lymphoma.

Based on the above responses, a series of trials confirmed drug activity in relapsed or refractory MM. This included the SUMMIT trial, a large multicenter, phase II trial of bortezomib as a single agent.[111] Patients were required to have refractory disease, and 202 patients were registered to the study. Bortezomib was administered at 1.3 mg/m² IV on days 1, 4, 8, and 11 every 21 days. In this refractory patient population with a median of six prior lines of treatment, bortezomib was effective, with an overall response rate of 35% and the median duration of response was 12 months. Adverse events (grade 3-4) included thrombocytopenia (31%), peripheral neuropathy (12%), neutropenia (14%), fatigue (12%), and anemia (8%). The frequency and severity of the diarrhea appeared to be dose dependent.

Following the SUMMIT trial, a second dose-response phase II study of bortezomib in MM was launched in a similar patient population, the CREST study,[112] with similar findings, though in patients who did not achieve at least a partial response, dexamethasone was added. In May 2003, based on the analysis of the SUMMIT and the CREST trials, the FDA granted accelerated approval to bortezomib for the treatment of MM patients who have received at least two prior therapies and have demonstrated disease progression on the last therapy.

The APEX study confirmed the efficacy of bortezomib in a randomized phase 3 trial.[113] This study assigned 669 patients with MM previously treated with at least one regimen to receive bortezomib, at a dose of 1.3 mg/m² IV on days 1, 4, 8, and 11 for eight 3-week cycles, followed by treatment on days 1, 8, 15, and 22 for three 5-week cycles versus high dose dexamethasone. The time to disease progression was significantly longer in the bortezomib arm, 6.22 months, compared to the dexamethasone arm, 3.49 months, (hazard ratio 0.55; $P < 0.001$). The ORR was 38% for bortezomib and 18% for dexamethasone ($P < 0.001$). Furthermore, treatment with bortezomib improved overall survival, 29.8 versus 23.7 months in the dexamethasone arm, even though there was significant crossover from the dexamethasone arm to the bortezomib arm.[114]

Bortezomib Combinations

In addition to its role in relapsed disease, bortezomib is now a standard component of therapy for newly-diagnosed patients. In patients who are not eligible for intensive therapy with high dose melphalan and autologous stem cell transplant, the VISTA trial showed the superiority of using bortezomib upfront.[115] In this phase III trial, investigators randomly assigned 682 patients to receive melphalan and prednisone either alone (MP) or with bortezomib (VMP). The time to progression among patients receiving VMP was 24 months compared to 16.6 months in the MP arm (HR 0.48; $P < 0.001$). Patients with a PR or better were 71% in the bortezomib group and 35% in the control group; CR rates were 30% and 4%, respectively ($P < 0.001$). An updated analysis of the trial showed a 31% reduced risk of death with VMP, with a median OS of 56.4 versus 43.1 months (HR 0.61, $P < 0.001$).[116] There were no significant differences in grade 4 events (28% and 27%, respectively) or treatment-related deaths (1% and 2%). However, grade 3 to 4 peripheral neuropathy occurred in 12.9% of patients in the bortezomib arm versus not observed in the MP group. Based on the findings in the VISTA trial, bortezomib was approved as initial therapy. Table 19.2 summarizes phase III trials using proteasome inhibitors such as bortezomib.

Bortezomib has been incorporated into induction treatment regimens used prior to autologous stem cell transplant. Motivated by in vitro data showing synergistic activity between bortezomib and the immunomodulatory drug lenalidomide,[121] bortezomib has been combined with lenalidomide and dexamethasone (RVD) in newly diagnosed patients and achieved, at the time, an unprecedented overall response rate of 100% in a phase II trial.[122] A recent phase III trial, SWOG S0777, confirmed this finding, demonstrating superior outcomes when bortezomib was added to lenalidomide and dexamethasone (RVD) compared to the standard of lenalidomide and dexamethasone (Rd).[117] RVD improved both progression free survival (PFS) 43 versus 30 months ($P = 0.0018$) and median overall survival 75 versus 64 months ($P = 0.025$). RVD is now a standard front-line regimen in the U.S. Other widely used combinations in newly diagnosed patients include combination of bortezomib with thalidomide and dexamethasone (VTD).[123] and (CyBorD).[124] A meta-analysis of several phase III trials showed that bortezomib-based inductions regimens compared to non-bortezomib regimens had superior response rates (post transplant near complete response rate or better, 38% versus 24%), median progression

TABLE
19.2   *Selected phase III trials of proteasome inhibitor in multiple myeloma*

Reference	Name of Trial	No. Prior Lines	Arm	N	PFS	HR	ORR (%)	≥VGPR (%)	≥CR (%)
San Miguel et al.[115]	VISTA	Newly diagnosed	VMP	344	24*	0.48	71		30
			MP	338	16.6		35		4
Durie et al.[117]	SWOG S0777	Newly diagnosed	VRd	264	43	0.712	82	28	16
			Rd	261	30		72	23	8
Richardson et al.[113]	APEX	≥1	V	333	6.22*	0.55	38		6
			D	336	3.49		18		1
San Miguel et al.[90]	PANORAMA 1	1 to 3	Pano-Vd	387	11.99	0.63	60.7		11
			Vd	381	8.08		54.6		6
Stewart et al.[48]	ASPIRE	1 to 3	KRd	396	26.3	0.69	87	70	32
			Rd	396	17.6		67	40	9
Dimopoulos et al.[118]	ENDEAVOR	1 to 3	Kd	464	18.7	0.53	77	54	13
			Vd	465	9.4		63	29	6
Moreau et al.[119]	TOURMALINE-MM1	1 to 3	IRd	360	20.6	0.74	78	48	12
			Rd	362	14.7		72	39	7
Palumbo et al.[120]	CASTOR	≥1	Vd-dara	251	NE	0.39	82.9	59.2	19.2
			Vd	247	7.2		63.2	29.1	9

D, dexamethasone; dara, daratumumab; I, ixazomib; K, carfilzomib; M, melphalan; P, prednisone; pano, panobinostat, R, lenalidomide; V, bortezomib.
*Time to progression.

free survival (35.9 28.6 months), and 3 year overall survival (79.7% versus 74.7%).[125] Bortezomib has also shown efficacy as maintenance therapy after autologous stem cell transplant.[126]

In addition to the synergism observed with immunomodulatory drugs like thalidomide and lenalidomide, bortezomib also adds to the effect of anthracyclines. The basis of this particular synergistic interaction is the observation that PIs transcriptionally induce the mitogen-activated protein kinase phosphatase-1 (MKP-1) phosphatases, a process that is anti-apoptotic through its inactivation of JNK, while anthracyclines like doxorubicin appear to downregulate MKP-1.[127,128] A phase III randomized study compared the combination of pegylated liposomal doxorubicin (PegLD; Doxil) plus bortezomib with bortezomib monotherapy in patients with relapsed or refractory MM.[129] Median time to progression was increased from 6.5 months for bortezomib to 9.3 months with the PegLD-bortezomib combination ($P = 0.000004$). The 15-month survival rate for PegLD-bortezomib was 76% compared with 65% for bortezomib alone ($P = 0.03$). The combination therapy was associated with a higher incidence of grade 3 to 4 myelosuppression, constitutional symptoms, and other toxicities such as hand-foot syndrome.

Histone deacetylase (HDAC) inhibitors such as vorinostat and now panobinostat are an important new class of drugs in oncology,[130] and bortezomib synergizes with this class of drugs. By increasing histone acetylation, HDAC inhibition leads to modulation of chromatin structure, transcriptional activation and other nuclear events (see Chapter 16). There are several classes of HDACs, and there are also non-histone substrates of HDACs in the cytoplasm through which HDAC inhibitors have additional effects. In MM, preclinical work with proteasome and HDAC inhibitors showed synergistic activity by disrupting proteasomal and aggresomal protein degradation

systems, leading to accumulation of polyubiquitinated proteins and activation of apoptosis.[87,131] This finding set the stage for the clinical development of HDAC inhibitors in MM as combination therapy, beginning with vorinostat and then panobinostat (LBH589), which are both pan HDAC inhibitors. Panobinostat is now approved for the treatment of relapsed MM, based on the results of PANORAMA-1, a phase III trial comparing panobinostat, bortezomib, and dexamethasone to bortezomib and dexamethasone in patients with 1 to 3 prior lines of therapy.[90] When panobinostat was evaluated in patients who received prior treatment with both bortezomib and an immunomodulatory drug and a median of two prior therapies, the median PFS was 10.6 months in the panobinostat arm versus 5.8 months in the control arm, and the ORR was also higher, 59% v 41%, respectively. However, significant adverse events included diarrhea and cardiac events such as arrhythmias in the panobinostat arm. This toxicity has motivated development of selective HDAC6 inhibitors such as ricolinostat and citarinostat.[132,133]

Overall, the introduction of newer, more effective combination treatments employing the proteasome inhibitor bortezomib has transformed MM care by significantly improving overall survival following disease relapse. For example, one study found that overall survival in patients who relapsed after 2000 had an overall survival of 23.9 months compared to 11.8 months in patients who relapsed prior to this time point.[134] Similarly, overall survival in MM from time of diagnosis has improved over the years, with median OS of 6.1 years in patients diagnosed from 2006 to 2010 compared to 2.5 years in patients diagnosed before 1996,[134,135] due to the introduction of proteasome inhibitors and immunomodulatory drugs as well as use of high dose melphalan and autologous stem cell transplant. Bortezomib continues to be a backbone of regimens with newer drugs. This includes combinations with the newest immunomodulatory drug pomalidomide,[136,137] the anti-SLAMF7 monoclonal antibody elotuzumab,[138] and the anti-CD38 monoclonal antibody daratumumab.[120]

Adverse Events with Bortezomib

Peripheral neuropathy is the principal side effect of bortezomib. In the initial SUMMIT and CREST phase II trials in patients with relapsed MM, peripheral neuropathy occurred in 35% of patients, including 13% where it was grade ≥ 3.[139] Generally, the peripheral neuropathy is reversible. In the APEX study, 64% of patients had improvement or resolution to baseline at a median of 110 days, and the reversibility was higher when dose modifications were used. The effectiveness of bortezomib did not appear to be affected by these dose modifications.

With additional clinical experience, the way bortezomib is given has changed from IV to subcutaneously (SC). This change was motivated by a randomized study of IV versus SC administration in 222 patients with relapsed disease after 1 to 3 prior lines of treatment.[140] Peripheral neuropathy was significantly less with the SC route, with grade ≥3 neuropathy of 6% compared to 12% (*P* = 0.026) with the conventional IV route. The ORR was the same in both groups, 42%. Pharmacokinetic studies showed that systemic exposure was equivalent with either route, though the peak drug concentration was lower with the SC route.[141] Given its improved tolerability and similar efficacy, the SC route is now approved by the FDA and has become standard.

Thrombocytopenia is the most common grade 3 to 4 adverse event with bortezomib. In the APEX trial, it occurred in 30% of patients. However, unlike the thrombocytopenia seen in traditional cytotoxic chemotherapy, the thrombocytopenia with bortezomib may be due to reversible effects on megakaryocyte function rather than direct cytotoxicity and is not cumulative.[142] Bortezomib is also associated with a significantly increased risk of herpes zoster. In the APEX trial, the incidence of herpes zoster was 13% compared to 5% (*P* = 0.0002).[143] Use of acyclovir or equivalent for prophylaxis of this infection is standard practice.[144]

In addition to changes in the route of administration, there is also increasing use of weekly bortezomib, motivated by weekly schedules in the upfront setting that showed similar efficacy and improved tolerability.[145,146] Consequently, over time, the practice has shifted from the twice/week, IV, 21 day schedule to increasing use of weekly bortezomib given SC (for example, on days 1, 8, 15, 22 on a 35 day schedule).[147]

Bortezomib in Other Diseases

AL Amyloidosis

AL amyloidosis is a rare plasma cell disorder associated with deposition of amyloid fibrils composed of fragments of monoclonal light chains in organs such as the heart and kidney and may lead to cardiac dysfunction and renal failure. Bortezomib plays an important role in the treatment of AL amyloidosis. A retrospective analysis of 94 patients with AL amyloidosis treated at three centers with bortezomib (with or without dexamethasone) showed a response in 71% of patients.[148] The majority of patients (81%) had one or more prior therapies, and responses were also associated with improvement in cardiac function. Bortezomib has also been combined with

cyclophosphamide and dexamethasone, producing rapid and deep responses. Response rates were 81.4% to 94%.[149,150]

Mantle Cell Lymphoma

Based on the activity seen in the phase I study, several small single-agent phase II study of bortezomib in patients with relapsed or refractory indolent B-cell lymphoma and mantle cell lymphoma (MCL) were conducted,[151,152] with responses ranging from 41% to 54% in mantle cell lymphoma. A larger multicenter phase II evaluated 155 patients with progressive MCL previously treated with at least one prior regimen.[153] All patients received bortezomib at a dose of 1.3 mg/m² on days 1, 4, 8, and 11 of each 3-week cycle. The ORR was 31% and median response duration was 9.3 months. The activity of bortezomib on MCL appeared to be independent of the number of prior regimens. Based on this study, in December 2006, the FDA approved bortezomib for the treatment of patients with MCL who have received at least one prior treatment for their disease, and it became the first drug specifically approved for MCL.[26]

Bortezomib has also been evaluated in newly-diagnosed MCL patients. A phase III study randomized 487 patients with newly diagnosed MCL who were not eligible for autologous stem cell transplant to the conventional arm of six to eight cycles of R-CHOP versus VR-CAP.[154] In VR-CAP, the vincristine in the R-CHOP regimen is replaced by bortezomib given 1.3 mg/m² IV on days 1, 4, 8, and 11. The VR-CAP regimen showed superior progression-free survival, 24.7 versus 14.4 months (HR 0.63, *P* <0.001). Median overall survival trended towards significant improvement in the VR-CAP arm, with median overall survival not reached versus 56.3 months (HR 0.8, *P* = 0.17). The bortezomib arm had more myelosuppression, with more grade ≥3 thrombocytopenia (57% versus 6%) and grade ≥3 neutropenia (85% versus 67%). However, there was no difference in bleeding episodes between either arm. The incidence of febrile neutropenia was similar (15% versus 14%). Rates of peripheral neuropathy were comparable in both arms.

Waldenström's Macroglobulinemia

Bortezomib has also become a component of treatment for the B cell lymphoma, Waldenström's macroglobulinemia. Bortezomib has been evaluated on the conventional twice weekly[155] and weekly schedule[156] in combination with dexamethasone and rituximab (BDR). In a phase II study in newly-diagnosed patients, the BDR regimen showed an 85% response rate and median progression free survival of 42 months.[157]

Solid Tumors

While initial studies in a range of solid tumors were promising, follow up studies including combinations did not demonstrate significant efficacy for bortezomib.[158] This has been attributed to the pharmacokinetics of bortezomib and decreased availability of bortezomib to solid tumors compared to its access to the bone marrow compartment.[92]

Carfilzomib

Carfilzomib (previously known as PR-171) is a second-generation tetrapeptide epoxyketone-based, irreversible proteasome inhibitor. By covalent, irreversible binding to the proteasome, carfilzomib produces more sustained inhibition of the proteasome, as synthesis of new proteasome complexes is required to overcome its effects.[27] It is a more potent agent and has greater selectivity for chymotrypsin-like protease β5 subunit and lower affinity for trypsin- and caspase-like proteases compared to bortezomib, which binds to the proteasome reversibly and where inhibition of other serine proteases may potentially account for the greater neurotoxicity of bortezomib.[19] Carfilzomib also remains cytotoxic to some cells that are resistant to bortezomib.[27]

Clinical Pharmacology

Following repeated doses of carfilzomib at 15 and 20 mg/m^2, systemic exposure (AUC) and half-life were similar on days 1 and 15 or 16 of cycle 1, suggesting no systemic accumulation.[159] At doses between 20 and 56 mg/m^2, there is a dose-dependent increase in exposure. The mean steady-state volume of distribution of a 20 mg/m^2 dose of carfilzomib is 28 L, indicating extensive penetration of all tissues except the brain. In vitro, the binding of carfilzomib to human plasma proteins averages 97%. Carfilzomib is rapidly and extensively metabolized through peptidase cleavage and epoxide hydrolysis as the principal pathways of metabolism. There is minimal metabolism through cytochrome P450-mediated mechanisms. Carfilzomib is rapidly cleared from the systemic circulation with a half-life elimination of ≤1 hour on day 1 of cycle 1 at doses ≥15 mg/m^2. In 24 hours, approximately 25% of the administered dose of carfilzomib is recovered in urine as metabolites.

Carfilzomib is primarily metabolized extrahepatically via peptidase and epoxide hydrolase activities, and as a result, the pharmacokinetic profiles of carfilzomib is unlikely to be affected by concomitant administration of cytochrome P450 inhibitors and inducers.[159,160] As demonstrated in the in vitro studies, carfilzomib showed modest direct and time-dependent inhibition of CYP3A in human liver microsomes. The rapid systemic clearance and short half-life of carfilzomib limit clinically significant drug-drug interactions. Carfilzomib is not expected to influence exposure of other drugs.

Carfilzomib in Patients with Renal and Hepatic Dysfunction

The pharmacokinetics of carfilzomib were studied in relapsed MM patients with normal renal function; mild, moderate or severe renal impairment; and patients with end stage renal disease requiring hemodialysis.[159,161,162] Exposure of carfilzomib (AUC and C$_{max}$) in patients with mild, moderate, and severe renal impairment was similar to those with normal renal function. No initial dose adjustment is required in patients with preexisting renal impairment. Relative to patients with normal renal function, ESRD patients on hemodialysis showed 33% higher carfilzomib AUC. Carfilzomib should be administered after dialysis.

Although infrequent, cases of carfilzomib-related acute renal injuries have been reported.[163] If renal toxicity occurs during treatment (serum creatinine ≥2 times baseline, creatinine clearance <15 mL/minute or creatinine clearance decreases to ≤50% of baseline, or patient requires dialysis), it is recommended to withhold the next dose and monitor renal function. If attributable to carfilzomib, the recommendation is to resume dosing when renal function has improved to within 25% of baseline; resuming with a dose reduction of 1 level.[159]

The pharmacokinetics of carfilzomib were studied in patients with relapsed or progressive advance malignancies with varying degrees of hepatic impairment: mild (bilirubin > 1 to 1.5 × ULN or AST > ULN) or moderate (bilirubin >1.5 to 3 × ULN) chronic hepatic impairment.[164] Compared to patients with normal hepatic function, patients with mild and moderate hepatic impairment had approximately 20% to 50% higher carfilzomib AUC. These increases were felt to be unlikely to be clinically significant because of the intrinsic pharmacokinetic variability of carfilzomib.[164] For patients with mild or moderate hepatic impairment, reducing the dose by 25% may be considered.[159] The pharmacokinetics of carfilzomib has not been evaluated in patients with severe hepatic impairment (bilirubin >3 × ULN and any AST).

Pharmacodynamics

Whether the level of proteasome inhibition is a function of peak plasma levels or total exposure to carfilzomib was explored in an animal model.[165] The level of target inhibition achieved in vivo was a function of the total dose administered but not C$_{max}$. The potent proteasome inhibition in a variety of tissues also reflected rapid and wide tissue distribution of carfilzomib after a single intravenous administration.

Suppression of proteasome chymotrypsin-like (CT-L) activity was observed when measured in blood 1 hour after the first dose of intravenous carfilzomib.[159] Doses of carfilzomib ≥ 15 mg/m^2 with or without lenalidomide and dexamethasone induced a ≥80% inhibition of the CT-L activity of the proteasome. Also, proteasome inhibition was maintained for ≥48 hours following the first dose of carfilzomib for each week of dosing.

Multiple Myeloma

A phase II trial, PX-171-003, evaluated carfilzomib as a single agent in heavily pre-treated MM patients.[166] Carfilzomib was given as an infusion at 20 mg/m^2 on days 1, 2, 8, 9, 15, 16 of a 28 day cycle; with cycle 2, the dose was increased to 27 mg/m^2. Patients were required to have had two or more prior regimens and prior treatment with bortezomib and an immunomodulatory drug. The patients in this trial had received a median of 5 prior lines of treatment, and the regimen showed an ORR of 23.7%. Based on the findings of this study, the FDA approved carfilzomib in July 2012 for patients with relapsed disease and who received at least two prior therapies, including bortezomib and an immunomodulatory drug, such as lenalidomide.[167]

Unlike bortezomib, peripheral neuropathy was less common and less severe, with grade 3 to 4 neuropathy occurring in 1.1% of patients. However, toxicities that occurred more frequently in carfilzomib included cardiac failure in 7% of patients. Dyspnea was reported in 35% of patients, including 5% experiencing grade 3 dyspnea.

In patients who are refractory to bortezomib, a phase I-II trial found that replacing bortezomib with carfilzomib was safe and effective.[168] This replacement strategy was tested across multiple combinations, including carfilzomib and dexamethasone, carfilzomib with pegylated liposomal doxorubicin, and carfilzomib with cyclophosphamide and ascorbic acid. The ORR across this heterogeneous population was 43.2%, showing that the substitution of bortezomib with carfilzomib can recover responses in bortezomib-refractory disease.

The ENDEAVOR trial compared carfilzomib with bortezomib in patients with relapsed disease.[118] This phase III study randomized patients with 1 to 3 prior lines of treatment to the combination of carfilzomib and dexamethasone versus bortezomib and dexamethasone. The dosing of carfilzomib was higher than the initial studies, ramping up from 20 to 56 mg/m². Bortezomib was given according to the traditional schedule of 1.3 mg/m² on days 1, 4, 8, 11 on a 21 day cycle with dexamethasone. Bortezomib was given either IV or SC by investigator choice; most patients (79%) received SC bortezomib throughout the study. The ORR was significantly higher in the carfilzomib arm, 77% versus 63% in the bortezomib arm ($P < 0.0001$), and median PFS was also higher, 18.7 versus 9.4 months ($P < 0.0001$). Of note, while 54% of patients had prior bortezomib, in a subgroup analysis, patients who were bortezomib-naïve also showed significantly improved PFS in the carfilzomib arm. Furthermore, treatment with carfilzomib improved overall survival, with a median of 47.6 months compared to 40 months in the bortezomib arm (HR 0.791, one sided $P = 0.01$).[169]

The incidence of grade 2 or greater peripheral neuropathy was significantly higher in the bortezomib group compared to the carfilzomib group, 32% versus 6% respectively; grade 3 or higher peripheral neuropathy was 8% versus 2%. Dose reductions due to adverse events were more common in the in the bortezomib group (48%) than in the carfilzomib group (23%), which may have compromised the true efficacy of bortezomib. Even though the majority of the patients received bortezomib SC, peripheral neuropathy continued to be an ongoing finding, and the majority of the dose reductions in the bortezomib group (62%) were due to peripheral neuropathy.

Additional notable differences in toxicity between the two groups included renal dysfunction. Acute renal failure, all grades, was higher in the carfilzomib arm than the bortezomib arm, 8% versus 5%; grade 3 or higher, 4% versus 3%. Hypertension, grade 3 or higher, was seen more frequently in carfilzomib compared to bortezomib, 9% versus 3%. Cardiac failure (which included cardiac failure, decreased ejection fraction, pulmonary edema), all grades, was more frequent in the carfilzomib group compared to the bortezomib group (8.2% versus 2.9%); grade 3 or higher (4.8% versus 1.8%). Of note, in a subset of patients in whom serial echocardiograms were performed, there was no difference in the degree of reduction in left ventricular function. Endothelial dysfunction has been proposed as a potential mechanism of the cardiovascular toxicity of carfilzomib.[170,171]

Carfilzomib Combinations

The ASPIRE trial was a phase III trial that evaluated the combination of carfilzomib with lenalidomide and dexamethasone (KRd) compared to lenalidomide and dexamethasone in relapsed MM.[48] Patients were eligible to participate if they received 1 to 3 prior lines of therapy. Prior lenalidomide and bortezomib treatment were permitted if there was no disease progression with these drugs; the majority of patients (80.2%) had not received prior lenalidomide therapy. Carfilzomib was given 20 mg/m² with ramp up to 27 mg/m² on the conventional schedule. From cycles 13 to 18, the second week of carfilzomib was omitted, and after cycle 18, carfilzomib was discontinued. Lenalidomide was given 25 mg on days 1 to 21 with dexamethasone 40 mg weekly; the same schedule of lenalidomide and dexamethasone was given in the control group. The ORR was significantly higher in the carfilzomib arm compared to the control

arm, 87.1% versus 66.7% ($P < 0.001$)), and similarly the carfilzomib arm had a higher complete response rate, 31.8% versus 9.3%. The median progression free survival was 26.3 versus 17.6 months ($P = 0.001$). The depth and duration of response in the treatment arm were unprecedented at the time (though the control group also had a high response rate), and serious adverse events were uncommon. However, grade 3 to 4 dyspnea (2.8%), hypertension (4.3%), and cardiac failure (3.8%) were higher in the carfilzomib group, showing a similar toxicity profile seen in previous studies, such as the ENDEAVOR trial. In July 2015, the FDA approved carfilzomib in combination with lenalidomide and dexamethasone in relapsed MM.

Carfilzomib has also been combined with the newer immunomodulatory drug pomalidomide, along with dexamethasone. A phase I study evaluated this regimen in patients with disease refractory to prior lenalidomide treatment.[172] A total of 32 patients were enrolled; they had received a median of 6 prior lines of treatment (range 2 to 12), and 100% were refractory to lenalidomide and 97% were refractory to bortezomib. Dosing of carfilzomib was similar to the ASPIRE study, 20 mg/m² with ramp up to 27 mg/m²; pomalidomide was 4 mg on days 1 to 21; and dexamethasone was given 40 mg weekly. The maximum tolerated dose was dose level 1, likely reflecting the extensive treatment history of this patient population. Toxicities included grade ≥ 3 anemia (19%), thrombocytopenia (22%), and neutropenia (44%). The ORR was 50% with a median PFS of 7.2 months, which is notable given that all patients were refractory to lenalidomide and nearly all were refractory to bortezomib. The regimen thus showed significant activity in a heavily-pretreated, double refractory cohort, with side effect profile typical for an IMiD and PI combination.

Weekly Carfilzomib

A practical consideration for carfilzomib is the twice/week schedule, especially given that patients may be on therapy for a prolonged duration. The CHAMPION-1 trial evaluated the safety and efficacy of giving carfilzomib *weekly*.[173] This phase I/II trial enrolled patients with 1 to 3 prior lines of treatment. Carfilzomib was given as a 30 minute infusion on days 1, 8, 15 with dexamethasone. All patients received carfilzomib 20 mg/m² on day 1; patients later received 45, 56, 70, or 88 mg/m² with subsequent doses. The 70 mg/m² dose level was determined to be the MTD. Grade 3 or higher adverse events were uncommon (most common, fatigue, 11%), and the ORR was 77% with a PFS of 12.6 months. Notably, cardiac adverse events were not seen with the higher doses of carfilzomib. The rate of grade ≥3 dyspnea was 5%, similar to previous studies. The weekly dosing schedule in the CHAMPION-1 trial (20/70) is being compared to the conventional twice/week schedule (20/27) in an ongoing phase III trial, ARROW (NCT02412878).

Ixazomib

Ixazomib, like bortezomib, is a reversible boronate-containing PI that preferentially binds the β5 subunit of the 20S proteasome with a measured IC_{50} (half maximal inhibitory concentration) of 3.4 nM.[28] At higher concentrations, it also binds the β1 and β2 sites. The major distinguishing feature of ixazomib among the PIs is its oral dosing. Even though the selectivity and potency of ixazomib were similar to that of bortezomib, the measured dissociation rate for ixazomib from the proteasome was approximately sixfold faster than that of bortezomib ($t_{1/2}$ of 18 and 110 min, respectively).[174] This is believed to contribute to the superior tissue penetration of ixazomib. In preclinical models, ixazomib had activity in bortezomib-resistant MM cells.[175]

Clinical Pharmacology

After oral administration, the median time to achieve peak ixazomib plasma concentrations is one hour. Its mean absolute bioavailability is 58%; high-fat meals have shown to decrease its AUC by 28% and Cmax by 69%. Ixazomib is 99% bound to plasma proteins and distributes into red blood cells with a blood-to-plasma ratio of 10. The steady-state volume of distribution is 543 L. The terminal half-life (t1/2) of ixazomib is 9.5 days and following weekly oral dosing, the accumulation ratio is determined to be twofold. Ixazomib is metabolized by hepatic CYP enzymes and non-CYP proteins. After administration of a single oral dose, 62% of the administered dose was excreted in urine (<3.5% as unchanged drug) and 22% in the feces.[176]

At clinically relevant ixazomib concentrations, no specific CYP isoform has shown to contribute predominantly to its metabolism.[177] At higher than clinical concentrations, however, there were multiple possible CYP isoforms involved in metabolism include CYP3A4, 1A2, 2B6, 2C8, 2D6, 2C19, and 2C9; with the estimated relative contribution being highest for CYP3A (42%). In a multiarm phase 1 drug-drug interactions studies in 88 patients with advanced solid tumors or lymphoma, rifampin, a potent CYP3A4 inducer, reduced plasma exposures of ixazomib by 74% and C_{max} by 54%. On the basis of these results, it is recommended that patients should avoid concomitant administration of strong CYP3A inducers with ixazomib.[176]

Ixazomib in Patients with Renal and Hepatic Dysfunction

The International Myeloma Working Group (IMWG) suggests that ixazomib, in combination with lenalidomide and dexamethasone, may be safely administered to patients with a creatinine clearance ≥ 30 mL/minute.[178] For patients with pre-existing renal impairment of creatinine clearance (<30 mL/minute) and for patients with ESRD requiring dialysis, it is recommended to reduce the initial dose to 3 mg once weekly on days 1, 8, and 15 of a 28-day treatment cycle. Ixazomib is not dialyzable and may be administered without regard to dialysis timing.[176]

No dosage adjustment is necessary for mild hepatic impairment (total bilirubin ≤ ULN and AST > ULN or total bilirubin >1 to 1.5 times ULN and any AST). For, moderate impairment (total bilirubin >1.5 to 3 times ULN) or severe (total bilirubin >3 times ULN), the recommendation is to reduce the initial dose to 3 mg once weekly on days 1, 8, and 15 of a 28-day treatment cycle.[176]

Multiple Myeloma

Phase I trials examined weekly[179] and twice/week dosing[180] of ixazomib as a single agent in MM patients with relapsed/refractory disease. In weekly dosing, ixazomib was given on days 1, 8, and 15 of a 28 cycle, and the twice/week dosing schedule was similar to bortezomib on a 21-day cycle. The MTD for the weekly dosing was 2.97 mg/m² and 2 mg/m² for twice/week schedule. Pharmacokinetic studies showed a long terminal half-life of 3.6 to 11.3 days, providing support for once/week dosing. In these studies, peripheral neuropathy was uncommon, with only one case of grade 3 peripheral neuropathy out of 60 patients in the weekly dosing cohort was observed. Rash was reported in 9% of weekly dosing and 40% of the twice/week dosing trials. The patients in both of these trials were heavily pretreated, with a median of four prior lines of treatment. The ORR for weekly ixazomib was 18% (and 27% at the MTD).

Ixazomib has also been studied in combination with lenalidomide and dexamethasone. The TOURMALINE-MM1 trial compared the combination of ixazomib with lenalidomide and dexamethasone (IRd) versus lenalidomide and dexamethasone (Rd) in a phase III, double blind, randomized study in 722 patients with relapsed disease and 1 to 3 prior lines of treatment.[181] This trial excluded patients who were refractory to prior PI- or lenalidomide-based treatment. The majority of patients (69%) had prior bortezomib treatment (but were not refractory to bortezomib), and only 12% had prior lenalidomide treatment. The median PFS was significantly higher in the IRd arm, 20.6 versus 14.7 months in the Rd arm ($P = 0.012$), and the ORR was higher with IRd 78.3% versus 71.5% ($P = 0.035$). The toxicity profile between both arms was generally similar, including peripheral neuropathy. However, rash was higher in the ixazomib arm versus the control arm, grade 3 to 4 rash 5% versus 2% in the control arm. As with other PIs, thrombocytopenia was also higher, grade 3 to 4 19% versus 9%.

Based on the findings in the TOURMALINE-MM1 study, the FDA approved ixazomib in November 2015 as part of a combination with lenalidomide and dexamethasone in patients with relapsed disease who have received at least one prior therapy. Ixazomib thus became the first approved oral proteasome inhibitor, and this increases the convenience and accessibility of PI for extended therapy.

Novel Proteasome Inhibitors

To overcome some of the potential mechanisms of resistance to bortezomib, the next generation of PIs such as marizomib and oprozomib have been developed and are in early clinical trials.

Marizomib

Marizomib (salinosporamide A; NPI-0052) is a β-lactone similar to clasto-lactacystin (Fig. 19.3) and is derived from the marine actinomycetes *Salinispora tropica*.[19,36] Compared to bortezomib and carfilzomib, marizomib is unique in irreversibly inhibiting all three activities of the proteasome enzyme activities.[37-40] Marizomib has shown strong synergistic activity in preclinical models,[182] such as with pomalidomide.[183]

Marizomib is currently being evaluated in clinical trials in MM and other advanced malignancies.[42,43] Marizomib was given intravenously according to two schedules, weekly on day 1, 8, 15 on a 4 week cycle or twice/week on days 1, 4, 8, 11 on a 3 week cycle. In the twice/week schedule, the patients had extensive prior history of treatment with a median of six prior lines of treatment, and the overall response rate was 11%. While marizomib was tolerated well without the degree of peripheral neuropathy or hematologic toxicity seen with other proteasome inhibitors, dose limiting toxicities included mental status change and gait disturbance. This may reflect the lipophilic structure of marizomib and its ability to cross the blood brain barrier, suggesting that it may play a role in disease involving the central nervous system. A case report of two patients with MM with central nervous system involvement improved with marizomib therapy.[184] It has been evaluated in malignant gliomas, and preclinical models show significant antitumor effect.[185]

Marizomib has also been evaluated in combination with pomalidomide and dexamethasone in a phase I study.[186] This study enrolled patients with 2 or more prior lines of treatment and who had received prior lenalidomide and bortezomib. This study enrolled 20 patients who were heavily pre-treated with a median of 5 prior lines of treatment and achieved an ORR of 64%; no DLTs were observed.

Oprozomib

Oprozomib (ONX-0912) is an orally bioavailable epoxyketone-based proteasome inhibitor under development. It is a truncated derivate of carfilzomib that maintains the selectivity, potency, and antitumor activity.[27] Based on encouraging preclinical activity,[187] oprozomib has been evaluated as a single agent and in combination with lenalidomide and dexamethasone or in combination with pomalidomide and dexamethasone. For example, a phase Ib/II trial evaluated oprozomib with dexamethasone in patients with 1 to 5 prior lines of therapy.[188] While this combination showed an ORR of 41.7%, gastrointestinal adverse events were notable in this trial (and in other oprozomib trials), with grade 3 diarrhea (21%) and nausea (10%).

Drug Resistance

Although the significant antitumor activity of bortezomib in MM patients has been extensively demonstrated, not all patients respond to therapy and most of the responders will ultimately relapse. The ability of bortezomib to overcome the poor prognosis of conventional, cytotoxic anti-MM therapies strongly suggests that sensitivity versus resistance to bortezomib is determined by different molecular mechanisms than those determining responsiveness to cytotoxic therapy.

Several studies have investigated gene expression profiles specific to MM patients treated with bortezomib, specifically in the phase 2 SUMMIT and CREST trials and the APEX phase 3 trial.[111,112] Such profiling revealed response and survival classifiers that were significantly associated with outcome via testing on independent data. In addition, predictive models and biologic correlates of response showed some specificity for bortezomib rather than dexamethasone.[189] While these studies provided interesting evidence regarding the molecular mechanisms behind bortezomib resistance, the heterogeneity of the patient population evaluated precluded a general application of these markers. Studies using acute lymphoblastic leukemia cell line models initially suggested that mutations in the proteasome β5 subunit (PSMB5) protein might play a role in bortezomib resistance.[190] However, the role of this mutation in MM has not been confirmed.[191,192]

Resistance to proteasome inhibitors may also be explained by decreased IRE1-XBP1 activity. IRE1 (inositol requiring enzyme 1) is a kinase and endoribonuclease which controls and activates the unfolded protein response through nonconventional splicing of the transcription factor XBP1 (X-box binding protein 1) to XBP1s,[193] and XBP1s is required for the secretory maturation of plasma cells.[194] Recently, it was shown that IRE1-XBP1 signaling is suppressed in bortezomib-refractory myeloma.[195] MM subpopulations consisting of XBP1s− preplasmablasts and earlier progenitors may be intrinsically resistant to proteasome inhibitors. These XBP1s− progenitors are less secretory, produce less immunoglobulin, and were consequently less susceptible to endoplasmic reticulum stress caused by proteasome inhibition. These findings suggest a tumor progenitor structure where these progenitor cells may be a reservoir of proteasome inhibitor resistance.

A novel approach for addressing resistance to proteasome inhibitors mediated by XBP1 is through the HIV protease inhibitor nelfinavir. In preclinical studies, nelfinavir can induce the unfolded protein response and IRE1.[196] A phase II trial of nelfinavir with bortezomib in multiple myeloma refractory to proteasome inhibitor (SAKK 39/13) showed a response rate of 65% in 34 patients.[197]

Additionally, generation of highly carfilzomib-resistant myeloma cell lines has shown up-regulation of the multidrug resistance (MDR) protein ABCB1.[198] This mechanism appears to be more operative in carfilzomib resistance than bortezomib resistance. Treatment with MDR inhibitors decreased carfilzomib resistance. Additionally, spliced XPB1 was also low, consistent with the previously described mechanisms of resistance. The HIV protease inhibitors nelfinavir and lopinavir could overcome resistance to carfilzomib mediated through ABCB1 by facilitating the mitochondrial permeability transition pore.[199]

Targeting other components of the UPP such as events upstream of the proteasome may be another path for enhancing proteasome inhibitor activity as well as overcoming resistance. Protein ubiquitination begins the process for tagging specific proteins for degradation by the proteasome. This is countered and regulated by deubiquitinating enzymes (DUBs) which are peptidases that remove the ubiquitin tag and thereby prevent protein degradation.[200,201] There are several families of DUBs, but of particular interest in MM are Rpn11 (also known as POH1 or PSMD14), UCHL5, and USP14, all of which are closely associated with the 19S regulatory subunit of the proteasome complex. USP14 and UCHL5 are more highly expressed in myeloma cells than in normal plasma cells, and in preclinical models, inhibition of USP14 and UCHL5 can overcome proteasome inhibitor resistance in MM.[202] VLX1570 is a USP14 inhibitor that is currently in clinical development in MM (NCT02372240).[203] Similarly, inhibition of the Rpn11 DUB can also block proteasome activity, induce apoptosis in MM cells, and overcome resistance to bortezomib.[204]

The ubiquitin receptor Rpn13 (also known as ADRM1) is another target under consideration. The Rpn13 ubiquitin receptor recognizes ubiquitinated proteins and interacts with the Rpn11 DUB enzyme. Rpn13 is highly expressed on MM cells, and inhibition of Rpn13 with the inhibitor RA190 decreases viability of MM cells and can overcome bortezomib resistance.[205] Additionally, RA190 can synergize with bortezomib, lenalidomide, or pomalidomide.

Finally, the next frontier in drug development may be developing strategies for promoting degradation of specific proteins. Recently, the mechanism of action of immunomodulatory drugs, a principal drug class in MM therapy comprised of members such as thalidomide, lenalidomide and pomalidomide, was elucidated (see also Chapter 20). These drugs bind to cereblon, a component of the E3 ubiquitin ligase complex, which then alters its substrate recognition and leads to ubiquitination and subsequent degradation of transcription factors IKZF1 (Ikaros) and IKZF3 (Aiolos) that are important for MM proliferation.[206,207] This unique mechanism can be engineered to target other proteins for disposal. Recently, a phthalamide was modified to bind to the transcriptional coactivator BRD4 and engage the cereblon E3 ubiquitin ligase complex, leading to the destruction of BRD4.[208] These new drugs, or "degronimids" may thus provide a pathway for addressing previously "untargetable" proteins like transcription factors. A similar approach was deployed with Proteolysis Targeting Chimera (PROTAC) technology, which in one example recruits either cereblon or Von Hippel Lindau E3 ligases to dispose of c-ABL and BCR-ABL.[209]

Conclusions

The proteasome plays a key role in both normal physiology and cancer pathogenesis. Given the unique features of MM cells and immunoglobulin synthesis, MM is highly sensitive to proteasome inhibition. This finding has ushered in a new class of drugs and three drugs which are in clinical use, beginning with bortezomib and then carfilzomib and ixazomib, transforming patient outcomes. There are ongoing efforts to optimize proteasome inhibition, through combinations and targeting other components of the ubiquitin-proteasome pathway.

Acknowledgments

We would like to acknowledge the authors of the previous edition of this chapter: Igor Espinoza-Delgado, Monica G. Chiaramonte, Richard D. Swerdlow, and John J. Wright.

References

1. Hoeller D, Hecker CM, Dikic I. Ubiquitin and ubiquitin-like proteins in cancer pathogenesis. *Nat Rev Cancer.* 2006;6:776-788.
2. Rubinsztein DC. The roles of intracellular protein-degradation pathways in neurodegeneration. *Nature.* 2006;443:780-786.
3. Chen ZJ. Ubiquitin signalling in the NF-kappaB pathway. *Nat Cell Biol.* 2005;7:758-765.
4. Reed SI. The ubiquitin-proteasome pathway in cell cycle control. *Results Probl Cell Differ.* 2006;42:147-181.
5. Huen MS, Chen J. The DNA damage response pathways: at the crossroad of protein modifications. *Cell Res.* 2008;18:8-16.
6. Kostova Z, Tsai YC, Weissman AM. Ubiquitin ligases, critical mediators of endoplasmic reticulum-associated degradation. *Semin Cell Dev Biol.* 2007;18:770-779.
7. Wang J, Maldonado MA. The ubiquitin-proteasome system and its role in inflammatory and autoimmune diseases. *Cell Mol Immunol.* 2006;3:255-261.
8. Eldridge AG, O'Brien T. Therapeutic strategies within the ubiquitin proteasome system. *Cell Death Differ.* 2010;17:4-13.
9. Vassilev LT, Vu BT, Graves B, et al. In vivo activation of the p53 pathway by small-molecule antagonists of MDM2. *Science.* 2004;303:844-848.
10. Adams J, Palombella VJ, Elliott PJ. Proteasome inhibition: a new strategy in cancer treatment. *Invest New Drugs.* 2000;18:109-121.
11. Holzl H, Kapelari B, Kellermann J, et al. The regulatory complex of Drosophila melanogaster 26S proteasomes. Subunit composition and localization of a deubiquitylating enzyme. *J Cell Biol.* 2000;150:119-130.
12. Kisselev AF, Akopian TN, Woo KM, et al. The sizes of peptides generated from protein by mammalian 26 and 20 S proteasomes. Implications for understanding the degradative mechanism and antigen presentation. *J Biol Chem.* 1999;274:3363-3371.
13. Nussbaum AK, Dick TP, Keilholz W, et al. Cleavage motifs of the yeast 20S proteasome beta subunits deduced from digests of enolase 1. *Proc Natl Acad Sci U S A.* 1998;95:12504-12509.
14. Voges D, Zwickl P, Baumeister W. The 26S proteasome: a molecular machine designed for controlled proteolysis. *Annu Rev Biochem.* 1999;68:1015-1068.
15. Ciechanover A. The ubiquitin-proteasome pathway: on protein death and cell life. *EMBO J.* 1998;17:7151-7160.
16. Lee DH, Goldberg AL. Proteasome inhibitors: valuable new tools for cell biologists. *Trends Cell Biol.* 1998;8:397-403.
17. Spataro V, Norbury C, Harris AL. The ubiquitin-proteasome pathway in cancer. *Br J Cancer.* 1998;77:448-455.
18. Zwickl P, Baumeister W, Steven A. Dis-assembly lines: the proteasome and related ATPase-assisted proteases. *Curr Opin Struct Biol.* 2000;10:242-250.
19. Moreau P, Richardson PG, Cavo M, et al. Proteasome inhibitors in multiple myeloma: 10 years later. *Blood.* 2012;120:947-959.
20. Demo SD, Kirk CJ, Aujay MA, et al. Antitumor activity of PR-171, a novel irreversible inhibitor of the proteasome. *Cancer Res.* 2007;67:6383-6391.
21. Dick LR, Fleming PE. Building on bortezomib: second-generation proteasome inhibitors as anti-cancer therapy. *Drug Discov Today.* 2010;15:243-249.
22. Adams J. The development of proteasome inhibitors as anticancer drugs. *Cancer Cell.* 2004;5:417-421.
23. Dou QP, Goldfarb RH. Bortezomib (millennium pharmaceuticals). *IDrugs.* 2002;5:828-834.
24. Lu S, Wang J. The resistance mechanisms of proteasome inhibitor bortezomib. *Biomark Res.* 2013;1:13.
25. Bross PF, Kane R, Farrell AT, et al. Approval summary for bortezomib for injection in the treatment of multiple myeloma. *Clin Cancer Res.* 2004;10:3954-3964.
26. Kane RC, Dagher R, Farrell A, et al. Bortezomib for the treatment of mantle cell lymphoma. *Clin Cancer Res.* 2007;13:5291-5294.
27. Allegra A, Alonci A, Gerace D, et al. New orally active proteasome inhibitors in multiple myeloma. *Leuk Res.* 2014;38:1-9.
28. Brayer J, Baz R. The potential of ixazomib, a second-generation proteasome inhibitor, in the treatment of multiple myeloma. *Ther Adv Hematol.* 2017;8:209-220.
29. Piva R, Ruggeri B, Williams M, et al. CEP-18770: A novel, orally active proteasome inhibitor with a tumor-selective pharmacologic profile competitive with bortezomib. *Blood.* 2008;111:2765-2775.
30. Kubiczkova L, Pour L, Sedlarikova L, et al. Proteasome inhibitors—molecular basis and current perspectives in multiple myeloma. *J Cell Mol Med.* 2014;18:947-961.
31. Fenteany G, Standaert RF, Lane WS, et al. Inhibition of proteasome activities and subunit-specific amino-terminal threonine modification by lactacystin. *Science.* 1995;268:726-731.
32. Corey EJ, Li WD. Total synthesis and biological activity of lactacystin, omuralide and analogs. *Chem Pharm Bull (Tokyo).* 1999;47:1-10.
33. Dick LR, Cruikshank AA, Grenier L, et al. Mechanistic studies on the inactivation of the proteasome by lactacystin: a central role for clasto-lactacystin beta-lactone. *J Biol Chem.* 1996;271:7273-7276.
34. Fenteany G, Standaert RF, Reichard GA, et al. A beta-lactone related to lactacystin induces neurite outgrowth in a neuroblastoma cell line and inhibits cell cycle progression in an osteosarcoma cell line. *Proc Natl Acad Sci U S A.* 1994;91:3358-3362.
35. Katagiri M, Hayashi M, Matsuzaki K, et al. The neuritogenesis inducer lactacystin arrests cell cycle at both G0/G1 and G2 phases in neuro 2a cells. *J Antibiot (Tokyo).* 1995;48:344-346.
36. Feling RH, Buchanan GO, Mincer TJ, et al. Salinosporamide A: a highly cytotoxic proteasome inhibitor from a novel microbial source, a marine bacterium of the new genus salinospora. *Angew Chem Int Ed Engl.* 2003;42:355-357.
37. Groll M, Huber R, Potts BC. Crystal structures of Salinosporamide A (NPI-0052) and B (NPI-0047) in complex with the 20S proteasome reveal important consequences of beta-lactone ring opening and a mechanism for irreversible binding. *J Am Chem Soc.* 2006;128:5136-5141.

38. Berkers CR, Verdoes M, Lichtman E, et al. Activity probe for in vivo profiling of the specificity of proteasome inhibitor bortezomib. *Nat Methods.* 2005;2:357-362.

39. Chauhan D, Catley L, Li G, et al. A novel orally active proteasome inhibitor induces apoptosis in multiple myeloma cells with mechanisms distinct from Bortezomib. *Cancer Cell.* 2005;8:407-419.

40. Groll M, Berkers CR, Ploegh HL, et al. Crystal structure of the boronic acid-based proteasome inhibitor bortezomib in complex with the yeast 20S proteasome. *Structure.* 2006;14:451-456.

41. Chauhan D, Singh A, Brahmandam M, et al. Combination of proteasome inhibitors bortezomib and NPI-0052 trigger in vivo synergistic cytotoxicity in multiple myeloma. *Blood.* 2008;111:1654-1664.

42. Harrison SJ, Mainwaring P, Price T, et al. Phase I clinical trial of marizomib (NPI-0052) in patients with advanced malignancies including multiple myeloma: study NPI-0052-102 final results. *Clin Cancer Res.* 2016;22:4559-4566.

43. Richardson PG, Zimmerman TM, Hofmeister CC, et al. Phase 1 study of marizomib in relapsed or relapsed and refractory multiple myeloma: NPI-0052-101 Part 1. *Blood.* 2016;127:2693-2700.

44. Hanada M, Sugawara K, Kaneta K, et al. Epoxomicin, a new antitumor agent of microbial origin. *J Antibiot (Tokyo).* 1992;45:1746-1752.

45. Kuhn DJ, Chen Q, Voorhees PM, et al. Potent activity of carfilzomib, a novel, irreversible inhibitor of the ubiquitin-proteasome pathway, against preclinical models of multiple myeloma. *Blood.* 2007;110:3281-3290.

46. Jagannath S, Vij R, Stewart AK, et al. Initial results of PX-171-003, an open-label, single-arm, phase ii study of carfilzomib (CFZ) in patients with relapsed and refractory multiple myeloma (MM). *Blood.* 2008;112:864.

47. O'Connor OA, Stewart AK, Vallone M, et al. A phase 1 dose escalation study of the safety and pharmacokinetics of the novel proteasome inhibitor carfilzomib (PR-171) in patients with hematologic malignancies. *Clin Cancer Res.* 2009;15:7085-7091.

48. Stewart AK, Rajkumar SV, Dimopoulos MA, et al. Carfilzomib, lenalidomide, and dexamethasone for relapsed multiple myeloma. *N Engl J Med.* 2015;372:142-152.

49. Orlowski RZ, Baldwin AS, Jr. NF-kappaB as a therapeutic target in cancer. *Trends Mol Med.* 2002;8:385-389.

50. Palombella VJ, Rando OJ, Goldberg AL, et al. The ubiquitin-proteasome pathway is required for processing the NF-kappa B1 precursor protein and the activation of NF-kappa B. *Cell.* 1994;78:773-785.

51. Ghosh S, May MJ, Kopp EB. NF-kappa B and Rel proteins: evolutionarily conserved mediators of immune responses. *Annu Rev Immunol.* 1998;16:225-260.

52. Dejardin E, Droin NM, Delhase M, et al. The lymphotoxin-beta receptor induces different patterns of gene expression via two NF-kappaB pathways. *Immunity.* 2002;17:525-535.

53. Derudder E, Dejardin E, Pritchard LL, et al. RelB/p50 dimers are differentially regulated by tumor necrosis factor-alpha and lymphotoxin-beta receptor activation: critical roles for p100. *J Biol Chem.* 2003;278:23278-23284.

54. Ghosh S, Karin M. Missing pieces in the NF-kappaB puzzle. *Cell.* 2002;109 Suppl:S81-S96.

55. Xiao G, Harhaj EW, Sun SC. NF-kappaB-inducing kinase regulates the processing of NF-kappaB2 p100. *Mol Cell.* 2001;7:401-409.

56. Basseres DS, Baldwin AS. Nuclear factor-kappaB and inhibitor of kappaB kinase pathways in oncogenic initiation and progression. *Oncogene.* 2006;25:6817-6830.

57. Burstein E, Duckett CS. Dying for NF-kappaB? Control of cell death by transcriptional regulation of the apoptotic machinery. *Curr Opin Cell Biol.* 2003;15:732-737.

58. Cilloni D, Martinelli G, Messa F, et al. Nuclear factor kB as a target for new drug development in myeloid malignancies. *Haematologica.* 2007;92:1224-1229.

59. Dutta J, Fan Y, Gupta N, et al. Current insights into the regulation of programmed cell death by NF-kappaB. *Oncogene.* 2006;25:6800-6816.

60. Jost PJ, Ruland J. Aberrant NF-kappaB signaling in lymphoma: mechanisms, consequences, and therapeutic implications. *Blood.* 2007;109:2700-2707.

61. Luo JL, Kamata H, Karin M. The anti-death machinery in IKK/NF-kappaB signaling. *J Clin Immunol.* 2005;25:541-550.

62. Bharti AC, Donato N, Singh S, et al. Curcumin (diferuloylmethane) down-regulates the constitutive activation of nuclear factor-kappa B and IkappaBalpha kinase in human multiple myeloma cells, leading to suppression of proliferation and induction of apoptosis. *Blood.* 2003;101:1053-1062.

63. Hideshima T, Chauhan D, Richardson P, et al. NF-kappa B as a therapeutic target in multiple myeloma. *J Biol Chem.* 2002;277:16639-16647.

64. Ni H, Ergin M, Huang Q, et al. Analysis of expression of nuclear factor kappa B (NF-kappa B) in multiple myeloma: downregulation of NF-kappa B induces apoptosis. *Br J Haematol.* 2001;115:279-286.

65. Hideshima T, Ikeda H, Chauhan D, et al. Bortezomib induces canonical nuclear factor-kappaB activation in multiple myeloma cells. *Blood.* 2009;114:1046-1052.

66. Xu C, Bailly-Maitre B, Reed JC. Endoplasmic reticulum stress: cell life and death decisions. *J Clin Invest.* 2005;115:2656-2664.

67. Kaneko M, Niinuma Y, Nomura Y. Activation signal of nuclear factor-kappa B in response to endoplasmic reticulum stress is transduced via IRE1 and tumor necrosis factor receptor-associated factor 2. *Biol Pharm Bull.* 2003;26:931-935.

68. Wu J, Kaufman RJ. From acute ER stress to physiological roles of the unfolded protein response. *Cell Death Differ.* 2006;13:374-384.

69. Bernales S, McDonald KL, Walter P. Autophagy counterbalances endoplasmic reticulum expansion during the unfolded protein response. *PLoS Biol.* 2006;4:e423.

70. Egger L, Schneider J, Rheme C, et al. Serine proteases mediate apoptosis-like cell death and phagocytosis under caspase-inhibiting conditions. *Cell Death Differ.* 2003;10:1188-1203.

71. Levine B, Kroemer G. Autophagy in the pathogenesis of disease. *Cell.* 2008;132:27-42.

72. Ogata M, Hino S, Saito A, et al. Autophagy is activated for cell survival after endoplasmic reticulum stress. *Mol Cell Biol.* 2006;26:9220-9231.

73. Fribley A, Zeng Q, Wang CY. Proteasome inhibitor PS-341 induces apoptosis through induction of endoplasmic reticulum stress-reactive oxygen species in head and neck squamous cell carcinoma cells. *Mol Cell Biol.* 2004;24:9695-9704.

74. Landowski TH, Megli CJ, Nullmeyer KD, et al. Mitochondrial-mediated disregulation of Ca^{2+} is a critical determinant of Velcade (PS-341/bortezomib) cytotoxicity in myeloma cell lines. *Cancer Res.* 2005;65:3828-3836.

75. Lee AH, Iwakoshi NN, Anderson KC, et al. Proteasome inhibitors disrupt the unfolded protein response in myeloma cells. *Proc Natl Acad Sci U S A.* 2003;100:9946-9951.

76. Nawrocki ST, Carew JS, Dunner K, Jr., et al. Bortezomib inhibits PKR-like endoplasmic reticulum (ER) kinase and induces apoptosis via ER stress in human pancreatic cancer cells. *Cancer Res.* 2005;65:11510-11519.

77. Obeng EA, Carlson LM, Gutman DM, et al. Proteasome inhibitors induce a terminal unfolded protein response in multiple myeloma cells. *Blood.* 2006;107:4907-4916.

78. Mandic A, Hansson J, Linder S, et al. Cisplatin induces endoplasmic reticulum stress and nucleus-independent apoptotic signaling. *J Biol Chem.* 2003;278:9100-9106.

79. Marcu MG, Doyle M, Bertolotti A, et al. Heat shock protein 90 modulates the unfolded protein response by stabilizing IRE1alpha. *Mol Cell Biol.* 2002;22:8506-8513.

80. Mimnaugh EG, Xu W, Vos M, et al. Simultaneous inhibition of hsp 90 and the proteasome promotes protein ubiquitination, causes endoplasmic reticulum-derived cytosolic vacuolization, and enhances antitumor activity. *Mol Cancer Ther.* 2004;3:551-566.

81. Hideshima T, Bradner JE, Wong J, et al. Small-molecule inhibition of proteasome and aggresome function induces synergistic antitumor activity in multiple myeloma. *Proc Natl Acad Sci U S A.* 2005;102:8567-8572.

82. Garcia-Mata R, Gao YS, Sztul E. Hassles with taking out the garbage: aggravating aggresomes. *Traffic.* 2002;3:388-396.

83. Bali P, Pranpat M, Bradner J, et al. Inhibition of histone deacetylase 6 acetylates and disrupts the chaperone function of heat shock protein 90: a novel basis for antileukemia activity of histone deacetylase inhibitors. *J Biol Chem.* 2005;280:26729-26734.

84. Kawaguchi Y, Kovacs JJ, McLaurin A, et al. The deacetylase HDAC6 regulates aggresome formation and cell viability in response to misfolded protein stress. *Cell.* 2003;115:727-738.

85. Santo L, Hideshima T, Kung AL, et al. Preclinical activity, pharmacodynamic, and pharmacokinetic properties of a selective HDAC6 inhibitor, ACY-1215, in combination with bortezomib in multiple myeloma. *Blood.* 2012;119:2579-2589.

86. Mitsiades CS, Mitsiades NS, McMullan CJ, et al. Transcriptional signature of histone deacetylase inhibition in multiple myeloma: biological and clinical implications. *Proc Natl Acad Sci U S A.* 2004;101:540-545.

87. Pei XY, Dai Y, Grant S. Synergistic induction of oxidative injury and apoptosis in human multiple myeloma cells by the proteasome inhibitor bortezomib and histone deacetylase inhibitors. *Clin Cancer Res.* 2004;10:3839-3852.

88. Yu C, Rahmani M, Conrad D, et al. The proteasome inhibitor bortezomib interacts synergistically with histone deacetylase inhibitors to induce apoptosis in Bcr/Abl+ cells sensitive and resistant to STI571. *Blood.* 2003;102:3765-3774.

89. Dimopoulos M, Siegel DS, Lonial S, et al. Vorinostat or placebo in combination with bortezomib in patients with multiple myeloma (VANTAGE 088): a multicentre, randomised, double-blind study. *Lancet Oncol.* 2013;14:1129-1140.

90. San-Miguel JF, Hungria VT, Yoon SS, et al. Panobinostat plus bortezomib and dexamethasone versus placebo plus bortezomib and dexamethasone in patients with relapsed or relapsed and refractory multiple myeloma: a multicentre, randomised, double-blind phase 3 trial. *Lancet Oncol.* 2014;15:1195-1206.

91. Orlowski M, Wilk S. Catalytic activities of the 20 S proteasome, a multicatalytic proteinase complex. *Arch Biochem Biophys.* 2000;383:1-16.

92. Manasanch EE, Orlowski RZ. Proteasome inhibitors in cancer therapy. *Nat Rev Clin Oncol.* 2017;14:417-433.

93. Imajoh-Ohmi S, Kawaguchi T, Sugiyama S, et al. Lactacystin, a specific inhibitor of the proteasome, induces apoptosis in human monoblast U937 cells. *Biochem Biophys Res Commun.* 1995;217:1070-1077.

94. Shah SA, Potter MW, McDade TP, et al. 26S proteasome inhibition induces apoptosis and limits growth of human pancreatic cancer. *J Cell Biochem.* 2001;82:110-122.

95. Bold RJ, Virudachalam S, McConkey DJ. Chemosensitization of pancreatic cancer by inhibition of the 26S proteasome. *J Surg Res.* 2001;100:11-17.

96. Pham LV, Tamayo AT, Yoshimura LC, et al. Inhibition of constitutive NF-kappa B activation in mantle cell lymphoma B cells leads to induction of cell cycle arrest and apoptosis. *J Immunol.* 2003;171:88-95.

97. An B, Goldfarb RH, Siman R, et al. Novel dipeptidyl proteasome inhibitors overcome Bcl-2 protective function and selectively accumulate the cyclin-dependent kinase inhibitor p27 and induce apoptosis in transformed, but not normal, human fibroblasts. *Cell Death Differ.* 1998;5:1062-1075.

98. Orlowski RZ, Eswara JR, Lafond-Walker A, et al. Tumor growth inhibition induced in a murine model of human Burkitt's lymphoma by a proteasome inhibitor. *Cancer Res.* 1998;58:4342-4348.

99. Adams J, Palombella VJ, Sausville EA, et al. Proteasome inhibitors: a novel class of potent and effective antitumor agents. *Cancer Res.* 1999;59:2615-2622.

100. Hideshima T, Mitsiades C, Akiyama M, et al. Molecular mechanisms mediating antimyeloma activity of proteasome inhibitor PS-341. *Blood.* 2003;101:1530-1534.

101. LeBlanc R, Catley LP, Hideshima T, et al. Proteasome inhibitor PS-341 inhibits human myeloma cell growth in vivo and prolongs survival in a murine model. *Cancer Res.* 2002;62:4996-5000.

102. Supko JG, Eder JP, Lynch TJ. Pharmacokinetics of gemcitabine and the proteasome inhibitor bortezomib (formerly PS-241) in adult patients with solid malignancies. *Proc Am Soc Clin Oncol.* 2003;20:A339.

103. Nix D, Pein C, Newman R. Clinical development of a proteasome inhibitor, PS-341, for the treatment of cancer. *Proc Am Soc Clin Oncol.* 2001;20:Abstract 339.

104. Venkatakrishnan K, Rader M, Ramanathan RK, et al. Effect of the CYP3A inhibitor ketoconazole on the pharmacokinetics and pharmacodynamics of bortezomib in patients with advanced solid tumors: a prospective, multi-center, open-label, randomized, two-way crossover drug-drug interaction study. *Clin Ther.* 2009;31 Pt 2:2444-2458.

105. Velcade Prescribing Information. 2017. Accessed December 8, 2017, at http://www.velcade.com/files/pdfs/velcade_prescribing_information.pdf.

106. Leal TB, Remick SC, Takimoto CH, et al. Dose-escalating and pharmacological study of bortezomib in adult cancer patients with impaired renal function: a National Cancer Institute Organ Dysfunction Working Group Study. *Cancer Chemother Pharmacol.* 2011;68:1439-1447.

107. LoRusso PM, Venkatakrishnan K, Ramanathan RK, et al. Pharmacokinetics and safety of bortezomib in patients with advanced malignancies and varying degrees of liver dysfunction: phase I NCI Organ Dysfunction Working Group Study NCI-6432. *Clin Cancer Res.* 2012;18:2954-2963.

108. Orlowski RZ, Stinchcombe TE, Mitchell BS, et al. Phase I trial of the proteasome inhibitor PS-341 in patients with refractory hematologic malignancies. *J Clin Oncol.* 2002;20:4420-4427.

109. Aghajanian C, Soignet S, Dizon DS, et al. A phase I trial of the novel proteasome inhibitor PS341 in advanced solid tumor malignancies. *Clin Cancer Res.* 2002;8:2505-2511.

110. Papandreou CN, Daliani DD, Nix D, et al. Phase I trial of the proteasome inhibitor bortezomib in patients with advanced solid tumors with observations in androgen-independent prostate cancer. *J Clin Oncol.* 2004;22:2108-2121.

111. Richardson PG, Barlogie B, Berenson J, et al. A phase 2 study of bortezomib in relapsed, refractory myeloma. *N Engl J Med.* 2003;348:2609-2617.

112. Jagannath S, Barlogie B, Berenson J, et al. A phase 2 study of two doses of bortezomib in relapsed or refractory myeloma. *Br J Haematol.* 2004;127:165-172.

113. Richardson PG, Sonneveld P, Schuster MW, et al. Bortezomib or high-dose dexamethasone for relapsed multiple myeloma. *N Engl J Med.* 2005;352:2487-2498.

114. Richardson PG, Sonneveld P, Schuster M, et al. Extended follow-up of a phase 3 trial in relapsed multiple myeloma: final time-to-event results of the APEX trial. *Blood.* 2007;110:3557-3560.

115. San Miguel JF, Schlag R, Khuageva NK, et al. Bortezomib plus melphalan and prednisone for initial treatment of multiple myeloma. *N Engl J Med.* 2008;359:906-917.

116. San Miguel JF, Schlag R, Khuageva NK, et al. Persistent overall survival benefit and no increased risk of second malignancies with bortezomib-melphalan-prednisone versus melphalan-prednisone in patients with previously untreated multiple myeloma. *J Clin Oncol.* 2013;31:448-455.

117. Durie BG, Hoering A, Abidi MH, et al. Bortezomib with lenalidomide and dexamethasone versus lenalidomide and dexamethasone alone in patients with newly diagnosed myeloma without intent for immediate autologous stem-cell transplant (SWOG S0777): a randomised, open-label, phase 3 trial. *Lancet.* 2017;389:519-527.

118. Dimopoulos MA, Moreau P, Palumbo A, et al. Carfilzomib and dexamethasone versus bortezomib and dexamethasone for patients with relapsed or refractory multiple myeloma (ENDEAVOR): a randomised, phase 3, open-label, multicentre study. *Lancet Oncol.* 2016;17:27-38.

119. Moreau P, Masszi T, Grzasko N, et al. Oral ixazomib, lenalidomide, and dexamethasone for multiple myeloma. *N Engl J Med.* 2016;374:1621-1634.

120. Palumbo A, Chanan-Khan A, Weisel K, et al. Daratumumab, bortezomib, and dexamethasone for multiple myeloma. *N Engl J Med.* 2016;375:754-766.

121. Mitsiades N, Mitsiades CS, Poulaki V, et al. Apoptotic signaling induced by immunomodulatory thalidomide analogs in human multiple myeloma cells: therapeutic implications. *Blood.* 2002;99:4525-4530.

122. Richardson PG, Weller E, Lonial S, et al. Lenalidomide, bortezomib, and dexamethasone combination therapy in patients with newly diagnosed multiple myeloma. *Blood.* 2010;116:679-686.

123. Moreau P, Hulin C, Macro M, et al. VTD is superior to VCD prior to intensive therapy in multiple myeloma: results of the prospective IFM2013-04 trial. *Blood.* 2016;127:2569-2574.

124. Kumar S, Flinn I, Richardson PG, et al. Randomized, multicenter, phase 2 study (EVOLUTION) of combinations of bortezomib, dexamethasone, cyclophosphamide, and lenalidomide in previously untreated multiple myeloma. *Blood.* 2012;119:4375-4382.

125. Sonneveld P, Goldschmidt H, Rosinol L, et al. Bortezomib-based versus nonbortezomib-based induction treatment before autologous stem-cell transplantation in patients with previously untreated multiple myeloma: a meta-analysis of phase III randomized, controlled trials. *J Clin Oncol.* 2013;31:3279-3287.

126. Sonneveld P, Schmidt-Wolf IG, van der Holt B, et al. Bortezomib induction and maintenance treatment in patients with newly diagnosed multiple myeloma: Results of the randomized phase III HOVON-65/GMMG-HD4 trial. *J Clin Oncol.* 2012;30(24):2946-2955.

127. Orlowski RZ, Small GW, Shi YY. Evidence that inhibition of p44/42 mitogen-activated protein kinase signaling is a factor in proteasome inhibitor-mediated apoptosis. *J Biol Chem.* 2002;277:27864-27871.

128. Small GW, Somasundaram S, Moore DT, et al. Repression of mitogen-activated protein kinase (MAPK) phosphatase-1 by anthracyclines contributes to their antiapoptotic activation of p44/42-MAPK. *J Pharmacol Exp Ther.* 2003;307:861-869.

129. Orlowski RZ, Nagler A, Sonneveld P, et al. Randomized phase III study of pegylated liposomal doxorubicin plus bortezomib compared with bortezomib alone in relapsed or refractory multiple myeloma: combination therapy improves time to progression. *J Clin Oncol.* 2007;25:3892-3901.

130. Minucci S, Pelicci PG. Histone deacetylase inhibitors and the promise of epigenetic (and more) treatments for cancer. *Nat Rev Cancer.* 2006;6:38-51.

131. Richardson PG, Mitsiades CS, Laubach JP, et al. Preclinical data and early clinical experience supporting the use of histone deacetylase inhibitors in multiple myeloma. *Leuk Res.* 2013;37:829-837.

132. Yee AJ, Bensinger WI, Supko JG, et al. Ricolinostat plus lenalidomide, and dexamethasone in relapsed or refractory multiple myeloma: a multicentre phase 1b trial. *Lancet Oncol.* 2016;17:1569-1578.

133. Vogl DT, Raje N, Jagannath S, et al. Ricolinostat, the first selective histone deacetylase 6 inhibitor, in combination with bortezomib and dexamethasone for relapsed or refractory multiple myeloma. *Clin Cancer Res.* 2017;23:3307-3315.

134. Kumar SK, Rajkumar SV, Dispenzieri A, et al. Improved survival in multiple myeloma and the impact of novel therapies. *Blood.* 2008;111:2516-2520.

135. Kumar SK, Dispenzieri A, Lacy MQ, et al. Continued improvement in survival in multiple myeloma: changes in early mortality and outcomes in older patients. *Leukemia.* 2014;28:1122-1128.

136. Richardson PG, Hofmeister CC, Raje NS, et al. Pomalidomide, bortezomib and low-dose dexamethasone in lenalidomide-refractory and proteasome inhibitor-exposed myeloma. *Leukemia.* 2017;31:2695-2701.

137. Paludo J, Mikhael JR, LaPlant BR, et al. Pomalidomide, bortezomib, and dexamethasone for patients with relapsed lenalidomide-refractory multiple myeloma. *Blood.* 2017;130:1198-1204.

138. Jakubowiak A, Offidani M, Pegourie B, et al. Randomized phase 2 study: elotuzumab plus bortezomib/dexamethasone vs bortezomib/dexamethasone for relapsed/refractory MM. *Blood.* 2016;127:2833-2840.

139. Richardson PG, Briemberg H, Jagannath S, et al. Frequency, characteristics, and reversibility of peripheral neuropathy during treatment of advanced multiple myeloma with bortezomib. *J Clin Oncol.* 2006;24:3113-3120.

140. Moreau P, Pylypenko H, Grosicki S, et al. Subcutaneous versus intravenous administration of bortezomib in patients with relapsed multiple myeloma: a randomised, phase 3, non-inferiority study. *Lancet Oncol.* 2010;12:431-440.

141. Moreau P, Karamanesht, II, Domnikova N, et al. Pharmacokinetic, pharmacodynamic and covariate analysis of subcutaneous versus intravenous administration of bortezomib in patients with relapsed multiple myeloma. *Clin Pharmacokinet.* 2012;51:823-829.

142. Lonial S, Waller EK, Richardson PG, et al. Risk factors and kinetics of thrombocytopenia associated with bortezomib for relapsed, refractory multiple myeloma. *Blood.* 2005;106:3777-3784.

143. Chanan-Khan A, Sonneveld P, Schuster MW, et al. Analysis of herpes zoster events among bortezomib-treated patients in the phase III APEX study. *J Clin Oncol.* 2008;26:4784-4790.

144. Vickrey E, Allen S, Mehta J, et al. Acyclovir to prevent reactivation of varicella zoster virus (herpes zoster) in multiple myeloma patients receiving bortezomib therapy. *Cancer.* 2009;115:229-232.

145. Reeder CB, Reece DE, Kukreti V, et al. Once- versus twice-weekly bortezomib induction therapy with CyBorD in newly diagnosed multiple myeloma. *Blood.* 2010;115:3416-3417.

146. Girnius SK, Lee S, Kambhampati S, et al. A Phase II trial of weekly bortezomib and dexamethasone in veterans with newly diagnosed multiple myeloma not eligible for or who deferred autologous stem cell transplantation. *Br J Haematol.* 2015;169:36-43.

147. O'Donnell EK, Laubach JP, Yee AJ, et al. A phase 2 study of modified lenalidomide, bortezomib and dexamethasone in transplant-ineligible multiple myeloma. *Br J Haematol.* 2018;May 8. doi: 10.1111/bjh.15261.

148. Kastritis E, Wechalekar AD, Dimopoulos MA, et al. Bortezomib with or without dexamethasone in primary systemic (light chain) amyloidosis. *J Clin Oncol.* 2010;28:1031-1037.

149. Venner CP, Lane T, Foard D, et al. Cyclophosphamide, bortezomib, and dexamethasone therapy in AL amyloidosis is associated with high clonal response rates and prolonged progression-free survival. *Blood.* 2012;119:4387-4390.

150. Mikhael JR, Schuster SR, Jimenez-Zepeda VH, et al. Cyclophosphamide-bortezomib-dexamethasone (CyBorD) produces rapid and complete hematologic response in patients with AL amyloidosis. *Blood.* 2012;119:4391-4394.

151. O'Connor OA, Wright J, Moskowitz C, et al. Phase II clinical experience with the novel proteasome inhibitor bortezomib in patients with indolent non-Hodgkin's lymphoma and mantle cell lymphoma. *J Clin Oncol.* 2005;23:676-684.

152. Goy A, Younes A, McLaughlin P, et al. Phase II study of proteasome inhibitor bortezomib in relapsed or refractory B-cell non-Hodgkin's lymphoma. *J Clin Oncol.* 2005;23:667-675.

153. Fisher RI, Bernstein SH, Kahl BS, et al. Multicenter phase II study of bortezomib in patients with relapsed or refractory mantle cell lymphoma. *J Clin Oncol.* 2006;24:4867-4874.

154. Robak T, Huang H, Jin J, et al. Bortezomib-based therapy for newly diagnosed mantle-cell lymphoma. *N Engl J Med.* 2015;372:944-953.

155. Treon SP, Ioakimidis L, Soumerai JD, et al. Primary therapy of Waldenstrom macroglobulinemia with bortezomib, dexamethasone, and rituximab: WMCTG clinical trial 05-180. *J Clin Oncol.* 2009;27:3830-3835.

156. Ghobrial IM, Hong F, Padmanabhan S, et al. Phase II trial of weekly bortezomib in combination with rituximab in relapsed or relapsed and refractory Waldenstrom macroglobulinemia. *J Clin Oncol.* 2010;28:1422-1428.

157. Dimopoulos MA, Garcia-Sanz R, Gavriatopoulou M, et al. Primary therapy of Waldenstrom macroglobulinemia (WM) with weekly bortezomib, low-dose dexamethasone, and rituximab (BDR): long-term results of a phase 2 study of the European Myeloma Network (EMN). *Blood.* 2013;122:3276-3282.

158. Huang Z, Wu Y, Zhou X, et al. Efficacy of therapy with bortezomib in solid tumors: a review based on 32 clinical trials. *Future Oncol.* 2014;10:1795-1807.

159. Kyprolis Prescribing Information. 2017. Accessed December 8, 2017, at http://pi.amgen.com/~/media/amgen/repositorysites/pi-amgen-com/kyprolis/kyprolis_pi.ashx.

160. Wang Z, Yang J, Kirk C, et al. Clinical pharmacokinetics, metabolism, and drug-drug interaction of carfilzomib. *Drug Metab Dispos.* 2013;41:230-237.

161. Quach H, White D, Spencer A, et al. Pharmacokinetics and safety of carfilzomib in patients with relapsed multiple myeloma and end-stage renal disease (ESRD): an open-label, single-arm, phase I study. *Cancer Chemother Pharmacol.* 2017;79:1067-1076.

162. Badros AZ, Vij R, Martin T, et al. Carfilzomib in multiple myeloma patients with renal impairment: pharmacokinetics and safety. *Leukemia.* 2013;27:1707-1714.

163. Jhaveri KD, Chidella S, Varghese J, et al. Carfilzomib-related acute kidney injury. *Clin Adv Hematol Oncol.* 2013;11:604-605.

164. Brown J, Plummer R, Bauer TM, et al. Pharmacokinetics of carfilzomib in patients with advanced malignancies and varying degrees of hepatic impairment: an open-label, single-arm, phase 1 study. *Exp Hematol Oncol.* 2017;6:27.

165. Yang J, Wang Z, Fang Y, et al. Pharmacokinetics, pharmacodynamics, metabolism, distribution, and excretion of carfilzomib in rats. *Drug Metab Dispos.* 2011;39:1873-1882.

166. Siegel DS, Martin T, Wang M, et al. A phase 2 study of single-agent carfilzomib (PX-171-003-A1) in patients with relapsed and refractory multiple myeloma. *Blood.* 2012;120:2817-2825.

167. Herndon TM, Deisseroth A, Kaminskas E, et al. U.S. Food and drug administration approval: carfilzomib for the treatment of multiple myeloma. *Clin Cancer Res.* 2013;19:4559-4563.

168. Berenson JR, Hilger JD, Yellin O, et al. Replacement of bortezomib with carfilzomib for multiple myeloma patients progressing from bortezomib combination therapy. *Leukemia.* 2014;28:1529-1536.

169. Dimopoulos MA, Goldschmidt H, Niesvizky R, et al. Carfilzomib or bortezomib in relapsed or refractory multiple myeloma (ENDEAVOR): an interim overall survival analysis of an open-label, randomised, phase 3 trial. *Lancet Oncol.* 2017;18:1327-1337.

170. Rosenthal A, Luthi J, Belohlavek M, et al. Carfilzomib and the cardiorenal system in myeloma: an endothelial effect? *Blood Cancer J.* 2016;6:e384.

171. Chari A, Hajje D. Case series discussion of cardiac and vascular events following carfilzomib treatment: possible mechanism, screening, and monitoring. *BMC Cancer.* 2014;14:915.

172. Shah JJ, Stadtmauer EA, Abonour R, et al. Carfilzomib, pomalidomide, and dexamethasone for relapsed or refractory myeloma. *Blood.* 2015;126:2284-2290.

173. Berenson JR, Cartmell A, Bessudo A, et al. CHAMPION-1: a phase 1/2 study of once-weekly carfilzomib and dexamethasone for relapsed or refractory multiple myeloma. *Blood.* 2016;127:3360-3368.

174. Kupperman E, Lee EC, Cao Y, et al. Evaluation of the proteasome inhibitor MLN9708 in preclinical models of human cancer. *Cancer Res.* 2010;70:1970-1980.

175. Chauhan D, Tian Z, Zhou B, et al. In vitro and in vivo selective antitumor activity of a novel orally bioavailable proteasome inhibitor MLN9708 against multiple myeloma cells. *Clin Cancer Res.* 2011;17:5311-5321.

176. Ninlaro Prescribing Information. 2017. at https://www.ninlarohcp.com/pdf/prescribing-information.pdf.

177. Gupta N, Hanley MJ, Venkatakrishnan K, et al. Effects of strong CYP3A inhibition and induction on the pharmacokinetics of ixazomib, an oral proteasome inhibitor: results of drug-drug interaction studies in patients with advanced solid tumors or lymphoma and a physiologically based pharmacokinetic analysis. *J Clin Pharmacol.* 2017;58:180-192.

178. Dimopoulos MA, Sonneveld P, Leung N, et al. International myeloma working group recommendations for the diagnosis and management of myeloma-related renal impairment. *J Clin Oncol.* 2016;34:1544-1557.

179. Kumar SK, Bensinger WI, Zimmerman TM, et al. Phase 1 study of weekly dosing with the investigational oral proteasome inhibitor ixazomib in relapsed/refractory multiple myeloma. *Blood.* 2014;124:1047-1055.

180. Richardson PG, Baz R, Wang M, et al. Phase 1 study of twice-weekly ixazomib, an oral proteasome inhibitor, in relapsed/refractory multiple myeloma patients. *Blood.* 2014;124:1038-1046.

181. Moreau P, Masszi T, Grzasko N, et al. Ixazomib, an investigational oral proteasome inhibitor (PI), in combination with lenalidomide and dexamethasone (IRd), significantly extends progression-free survival (PFS) for patients (Pts) with relapsed and/or refractory multiple myeloma (RRMM): The phase 3 tourmaline-MM1 study (NCT01564537). *Blood.* 2015;126:Abstract 727.

182. Ventii KH, Wilkinson KD. Protein partners of deubiquitinating enzymes. *Biochem J.* 2008;414:161-175.

183. Das DS, Ray A, Song Y, et al. Synergistic anti-myeloma activity of the proteasome inhibitor marizomib and the IMiD((R)) immunomodulatory drug pomalidomide. *Br J Haematol.* 2015;171:798-812.

184. Badros A, Singh Z, Dhakal B, et al. Marizomib for central nervous system-multiple myeloma. *Br J Haematol.* 2017;177:221-225.

185. Di K, Lloyd GK, Abraham V, et al. Marizomib activity as a single agent in malignant gliomas: ability to cross the blood-brain barrier. *Neuro Oncol.* 2016;18:840-848.

186. Spencer A, Harrison S, Zonder J, et al. A phase 1 clinical trial evaluating marizomib, pomalidomide and low-dose dexamethasone in relapsed and refractory multiple myeloma (NPI-0052-107): final study results. *Br J Haematol.* 2017;180:41-51.

187. Shah J, Niesvizky R, Stadtmauer E, et al. Oprozomib, pomalidomide, and dexamethasone (OPomd) in patients (Pts) with relapsed and/or refractory multiple myeloma (RRMM): initial results of a phase 1b study (NCT01999335). *Blood.* 2015;126:Abstract 378.

188. Hari PN, Shain KH, Voorhees PM, et al. Oprozomib and dexamethasone in patients with relapsed and/or refractory multiple myeloma: Initial results from the dose escalation portion of a phase 1b/2, multicenter, open-label study. *Blood.* 2014;124:Abstract 3453.

189. Mulligan G, Mitsiades C, Bryant B, et al. Gene expression profiling and correlation with outcome in clinical trials of the proteasome inhibitor bortezomib. *Blood.* 2007;109:3177-3188.

190. Oerlemans R, Franke NE, Assaraf YG, et al. Molecular basis of bortezomib resistance: proteasome subunit beta5 (PSMB5) gene mutation and overexpression of PSMB5 protein. *Blood.* 2008;112:2489-2499.

191. Politou M, Karadimitris A, Terpos E, et al. No evidence of mutations of the PSMB5 (beta-5 subunit of proteasome) in a case of myeloma with clinical resistance to Bortezomib. *Leuk Res.* 2006;30:240-241.

192. Wang L, Kumar S, Fridley BL, et al. Proteasome beta subunit pharmacogenomics: gene resequencing and functional genomics. *Clin Cancer Res.* 2008;14:3503-3513.

193. Walter P, Ron D. The unfolded protein response: from stress pathway to homeostatic regulation. *Science.* 2011;334:1081-1086.

194. Reimold AM, Iwakoshi NN, Manis J, et al. Plasma cell differentiation requires the transcription factor XBP-1. *Nature.* 2001;412:300-307.

195. Leung-Hagesteijn C, Erdmann N, Cheung G, et al. Xbp1s-negative tumor B cells and pre-plasmablasts mediate therapeutic proteasome inhibitor resistance in multiple myeloma. *Cancer Cell.* 2013;24:289-304.

196. Kraus M, Bader J, Overkleeft H, et al. Nelfinavir augments proteasome inhibition by bortezomib in myeloma cells and overcomes bortezomib and carfilzomib resistance. *Blood Cancer J.* 2013;3:e103.

197. Driessen C, Müller R, Novak U, et al. The HIV protease inhibitor nelfinavir in combination with bortezomib and dexamethasone (NVd) has excellent activity in patients with advanced, proteasome inhibitor-refractory multiple myeloma: A multicenter phase II trial (SAKK 39/13). *Blood.* 2016;128:487.

198. Soriano GP, Besse L, Li N, et al. Proteasome inhibitor-adapted myeloma cells are largely independent from proteasome activity and show complex proteomic changes, in particular in redox and energy metabolism. *Leukemia.* 2016;30:2198-2207.

199. Besse A, Stolze SC, Rasche L, et al. Carfilzomib resistance due to ABCB1/MDR1 overexpression is overcome by nelfinavir and lopinavir in multiple myeloma. *Leukemia.* 2017;32:391-401.

200. Goldberg AL. Protein degradation and protection against misfolded or damaged proteins. *Nature.* 2003;426:895-899.

201. Harrigan JA, Jacq X, Martin NM, et al. Deubiquitylating enzymes and drug discovery: emerging opportunities. *Nat Rev Drug Discov.* 2017;17:57-78.

202. Tian Z, D'Arcy P, Wang X, et al. A novel small molecule inhibitor of deubiquitylating enzyme USP14 and UCHL5 induces apoptosis in multiple myeloma and overcomes bortezomib resistance. *Blood.* 2014;123:706-716.

203. Wang X, Mazurkiewicz M, Hillert EK, et al. The proteasome deubiquitinase inhibitor VLX1570 shows selectivity for ubiquitin-specific protease-14 and induces apoptosis of multiple myeloma cells. *Sci Rep.* 2016;6:26979.

204. Song Y, Li S, Ray A, et al. Blockade of deubiquitylating enzyme Rpn11 triggers apoptosis in multiple myeloma cells and overcomes bortezomib resistance. *Oncogene.* 2017;36:5631-5638.

205. Song Y, Ray A, Li S, et al. Targeting proteasome ubiquitin receptor Rpn13 in multiple myeloma. *Leukemia.* 2016;30:1877-1886.

206. Kronke J, Udeshi ND, Narla A, et al. Lenalidomide causes selective degradation of IKZF1 and IKZF3 in multiple myeloma cells. *Science.* 2014;343:301-305.

207. Lu G, Middleton RE, Sun H, et al. The myeloma drug lenalidomide promotes the cereblon-dependent destruction of Ikaros proteins. *Science.* 2014;343:305-309.

208. Winter GE, Buckley DL, Paulk J, et al. Drug development. Phthalimide conjugation as a strategy for in vivo target protein degradation. *Science.* 2015;348:1376-1381.

209. Lai AC, Toure M, Hellerschmied D, et al. Modular PROTAC design for the degradation of oncogenic BCR-ABL. *Angew Chem Int Ed Engl.* 2016;55:807-810.

Thalidomide and its Analogs in the Treatment of Hematologic Malignancies, Including Multiple Myeloma, and Solid Tumors

Jacob Laubach, Constantine S. Mitsiades, and Bruce A. Chabner

Discovery and Mode of Action of Thalidomide

Thalidomide was originally developed in the 1950s for the treatment of pregnancy-associated morning sickness. However, its extensive over-the-counter marketing in Europe led to tragic consequences of teratogenecity[1–3] and its subsequent withdrawal from the market.[4,5] The teratogenic properties of thalidomide raised the hypothesis that the potent inhibitory effects of thalidomide on growing fetal tissues might be redirected toward inhibiting cancer growth.[6] In fact, in the early 1960s, a trial of thalidomide for 71 patients with advanced cancers reported resolution of a pulmonary metastasis in a patient with renal cell carcinoma (RCC).[7] In the second trial in 21 patients with various types of advanced cancer (including two patients with multiple myeloma [MM]), thalidomide at 600 to 2,000 mg daily doses, palliated symptoms in approximately one third of patients, slowed tumor growth in 2 patients.[8] However, these results were not deemed sufficiently encouraging to warrant further clinical development efforts, until evidence emerged of its immune-modulatory actions[9,10] and its beneficial effects in treating erythema nodosum leprosum (ENL),[11] Behçet's disease,[12] graft versus host disease (GVHD),[13] and oral ulcers and wasting associated with HIV infection.[14,15] This reemergence of thalidomide was reflected by its Food and Drug Administration (FDA) approval in 1998 for the short-term treatment of cutaneous manifestations of moderate to severe ENL, together with its use as maintenance therapy to prevent recurrence of cutaneous ENL.[9] This FDA approval was of critical importance for the clinical applications of thalidomide not only because the drug has since become a treatment of choice for ENL but also because the approval allowed for off-label uses of this medication in other disease states in which the immunomodulatory and antiangiogenic properties of thalidomide might be beneficial.[9,16–18] To prevent any occurrence of teratogenic effects, thalidomide is now administered under strict guidelines to prevent fetal exposure to this medication.[17]

The interest in thalidomide as an anticancer drug was rekindled in the 1990s with the realization that tumor-associated vasculature is an important therapeutic target in a broad range of neoplasias and that thalidomide and its metabolites possess substantial antiangiogenic properties in a wide range of in vivo and in vitro models of neovascularization.[16,19–28] Indeed, thalidomide inhibited angiogenesis induced by basic fibroblast growth factor (bFGF) in the rabbit cornea micropocket assay or by vascular endothelial growth factor (VEGF) in a murine model of corneal vascularization.[16,27] Thalidomide was thus evaluated for the treatment of various neoplasias.[29] Of particular note was the well-chronicled decision to test thalidomide, at the suggestion of an especially enlightened wife of an MM patient at the University of Arkansas, where clinical benefit in two of three patients led to a larger phase II effort.[30] Extensive clinical trials confirmed activity of thalidomide-based therapy for MM and led to studies in other hematologic malignancies and solid tumors. Despite progress in its use and the fact that thalidomide is not associated with the classical pattern of toxicities seen with conventional DNA- or microtubule-targeting chemotherapeutics, this drug is not devoid of adverse effects. This realization led to clarification of the novel mechanism of action of thalidomide analogs (referred to as "ImmunoModulatory Thalidomide Derivatives" or IMIDs) and the design of analogs with improved clinical activity and reduced side effects.

In this chapter, we present a comprehensive review of the pharmacology of thalidomide and its analogs, a description of preclinical studies that illuminate the complex mechanisms of the action of thalidomide, and a brief overview of clinical trials of IMIDs in MM, and in other malignancies.

Mechanism of Action of Thalidomide and Analogs

It was originally hypothesized that the teratogenic and antitumor effects of thalidomide have common underlying mechanistic denominator(s), such as the antiangiogenic or immunostimulatory effect(s) of these compounds. Through protein affinity purification using particles covalently bound to thalidomide, Handa's laboratory first documented that thalidomide binds to a unique substrate, the E3 ubiquitin ligase cereblon, and alters its specificity in a manner that leads to ubiquitination and proteasomal degradation of neosubstrates, including the transcription factors Ikaros and Aiolos,[31] which typically do not interact with cereblon. There is now strong evidence that depletion of these proteins can account for the anti-MM effects of IMIDs[31–33] (Fig. 20.1).

Regarding the other antitumor actions of IMIDs, lenalidomide is uniquely active in patients with the 5q-myelodysplasic syndrome

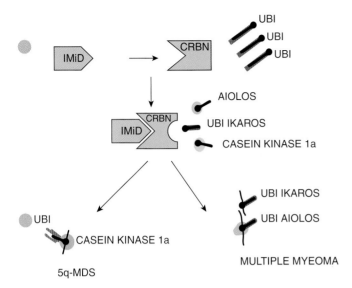

FIGURE **20.1** Interaction of IMiDs with cereblon (CRBN), an E3 ligase, altering the substrate selectivity of the enzyme and leading to the attachment of ubiquitin to transcription factors Ikaros and Aiolos, as well as casein kinase 1a, and other neosubstrates. These ubiquitinated substrates are then degraded, leading to beneficial effects in multiple myeloma and 5q-myelodysplasia (MDS).

(MDS); engagement of cereblon by lenalidomide induces the binding of the E3 ligase to casein kinase 1a, which is located in the deleted 5q-region of chromosome 5, and is therefore haplodeficient in these patients. The degradation of casein kinase 1a activates p53 and leads to apoptosis.[31]

A number of factors lend uncertainty as to whether other known effects on the immune system and on stromal-tumor interactions may contribute to its antitumor activity, and indeed whether these actions result from drug-CRBN interaction. These factors include (a) the preclinical in vitro and in vivo studies of thalidomide necessary to dissect its mechanisms of action are difficult to perform and interpret because of the enantiomeric interconversion and spontaneous cleavage of the drug to multiple metabolites in vivo,[34] many of which have been incompletely characterized; (b) the in vivo activity of thalidomide likely requires metabolic activation by the liver, a finding that may account at least in part for the discordance between the modest, at best, activity of thalidomide in in vitro assays of antitumor activity[28,35] and its potent in vivo effect; (c) the metabolic, immunologic, and antiangiogenic actions in preclinical studies of members of the thalidomide class are quite complex, and their possible relevance to anticancer therapy in humans is difficult to discern; (d) although it is now documented that thalidomide and its derivatives bind to CRBN, their chemical structures does not offer readily recognizable clues to confirm or refute the existence of other possible intracellular molecular targets that might fully explain its clinical activity or profile of adverse events; and (e) the species-specific differences in the metabolism and other pharmacokinetic properties of thalidomide complicate the extrapolation of in vivo data from many animal models to the clinical setting in humans.[27]

A wealth of mechanistic information has been acquired in MM, mainly because this is the disease setting in which this drug class has demonstrated its most impressive clinical activity. Despite the modest activity of thalidomide in antitumor assays in vitro,[35] this drug is currently considered to confer its in vivo anti-MM effects via at least four distinct, but potentially complementary, actions: (a) direct antiproliferative/proapoptotic antitumor effect,[35] probably mediated by one or more of its in vivo metabolites[36]; (b) indirect targeting of tumor cells by abrogation of protective effects conferred to MM tumor cells by bone marrow stromal cells (BMSCs) via paracrine or autocrine secretion of cytokines and growth factor or via cell adhesion molecule-mediated interactions[35]; (c) antiangiogenic effects; and (d) immunomodulatory effects, which contribute to enhanced antitumor immune response.[37]

Direct Antitumor Activity

The notion that thalidomide possesses direct antitumor effects in MM and other diseases is inferred from preclinical and clinical studies. Although the in vitro effect of thalidomide on proliferation and viability of MM cells is relatively modest in short-term assays,[35] thalidomide derivatives, such as lenalidomide (Revlimid, CC-5013), and pomalidomide (CC-4047, Actimid, later called pomalidomide),[35,36] have far more potent in vitro antiproliferative and proapoptotic properties. These effects were assayed in the absence of any other cell type (e.g., stromal, endothelial, immune, or liver cells),[35,36] suggesting that thalidomide and its metabolites may confer direct in vivo anticancer effects. The precise mechanism(s) for this direct effect has since been clarified by the demonstration that IMiDs as a class bind to the E3 ligase cereblon (CRBN), and alter its specificity in a manner that leads to ubiquitination and proteasomal degradation of proteins the stability of which is not otherwise regulated by CRBN.[32,33] The two main MM-relevant neosubstrates of CRBN are the transcription factors IKZF1 and IKZF3 (also referred to as *Ikaros* and *Aiolos*). In contrast to their roles in other lineages (e.g., myeloid or T lymphocytes), IKZF1 and IKZF3 reportedly function as positive regulators of MM cell proliferation and survival, so their IMID-mediated depletion is congruent with and can account for at least part of the direct, cell autonomous, anti-MM activity of these agents. Other neosubstrates of CRBN have been described, but it is either unclear if they contribute to the anti-MM activity of IMiDs (e.g., ZFP91[38] or have relevance to the activity of lenalidomide in 5q-MDS (e.g., casein kinase 1A [CSNK1A1]),[39] or have a link with the general properties of these drugs but may not mediate their preferential antineoplastic activity in these specific disorders.[40] Discovery of the CRBN-IMiD interaction has led to a new strategy to identify new compounds, which interact with CRBN to degrade specific neosubstrates. In fact, it has been proposed that thalidomide and its derivatives should be referred to as "CRBN-binding agents," to better reflect the central role of this E3 ligase in their mechanism of action.

IMiDs have a panoply of additional immunomodulatory and antiangiogenic effects, which may contribute to either the antitumor or side effect profile of individual agents. Clinically relevant concentrations of thalidomide derivatives, such as lenalidomide and pomalidomide, suppress the transcriptional activity of NF-κB in MM cells.[36,41] NF-κB is a protective responder to DNA damage, suppressing apoptosis by promoting the expression of intracellular antiapoptotic molecules that antagonize the toxic effects of corticosteroids and chemotherapeutic drugs, and perhaps accounting for.[36,41,42] NF-κB protects cells from the proapoptotic effects of steroids or cytotoxic chemotherapeutics;[36,41,42] the apparent benefits of IMIDs with dexamethasone or cytotoxic chemotherapeutics may result from suppression of NF-κB.[43–51]

Stroma-Tumor Interactions

Thalidomide and its analogues modulate the adhesive interactions of MM cells with BMSCs.[52] MM cells adhere to BMSCs and trigger their secretion of proliferative/antiapoptotic cytokines (e.g., interleukin [IL]-6).[53–55] This event is mainly paracrine, is mediated by transcriptional activation of NF-κB in BMSCs,[54] and dampens the sensitivity of MM cells to dexamethasone or cytotoxic chemotherapy.[56] Thalidomide/IMiD blocks this MM-stromal paracrine interaction, significantly inhibits proliferation, and lessens drug resistance of MM cells in the BM microenvironment.

Inhibition of Cytokine Production and Antiangiogenic Action

Thalidomide also inhibits TNF-α production, while leaving the patient's immune system otherwise intact.[57] Thus, thalidomide is useful in various inflammatory disorders characterized by increased TNF-α secretion, such as ENL, mycobacterium tuberculosis infection, GVHD, and cancer- and HIV-related cachexia.

The precise mechanism mediating thalidomide-induced inhibition of TNF-α activity is not fully understood, but is apparently distinct from those of other TNF-α inhibitors, such as pentoxifylline and dexamethasone.[58,59] Thalidomide may accelerate the degradation of TNF-α mRNA, thereby substantially (but not necessarily completely) suppressing the tumor-stimulating action of TNF-α protein.[58,60] Interestingly, thalidomide can decrease the binding of the transcription factor NF-κB to its consensus DNA-binding sites, which include not only the actual TNF-α gene[61] but also other genes modulated by TNF-α, in an NF-κB–dependent fashion.[36] Even the antiangiogenic properties of thalidomide may be mediated, at least in part, by inhibition of TNF-α signaling, in view of the proangiogenic effects of TNF-α itself.[16] However, the absence of a major effect of TNF-α in experimental models of angiogenesis and the inability of (at least some) potent TNF-α inhibitors to directly influence angiogenesis suggest that thalidomide's antiangiogenic effects cannot be attributed to TNF-α inhibition alone.[16,27]

Thalidomide and its analogs suppress the production of cytokines that regulate tumor cell proliferation and osteoclast function, including IL-6, IL-1β, IL-10, and TNF-α.[62] Thalidomide also decreases the secretion of VEGF, IL-6, and bFGF by MM and/or BM stromal cells.[16,27,63–65] These mechanisms are summarized in Figure 20.2.

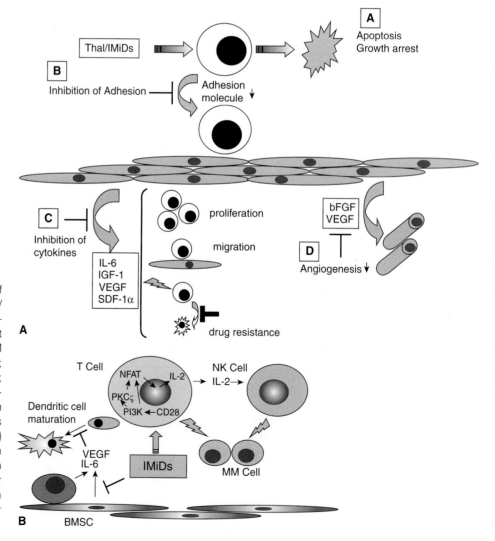

Figure 20.2 A. Antitumor activity of Thal/IMiDs in the bone marrow (BM) milieu. Thal/IMiDs (A) induce G1 growth arrest and/or apoptosis in MM cell lines and patient cells resistant to conventional chemotherapy; (B) inhibit MM cell adhesion to BM stroma and stem cells (SCs); (C) decrease cytokine production and sequelae; (D) decrease angiogenesis, in the BM microenvironment. **B.** Mechanisms of action of IMiDs in augmentation of host immune response. IMiDs augment differentiation of dendritic cells (DC) by inhibiting secretion of IL-6 and VEGF from multiple myeloma (MM) or bone marrow stem cells (BMSCs). IMiDs also stimulate natural killer (NK) cell activity by triggering IL-2 secretion from T cells mediated by CD28/PI3-K/NF-AT2 (nuclear factor of activated T cells) signaling pathway.

Immunomodulation

While IMIDs as a class have a broad range of effects on immune function, the precise effect of thalidomide on immune effector cells and their role in antitumor activity of these compounds is unclear.[66–68] Thalidomide stimulates T-cell responses against tumor cells, and this may be due to the fact that IKZF1 suppresses in T cells the production of and response to IL-2.[69] It is possible, however, that the impact of thalidomide on immune cells is subtype and context specific, as there have been reports that it may inhibit proliferation of already stimulated lymphocytes.[65–68,70]

Prior to the identification of CRBN as a key target for thalidomide and IMIDs, it had been reported that thalidomide modifies the expression patterns of cell adhesion molecules on leukocytes, inhibits neutrophil chemotaxis, and inhibits TNF-α signaling and production, enhances synthesis of IL-2, and inhibits IL-6.[54,71–74] However, in retrospect, it is not clear if these observations are generalizable to all forms of immune cell populations with antitumor properties, and perhaps with the exception of IL-2 and IL-12 production, the contribution of these molecular events to the immunostimulatory activity of IMIDs has not been fully examined.

Of particular relevance to MM, thalidomide and its analogs augment natural killer (NK) cell-mediated cytotoxicity against MM cells.[37] Thalidomide and IMIDs have been reported to act as costimulators that can trigger proliferation of anti–CD3-stimulated T cells from MM patients, accompanied by an increase in interferon-γ and IL-12 secretion. Importantly, treatment of patient peripheral blood mononuclear cells (PBMCs) with thalidomide or other IMIDs enhanced their ability to lyse autologous MM cells. Furthermore, in MM patients, thalidomide stimulated an increase in circulating CD3-CD56$^+$ NK cells.[37]

Pharmacology of Thalidomide

Thalidomide or α-N-phthalimido-glutarimide ($C_{13}O_4N_2H_9$, molecular weight of 258.2)[75] is a glutamic acid derivative, which contains two amide rings and a single chiral center (Fig. 20.3).[75] The key features for thalidomide are shown in Table 20.1. The currently available formulation of thalidomide consists, at physiologic pH, of a nonpolar racemic mixture of S(−) and R(+) isomers, which are cell membrane permeable.[75,87,88] The S isomer has been associated with the teratogenicity of thalidomide, while the R isomer has been linked with the sedative properties of the drug.[27,87,88] Because of rapid interconversion of these two isomers at physiologic pH in vivo, efforts to generate formulations of only the R isomer have failed to neutralize the teratogenic potential of thalidomide.[89]

Pharmacokinetics

The standard dose of thalidomide is 400 mg per daily, orally. The pharmacokinetics properties of thalidomide are variable, with the $t_{1/2}$ of parent compound in plasma falling in the range of 4 to 9 hours.[35] Dose reduction is indicated for progressive neuropathy or excessive sedation.

Absorption

Oral administration of thalidomide in mice and in humans demonstrated a similar pharmacokinetic pattern, with approximately 4-hour (range 3 to 6 hours) mean time to reach peak concentration in humans (t_{max}) after a thalidomide dose of 200 mg.[90–92] While the area under the curve (AUC) of concentration x time correlates with the thalidomide dose, the maximum concentration (C_{max}) is highly variable reflecting the variability of GI absorption, especially for doses in the range of 200 mg or below.[77,93] Correction for ideal body weight or body surface area does not lessen the variability.[90,91]

Distribution

In animal studies, thalidomide is widely distributed throughout most tissues[78] without significant drug binding by plasma proteins.[91,92] Thalidomide is detected in semen of patients after a period of 4 weeks of therapy.[79]

Metabolism

Thalidomide undergoes rapid and spontaneous nonenzymatic hydrolytic cleavage at physiologic pH (Fig. 20.3), generating up to 50 metabolites, 5 of which are considered to be primary metabolites.[28,78,80,89] The majority of these metabolites are unstable and their rapid degradation under physiologic conditions has complicated their characterization.[80] Although in vitro studies in rat cells suggested that thalidomide induces cytochrome (CYP) isoenzymes, subsequent evaluation of single- or multiple-dose pharmacokinetic parameters of oral thalidomide at 200 mg daily in healthy volunteers showed that thalidomide does not inhibit or induce its own metabolism over a 21-day period or longer in humans.[81,82] Only about 20% of the drug undergoes hydroxylative metabolism via the hepatic CYP2C19 isoenzyme.[83–85]

It is not clear whether any of the metabolites have biological activity. Significant intraspecies differences in the patterns of metabolism of thalidomide in mice versus humans[94–96] may explain the lack of teratogenicity in mice but the major phocomelias in humans[1–5] and why, in immunodeficient mouse models of MM, thalidomide exhibited antitumor activity only after xenotransplantation of human liver into the mice.[97]

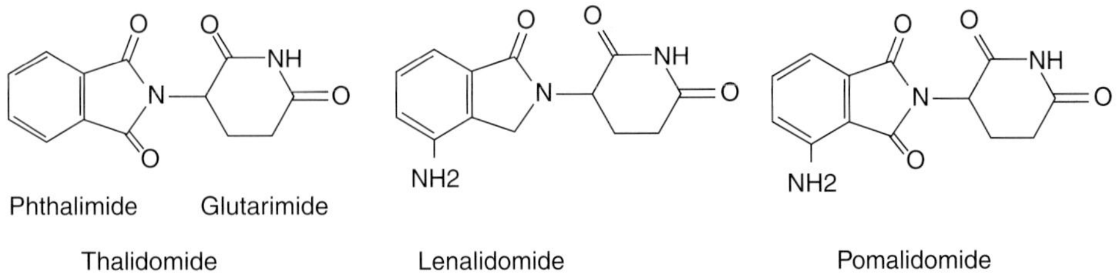

Phthalimide   Glutarimide

Thalidomide   Lenalidomide   Pomalidomide

FIGURE **20.3** Structures of thalidomide and its analogs.

TABLE

20.1 *Key features of thalidomide and analogues*

	Lenalidomide[86]	Thalidomide[77–85]	Pomalidomide[76]
Mechanism of action	Same as thalidomide, but overall higher potency	Interacts with cereblon to degrade key prosurvival proteins Blockade of tumor cell-stroma interactions Inhibition of cytokine production, including TNF-α and VEGF Immune-modulating, with stimulation of T-cell and NK cell activity	Same as thalidomide
Clinical pharmacology	Rapid absorption with T^max at 0.6–1.5 h Food decreases bioavailability AUC dose proportional over clinical range $t_{1/2}$ in plasma: 3 h. With moderate to severe renal impairment, 9–16 h Metabolism: Not a substrate of hepatic metabolic enzymes; unchanged lenalidomide is predominant circulating compound Elimination: 80% eliminated through urinary excretion of unchanged drug ***See text for dose adjustments in renal failure***	Oral bioavailability: Rapid absorption with time to peak plasma concentration at 4 h $t_{1/2}$ in plasma: 4.1–18.3 h Metabolism: Rapid, spontaneous nonenzymatic hydrolytic cleavage. Limited metabolism via CYP2C19 hydroxylation Elimination: Primarily through metabolism	Peak absorption at 3 h. AUC is dose proportional over clinical range $t_{1/2}$ in plasma: 7.5 h Metabolism: Spontaneous hydrolysis and hydroxylation by CYP2A1 and CYP 3A4 Elimination: Metabolism as above No dose adjustment for renal dysfunction
FDA indications	Relapsed/refractory multiple myeloma Low-risk or intermediate-1–risk myelodysplastic syndrome associated with 5q cytogenetic abnormality	Newly diagnosed and relapsed/refractory multiple myeloma Cutaneous erythema nodosum leprosum	Relapsed/refractory MM after lenalidomide and a proteasome inhibitor
Dosage	Multiple myeloma: 25 mg daily days 1–21 of 28-d cycle Myelodysplastic syndrome: 10 mg once daily Dose adjustment for CCr (mL/min): >50–80<: no change >30–50<: 10 mg/d <30: 15 mg q.o.d. End stage renal disease: 5 mg/d	100–200 mg once daily	4 mg/d, days 1–21 of 28-d cycle Decrease dose 50% in the presence of severe hepatic dysfunction. Give 25% dose after renal dialysis.
Drug interactions	The toxicity of anti-TNF agents such as abatacept, anakinra, canakinumab, and certolizumab may be enhanced by lenalidomide	The toxicity of anti-TNF agents such as abatacept, anakinra, canakinumab, and certolizumab may be enhanced by thalidomide	CYP inducers/inhibitors will alter pharmacokinetics
Common toxicities	Fatigue, diarrhea and/or constipation, rash, muscle cramps, cytopenias. Deep vein thrombosis 5%–10% (esp. with dexamethasone)	Fatigue, sedation, constipation, rash, peripheral neuropathy, leukopenia, venous thromboembolic events	Same as lenalidomide; also hepatic enzyme elevation, and rarely necrosis, peripheral neuropathy and confusional states, rarely tumor lysis
Warnings and precautions	FDA mandated remediation program. See thalidomide	FDA mandated remediation program. Thalidomide is a known teratogen and pregnancy should be avoided throughout therapy. Thalidomide should be used with caution in patients at risk for venous thromboembolic disease. Neuropathy can be permanent. Caution is advised when administering to patients with history of cardiovascular disease	FDA mandated remediation program. See thalidomide

Clearance

The primary mechanism of elimination of thalidomide occurs through spontaneous hydrolysis in all body fluids, with an apparent mean clearance of 10 L/h for the (R)-enantiomer and 21 L/h for the (S)-enantiomer in adult subjects.[34] This leads to higher blood concentrations of the (R)-enantiomer compared to those of the (S)-enantiomer. Thalidomide and its metabolites are rapidly excreted in the urine, while the nonabsorbed portion of the drug is excreted unchanged in feces, but clearance is primarily nonrenal, with mean terminal half-lives of the R and S isomers measured in healthy male human volunteers at 4.6 and 4.8 hours, respectively.[78,91,93] After a single dose (200 mg daily), minimal amounts of intact drug are excreted in urine over a 24-hour period.[91] Studies of both single and multiple dosing of thalidomide in elderly prostate cancer patients showed significantly longer half-life at higher dose (1,200 mg daily) versus lower doses (200 mg daily).[90] Conversely, no effect of increased age on elimination half-life was identified in the age range of 55 to 80 years.[90]

The effect of hepatic dysfunction on drug clearance has not been evaluated.

Drug Interactions

Systematic characterization of interactions between thalidomide and other drugs has not been conducted, with the exception of studies that showed a lack of significant interaction with oral contraceptives.[98] Animal studies indicated that thalidomide enhances the sedative effects of barbiturates and alcohol, as well as the catatonic effects of chlorpromazine and reserpine.[99] Conversely, the CNS stimulatory effects of medications such as methamphetamine and methylphenidate counteract the depressant effects of thalidomide.[99]

Adverse Effects

Generally, thalidomide is well tolerated at doses below 200 mg daily. Sedation and constipation are the most common adverse effects.[30,98,100,101]

The most serious adverse effect is a dose- and time-dependent peripheral sensory neuropathy.[102] Thromboembolic events (deep vein thrombosis with embolism, arterial occlusions) are increased in frequency in thalidomide-treated patients, particularly when thalidomide is used in combination with steroids and with anthracycline-based chemotherapy. In fact, thromboembolic complications, which rarely occur with single-agent thalidomide, initially led to closure of studies evaluating the regimen of thalidomide, liposomal doxorubicin, and dexamethasone.[103,104] Cardiovascular side effects associated with thalidomide include bradycardia and hypotension. The risk of adverse cardiovascular events with thalidomide treatment is higher among elderly patients with coronary disease who received multiple antihypertensive medications. Comprehensive guidelines from the International Myeloma Working Group (IMWG)[105] have been addressing the specific indications for prophylactic anticoagulation, recommending aspirin use for patients with one or no risk factor for venous thromboembolism; low molecular weight heparin (LMWH) equivalent to enoxaparin 40 mg per day; for those with two or more risk factors related to the patient herself/himself or the myeloma therapy administered; and LMWH also recommended for all patients receiving concurrent

high-dose dexamethasone or doxorubicin-based regimens, while warfarin targeting a INR of 2 to 3 is recommended as an alternative to LMWH.

Pulmonary hypertension has been reported in association with thalidomide.[106]

Peripheral neuropathy occurs in 10% to 30% of patients,[30,31,107] and is characterized as asymmetric, painful, peripheral paresthesia with sensory loss,[18,108–112] often presenting with numbness of the toes and feet, muscle cramps, weakness, signs of pyramidal tract dysfunction, or carpal tunnel syndrome.[18,75,108–112] The risk of developing peripheral neuropathy increases with higher cumulative doses of the drug, especially in elderly patients.[75] Although clinical improvement occurs following discontinuation of the drug, a degree of sensory loss may be permanent.[108–112]

Particular caution and careful monitoring are necessary when cancer patients with a prior history of neuropathy are treated with thalidomide alone or in combination with other agents associated with development of neuropathy, especially since there has been little progress in defining effective strategies for alleviation of neuropathic symptoms.

Because of its potential to cause embryo-fetal toxicity, a Black Box Warning accompanied approval of thalidomide and the other approved IMiDs, and indicates that these drugs are contraindicated in pregnancy, and mandates that women of reproductive potential must use two forms of contraception or abstinence during and for 4 weeks after stopping these agents. The drug label should be consulted prior to use.

Pharmacology of Lenalidomide (Revlimid)

In an attempt to circumvent the toxicity profile of thalidomide, several laboratories have developed analogs that preserve and even expand thalidomide antitumor activity. The first and most successful of these is lenalidomide (or 3-[4′aminoisoindoline-1′-one]-1-piperidine-2,6-dione) (Fig. 20.3), a 4-amino analog, also lacking the phthalimide ring carbonyl, a much more stable structure in aqueous solution. The key features for lenalidomide are shown in Table 20.1. It preserves the essential interaction with cereblon, and exhibits a constellation of additional pharmacological properties, including stimulation of T cells and NK cells, inhibition of angiogenesis and tumor cell proliferation, as well as modulation of hematopoietic stem cell differentiation[35–37,62,113] and has important activity in MM, Waldenström's macroglobulinemia, lymphomas, and in the 5q-variant of the myelodysplastic syndrome (MDS). Preclinical data suggested that it would have more potent activity than thalidomide, less toxicity, and would lack teratogenic effects. For MM, a 25-mg daily dose is indicated, while for myelodysplasia, the indicated dose is 10 mg per day, with modifications for renal dysfunction. The drug is rapidly absorbed following oral administration, with peak plasma levels occurring between 0.6 and 1.5 hours postdose.[114,115] Coadministration with food delays absorption somewhat but does not alter its bioavailability. The drug is composed of R- and S-isomers that rapidly interconvert, and are found in roughly equal concentrations in plasma. The C_{max} and AUC values of total lenalidomide increase proportionately with increasing dose, both over a single-dose range of 5 to 400 mg. Steady-state

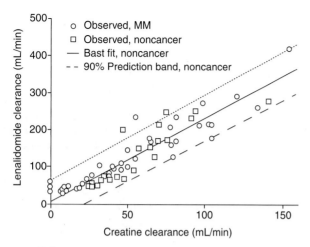

Figure **20.4** Correlation of area under the curve (AUC) of lenalidomide in plasma and creatinine clearance (CCr) of subjects. The *solid line* is the best fit line of linear regression, and the *dotted line* indicates the 90% predicted interval of best fit for patients without cancer. (From Chen N, Zhou S, Palmisano M. Clinical pharmacokinetics and pharmacodynamics of lenalidomide. *Clin Pharmacokinet.* 2017;56:139-152, with permission.)

levels of lenalidomide are achieved by the 4th day of administration, and there is no evidence of disproportionate drug accumulation with multiple dosing. About 70% of an oral dose is excreted by the kidney, clearance correlating closely with creatinine clearance (Fig. 20.4). Lenalidomide can be safely administered in full doses to patients with mild renal impairment (CCr > 50 to <80 mL/min), but for patients with moderate (>30 to 50 < mL/min) or severe renal impairment (<30 mL/min) or those with end-stage renal disease on dialysis, reduced doses should be given as indicated in Table 20.1 according to International Myeloma Working group guidelines.[115] No significant drug interactions have been reported. Regarding pharmacodynamics, a strong relationship exists between the AUC of lenalidomide and neutropenia/thrombocytopenia.

Adverse Effects of Lenalidomide

Some of the main side effects observed with thalidomide, including sedation, constipation, and peripheral neuropathy, occur infrequently in patients receiving lenalidomide. Myelosuppression is the most common high-grade toxicity associated with the regimen of lenalidomide and dexamethasone in relapsed MM.[116,117] Venous thromboembolism occurs rarely with single-agent lenalidomide,[118,119] but the risk increases in regimens that include dexamethasone.[116,117] Rash occurs in up to 30% of patients who receive lenalidomide and can be morbilliform, urticarial, dermatitic, or acneiform.[118–120] The rash is typically mild and transient and resolves with either short-term topical corticosteroid therapy or temporary discontinuation of the drug. Lenalidomide impairs stem cell collection,[121–123] but successful stem mobilization has been consistently achieved with cyclophosphamide and filgrastim pretreatment.

Lenalidomide may cause a dramatic swelling of lymph nodes, and tumor lysis, in patients with CLL, a phenomenon referred to as the tumor flare reaction. The reaction is particularly common in patients with renal dysfunction receiving a 20- to 25-mg/d dose. Pretreatment allopurinol and hydration are indicated in these patients.

Pharmacology of Pomalidomide

Pomalidomide (Fig. 20.3), a 4-amino analog of thalidomide, also a stable structure, achieved FDA approval for relapsed/refractory MM in 2013 in a regimen of 4 mg/d for days 1 to 21 in a 28-day cycle. These studies indicated that the orally administered drug is well absorbed, has a mean C_{max} of 13 ng/mL, an AUC of 189 ng × h/mL, and a t_{max} of 3 hours after a 4-mg dose. The $t_{1/2}$ of parent compound is 7.5 hours. The AUC is dose proportional in the clinical dose range. 5-Hydroxy pomalidomide, the primary metabolite, is formed by CYP1A2 and CYP 3A4. The parent compound also undergoes hydrolysis of its glutarimide ring, as well as cleavage of the glutarimide ring from its partner, 3-aminophthalimido ring. None of the metabolites or hydrolysis products have significant antitumor activity.[124] Dose modification is not necessary for renal dysfunction.

The main adverse events observed in patients receiving pomalidomide include neutropenia in 50% of those treated, (particularly in heavily pretreated patients receiving higher doses of pomalidomide), thrombocytopenia, and anemia; fatigue and thromboembolic events occur in low (<5%) rates in patients receiving pomalidomide alone, and higher (up to approximately 25%) in patients receiving the dexamethasone combination.[125] Prophylaxis with aspirin is deemed as a reasonable approach to prevent thromboembolic events. Pomalidomide can infrequently (approximately 1%) cause acute noninfectious pneumonitis,[126] which is typically responsive to corticosteroids. Rarely, serious hepatotoxicity has led to liver failure, including fatalities. Liver function tests should be monitored and treatment suspended in patients with elevated values. Hypersensitivity reactions, including rash, fever, and exfoliative dermatitis, may occur. Tumor lysis syndrome is seen in patients with high tumor burden.

Doses should be reduced by 25% in patients on hemodialysis for end-stage renal disease, and in patients with mild to moderate hepatic dysfunction, and by 50% in the presence of severe hepatic dysfunction.

Clinical Studies of Thalidomide and Its Derivatives in Multiple Myeloma

Rationale for Use of Thalidomide in MM

When thalidomide was first tested clinically in MM in the late 1990s, standard MM therapy was based almost exclusively on glucocorticoids and DNA damaging chemotherapy (including high-dose melphalan with stem cell transplant)[127,128] and novel therapeutic modalities, departing from this conventional framework, were needed to improve clinical outcomes. Thalidomide was considered as a candidate for such a role, because it inhibits angiogenesis,[16] which was recognized in the mid- to late-1990s as a key hallmark of tumor biology in vivo and a putative therapeutic target in its own right.[100] Bone marrow sinusoids in normal individuals have extensive networks of vascular support, but the homing to marrow of malignant cells from MM cells or other hematologic neoplasias is associated with a further increase in BM microvascular density, particularly in cases with poor prognosis or advanced relapsed/refractory disease.[26,31,100,129–134]

In light of the recent knowledge on the role of CRBN and its neosubstrates on the effects of thalidomide and its derivatives on MM and T cells, it is less clear how much the proposed antiangiogenic effect actually contributes to the clinical activity of thalidomide. However, this effect was a strong component of the initial rationale of exploring the use of thalidomide in MM and other hematologic neoplasias.

Thalidomide in Relapsed and Refractory MM

Thalidomide therapy for advanced refractory MM was initiated after initial experience in three patients treated at the University of Arkansas, Little Rock. This prompted a phase II study of single-agent thalidomide in 84 patients who had relapsed and refractory MM,[31] and were heavily pretreated based on the standard-of-care regimens available that time (e.g., 90% of patients had relapsed after receiving high-dose chemotherapy) and high proportion of patients with at least one feature associated with adverse prognosis to those standard-of-care regimens, including deletion of chromosome 13[31,135]; greater than 50% infiltration of BM by malignant plasma cells; or plasma cell labeling index greater than 1% (which signifies increased proliferative rate of MM cells). Patients received a starting dose of 200 mg at nighttime, with subsequent dose escalations by 200 mg every 2 weeks, to a maximum of 800 mg. In this study, a large percentage of patients attained higher daily doses of thalidomide (up to 400, 600, and 800 mg/d in 86%, 68%, and 55% of patients, respectively). It should be noted though that subsequent studies have in general administered thalidomide at lower doses (e.g., 200 mg/d or lower), especially in the context of combination with other anti-MM drugs, in order to decrease the rate of severe adverse events and allow patients to stay on treatment for longer periods of time.

In this first thalidomide trial in MM, response was defined as ≥25% reduction in serum or urine levels of paraprotein and was seen in 27 patients (32%); 8 patients exhibited ≥90% decrease in serum or urine paraprotein level; median time to response was approximately 2 months; and 78% of responding patients had decreased plasma cell infiltration of BM and increased hemoglobin values were observed. Notably, BM microvascular density was not significantly decreased, even among those who responded to treatment. At that time, this observation was not considered to override the initial rationale for thalidomide use on the basis of its antiangiogenic potential.

In this initial thalidomide trial in MM, adverse events were reported to be mild to moderate, with incidence at higher dose levels. Constipation was frequent, but manageable with administration of laxatives. Peripheral neuropathy was reported in 12% and 28% in patients receiving 200 and 800 mg daily dose, respectively. Other mild to moderate side effects included weakness, fatigue, and somnolence. More severe adverse events were infrequent (occurring in ≤10% of patients), and hematologic effects were rare. For instance, significant leukopenia, anemia, and/or thrombocytopenia were reported in less than 5% of patients. One responding patient died suddenly on day 37 of treatment, most likely due to sepsis, but a possible relationship to thalidomide could not be ruled out. After 12 months of follow-up, Kaplan-Meier estimates of the mean EFS and OS for all patients were 22% and 58%, respectively.

Given that therapeutic options were quite limited for this patient population at the time of that trial, its results created a paradigm shift for the myeloma therapy, led to subsequent studies

from other centers (e.g., a phase II trial at the MD Anderson Cancer Center[103,136]), which confirmed the anti-MM activity of single-agent thalidomide, provided the impetus for trials combining thalidomide with other therapies, and examined the role of thalidomide or its combinations, in earlier stages of the disease.

Thalidomide-based combination regimens were explored with the intent to capitalize on the different mechanisms of action and nonoverlapping toxicities of thalidomide versus other drug classes and, importantly, the potential for additive or even synergistic anti-MM effect. Initially, these regimens primarily included conventional agents, for example, chemotherapy and dexamethasone, including the combination of thalidomide with dexamethasone, cyclophosphamide, etoposide, and cisplatin, the combination of dexamethasone, thalidomide, and 4 days of continuous-infusion cisplatin, doxorubicin, cyclophosphamide, and etoposide (DTPACE)[137]; combination of dexamethasone and clarithromycin with low-dose thalidomide,[49] although the effect of clarithromycin appears to involve a change in the metabolism of dexamethasone, rather than potentiation of thalidomide activity per se; and combination of melphalan, thalidomide, and prednisone (MPT).[138] Eventually, when proteasome inhibitors, such as bortezomib emerged, additional combinations were developed, incorporating both of these new class of drugs, such as bortezomib, thalidomide, dexamethasone,[139] (VTD); bortezomib, melphalan-prednisone, thalidomide (VMPT)[140]; bortezomib, dexamethasone, thalidomide, cisplatin, doxorubicin, cyclophosphamide, and etoposide (VDT-PACE)[141–143] and other more complex regimens.

Some of these combinations, which were initially developed in advanced, relapsed/refractory MM, were eventually tested in earlier lines of therapy, including newly diagnosed MM and the setting of maintenance therapy after autologous stem cell transplantation. For example, several randomized studies compared MPT versus melphalan and prednisone (MP) a previous standard of care in MM, and demonstrated the superiority of MPT in transplant-ineligible newly diagnosed MM.[138,144,145]

For the transplant-eligible newly diagnosed patients, melphalan-containing induction therapies are avoided due to the toxic effect of melphalan on hematopoietic stem cells. By contrast, given its lack of myelotoxicity, thalidomide and dexamethasone (Thal-Dex) represents a good option in this context. In fact, based on a phase III study on 470 previously untreated MM patients, Thal-Dex was superior to dexamethasone alone in terms of both ORR (63% versus 46%) and TTP (median 22.6 months versus 6.5 months),[146] without a difference in OS at the time of publication of the corresponding study. In that study, as well as others with this doublet combination, Thal-Dex treated patients exhibited higher frequency of venous thromboembolic events, such as deep vein thrombosis (DVT) and pulmonary embolism (PE), compared to historical experience with dexamethasone alone or the clinical studies of thalidomide monotherapy. As explained in a previous section of this chapter, this hypercoagulability on combination with dexamethasone, and potentially other drugs, has been observed with other members of the thalidomide class, including lenalidomide. It is conceivable that thalidomide and its metabolites cause a modest increase in the degree of therapy-associated hypercoagulability, which is significantly enhanced when the drug is combined with other agents, with potential agents, with prothrombotic properties, or capable of triggering vascular endothelial stress.[104,147]

Several randomized clinical trials have evaluated the role of thalidomide in the maintenance therapy after autologous stem cell transplant (ASCT) for select patients[148–150]: patients who received thalidomide-containing maintenance therapy experienced longer progression-free (in all 4 studies) and overall survival (in three of the four studies), a result supported by 2 separate meta-analyses.[151,152] It is notable though that in the study by Attal et al., the benefit of thalidomide maintenance therapy was observed in patients who did not achieve at least a very good partial remission (VGPR) with induction and ASCT.[148] In addition, in the study by Barlogie and colleagues, the median survival following relapse was shorter among patients who received thalidomide as part of therapy.[149] These considerations, as well as the cumulative toxicities associated with thalidomide maintenance, particularly peripheral neuropathy, and likely played a key role why lenalidomide, which does not cause neuropathy, became the main member of the thalidomide class used in the maintenance setting.

In the United States and many Western countries, thalidomide use for MM treatment has been largely replaced by lenalidomide or pomalidomide. It is notable though that in countries with resource-challenged healthcare systems, use of thalidomide and its combinations are still important therapeutic options worldwide.

Lenalidomide

Rationale for Its Use in MM

Thalidomide-based therapies achieve higher response rates and longer progression-free survival (PFS) and overall survival (OS), compared to regimens with single-agent thalidomide era. However, thalidomide has substantial adverse events (sedation, neuropathy), especially at higher doses or with longer-term treatment. Some of these toxicities can generally be managed through preemptive dose reductions, careful patient selection, and comprehensive monitoring of patients. However, clinical investigators soon realized that some thalidomide analogs may retain or even surpass the anti-MM activity of their parent compound while exhibiting less toxicity (neuropathy and sedation).[119]

The original efforts to develop thalidomide analogs yielded two classes of derivatives, the phosphodiesterase type 4 inhibitors, which inhibit TNF-α signaling but have little effect on T-cell activation (the so-called selective cytokine inhibitory drugs or SelCids), and another group of nonphosphodiesterase type 4 inhibitors, known as IMiDs, which not only inhibit TNF-α but also markedly stimulate T-cell proliferation and interferon-gamma production. Lenalidomide and pomalidomide are members of the IMiD class of drugs.

Lenalidomide in Relapsed MM

Building on the clinical success of thalidomide and preclinical studies, which showed that IMiDs, including lenalidomide (initially referred to as CC-5013), exhibit greater potency than thalidomide, a phase I dose escalation study of this agent was performed in patients with relapsed or refractory MM.[119] The study identified grade 3 myelosuppression beyond day 28 in all patients treated at the 50 mg/d dose level, but dose reduction to 25 mg/d was well tolerated, and therefore this dose was considered to represent the maximal tolerated dose (MTD) for lenalidomide. Unlike thalidomide use, no

significant somnolence, constipation, or neuropathy was seen in any cohort of that study. Best responses of at least 25% reduction in paraprotein occurred in 71% (17 of 24), including 46% (n=11) patients who had received prior thalidomide.[119]

After these encouraging results, a phase II multicenter randomized controlled open-label study compared oral lenalidomide at 30 mg once daily or 15 mg twice daily for a total of six cycles, each comprising 3 weeks on therapy and 1 week off. The trial documented that the 30-mg once daily dose is better tolerated than the twice daily regimen and is highly active, with a response rate of approximately 35% and a manageable adverse event profile. Notably, when dexamethasone was added to lenalidomide, responses were seen in about 40% of cases.[118]

This observation about the increased response rate in combination with dexamethasone, combined with similar prior experience with thalidomide-dexamethasone combinations led to two international phase III studies of dexamethasone (40 mg days 1 to 4, 9 to 12, and 17 to 20 during the first four cycles and on days 1 to 4 of subsequent cycles) plus lenalidomide (25 mg/d on days 1 to 21 of a 28-day cycle) or placebo in relapsed MM, the North American MM-009[116] and the European/Israeli/Australian MM-010 study.[117] Median TTP, the primary end point of the study, overall response rates, and CR rates, as well as median OS were superior with lenalidomide-dexamethasone (LD) as compared to dexamethasone in both studies. These results led to the approval of lenalidomide/dexamethasone in relapsed MM by both the FDA and the European Medicines Agency (EMEA).

Similar to the clinical development of thalidomide, the clinical success of lenalidomide in advanced MM, eventually led to clinical studies in the newly diagnosed and maintenance settings, as well as efforts to develop additional lenalidomide-containing combination regimens.

In a randomized phase III study in previously untreated MM, 445 patients received lenalidomide (25 mg days 1 to 21 of each 28-day cycle) combined with high-dose dexamethasone (LD) (40 mg days 1 to 4, 9 to 12, and 17 to 20) of low-dose dexamethasone (Ld) (40 mg days 1, 8, 15, and 22): LD treatment led to superior response rates than Ld, but significantly higher 1-year OS was observed in the Ld arm (96% versus 87%).[153] This result presumably occurred because of increased adverse events related to the higher doses of corticosteroids, in particular, venous thromboembolic events, and serious infections.

A randomized phase 3 trial compared, in transplant-ineligible newly diagnosed MM patients, the combination of lenalidomide and dexamethasone in 28-day cycles until disease progression versus the same combination for 72 weeks (18 cycles) or to MPT for 72 weeks. In that study, continuous lenalidomide-dexamethasone had longer progression-free survival versus MPT, and demonstrated an overall survival benefit at the interim analysis.[154]

Another lenalidomide-containing regimen evaluated for frontline therapy in MM included melphalan, prednisone, and lenalidomide (MPR), which was studied in elderly, transplant-ineligible MM patients. After a phase I study which established the MTD (melphalan 0.18 mg/kg days 1 to 4, prednisone 2 mg/kg days 1 to 4, and lenalidomide 10 mg days 1 to 21 of each 28-day cycle) for this regimen,[155] a randomized clinical trial demonstrated superior PFS with MPR followed by lenalidomide maintenance versus MPR without lenalidomide maintenance or MP alone.[156]

Lenalidomide maintenance initiated after autologous SCT was examined in 2 randomized placebo-controlled clinical trials by CALGB[157] and the IFM group.[158] Lenalidomide maintenance significantly prolonged the progression-free survival in both trials, and improved overall survival in the CALGB study.[157] A third open-label randomized phase 3 study in patients with newly diagnosed MM compared high-dose melphalan (200 mg/m^2) plus autologous SCT versus MPR; and also compared lenalidomide maintenance therapy versus no maintenance therapy. PFS and OS were significantly longer with high-dose melphalan plus SCT versus MPR. PFS was also significantly longer with lenalidomide maintenance than with no maintenance, but the increase in 3-year OS rate was not statistically significant (88.0% versus 79.2%). A meta-analysis of these randomized trials[159] concluded that lenalidomide maintenance after SCT was associated with substantial improvement in OS.

It is notable though that all these randomized studies pointed to more adverse events and an increase in second primary cancers with Len maintenance. On aggregate though, lenalidomide maintenance was associated with lower cumulative incidence rates of not only progression or death as a result of myeloma but also death from any cause, which is inclusive of second primary cancers. This in turn implied that despite the increased rate in second primary cancers was not sufficient to overturn the substantial benefit to patients. These considerations led in 2017 to the U.S. Food and Drug Administration approval of lenalidomide as maintenance therapy after autologous SCT for MM.

Lenalidomide-Bortezomib-Dexamethasone (RVD) Combinations: a Key Backbone for MM Therapy

The combination of lenalidomide-bortezomib-dexamethasone (RVD) holds a special position in the discussion about lenalidomide-based combinations and more broadly the role of IMIDs in the therapeutic management of MM. This combination was first informed by preclinical studies, which observed that lenalidomide and pomalidomide (referred to at the time as IMID3/CC5013 and IMID1/CC4047) could enhance the in vitro anti-MM activity of bortezomib.[36] The initial reaction by many corners of the MM field was that these interesting preclinical observations were otherwise not applicable to the clinical setting: for instance, the prevailing notion at the time was that thalidomide derivatives exhibit their anti-MM activity through primarily cell nonautonomous mechanisms and that direct antiproliferative/proapoptotic effects of these agents had a limited contribution to the overall clinical activity of this drug class. There was also a concern, in the early days of clinical development of proteasome inhibitors and IMIDs, that these 2 drug classes would not be good combination partners. The fact that proteasome inhibitors could cause immunosuppressive effects (e.g., suppression of antigen presentation in dendritic cells) that would thwart the immune-stimulatory effects of IMIDs. As more clinical experience accumulated for both classes of drugs and proteasome inhibitors were clearly documented to have limited and manageable immunosuppressive effects (e.g., herpes zoster viral reactivation), clinical trials of this combination were initiated.

The first RVD trial was a phase I dose-escalation study in patients with relapsed or refractory MM.[160] Patients received lenalidomide

(5, 10, or 15 mg/d on days 1 through 14 of 21-day cycles) and bortezomib (1.0 or 1.3 mg/m^2 on days 1, 4, 8, and 11 of each cycle). Dexamethasone (20 or 40 mg on days 1, 2, 4, 5, 8, 9, 11, and 12) was added for progressive disease after two cycles. The study documented that lenalidomide-bortezomib, with or without Dex, was well tolerated. Reversible neutropenia, thrombocytopenia, anemia, and leukopenia were the most common treatment-related grades 3 to 4 toxicities. Among 36 response-evaluable patients, 61% achieved minimal response (>25% paraprotein reduction or better), while 83% of patients who had dexamethasone added achieved stable disease or better. Median overall survival was 37 months. This promising clinical activity led to a phase II trial of RVD in the relapsed/refractory setting[161] and a phase I/II study in newly diagnosed MM.[162]

In the multicenter phase II RVD trial in relapsed/refractory MM[161], 64 patients received up to eight 21-day cycles of bortezomib 1.0 mg/m^2, lenalidomide 15 mg/d, and dexamethasone 40/20 mg/d (cycles 1 to 4) and 20/10 mg/d (cycles 5 to 8) (days of/after bortezomib dosing). Responding patients could receive maintenance therapy. This study confirmed the tolerability of this regimen and its activity against patients with previous exposure to bortezomib and/or thalidomide/IMIDs or with various adverse prognostic features: 64% of patients had partial response or better, and the median duration of response was 8.7 months. Median progression-free and overall survivals were 9.5 and 30 months, respectively (median follow-up: 44 months).

In the newly diagnosed setting,[162] the phase I/II trial determined the phase 2 dosing of RVD to be bortezomib 1.3 mg/m^2, lenalidomide 25 mg, and dexamethasone 20 mg. The adverse effect profile was concordant with the studies in relapsed/refractory patients. Rate of partial response or better was 100% in both the phase 2 population and overall, with 74% and 67% each achieving very good partial response or better, while the estimated 18-month progression-free and overall survival for the combination treatment with/without transplantation were 75% and 97%, respectively. Lenalidomide-bortezomib-dexamethasone demonstrates favorable tolerability and is highly effective in the treatment of newly diagnosed myeloma.

The pronounced activity of RVD in the newly diagnosed setting prompted extensive studies of its role as a backbone combination for more complex regimens, as well as an induction regimen prior to autologous SCT. Indeed, RVD became the basis for regimens such as RVD plus pegylated liposomal doxorubicin[163]; or RVD plus cyclophosphamide.[164,165] These RVD-based regimens shared with RVD very high rates of durable responses, although with higher rates of adverse events. Given that RVD by itself achieves partial response rates exceeding 90% in newly diagnosed patients, it is difficult to establish that RVD combinations plus chemotherapy are more efficacious, and given the considerations about the adverse events, RVD itself was regard, as an attractive option for cytotoxic chemotherapy-free induction regimens for transplant-eligible newly diagnosed patients.

Two randomized clinical trials have examined the role of RVD with versus without autologous SCT, namely the IFM2009 study[166] and a parallel effort in the United States. The results of the first study indicate that RVD combined with SCT achieves a median progression-free survival of 50 months, and greater than 80% of patients are still alive after 5 years of follow-up. After 5+ years of follow-up in this study, patients who were randomized to the RVD-only arm had similar overall survival as the patients in the RVD plus ASCT arm. In addition, the difference in progression-free survival between patients in the RVD plus ASCT versus RVD-only arm of the study was less pronounced among patients who had achieved negativity for minimal residual disease (MRD-negative status). These latter observations, which will be further validated and expanded in the ongoing US-based study, which will provide insights on the potential scenario that, for at least a subset of MM patients who are receiving only RVD treatment, some key parameters of clinical benefit achieved with this treatment may be in the same order of magnitude as those observed in patients receiving RVD plus ASCT.

The results of the studies further support the significance of the RVD regimen, in particular and more broadly the concept of combining proteasome inhibitors and thalidomide derivatives, which is not considered an essential "backbone" for the treatment of MM. Indeed, while RVD has not received so far FDA approval, it has represented a de facto standard of care regimen for many years, especially in the United States. Importantly, the major clinical impact of these combinations provided a framework for the rapid clinical development of other combinations incorporating bortezomib or next generation proteasome inhibitors (e.g., carfilzomib, ixazomib) with lenalidomide or pomalidomide.

For example, the combinations of carfilzomib-lenalidomide-dexamethasone (CRD)[167], ixazomib-lenalidomide-dexamethasone[166-168] have both achieved US FDA approval the basis of randomized trials documenting superiority of these combinations to the doublet of lenalidomide plus dexamethasone. These approvals occurred only within a few years after the corresponding phase I studies of these combinations, in large part because the clinical development of these active regimens was build on the blueprint provided by the success of RVD in improving the outcomes of MM patients.

The clinical development and regulatory approval in the United States and other countries for pomalidomide also established a framework to substitute this IMID for lenalidomide, in various triplet combinations with proteasome inhibitors and glucocorticoids. Further phase I or II studies have examined the safety and efficacy of pomalidomide, bortezomib, and dexamethasone (PVD),[169,170] pomalidomide, ixazomib, and dexamethasone (PID),[168] and carfilzomib, pomalidomide, and dexamethasone.[169] All of these regimens exhibit activity against advanced MM. The newer members of the proteasome inhibitor or IMID classes exhibit substantial clinical activity in cases of patients with resistance or prior exposure to earlier versions of the same drug classes. It is therefore plausible that some of these regimens will become widely used in the context of resistance or prior exposure to RVD and more broadly in earlier lines of treatment.

The Impact of Novel Immunotherapies for MM on the Clinical Uses of lenalidomide and Other IMIDs

An important consideration in designing future regimens combining proteasome inhibitors with lenalidomide or other IMIDs is the emergence of novel monoclonal antibodies, such as the anti-CD38 antibodies daratumumab and isatuximab, and bispecific antibodies (Chapter 29), and CAR-T cells (Chapter 31). Because of their immune-stimulatory properties, lenalidomide and other IMIDs are considered promising partners for combination regimens with novel immunotherapies for MM. For example, daratumumab was FDA-approved in combination with lenalidomide and dexamethasone, based on the results of the POLLUX trial.[170] Similar studies combining lenalidomide or other IMIDs with other anti-CD38 antibodies (e.g., isatuximab) or antibodies against other targets (e.g., BCMA, immune check-points) are in progress.

Pomalidomide

Pomalidomide (previously referred to as CC-4047 or IMID1) is the second clinically useful immunomodulatory thalidomide derivative. Its clinical development followed a path similar to lenalidomide, with phase I testing as single agent or combined with dexamethasone in the relapsed and refractory setting,[171,172] phase II studies in combination with dexamethasone, and phase III data documenting the superior efficacy of pomalidomide plus dexamethasone versus dexamethasone alone.

Phase I studies established 2 mg/d continuous dosing, and 4 mg/d for 21 days of a 28-day cycle as safe doses and schedules, and showed a significant level of activity against relapsed or refractory MM. Rash, neutropenia, and occasional deep vein thromboses were notable adverse events.[171,172]

Phase II studies confirmed the safety and efficacy of oral pomalidomide (at 2 mg daily on days 1 to 28 of a 28-day cycle) plus oral dexamethasone (40 mg daily on days 1, 8, 15, and 22 of each cycle),[173] and addressed the outcomes with 2 different pomalidomide doses (4 mg versus 2 mg)[174]; the use of oral pomalidomide (4 mg) on days 1 to 21 (arm 21/28) versus continuously (arm 28/28) over a 28-day cycle, plus dexamethasone given weekly[175]; or the safety and efficacy of pomalidomide (4 mg/d on days 1 to 21 of each 28-day cycle) with versus without low-dose dexamethasone (40 mg/wk) in patients who had received ≥2 prior therapies (including lenalidomide and bortezomib) and had progressed within 60 days of their last therapy.[176] The aggregate conclusion from these studies was that combining oral pomalidomide with low-dose dexamethasone was a safe and effective regimen for relapsed and refractory MM, including patients refractory to both bortezomib and lenalidomide, and that a 4-mg/d pomalidomide dosing for 21 of 28 days of each cycle of treatment was the best option for further evaluation in randomized trials.

Pomalidomide gained regulatory approval based on a randomized open-label phase 3 trial (MM-003) of pomalidomide plus low-dose dexamethasone versus high-dose dexamethasone alone for patients with relapsed and refractory MM, who had failed at least two previous treatments of bortezomib and lenalidomide.[177] Patients were randomized in a 2:1 ratio between pomalidomide plus low-dose dexamethasone versus high-dose dexamethasone (40 mg/d on days 1 to 4, 9 to 12, and 17 to 20, orally) until disease progression or unacceptable toxicity. Randomization was performed in a stratified manner to ensure balance between the 2 arms in terms of age (≤75 years versus >75 years), disease population (refractory versus relapsed and refractory versus bortezomib intolerant), and number of previous treatments (two versus more than two).

Patients in the pomalidomide arm had longer median PFS (4.0 months versus 1.9 months), higher rates of grade 3 to 4 neutropenia (48% versus 16%), and pneumonia (13% versus 8%), and had similar (4% versus 5%) rates of treatment-related adverse events leading to death. Analyses performed with a two-stage Weibull method to adjust for the crossover of patients from the control arm to pomalidomide-based therapy identified that the adjusted median OS was 5.7 months versus 12.7 months, respectively.[178]

Since the FDA approval of pomalidomide-dexamethasone, and similarly to the experience with thalidomide- and especially lenalidomide-based combinations, the pomalidomide-dexamethasone doublet has become incorporated into several different regimens, including not only the previously outlined pomalidomide-bortezomib-dexamethasone (PVD)[179] but also other regimens. For instance, ixazomib, pomalidomide, and dexamethasone[168]; carfilzomib, pomalidomide, and dexamethasone[180]; marizomib, pomalidomide, and low-dose dexamethasone[181]; pomalidomide, dexamethasone, and pegylated liposomal doxorubicin[182]; daratumumab, pomalidomide, and dexamethasone[183]; pembrolizumab, pomalidomide, and low-dose dexamethasone[184]; and pomalidomide, cyclophosphamide, and dexamethasone.[185]

Most of these regimens have been tested so far in relapsed/refractory MM, but given their activity and tolerability, it is expected that at least some of them will be transitioned to earlier lines of therapy in the near future.

Clinical Studies of Thalidomide and Its Derivatives in Neoplasias Beyond MM

Therapeutic agents inducing antiangiogenic and immune-stimulatory effects can in principle exhibit clinical activities that extend to a broad range of tumors. For this reason, thalidomide and its derivatives were tested clinically against diverse neoplasias beyond myeloma, including both hematologic malignancies and solid tumors. However, in only few of these clinical settings has thalidomide or its derivatives demonstrated meaningful clinical activity.

Outside of MM, the 5q-myelodysplastic syndrome (MDS) is the clinical setting in which lenalidomide and to a lesser extent thalidomide (but not pomalidomide) have demonstrated the most consistent and pronounced clinical activity. Because BM biopsies of at least some cases of MDS exhibit increased angiogenesis, thalidomide was tested in MDS; clinical responses were reported in two of five thalidomide-treated MDS patients, with concomitant decreases in FGF and VEGF in responders.[186] In larger studies of 83, 30, and 34 MDS patients, hematologic improvement (e.g., transfusion independence) was observed in approximately 30% of evaluable patients for the first two trials and 65% in the third trial.[187–189] Higher platelet counts and lower blast percentage at baseline appeared to be associated with a higher probability of response to thalidomide. Additional studies documented normalization of counts, with cytogenetic responses, in three thalidomide-treated patients with MDS.[190] However, improvement in nonerythroid lineages was not commonly seen,[187] and dose escalation beyond 200 mg daily did not necessarily confer better hematological responses, but led to cumulative neurological toxicity and extensive early patient withdrawal from the study due to toxicity.[191] When combined with darbepoetin

treatment for MDS, thalidomide was associated with increased thromboembolic events in a small study.[192] For those patients who tolerated thalidomide use and completed a minimum of 12 weeks' treatment, the erythropoietic response rate was 29%, with median time to erythroid response of 16 weeks[187]; therefore, prolonged drug treatment appeared necessary to maximize hematological benefit. Subsequent studies confirmed that thalidomide can lower transfusion requirements, but due to the need for its prolonged administration, thalidomide use was deemed to be more suitable for patients with lower risk disease.[188,193,194]

The encouraging clinical experience with thalidomide in MDS, and the favorable profile of manageable side effects of thalidomide derivatives in MM, provided a strong rationale for evaluating lenalidomide in MDS patients.[195–198] An early study of 25 MDS patients with symptomatic or transfusion-dependent anemia reported that 62% of patients who completed 8 or more weeks of lenalidomide treatment had erythroid response (International Working Group [IWG]) and 12 patients experiencing sustained transfusion independence or rise in hemoglobin levels by 2 g/dL or greater.[195–198] Improvement in hematopoietic function was better among patients with low-risk or intermediate(int)-1–risk MDS, with 15 of 21 (71%) experiencing hematological benefit. Erythroid responses to lenalidomide were associated with complete or partial (>50%) reduction in the proportion of abnormal metaphases in 9 of 13 informative patients, as well as improved primitive progenitor outgrowth, and reduced grade of cytological dysplasia. Myeloid and platelet toxicity was dose limiting, but occurred at all dose levels depending upon cumulative drug exposure, necessitating either dose reduction or treatment interruption. These preliminary data suggested that lenalidomide represented a promising oral agent in MDS patients.

The clinical benefit of lenalidomide in MDS is confined to patients with chromosome 5q deletion. In a pivotal study involving 148 patients with 5q-MDS who received lenalidomide 10 mg daily days 1 to 21 or daily in a 28-day cycle, the need for red blood cell transfusion decreased in 76% of patients and transfusions were no longer necessary in 67%.[199] Complete resolution of cytogenetic abnormalities occurred in 36% of patients. Therapy was well tolerated, with neutropenia and thrombocytopenia being the most common high-grade toxicities. These impressive results have been confirmed in other studies of lenalidomide in MDS with 5q deletion.[200] Lenalidomide thus now represents a standard of care for individuals with low-risk and int-1–risk MDS with 5q deletion.

Primary Myelofibrosis

The increased microvascular density in the BM of patients with primary myelofibrosis (MF)[201] also prompted evaluation of thalidomide in this clinical setting. Several studies reported[202–211] that thalidomide offers, in variable percentages of patients, improvement in hematologic parameters, including increased platelet counts and hemoglobin levels, decrease in spleen size (though usually of moderate degree), increased BM megakaryopoiesis, as well as decreased BM angiogenesis.[203] Interestingly, however, some of the patients treated with 200 to 400 mg/d developed significant myeloproliferative reactions, including marked leukocytosis and thrombocytosis of unknown mechanism.[205,206] On the other hand, more than 60% of patients discontinued the drug within 6 months of starting thalidomide therapy due to side effects and almost 20% of patients had myeloproliferative reactions with leukocytosis and/or thrombocytosis. However, thalidomide appeared to maintain its clinical activity in primary MF even when daily thalidomide dose was reduced to as low as 50 mg, while most of the side effects appeared to occur at higher doses, suggesting that lower dosing may improve the therapeutic ratio. Furthermore, it appears that combination of low-dose thalidomide (50 mg daily) with oral prednisone (starting at 0.5 mg/kg/d and tapered over 3 months) is not only well tolerated but also leads to durable objective responses, including improvement in anemia, thrombocytopenia, or spleen size in some patients.[210,212]

Lenalidomide in combination with prednisone appears to be active in this disease entity. In a study involving 40 patients with MF who received lenalidomide 10 mg daily days 1 to 21 of a 28-day cycle for six cycles, the rate of partial response by IWG for Myelofibrosis Research and Treatment (IWG-MRT) was 7.5% and of clinical response, 23%.[211] Anemia and splenomegaly improved in 30% and 42% of patients, respectively. Based on a randomized phase II study, pomalidomide too appears to be active in the setting of primary MF.[206]

The clinical results observed with thalidomide and its analogs in MM raised the possibility that MM is more thalidomide responsive than other neoplasias because of characteristics intrinsic to the plasma cell lineage. This also suggested by extension that thalidomide may also be active against other plasma cell dyscrasias, including Waldenström's macroglobulinemia (WM). Indeed, single-agent thalidomide, administered in the context of a small phase II study, led to a 25% response rate in WM,[213] while a combination of low-dose thalidomide (200 mg daily), dexamethasone (40 mg once weekly), and clarithromycin (500 mg bid) showed activity.[44] Lenalidomide in conjunction with rituximab was subsequently evaluated in WM.[214] However, the regimen unexpectedly led to clinically significant anemia in 13 of 16 patients enrolled and response to therapy was inferior to that historically seen with thalidomide-containing regimens. In primary systemic amyloidosis, a phase I/II trial of single-agent thalidomide showed hematologic improvement in 5 of 11 patients and disease stabilization in 3 patients.[215] However, as in other reports, substantial toxicities were observed, especially at higher doses of thalidomide.[144,216] In contrast to experience with the agent in WM, lenalidomide therapy in AL amyloidosis has generated encouraging results in early phase clinical trials. In a phase II study involving patients with AL amyloidosis, lenalidomide 15 mg daily days 1 to 21 of a 28-day cycle produced an ORR of 60% and a CR rate of 24%.[186]

In the early stages of clinical development of thalidomide for oncologic indications, clinical or preclinical studies suggested that diseases such as acute myelogenous leukemia,[193,194] chronic lymphocytic leukemia, non-Hodgkin's lymphoma, Kaposi's sarcoma,[217] or renal cell carcinoma may be settings where thalidomide itself of IMIDs may potentially provide clinical benefit. For instance, some favorable clinical responses were observed with single-agent thalidomide in AML[193,194]; low-dose thalidomide plus 5-azacytidine in the treatment of AML arising from prior MDS[187]; lenalidomide in AML[218,219]; single-agent lenalidomide in relapsed and refractory CLL (with ORR on the order of 30%)[220]; or single-agent lenalidomide in relapsed or refractory NHL.[221] However, for most of these neoplasias, thalidomide or its derivatives are not routinely used

clinically, either because additional clinical studies did not detect an efficacy signal sufficient to warrant the administration of these agents or because of side effects, for example, the tumor flare syndrome with lenalidomide treatment in CLL, with clinical findings such as fever, rash, and rapid lymph node enlargement.[222]

Conclusion

Despite the tragic teratogenic effects associated with thalidomide in its initial clinical application, careful oversight and monitoring have allowed for its reemergence in the treatment of various diseases, wherein its diverse immunomodulatory, protein degradative, and antiangiogenic properties are beneficial. Importantly, through a combination of preclinical study, serendipity, and thoughtful clinical development, thalidomide has become more than a promising agent; thalidomide and its derivatives are now an integral part of the management of MM, MDS, and nonmalignant conditions (ENL). The development of lenalidomide and pomalidomide, which exhibit more refined biological properties and attenuated side effects, has led to new clinical applications of this drug class in both MM and other diseases. It may in fact be appropriate to redefine our thinking about thalidomide analogues, and view them not as an incremental variation over their parent compound but as a diverse group of structurally related, but functionally distinct agents, as clearly shown by their different pharmacological and clinical properties. While major recent progress has takes place in terms of better understanding the molecular basis for the mechanisms of action (e.g., cereblon interaction, antiangiogenic effects, stromal adhesive interactions, or immunomodulatory properties) of this drug class, it is still uncertain how these properties contribute to their multiple clinical actions, and their antitumor activity against MM and other hematologic disorders. The emergence and refinement of this drug class in combination with dexamethoasone and with new or established proteosome inhibitors,[223–226] have provided a remarkable paradigm for development of new cancer treatments.

Acknowledgments

The authors are grateful for the assistance of Jeffrey Sorrell in preparing this manuscript.

References

1. Somers GS. Thalidomide and congenital abnormalities. *Lancet.* 1962;1(7235): 912-913.
2. Speirs AL. Thalidomide and congenital abnormalities. *Lancet.* 1962;1(7224): 303-305.
3. Yang TJ, Yang TS, Liang HM. Thalidomide and congenital abnormalities. *Lancet.* 1963;1(7280):552-553.
4. Lenz W. The susceptible period for thalidomide malformations in man and monkey. *Ger Med Mon.* 1968;13(4):197-198.
5. Lenz W. Malformations caused by drugs in pregnancy. *Am J Dis Child.* 1966;112(2):99-106.
6. Rogerson G. Thalidomide and congenital abnormalities. *Lancet.* 1962;1:691.
7. Grabstald H, Golbey R. Clinical experiences with thalidomide in patients with cancer. *Clin Pharmacol Ther.* 1965;6:298-302.

8. Olson KB, Hall TC, Horton J, Khung CL, Hosley HF. Thalidomide (N-phthaloylglutamimide) in the treatment of advanced cancer. *Clin Pharmacol Ther.* 1965;6:292-297.

9. Hales BF. Thalidomide on the comeback trail. *Nat Med.* 1999;5(5):489-490.

10. Moller DR, Wysocka M, Greenlee BM, et al. Inhibition of IL-12 production by thalidomide. *J Immunol.* 1997;159(10):5157-5161.

11. Sheskin J. Thalidomide in the treatment of lepra reactions. *Clin Pharmacol Ther.* 1965;6:303-306.

12. Hamuryudan V, Mat C, Saip S, et al. Thalidomide in the treatment of the mucocutaneous lesions of the Behcet syndrome. A randomized, double-blind, placebo-controlled trial. *Ann Intern Med.* 1998;128(6):443-450.

13. Parker PM, Chao N, Nademanee A, et al. Thalidomide as salvage therapy for chronic graft-versus-host disease. *Blood.* 1995;86(9):3604-3609.

14. Reyes-Teran G, Sierra-Madero JG, Martinez del Cerro V, et al. Effects of thalidomide on HIV-associated wasting syndrome: a randomized, double-blind, placebo-controlled clinical trial. *AIDS.* 1996;10(13):1501-1507.

15. Jacobson JM, Greenspan JS, Spritzler J, et al. Thalidomide for the treatment of oral aphthous ulcers in patients with human immunodeficiency virus infection. National Institute of Allergy and Infectious Diseases AIDS Clinical Trials Group. *N Engl J Med.* 1997;336(21):1487-1493.

16. D'Amato RJ, Loughnan MS, Flynn E, Folkman J. Thalidomide is an inhibitor of angiogenesis. *Proc Natl Acad Sci U S A.* 1994;91(9):4082-4085.

17. Zeldis JB, Williams BA, Thomas SD, Elsayed ME. S.T.E.P.S.: a comprehensive program for controlling and monitoring access to thalidomide. *Clin Ther.* 1999;21(2):319-330.

18. Stirling DI. Thalidomide and its impact in dermatology. *Semin Cutan Med Surg.* 1998;17(4):231-242.

19. Folkman J. Tumor angiogenesis: therapeutic implications. *N Engl J Med.* 1971;285(21):1182-1186.

20. Weidner N, Semple JP, Welch WR, Folkman J. Tumor angiogenesis and metastasis—correlation in invasive breast carcinoma. *N Engl J Med.* 1991;324(1):1-8.

21. Weidner N, Folkman J, Pozza F, et al. Tumor angiogenesis: a new significant and independent prognostic indicator in early-stage breast carcinoma. *J Natl Cancer Inst.* 1992;84(24):1875-1887.

22. Weidner N, Carroll PR, Flax J, Blumenfeld W, Folkman J. Tumor angiogenesis correlates with metastasis in invasive prostate carcinoma. *Am J Pathol.* 1993;143(2):401-409.

23. Hlatky L, Tsionou C, Hahnfeldt P, Coleman CN. Mammary fibroblasts may influence breast tumor angiogenesis via hypoxia-induced vascular endothelial growth factor up-regulation and protein expression. *Cancer Res.* 1994;54(23):6083-6086.

24. Folkman J. Angiogenesis in cancer, vascular, rheumatoid and other disease. *Nat Med.* 1995;1(1):27-31.

25. Folkman J. Seminars in medicine of the Beth Israel Hospital, Boston. Clinical applications of research on angiogenesis. *N Engl J Med.* 1995;333(26):1757-1763.

26. Perez-Atayde AR, Sallan SE, Tedrow U, Connors S, Allred E, Folkman J. Spectrum of tumor angiogenesis in the bone marrow of children with acute lymphoblastic leukemia. *Am J Pathol.* 1997;150(3):815-821.

27. Kenyon BM, Browne F, D'Amato RJ. Effects of thalidomide and related metabolites in a mouse corneal model of neovascularization. *Exp Eye Res.* 1997;64(6):971-978.

28. Bauer KS, Dixon SC, Figg WD. Inhibition of angiogenesis by thalidomide requires metabolic activation, which is species-dependent. *Biochem Pharmacol.* 1998;55(11):1827-1834.

29. Marx GM, Pavlakis N, McCowatt S, et al. Phase II study of thalidomide in the treatment of recurrent glioblastoma multiforme. *J Neurooncol.* 2001;54(1):31-38.

30. Singhal S, Mehta J, Desikan R, et al. Antitumor activity of thalidomide in refractory multiple myeloma. *N Engl J Med.* 1999;341(21):1565-1571.

31. Ito T, Handa H. Cereblon and its downstream substrates as molecular targets of immunomodulatory drugs. *Int J Haematol.* 2016;104:293-299.

32. Krönke J, Udeshi ND, Narla A, et al. Lenalidomide causes selective degradation of IKZF1 and IKZF3 in multiple myeloma cells. *Science.* 2014;3436168:301-305.

33. Lu G, Middleton RE, Sun H, et al. The myeloma drug lenalidomide promotes the cereblon-dependent destruction of Ikaros proteins. *Science.* 2014;343(6168):305-309.

34. Eriksson T, Bjorkman S, Hoglund P. Clinical pharmacology of thalidomide. *Eur J Clin Pharmacol.* 2001;57(5):365-376.

35. Hideshima T, Chauhan D, Shima Y, et al. Thalidomide and its analogs overcome drug resistance of human multiple myeloma cells to conventional therapy. *Blood.* 2000;96(9):2943-2950.

36. Mitsiades N, Mitsiades CS, Poulaki V, et al. Apoptotic signaling induced by immunomodulatory thalidomide analogs in human multiple myeloma cells: therapeutic implications. *Blood.* 2002;99(12):4525-4530.

37. Davies FE, Raje N, Hideshima T, et al. Thalidomide and immunomodulatory derivatives augment natural killer cell cytotoxicity in multiple myeloma. *Blood.* 2001;98(1):210-216.

38. An J, Ponthier CM, Sack R, et al. pSILAC mass spectrometry reveals ZFP91 as IMiD-dependent substrate of the CRL4(CRBN) ubiquitin ligase. *Nat Commun* 2017;8:15398.

39. Kronke J, Fink EC, Hollenbach PW, et al. Lenalidomide induces ubiquitination and degradation of CK1alpha in del(5q) MDS. *Nature.* 2015;523(7559):183-188.

40. Eichner R, Heider M, Fernandez-Saiz V, et al. Immunomodulatory drugs disrupt the cereblon-CD147-MCT1 axis to exert antitumor activity and teratogenicity. *Nat Med.* 2016;22(7):735-743.

41. Mitsiades N, Mitsiades CS, Poulaki V, et al. Biologic sequelae of nuclear factor-kappaB blockade in multiple myeloma: therapeutic applications. *Blood.* 2002;99(11):4079-4086.

42. Hideshima T, Chauhan D, Richardson P, et al. NF-kappa B as a therapeutic target in multiple myeloma. *J Biol Chem.* 2002;277(19):16639-16647.

43. Dimopoulos MA, Anagnostopoulos A. Thalidomide in relapsed/refractory multiple myeloma: pivotal trials conducted outside the United States. *Semin Hematol.* 2003;40(4 suppl 4):8-16.

44. Coleman M, Leonard J, Lyons L, Szelenyi H, Niesvizky R. Treatment of Waldenstrom's macroglobulinemia with clarithromycin, low-dose thalidomide, and dexamethasone. *Semin Oncol.* 2003;30(2):270-274.

45. Srkalovic G, Elson P, Trebisky B, Karam MA, Hussein MA. Use of melphalan, thalidomide, and dexamethasone in treatment of refractory and relapsed multiple myeloma. *Med Oncol.* 2002;19(4):219-226.

46. Rajkumar SV, Hayman S, Gertz MA, et al. Combination therapy with thalidomide plus dexamethasone for newly diagnosed myeloma. *J Clin Oncol.* 2002;20(21):4319-4323.

47. Garcia-Sanz R, Gonzalez-Fraile MI, Sierra M, Lopez C, Gonzalez M, San Miguel JF. The combination of thalidomide, cyclophosphamide and dexamethasone (ThaCyDex) is feasible and can be an option for relapsed/refractory multiple myeloma. *Hematol J.* 2002;3(1):43-48.

48. Garcia-Sanz R, Gonzalez-Porras JR, Hernandez JM, et al. The oral combination of thalidomide, cyclophosphamide and dexamethasone (ThaCyDex) is effective in relapsed/refractory multiple myeloma. *Leukemia.* 2004;18(4):856-863.

49. Coleman M, Leonard J, Lyons L, et al. BLT-D (clarithromycin [Biaxin], low-dose thalidomide, and dexamethasone) for the treatment of myeloma and Waldenstrom's macroglobulinemia. *Leuk Lymphoma.* 2002;43(9):1777-1782.

50. Alexanian R, Weber D, Giralt S, Delasalle K. Consolidation therapy of multiple myeloma with thalidomide-dexamethasone after intensive chemotherapy. *Ann Oncol.* 2002;13(7):1116-1119.

51. Palumbo A, Giaccone L, Bertola A, et al. Low-dose thalidomide plus dexamethasone is an effective salvage therapy for advanced myeloma. *Haematologica.* 2001;86(4):399-403.

52. Geitz H, Handt S, Zwingenberger K. Thalidomide selectively modulates the density of cell surface molecules involved in the adhesion cascade. *Immunopharmacology.* 1996;31(2-3):213-221.

53. Uchiyama H, Barut BA, Mohrbacher AF, Chauhan D, Anderson KC. Adhesion of human myeloma-derived cell lines to bone marrow stromal cells stimulates interleukin-6 secretion. *Blood.* 1993;82(12):3712-3720.

54. Chauhan D, Uchiyama H, Akbarali Y, et al. Multiple myeloma cell adhesion-induced interleukin-6 expression in bone marrow stromal cells involves activation of NF-kappa B. *Blood.* 1996;87(3):1104-1112.

55. Hallek M, Bergsagel PL, Anderson KC. Multiple myeloma: increasing evidence for a multistep transformation process. *Blood.* 1998;91(1):3-21.

56. Damiano JS, Cress AE, Hazlehurst LA, Shtil AA, Dalton WS. Cell adhesion mediated drug resistance (CAM-DR): role of integrins and resistance to apoptosis in human myeloma cell lines. *Blood.* 1999;93(5):1658-1667.

57. Dunzendorfer S, Schratzberger P, Reinisch N, Kahler CM, Wiedermann CJ. Effects of thalidomide on neutrophil respiratory burst, chemotaxis, and transmigration of cytokine- and endotoxin-activated endothelium. *Naunyn Schmiedebergs Arch Pharmacol.* 1997;356(5):529-535.

58. Moreira AL, Sampaio EP, Zmuidzinas A, Frindt P, Smith KA, Kaplan G. Thalidomide exerts its inhibitory action on tumor necrosis factor alpha by enhancing mRNA degradation. *J Exp Med.* 1993;177(6):1675-1680.

59. Calderon P, Anzilotti M, Phelps R. Thalidomide in dermatology. New indications for an old drug. *Int J Dermatol.* 1997;36(12):881-887.

60. Sampaio EP, Sarno EN, Galilly R, Cohn ZA, Kaplan G. Thalidomide selectively inhibits tumor necrosis factor alpha production by stimulated human monocytes. *J Exp Med.* 1991;173(3):699-703.

61. Turk BE, Jiang H, Liu JO. Binding of thalidomide to alpha1-acid glycoprotein may be involved in its inhibition of tumor necrosis factor alpha production. *Proc Natl Acad Sci U S A.* 1996;93(15):7552-7556.

62. Corral LG, Haslett PA, Muller GW, et al. Differential cytokine modulation and T cell activation by two distinct classes of thalidomide analogues that are potent inhibitors of TNF-alpha. *J Immunol.* 1999;163(1):380-386.

63. Gupta D, Treon SP, Shima Y, et al. Adherence of multiple myeloma cells to bone marrow stromal cells upregulates vascular endothelial growth factor secretion: therapeutic applications. *Leukemia.* 2001;15(12):1950-1961.

64. Kotoh T, Dhar DK, Masunaga R, et al. Antiangiogenic therapy of human esophageal cancers with thalidomide in nude mice. *Surgery.* 1999;125(5):536-544.

65. Hastings RC, Trautman JR, Enna CD, Jacobson RR. Thalidomide in the treatment of erythema nodosum leprosum. With a note on selected laboratory abnormalities in erythema nodosum leprosum. *Clin Pharmacol Ther.* 1970;11(4):481-487.

66. Fernandez LP, Schlegel PG, Baker J, Chen Y, Chao NJ. Does thalidomide affect IL-2 response and production? *Exp Hematol.* 1995;23(9):978-985.

67. Keenan RJ, Eiras G, Burckart GJ, et al. Immunosuppressive properties of thalidomide. Inhibition of in vitro lymphocyte proliferation alone and in combination with cyclosporine or FK506. *Transplantation.* 1991;52(5): 908-910.

68. Moncada B, Baranda ML, Gonzalez-Amaro R, Urbina R, Loredo CE. Thalidomide—effect on T cell subsets as a possible mechanism of action. *Int J Lepr Other Mycobact Dis.* 1985;53(2):201-205.

69. Avitahl N, Winandy S, Friedrich C, Jones B, Ge Y, Georgopoulos K. Ikaros sets thresholds for T cell activation and regulates chromosome propagation. *Immunity.* 1999;10(3):333-343.

70. Shannon EJ, Ejigu M, Haile-Mariam HS, Berhan TY, Tasesse G. Thalidomide's effectiveness in erythema nodosum leprosum is associated with a decrease in CD4+ cells in the peripheral blood. *Lepr Rev.* 1992;63(1):5-11.

71. Haslett P, Hempstead M, Seidman C, et al. The metabolic and immunologic effects of short-term thalidomide treatment of patients infected with the human immunodeficiency virus. *AIDS Res Hum Retroviruses.* 1997;13(12):1047-1054.

72. Nogueira AC, Neubert R, Helge H, Neubert D. Thalidomide and the immune system. 3. Simultaneous up- and down-regulation of different integrin receptors on human white blood cells. *Life Sci.* 1994;55(2): 77-92.

73. Rowland TL, McHugh SM, Deighton J, Dearman RJ, Ewan PW, Kimber I. Differential regulation by thalidomide and dexamethasone of cytokine expression in human peripheral blood mononuclear cells. *Immunopharmacology.* 1998;40(1):11-20.

74. Shannon EJ, Sandoval F. Thalidomide increases the synthesis of IL-2 in cultures of human mononuclear cells stimulated with Concanavalin-A, Staphylococcal enterotoxin A, and purified protein derivative. *Immunopharmacology.* 1995;31(1):109-116.

75. Tseng S, Pak G, Washenik K, Pomeranz MK, Shupack JL. Rediscovering thalidomide: a review of its mechanism of action, side effects, and potential uses. *J Am Acad Dermatol.* 1996;35(6):969-979.

76. Li Y, Xu Y, Liu L, et al. Population pharmacokinetics of pomalidomide. *J Clin Pharmacol.* 2015;55:563-572.

77. Lutwak-Mann C, Schmid K, Keberle H. Thalidomide in rabbit semen. *Nature.* 1967;214(5092):1018-1020.

78. Tanaka A, Hasegawa A, Urakubo G. Metabolic fate of thalidomide in rats. *Chem Pharm Bull (Tokyo).* 1965;13(10):1263-1265.

79. Teo SK, Harden JL, Burke AB, et al. Thalidomide is distributed into human semen after oral dosing. *Drug Metab Dispos.* 2001;29(10):1355-1357.

80. Schumacher H, Smith RL, Williams RT. The metabolism of thalidomide: the spontaneous hydrolysis of thalidomide in solution. *Br J Pharmacol Chemother.* 1965;25(2):324-337.

81. Aweeka F, Trapnell C, Chernoff M, et al. Pharmacokinetics and pharmacodynamics of thalidomide in HIV patients treated for oral aphthous ulcers: ACTG protocol 251. AIDS Clinical Trials Group. *J Clin Pharmacol.* 2001;41(10):1091-1097.

82. Wohl DA, Aweeka FT, Schmitz J, et al. Safety, tolerability, and pharmacokinetic effects of thalidomide in patients infected with human immunodeficiency virus: AIDS Clinical Trials Group 267. *J Infect Dis.* 2002;185(9):1359-1363.

83. Scheffler MR, Colburn W, Kook KA, Thomas SD. Thalidomide does not alter estrogen-progesterone hormone single dose pharmacokinetics. *Clin Pharmacol Ther.* 1999;65(5):483-490.

84. Tsambaos D, Bolsen K, Georgiou S, Monastirli A, Goerz G. Effects of oral thalidomide on rat liver and skin microsomal P450 isozyme activities and on urinary porphyrin excretion: interaction with oral hexachlorobenzene. *Arch Dermatol Res.* 1994;286(6):347-349.

85. Wiener H, Krivanek P, Tuisl E, Kolassa N. Induction of drug metabolism in the rat by taglutimide, a sedative-hypnotic glutarimide derivative. *Eur J Drug Metab Pharmacokinet.* 1980;5(2):93-97.

86. Chen N, Zhou S, Palmisano M. Clinical pharmacokinetics and pharmacodynamics of lenalidomide. *Clin Pharmacokinet.* 2017;56:139-152.

87. Reist M, Carrupt PA, Francotte E, Testa B. Chiral inversion and hydrolysis of thalidomide: mechanisms and catalysis by bases and serum albumin, and chiral stability of teratogenic metabolites. *Chem Res Toxicol.* 1998;11(12):1521-1528.

88. Muller GW, Chen R, Huang SY, et al. Amino-substituted thalidomide analogs: potent inhibitors of TNF-alpha production. *Bioorg Med Chem Lett.* 1999;9(11):1625-1630.

89. Eriksson T, Bjorkman S, Roth B, Fyge A, Hoglund P. Stereospecific determination, chiral inversion in vitro and pharmacokinetics in humans of the enantiomers of thalidomide. *Chirality.* 1995;7(1):44-52.

90. Figg WD, Raje S, Bauer KS, et al. Pharmacokinetics of thalidomide in an elderly prostate cancer population. *J Pharm Sci.* 1999;88(1):121-125.

91. Chen TL, Vogelsang GB, Petty BG, et al. Plasma pharmacokinetics and urinary excretion of thalidomide after oral dosing in healthy male volunteers. *Drug Metab Dispos.* 1989;17(4):402-405.

92. Piscitelli SC, Figg WD, Hahn B, Kelly G, Thomas S, Walker RE. Single-dose pharmacokinetics of thalidomide in human immunodeficiency virus-infected patients. *Antimicrob Agents Chemother.* 1997;41(12):2797-2799.

93. Teo SK, Colburn WA, Thomas SD. Single-dose oral pharmacokinetics of three formulations of thalidomide in healthy male volunteers. *J Clin Pharmacol.* 1999;39(11):1162-1168.

94. Lu J, Helsby N, Palmer BD, et al. Metabolism of thalidomide in liver microsomes of mice, rabbits, and humans. *J Pharmacol Exp Ther.* 2004;310(2):571-577.

95. Lu J, Palmer BD, Kestell P, et al. Thalidomide metabolites in mice and patients with multiple myeloma. *Clin Cancer Res.* 2003;9(5):1680-1688.

96. Chung F, Lu J, Palmer BD, et al. Thalidomide pharmacokinetics and metabolite formation in mice, rabbits, and multiple myeloma patients. *Clin Cancer Res.* 2004;10(17):5949-5956.

97. Yaccoby S, Johnson CL, Mahaffey SC, Wezeman MJ, Barlogie B, Epstein J. Antimyeloma efficacy of thalidomide in the SCID-hu model. *Blood.* 2002;100(12):4162-4168.

98. Trapnell CB, Donahue SR, Collins JM, Flockhart DA, Thacker D, Abernethy DR. Thalidomide does not alter the pharmacokinetics of ethinyl estradiol and norethindrone. *Clin Pharmacol Ther.* 1998;64(6):597-602.

99. Somers GF. Pharmacological properties of thalidomide (alpha-phthalimido glutarimide), a new sedative hypnotic drug. *Br J Pharmacol Chemother.* 1960;15:111-116.

100. Eisen T, Boshoff C, Mak I, et al. Continuous low dose thalidomide: a phase II study in advanced melanoma, renal cell, ovarian and breast cancer. *Br J Cancer.* 2000;82(4):812-817.

101. Eisen TG. Thalidomide in solid tumors: the London experience. *Oncology (Williston Park).* 2000;14(12 suppl 13):17-20.

102. Richardson P, Schlossman R, Jagannath S, et al. Thalidomide for patients with relapsed multiple myeloma after high-dose chemotherapy and stem cell transplantation: results of an open-label multicenter phase 2 study of efficacy, toxicity, and biological activity. *Mayo Clin Proc.* 2004;79(7):875-882.

103. Weber D, Rankin K, Gavino M, Delasalle K, Alexanian R. Thalidomide alone or with dexamethasone for previously untreated multiple myeloma. *J Clin Oncol.* 2003;21(1):16-19.

104. Osman K, Comenzo R, Rajkumar SV. Deep venous thrombosis and thalidomide therapy for multiple myeloma. *N Engl J Med.* 2001;344(25):1951-1952.

105. Palumbo A, Rajkumar SV, Dimopoulos MA, et al. Prevention of thalidomide- and lenalidomide-associated thrombosis in myeloma. *Leukemia.* 2008;22(2):414-423.

106. Younis TH, Alam A, Paplham P, Spangenthal E, McCarthy P. Reversible pulmonary hypertension and thalidomide therapy for multiple myeloma. *Br J Haematol.* 2003;121(1):191-192.

107. Figg WD, Dahut W, Duray P, et al. A randomized phase II trial of thalidomide, an angiogenesis inhibitor, in patients with androgen-independent prostate cancer. *Clin Cancer Res.* 2001;7(7):1888-1893.

108. Mellin GW, Katzenstein M. The saga of thalidomide. Neuropathy to embryopathy, with case reports of congenital anomalies. *N Engl J Med.* 1962;267:1238-1244.

109. Aronson IK, Yu R, West DP, Van den Broek H, Antel J. Thalidomide-induced peripheral neuropathy. Effect of serum factor on nerve cultures. *Arch Dermatol.* 1984;120(11):1466-1470.

110. Briani C, Zara G, Rondinone R, et al. Thalidomide neurotoxicity: prospective study in patients with lupus erythematosus. *Neurology.* 2004;62(12):2288-2290.

111. Clemmensen OJ, Olsen PZ, Andersen KE. Thalidomide neurotoxicity. *Arch Dermatol.* 1984;120(3):338-341.

112. Fullerton PM, O'Sullivan DJ. Thalidomide neuropathy: a clinical electrophysiological, and histological follow-up study. *J Neurol Neurosurg Psychiatry.* 1968;31(6):543-551.

113. Corral LG, Kaplan G. Immunomodulation by thalidomide and thalidomide analogues. *Ann Rheum Dis.* 1999;58(suppl 1):I107-I113.

114. Noormohamed FH, Youle MS, Higgs CJ, et al. Pharmacokinetics and hemodynamic effects of single oral doses of thalidomide in asymptomatic human immunodeficiency virus-infected subjects. *AIDS Res Hum Retroviruses.* 1999;15(12):1047-1052.

115. Dimopoulos MA, Sonneveld P, Leung N, et al. International Myeloma Working Group recommendations for the diagnosis and management of myeloma-related renal impairment. *J Clin Oncol.* 2016;34(13):1544-1557.

116. Weber DM, Chen C, Niesvizky R, et al. Lenalidomide plus dexamethasone for relapsed multiple myeloma in North America. *N Engl J Med.* 2007;357(21):2133-2142.

117. Dimopoulos M, Spencer A, Attal M, et al. Lenalidomide plus dexamethasone for relapsed or refractory multiple myeloma. *N Engl J Med.* 2007;357(21):2123-2132.

118. Richardson P, Jagannath S, Hussein M, et al. Safety and efficacy of single-agent lenalidomide in patients with relapsed and refractory multiple myeloma. *Blood.* 2009;114(4):772-778.

119. Richardson PG, Schlossman RL, Weller E, et al. Immunomodulatory drug CC-5013 overcomes drug resistance and is well tolerated in patients with relapsed multiple myeloma. *Blood.* 2002;100(9):3063-3067.

120. Sviggum HP, Davis MD, Rajkumar SV, Dispenzieri A. Dermatologic adverse effects of lenalidomide therapy for amyloidosis and multiple myeloma. *Arch Dermatol.* 2006;142(10):1298-1302.

121. Kumar S, Dispenzieri A, Lacy MQ, et al. Impact of lenalidomide therapy on stem cell mobilization and engraftment post-peripheral blood stem cell transplantation in patients with newly diagnosed myeloma. *Leukemia.* 2007;21(9):2035-2042.

122. Mazumder A, Kaufman J, Niesvizky R, Lonial S, Vesole D, Jagannath S. Effect of lenalidomide therapy on mobilization of peripheral blood stem cells in previously untreated multiple myeloma patients. *Leukemia.* 2008;22(6):1280-1281; author reply 1281-1282.

123. Paripati H, Stewart AK, Cabou S, et al. Compromised stem cell mobilization following induction therapy with lenalidomide in myeloma. *Leukemia.* 2008;22(6):1282-1284.

124. Hoffmann M, Kasserra C, Reyes J, et al. Absorption, metabolism and excretion of [14C]pomalidomide in humans following oral administration. *Cancer Chemother Pharmacol.* 2013;71(2):489-501.

125. Carrier M, Le Gal G, Tay J, Wu C, Lee AY. Rates of venous thromboembolism in multiple myeloma patients undergoing immunomodulatory therapy with thalidomide or lenalidomide: a systematic review and meta-analysis. *J Thromb Haemost.* 2011;9(4):653-663.

126. McCurdy AR, Lacy MQ. Pomalidomide and its clinical potential for relapsed or refractory multiple myeloma: an update for the hematologist. *Ther Adv Hematol.* 2013;4(3):211-216.

127. Anderson KC, Hamblin TJ, Traynor A. Management of multiple myeloma today. *Semin Hematol.* 1999;36(1 suppl 3):3-8.

128. Stevenson F, Anderson KC. Introduction: immunotherapy for multiple myeloma—insights and advances. *Semin Hematol.* 1999;36(1 suppl 3):1-2.

129. Vacca A, Ribatti D, Roncali L, et al. Bone marrow angiogenesis and progression in multiple myeloma. *Br J Haematol.* 1994;87(3):503-508.

130. Vacca A, Di Loreto M, Ribatti D, et al. Bone marrow of patients with active multiple myeloma: angiogenesis and plasma cell adhesion molecules LFA-1, VLA-4, LAM-1, and CD44. *Am J Hematol.* 1995;50(1):9-14.

131. Ribatti D, Vacca A, Nico B, et al. Bone marrow angiogenesis and mast cell density increase simultaneously with progression of human multiple myeloma. *Br J Cancer.* 1999;79(3-4):451-455.

132. Munshi NC, Wilson C. Increased bone marrow microvessel density in newly diagnosed multiple myeloma carries a poor prognosis. *Semin Oncol.* 2001;28(6):565-569.

133. Rajkumar SV, Fonseca R, Witzig TE, Gertz MA, Greipp PR. Bone marrow angiogenesis in patients achieving complete response after stem cell transplantation for multiple myeloma. *Leukemia.* 1999;13(3):469-472.

134. Nguyen M, Tran C, Barsky S, et al. Thalidomide and chemotherapy combination. *Int J Oncol.* 1997;10(5):965-969.

135. Barlogie B, Desikan R, Eddlemon P, et al. Extended survival in advanced and refractory multiple myeloma after single-agent thalidomide: identification of prognostic factors in a phase 2 study of 169 patients. *Blood.* 2001;98(2):492-494.

136. Alexanian R, Weber D, Anagnostopoulos A, Delasalle K, Wang M, Rankin K. Thalidomide with or without dexamethasone for refractory or relapsing multiple myeloma. *Semin Hematol.* 2003;40(4 suppl 4):3-7.

137. Lee CK, Barlogie B, Munshi N, et al. DTPACE: an effective, novel combination chemotherapy with thalidomide for previously treated patients with myeloma. *J Clin Oncol.* 2003;21(14):2732-2739.

138. Palumbo A, Bringhen S, Caravita T, et al. Oral melphalan and prednisone chemotherapy plus thalidomide compared with melphalan and prednisone alone in elderly patients with multiple myeloma: randomised controlled trial. *Lancet.* 2006;367(9513):825-831.

139. Ciolli S, Leoni F, Gigli F, Rigacci L, Bosi A. Low dose Velcade, thalidomide and dexamethasone (LD-VTD): an effective regimen for relapsed and refractory multiple myeloma patients. *Leuk Lymphoma.* 2006;47(1):171-173.

140. Palumbo A, Ambrosini MT, Benevolo G, et al. Bortezomib, melphalan, prednisone, and thalidomide for relapsed multiple myeloma. *Blood.* 2007;109(7):2767-2772.

141. Barlogie B, Anaissie E, van Rhee F, et al. Incorporating bortezomib into upfront treatment for multiple myeloma: early results of total therapy 3. *Br J Haematol.* 2007;138(2):176-185.

142. van Rhee F, Bolejack V, Hollmig K, et al. High serum-free light chain levels and their rapid reduction in response to therapy define an aggressive multiple myeloma subtype with poor prognosis. *Blood.* 2007;110(3):827-832.

143. Lakshman A, Singh PP, Rajkumar SV, et al. Efficacy of VDT PACE-like regimens in treatment of relapsed/refractory multiple myeloma. *Am J Hematol.* 2018;93(2):179-186.

144. Facon T, Mary JY, Hulin C, et al. Melphalan and prednisone plus thalidomide versus melphalan and prednisone alone or reduced-intensity autologous stem cell transplantation in elderly patients with multiple myeloma (IFM 99-06): a randomised trial. *Lancet.* 2007;370(9594):1209-1218.

145. Avet-Loiseau H, Attal M, Moreau P, et al. Genetic abnormalities and survival in multiple myeloma: the experience of the Intergroupe Francophone du Myelome. *Blood.* 2007;109(8):3489-3495.

146. Rajkumar SV, Rosinol L, Hussein M, et al. Multicenter, randomized, double-blind, placebo-controlled study of thalidomide plus dexamethasone compared with dexamethasone as initial therapy for newly diagnosed multiple myeloma. *J Clin Oncol.* 2008;26(13):2171-2177.

147. Rosovsky R, Hong F, Tocco D, et al. Endothelial stress products and coagulation markers in patients with multiple myeloma treated with lenalidomide plus dexamethasone: an observational study. *Br J Haematol.* 2013;160(3):351-358.

148. Attal M, Harousseau JL, Leyvraz S, et al. Maintenance therapy with thalidomide improves survival in patients with multiple myeloma. *Blood.* 2006;108(10):3289-3294.

149. Barlogie B, Tricot G, Anaissie E, et al. Thalidomide and hematopoietic-cell transplantation for multiple myeloma. *N Engl J Med.* 2006;354(10):1021-1030.

150. Spencer A, Prince HM, Roberts AW, et al. Consolidation therapy with low-dose thalidomide and prednisolone prolongs the survival of multiple myeloma patients undergoing a single autologous stem-cell transplantation procedure. *J Clin Oncol.* 2009;27(11):1788-1793.

151. Morgan GJ, Gregory WM, Davies FE, et al. The role of maintenance thalidomide therapy in multiple myeloma: MRC Myeloma IX results and meta-analysis. *Blood.* 2012;119(1):7-15.

152. Kagoya Y, Nannya Y, Kurokawa M. Thalidomide maintenance therapy for patients with multiple myeloma: meta-analysis. *Leuk Res.* 2012;36(8):1016-1021.

153. Rajkumar SV, Jacobus S, Callander NS, et al. Lenalidomide plus high-dose dexamethasone versus lenalidomide plus low-dose dexamethasone as initial therapy for newly diagnosed multiple myeloma: an open-label randomised controlled trial. *Lancet Oncol.* 2010;11(1):29-37.

154. Benboubker L, Dimopoulos MA, Dispenzieri A, et al. Lenalidomide and dexamethasone in transplant-ineligible patients with myeloma. *N Engl J Med.* 2014;371(10):906-917.

155. Palumbo A, Falco P, Corradini P, et al. Melphalan, prednisone, and lenalidomide treatment for newly diagnosed myeloma: a report from the GIMEMA–Italian Multiple Myeloma Network. *J Clin Oncol.* 2007;25(28):4459-4465.

156. Palumbo A, Hajek R, Delforge M, et al. Continuous lenalidomide treatment for newly diagnosed multiple myeloma. *N Engl J Med.* 2012;366(19):1759-1769.

157. McCarthy PL, Owzar K, Hofmeister CC, et al. Lenalidomide after stem-cell transplantation for multiple myeloma. *N Engl J Med.* 2012;366(19):1770-1781.

158. Attal M, Lauwers-Cances V, Marit G, et al. Lenalidomide maintenance after stem-cell transplantation for multiple myeloma. *N Engl J Med.* 2012;366(19):1782-1791.

159. McCarthy PL, Holstein SA, Petrucci MT, et al. Lenalidomide maintenance after autologous stem-cell transplantation in newly diagnosed multiple myeloma: a meta-analysis. *J Clin Oncol.* 2017;35(29):3279-3289.

160. Richardson PG, Weller E, Jagannath S, et al. Multicenter, phase I, dose-escalation trial of lenalidomide plus bortezomib for relapsed and relapsed/refractory multiple myeloma. *J Clin Oncol.* 2009;27(34):5713-5719.

161. Richardson PG, Xie W, Jagannath S, et al. A phase 2 trial of lenalidomide, bortezomib, and dexamethasone in patients with relapsed and relapsed/refractory myeloma. *Blood.* 2014;123(10):1461-1469.

162. Richardson PG, Weller E, Lonial S, et al. Lenalidomide, bortezomib, and dexamethasone combination therapy in patients with newly diagnosed multiple myeloma. *Blood.* 2010;116(5):679-686.

163. Jakubowiak AJ, Griffith KA, Reece DE, et al. Lenalidomide, bortezomib, pegylated liposomal doxorubicin, and dexamethasone in newly diagnosed multiple myeloma: a phase 1/2 Multiple Myeloma Research Consortium trial. *Blood.* 2011;118(3):535-543.

164. Kumar S, Flinn I, Richardson PG, et al. Randomized, multicenter, phase 2 study (EVOLUTION) of combinations of bortezomib, dexamethasone, cyclophosphamide, and lenalidomide in previously untreated multiple myeloma. *Blood.* 2012;119(19):4375-4382.

165. Kumar SK, Flinn I, Noga SJ, et al. Bortezomib, dexamethasone, cyclophosphamide and lenalidomide combination for newly diagnosed multiple myeloma: phase 1 results from the multicenter EVOLUTION study. *Leukemia.* 2010;24(7):1350-1356.

166. Attal M, Lauwers-Cances V, Hulin C, et al. Lenalidomide, bortezomib, and dexamethasone with transplantation for myeloma. *N Engl J Med.* 2017;376(14):1311-1320.

167. Stewart AK, Rajkumar SV, Dimopoulos MA, et al. Carfilzomib, lenalidomide, and dexamethasone for relapsed multiple myeloma. *N Engl J Med.* 2015;372(2):142-152.

168. Krishnan A, Kapoor P, Palmer JM, et al. Phase I/II trial of the oral regimen ixazomib, pomalidomide, and dexamethasone in relapsed/refractory multiple myeloma. *Leukemia.* doi: 10.1080/21645515.2018.146182.

169. Bringhen S, Mina R, Cafro AM, et al. Once-weekly carfilzomib, pomalidomide, and low-dose dexamethasone for relapsed/refractory myeloma: a phase I/II study. *Leukemia.* doi: 10.1038/s41375-018-0024-1.

170. Dimopoulos MA, Oriol A, Nahi H, et al. Daratumumab, lenalidomide, and dexamethasone for multiple myeloma. *N Engl J Med.* 2016;375(14):1319-1331.

171. Schey SA, Fields P, Bartlett JB, et al. Phase I study of an immunomodulatory thalidomide analog, CC-4047, in relapsed or refractory multiple myeloma. *J Clin Oncol.* 2004;22(16):3269-3276.

172. Richardson PG, Siegel D, Baz R, et al. Phase 1 study of pomalidomide MTD, safety, and efficacy in patients with refractory multiple myeloma who have received lenalidomide and bortezomib. *Blood.* 2013;121(11):1961-1967.

173. Lacy MQ, Hayman SR, Gertz MA, et al. Pomalidomide (CC4047) plus low-dose dexamethasone as therapy for relapsed multiple myeloma. *J Clin Oncol.* 2009;27(30):5008-5014.

174. Lacy MQ, Allred JB, Gertz MA, et al. Pomalidomide plus low-dose dexamethasone in myeloma refractory to both bortezomib and lenalidomide: comparison of 2 dosing strategies in dual-refractory disease. *Blood.* 2011;118(11):2970-2975.

175. Leleu X, Attal M, Arnulf B, et al. Pomalidomide plus low-dose dexamethasone is active and well tolerated in bortezomib and lenalidomide-refractory multiple myeloma: Intergroupe Francophone du Myelome 2009-02. *Blood.* 2013;121(11):1968-1975.

176. Richardson PG, Siegel DS, Vij R, et al. Pomalidomide alone or in combination with low-dose dexamethasone in relapsed and refractory multiple myeloma: a randomized phase 2 study. *Blood.* 2014;123(12):1826-1832.

177. San Miguel J, Weisel K, Moreau P, et al. Pomalidomide plus low-dose dexamethasone versus high-dose dexamethasone alone for patients with relapsed and refractory multiple myeloma (MM-003): a randomised, open-label, phase 3 trial. *Lancet Oncol.* 2013;14(11):1055-1066.

178. Morgan G, Palumbo A, Dhanasiri S, et al. Overall survival of relapsed and refractory multiple myeloma patients after adjusting for crossover in the MM-003 trial for pomalidomide plus low-dose dexamethasone. *Br J Haematol.* 2015;168(6):820-823.

179. Paludo J, Mikhael JR, LaPlant BR, et al. Pomalidomide, bortezomib, and dexamethasone for patients with relapsed lenalidomide-refractory multiple myeloma. *Blood.* 2017;130(10):1198-1204.

180. Shah JJ, Stadtmauer EA, Abonour R, et al. Carfilzomib, pomalidomide, and dexamethasone for relapsed or refractory myeloma. *Blood.* 2015;126(20):2284-2290.

181. Spencer A, Harrison S, Zonder J, et al. A phase 1 clinical trial evaluating marizomib, pomalidomide and low-dose dexamethasone in relapsed and refractory multiple myeloma (NPI-0052-107): final study results. *Br J Haematol.* 2018;180(1):41-51.

182. Cohen A, Spektor TM, Stampleman L, et al. Safety and efficacy of pomalidomide, dexamethasone and pegylated liposomal doxorubicin for patients with relapsed or refractory multiple myeloma. *Br J Haematol.* 2018;180(1):60-70.

183. Chari A, Suvannasankha A, Fay JW, et al. Daratumumab plus pomalidomide and dexamethasone in relapsed and/or refractory multiple myeloma. *Blood.* 2017;130(8):974-981.

184. Badros A, Hyjek E, Ma N, et al. Pembrolizumab, pomalidomide, and low-dose dexamethasone for relapsed/refractory multiple myeloma. *Blood.* 2017;130(10):1189-1197.

185. Baz RC, Martin TG, 3rd, Lin HY, et al. Randomized multicenter phase 2 study of pomalidomide, cyclophosphamide, and dexamethasone in relapsed refractory myeloma. *Blood.* 2016;127(21):2561-2568.

186. Bertolini F, Mingrone W, Alietti A, et al. Thalidomide in multiple myeloma, myelodysplastic syndromes and histiocytosis. Analysis of clinical results and of surrogate angiogenesis markers. *Ann Oncol.* 2001;12(7):987-990.

187. Raza A, Meyer P, Dutt D, et al. Thalidomide produces transfusion independence in long-standing refractory anemias of patients with myelodysplastic syndromes. *Blood.* 2001;98(4):958-965.

188. Zorat F, Shetty V, Dutt D, et al. The clinical and biological effects of thalidomide in patients with myelodysplastic syndromes. *Br J Haematol.* 2001;115(4):881-894.

189. Strupp C, Germing U, Aivado M, Misgeld E, Haas R, Gattermann N. Thalidomide for the treatment of patients with myelodysplastic syndromes. *Leukemia.* 2002;16(1):1-6.

190. Strupp C, Hildebrandt B, Germing U, Haas R, Gattermann N. Cytogenetic response to thalidomide treatment in three patients with myelodysplastic syndrome. *Leukemia.* 2003;17(6):1200-1202.

191. Moreno-Aspitia A, Colon-Otero G, Hoering A, et al. Thalidomide therapy in adult patients with myelodysplastic syndrome. A North Central Cancer Treatment Group phase II trial. *Cancer.* 2006;107(4):767-772.

192. Steurer M, Sudmeier I, Stauder R, Gastl G. Thromboembolic events in patients with myelodysplastic syndrome receiving thalidomide in combination with darbepoietin-alpha. *Br J Haematol.* 2003;121(1):101-103.

193. Steins MB, Bieker R, Padro T, et al. Thalidomide for the treatment of acute myeloid leukemia. *Leuk Lymphoma.* 2003;44(9):1489-1493.

194. Steins MB, Padro T, Bieker R, et al. Efficacy and safety of thalidomide in patients with acute myeloid leukemia. *Blood.* 2002;99(3):834-839.

195. List AF. New approaches to the treatment of myelodysplasia. *Oncologist.* 2002;7(suppl 1):39-49.

196. Melchert M, Kale V, List A. The role of lenalidomide in the treatment of patients with chromosome 5q deletion and other myelodysplastic syndromes. *Curr Opin Hematol.* 2007;14(2):123-129.

197. Melchert M, List A. Targeted therapies in myelodysplastic syndrome. *Semin Hematol.* 2008;45(1):31-38.

198. Melchert M, Williams C, List A. Remitting activity of lenalidomide in treatment-induced myelodysplastic syndrome. *Leukemia.* 2007;21(7):1576-1578.

199. List A, Kurtin S, Roe DJ, et al. Efficacy of lenalidomide in myelodysplastic syndromes. *N Engl J Med.* 2005;352(6):549-557.

200. List A, Dewald G, Bennett J, et al. Lenalidomide in the myelodysplastic syndrome with chromosome 5q deletion. *N Engl J Med.* 2006;355(14):1456-1465.

201. Ponce CC, de Lourdes Lopes Ferrari Chauffaille M, Ihara SS, Silva MR. Increased angiogenesis in primary myelofibrosis: latent transforming growth factor-beta as a possible angiogenic factor. *Rev Bras Hematol Hemoter.* 2014;36(5):322-328.

202. Mesa RA, Hanson CA, Rajkumar SV, Schroeder G, Tefferi A. Evaluation and clinical correlations of bone marrow angiogenesis in myelofibrosis with myeloid metaplasia. *Blood.* 2000;96(10):3374-3380.

203. Elliott MA, Mesa RA, Li CY, et al. Thalidomide treatment in myelofibrosis with myeloid metaplasia. *Br J Haematol.* 2002;117(2):288-296.

204. Piccaluga PP, Visani G, Pileri SA, et al. Clinical efficacy and antiangiogenic activity of thalidomide in myelofibrosis with myeloid metaplasia. A pilot study. *Leukemia.* 2002;16(9):1609-1614.

205. Barosi G, Grossi A, Comotti B, Musto P, Gamba G, Marchetti M. Safety and efficacy of thalidomide in patients with myelofibrosis with myeloid metaplasia. *Br J Haematol.* 2001;114(1):78-83.

206. Tefferi A, Elliot MA. Serious myeloproliferative reactions associated with the use of thalidomide in myelofibrosis with myeloid metaplasia. *Blood.* 2000;96(12):4007.

207. Marchetti M, Barosi G, Balestri F, et al. Low-dose thalidomide ameliorates cytopenias and splenomegaly in myelofibrosis with myeloid metaplasia: a phase II trial. *J Clin Oncol.* 2004;22(3):424-431.

208. Merup M, Kutti J, Birgergard G, et al. Negligible clinical effects of thalidomide in patients with myelofibrosis with myeloid metaplasia. *Med Oncol.* 2002;19(2):79-86.

209. Barosi G, Elliott M, Canepa L, et al. Thalidomide in myelofibrosis with myeloid metaplasia: a pooled-analysis of individual patient data from five studies. *Leuk Lymphoma.* 2002;43(12):2301-2307.

210. Mesa RA, Steensma DP, Pardanani A, et al. A phase 2 trial of combination low-dose thalidomide and prednisone for the treatment of myelofibrosis with myeloid metaplasia. *Blood.* 2003;101(7):2534-2541.

211. Quintas-Cardama A, Kantarjian HM, Manshouri T, et al. Lenalidomide plus prednisone results in durable clinical, histopathologic, and molecular responses in patients with myelofibrosis. *J Clin Oncol.* 2009;27(28):4760-4766.

212. Mesa RA, Elliott MA, Schroeder G, Tefferi A. Durable responses to thalidomide-based drug therapy for myelofibrosis with myeloid metaplasia. *Mayo Clin Proc.* 2004;79(7):883-889.

213. Dimopoulos MA, Tsatalas C, Zomas A, et al. Treatment of Waldenstrom's macroglobulinemia with single-agent thalidomide or with the combination of clarithromycin, thalidomide and dexamethasone. *Semin Oncol.* 2003;30(2):265-269.

214. Treon SP, Soumerai JD, Branagan AR, et al. Lenalidomide and rituximab in Waldenstrom's macroglobulinemia. *Clin Cancer Res.* 2009;15(1):355-360.

215. Seldin DC, Choufani EB, Dember LM, et al. Tolerability and efficacy of thalidomide for the treatment of patients with light chain-associated (AL) amyloidosis. *Clin Lymphoma.* 2003;3(4):241-246.

216. Dispenzieri A, Lacy MQ, Rajkumar SV, et al. Poor tolerance to high doses of thalidomide in patients with primary systemic amyloidosis. *Amyloid.* 2003;10(4):257-261.

217. Little RF, Wyvill KM, Pluda JM, et al. Activity of thalidomide in AIDS-related Kaposi's sarcoma. *J Clin Oncol.* 2000;18(13):2593-2602.

218. Basile FG. Durable clinical and cytogenetic remission in an elderly patient with relapsed acute myeloid leukemia treated with low-dose lenalidomide. *Leuk Lymphoma.* 2009;50(4):653-655.

219. Penarrubia MJ, Silvestre LA, Conde J, Cantalapiedra A, Garcia Frade LJ. Hematologic and cytogenetic response to lenalidomide in de novo acute myeloid leukemia with chromosome 5q deletion. *Leuk Res.* 2009;33(6): e8-e9.

220. Chanan-Khan A, Miller KC, Musial L, et al. Clinical efficacy of lenalidomide in patients with relapsed or refractory chronic lymphocytic leukemia: results of a phase II study. *J Clin Oncol.* 2006;24(34):5343-5349.

221. Witzig TE, Wiernik PH, Moore T, et al. Lenalidomide oral monotherapy produces durable responses in relapsed or refractory indolent non-Hodgkin's lymphoma. *J Clin Oncol.* 2009;27(32):5404-5409.

222. Aue G, Njuguna N, Tian X, et al. Lenalidomide-induced upregulation of CD80 on tumor cells correlates with T-cell activation, the rapid onset of a cytokine release syndrome and leukemic cell clearance in chronic lymphocytic leukemia. *Haematologica.* 2009;94(9):1266-1273.

223. Kumar SK, Berdeja JG, Niesvizky R, et al. Safety and tolerability of ixazomib, an oral proteasome inhibitor, in combination with lenalidomide and dexamethasone in patients with previously untreated multiple myeloma: an open-label phase 1/2 study. *Lancet Oncol.* 2014;15(13):1503-1512.

224. Kumar S, Moreau P, Hari P, et al. Management of adverse events associated with ixazomib plus lenalidomide/dexamethasone in relapsed/refractory multiple myeloma. *Br J Haematol.* 2017;178(4):571-582.

225. Moreau P, Masszi T, Grzasko N, et al. Oral ixazomib, lenalidomide, and dexamethasone for multiple myeloma. *N Engl J Med.* 2016;374(17): 1621-1634.

226. Richardson PG, Hofmeister CC, Raje NS, et al. Pomalidomide, bortezomib and low-dose dexamethasone in lenalidomide-refractory and proteasome inhibitor-exposed myeloma. *Leukemia.* 2017;31(12):2695-2701.

Targeted Therapy in Non–Small Cell Lung Cancer

Harper G. Hubbeling, Jessica J. Lin, Justin F. Gainor, Ibiayi Dagogo-Jack, and Alice T. Shaw

The treatment of advanced non–small cell lung cancer (NSCLC) underwent a major paradigm shift with the advent of small-molecule targeted therapy. Since the initial description of oncogenic activating mutations in the epidermal growth factor receptor (*EGFR*) gene in 2004, more than 10 potentially actionable driver gene alterations have been discovered in NSCLC (Figs. 21.1 and 21.2).[1] In tandem, rapid clinical development of molecularly targeted agents has led to U.S. Food and Drug Administration (FDA)–approved kinase inhibitors now available for use in EGFR-, ALK-, ROS1-, and BRAF-driven lung cancers (see Figs. 21.3 and 21.4). These inhibitors are typically highly effective in appropriately selected patient populations, with response rates of 60% to 85% in the first-line setting. Thus, targeted therapy has become a cornerstone of advanced NSCLC treatment in select molecular subsets. However, drug resistance has proven to be a universal barrier limiting the success of targeted therapy, with most responses lasting less than

1 to 2 years.[2] A detailed understanding of the mechanisms underlying drug resistance is essential to maximize the clinical benefit derived from targeted therapy.

Here, we review the targeted agents available in advanced NSCLC, both approved and investigational. We discuss the clinical indications, pharmacokinetic properties, and toxicity profiles of these agents. In addition, we provide an overview of the known mechanisms of resistance and efforts to overcome drug resistance.

Epidermal Growth Factor Receptor Mutation

EGFR belongs to the ErbB family of transmembrane receptor tyrosine kinases (RTKs). When activated by its ligands (EGF, TGFa, amphiregulin, and epiregulin), EGFR stimulates the growth and differentiation of epithelial cells. *EGFR* mutations are found in

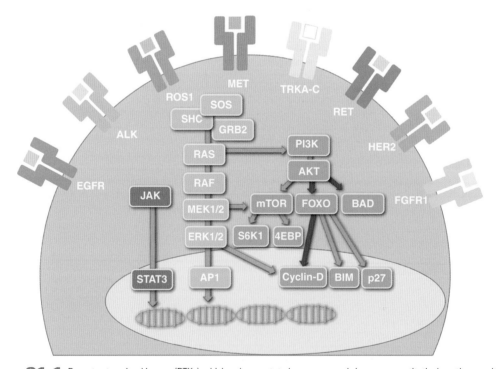

FIGURE **21.1** Receptor tyrosine kinases (RTKs) which, when mutated or rearranged, become constitutively active resulting in deregulation of MAPK, PI3K, and JAK/STAT pathway signaling driving oncogenesis in non–small cell lung cancer. Genetic alterations in the RTKs pictured lead to oncogene addiction and thus are ideal targets for inhibition with small molecules. *Yellow arrows* indicate a stimulatory effect, while *red arrows* indicate inhibition. (Adapted from Lin JJ, Riely GJ, Shaw AT. Targeting ALK: Precision Medicine Takes on Drug Resistance. *Cancer Discov.* 2017;7(2):137-155. Copyright © 2017 American Association for Cancer Research. With permission from AACR.)

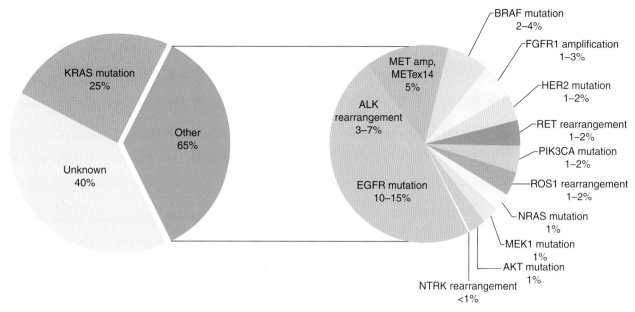

Figure 21.2 Frequency of driver mutations in lung adenocarcinoma. Frequency may vary depending on race, smoking status, gender, and age. amp, amplification; METex14, MET exon 14 skipping. (Modified and updated from Lin JJ, Shaw AT. Resisting resistance: targeted therapies in lung cancer. *Trends Cancer*. 2016;2(7):350-364 with FGFR1 amplification frequency from Weiss J, Sos ML, Seidel D, et al. Frequent and focal FGFR1 amplification associates with therapeutically tractable FGFR1 dependency in squamous cell lung cancer. *Sci Transl Med*. 2010;2(62):62ra93; Dutt A, Ramos AH, Hammerman PS, et al. Inhibitor-sensitive FGFR1 amplification in human non-small cell lung cancer. *PLoS One*. 2011;6(6):e20351.)

10% to 15% of NSCLC in the United States and are associated with Asian race, lack of tobacco exposure, and adenocarcinoma histology.[1,3–5] The most common *EGFR* mutations—a small in-frame deletion in exon 19 (exon 19 del) leading to elimination of an LREA motif, and L858R, a point mutation in exon 21—confer sensitivity to EGFR tyrosine kinase inhibitors (TKIs).[6,7] To date, three distinct generations of EGFR inhibitors have been developed (Table 21.1). Multiple phase III trials have consistently demonstrated superior efficacy and tolerability of EGFR-directed agents as compared to platinum-based chemotherapy in *EGFR*-mutant NSCLC (Table 21.2).[8–10] These studies ultimately led to the FDA approval of three EGFR TKIs (erlotinib, gefitinib, and afatinib) for first-line use in advanced, *EGFR*-mutant NSCLC. More broadly, these studies also established the importance of routine genotyping for *EGFR* mutations in advanced, nonsquamous NSCLC.

First-Generation EGFR Inhibitors

Erlotinib

Erlotinib is a potent, ATP-competitive inhibitor of EGFR. Erlotinib was approved for first-line use in *EGFR*-mutant NSCLC in 2013 after two phase III trials demonstrated significantly improved median progression-free survival (PFS) with erlotinib compared to standard chemotherapy in stage IIIB/IV *EGFR*-mutant NSCLC (9.7 versus 5.2 months [EURTAC] and 13.1 versus 4.6 months [OPTIMAL]; both $P < 0.0001$).[10,11] Both trials were notable for remarkable response rates to erlotinib (64% and 83% overall response rate [ORR], respectively); a significant improvement in quality of life with erlotinib therapy was also noted in the OPTIMAL trial.[10,11] More recently, erlotinib-based combinations have been

INHIBITORS								
EGFR	ALK	ROS1	BRAF	MET	TRKA-C	RET	HER2	FGFR1
Erlotinib	**Crizotinib**	**Crizotinib**	**Dabrafenib***	Crizotinib	Entrectinib	Vandetanib	Afatinib	Brivanib
Gefitinib	**Ceritinib**	Ceritinib	**Trametinib***	Capmatinib	Larotrectinib	Lenvatinib	Dacomitinib	Cediranib
Afatinib	**Alectinib**	Entrectinib	Vemurafenib	Cabozantinib	DS-6051b	Cabozantinib	Neratinib	Dovitinib
Osimertinib	**Brigatinib**	Lorlatinib		Tepotinib	Belizatinib	Sunitinib	Lapatinib	Lucitanib
Nazartinib	Lorlatinib	DS-6051b		Tivantinib	PLX7486	Sorafenib	Pyrotinib	Nintedanib
Olmutinib	TPX-0005	TPX-0005		AMG337	DCC701	Apatinib		AZD4547
PF-06747775	Ensartinib	Cabozantinib		Savolitinib	MGCD516	Ponatinib		BGJ398
				Glesatinib	AZD7451	Alectinib		Debio-1347
				AMG208		BLU-667		JNJ-42756493
				Merestinib		LOXO-292		LY2874455
				Altiratinib				
				Golvatinib				

Figure 21.3 Targeted small-molecule inhibitors in clinical use or undergoing clinical testing in non–small cell lung cancer (NSCLC). **Inhibitors in bold have received U.S. Food and Drug Administration (FDA) approval.** Antibodies being evaluated for the driver alterations are not shown in this table. *Dabrafenib and trametinib received FDA approval for combined use in BRAF-mutant NSCLC. (Modified and updated from Lin JJ, Shaw AT. Resisting resistance: targeted therapies in lung cancer. *Trends Cancer*. 2016;2(7):350-364.)

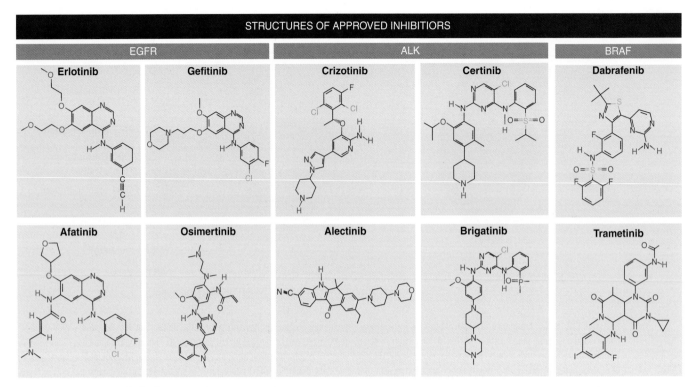

FIGURE **21.4** Structures of small-molecule inhibitors approved for use in non–small cell lung cancer. Available from PubChem: https://pubchem.ncbi.nlm.nih.gov/search/search.cgi.

explored. For example, in a randomized phase II study conducted in Japan, the combination of erlotinib with the vascular endothelial growth factor (VEGF) inhibitor bevacizumab has recently been shown to result in a significantly improved PFS compared with erlotinib alone in patients with *EGFR*-mutant NSCLC (16.0 versus 9.7 months with erlotinib alone, *P* = 0.0015), leading to regulatory approval for this combination in Europe.[12] Confirmatory phase II and III studies are now ongoing.[13]

Pharmacokinetics

The oral absorption of erlotinib is approximately 60%; bioavailability increases with concurrent food intake reaching 100% absorption and decreases by approximately 50% in the setting of proton pump inhibitor use.[14] Erlotinib reaches peak plasma levels (t_{max}) at 4 hours after dosing and has superior central nervous system (CNS) penetration compared with gefitinib, though still limited (CSF-to-plasma ratio of 0.03 and 0.01 for erlotinib and gefitinib, respectively).[15,16] Predominantly plasma protein bound, erlotinib has an apparent volume of distribution (V_D) of 232 L and a half-life ($t_{1/2}$) of 36 hours.[14] Erlotinib is metabolized primarily by hepatic CYP3A4 and to a lesser extent by CYP1A2 and CYP1A1.[14] Accordingly, plasma levels can vary dramatically with the use of CYP3A4 inducers or inhibitors; INR should be monitored closely in patients on warfarin.[14] Smoking increases the clearance rate of erlotinib by 24% and may decrease its antitumor effects.[14]

Toxicity

Diarrhea, rash, anorexia, and fatigue are the most common adverse events (AEs) observed in patients taking erlotinib, though these are generally grades 1 to 2.[10] Due to the abundant expression of EGFR within the epidermis and the role of EGFR in epidermal homeostasis, cutaneous toxicity is characteristic of EGFR

inhibition.[17] In addition to rash, dermatologic toxicities can manifest as xerosis, mucositis, photosensitivity, and changes in hair/nails.[17] Most AEs are tolerable when managed with supportive medications and dose reduction. Severe AEs seen rarely include hepatic dysfunction (~5%), interstitial lung disease (ILD) (0.6% to 2.2%), and gastrointestinal perforation (0.1% to 1%).[18,19] For management of EGFR TKI–induced ILD, see Gefitinib Toxicity below.

Gefitinib

Gefitinib, like erlotinib, competitively inhibits EGFR ATP binding. In cellular assays, gefitinib is less potent than erlotinib (IC_{50} of 20 to 80 nM versus 2 nM, respectively).[20] Gefitinib received FDA approval for the first-line management of *EGFR*-mutant NSCLC in 2015 after two phase III trials demonstrated improvements in PFS compared with platinum-doublet chemotherapy in stage IIIB/IV *EGFR*-mutant NSCLC (9.2 versus 6.3 months, *P* < 0.0001 [WJTOG3405]; 10.8 months versus 5.4 months, *P* < 0.001 [C000000376]).[4,8] Comparisons of gefitinib and erlotinib have not demonstrated a difference in efficacy.[21,22]

Pharmacokinetics

Gefitinib has 60% oral absorption unaffected by food intake and reaches peak plasma concentrations within 3 to 7 hours of dosing.[23] The V_D of gefitinib is 1,400 L, and CSF-to-plasma ratio is low at approximately 0.01.[15] Mean terminal $t_{1/2}$ is 41 hours, and metabolism is primarily via hepatic CYP3A4. Accordingly, CYP3A4 inducers and inhibitors may alter gefitinib plasma concentrations and efficacy. Patients using warfarin should be monitored closely for INR elevation. Additionally, drugs that cause sustained elevations in gastric pH to ≥5 (e.g., ranitidine) reduce mean gefitinib area under the curve (AUC) by 47%.[23]

TABLE
21.1   *Key features of approved EGFR inhibitors*

	Mechanism of Action	$t_{1/2}$ (hours)	CSF:plasma[a]	CNS Efflux	Clearance Mechanism	Common Toxicity (>25% incidence)	Drug Interactions
First Generation EGFR Inhibitors							
Erlotinib[b]	• Quinazoline-based tyrosine kinase inhibitors • Selective for WT EGFR • Bind WT EGFR intracellular catalytic domain • Reversible/noncovalent	36	0.03 to 0.06	• P-gp and BCRP substrate	• CYP3A4	• Cutaneous • Diarrhea • Anorexia[b] • Fatigue[b] • Dyspnea[b] • Cough[b] • Nausea[b]	• CYP3A4 inhibitors increase exposure • CYP3A4 inducers decrease exposure • CYP1A2 inducers decrease exposure[b] • PPIs block absorption • Smoking increases clearance[b]
Gefitinib		41	0.01		• CYP1A1/2[b]		
Second-Generation EGFR Inhibitors							
Afatinib	• Quinazoline-based tyrosine kinase inhibitor • Pan-ErbB inhibitor • Binds WT EGFR intracellular catalytic domain • Irreversible/covalent	37	<0.01	• P-gp and BCRP substrate	• Excreted unchanged in feces	• Diarrhea • Rash • Stomatitis • Dry skin • Paronychia • Anorexia	• P-gp inhibitors increase exposure • P-gp inducers decrease exposure
Third-Generation EGFR Inhibitors							
Osimertinib	• Pyrimidine-based tyrosine kinase inhibitor • Selective for mutant EGFR; limited affinity for WT EGFR • Binds to Cys797 at the edge of EGFR ATP binding pocket • Irreversible/covalent	48	0.16	• P-gp and BCRP substrate	• CYP3A4/5	• Diarrhea • Rash • Dry skin • Nail toxicity	• CYP3A inhibitors increase exposure • CYP3A inducers decrease exposure

[a]Approximate ratio of CSF to plasma drug concentration based on available clinical data.
[b]Attributes unique to erlotinib. With regard to toxicities; these toxicities may also be observed in patients on gefitinib, however at <25% incidence.
EGFR, epidermal growth factor receptor; $t_{1/2}$, median terminal half-life; CSF, cerebrospinal fluid; CNS, central nervous system; WT, wild-type; P-gp, P-glycoprotein; BCRP, breast cancer resistance protein; CYP3A4, cytochrome P450 3A4; CYP1A1/2, cytochrome P450 1A1/2; PPIs, proton pump inhibitors; Cys, cysteine; ATP, adenosine triphosphate.

TABLE

21.2   *Clinical trials and resistance mechanisms for approved EGFR inhibitors*

Select Trials (phase, line)		No. of Patients	ORR (%)	PFS (months)	On-Target Resistance	Off-Target Resistance
First- and Second-Generation EGFR Inhibitors						
Erlotinib	CTONG-0802 (III, 1L)	165	83	13.1	• *EGFR* T790M	• *HER2* amplification
	EURTAC (III, 1L)	173	64	9.7	• *EGFR* amplification	• *MET* amplification/ HGF overexpression
Gefitinib	WJTOG3405 (III, 1L)	172	62	9.2		• *PIK3CA* mutation
	C000000376 (III, 1L)	230	74	10.8		• *BRAF* mutation
Afatinib	LUX-Lung 3 (III, 1L)	345	56	13.6		• EMT
	LUX-Lung 6 (III, 1L)	364	67	11.0		• SCLC transformation
	LUX-Lung 7 (II, 1L)	319	72.5	11.0		
Third-Generation EGFR Inhibitors						
Osimertinib	FLAURA (III, 1L)	674	80	18.9	• *EGFR* C797S	• *HER2* amplification
	NCT01802632 (I, 2L)	253	61	9.6	• *EGFR* L718Q	• *MET* amplification
	AURA-3 (III, 2L)	419	71	10.1	• *EGFR* T790M loss	• *KRAS* mutation
					• *EGFR* amplification	• *BRAF* mutation
						• SCLC transformation

EGFR, epidermal growth factor receptor; No., number; ORR, objective response rate; PFS, progression-free survival; 1L, first-line; 2L, second-line; HER2, receptor tyrosine-protein kinase erbB-2; MET, hepatocyte growth factor receptor; EMT, epithelial-to-mesenchymal transition; SCLC, small cell lung cancer.
Modified and updated from Lovly CM, Iyengar P, Gainor JF. Managing resistance to EGFR- and ALK-targeted therapies. *Am Soc Clin Oncol Educ Book.* 2017;37:607-618.

Toxicity

The most frequent AEs on gefitinib are rash, diarrhea, dry skin, and elevated aspartate aminotransferase or alanine aminotransferase.[4,8] As with erlotinib, gefitinib-induced cutaneous toxicities can generally be managed with vigilant supportive care in collaboration with local care providers including treatment with topical corticosteroids and antibiotics (e.g., erythromycin, metronidazole). More severe cutaneous toxicity may require oral antibiotic treatment (e.g., doxycycline, minocycline), drug interruptions as necessary, and rarely drug discontinuation. Hepatic toxicity can be severe and occurs more frequently with gefitinib than with erlotinib.[18,24] Periodic liver function testing is warranted for patients on gefitinib as hepatic toxicity can be asymptomatic. ILD can occur acutely in 0.3% to 2% of patients receiving gefitinib; because up to one third of cases are fatal, monitoring of respiratory symptoms is crucial.[23] Radiographically confirmed ILD requires immediate discontinuation of gefitinib, treatment with oxygen therapy when indicated, and initiation of corticosteroids.[25]

Second-Generation EGFR Inhibitors

Afatinib

Second-generation EGFR inhibitors, including afatinib, are pan-ErbB inhibitors that bind irreversibly to EGFR, in contrast to first-generation EGFR inhibitors, which bind EGFR reversibly. Afatinib received FDA approval in 2013 based on phase III data from LUX-Lung 3 showing a significant improvement in median PFS with afatinib as compared to chemotherapy in stage IIIB/IV *EGFR*-mutant NSCLC patients (13.6 versus 6.9 months, $P = 0.001$).[9] This finding

was subsequently recapitulated in an Asian cohort in the LUX-Lung 6 trial.[26] Of note, while there was no overall survival (OS) difference noted in the intention-to-treat populations for either trial, pooled analysis of LUX-Lung 3 and LUX-Lung 6 revealed an OS benefit for afatinib compared with chemotherapy in patients with EGFR exon 19 del (31.7 versus 20.7 months, $P = 0.0001$), which was not observed in patients with L858R.[27] LUX-Lung 7, a recent randomized phase II study comparing gefitinib with afatinib as first-line therapy for *EGFR*-mutant NSCLC, showed an improved response rate with afatinib (72.5% versus 56%, $P = 0.0018$) as well as a modest absolute improvement in PFS (median 11.0 versus 10.9 months, HR 0.74 [95% CI 0.57 to 0.95], $P = 0.0178$); however, there was no significant difference in OS, including the exon 19 del subset.[28]

Pharmacokinetics

Afatinib should be taken at least 1 hour before or 3 hours after meals due to reduced exposure when ingested concurrently with high-fat food. Peak plasma concentration of afatinib is reached within 2 to 5 hours. Afatinib is approximately 95% plasma protein bound and has a high apparent V_D (2,770 L) indicative of significant tissue distribution. Mean terminal $t_{1/2}$ is approximately 37 hours permitting daily dosing. Afatinib metabolism is minimal with unchanged drug predominantly excreted in feces. Notably, due to this minimal metabolism and in particular due to negligible CYP-mediated metabolism, afatinib is less prone to drug interactions than the first-generation EGFR TKIs. Afatinib is a substrate of P-glycoprotein (P-gp), a key efflux transporter located at the blood-brain barrier (BBB). Therefore, caution should be taken with concomitant use of strong P-gp modulators.

Toxicity

The most common overall and grade 3 to 4 afatinib-related AEs are diarrhea (overall: 88% to 95%; grade 3 to 4: 5% to 14%) and rash (overall: 81% to 89%; grade 3 to 4: 14% to 16%).[9,26] Dermatologic toxicities commonly observed on afatinib include dry skin, stomatitis, mucositis, and nail changes.[9,26] Rates of diarrhea and rash appear to be higher in patients on afatinib as compared with gefitinib or erlotinib.[24] Increased rates of grade 3 to 4 diarrhea, rash, and fatigue on afatinib may result in more frequent dose reduction (42% with afatinib versus 2% with gefitinib).[28]

Resistance to First- and Second-Generation EGFR Inhibitors

Despite initial response to erlotinib, gefitinib, or afatinib, patients typically develop resistance within 1 to 2 years of treatment initiation.[8-10] Approximately 60% of resistance to first-and second-generation EGFR inhibitors is due to a secondary mutation in the EGFR kinase domain at the gatekeeper residue, T790M.[29-31] EGFR T790M is detected with 60% to 77% sensitivity in plasma.[32,33] T790M-mediated resistance is thought to be predominantly due to increased kinase affinity for ATP; steric hindrance may also contribute.[34] In vitro studies have demonstrated that T790M arises both through selection of pre-existing clones and de novo acquisition.[35] Of the first-and second-generation EGFR inhibitors, afatinib alone demonstrated activity against EGFR T790M in vitro; however, unfortunately significant toxicity secondary to afatinib's activity against wild-type EGFR has precluded this agent's use in patients with EGFR T790M–mutant NSCLC.[36] EGFR amplification is an additional target-dependent mechanism of resistance to EGFR TKIs. Off-target (i.e., not pertaining to the targetable EGFR driver alteration) resistance mechanisms to first-and second-generation EGFR inhibition have also been described. These include upregulation of bypass signaling pathways, which can be mediated by amplification of MET or HER2, and PIK3CA mutations. Histologic changes, such as epithelial-to-mesenchymal transition (EMT) and small cell transformation, have also been described as mechanisms of resistance to EGFR inhibitors.[29,30,37] The CNS is a site of particular importance in first-and second-generation EGFR TKI resistance due to the limited BBB penetration of these agents.

Third-Generation EGFR Inhibitors

Osimertinib

Osimertinib, an irreversible inhibitor of EGFR that covalently binds to the C797 residue, selectively inhibits mutated EGFR (including exon 19 deletions, the L858R substitution, and T790M) with more than 100-fold greater potency against mutated EGFR than the wild-type enzyme. In a phase I study, osimertinib demonstrated a 61% ORR and 9.6-month median PFS in patients with T790M-mutant NSCLC post-progression on erlotinib, gefitinib, or afatinib, with significantly reduced efficacy in a T790M-negative cohort (ORR, 26%; median PFS, 3.4 months).[38] These findings led to the FDA's accelerated approval of osimertinib in EGFR T790M–mutant NSCLC patients who previously progressed on/after EGFR TKI therapy, in 2015. Subsequently, in an international phase III trial, AURA 3, osimertinib was shown to

be superior to platinum chemotherapy in EGFR TKI–pretreated patients with EGFR T790M NSCLC (ORR, 71% versus 31%; median PFS, 10.1 versus 4.4 months).[39] Notably, because osimertinib has excellent CNS penetration, its clinical benefit extends to patients with CNS metastases (intracranial [IC]-ORR of 70% in EGFR TKI–pretreated T790M-mutant NSCLC patients with one or more measurable CNS metastases).[40] Given the significant activity of osimertinib among patients previously treated with EGFR inhibitors, there has been considerable interest in evaluating this agent in the treatment-naïve setting. Preliminary results from a phase III trial comparing osimertinib to erlotinib or gefitinib in the first-line setting showed improved PFS with osimertinib in EGFR-mutant NSCLC patients with and without CNS involvement (FLAURA, median PFS 18.9 versus 10.2 months, HR 0.46, $P < 0.0001$; subcohort with CNS metastases, median PFS 15.2 versus 9.6 months, HR 0.47, $P = 0.0009$).[41]

Pharmacokinetics

Osimertinib is absorbed slowly and can take up to 24 hours to reach maximal plasma concentrations (median t_{max}: 6 hours).[42] Food has minimal effect on exposure. Once absorbed, osimertinib is extensively distributed (V_D: 1,192 L). The CSF-to-plasma ratio of osimertinib is high compared to earlier-generation EGFR inhibitors (2.2 one hour post dose).[43] Osimertinib has a long half-life (approximately 50 hours) and is metabolized predominantly by hepatic CYP3A4/5.[44] AZ5104 is an active metabolite of osimertinib that circulates at 10% of osimertinib exposure and has comparable pharmacokinetic properties to osimertinib.

Toxicity

The most common AEs observed with osimertinib are diarrhea, dry skin, rash, paronychia, and anorexia.[39] Osimertinib incurs lower rates of grade 3 and 4 AEs relative to earlier-generation EGFR TKIs (34% versus 45% incidence of grade ≥3 AEs for osimertinib and erlotinib/gefitinib, respectively) as well as less frequent drug discontinuation due to toxicity (incidence: 13.3% versus 18.1%).[41] ILD and QT prolongation both occur in approximately 4% of patients on osimertinib and can be severe.[39]

EGFR T790M–Selective Inhibitors Under Investigation

Beyond osimertinib, T790M-selective TKIs being evaluated in clinical trials include **olmutinib (BI1482694/HM61713), nazartinib (EGF816),** and **PF-06747775**. Based on preliminary analysis of an early-phase study, olmutinib leads to objective responses in 56% of patients with EGFR T790M–mutant tumors after progression on a first-line EGFR TKI, with a median duration of response (DOR) of 8.3 months.[45] Notably, in experimental models, nazartinib has shown efficacy against NSCLC with EGFR exon 20 insertion, an aberration insensitive to all clinically available EGFR TKIs.[46] Preliminary results from a phase I dose escalation study of nazartinib in advanced EGFR T790M–mutant NSCLC demonstrated tolerability and found a 44% ORR (56/127) and 9.2-month median PFS.[47] A phase I/II trial of PF-06747775 in EGFR-mutant advanced NSCLC patients with or without T790M is ongoing (NCT02349633).

Resistance to Third-Generation EGFR Inhibitors

As with first-and second-generation EGFR TKIs, resistance to osimertinib and other T790M-selective TKIs eventually emerges and limits efficacy. Mechanisms of resistance to third-generation EGFR TKIs are currently undergoing characterization; available data are limited to case reports and small case series. C797S and L718Q mutations in *EGFR* have been identified as tertiary mutations driving on-target resistance to osimertinib, though the frequency of these mutations remains to be determined.[48–50] Loss of *EGFR* T790M has also been described as an on-target cause of resistance.[51] Off-target resistance mechanisms identified include *HER2* or *MET* amplification.[52,53] *BRAF* and *KRAS* mutations have also been found to be potential drivers of clinical resistance to osimertinib, consistent with preclinical models of osimertinib resistance.[51,54,55] Finally, small cell transformation has been observed after progression on osimertinib.[56,57]

Combination Therapy and Fourth-Generation EGFR Inhibition

While there are currently no FDA-approved targeted therapies for patients who progress on or after a third-generation EGFR TKI, several clinical trials are investigating novel therapeutic options for this cohort. TATTON (NCT02143466) is a phase Ib trial investigating the combination of osimertinib and MEK or MET inhibition (selumetinib or savolitinib, respectively) based on compelling preclinical evidence for dual EGFR/MAPK or EGFR/MET inhibition.[53,54,58] Osimertinib is also undergoing phase I investigation in combination with the BCL2 inhibitor navitoclax (NCT02520778), based on in vitro data demonstrating restoration of EGFR TKI sensitivity with BCL2 inhibition.[35] Depending on the allelic context of resistance mutations (i.e., whether acquired EGFR mutations are in cis versus trans), cross-generation EGFR TKI combinations have demonstrated efficacy. For example, *EGFR*-mutant models with *EGFR* C797S and T790M in trans are sensitive to combined gefitinib and osimertinib.[59–61] Of note, the combination of gefitinib and osimertinib is also being explored in the treatment-naïve setting (NCT03122717).

Finally, a fourth generation of EGFR TKIs, distinguished from their predecessors by an allosteric mechanism of action, is currently under development. These inhibitors have not reached clinical testing; however, preclinical results have been promising. One such inhibitor, EAI045, can overcome *EGFR* L858R/T790M and triple-mutant *EGFR* L858R/T790M/C797S in combination with the EGFR monoclonal antibody cetuximab in mouse models.[62]

Anaplastic Lymphoma Kinase Rearrangement

Anaplastic lymphoma kinase (ALK), an RTK belonging to the insulin receptor superfamily, was first reported as an oncogene in NSCLC in 2007.[63] In lung cancer, *ALK* is most frequently fused to the echinoderm microtubule–associated protein-like 4 (*EML4*) gene. Numerous other partner proteins have been identified, including TFG, KIF5B, and KLC1.[64–66] *ALK* rearrangements are detected in 3% to 7% of NSCLC cases and are associated with younger age at diagnosis, never- or light smoking history, and more advanced stage at presentation.[67] *ALK*-rearranged NSCLC is highly

sensitive to ALK-directed therapies. Since 2007, three generations of small-molecule ALK TKIs have been developed, each successively more selective and potent than the last (Table 21.3). The optimal sequence of these agents to overcome resistance and maximize clinical benefit is under investigation (Table 21.4).

First-Generation ALK Inhibitors

Crizotinib

Crizotinib, a TKI with activity against c-MET, ALK, and ROS1, was the first TKI approved by the FDA for use in advanced *ALK*-rearranged NSCLC in 2011.[68] Two randomized trials comparing crizotinib to chemotherapy in the first-and second-line setting demonstrated a superior PFS with crizotinib compared to chemotherapy (PROFILE 1014, first-line, median PFS 10.9 versus 7.0 months [$P < 0.001$]; PROFILE 1007, second-line, median PFS 7.7 versus 3.0 months [$P < 0.001$]).[69,70] Crizotinib's efficacy is limited by its CNS penetration, which, while superior to that achieved with standard chemotherapy (IC-ORR 77% versus 28% for crizotinib and chemotherapy, respectively), is notably inferior to subsequent generations of ALK TKIs (IC-ORR 50% versus 81% for crizotinib and alectinib in the ALEX study, respectively).[69,71,72] Crizotinib is the standard of care for *ROS1*-rearranged NSCLC and is under active investigation for MET-driven NSCLC (see ROS1 and MET sections).

Pharmacokinetics

Crizotinib is orally bioavailable with a median time to maximal plasma concentration of 4 hours and a mean terminal $t_{1/2}$ of 42 hours at the standard dose of 250 mg twice a day. It is a substrate and moderate inhibitor of CYP3A with extensive hepatic metabolism; 2.3% of drug is excreted in the urine unchanged. While severe hepatic impairment should impact crizotinib metabolism, this remains unstudied, and at a total bilirubin of ≤2.1 mg/dL and AST ≤ 124 U/L, crizotinib metabolism is not significantly affected. Severe renal impairment has been shown to significantly increase crizotinib's AUC_{inf} and C_{max}.[73] Crizotinib is a substrate of P-gp, limiting its ability to cross the BBB, resulting in a low ratio of CSF to plasma drug concentration (0.06% to 0.26%).[71,74,75]

Toxicity

Crizotinib is generally well tolerated. The most frequent crizotinib-related AEs include visual disturbance, nausea/vomiting, diarrhea, constipation, fatigue, and peripheral edema, all of which tend to be mild, grade 1 events.[68,76]

Resistance to First-Generation ALK Inhibitors

Despite an initial response to crizotinib, patients generally relapse within 1 to 2 years.[69] As compared to resistance after progression on more potent, second-generation ALK TKIs, resistance to crizotinib is less frequently driven by secondary mutations within the ALK tyrosine kinase domain (20% to 30% with crizotinib versus 50% to 60% with second-generation TKIs).[77] The spectrum of secondary *ALK* mutations observed in crizotinib-resistant cases is broad (Table 21.4).[77] This resistance pattern likely reflects inadequate crizotinib potency and/or unfavorable pharmacokinetics leading to ineffective suppression of resistance mutations, many of which can be overcome by next-generation ALK TKIs. Secondary

TABLE

21.3 *Key features of approved ALK inhibitors*

	Mechanism of Action	$t_{1/2}$ (hours)	CSF:plasma[a]	CNS Efflux	Clearance Mechanism	Common Toxicity (>25% incidence)	Drug Interactions
First Generation ALK inhibitors							
Crizotinib	• Aminopyridine tyrosine kinase inhibitor • Inhibits ALK, ROS1, and MET	42	<0.003	• P-gp substrate	• CYP3A4/5	• Visual disturbance • Vomiting • Nausea • Diarrhea • Constipation • Abdominal pain • Edema • Dysgeusia • LFT elevation • Hypophosphatemia	• CYP3A inhibitors/ inducers affect exposure • CYP3A substrates affected by crizotinib
Second Generation ALK inhibitors							
Ceritinib	• Bis-anilino pyrimidine tyrosine kinase inhibitor • Inhibits ALK, ROS1, IGF1R, and IR	40		• P-gp substrate	• CYP3A4/5	• Diarrhea • Nausea • Vomiting • Abdominal pain • Constipation • Fatigue • Decreased appetite • Anemia • LFT elevation • Creatinine elevation • Hyperglycemia • Hypophosphatemia • Lipase elevation	• CYP3A inhibitors/ inducers increase exposure • CYP3A substrates affected by ceritinib • CYP2C9 substrates affected by ceritinib
Alectinib	• Tetracyclic tyrosine kinase inhibitor • Inhibits ALK, RET, LTK, and GAK	33	0.75		• CYP3A4	• Fatigue • Constipation • Edema • Myalgia • LFT elevation • CPK elevation • Hyperglycemia • Hypocalcemia • Hypophosphatemia • Creatinine elevation • Anemia	
Brigatinib	• Aminopyrimidine tyrosine kinase inhibitor • Inhibits ALK and ROS1	25		• P-gp & BCRP substrate	• CYP3A4 • CYP2C8	• Nausea • Diarrhea • Headache • Fatigue • Cough • CPK elevation	• CYP3A inhibitors/ inducers affect exposure • CYP3A substrates affected by brigatinib

[a]Approximate ratio of CSF to plasma drug concentration based on available clinical data.
ALK, anaplastic lymphoma kinase; $t_{1/2}$, median terminal half-life; CSF, cerebrospinal fluid; CNS, central nervous system; MET, hepatocyte growth factor receptor; P-gp, P-glycoprotein; CYP3A4/5, cytochrome P450 3A4/5; LFT, liver function test; IGF1R, insulin-like growth factor 1 receptor; IR, insulin receptor; CYP2C8, cytochrome P450 2C8; RET, RET proto-oncogene; LTK, leukocyte tyrosine kinase; GAK, cyclin G–associated kinase; CPK, creatine phosphokinase.

TABLE

21.4   *Clinical trials and resistance mechanisms for approved ALK inhibitors*

	Select Trials (phase, line)	No. of Patients	ORR (%)	PFS (months)	On-Target Resistance	Off-Target Resistance
First Generation ALK inhibitors						
Crizotinib	PROFILE 1014 (III, 1L)	343	74	10.9	• *ALK* L1196M	• EGFR activation
	PROFILE 1007 (III, 2L)	347	65	7.7	• *ALK* G1269A	• MAPK activation
					• *ALK* G1202R	• *c-KIT* amplification
					• *ALK* D1203N	• SCF overexpression
					• *ALK* S1206C/Y	• SRC activation
					• *ALK* 1151Tins	• IGF-1R activation
					• *ALK* L1152R	• HER2/3 activation
					• *ALK* C1156Y	• PKC activation
					• *ALK* I1171T/N/S	• SCLC transformation
					• *ALK* F1174L	
					• *ALK* E1210K	
					• *ALK* V1180L	
					• *ALK* amplification	
Second-Generation ALK Inhibitors						
Ceritinib	ASCEND-4 (III, 1L)	376	72.5	16.6	• *ALK* G1202R[a,b,c]	• MAPK activation
	ASCEND-1 (I, 2L)	163	56	6.9	• *ALK* I1151Tins[a]	• SRC activation
	ASCEND-2 (II, 2L)	140	38.6	5.7	• *ALK* L1152P/R[a]	• *PIK3CA* mutation
	ASCEND-5 (III, 2L)	231	39.1	5.4	• *ALK* C1156Y/T[a]	• *MET* amplification
Alectinib	ALEX (III, 1L)	303	82.9	25.7	• *ALK* F1174C/L/V[a]	• EMT
	J-ALEX (III, 1L)	207	85.4	NR	• *ALK* I1171T/N/S[b]	
	NP28761 (II, 2L)	87	48	8.1	• *ALK* V1180L[b]	
	NP28673 (II, 2L)	138	50	8.9	• *ALK* E1210K/S1206C[c]	
Brigatinib	NCT02737501 (III, 1L)	270	—	—	• *ALK* E1210K/	
	ALTA (II, 2L)	222	54	12.9	D1203N[c]	
	NCT01449461 (I/II, 2L)	79	62	13.2		

[a]Confers resistance to ceritinib.
[b]Confers resistance to alectinib.
[c]Confers resistance to brigatinib.
ALK, anaplastic lymphoma kinase; No., number; ORR, overall response rate; PFS, progression-free survival; 1L, first-line; 2L, second-line; EGFR, epithelial growth factor receptor; MAPK, mitogen-activated protein kinase; c-KIT, stem cell growth factor receptor; SCF, stem cell factor; SRC, SRC proto-oncogene; IGF-1R, insulin-like growth factor 1 receptor; HER2/3, receptor tyrosine-protein kinase erbB-2/3; PKC, protein kinase C; SCLC, small cell lung cancer; NR, not reached; MET, hepatocyte growth factor receptor; EMT, epithelial-to-mesenchymal transition.
Modified from Lovly CM, Iyengar P, Gainor JF. Managing resistance to EGFR- and ALK-targeted therapies. *Am Soc Clin Oncol Educ Book.* 2017;37:607-618. Reprinted with permission. Copyright © 2017 American Society of Clinical Oncology. All rights reserved.

ALK mutations detected post-crizotinib include mutations in the ATP-binding pocket causing steric hindrance of crizotinib binding (most commonly L1196M, the analogue of T790M in *EGFR*, and G1296A), mutations in the solvent exposed kinase region thought to decrease crizotinib binding affinity (G1202R, D1203N, and S1206C/Y), and others including 1151Tins, L1152R, C1156Y, I1171T/N/S, F1174L, E1210K, and V1180L.[78–81] *ALK* amplification can also cause on-target resistance to crizotinib and is seen in approximately 10% of cases.[77]

Off-target mechanisms of crizotinib resistance include EGFR activation, *c-KIT* amplification, SCF overexpression, IGF-1R activation, SRC activation, activating mutations in *KRAS*, and small cell transformation.[79,82–85] Notably, the majority of NSCLC cases progressing on/after crizotinib respond to a second-generation

ALK inhibitor, even in the absence of an *ALK* resistance mutation, suggesting retained ALK dependency post crizotinib. Again, this likely reflects the inadequate suppression of the oncogenic *ALK* fusion by crizotinib.

Second-Generation ALK Inhibitors

Ceritinib

Ceritinib potently inhibits ALK in vitro with an IC_{50} in enzymatic assays that is 20-fold lower than crizotinib.[86] Ceritinib retains activity against many crizotinib-resistant mutations, including L1196M, S1206C/Y, G1269A/S as well as V1180L, and I1171T/N/S.[87] Notably, ceritinib cannot overcome the solvent front mutation G1202R. Ceritinib was approved for second-line use in 2014 based on a phase I multicenter trial (ASCEND-1: 56% ORR in crizotinib-treated patients, median PFS 7.0 months).[88] Subsequently, the superiority of ceritinib over chemotherapy as second-line therapy in advanced *ALK*-rearranged NSCLC was confirmed by the phase III ASCEND-5 trial (median PFS 5.4 versus 1.6 months, $P < 0.001$).[89] Recently, positive results from ASCEND-4, a phase III trial comparing ceritinib and chemotherapy in untreated *ALK*-rearranged NSCLC (median PFS 16.6 versus 8.1 months, $P < 0.00001$), led to FDA approval of ceritinib as first-line therapy.[90] While ceritinib does have some CNS activity (35% IC-ORR and median IC-DOR of 6.9 months in ASCEND-5), median PFS of first-line ceritinib was only 10.7 months in patients with brain metastases at baseline, as compared to 26.3 months in patients without brain metastases.[89,90] These findings and others suggest that ceritinib, which is a substrate of P-gp, has limited intracranial activity.

Pharmacokinetics

At the standard dose of 750 mg daily, maximum ceritinib plasma concentration is reached at 6 hours; terminal $t_{1/2}$ is approximately 40 hours. Ceritinib is metabolized primarily by CYP3A and should not be taken concurrently with CYP3A inhibitors due to their significant affect on ceritinib AUC.[91] Like crizotinib, ceritinib is a substrate of P-gp.

Toxicity

Ceritinib has significant predominantly gastrointestinal toxicity at standard dosing of 750 mg taken under fasting conditions. The majority of patients experience nausea, diarrhea, or vomiting on ceritinib, often requiring dose interruption or reduction; elevation of transaminases and lipase is also commonly observed and can be severe.[88,90,92,93] Of note, a food-effect study (ASCEND-8) suggests that taking 450 mg daily with food may significantly ameliorate ceritinib's GI adverse effects while achieving similar steady-state levels as the 750-mg daily fasting dosing.[94] Rare but significant AEs on ceritinib include pneumonitis, QT prolongation, and bradycardia.[91]

Alectinib

Alectinib is a highly potent (IC_{50} 2 nM, in vitro kinase assay), selective ALK inhibitor notable for its CNS activity and efficacy against many secondary mutations responsible for crizotinib resistance, including L1196M, G1269A, C1156Y, F1174L, L1152P/R, and S1206C/Y.[95] Like ceritinib, alectinib is inactive against *ALK* G1202R. Alectinib was FDA approved in 2015 for second-line use in *ALK*-rearranged patients post-progression on crizotinib based on two single-arm phase II trials demonstrating promising systemic and intracranial activity in this setting (ORR 38% to 44%, 60% CNS specific; DOR 7.5 to 11.2 months, 9.1 months in the CNS).[96,97] Subsequently, two randomized phase III trials (J-ALEX and global ALEX), comparing alectinib to crizotinib as first-line TKI therapy for advanced *ALK*-rearranged NSCLC, have shown superior efficacy and lower toxicity with alectinib (ALEX: median PFS 25.7 versus 10.4 months, HR for disease progression or death 0.47, [95% CI 0.34 to 0.65], $P < 0.001$) and impressive CNS efficacy (ALEX: 81% IC-ORR and median IC-DOR of 17.5 months).[72,98] Alectinib currently has FDA breakthrough therapy designation for first-line use in advanced *ALK*-rearranged NSCLC and may soon supplant crizotinib as the standard of care in this setting.

Pharmacokinetics

Alectinib has moderate bioavailability, maximized when absorbed concurrently with food, and reaches peak plasma concentration by 4 hours.[99] CYP3A is responsible for the primary metabolism of alectinib to its major metabolite, M4, which is in turn also metabolized by CYP3A.[99] Alectinib and M4 are similarly potent inhibitors of ALK, present at a metabolite to parent ratio of 0.4 and with effective $t_{1/2}$ of 33 and 31 hours, respectivly.[99] Unlike crizotinib and ceritinib, alectinib is not a substrate of P-gp, contributing to its effective BBB penetration.[100]

Toxicity

AEs observed on alectinib have been predominantly mild (grade 1) and include fatigue, edema, constipation, myalgias, dysgeusia, photosensitivity, and creatine phosphokinase (CPK) elevation. Notably, GI toxicity is observed at a lower frequency than seen in patients on crizotinib or ceritinib.[95]

Brigatinib

Brigatinib is a potent inhibitor of ALK with a broad spectrum of activity against crizotinib resistance mutations. While preclinical data suggested that brigatinib might be active against G1202R and one clinical case of brigatinib response in G1202R-mutant NSCLC has been confirmed, both structural modeling studies and clinical analysis of resistant specimens suggest that brigatinib's activity against G1202R is limited.[77,101–103] Brigatinib was approved for use in crizotinib-refractory *ALK*-rearranged NSCLC in 2017 on the basis of the phase II ALTA trial (ORR 54%; median PFS 12.9 months).[102] IC-ORR of 67% in ALTA with an unreached IC-DOR in intracranial responders support the intracranial efficacy of brigatinib. A phase III study of brigatinib versus crizotinib as first-line therapy for advanced *ALK*-rearranged NSCLC is ongoing (NCT02737501).

Pharmacokinetics

Brigatinib is orally bioavailable and reaches peak plasma concentration by 3 hours. Brigatinib's AUC is not significantly affected by coadministration with food. It is 66% bound by plasma proteins. Brigatinib has a mean elimination $t_{1/2}$ of 25 hours and is metabolized by CYP2C8 and CYP3A4 in vitro, prompting recommendations to avoid concomitant use of strong CYP3A inhibitors. While mild hepatic and renal impairment have no clinically meaningful impact on the pharmacokinetics of brigatinib, moderate-to-severe impairment remains unstudied. Brigatinib is a substrate of P-gp.[104]

Toxicity

Brigatinib is generally well tolerated. The most common treatment-related AEs are fatigue, nausea, diarrhea, headache, and cough. Serious AEs reported include dyspnea, hypoxia, pneumonia, pulmonary embolism, and pyrexia. Early-onset pulmonary events including hypoxia and dyspnea were noted in 14% of patients starting at a 180-mg dose of brigatinib; pulmonary events were noted in only 2% of patients treated with a 7-day 90-mg lead-in to 180-mg daily dosing as used in the ALTA trial.[105] Of note, these early pulmonary events can be severe and life-threatening, so close monitoring of patients during the first week of therapy is warranted.

Resistance to Second-Generation ALK Inhibitors

Compared to crizotinib, resistance to second-generation ALK TKIs is more frequently attributable to a secondary mutation in *ALK* with a narrower spectrum of mutations capable of driving resistance; this difference may reflect greater potency against the target kinase relative to crizotinib.[77] *ALK* G1202R is the most frequently observed *ALK* mutation after progression on all second-generation ALK TKIs.[77] However, each ALK inhibitor has a unique spectrum of activity against different mutant ALK kinases. For example, I1171T/N/S and V1180L mutations confer resistance to alectinib but retain sensitivity to ceritinib and other next-generation TKIs.[77,106] Ceritinib is uniquely vulnerable to F1174C/L/V, a crizotinib resistance mutation overcome by alectinib.[107,108]

Compound mutations in *ALK* can arise, causing resistance to more potent inhibitors as patients undergo sequential ALK TKI therapies. For instance, E1210K+S1206C and E1210K+D1203N have been reported to confer resistance to brigatinib. In a study using whole exome sequencing of serial resistance biopsies to perform clonal analysis, an *ALK*[E1210K] subclone was found to emerge during crizotinib therapy, which later expanded on brigatinib therapy and acquired compound mutations with S1206C and D1203N.[77] This case illustrates the broader challenge of increasingly resistant compound mutations arising after sequential TKI therapy, which, with further study, may have implications for guiding optimal sequencing of ALK TKIs.

Reported off-target mechanisms of resistance to second-generation ALK TKIs include mutations in *PIK3CA* and *MAP2K1*, SRC activation, *MET* amplification, and EMT and small cell transformation.[77,109–111] Notably, reactivation of the mitogen-activated protein kinase (MAPK) pathway causing ALK TKI resistance can be reversed with MEK inhibition in vitro; the combination of ALK TKIs and MEK inhibitors is currently being explored in two separate phase I/II trials (NCT03087448 and NCT03202940).[112]

ALK Inhibitors Under Development

Lorlatinib (PF-06463922)

Lorlatinib is a highly selective and potent dual ALK/ROS1 inhibitor active against all known single *ALK* resistance mutations. This activity notably includes G1202R, distinguishing lorlatinib from second-generation ALK TKIs.[113] In vitro data suggest that lorlatinib will also be an efficacious inhibitor of some compound *ALK* mutations emerging after sequential first-and second-generation ALK TKI therapy (e.g., D1203N+E1210K and D1203N+F1174C).[77]

Lorlatinib is a cyclic 2-aminopyridine derivative originally selected as a low efflux substrate from cell lines overexpressing P-gp.[114] Lorlatinib's anticipated CNS efficacy has been borne out by preliminary clinical data from the phase I portion of an ongoing phase I/II trial (NCT01970865), which demonstrated an IC-ORR of 39%, ORR of 46%, and median PFS of 11.4 months in all patients and remarkably similar results in the subcohort pretreated with two or more ALK TKIs (ORR 42%; median PFS 9.2 months).[115] Hypercholesterolemia was the most common all-grade and grade 3 to 4 AE observed in dose escalation testing with hypertriglyceridemia and peripheral edema also commonly observed. Reversible CNS effects are also seen on lorlatinib including neurocognitive disorders and mood lability as well as peripheral neuropathy.[115]

Lorlatinib was granted FDA breakthrough therapy designation for advanced previously treated *ALK*-rearranged NSCLC in 2017.

While no single *ALK* secondary mutation has been found to confer resistance to lorlatinib, a compound C1156Y+L1198F mutation was detected in a patient relapsing after C1156Y-driven resistance to crizotinib, followed by sequential treatment with ceritinib and lorlatinib.[116] Remarkably, C1156Y+L1198F was shown to resensitize cancer cells to crizotinib in this case. In one series of ceritinib-resistant, patient-derived cell lines, the absence of *ALK* resistance mutations was found to be highly predictive of lorlatinib resistance, suggesting that loss of ALK dependency, rather than drug evasion by compound mutation, may prove to be the largest obstacle to lorlatinib.[77] Thus, at least in certain cases, ALK independence may thwart the ability of lorlatinib to salvage relapse on second-generation TKIs.

Ensartinib (X-396)

Ensartinib is a small-molecule TKI targeting ALK, ROS1, MET, and AXL. Ensartinib has completed phase I/II testing and is currently undergoing phase III testing versus crizotinib for treatment of TKI-naïve *ALK*-rearranged NSCLC (NCT02767804).[113] Preliminary results from the phase I/II trial of 225-mg daily ensartinib showed responses in 77% (7/9) crizotinib-naïve patients and 73% (16/22) crizotinib-treated patients with 53% CNS response across both groups.[117] Most treatment-related AEs observed were mild with rash, nausea, vomiting, fatigue, and pruritus occurring most frequently. Ensartinib is effective against C1156Y/T and L1196M, but not against ALK G1202R; resistance mechanisms have not yet been reported.

TPX-0005

TPX-0005 is a multitargeted inhibitor of ALK, ROS1, and TRK kinases. This TKI was specifically designed to overcome resistance mutations, including the solvent front mutation *ALK* G1202R. Preclinical data suggest that TPX-0005 may also inhibit SRC and FAK, both of which may play a role in off-target resistance to TKIs. A phase I study of TPX-0005 is currently enrolling in the United States and Republic of Korea (NCT03093116).

ROS1 Translocation

ROS1 is an orphan RTK with significant sequence homology to ALK. *ROS1* rearrangements were first discovered in NSCLC in 2007 and have since been identified in 1% to 2% of NSCLC.[118] Similar to *ALK*-rearranged NSCLC, *ROS1*-rearranged NSCLC is associated with younger age, never-or light smoking history, and adenocarcinoma histology.[119] Fourteen distinct *ROS1* fusion partners have been identified, most commonly *CD74*.[120] Due to the rarity of *ROS1*-rearranged NSCLC, phase III comparisons of targeted therapy and chemotherapy have not been feasible, though phase I/II studies and retrospective evidence strongly suggest that ROS1 targeted therapies are superior to chemotherapy.[121]

Crizotinib

Crizotinib (see ALK section) is the only ROS1-directed inhibitor that is FDA approved to date. Crizotinib gained FDA approval for advanced *ROS1*-rearranged NSCLC in 2016 based on remarkable efficacy in a phase I expansion cohort (ORR 72%; median PFS

19.2 months).[122] Of note, subsequent phase II and retrospective data suggest somewhat more modest but still impressive efficacy (median PFS 9 to 13.4 months).[123–125]

In contrast to *ALK*, crizotinib resistance in *ROS1*-rearranged patients is predominantly on-target and attributable to mutations concentrated in a narrow segment of the kinase. This likely reflects the greater potency of crizotinib for ROS1 compared to ALK.[121] *ROS1* G2032R, a solvent front mutation, which is analogous to *ALK* G1202R and causes steric hindrance to crizotinib binding, was found to underlie up to 50% of on-target crizotinib resistance in a recent study.[121,126] Other on-target resistance mutations reported include D2033N, S1986Y/F, L2026M, and L1951R.[127] Off-target resistance mechanisms to crizotinib have also been reported in *ROS1*-rearranged lung cancer, namely, upregulation of bypass signaling pathways including EGFR, RAS, and KIT.[128–130]

ROS1 Inhibitors Under Development

Beyond crizotinib, phase II data have also been reported for **ceritinib** (see ALK section) in *ROS1*-rearranged NSCLC. A multicenter Korean study of ceritinib in heavily pretreated but crizotinib-naïve patients showed a 67% ORR and 19.3-month median PFS.[92] However, ceritinib's efficacy must be weighed against its toxicities, including high rates of diarrhea, nausea, anorexia, and vomiting that can limit tolerability and prevent continuous dosing. Furthermore, the utility of ceritinib is likely confined to the crizotinib-naïve setting given preclinical data showing a lack of activity against crizotinib resistance mutations including G2032R, D2033N, L1951R, and S1986Y/F and clinical data showing no responses among a handful of crizotinib-treated, *ROS1*-rearranged NSCLC patients.[92,131–133]

Several other ROS1-active agents under development also have unclear utility in the setting of G2032R. **Entrectinib** (see NTRK section) is a CNS-penetrant TKI currently in phase II investigation in *ROS1*-rearranged NSCLC after promising phase I results in crizotinib-naïve patients (86% ORR; 19-month median PFS).[134] However, entrectinib has failed to demonstrate preclinical efficacy against G2032R, and six patients previously treated with crizotinib did not respond to entrectinib.[134–136] **Lorlatinib**, also undergoing phase II testing in *ROS1*-rearranged NSCLC (NCT01970865), is active against *ROS1* resistance mutations L2026M and D2033 in vitro and clinically inhibits S1986Y/F.[132,137] However, lorlatinib may have suboptimal activity against *ROS1* G2032R based on cellular assays.[137]

Several ROS1-directed agents have demonstrated preclinical potential to inhibit G2032R. **DS-6051b** is an inhibitor of ROS1 and NTRK undergoing phase I testing in *ROS1*-rearranged NSCLC (NCT02279433). Preliminary results from a phase I study of DS-6051b in mixed crizotinib-treated and crizotinib-naïve *ROS1*-rearranged NSCLC patients reported partial response in 4/7 patients; mutation status of responders has not been reported.[138] **TPX-0005** (see ALK section) is a multitargeted TKI under development (NCT03093116) and is notable for its small size and low-nanomolar activity against G2032R in vitro. Finally, **cabozantinib**, a multikinase inhibitor of multiple targets including VEGFR2, MET, RET, KIT, AXL, and FLT3, is active against *ROS1* G2032R and D1203N in cellular assays.[127,133] Based on case reports, cabozantinib may have clinical efficacy in *ROS1*-rearranged NSCLC, including in the setting of crizotinib resistance due to solvent front

mutations.[131,133] However, the potential benefit of cabozantinib in this context will need to be weighed against its significant toxicities, including palmar-plantar rash, fatigue, diarrhea, LFT elevation, nausea, thrombocytopenia, proteinuria, oral mucositis, hypertension, and elevated lipase.[139] An ongoing phase II trial (NCT01639508) is assessing cabozantinib's efficacy in advanced NSCLC harboring *RET*, *ROS1*, or *NTRK* fusions, as well as increased MET or AXL activity.

BRAF Mutation

BRAF, in contrast to the transmembrane kinases discussed above, is a cytosolic signaling molecule downstream of KRAS and is a serine/threonine kinase. *BRAF* mutations, detected in approximately 2% to 4% of lung cancers, tend to occur in smokers with adenocarcinoma and lead to constitutive activation of the MAPK signaling pathway.[140,141] In contradistinction to melanoma, non-V600 and V600 mutations occur at comparable frequencies in lung cancer.[141] The prognostic significance of V600E remains to be established, with studies to date showing contradicting PFS and OS results likely due to small patient numbers.[142,143] *BRAF* mutations beyond V600E have been less well characterized both in terms of biology and drug sensitivity; these include kinase-activating mutations (G469A/V, K601E, L597R) and kinase-inactivating mutations (D594G and G466V).[141]

BRAF Inhibitors

Vemurafenib and **dabrafenib** are ATP-competitive kinase inhibitors designed specifically to target V600E-mutated BRAF. Both have shown clinical efficacy in phase II studies of V600E-selected NSCLC: ORR and median PFS of 42% and 7.3 months for vemurafenib ($n = 20$, 18/20 V600E) and 33% and 5.5 months for dabrafenib ($n = 78$, all V600E).[144,145] The modest success obtained with single-agent BRAF inhibition may be due to a compensatory increase in BRAF-independent RAS signaling.[146,147] Consistent with this proposed feedback mechanism and in line with previous observations in melanoma, a phase II study of dabrafenib combined with the allosteric MEK1/2 inhibitor trametinib in pretreated *BRAF* V600E NSCLC patients showed a remarkable increase in efficacy compared to that achieved with dabrafenib alone (ORR 63%; median PFS 9.7 months).[148,149] In a separate cohort of this phase II study, the combination achieved an ORR of 61.1% among 36 treatment-naïve patients. Although the median PFS had not been reached at 9 months follow-up, 59% had responses lasting longer than 6 months. Based on the findings from this multicohort phase II study, the combination of **dabrafenib/trametinib** gained FDA approval for treatment of *BRAF* V600E–mutant NSCLC in June 2017. Notably, the approval does not specify line of treatment.

Pharmacokinetics

The pharmacokinetic profile of vemurafenib is notable for rapid oral absorption and significant accumulation with a long $t_{1/2}$ of approximately 57 hours. Vemurafenib is primarily eliminated by the liver; mild-to-moderate hepatic or renal impairment do not necessitate dose reduction. Vemurafenib is a CYP3A4 substrate and inducer, a moderate CYP1A2 inhibitor, and a P-gp/BRCP substrate and inhibitor.[150] Similar to vemurafenib, dabrafenib has high oral bioavailability indicative of extensive absorption and low first-pass intestinal and hepatic metabolism.[151] Biliary secretion is the major excretion pathway for dabrafenib and its metabolites.[151] Dabrafenib itself has a shorter median terminal $t_{1/2}$ (5 hours); however, dabrafenib's major circulating metabolites (hydroxy-, carboxy-, and desmethyl-dabrafenib) have estimated half-lives of >24 hours and accumulate significantly.[152] Dabrafenib can alter exposure to drugs metabolized by the CYP2C family, and inhibition of CYP2C8/CYP3A can alter exposure to dabrafenib.[153]

Trametinib has rapid, effective oral absorption (72% bioavailability, t_{max} 1.5 hours) and is 97% plasma protein bound (Vc/F 214 L).[154] Trametinib is not a CYP substrate and is metabolized predominantly by deacetylation with a $t_{1/2}$ of approximately 4 days.

Toxicity

BRAF inhibition causes a spectrum of cutaneous AEs including rash, pruritus, hyperkeratosis, papilloma, dry skin, palmar-plantar erythrodysesthesia, and, most notably, secondary cutaneous malignancies including squamous cell carcinoma (SCC), basal cell carcinoma, and keratoacanthoma.[144,145] Cutaneous SCC is observed in 12% to 23% of NSCLC patients on single-agent vemurafenib or dabrafenib; notably, noncutaneous SCC occurs, though rarely.[144,145] Common noncutaneous AEs attributable to BRAF inhibition include pyrexia, arthralgia, and fatigue.[144] Like single-agent therapy, combined dabrafenib/trametinib has significant but manageable toxicity, with grade 3 to 4 AEs seen in approximately 50% of patients; pyrexia and GI toxicity are commonly observed.[149] Combined BRAF/MEK inhibition may reduce AEs related to increased MAPK signaling such as cutaneous SCC and keratoacanthoma.[148,155]

Mechanisms of Resistance

Mechanisms mediating resistance to BRAF inhibition in NSCLC are unknown given the short duration of use of these drugs in NSCLC. However, mechanisms underlying resistance to BRAF inhibition observed in melanoma are heterogeneous and include reactivation of the MAPK pathway via *BRAF* amplification or *de novo NRAS*, *KRAS*, and *MAP2K1/2* mutations, as well as non-MAPK pathway changes such as adaptive activation of the PI3K-PTEN-AKT cascade.[155–157] Notably, combined inhibition of BRAF and MEK may delay the development of acquired resistance to therapy.[148]

MET Mutation and Amplification

MET, the hepatocyte growth factor receptor, is an RTK that mediates wound healing and regulates cell survival, growth, and motility.[158] Activation of MET signaling can be caused by diverse mechanisms including protein overexpression, gene amplification, mutation, or rearrangement.[158] MET deregulation is implicated in multiple malignancies including NSCLC where it is both a primary oncogenic driver and a cause of acquired resistance to targeted therapy (see EGFR and ALK sections).[158] Since the discovery of MET deregulation in NSCLC in the 1990s, there have been multiple unsuccessful phase III studies exploring MET inhibitors in MET-overexpressed NSCLC.[159,160] These studies were likely limited by the heterogeneous mechanisms leading to MET overexpression. A recent shift in focus toward evaluating MET-directed therapies for

lung cancers harboring genetic alterations that create an oncogene-addicted state, namely, high-level *MET* amplification and splice alterations that lead to exon 14 skipping, has yielded more promising results. *MET* exon 14 skipping (*MET*ex14), an alteration that protects MET from ubiquitin-mediated degradation, is present in ~3% of NSCLC. *MET*ex14 is enriched in sarcomatoid tumors, is associated with older age at diagnosis, occurs in both smokers and never-smokers, and may coexist with *MET* amplification.[158,161,162] High-level *MET* amplification (defined as a ratio of MET/CEP7 ≥ 5) is less common, can occur independent of *MET*ex14, and may be enriched in smokers and patients with sarcomatoid carcinoma.[163]

MET Inhibitors Under Investigation

Small-molecule inhibitors of MET developed to date include multikinase inhibitors—**crizotinib, cabozantinib, glesatinib, AMG208, merestinib, altiratinib, and golvatinib**—and MET-selective inhibitors—**capmatinib, tepotinib, tivantinib, AMG337, and savolitinib**.[164] Although there are no FDA-approved therapies for selective targeting of MET, several reports of durable response to crizotinib or cabozantinib in patients with NSCLC harboring *MET*ex14 or high-level *MET* amplification have been published.[165–167] Furthermore, several ongoing studies are exploring multikinase and MET-selective inhibitors in this population. Preliminary results from an expansion cohort of the PROFILE 1001 phase I study demonstrated a 44% ORR in 18 patients with *MET*ex14 NSCLC. Treatment-related AEs were consistent with those observed for *ALK*-and *ROS1*-rearranged patients treated with crizotinib (see ALK section).[164] It is anticipated that MET-selective inhibitors will be better tolerated than multikinase inhibitors. Indeed, selective inhibition of MET is well tolerated overall, with common AEs including nausea, anorexia, and fatigue.[166] Edema, often of the extremities and, in some cases, anasarca, is a toxicity characteristic of MET inhibitors, though the mechanism is unknown.

Similar to other TKIs, secondary kinase domain mutations are implicated in resistance to MET TKIs. *MET* D1228N, G1163R, and Y1230C/H mutations have been reported in the setting of crizotinib resistance in patients with *MET*ex14.[167–169] Both D1228 and Y1230 are important residues in the stabilization of the unique autoinhibitory conformation of MET, with Y1230 directly interacting (via π-stacking) with the aromatic ring of crizotinib and other type I MET inhibitors (e.g., capmatinib, tepotinib, savolitinib, AMG337). Type II MET inhibitors (e.g., cabozantinib, glesatinib, merestinib) do not bind the autoinhibitory conformation of MET but rather the ATP adenine-binding site, suggesting that they might have activity against D1228 and Y1230.[169] Indeed, a recent study reported suppression of Y1230 mutations in a patient who achieved a mixed response to glesatinib after progression on crizotinib.[169] Notably, the patient developed a *MET* 1195V mutation at resistance. The 1195V variant is predicted to affect both type I and II inhibitor binding by destabilizing the autoinhibited activation loop confirmation and altering the shape of the hydrophobic pocket. In addition to these clinically observed mutations, mutations involving the F1200 residue are expected to confer global resistance to type I and II inhibitors based on preclinical and structural studies. Interestingly, resistance to the combination of an EGFR TKI and a type I MET TKI appears to be similarly driven by acquisition of *MET* resistance mutations.[170,171]

Neurotrophic Receptor Tyrosine Kinase Rearrangement

Rearrangement of the neurotrophic receptor tyrosine kinase (*NTRK1*) gene, which encodes the TRKA kinase involved in neuronal development, occurs at a low frequency in numerous solid malignancies including colon, thyroid, melanoma, glioblastoma, and AML. *NTRK1* rearrangement was discovered in NSCLC in 2013, where it is a rare oncogenic driver, identified at a frequency of 0.1% (1/1,378) in one study.[172,173] Fusion partners of *NTRK1* reported in NSCLC include *SQSTM1*, *MPRIP*, *TPR*, and *CD74*.[174,175] Due to both the recent discovery and low frequency of *NTRK1* rearrangements in NSCLC, clinical testing of TRK inhibition in this setting is relatively nascent.

NTRK Inhibitors Under Investigation

Larotrectinib (LOXO-101)

Larotrectinib is a highly selective and potent pan-TRK TKI with no significant inhibitory activity outside of the TRK family. Larotrectinib is currently undergoing phase II testing in advanced solid tumors harboring TRKA, TRKB, and TRKC fusion proteins (NCT02576431) and has received FDA breakthrough therapy designation in this setting for the treatment of adult and pediatric patients.[176] A recent combined analysis of three small phase I and II trials of larotrectinib in diverse *NTRK1-3*–rearranged malignancies including five lung cancer patients showed a response rate of 78% and DOR of up to 23 months.[177] Larotrectinib is orally bioavailable with high plasma exposure and little accumulation with a $t_{1/2}$ of approximately 160 minutes. The drug is generally well tolerated with common AEs including grade 1 to 2 fatigue, dizziness, nausea, and anemia.[175,177]

Entrectinib (RXDX-101)

Entrectinib is a multikinase inhibitor with activity against ALK, ROS1, and TRKA-C.[173] After promising results from a phase I study in *NTRK*-, *ROS1*-, and *ALK*-rearranged solid tumors (ORR of 100% [3/3], 86%, and 57%, respectively, with a 63% [5/8] IC-ORR across all groups), entrectinib also received FDA breakthrough therapy designation for the same indication as larotrectinib. Notably, a patient with *SQSTM1-NTRK1*–fused NSCLC treated with entrectinib experienced a durable response of over 6 months and a complete and durable response in the CNS.[173] An ongoing phase II basket trial in solid malignancies with *NTRK1-3*, *ALK*, and *ROS1* rearrangements is actively recruiting patients (NCT02568267). Entrectinib has an estimated $t_{1/2}$ of 20 to 22 hours at the standard 600-mg daily dose. Dose reduction was required due to toxicity in 15% of patients, with common AEs including fatigue, dysgeusia, paresthesias, nausea, and myalgias. Severe AEs reported included fatigue, cognitive disturbance, and eosinophilic myocarditis.[134]

Multiple other inhibitors with TRK activity are undergoing clinical evaluation, including **cabozantinib** (NCT01639508, see ROS1 section)**, DS-6051b** (NCT02675491), **TPX-0005** (NCT03093116), **belizatinib** (NCT02048488), **PLX7486** (NCT01804530), **DCC2701** (NCT02228811), and **MGCD516** (NCT02219711).

Mechanisms of Resistance to TRK Inhibition

Two mechanisms of resistance to TRKA inhibition have been reported clinically.[178–180] *NTRK1* G595R and G667C mutations (analogous to *ALK* G1202R and G1269A, respectively) were found in an *LMNA-NTRK1*–rearranged colorectal cancer patient progressing on entrectinib, mutations that have been shown to emerge preclinically on high- and low-dose entrectinib, respectively.[178,179,181] Of note, G667C, but not G595R, could be overcome with subsequent exposure to larotrectinib. **LOXO-195** is a new highly selective and potent pan-TRK inhibitor designed to be active against *NTRK1* G595R–mutant cells. LOXO-195 induced a 6-month response in a patient with *LMNA-NTRK1* fusion colorectal cancer with the G595R resistance mutation.[175,180] A patient with *ETV6-NTRK3*–rearranged mammary analogue secretory carcinoma was found to have a G623R mutation in the kinase ATP-binding pocket of *NTRK3*, which is structurally analogous to *NTRK1* G595R, *ALK* G1202R, and *ROS1* G2032R.[179]

RET Rearrangement

The rearranged during transfection (*RET*) gene encodes an RTK that normally functions in renal organogenesis and enteric nervous system development.[118] Initially discovered as an oncogenic driver in NSCLC in 2012, *RET* rearrangements are detected in 1% to 2% of NSCLC, typically associated with younger age, minimal smoking, and adenocarcinoma or adenosquamous carcinoma.[119,182] *KIF5B* is the most common *RET* fusion partner in NSCLC; others include *CCDC6*, *NCOA4*, *CLIP1*, *ERC1*, and *TRIM33*.[139,183,184]

Multikinase Inhibitors with RET Activity Under Investigation

To date, there are no FDA-approved RET inhibitors available for use in advanced *RET*-rearranged NSCLC. However, several multikinase inhibitors have shown RET activity in vitro and are in early-phase testing in *RET*-rearranged NSCLC. These include **vandetanib, lenvatinib, cabozantinib, sunitinib, sorafenib, apatinib, ponatinib,** and **alectinib.**[119]

Phase II, single-arm study results have been published for cabozantinib and vandetanib. Among 25 evaluable patients with *RET*-rearranged NSCLC, **cabozantinib** led to an ORR of 28% and a median PFS of 5.5 months.[139] Notably, dose reductions were required in 73% of patients due to intolerable drug-related toxicities, including palmar-plantar erythrodysesthesia, fatigue, and diarrhea. **Vandetanib** has been tested in two independent phase II studies (each with 17 evaluable *RET*-rearranged NSCLC patients), demonstrating an ORR of 18% to 47% and a median PFS of 4.5 to 4.7 months.[185,186] Additionally, preliminary results were recently presented from a phase II study of **lenvatinib** in 25 patients with *RET*-rearranged NSCLC, with an ORR of 16%.[187]

Collectively, these data suggest that the currently available multikinase inhibitors have limited efficacy against *RET*-rearranged NSCLC, with an ORR that tends to be significantly lower than what is observed with EGFR- or ALK-directed therapies in *EGFR*-mutant or *ALK*-rearranged lung cancer. Indeed, in one retrospective analysis evaluating an international multicenter registry of *RET*-rearranged lung cancer patients, responses to multikinase inhibitors (including cabozantinib, vandetanib, sunitinib, lenvatinib, and nintedanib) were seen in 26% of 50 evaluable patients, with a median PFS of only 2.3 months.[188]

RET-Selective Inhibitors in Development

The relatively limited activity of these TKIs may be due to their suboptimal anti-RET activity at doses used in the clinic. This, in turn, may be secondary to their relatively low potency against RET, and/or the toxicities—for example, related to KDR inhibition—that hamper chronic dosing. Here, the development of highly RET-potent and RET-selective inhibitors will prove critical.

A number of RET-selective and RET-potent inhibitors are now entering early-phase testing. **BLU-667** and **LOXO-292** are orally available TKIs designed to specifically target RET while sparing closely related kinases such as KDR. Both have entered phase I testing (NCT03037385, NCT03157128); safety and efficacy data are not available at the time of this publication.

Combination Therapy in RET

The efficacy of RET-targeted therapies may, alternatively, be limited due to concomitant molecular alterations present in the tumor, necessitating the design of combination regimens in order to achieve clinically meaningful and durable activity. One combination strategy under development is **vandetanib plus everolimus**, an inhibitor of mTOR. mTOR, downstream of PI3K and AKT, is a key mediator of RET-driven cell growth.[189] In addition, everolimus may modulate P-gp–mediated drug efflux to improve the BBB penetration of vandetanib.[190] Results from a phase I study of vandetanib and everolimus were promising: Among six patients with *RET*-rearranged NSCLC, responses were reported in 83%, with CNS responses in 100% of patients with brain metastases.[191]

ERBB2 Mutation

Mutations in *ERBB2*—the gene encoding HER2—were discovered as an oncogenic driver in NSCLC in 2004.[192] Identified in 1% to 2% of NSCLC, *ERBB2* mutations are predominantly in-frame insertions in exon 20, analogous to *EGFR* exon 20 insertion mutations.[119,193–195] The most commonly reported *ERBB2* mutation is a YVMA insertion at codon 775; point mutations such as L755S and G776C have also been described.[196] *ERBB2* mutation occurs independently of *ERBB2* amplification or overexpression in NSCLC.[195–197]

HER2-Targeted Agents Under Investigation

A potential role for HER2-directed therapies in *ERBB2*-mutant NSCLC has been suggested by a number of small phase II studies, retrospective analyses, and case reports. In a retrospective analysis of the European cohort with *ERBB2* mutations (EUHER2), **trastuzumab** (a HER2 monoclonal antibody) in combination with chemotherapy led to an ORR of 50% and disease control rate (DCR) of 75%, with a median PFS of 5.1 months.[198] By comparison, the ORR, DCR, and median PFS with **afatinib**, a dual HER2/EGFR TKI (see EGFR section), in this retrospective series were 18.2%, 63.7%, and 3.9 months, respectively.[198] In a small phase II study, afatinib led to objective response in 0 of 7 *ERBB2*-mutant patients, with disease control in 5 of 7 patients (71%).[199] Another pan-HER

TKI, **dacomitinib**, showed an ORR of 12% (3/26) in a phase II study that included 26 *ERBB2*-mutant NSCLC patients.[200]

The modest success achieved with single agents, coupled with preclinical data suggesting synergy with combined HER2/mTOR inhibition, led to a phase I trial of **neratinib** (pan-HER TKI) plus **temsirolimus** (mTOR inhibitor), which reported a 29% ORR (2/7).[201,202] Based on these results, a phase II randomized study of neratinib with or without temsirolimus was initiated. The ORR with neratinib alone was 0%, versus 14% with the combination therapy.[203] The reasons for the differential responses seen with the HER2-directed TKIs are unclear, although the data collectively suggest that a single-agent TKI may not provide sufficient antitumor activity in *ERBB2*-mutant disease.

Most recently, preliminary results from a phase II basket trial of ado-trastuzumab emtansine (**T-DM1**) in *ERBB2*-mutant NSCLC were presented. Responses were seen in 44% (8/18) with a median PFS of 4 months.[204] Overall, these findings highlight the need to develop better HER2-directed agents with more durable clinical activity.

Fibroblast Growth Factor Receptor 1 Amplification

The fibroblast growth factor receptor (FGFR) family, composed of 4 RTKs and 22 ligands, regulates multiple physiologic processes including embryogenesis, angiogenesis, immunity, and metabolism.[205] Deregulation of FGFR kinases can be caused by point mutation, rearrangement, or amplification and has been implicated in the pathogenesis of diverse malignancies.[206] Moreover, FGFR pathway activation has been shown to mediate resistance to multiple targeted therapies (e.g., BRAF, HER2, MET, and EGFR).[207,208] Among the FGFR alterations identified in lung cancer, *FGFR1* amplification, which occurs in 10% to 25% of SCCs of the lung, is the most prevalent.[119] Preclinical data indicate that *FGFR1* amplification can, but does not always, confer dependence on FGFR1 signaling and corresponding sensitivity to its inhibition.[209–211] As the genetic alterations identified in squamous cell lung cancer to date have evaded targeted approaches, the frequency of *FGFR* alterations has generated significant interest. However, the modest clinical efficacy of single-agent FGFR1 inhibition described below suggests a complex and as of yet incompletely understood biology.

FGFR Inhibitors Under Investigation

The first generation of FGFR TKIs was composed of repurposed multikinase VEGFR inhibitors with low potency FGFR inhibition (e.g., **brivanib, cediranib, dovitinib, lucitanib,** and **nintedanib**).[212] A second generation of more selective FGFR inhibitors includes FGFR1/2/3 inhibitors **AZD4547, BGJ398,** and **Debio-1347** and pan-FGFR inhibitors **JNJ-42756493, LY2874455,** and **FIIN-2**.[213] Phase I studies of AZD4547 and BGJ398 in heavily pretreated *FGFR1*-amplified squamous cell lung cancer patients have demonstrated manageable toxicity with predominantly gastrointestinal and dermatologic AEs.[140,214] Hyperphosphatemia, a known class effect due to the role of FGFR in renal phosphate excretion, was also observed.[140,214,215] Unfortunately, preliminary efficacy has been disappointing with ORRs of 8% (2/15) and 11% (4/38) for AZD4547 and BGJ398, respectively.[140,214]

Mechanisms of Resistance

Discrepancy between the relative levels of *FGFR1* gene amplification and protein expression has raised concern that FISH-based molecular enrichment strategies may not result in ideal selection of patients for FGFR-directed therapies.[209,211] Furthermore, preclinical studies have shown that cell lines with equivalent levels of FGFR protein expression can have differential sensitivity to FGFR1 inhibition, suggesting that refining the identification of true (i.e., protein level) *FGFR1* amplification may not ultimately provide a biomarker for FGFR1 dependence.[216,217] Notably, *FGFR1*-amplified tumors have increased expression of neighboring genes on the 8p12 amplicon, raising the possibility that codependence may underlie primary resistance to FGFR1 inhibition in some cases.[218] In contrast, coamplification of *MYC*, found in 40% of *FGFR1*-amplified squamous cell lung cancer, may increase sensitivity to FGFR1 inhibition.[219,220]

While primary resistance is arguably the greatest obstacle to clinical efficacy for FGFR1 inhibitors, secondary resistance does emerge, both via alterations in the FGFR kinase and activation of bypass or downstream signaling. Activation of MET and MAPK signaling have been shown to be sufficient to circumvent FGFR dependency in several cancer cell lines.[221,222] In the preclinical setting, the combination of crizotinib and BGJ398 proved effective in suppressing growth of an *FGFR1*-amplified cell line that developed resistance to FGFR inhibition via MET upregulation.[223] Within the FGFR1 kinase, V561M, a gatekeeper residue mutation, confers resistance to lucitanib and BGJ398 while retaining sensitivity to AZD4547.[210,223–226] **FIIN2** and **FIIN3** are covalent FGFR1-4 inhibitors selected for development based on their potency against the *FGFR* gatekeeper mutation.[226] Further development and clinical testing of highly potent covalent selective FGFR inhibitors (e.g., **TAS120** and **PRN1371**) are currently underway.[227,228]

References

1. Lynch TJ, Bell DW, Sordella R, et al. Activating mutations in the epidermal growth factor receptor underlying responsiveness of non-small-cell lung cancer to gefitinib. *N Engl J Med.* 2004;350(21):2129-2139.
2. Swanton C, Govindan R. Clinical implications of genomic discoveries in lung cancer. *N Engl J Med.* 2016;374(19):1864-1873.
3. Pao W, Miller V, Zakowski M, et al. EGF receptor gene mutations are common in lung cancers from "never smokers" and are associated with sensitivity of tumors to gefitinib and erlotinib. *Proc Natl Acad Sci U S A.* 2004;101(36):13306-13311.
4. Maemondo M, Inoue A, Kobayashi K, et al. Gefitinib or chemotherapy for non-small-cell lung cancer with mutated EGFR. *N Engl J Med.* 2010;362(25):2380-2388.
5. Piotrowska Z, Sequist LV. Treatment of EGFR-mutant lung cancers after progression in patients receiving first-line egfr tyrosine kinase inhibitors: a review. *JAMA Oncol.* 2016;2(7):948-954.
6. Lovly CM, Iyengar P, Gainor JF. Managing resistance to EGFR- and ALK-targeted therapies. *Am Soc Clin Oncol Educ Book.* 2017;37:607-618.
7. Kris MG, Johnson BE, Berry LD, et al. Using multiplexed assays of oncogenic drivers in lung cancers to select targeted drugs. *JAMA.* 2014;311(19):1998-2006.
8. Mitsudomi T, Morita S, Yatabe Y, et al. Gefitinib versus cisplatin plus docetaxel in patients with non-small-cell lung cancer harbouring mutations of the epidermal growth factor receptor (WJTOG3405): an open label, randomised phase 3 trial. *Lancet Oncol.* 2010;11(2):121-128.
9. Sequist LV, Yang JC, Yamamoto N, et al. Phase III study of afatinib or cisplatin plus pemetrexed in patients with metastatic lung adenocarcinoma with EGFR mutations. *J Clin Oncol.* 2013;31(27):3327-3334.
10. Rosell R, Carcereny E, Gervais R, et al. Erlotinib versus standard chemotherapy as first-line treatment for European patients with advanced EGFR mutation-positive non-small-cell lung cancer (EURTAC): a multicentre, open-label, randomised phase 3 trial. *Lancet Oncol.* 2012;13(3):239-246.
11. Zhou C, Wu YL, Chen G, et al. Erlotinib versus chemotherapy as first-line treatment for patients with advanced EGFR mutation-positive non-small-cell lung cancer (OPTIMAL, CTONG-0802): a multicentre, open-label, randomised, phase 3 study. *Lancet Oncol.* 2011;12(8):735-742.
12. Rosell R, Dafni U, Felip E, et al. Erlotinib and bevacizumab in patients with advanced non-small-cell lung cancer and activating EGFR mutations (BELIEF): an international, multicentre, single-arm, phase 2 trial. *Lancet Respir Med.* 2017;5(5):435-444.
13. Seto T, Kato T, Nishio M, et al. Erlotinib alone or with bevacizumab as first-line therapy in patients with advanced non-squamous non-small-cell lung cancer harbouring EGFR mutations (JO25567): an open-label, randomised, multicentre, phase 2 study. *Lancet Oncol.* 2014;15(11):1236-1244.
14. Johnson JR, Cohen M, Sridhara R, et al. Approval summary for erlotinib for treatment of patients with locally advanced or metastatic non-small cell lung cancer after failure of at least one prior chemotherapy regimen. *Clin Cancer Res.* 2005;11(18):6414-6421.
15. Togashi Y, Masago K, Masuda S, et al. Cerebrospinal fluid concentration of gefitinib and erlotinib in patients with non-small cell lung cancer. *Cancer Chemother Pharmacol.* 2012;70(3):399-405.
16. Broniscer A, Panetta JC, O'Shaughnessy M, et al. Plasma and cerebrospinal fluid pharmacokinetics of erlotinib and its active metabolite OSI-420. *Clin Cancer Res.* 2007;13(5):1511-1515.
17. Macdonald JB, Macdonald B, Golitz LE, LoRusso P, Sekulic A. Cutaneous adverse effects of targeted therapies: Part I: inhibitors of the cellular membrane. *J Am Acad Dermatol.* 2015;72(2):203-218; quiz 219-220.
18. Takeda M, Okamoto I, Nakagawa K. Pooled safety analysis of EGFR-TKI treatment for EGFR mutation-positive non-small cell lung cancer. *Lung Cancer.* 2015;88(1):74-79.
19. Gass-Jégu F, Gschwend A, Gairard-Dory AC, et al. Gastrointestinal perforations in patients treated with erlotinib: a report of two cases with fatal outcome and literature review. *Lung Cancer.* 2016;99:76-78.
20. Wakeling AE, Guy SP, Woodburn JR, et al. ZD1839 (Iressa): an orally active inhibitor of epidermal growth factor signaling with potential for cancer therapy. *Cancer Res.* 2002;62(20):5749-5754.
21. Yang J, Zhou Q, Yan HH, et al. A randomized controlled trial of erlotinib versus gefitinib in advanced non-small-cell lung cancer harboring EGFR mutations (CTONG0901) [Abstr 16.13]. *16th World Conference on Lung Cancer; Denver, CO, USA; Sept 6–9, 2015.*
22. Lim SH, Lee JY, Sun JM, Ahn JS, Park K, Ahn MJ. Comparison of clinical outcomes following gefitinib and erlotinib treatment in non-small-cell lung cancer patients harboring an epidermal growth factor receptor mutation in either exon 19 or 21. *J Thorac Oncol.* 2014;9(4):506-511.
23. Cohen MH, Williams GA, Sridhara R, et al. United States Food and Drug Administration drug approval summary: gefitinib (ZD1839; Iressa) tablets. *Clin Cancer Res.* 2004;10(4):1212-1218.
24. Ding PN, Lord SJ, Gebski V, et al. Risk of treatment-related toxicities from EGFR tyrosine kinase inhibitors: a meta-analysis of clinical trials of gefitinib, erlotinib, and afatinib in advanced EGFR-mutated non-small cell lung cancer. *J Thorac Oncol.* 2017;12(4):633-643.
25. Hong D, Zhang G, Zhang X, Lian X. Pulmonary toxicities of gefitinib in patients with advanced non-small-cell lung cancer: a meta-analysis of randomized controlled trials. *Medicine (Baltimore).* 2016;95(9):e3008.
26. Wu YL, Zhou C, Hu CP, et al. Afatinib versus cisplatin plus gemcitabine for first-line treatment of Asian patients with advanced non-small-cell lung cancer harbouring EGFR mutations (LUX-Lung 6): an open-label, randomised phase 3 trial. *Lancet Oncol.* 2014;15(2):213-222.
27. Yang JC, Wu YL, Schuler M, et al. Afatinib versus cisplatin-based chemotherapy for EGFR mutation-positive lung adenocarcinoma (LUX-Lung 3 and LUX-Lung 6): analysis of overall survival data from two randomised, phase 3 trials. *Lancet Oncol.* 2015;16(2):141-151.
28. Paz-Ares L, Tan EH, O'Byrne K, et al. Afatinib versus gefitinib in patients with EGFR mutation-positive advanced non-small-cell lung cancer: overall survival data from the phase IIb LUX-Lung 7 trial. *Ann Oncol.* 2017;28(2):270-277.
29. Sequist LV, Waltman BA, Dias-Santagata D, et al. Genotypic and histological evolution of lung cancers acquiring resistance to EGFR inhibitors. *Sci Transl Med.* 2011;3(75):75ra26.

30. Yu HA, Arcila ME, Rekhtman N, et al. Analysis of tumor specimens at the time of acquired resistance to EGFR-TKI therapy in 155 patients with EGFR-mutant lung cancers. *Clin Cancer Res.* 2013;19(8):2240-2247.

31. Campo M, Gerber D, Gainor JF, et al. Acquired resistance to first-line afatinib and the challenges of prearranged progression biopsies. *J Thorac Oncol.* 2016;11(11):2022-2026.

32. Jenkins S, Yang JC, Ramalingam SS, et al. Plasma ctDNA analysis for detection of the EGFR T790M mutation in patients with advanced non-small cell lung cancer. *J Thorac Oncol.* 2017;12(7):1061-1070.

33. Sacher AG, Paweletz C, Dahlberg SE, et al. Prospective validation of rapid plasma genotyping for the detection of EGFR and KRAS mutations in advanced lung cancer. *JAMA Oncol.* 2016;2(8):1014-1022.

34. Yun CH, Mengwasser KE, Toms AV, et al. The T790M mutation in EGFR kinase causes drug resistance by increasing the affinity for ATP. *Proc Natl Acad Sci U S A.* 2008;105(6):2070-2075.

35. Hata AN, Niederst MJ, Archibald HL, et al. Tumor cells can follow distinct evolutionary paths to become resistant to epidermal growth factor receptor inhibition. *Nat Med.* 2016;22(3):262-269.

36. Li D, Ambrogio L, Shimamura T, et al. BIBW2992, an irreversible EGFR/HER2 inhibitor highly effective in preclinical lung cancer models. *Oncogene.* 2008;27(34):4702-4711.

37. Takezawa K, Pirazzoli V, Arcila ME, et al. HER2 amplification: a potential mechanism of acquired resistance to EGFR inhibition in EGFR-mutant lung cancers that lack the second-site EGFRT790M mutation. *Cancer Discov.* 2012;2(10):922-933.

38. Jänne PA, Yang JC, Kim DW, et al. AZD9291 in EGFR inhibitor-resistant non-small-cell lung cancer. *N Engl J Med.* 2015;372(18):1689-1699.

39. Mok TS, Wu YL, Ahn MJ, et al. Osimertinib or platinum-pemetrexed in EGFR T790M-positive lung cancer. *N Engl J Med.* 2017;376(7):629-640.

40. Mok T, Ahn MJ, Han JY et al. CNS response to osimertinib in patients (pts) with T790M-positive advanced NSCLC: data from a randomized phase III trial (AURA3). *J Clin Oncol.* 2017;35(suppl 15):9005-9005.

41. Ramalingam S, Reungwetwattana T, Chewaskulyong B, et al. Osimertinib vs standard of care (SoC) EGFR-TKI as first-line therapy in patients (pts) with EGFRm advanced NSCLC: FLAURA. *Presented at: 2017 ESMO Congress; Madrid, Spain; September 9-12, 2017. Abstract LBA2_PR.*

42. Planchard D, Brown KH, Kim DW, et al. Osimertinib Western and Asian clinical pharmacokinetics in patients and healthy volunteers: implications for formulation, dose, and dosing frequency in pivotal clinical studies. *Cancer Chemother Pharmacol.* 2016;77(4):767-776.

43. Ballard P, Yates JW, Yang Z, et al. Preclinical comparison of osimertinib with other EGFR-TKIs in EGFR-mutant NSCLC brain metastases models, and early evidence of clinical brain metastases activity. *Clin Cancer Res.* 2016;22(20):5130-5140.

44. Brown K, Comisar C, Witjes H, et al. Population pharmacokinetics and exposure-response of osimertinib in patients with non-small cell lung cancer. *Br J Clin Pharmacol.* 2017;83(6):1216-1226.

45. Park K, Lee J-S, Lee KH, et al. BI 1482694 (HM61713), an EGFR mutant-specific inhibitor, in T790M+ NSCLC: efficacy and safety at the RP2D *J Clin Oncol.* 2016;34(suppl; abstr 9055).

46. Jia Y, Juarez J, Li J, et al. EGF816 exerts anticancer effects in non-small cell lung cancer by irreversibly and selectively targeting primary and acquired activating mutations in the EGF receptor. *Cancer Res.* 2016;76(6):1591-1602.

47. Tan DS, Yang JC, Leighl NB, et al. Updated results of a phase I study of EGF816, a third-generation, mutant-selective EGFR tyrosine kinase inhibitor, in advanced non-small cell lung cancer harboring T790M. *J Clin Oncol.* 2016;34(suppl; abstr 9044).

48. Yu HA, Tian SK, Drilon AE, et al. Acquired resistance of EGFR-mutant lung cancer to a T790M-specific egfr inhibitor: emergence of a third mutation (C797S) in the EGFR tyrosine kinase domain. *JAMA Oncol.* 2015;1(7):982-984.

49. Thress KS, Paweletz CP, Felip E, et al. Acquired EGFR C797S mutation mediates resistance to AZD9291 in non-small cell lung cancer harboring EGFR T790M. *Nat Med.* 2015;21(6):560-562.

50. Bersanelli M, Minari R, Bordi P, et al. L718Q mutation as new mechanism of acquired resistance to AZD9291 in EGFR-mutated NSCLC. *J Thorac Oncol.* 2016;11(10):e121-123.

51. Piotrowska Z, Stirling K, Heist R, et al. Heterogeneity and variation in resistance mechanisms among 223 epidermal growth factor receptor-mutant

52. Planchard D, Loriot Y, André F, et al. EGFR-independent mechanisms of acquired resistance to AZD9291 in EGFR T790M-positive NSCLC patients. *Ann Oncol.* 2015;26(10):2073-2078.

53. Piotrowska Z, Thress K, Mooradian MJ, et al. MET amplification (amp) is a major resistance mechanism to osimertinib. *J Clin Oncol.* 2017;35(15, suppl; abstr 9020).

54. Eberlein CA, Stetson D, Markovets AA, et al. Acquired resistance to the mutant-selective EGFR inhibitor AZD9291 is associated with increased dependence on RAS signaling in preclinical models. *Cancer Res.* 2015;75(12):2489-2500.

55. Ortiz-Cuaran S, Scheffler M, Plenker D, et al. Heterogeneous mechanisms of primary and acquired resistance to third-generation EGFR inhibitors. *Clin Cancer Res.* 2016;22(19):4837-4847.

56. Li L, Wang H, Li C, Wang Z, Zhang P, Yan X. Transformation to small-cell carcinoma as an acquired resistance mechanism to AZD9291: a case report. *Oncotarget.* 2017;8(11):18609-18614.

57. Marcoux N, Piotrowska Z, Farago AF, et al. Clinical outcomes for EGFR-mutant adenocarcinomas that transform to small cell lung cancer. *Ann Oncol.* 2017;28(suppl 5).

58. Tricker EM, Xu C, Uddin S, et al. Combined EGFR/MEK inhibition prevents the emergence of resistance in EGFR-mutant lung cancer. *Cancer Discov.* 2015;5(9):960-971.

59. Arulananda S, Do H, Musafer A, Mitchell P, Dobrovic A, John T. Combination osimertinib and gefitinib in C797S and T790M EGFR mutated non-small-cell lung cancer. *J Thorac Oncol.* 2017;12(11):1728-1732.

60. Niederst MJ, Hu H, Mulvey HE, et al. The allelic context of the C797S mutation acquired upon treatment with third-generation EGFR inhibitors impacts sensitivity to subsequent treatment strategies. *Clin Cancer Res.* 2015;21(17):3924-3933.

61. Chic N, Mayo-de-Las-Casas C, Reguart N. Successful treatment with gefitinib in advanced non-small cell lung cancer after acquired resistance to osimertinib. *J Thorac Oncol.* 2017;12(6):e78-e80.

62. Jia Y, Yun CH, Park E, et al. Overcoming EGFR(T790M) and EGFR(C797S) resistance with mutant-selective allosteric inhibitors. *Nature.* 2016;534(7605):129-132.

63. Soda M, Choi YL, Enomoto M, et al. Identification of the transforming EML4-ALK fusion gene in non-small-cell lung cancer. *Nature.* 2007;448(7153):561-566.

64. Rikova K, Guo A, Zeng Q, et al. Global survey of phosphotyrosine signaling identifies oncogenic kinases in lung cancer. *Cell.* 2007;131(6):1190-1203.

65. Takeuchi K, Choi YL, Togashi Y, et al. KIF5B-ALK, a novel fusion oncokinase identified by an immunohistochemistry-based diagnostic system for ALK-positive lung cancer. *Clin Cancer Res.* 2009;15(9):3143-3149.

66. Togashi Y, Soda M, Sakata S, et al. KLC1-ALK: a novel fusion in lung cancer identified using a formalin-fixed paraffin-embedded tissue only. *PLoS One.* 2012;7(2):e31323.

67. Shaw AT, Yeap BY, Mino-Kenudson M, et al. Clinical features and outcome of patients with non-small-cell lung cancer who harbor EML4-ALK. *J Clin Oncol.* 2009;27(26):4247-4253.

68. Shaw AT, Engelman JA. ALK in lung cancer: past, present, and future. *J Clin Oncol.* 2013;31(8):1105-1111

69. Shaw AT, Kim DW, Nakagawa K, et al. Crizotinib versus chemotherapy in advanced ALK-positive lung cancer. *N Engl J Med.* 2013;368(25):2385-2394.

70. Solomon BJ, Mok T, Kim DW, et al. First-line crizotinib versus chemotherapy in ALK-positive lung cancer. *N Engl J Med.* 2014;371(23):2167-2177.

71. Costa DB, Kobayashi S, Pandya SS, et al. CSF concentration of the anaplastic lymphoma kinase inhibitor crizotinib. *J Clin Oncol.* 2011;29(15):e443-445.

72. Peters S, Camidge DR, Shaw AT, et al. Alectinib versus crizotinib in untreated ALK-positive non-small-cell lung cancer. *N Engl J Med.* 2017;377(9):829-838.

73. Wang E, Nickens DJ, Bello A, et al. Clinical implications of the pharmacokinetics of crizotinib in populations of patients with non-small cell lung cancer. *Clin Cancer Res.* 2016;22(23):5722-5728.

74. Metro G, Lunardi G, Floridi P, et al. CSF concentration of crizotinib in two ALK-positive non-small-cell lung cancer patients with CNS metastases deriving clinical benefit from treatment. *J Thorac Oncol.* 2015;10(5):e26-27.

non-small cell lung cancer patients with >1 post-resistance biopsy. *Int J Radiat Oncol Biol Phys.* 2017;98(1):220.

75. Katayama R, Sakashita T, Yanagitani N, et al. P-glycoprotein mediates ceritinib resistance in anaplastic lymphoma kinase-rearranged non-small cell lung cancer. *EBioMedicine*. 2016;3:54-66.

76. Dagogo-Jack I, Shaw AT, Riely GJ. Optimizing treatment for patients with anaplastic lymphoma kinase-positive lung cancer. *Clin Pharmacol Ther*. 2017;101(5):625-633.

77. Gainor JF, Dardaei L, Yoda S, et al. Molecular mechanisms of resistance to first-and second-generation ALK inhibitors in ALK-rearranged lung cancer. *Cancer Discov*. 2016;6(10):1118-1133.

78. Choi YL, Soda M, Yamashita Y, et al. EML4-ALK mutations in lung cancer that confer resistance to ALK inhibitors. *N Engl J Med*. 2010;363(18):1734-1739.

79. Katayama R, Shaw AT, Khan TM, et al. Mechanisms of acquired crizotinib resistance in ALK-rearranged lung cancers. *Sci Transl Med*. 2012;4(120):120ra117.

80. Matikas A, Kentepozidis N, Georgoulias V, Kotsakis A. Management of resistance to crizotinib in anaplastic lymphoma kinase-positive non-small-cell lung cancer. *Clin Lung Cancer*. 2016;17(6):474-482.

81. Dagogo-Jack I, Shaw AT. Crizotinib resistance: implications for therapeutic strategies. *Ann Oncol*. 2016;27(suppl 3):iii42-iii50.

82. Sasaki T, Koivunen J, Ogino A, et al. A novel ALK secondary mutation and EGFR signaling cause resistance to ALK kinase inhibitors. *Cancer Res*. 2011;71(18):6051-6060.

83. Doebele RC, Pilling AB, Aisner DL, et al. Mechanisms of resistance to crizotinib in patients with ALK gene rearranged non-small cell lung cancer. *Clin Cancer Res*. 2012;18(5):1472-1482.

84. Cha YJ, Cho BC, Kim HR, Lee HJ, Shim HS. A case of ALK-rearranged adenocarcinoma with small cell carcinoma-like transformation and resistance to crizotinib. *J Thorac Oncol*. 2016;11(5):e55-e58.

85. Miyamoto S, Ikushima S, Ono R, et al. Transformation to small-cell lung cancer as a mechanism of acquired resistance to crizotinib and alectinib. *Jpn J Clin Oncol*. 2016;46(2):170-173.

86. Metro G, Tazza M, Matocci R, Chiari R, Crin ÚL. Optimal management of ALK-positive NSCLC progressing on crizotinib. *Lung Cancer*. 2017;106:58-66.

87. Katayama R, Friboulet L, Koike S, et al. Two novel ALK mutations mediate acquired resistance to the next-generation ALK inhibitor alectinib. *Clin Cancer Res*. 2014;20(22):5686-5696.

88. Shaw AT, Kim DW, Mehra R, et al. Ceritinib in ALK-rearranged non-small-cell lung cancer. *N Engl J Med*. 2014;370(13):1189-1197.

89. Shaw AT, Kim TM, Crinò L, et al. Ceritinib versus chemotherapy in patients with ALK-rearranged non-small-cell lung cancer previously given chemotherapy and crizotinib (ASCEND-5): a randomised, controlled, open-label, phase 3 trial. *Lancet Oncol*. 2017;18(7):874–886.

90. Soria JC, Tan DS, Chiari R, et al. First-line ceritinib versus platinum-based chemotherapy in advanced ALK-rearranged non-small-cell lung cancer (ASCEND-4): a randomised, open-label, phase 3 study. *Lancet*. 2017;389(10072):917-929.

91. Mok TSK, Crino L, Felip E, et al. The accelerated path of ceritinib: translating pre-clinical development into clinical efficacy. *Cancer Treat Rev*. 2017;55:181-189.

92. Lim SM, Kim HR, Lee JS, et al. Open-label, multicenter, phase II study of ceritinib in patients with non-small-cell lung cancer harboring ROS1 rearrangement. *J Clin Oncol*. 2017;35(23):2613-2618.

93. Crinò L, Ahn MJ, De Marinis F, et al. Multicenter phase II study of whole-body and intracranial activity with ceritinib in patients with ALK-rearranged non-small-cell lung cancer previously treated with chemotherapy and crizotinib: results from ASCEND-2. *J Clin Oncol*. 2016;34(24):2866-2873.

94. Cho BC, Kim DW, Bearz A, et al. ASCEND-8: a randomized phase 1 study of ceritinib 450 mg or 600 mg taken with a low-fat meal versus 750 mg in fasted state in patients with anaplastic lymphoma kinase (ALK)-rearranged metastatic non-small cell lung cancer (NSCLC). *J Thorac Oncol*. 2017;12(9):1357-1367.

95. Katayama R, Lovly CM, Shaw AT. Therapeutic targeting of anaplastic lymphoma kinase in lung cancer: a paradigm for precision cancer medicine. *Clin Cancer Res*. 2015;21(10):2227-2235.

96. Shaw AT, Gandhi L, Gadgeel S, et al. Alectinib in ALK-positive, crizotinib-resistant, non-small-cell lung cancer: a single-group, multicentre, phase 2 trial. *Lancet Oncol*. 2016;17(2):234-242.

97. Ou SH, Ahn JS, De Petris L, et al. Alectinib in crizotinib-refractory ALK-rearranged non-small-cell lung cancer: a phase II global study. *J Clin Oncol*. 2016;34(7):661-668.

98. Hida T, Nokihara H, Kondo M, et al. Alectinib versus crizotinib in patients with ALK-positive non-small-cell lung cancer (J-ALEX): an open-label, randomised phase 3 trial. *Lancet*. 2017;390(10089):29-39.

99. Morcos PN, Cleary Y, Guerini E, et al. Clinical drug-drug interactions through cytochrome P450 3A (CYP3A) for the selective ALK inhibitor alectinib. *Clin Pharmacol Drug Dev*. 2017;6(3):280-291.

100. Kodama T, Hasegawa M, Takanashi K, Sakurai Y, Kondoh O, Sakamoto H. Antitumor activity of the selective ALK inhibitor alectinib in models of intracranial metastases. *Cancer Chemother Pharmacol*. 2014;74(5):1023-1028.

101. Zhang S, Anjum R, Squillace R, et al. The potent ALK inhibitor brigatinib (AP26113) overcomes mechanisms of resistance to first-and second-generation ALK inhibitors in preclinical models. *Clin Cancer Res*. 2016;22(22):5527-5538.

102. Kim DW, Tiseo M, Ahn MJ, et al. Brigatinib in patients with crizotinib-refractory anaplastic lymphoma kinase-positive non-small-cell lung cancer: a randomized, multicenter phase II trial. *J Clin Oncol*. 2017;35(22):2490-2498.

103. Shaw AT, Bauer TM, Felip E, et al. Clinical activity and safety of PF-06463922 from a dose escalation study in patients with advanced ALK+ or ROS1+ NSCLC. *J Clin Oncol*. 2015;33(suppl; abstr 8018).

104. Gettinger SN, Bazhenova LA, Langer CJ, et al. Activity and safety of brigatinib in ALK-rearranged non-small-cell lung cancer and other malignancies: a single-arm, open-label, phase 1/2 trial. *Lancet Oncol*. 2016;17(12):1683-1696.

105. Passaro A, Lazzari C, Karachaliou N, et al. Personalized treatment in advanced ALK-positive non-small cell lung cancer: from bench to clinical practice. *Onco Targets Ther*. 2016;9:6361-6376.

106. Ou SH, Greenbowe J, Khan ZU, et al. I1171 missense mutation (particularly I1171N) is a common resistance mutation in ALK-positive NSCLC patients who have progressive disease while on alectinib and is sensitive to ceritinib. *Lung Cancer*. 2015;88(2):231-234.

107. Ou SH, Milliken JC, Azada MC, Miller VA, Ali SM, Klempner SJ. ALK F1174V mutation confers sensitivity while ALK I1171 mutation confers resistance to alectinib. The importance of serial biopsy post progression. *Lung Cancer*. 2016;91:70-72.

108. Friboulet L, Li N, Katayama R, et al. The ALK inhibitor ceritinib overcomes crizotinib resistance in non-small cell lung cancer. *Cancer Discov*. 2014;4(6):662-673.

109. Gouji T, Takashi S, Mitsuhiro T, Yukito I. Crizotinib can overcome acquired resistance to CH5424802: is amplification of the MET gene a key factor? *J Thorac Oncol*. 2014;9(3):e27-e28.

110. Fujita S, Masago K, Katakami N, Yatabe Y. Transformation to SCLC after treatment with the ALK inhibitor alectinib. *J Thorac Oncol*. 2016;11(6):e67-e72.

111. Lin JJ, Shaw AT. Resisting resistance: targeted therapies in lung cancer. *Trends Cancer*. 2016;2(7):350-364.

112. Hrustanovic G, Olivas V, Pazarentzos E, et al. RAS-MAPK dependence underlies a rational polytherapy strategy in EML4-ALK-positive lung cancer. *Nat Med*. 2015;21(9):1038-1047.

113. Lin JJ, Riely GJ, Shaw AT. Targeting ALK: precision medicine takes on drug resistance. *Cancer Discov*. 2017;7(2):137-155.

114. Awad MM, Shaw AT. ALK inhibitors in non-small cell lung cancer: crizotinib and beyond. *Clin Adv Hematol Oncol*. 2014;12(7):429-439.

115. Solomon BJ, Bauer TM, Felip E, et al. Safety and efficacy of lorlatinib (PF-06463922) from the dose escalation component of a study in patients with advanced ALK+ or ROS1+ non-small cell lung cancer (NSCLC). *J Clin Oncol*. 2016;34(suppl; abstr 9009).

116. Shaw AT, Friboulet L, Leshchiner I, et al. Resensitization to crizotinib by the lorlatinib ALK resistance mutation L1198F. *N Engl J Med*. 2016;374(1):54-61.

117. Horn L, Wakelee H, Reckamp KL, et al. MINI01.02: response and plasma genotyping from phase I/II trial of ensartinib (X-396) in patients (pts) with ALK+ NSCLC: topic: medical oncology. *J Thorac Oncol*. 2016;11(11S):S256-S257.

118. Gainor JF, Shaw AT. Novel targets in non-small cell lung cancer: ROS1 and RET fusions. *Oncologist*. 2013;18(7):865-875.

119. Hirsch FR, Suda K, Wiens J, Bunn PA. New and emerging targeted treatments in advanced non-small-cell lung cancer. *Lancet.* 2016;388(10048):1012-1024.

120. Zhu VW, Upadhyay D, Schrock AB, Gowen K, Ali SM, Ou SH. TPD52L1-ROS1, a new ROS1 fusion variant in lung adenosquamous cell carcinoma identified by comprehensive genomic profiling. *Lung Cancer.* 2016;97:48-50.

121. Dagogo-Jack I, Shaw AT. Expanding the roster of ROS1 inhibitors. *J Clin Oncol.* 2017;35(23):2595-2597.

122. Shaw AT, Ou SH, Bang YJ, et al. Crizotinib in ROS1-rearranged non-small-cell lung cancer. *N Engl J Med.* 2014;371(21):1963-1971.

123. Mazières J, Zalcman G, Crinù L, et al. Crizotinib therapy for advanced lung adenocarcinoma and a ROS1 rearrangement: results from the EUROS1 cohort. *J Clin Oncol.* 2015;33(9):992-999.

124. Moro-Sibilot D, Faivre L, Zalcman G et al. Crizotinib in patients with advanced ROS1-rearranged non-small cell lung cancer (NSCLC) Preliminary results of the ASCé phase II trial. *J Clin Oncol.* 2015;33(suppl; abstr 8065).

125. Goto K, Yang JCH, Kim DW et al. Phase II study of crizotinib in East Asian patients with ROS1-positive advanced non-small cell lung cancer. *J Clin Oncol.* 2016;34(suppl; abstr 9022).

126. Awad MM, Engelman JA, Shaw AT. Acquired resistance to crizotinib from a mutation in CD74-ROS1. *N Engl J Med.* 2013;369(12):1173.

127. Lin JJ, Shaw AT. Recent advances in targeting ROS1 in lung cancer. *J Thorac Oncol.* 2017;12(11):1611-1625.

128. Davies KD, Mahale S, Astling DP, et al. Resistance to ROS1 inhibition mediated by EGFR pathway activation in non-small cell lung cancer. *PLoS One.* 2013;8(12):e82236.

129. Dziadziuszko R, Le AT, Wrona A, et al. An activating KIT mutation induces crizotinib resistance in ROS1-positive lung cancer. *J Thorac Oncol.* 2016;11(8):1273-1281.

130. Cargnelutti M, Corso S, Pergolizzi M, et al. Activation of RAS family members confers resistance to ROS1 targeting drugs. *Oncotarget.* 2015;6(7):5182-5194.

131. Katayama R, Kobayashi Y, Friboulet L, et al. Cabozantinib overcomes crizotinib resistance in ROS1 fusion-positive cancer. *Clin Cancer Res.* 2015;21(1):166-174.

132. Facchinetti F, Loriot Y, Kuo MS, et al. Crizotinib-resistant ROS1 mutations reveal a predictive kinase inhibitor sensitivity model for ROS1-and ALK-rearranged lung cancers. *Clin Cancer Res.* 2016;22(24):5983-5991.

133. Drilon A, Somwar R, Wagner JP, et al. A novel crizotinib-resistant solvent-front mutation responsive to cabozantinib therapy in a patient with ROS1-rearranged lung cancer. *Clin Cancer Res.* 2016;22(10):2351-2358.

134. Drilon A, Siena S, Ou SI, et al. Safety and antitumor activity of the multi-targeted Pan-TRK, ROS1, and ALK inhibitor entrectinib: combined results from two phase I trials (ALKA-372-001 and STARTRK-1). *Cancer Discov.* 2017;7(4):400-409.

135. Ardini E, Menichincheri M, Banfi P, et al. Entrectinib, a Pan-TRK, ROS1, and ALK inhibitor with activity in multiple molecularly defined cancer indications. *Mol Cancer Ther.* 2016;15(4):628-639.

136. Chong CR, Bahcall M, Capelletti M, et al. Identification of existing drugs that effectively target NTRK1 and ROS1 rearrangements in lung cancer. *Clin Cancer Res.* 2017;23(1):204-213.

137. Zou HY, Li Q, Engstrom LD, et al. PF-06463922 is a potent and selective next-generation ROS1/ALK inhibitor capable of blocking crizotinib-resistant ROS1 mutations. *Proc Natl Acad Sci U S A.* 2015;112(11):3493-3498.

138. Nosaki K, Fujiwara Y, Takeda M, et al. Phase I study of DS-6051b, a ROS1/NTRK inhibitor, in Japanese subjects with advanced solid tumors harboring either a ROS1 or NTRK fusion gene. *J Thorac Oncol.* 2017;12(1):S1069.

139. Drilon A, Rekhtman N, Arcila M, et al. Cabozantinib in patients with advanced RET-rearranged non-small-cell lung cancer: an open-label, single-centre, phase 2, single-arm trial. *Lancet Oncol.* 2016;17(12):1653-1660.

140. Paik PK, Shen R, Berger MF, et al. A phase 1b open label multicentre study of AZD4547 in patients with advanced squamous cell lung cancers. *Clin Cancer Res.* 2017.

141. Baik CS, Myall NJ, Wakelee HA. Targeting BRAF-mutant non-small cell lung cancer: from molecular profiling to rationally designed therapy. *Oncologist.* 2017;22(7):786-796.

142. Marchetti A, Felicioni L, Malatesta S, et al. Clinical features and outcome of patients with non-small-cell lung cancer harboring BRAF mutations. *J Clin Oncol.* 2011;29(26):3574-3579.

143. Cardarella S, Ogino A, Nishino M, et al. Clinical, pathologic, and biologic features associated with BRAF mutations in non-small cell lung cancer. *Clin Cancer Res.* 2013;19(16):4532-4540.

144. Hyman DM, Puzanov I, Subbiah V, et al. Vemurafenib in multiple nonmelanoma cancers with BRAF V600 mutations. *N Engl J Med.* 2015;373(8):726-736.

145. Planchard D, Kim TM, Mazieres J, et al. Dabrafenib in patients with BRAF(V600E)-positive advanced non-small-cell lung cancer: a single-arm, multicentre, open-label, phase 2 trial. *Lancet Oncol.* 2016;17(5):642-650.

146. Prahallad A, Sun C, Huang S, et al. Unresponsiveness of colon cancer to BRAF(V600E) inhibition through feedback activation of EGFR. *Nature.* 2012;483(7387):100-103.

147. Corcoran RB, Ebi H, Turke AB, et al. EGFR-mediated re-activation of MAPK signaling contributes to insensitivity of BRAF mutant colorectal cancers to RAF inhibition with vemurafenib. *Cancer Discov.* 2012;2(3):227-235.

148. Long GV, Flaherty KT, Stroyakovskiy D, et al. Dabrafenib plus trametinib versus dabrafenib monotherapy in patients with metastatic BRAF V600E/K-mutant melanoma: long-term survival and safety analysis of a phase 3 study. *Ann Oncol.* 2017;28(7):1631-1639.

149. Planchard D, Besse B, Groen HJ, et al. Dabrafenib plus trametinib in patients with previously treated BRAF(V600E)-mutant metastatic non-small cell lung cancer: an open-label, multicentre phase 2 trial. *Lancet Oncol.* 2016;17(7):984-993.

150. Zhang W, Heinzmann D, Grippo JF. Clinical pharmacokinetics of vemurafenib. *Clin Pharmacokinet.* 2017;56(9):1033-1043.

151. Ellens H, Johnson M, Lawrence SK, Watson C, Chen L, Richards-Peterson LE. Prediction of the transporter-mediated drug-drug interaction potential of dabrafenib and its major circulating metabolites. *Drug Metab Dispos.* 2017;45(6):646-656.

152. Falchook GS, Long GV, Kurzrock R, et al. Dose selection, pharmacokinetics, and pharmacodynamics of BRAF inhibitor dabrafenib (GSK2118436). *Clin Cancer Res.* 2014;20(17):4449-4458.

153. Suttle AB, Grossmann KF, Ouellet D, et al. Assessment of the drug interaction potential and single-and repeat-dose pharmacokinetics of the BRAF inhibitor dabrafenib. *J Clin Pharmacol.* 2015;55(4):392-400.

154. *United States Food and Drug Administration Highlights of Prescribing Information: Trametinib (Mekinist) tablets.* 2013.

155. Rivalland G, Mitchell P. Combined BRAF and MEK inhibition in BRAF-mutant NSCLC. *Lancet Oncol.* 2016;17(7):860-862.

156. Caparica R, de Castro G, Gil-Bazo I, et al. BRAF mutations in non-small cell lung cancer: has finally Janus opened the door? *Crit Rev Oncol Hematol.* 2016;101:32-39.

157. Rudin CM, Hong K, Streit M. Molecular characterization of acquired resistance to the BRAF inhibitor dabrafenib in a patient with BRAF-mutant non-small-cell lung cancer. *J Thorac Oncol.* 2013;8(5):e41-42.

158. Salgia R. MET in lung cancer: biomarker selection based on scientific rationale. *Mol Cancer Ther.* 2017;16(4):555-565.

159. Spigel DR, Edelman MJ, O'Byrne K, et al. Results from the phase III randomized trial of onartuzumab plus erlotinib versus erlotinib in previously treated stage IIIB or IV non-small-cell lung cancer: METLung. *J Clin Oncol.* 2017;35(4):412-420.

160. Scagliotti G, von Pawel J, Novello S, et al. Phase III multinational, randomized, double-blind, placebo-controlled study of tivantinib (ARQ 197) plus erlotinib versus erlotinib alone in previously treated patients with locally advanced or metastatic nonsquamous non-small-cell lung cancer. *J Clin Oncol.* 2015;33(24):2667-2674.

161. Awad MM, Oxnard GR, Jackman DM, et al. MET exon 14 mutations in non-small-cell lung cancer are associated with advanced age and stage-dependent MET genomic amplification and c-Met overexpression. *J Clin Oncol.* 2016;34(7):721-730.

162. Frampton GM, Ali SM, Rosenzweig M, et al. Activation of MET via diverse exon 14 splicing alterations occurs in multiple tumor types and confers clinical sensitivity to MET inhibitors. *Cancer Discov.* 2015;5(8):850-859.

163. Tong JH, Yeung SF, Chan AW, et al. MET amplification and exon 14 splice site mutation define unique molecular subgroups of non-small cell lung carcinoma with poor prognosis. *Clin Cancer Res.* 2016;22(12):3048-3056.

164. Drilon A, Cappuzzo F, Ou SI, Camidge DR. Targeting MET in lung cancer: will expectations finally be MET? *J Thorac Oncol.* 2017;12(1):15-26.

165. Caparica R, Yen CT, Coudry R, et al. Responses to crizotinib can occur in high-level MET-amplified non-small cell lung cancer independent of MET exon 14 alterations. *J Thorac Oncol.* 2017;12(1):141-144.

166. Schuler MH, Berardi R, Lim W, et al. Phase (Ph) I study of the safety and efficacy of the cMET inhibitor capmatinib (INC280) in patients (pts) with advanced cMET+ non-small cell lung cancer (NSCLC). *J Clin Oncol.* 2016;34:9067 (s).

167. Heist RS, Sequist LV, Borger D, et al. Acquired resistance to crizotinib in NSCLC with MET exon 14 skipping. *J Thorac Oncol.* 2016;11(8): 1242-1245.

168. Ou SI, Young L, Schrock AB, et al. Emergence of preexisting METY1230C mutation as a resistance mechanism to crizotinib in NSCLC with MET exon 14 skipping. *J Thorac Oncol.* 2017;12(1):137-140.

169. Engstrom L, Aranda R, Lee M, et al. Glesatinib exhibits antitumor activity in lung cancer models and patients harboring MET exon 14 mutations and overcomes mutation-mediated resistance to type I MET inhibitors in nonclinical models. *Clin Cancer Res.* 2017;23(21):6661-6672.

170. Li A, Yang JJ, Zhang XC, et al. Acquired METY1248H and D1246N mutations mediate resistance to MET inhibitors in non-small cell lung cancer. *Clin Cancer Res.* 2017;23(16):4929-4937.

171. Bahcall M, Sim T, Paweletz CP, et al. Acquired METD1228V mutation and resistance to MET inhibition in lung cancer. *Cancer Discov.* 2016;6(12):1334-1341.

172. Vaishnavi A, Le AT, Doebele RC. TRKing down an old oncogene in a new era of targeted therapy. *Cancer Discov.* 2015;5(1):25-34.

173. Farago AF, Le LP, Zheng Z, et al. Durable clinical response to entrectinib in NTRK1-rearranged non-small cell lung cancer. *J Thorac Oncol.* 2015;10(12):1670-1674.

174. Vaishnavi A, Capelletti M, Le AT, et al. Oncogenic and drug-sensitive NTRK1 rearrangements in lung cancer. *Nat Med.* 2013;19(11):1469-1472.

175. Hong DS, Farago AF, Brose MS et al. Clinical safety and activity from a phase 1 study of LOXO-101, a selective TRKA/B/C inhibitor, in solid-tumor patients with NTRK gene fusions. *American Association for Cancer Research 2016 Annual Meeting*; 2016.

176. Passiglia F, Caparica R, Giovannetti E, et al. The potential of neurotrophic tyrosine kinase (NTRK) inhibitors for treating lung cancer. *Expert Opin Investig Drugs.* 2016;25(4):385-392.

177. Hyman DM, Laetsch TW, Kummar S, et al. The efficacy of larotrectinib (LOXO-101), a selective tropomyosin receptor kinase (TRK) inhibitor, in adult and pediatric TRK fusion cancers. *J Clin Oncol.* 2017;35(suppl; abstr LBA2501).

178. Russo M, Misale S, Wei G, et al. Acquired resistance to the TRK inhibitor entrectinib in colorectal cancer. *Cancer Discov.* 2016;6(1):36-44.

179. Drilon A, Li G, Dogan S, et al. What hides behind the MASC: clinical response and acquired resistance to entrectinib after ETV6-NTRK3 identification in a mammary analogue secretory carcinoma (MASC). *Ann Oncol.* 2016;27(5):920-926.

180. Drilon A, Nagasubramanian R, Blake JF, et al. A next-generation TRK kinase inhibitor overcomes acquired resistance to prior TRK kinase inhibition in patients with TRK fusion-positive solid tumors. *Cancer Discov.* 2017;7(9):963-972.

181. Fuse MJ, Okada K, Oh-Hara T, Ogura H, Fujita N, Katayama R. Mechanisms of resistance to NTRK inhibitors and therapeutic strategies in NTRK1-rearranged cancers. *Mol Cancer Ther.* 2017;16(10):2130-2143.

182. Lipson D, Capelletti M, Yelensky R, et al. Identification of new ALK and RET gene fusions from colorectal and lung cancer biopsies. *Nat Med.* 2012;18(3):382-384.

183. Wang R, Hu H, Pan Y, et al. RET fusions define a unique molecular and clinicopathologic subtype of non-small-cell lung cancer. *J Clin Oncol.* 2012;30(35):4352-4359.

184. Drilon A, Wang L, Hasanovic A, et al. Response to cabozantinib in patients with RET fusion-positive lung adenocarcinomas. *Cancer Discov.* 2013;3(6):630-635.

185. Lee SH, Lee JK, Ahn MJ, et al. Vandetanib in pretreated patients with advanced non-small cell lung cancer-harboring RET rearrangement: a phase II clinical trial. *Ann Oncol.* 2017;28(2):292-297.

186. Yoh K, Seto T, Satouchi M, et al. Vandetanib in patients with previously treated RET-rearranged advanced non-small-cell lung cancer (LURET): an open-label, multicentre phase 2 trial. *Lancet Respir Med.* 2017;5(1):42-50.

187. Velcheti V, Hida T, Reckamp KL, et al. Phase 2 study of lenvatinib (LN) in patients (Pts) with *RET* fusion-positive adenocarcinoma of the lung. *Ann Oncol.* 2016;27(suppl. 6):1204PD.

188. Gautschi O, Milia J, Filleron T, et al. Targeting RET in patients with RET-rearranged lung cancers: results from the global, multicenter RET registry. *J Clin Oncol.* 2017;35(13):1403-1410.

189. Gild ML, Landa I, Ryder M, Ghossein RA, Knauf JA, Fagin JA. Targeting mTOR in RET mutant medullary and differentiated thyroid cancer cells. *Endocr Relat Cancer.* 2013;20(5):659-667.

190. Minocha M, Khurana V, Qin B, Pal D, Mitra AK. Co-administration strategy to enhance brain accumulation of vandetanib by modulating P-glycoprotein (P-gp/Abcb1) and breast cancer resistance protein (Bcrp1/Abcg2) mediated efflux with m-TOR inhibitors. *Int J Pharm.* 2012;434(1-2):306-314.

191. Cascone T, Subbiah V, Hess KR, et al: Significant systemic and CNS activity of RET inhibitor vandetanib combined with mTOR inhibitor everolimus in patients with advanced NSCLC with RET fusion. *Proc Am Soc Clin Oncol.* 2016;34.

192. Ricciardi GR, Russo A, Franchina T, et al. NSCLC and HER2: between lights and shadows. *J Thorac Oncol.* 2014;9(12):1750-1762.

193. Shigematsu H, Takahashi T, Nomura M, et al. Somatic mutations of the HER2 kinase domain in lung adenocarcinomas. *Cancer Res.* 2005;65(5):1642-1646.

194. Tomizawa K, Suda K, Onozato R, et al. Prognostic and predictive implications of HER2/ERBB2/neu gene mutations in lung cancers. *Lung Cancer.* 2011;74(1):139-144.

195. Mazières J, Peters S, Lepage B, et al. Lung cancer that harbors an HER2 mutation: epidemiologic characteristics and therapeutic perspectives. *J Clin Oncol.* 2013;31(16):1997-2003.

196. Arcila ME, Chaft JE, Nafa K, et al. Prevalence, clinicopathologic associations, and molecular spectrum of ERBB2 (HER2) tyrosine kinase mutations in lung adenocarcinomas. *Clin Cancer Res.* 2012;18(18):4910-4918.

197. Li BT, Ross DS, Aisner DL, et al. HER2 amplification and HER2 mutation are distinct molecular targets in lung cancers. *J Thorac Oncol.* 2016;11(3):414-419.

198. Mazières J, Barlesi F, Filleron T, et al. Lung cancer patients with HER2 mutations treated with chemotherapy and HER2-targeted drugs: results from the European EUHER2 cohort. *Ann Oncol.* 2016;27(2):281-286.

199. De Grève J, Moran T, Graas MP, et al. Phase II study of afatinib, an irreversible ErbB family blocker, in demographically and genotypically defined lung adenocarcinoma. *Lung Cancer.* 2015;88(1):63-69.

200. Kris MG, Camidge DR, Giaccone G, et al. Targeting HER2 aberrations as actionable drivers in lung cancers: phase II trial of the pan-HER tyrosine kinase inhibitor dacomitinib in patients with HER2-mutant or amplified tumors. *Ann Oncol.* 2015;26(7):1421-1427.

201. Perera SA, Li D, Shimamura T, et al. HER2YVMA drives rapid development of adenosquamous lung tumors in mice that are sensitive to BIBW2992 and rapamycin combination therapy. *Proc Natl Acad Sci U S A.* 2009;106(2):474-479.

202. Gandhi L, Bahleda R, Tolaney SM, et al. Phase I study of neratinib in combination with temsirolimus in patients with human epidermal growth factor receptor 2-dependent and other solid tumors. *J Clin Oncol.* 2014;32(2):68-75.

203. Gandhi L, Besse B, Mazieres J, et al. Neratinib + temsirolimus in HER2-mutant lung cancers: an international, randomized phase II study. *17th World Conference on Lung Cancer. Mini Oral Session 4302.* 2016.

204. Li BT, Shen R, Buonocore D, et al. Ado-trastuzumab emtansine in patients with *HER2* mutant lung cancers: Results from a phase II basket trial. *J Clin Oncol.* 2017;35(suppl; abstr 8510).

205. Turner N, Grose R. Fibroblast growth factor signalling: from development to cancer. *Nat Rev Cancer.* 2010;10(2):116-129.

206. Shaw AT, Hsu PP, Awad MM, Engelman JA. Tyrosine kinase gene rearrangements in epithelial malignancies. *Nat Rev Cancer.* 2013;13(11):772-787.

207. Terai H, Soejima K, Yasuda H, et al. Activation of the FGF2-FGFR1 autocrine pathway: a novel mechanism of acquired resistance to gefitinib in NSCLC. *Mol Cancer Res.* 2013;11(7):759-767.

208. Desai A, Menon SP, Dy GK. Alterations in genes other than EGFR/ALK/ROS1 in non-small cell lung cancer: trials and treatment options. *Cancer Biol Med.* 2016;13(1):77-86.

209. Zhang J, Zhang L, Su X, et al. Translating the therapeutic potential of AZD4547 in FGFR1-amplified non-small cell lung cancer through the use of patient-derived tumor xenograft models. *Clin Cancer Res.* 2012;18(24):6658-6667.

210. Weiss J, Sos ML, Seidel D, et al. Frequent and focal FGFR1 amplification associates with therapeutically tractable FGFR1 dependency in squamous cell lung cancer. *Sci Transl Med.* 2010;2(62):62ra93.

211. Wynes MW, Hinz TK, Gao D, et al. FGFR1 mRNA and protein expression, not gene copy number, predict FGFR TKI sensitivity across all lung cancer histologies. *Clin Cancer Res.* 2014;20(12):3299-3309.

212. Desai A, Adjei AA. FGFR signaling as a target for lung cancer therapy. *J Thorac Oncol.* 2016;11(1):9-20.

213. Katoh M. FGFR inhibitors: effects on cancer cells, tumor microenvironment and whole-body homeostasis (review). *Int J Mol Med.* 2016;38(1):3-15.

214. Nogova L, Sequist LV, Perez Garcia JM, et al. Evaluation of BGJ398, a fibroblast growth factor receptor 1–3 kinase inhibitor, in patients with advanced solid tumors harboring genetic alterations in fibroblast growth factor receptors: results of a global phase I, dose-escalation and dose-expansion study. *J Clin Oncol.* 2017;35(2):157-165.

215. Wöhrle S, Bonny O, Beluch N, et al. FGF receptors control vitamin D and phosphate homeostasis by mediating renal FGF-23 signaling and regulating FGF-23 expression in bone. *J Bone Miner Res.* 2011;26(10):2486-2497.

216. Weeden CE, Solomon B, Asselin-Labat ML. FGFR1 inhibition in lung squamous cell carcinoma: questions and controversies. *Cell Death Discov.* 2015;1:15049.

217. Dutt A, Ramos AH, Hammerman PS, et al. Inhibitor-sensitive FGFR1 amplification in human non-small cell lung cancer. *PLoS One.* 2011;6(6):e20351.

218. Rooney C, Geh C, Williams V, et al. Characterization of FGFR1 locus in sqNSCLC reveals a broad and heterogeneous amplicon. *PLoS One.* 2016;11(2):e0149628.

219. Malchers F, Dietlein F, Schöttle J, et al. Cell-autonomous and non-cell-autonomous mechanisms of transformation by amplified FGFR1 in lung cancer. *Cancer Discov.* 2014;4(2):246-257.

220. Lockwood W, Politi K. MYCxing it up with FGFR1 in squamous cell lung cancer. *Cancer Discov.* 2014;4(2):152-154.

221. Harbinski F, Craig VJ, Sanghavi S, et al. Rescue screens with secreted proteins reveal compensatory potential of receptor tyrosine kinases in driving cancer growth. *Cancer Discov.* 2012;2(10):948-959.

222. Kim SM, Kim H, Yun MR, et al. Activation of the Met kinase confers acquired drug resistance in FGFR-targeted lung cancer therapy. *Oncogenesis.* 2016;5(7):e241.

223. Malchers F, Ercanoglu MS, Schütte D, et al. Mechanisms of primary drug resistance in FGFR1 amplified lung cancer. *Clin Cancer Res.* 2017;23(18):5527-5536.

224. Sohl CD, Ryan MR, Luo B, Frey KM, Anderson KS. Illuminating the molecular mechanisms of tyrosine kinase inhibitor resistance for the FGFR1 gatekeeper mutation: the Achilles' heel of targeted therapy. *ACS Chem Biol.* 2015;10(5):1319-1329.

225. Liang D, Chen Q, Guo Y, Zhang T, Guo W. Insight into resistance mechanisms of AZD4547 and E3810 to FGFR1 gatekeeper mutation via theoretical study. *Drug Des Devel Ther* 2017;11:451-461.

226. Tan L, Wang J, Tanizaki J, et al. Development of covalent inhibitors that can overcome resistance to first-generation FGFR kinase inhibitors. *Proc Natl Acad Sci U S A.* 2014;111(45):E4869-E4877.

227. Li X, Guise CP, Taghipouran R, et al. 2-Oxo-3,4-dihydropyrimido[4, 5-D]pyrimidinyl derivatives as new irreversible pan fibroblast growth factor receptor (FGFR) inhibitors. *Eur J Med Chem.* 2017;135:531-543.

228. Brameld KA, Owens TD, Verner E, et al. Discovery of the irreversible covalent FGFR inhibitor 8-(3-(4-acryloylpiperazin-1-yl)propyl)-6-(2,6-dichloro-3,5-dimethoxyphenyl)-2-(methylamino)pyrido[2,3-D]pyrimidin-7(8H)-one (PRN1371) for the treatment of solid tumors. *J Med Chem.* 2017;60(15):6516-6527.

MAP Kinase Pathway

Douglas B. Johnson and Keith T. Flaherty

Cancer is a disorder driven by somatic genomic alterations. These alterations, acting alone or in concert, drive a variety of cell changes ultimately leading toward cancer, including unrestrained cellular proliferation, removal of cell cycle checkpoints, immune evasion, acquisition of invasiveness, and diminished apoptosis. In particular, activation of core cell signaling networks through mutational processes, such as the mitogen-activated protein kinase (MAPK) pathway, is a critical driver of cancer development and progression. Overdependence upon MAPK signaling, however, has proven to be some cancers' "Achilles heel," leading to opportunities for pharmacologic attack.

MAPK Pathway Overview

The MAPK pathway is comprised of several canonical members. In normal cells, this signal transduction pathway mediates numerous intracellular processes, including proliferation, hormone responses, and differentiation. In the physiologic state, growth factors bind to extracellular receptor tyrosine kinases (RTKs), triggering RTK autophosphorylation, dimerization, and activation. This, in turn, leads to adaptor molecule recruitment (including grb2 and shc), which then recruit guanine nucleotide exchange factors (GEFs), that mediated rat sarcoma homolog (RAS) protein activation.[1] These RAS proteins are GTPases that transduce signals from RTKs to downstream MAPK partners as well as other signaling pathways. The three different homologous RAS proteins, Kirsten, Harvey, and neuroblastoma RAS, function similarly and are affected by distinct mutation patterns in different cancers (see MAPK pathway in cancer section below). In the physiologic state, these proteins are activated by GEFs and suppressed by GTPase-activating proteins (GAPs) such as neurofibromin-1 (NF1, which may also be affected in cancer). RAS activation not only triggers MAPK signaling but parallel cell signaling networks such as the PI3K-AKT pathways.

Following RAS phosphorylation, rapidly accelerated fibrosarcoma (RAF) proteins are activated to form homo-or heterodimers among the three different RAF isoforms (ARAF, BRAF, and CRAF). These dimers then bind to and phosphorylate mitogen-activated protein extracellular signal–regulated kinase kinase (MEK), which then activates mitogen-activated extracellular signal–regulated kinase (ERK) in a signaling cascade. ERK then mediates cell survival and proliferation in the nucleus and also provides negative upstream feedback to attenuate further pathway activation (Fig. 22.1).

MAPK Pathway in Cancer

Mutations affecting genes encoding MAPK pathway members are highly prevalent across the cancer landscape. These mutations activate constitutive MAPK signaling, leading to unrestrained cell growth and proliferation. *RAS* mutations represent the most common oncogenic mutation and are present in nearly one third of all cancers. *RAS*-mutated cancers include pancreas adenocarcinoma (*KRAS* mutated in 95%), lung adenocarcinoma (*KRAS* 20%), colon adenocarcinoma (*KRAS* 50%, *NRAS* 5%), melanoma (*NRAS* 20%), urothelial bladder cancer (*HRAS* 15%), head and neck squamous cell carcinoma (*HRAS* 10%), acute myeloid leukemia (*NRAS* 10%), thyroid cancer (*NRAS* 10%), and many others at lower frequencies.[2] *RAS* mutations typically occur at codons 12, 13, and 61, with codons 12 and 13 primarily involved for *KRAS* mutations and codon 61 affected in *NRAS*. Mutant *NRAS* produces both MAPK activation and also PI3K/AKT and Ral-GDS pathway signaling. CRAF appears to be comparably important in transducing MAPK signaling downstream to other pathway members in the context of *RAS* mutations. Although MAP kinase pathway dependence has been clearly demonstrated in some *RAS*-mutated model systems and responses have been seen to single-agent MAP kinase pathway targeted therapy, predicting unique dependence on the MAP kinase pathway versus other RAS effector pathways has been elusive.[3]

Mutations in *BRAF* are also common, occurring in melanoma and thyroid cancer (both approximately 50%), colorectal

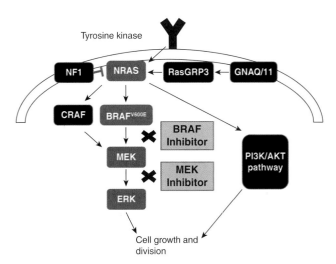

Tyrosine kinase

NF1 — NRAS — RasGRP3 — GNAQ/11

CRAF — BRAF^V600E

BRAF Inhibitor

MEK

MEK Inhibitor

ERK

PI3K/AKT pathway

Cell growth and division

FIGURE 22.1 Overview of MAP kinase pathway.

adenocarcinoma (10%), lung adenocarcinoma (5% to 10%), and a low frequency of numerous other malignancies.[2] The most common site of *BRAF* mutations is at the 600th codon, with an amino acid substitution of valine to glutamine (V600E) or lysine (V600K). The V600 mutation eliminates the need for upstream activation by RAS and mitigates the need for dimerization, thus producing constitutive MAPK signaling. Other non-V600 mutations have also been identified at lower frequencies that also activate MAPK signaling to varying degrees. Finally, fusions and intragenic deletions may activate BRAF by removing the regulatory RAS-binding domain, allowing for unopposed kinase activity. More so than *RAS*-mutated tumors, V600 *BRAF*–mutated tumors appear to be the most MAP kinase pathway dependent among the genetically defined subpopulations of cancer.

A number of other low-frequency mutations also produce constitutive MAPK signaling. CRAF and MEK mutations, as well as CRAF (*RAF1*) fusions, also occur at very low frequencies in several cancers. Mutations in the G-protein encoding genes *GNAQ* and *GNA11* are hallmarks of uveal melanoma and several other rare melanocytic tumors (blue nevi, central nervous system melanocytomas) and rarely occur in other melanoma subtypes.[4,5] These mutations are essentially specific to melanocytic tumors and produce MAPK signaling independent of other classic melanoma mutations (*BRAF* and *NRAS*). *GNAQ* and *GNA11* mutations are activating and drive unopposed G-protein signaling cascade activation, which activates MAPK signaling through RasGRP3 activation via protein kinase C (PKC)-dependent and PKC-independent mechanisms.[6]

Interestingly, another relatively commonly mutated gene affecting the MAPK pathway is *NF1*, the negative regulator (GEF) of RAS. Germ-line mutations in this gene are responsible for the genetic syndrome of neurofibromatosis type 1, characterized by pigmented macules (café au lait macules), freckling, neurofibromas, optic pathway gliomas, and malignant peripheral nerve sheath tumors. In melanomas and other cancers, somatic inactivating point mutations or large deletions across the gene may cause truncated or nonfunctional proteins, leading to unrestrained RAS activation. *NF1* mutations are observed most often in melanoma (15%), glioblastoma (15%), lung squamous cell carcinoma (15%), lung adenocarcinoma (10%), breast cancer (5%), and others.[2] In melanoma, *NF1* mutations are frequently accompanied by other mutations activating the MAPK pathway including atypical *BRAF* or *NRAS* mutations, suggesting that *NF1* loss may provide a relatively incomplete trigger of MAPK signaling.[7]

For each of these MAP kinase pathway–activating oncogenes, inhibition of the pathway is likely to be an important component of combination therapeutic regimens. However, for some, single-agent efficacy has been well documented and now incorporated into standard of care.

Inhibitors of Mutant BRAF in Melanoma

The discovery that approximately half of all melanomas harbored a *BRAF* V600 mutation triggered an intense interest in developing a clinically active inhibitor of the mutated BRAF oncoprotein. The earliest studies evaluated the multikinase inhibitor sorafenib, which ostensibly possessed BRAF inhibitory properties as demonstrated in cell line and in vivo experiments. Overall activity was disappointing,

though, both as a single agent and in combination with cytotoxic chemotherapy. For example, a phase III study compared carboplatin, paclitaxel, and sorafenib with carboplatin and paclitaxel alone in 823 patients with advanced melanoma.[8] No difference in overall or progression-free survival or response rate was observed in this study, either in the unselected population or in the *BRAF* mutation group. Although rare responses were observed with sorafenib monotherapy, these were later attributed to the antiangiogenic properties of the agent and also did not seem to correlate with *BRAF* mutation status. Other, BRAF/multikinase inhibitors also demonstrated suboptimal activity despite excellent preclinical rationale, including RAF-265.[9] This lack of activity spurred the search for more active, mutant-specific BRAF inhibitors.

Vemurafenib (PLX4032 and RG7204, Table 22.1) was initially identified using crystallography-guided approaches to bind mutant *BRAF* preferentially, although relatively potent inhibition of both wild-type BRAF and CRAF was also observed.[10] In preclinical models, dose-dependent inhibition of exclusively *BRAF* mutant cell lines and xenografts was observed, with no obvious effects on *BRAF* wild-type models. In initial patient studies, a crystalline formulation was given, which did provide modest ERK inhibition but had suboptimal bioavailability and was not associated with clinical responses. The drug was reformulated as a microprecipitated bulk powder, which resulted in increased bioavailability and drug exposures.

The initial phase I trial of vemurafenib was conducted in unselected melanoma patients.[11] After five patients with *BRAF* wild-type melanoma failed to respond to therapy in the dose escalation phase, an expansion cohort was limited to patients with *BRAF* V600E mutant melanoma. In the expansion phase, 32 patients received the recommended phase II dose (RP2D) of 960 mg twice daily. Of these patients, 81% had at least partial or complete responses, and a median progression-free survival of approximately 7 months was observed. Moreover, patients frequently derived benefit even hours to days after starting therapy, and patients with highly impaired functional status had remarkable improvements (Fig. 22.2).

TABLE 22.1	*Key features of vemurafenib pharmacology*
Mechanism of Action	**Inhibition of Serine-Threonine Kinase BRAF, Including BRAF V600**
Metabolism	Metabolized by CYP3A4
Pharmacokinetics	Elimination $t_{1/2}$ = 57 h
Elimination	Fecal (94%), urine (1%)
Drug interactions	Moderate CYP1A2 inhibitor
	Weak CYP2D6 inhibitor
	CYP3A4 inducer
Toxicity	Cutaneous squamous cell carcinomas
	Phototoxicity
	Liver laboratory abnormalities
	Arthralgia
	Nausea/vomiting
Precautions	Strong CYP3A4 inhibitors or inducers should be used with caution

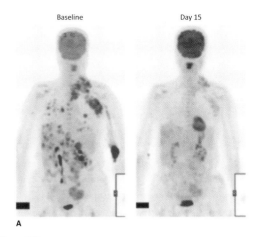

Baseline   Day 15

A

Best Overall Response

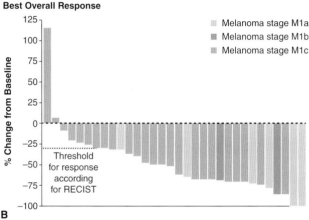

Melanoma stage M1a
Melanoma stage M1b
Melanoma stage M1c

B

FIGURE 22.2 Activity of the BRAF inhibitor vemurafenib demonstrating rapid response in a patient (**panel A**) and frequent responses across treated patients. Source: Inhibition of mutated, activated BRAF in metastatic melanoma. (From Flaherty KT, Puzanov I, Kim KB, et al. Inhibition of mutated, activated BRAF in metastatic melanoma. *N Engl J Med.* 2010;363(9):809-819. Copyright © 2010 Massachusetts Medical Society. Reprinted with permission from Massachusetts Medical Society.)

A follow-up phase II study was conducted to further evaluate the efficacy of vemurafenib in metastatic melanoma. Among 328 patients screened for study entry, 132 patients received therapy, including 122 with *BRAF*V600E and 10 with *BRAF*V600K mutations. Of these, a confirmed objective response rate of 53% was observed, with a median progression-free survival of 6.8 months and a median overall survival of 15.9 months. Landmark analyses of overall survival at 6, 12, and 18 months were 77%, 58%, and 43%, respectively.

Finally, a pivotal phase III study compared vemurafenib with dacarbazine in 675 previously untreated patients with metastatic, *BRAF*V600E–mutated melanoma.[12] The overall survival at 6 months was dramatically improved in the vemurafenib group (84% versus 64%; hazard ratio for death of 0.37, $P < 0.001$). Response rates were also similarly improved in the vemurafenib group (48% versus 5%). Vemurafenib received regulatory approval in 2011.

Dabrafenib (GSK2118436, Table 22.2) is a selective inhibitor of mutant *BRAF*. Following preclinical validation, a phase I study of patients with various solid tumors was performed, including 156 with metastatic melanoma.[13] Among 36 patients with *BRAF* V600 mutant melanoma who received the recommended phase II dose, 18 had confirmed responses (50%). This study also noted responses in patients with other *BRAF* mutant solid tumors, including cancers of the lung, thyroid, ovary, and colon, as well as in melanoma

TABLE 22.2 Key features of dabrafenib pharmacology

Mechanism of Action	Inhibition of Serine-Threonine Kinase BRAF, Including BRAF V600
Metabolism	Metabolized by CYP2C8 and CYP3A4
Pharmacokinetics	Terminal $t_{1/2}$ = 8 h
Elimination	Fecal (71%), urine (23%)
Drug interactions	Moderate CYP1A2 inhibitor
	Weak CYP2D6 inhibitor
	CYP3A4 inducer
Toxicity	Cutaneous squamous cell carcinomas
	Pyrexia (fever)
	Uveitis/iritis
	Arthralgia
	Rash
Precautions	Avoid use of strong CYP3A4 or CYP2C8 inducers/inhibitors
	Closely observe patients with G6PD deficiency
	Gastrointestinal acid altering drugs may decrease bioavailability

patients with *BRAF*V600K mutations. Further, activity was noted in patients with small (<1.5 cm), untreated brain metastases, with all patients experiencing some decrease in the size of brain metastases.

A follow-up phase II study evaluated dabrafenib in two cohorts of patients with brain metastases: Cohort A consisted of 89 patients with previously untreated brain metastases, and Cohort B included 83 patients who progressed on prior local therapies (e.g., radiation or surgery).[14] Intracranial responses were observed in 39% and 30% of patients in each cohort, respectively. The median progression-free survival was approximately 16 weeks, irrespective of cohort assignment or mutation status (*BRAF*V600E versus V600K). Overall, this approach appeared to be fairly safe; while 6% of patients experienced intracranial hemorrhage, this was observed due to treatment in only one case with the remainder attributed to progressive disease.

Finally, a phase III study randomized 250 patients with metastatic *BRAF* mutant melanoma, in a 3:1 fashion, to either dabrafenib or dacarbazine. Dabrafenib substantially improved progression-free survival compared with dacarbazine (median 5.1 versus 2.7 months, hazard ratio 0.30, $P < 0.001$). Overall survival was not significantly different, although the study was not powered to evaluate a survival difference and crossover from chemotherapy to dabrafenib was permitted. Based on these studies, dabrafenib became the second BRAF inhibitor approved for advanced, *BRAF* V600 mutant melanoma in 2013.

BRAF Inhibition in Other Cancers

*BRAF*V600 mutations are present at various frequencies in a variety of cancers and thus present therapeutic targets in these diseases as well. These include papillary thyroid cancer (approximately 60%), colorectal adenocarcinoma (10% to 20%), lung adenocarcinoma (up to 5%), and a low frequency of other solid tumors (including sarcomas, cholangiocarcinomas, and central nervous system cancers). Interestingly, the blood disorders hairy cell leukemia, Erdheim-Chester disease, and Langerhans cell histiocytosis also harbor high rates of *BRAF* V600E mutations.

To evaluate the activity of BRAF inhibition in these populations, a histology agnostic, so-called "basket" study of patients with advanced nonmelanoma cancers with *BRAF* V600 mutations was performed. This phase II study enrolled 122 patients, including those with colorectal cancer ($n = 37$), non–small cell lung cancer (NSCLC) ($n = 20$), Erdheim-Chester or Langerhans cell histiocytosis (ECD/LCH; $n = 18$), cholangiocarcinoma ($n = 8$), primary brain tumors ($n = 7$), and multiple myeloma ($n = 5$).[15] NSCLC patients experienced a 42% response rate with a median progression-free survival of 7.3 months, not dissimilar to the activity observed in melanoma. Patients with ECD/LCH similarly had a 43% response rate with no patients having progressed at a median of 5.3 months' follow-up duration. Isolated responses were also observed in anaplastic pleomorphic xanthoastrocytoma (3 of 4), anaplastic thyroid cancer (2 of 7), cholangiocarcinoma (1 of 8), salivary duct cancer, soft tissue sarcoma, and ovarian cancer. By contrast, no patients with multiple myeloma ($n = 5$) or colon cancer responded to vemurafenib monotherapy. An extension cohort permitted the combination of vemurafenib and cetuximab in 26 patients with colorectal cancer; 1 patient had a confirmed objective response (4% response rate), and approximately half had some degree of tumor regression not reaching the criteria for partial responses. A separate study showed that the combination of dabrafenib and trametinib in *BRAF* V600 mutant colon cancer also had somewhat suboptimal activity, demonstrating 5 responses among 43 treated patients (12%).[16]

A separate report detailed two phase II studies that evaluated the activity of vemurafenib in hairy cell leukemia that progressed on purine analogue therapy.[17] Remarkable 100% and 96% response rates (24 of 24 patients and 25 of 26 patients) were reported. In the Italian trial, a median progression-free survival of 19 months was reported for those experiencing a complete response but only 6 months for those with partial responses. In the American trial, 1-year progression-free and overall survival rates were 73% and 91%, respectively. These studies collectively suggest that BRAF inhibition is active in many *BRAF* V600 mutant cancers but has variable utility, which appears tumor type–specific.

Toxicity of BRAF Inhibitors

Single-agent BRAF inhibitors have produced fairly stereotypical toxicity profiles. Extended follow-up from the phase III study of vemurafenib reported the following grade 3 to 4 adverse events: cutaneous squamous cell carcinomas (cuSCCs; 19%), cutaneous keratoacanthomas (10%), rash (9%), and elevated liver function tests (11%).[18] Other common low-grade events included phototoxicity, arthralgias, fatigue, and nausea. Vemurafenib was discontinued in 7% due to adverse events. Relatively similar toxicities were observed with dabrafenib, although cuSCCs appeared to be less frequent (grade 3 to 4: 9%) and pyrexia was more common (any grade 25% and grade 3 2%).[19]

Single-agent BRAF inhibitors produce toxicities, in part, for a unique reason. While these mutant-specific BRAF inhibitors quench MAPK signaling in *BRAF* mutant cells, they paradoxically increase pathway signaling in BRAF wild-type cells. This, in part, explains why these agents do not induce toxicities characteristic of MAPK inhibition of MEK or ERK inhibitors (discussed below but includes hypoproliferative rash, cardiomyopathy). This effect is mediated by more efficient autodimerization between two BRAF proteins or between BRAF and CRAF. Of particular clinical importance, premalignant lesions harboring *RAS* mutations are stimulated by this paradoxical effect. In fact, most cuSCCs that occur on BRAF inhibition were found to have *HRAS* mutations.[20] This effect led to concerns that other, more lethal malignancies might be unmasked. One particularly provocative case of *RAS*-mutated chronic myelomonocytic leukemia occurred in a patient with advanced melanoma on vemurafenib therapy.[21] Rising leukocyte counts temporally correlated with vemurafenib therapy and decreased when treatment was held. Further, addition of a MEK inhibitor resulted in durable disease control for both malignancies.[22] Otherwise, very little evidence of increased incidence of *RAS* mutant, visceral noncutaneous malignancies has been uncovered.

MEK Inhibitors

While MEK (*MAP2K*) mutations are relatively infrequent in cancers, this molecule serves as a key hub of MAPK signaling. Further, since it lies downstream of both RAF and RAS, it was hoped that inhibiting MEK would have powerful effects in cancers with diverse mechanisms of MAPK activation, including *RAS* mutations. Initial efforts with early MEK inhibitors proved to produce poorly tolerated side effects, including rash and ocular effects. Later-generation MEK inhibitors, however, have provided more promising efficacy and tolerability.

Trametinib (GSK-1120212, JTP-74057, Table 22.3), an allosteric inhibitor of MEK1 and MEK2, was initially tested in a phase I study.[23] A dose-finding phase identified 2-mg daily continuous dosing as the recommended phase 2 dose. Following this, a separate cohort of patients with *KRAS*-or *BRAF*-mutated melanoma, pancreatic, non–small cell lung, or colorectal cancers (or other *BRAF*-mutated cancers) was accrued. Two of 26 patients with pancreatic cancer (8%), 2 of 30 patients with NSCLC (7%), and no patients with colorectal cancer responded to treatment. With the exception of colon cancer, approximately half of patients had at least some degree of tumor shrinkage, suggesting that MEK inhibition might be a key building block for future combination therapies. A separate report detailed the activity of trametinib in 81 patients with melanoma.[24] Among 30 patients with *BRAF* V600 mutant melanoma naïve to BRAF inhibitors, 10 confirmed responses were observed (33% response rate). By contrast, 0 of 6 patients with prior BRAF inhibitors, 0 of 7 with *NRAS* mutations, 0 of 16 with uveal melanoma, and 4 of 39 (10%) with *BRAF/NRAS* wild-type melanoma experienced objective responses to therapy. Temporary stable disease and tumor regression not meeting the threshold for responses were observed in all of these subgroups.

A randomized phase III study of trametinib versus dacarbazine or paclitaxel was then conducted in 322 patients with advanced *BRAF* V600–mutated melanoma.[25] Patients were randomized in a

TABLE

22.3 *Key features of trametinib pharmacology*

Mechanism of Action	Reversible Inhibitor of MEK1/2 Activation and Kinase Activity
Metabolism	Deacetylation
Pharmacokinetics	Elimination $t_{1/2}$ = 3.9 to 4.8 d
Elimination	Fecal (>80%), urine (<20%)
Drug interactions	None (when used as monotherapy)
Toxicity	Cardiomyopathy
	Pyrexia (fever)[a]
	Ocular toxicity (retinal pigment epithelial detachment, blurred vision)
	Hemorrhage[a]
	Venous thromboembolism[a]
	Rash
	Diarrhea
	Lymphedema

[a]When used in combination with dabrafenib.

2:1 fashion and crossover was permitted. Median progression-free survival was improved with trametinib (4.8 versus 1.5 months, hazard ratio 0.45, $P < 0.001$). Interestingly, despite crossover, overall survival was also improved with trametinib (81% versus 67% at 6 months; $P = 0.01$). The most common toxicities observed were acneiform rash, diarrhea, peripheral edema, and occasional reversible decreases in cardiac ejection fraction and ocular effects. Chorioretinopathy, a major complication of earlier MEK inhibitors, was not observed in this study. The FDA approved the use of trametinib in advanced *BRAF* V600–mutated melanoma in 2013.

Although BRAF inhibitors and MEK inhibitors have never been directly compared in the BRAF V600 mutant melanoma population, large phase III trial data clearly indicate a lower objective response rate for MEK inhibitors versus BRAF inhibitors. While preclinical evidence suggests that BRAF and MEK are equally viable points of therapeutic intervention in these tumors, it appears that the MAP kinase pathway inhibition produced by MEK inhibitors in normal tissue mediates toxicity and limits tolerable drug exposures in a way that prohibits the same degree of pathway inhibition in tumor cells that can be achieved with BRAF inhibitors that paradoxically activate the MAP kinase pathway in other tissues.

A number of other MEK inhibitors are in various stages of development. Selumetinib (AZD6244) is an allosteric MEK1/2 inhibitor that has demonstrated initially promising results in several cancers. In combination with docetaxel, selumetinib improved progression-free survival versus docetaxel alone in a small study of 87 patients with previously treated *KRAS* mutant NSCLC (median 5.3 months versus 2.1 months, $P = 0.01$) with a nonstatistically significant trend to improve overall survival.[26] Unfortunately, a phase III study did not confirm this benefit (unpublished, press release only).

In uveal melanoma, selumetinib improved progression-free survival compared with chemotherapy (median 16 weeks versus 7 weeks), although overall survival was not improved.[27] This study generated significant enthusiasm for MEK inhibition in uveal melanoma, a cancer without other active therapeutic strategies. Unfortunately, subsequent (and unpublished) studies evaluating trametinib in this setting have been unimpressive, tempering the enthusiasm for MEK inhibition in uveal melanoma. Further, selumetinib plus dacarbazine improved progression-free survival compared with dacarbazine alone in *BRAF* V600 mutant melanoma, but again no improvement in overall survival was observed.[28] Interestingly, however, selumetinib has demonstrated dramatic activity in another condition with MAPK pathway mutations: neurofibromatosis type I. In a small study, 71% of children with plexiform neurofibromas experienced partial responses to therapy, suggesting this agent may be a powerful tool in a subset of patients with this condition.[29] Binimetinib (MEK162), another MEK1/2 inhibitor, was compared with dacarbazine in advanced *NRAS* mutant melanoma after an initial response rate of 20% was noted in early studies.[3] Median progression-free survival was modestly improved with binimetinib (2.8 versus 1.5 months, $P < 0.001$), as was response rate (15% versus 7%). No improvement in overall survival was observed.[30]

One other genetic subset with compelling rationale for MEK inhibition is atypical, non–V600 *BRAF* mutations. Several studies have reported impressive clinical responses, primarily in melanoma, in these patients. In particular, the *BRAF* L597 and K601 mutations have demonstrated sensitivity, along with several *BRAF* fusions.[31,32] Currently, the NCI-MATCH study is evaluating trametinib across cancers with these atypical *BRAF* mutations or fusions.

These and several other MEK inhibitors are in development as single agents and in combination with other agents (see "Future directions"). These studies demonstrate that single-agent MEK inhibition produces relatively modest clinical benefits for patients with *NRAS* or *KRAS* mutant cancers. The strong signals toward activity suggest that combination therapy may provide more substantial clinical activity if optimal combinatorial partners can be identified.

Combined BRAF and MEK Inhibition

While the clinical activity of both BRAF and MEK inhibitors as single agents was impressive in melanoma patients and represented a major step forward, the respective median progression-free survival values of approximately 7 and 5 months clearly needed improvement. Genetic, transcriptomic, and proteomic studies (see "Resistance" section) demonstrated both genetic and nongenetic alterations in resistant tumors driving persistent MAPK signaling. Thus, attempts to more thoroughly abrogate MAPK pathway activity with combination BRAF and MEK inhibition were undertaken.

An initial phase I/II study was performed to evaluate the combination of dabrafenib and trametinib in patients with *BRAF* V600 mutations. Following dose finding, a randomized phase II study compared two different doses of combination therapy with single-agent dabrafenib.[33] In this study, the combination at full single-agent doses (dabrafenib 150 mg twice daily and trametinib 2 mg daily) produced a superior response rate (76% versus 54%, $P = 0.03$) and superior median progression-free survival (9.4 versus 5.8 months; hazard ratio 0.39; $P < 0.001$) compared with monotherapy. The combination of dabrafenib and trametinib received accelerated FDA approval based on the clear benefits of this combination in 2014, despite the relatively small study size.

The toxicity profile of combined BRAF and MEK inhibition represents a notable case study in cell signaling biology. The incidence of serious adverse events was similar between arms, but the types of events were distinct: Monotherapy was associated with more cuSCCs (all grades 19% versus 7%), whereas combination therapy had a higher rate of pyrexia (all grades 71% versus 26%). While pyrexia was frequent, most patients were able to continue therapy after dose reduction, interruption, or other supportive care. Gastrointestinal and classical MEK inhibitor–associated toxicities (cardiac and ocular events) were also more frequent in the combination but were generally of low grade. Interestingly, cutaneous events were quite low with the combination, despite the high incidence with both BRAF inhibitor monotherapy (cuSCCs, keratoacanthomas) and MEK inhibitor monotherapy (acneiform rash). This "canceling-out" effect has been attributed to divergent effects on MAPK signaling in BRAF WT keratinocytes by the two agents. Specifically, BRAF inhibitors paradoxically promote MAPK signaling and lead to hyperproliferative lesions, whereas MEK inhibitors inhibit the pathway, leading to hypoproliferation.

A subset of this study permitted patients who had previously progressed on BRAF inhibitor monotherapy to evaluate whether sequencing monotherapy and combination therapy might prove effective. In this BRAF inhibitor–refractory population, the median progression-free survival was 3.6 months and the response rate was 15%.[34] Patients who had received and benefited from BRAF inhibition for greater than 6 months seemed to derive most of the benefit, compared with those who more rapidly progressed (median progression-free survival 3.9 versus 1.8 months; response rate 26% versus 0%). Two studies attempted to assess whether particular molecular features of resistance could predict who would benefit from this approach and did not find obvious candidates.[35,36] Thus, this type of sequenced approach is generally not favored, and combination therapy up-front remains the standard.

Two follow-up phase III studies confirmed the benefits of first-line dabrafenib and trametinib therapy. The COMBI-D study randomized 423 patients with *BRAF* V600–mutated melanoma to either dabrafenib + trametinib or dabrafenib + placebo.[19] Combination therapy resulted in improved overall survival (median 25.1 versus 18.7 months, hazard ratio 0.71; $P = 0.01$), as well as improved progression-free survival (median 11 versus 9.9 months, hazard ratio 0.67, $P < 0.001$). Grade 3 or 4 adverse events occurred in 32% and 31% of patients receiving combination therapy or monotherapy, respectively, with similar profiles as observed in earlier studies. The COMBI-v study randomized 704 patients to dabrafenib + trametinib or vemurafenib and showed similar results overall.[37] Combination therapy was associated with improved overall survival at 12 months (72% versus 65%, hazard ratio 0.69; $P = 0.005$) and improved progression-free survival (median 11.4 versus 7.3 months, hazard ratio 0.56; $P < 0.001$) compared with vemurafenib monotherapy. Similarly, rates of severe adverse events were in line with prior reports, and cuSCCs only occurred in 1% of patients

treated with the combination. These studies, in conjunction with the prior phase II study, established dabrafenib + trametinib as the preferred, frontline targeted therapy option as opposed to BRAF or MEK inhibitor monotherapy.

A phase II trial also evaluated dabrafenib and trametinib in metastatic *BRAF* V600 mutant colon cancer.[16] Among 43 patients, only 5 (12%) experienced objective responses, substantially lower than in melanoma and seemingly only marginally better than vemurafenib monotherapy.[15] Two preclinical studies suggested a reason for this divergent activity across tumor types. In colon cancer, BRAF inhibition triggers feedback activation of EGFR signaling, which induces therapeutic resistance but could be counteracted by EGFR inhibition.[38,39] A number of other trials are ongoing to evaluate dabrafenib and trametinib in *BRAF* mutant thyroid cancers (NCT01723202) and other rare *BRAF* mutant tumors (NCT02034110). The National Cancer Institute MATCH trial (NCT02465060) is also evaluating this combination across *BRAF* V600 mutant cancers.

A second combination of BRAF and MEK inhibitors, vemurafenib (960 mg daily) and cobimetinib (GDC-0973; 60 mg daily for 21 of 28 days, Table 22.4), has also been developed. A phase IB trial initially evaluated this combination in 63 patients naïve to previous BRAF or MEK inhibitors and reported an 87% rate of confirmed objective responses, with a median progression-free survival of 13.7 months.[40] Similar to prior studies, patients who previously progressed on BRAF inhibitors had a lower response rate (15%). A follow-up phase III study randomized 495 patients with metastatic melanoma to either

TABLE 22.4	*Key features of cobimetinib pharmacology*
Mechanism of Action	**Reversible Inhibitor of MEK1/2**
Metabolism	Metabolized by CYP3A oxidation UGT2B7 glucuronidation
Pharmacokinetics	Mean elimination $t_{1/2}$ = 44 h
Elimination	Fecal (76%), urine (18%)
Drug interactions	Substrate of CYP3A
Toxicity[a]	Cardiomyopathy
	Rash and photosensitivity
	Ocular toxicity (retinopathy, retinal vein occlusion)
	Hemorrhage
	Nausea/vomiting
	Hepatotoxicity
	Diarrhea
	Hypertension
Precautions	Avoid use of strong CYP3A inducers/inhibitors
	Closely observe patients with G6PD deficiency
	Gastrointestinal acid altering drugs may decrease bioavailability

[a]When used in combination with vemurafenib.

vemurafenib plus cobimetinib or vemurafenib alone.[41] The combination produced an improvement in line with that demonstrated with dabrafenib and trametinib: improved progression-free survival (median 9.9 versus 6.2 months; $P < 0.001$), improved response rate (68% versus 45%; $P < 0.001$), and a trend toward improved overall survival at 9 months (81% versus 73%). The combination caused a higher frequency of grade 3+ adverse events (65% versus 59%), particularly including gastrointestinal events, rash, and increased liver function tests. In contrast to dabrafenib and trametinib, however, fever was rare (grade 3 to 4 in 2%). The combination of vemurafenib and cobimetinib received FDA approval in 2015.

A third combination regimen has also been developed, although this regimen is not FDA approved to date. Encorafenib (LGX818), a highly potent BRAF inhibitor in combination with binimetinib, was compared with either single-agent encorafenib or vemurafenib in a 1:1:1 fashion in patients with metastatic *BRAF* V600 mutant melanoma. Interestingly, encorafenib monotherapy performed unexpectedly well, and the combination improved outcomes in a nonstatistically significant fashion (hazard ratio 0.75, $P = 0.051$). However, the combination dramatically improved outcomes over single-agent vemurafenib, with an impressive median progression-free survival (14.9 versus 7.3 months, hazard ratio 0.54; $P < 0.001$). Similarly, single-agent encorafenib produced improved progression-free survival compared with vemurafenib. Grade 3 to 4 adverse events were not increased with the combination (58% versus 66% and 63%), and median time to first grade 3 to 4 toxicity was longer with the combination (2.5 versus 0.4 and 1.3 months).

Currently, it is not clear which of the two (or perhaps eventually three) FDA-approved BRAF and MEK inhibitors have superior efficacy profiles, and most investigators view these regimens as roughly equivalent. Thus, therapy can be selected based on toxicity profile, patient preference, clinician familiarity, and dosing schedule. If resistance develops to one regimen, it is not generally recommended to switch directly to the other regimen, given overlapping mechanisms of efficacy and resistance. Interestingly, however, responses have been observed with BRAF + MEK inhibitor retreatment following a treatment break. One prospective study evaluated 25 patients with progressive disease on BRAF/MEK inhibitors who had been off therapy for at least 12 weeks.[42] Partial responses were observed in 8 patients (32%) with another 10 (40%) demonstrating stable disease. Targeted therapy retreatment may be a viable option in this population.

Resistance to BRAF Inhibition

Intrinsic resistance (lack of an initial response) and more commonly acquired resistance (response followed by disease progression) occur in most patients, limiting long-term therapeutic benefits (Fig. 22.3). A number of major efforts have been undertaken to characterize the mechanisms of this resistance.

Intrinsic resistance, defined here as primary disease progression without any tumor shrinkage, remains somewhat poorly understood. This phenomenon occurs in about 10% of patients who receive single-agent BRAF inhibitors, and almost no patients are treated with combination BRAF/MEK inhibition. Several provocative studies have identified distinct transcriptomic profiles in

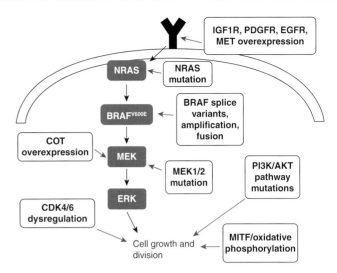

FIGURE 22.3 Overview of mechanisms of resistance to MAP kinase pathway inhibitors.

intrinsic resistance.[43,44] Tumors and cell lines that were poorly sensitive to BRAF inhibition tended to have high levels of AXL compared with MITF. MITF, the master transcriptional regulator of melanoma antigen expression, has been described as highly expressed in melanomas particularly dependent upon MAPK signaling. AXL, on the other hand, may represent a marker for alternative cell signaling pathways and lack of MAPK signaling; thus, melanomas with a low MITF/AXL ratio likely possess low levels of MAPK dependence and inability to response to pathway inhibition.

In addition to the true refractory population, several genomic and nongenomic features present in the pretreatment tumor appear to limit the duration and quality of therapeutic responses. These changes largely involve persistent or downstream activation of MAPK signaling (including *MEK1* mutations)[45] or alternative cell signaling pathways (including through MET activation[46,47] or *PTEN* mutations).[48] Mutations or overexpression of other genes affecting MAPK signaling, such as *NF1*, *COT*, *CDKN2A*, and *CCND1*, likely also contributes to primary resistance, but these have been less well validated.[49]

Acquired or adaptive resistance to BRAF inhibitors is a more prevalent clinical problem. The conventional dogma surrounding these agents has been that all patients inevitably develop acquired resistance and ultimately experience disease progression. However, a small group of patients (approximately 10% to 20%) obtain durable therapeutic benefits lasting for many years.[50] Several pretreatment clinical characteristics seem to predict these durable responses. In a pooled analysis of 617 patients who received dabrafenib and trametinib in randomized studies, patients with normal LDH and melanoma involving fewer than three organ sites experienced a 2-year progression-free survival of 46% and 2-year overall survival of 75%.[51] This contrasted with patients with LDH values of more than twice the upper limit of normal, who had 2-year progression-free and overall survival of 2% and 7%, respectively. Patients who remain in response at 2 to 3 years have had more long-term, sustained responses. Identifying both clinical and molecular biomarkers of such exceptional responding patients remains a major goal.

Despite these outstanding and durable responses in a minority of patients, acquired resistance still limits therapeutic benefits in most patients and has been the subject of intensive research interest. Using pretreatment and postprogression biopsies, researchers have characterized a diverse and sometimes confusing array of molecular changes driving resistance, which are only briefly described here. Tumor heterogeneity also complicates interpretation of these results. In contrast to other tumors, such as *EGFR* mutant lung cancer and chronic myeloid leukemias, second site mutations in the target gene (*BRAF* in this case) were not identified. Instead, acquired changes have largely fallen into three groups: those reactivating MAPK signaling (mutations in *NRAS* and *MEK1/2*, *BRAF* amplification or alternative splicing, *COT* overexpression), those activating alternative signaling pathways (MET overexpression, upstream receptor tyrosine kinase activation, PTEN/PI3K/AKT pathway mutations), and nongenomic, immune, or metabolic changes (T-cell exhaustion, loss of antigen presentation, oxidative phosphorylation addiction).[48,52-55]

Most initial studies profiled resistance to BRAF inhibitor monotherapy, but several efforts have subsequently assessed resistance to BRAF + MEK inhibition. The spectrum of changes driving resistance to combination therapy appears similar to those occurring on monotherapy but typically involves multiple genomic changes functioning in concert.[56-58] For example, *NRAS* mutations and *BRAF* hyperamplification may occur in the same sample in combination therapy resistance. Disconcertingly, studies that sequenced multiple tumors in the same patient revealed that resistance mechanisms were extremely heterogeneous within patients, often with totally distinct genomic alterations across tumors. Several patients, with up to 10 tumors sequenced, suggested that branched chain evolution occurs in response to BRAF inhibitor therapy.[48,52] These findings have produced some degree of pessimism that a single drug, administered at resistance, could overcome these diverse genomic and nongenomic drivers. Nonetheless, a number of studies are ongoing to test agents that block MAPK and/or PI3K pathway signaling in resistant melanomas (see *Experimental Approaches* section).

One other intriguing finding from these studies showed that some melanomas become "addicted" to the presence of MAPK inhibitors.[56,59] Intermittent or pulsed dosing forestalled resistance in some models, leading to interest in using this approach in routine clinical practice. A cooperative group clinical trial is currently testing whether intermittent dabrafenib and trametinib treatment is superior to continuous therapy. While this practice is not the standard of care at this point, many clinicians will use intermittent treatment schedules for patients who experience cumulative toxicities (e.g., 10 days on and 4 days off). Responses following a treatment break (and intervening therapies) have been described, suggesting the possibility of melanoma drug addiction.[42]

Experimental Approaches

ERK Inhibition

RAS, RAF, and MEK ultimately signal downstream to a common final pathway member: ERK. Resistant tumors are characterized by reactivated ERK signaling in most cases. Blocking this molecule would potentially abolish the key pathway mediator of MAPK

signaling and thus theoretically reverse or prevent resistance in a variety of tumors harboring RAS or RAF mutations. Initially, it was presumed that ERK inhibition would produce very similar biochemical effects as MEK inhibitors. More recently, developing ERK inhibitors has gained interest for two primary reasons.[60] First, despite MEK or BRAF/MEK inhibition in *BRAF* mutant melanomas, activation of ERK signaling still occurs in most resistant tumors. Second, directly targeting ERK may enhance negative feedback loops and thereby further extinguish pathway activation.

The ERK inhibitor SCH772984 has been characterized most thoroughly in preclinical experiments and potently inhibits ERK1 and ERK2.[61] This agent both directly inhibits ERK kinase activity and prevents phosphorylation of ERK by MEK. These effects result in apoptosis and tumor regression in animal models of *BRAF* or *RAS* mutant cancers and reverse established resistance to BRAF/MEK inhibitor treated models. Ulixertinib (BVD-523) has produced the most clinical data, reporting a phase I study with a 108 patient expansion cohort. Among 83 evaluable patients, 9 (11%) experienced partial responses lasting for 2 to 24 months. Patients who responded included *NRAS* mutant and refractory *BRAF* mutant melanomas, as well as *BRAF* mutant lung cancer and glioblastoma, cholangiocarcinoma, and head and neck squamous cell carcinomas with atypical *BRAF* mutations.[62] No treatment-related deaths occurred, but 32% of patients required dose reductions, due to the occurrence of rash, diarrhea, fatigue, and nausea. It remains unclear whether these disappointing results are due to a conceptual exaggeration of the importance of ERK in melanoma resistance or a failure of the inhibitor to reach its target.

Another intriguing approach to inhibiting ERK involves a scaffolding protein IQGAP1. This protein facilitates assembly of MAPK proteins and is necessary for RAS-driven tumorigenesis in some tumor models. IQGAP-1 binds to ERK through its WW domain, and knockout of this region disrupted MAPK signaling. Administering an inactivated form of the WW domain peptide inhibited IQGAP1-ERK binding and blocked RAS and RAF-driven tumorigenesis as well as reversing BRAF inhibitor resistance.[63] While this approach is intriguing, this type of peptide therapy remains unproven in human cancer treatment.

Dimer-Disrupting RAF Inhibitors

The next-generation agents are also known as "paradox-breakers." As mentioned in the BRAF inhibitor section, BRAF inhibitors potently extinguish MAPK signaling in *BRAF* V600 mutant cells by binding mutant BRAF and disrupting downstream signaling. Paradoxically, in wild-type cells, these agents activate MAPK signaling. While this phenomenon has not been definitively explained, evidence suggests that conformational changes induced by BRAF inhibitors enhance wild-type BRAF dimerization, either through BRAF-BRAF or BRAF-CRAF interactions.[60] Ultimately, enhanced dimerization may lead to unmasking of latent malignancies and promotion of resistance to BRAF inhibition; thus, disrupting these dimers may counterbalance the drawbacks of BRAF inhibitors.

A series of compounds, including the most advanced PLX8394, have been developed as dimer-disrupting BRAF inhibitors. In cell line systems, these agents had no effect on HRAS mutant squamous cell carcinoma lines and reversed some mechanisms of resistance to

BRAF inhibitors.[64] Notably, this agent was also active in *BRAF* V600 mutant lung adenocarcinoma models, and resistance to therapy occurred through EGFR-mediated MTOR signaling.[65] This agent is currently in early-phase clinical trials testing the agent in multiple *BRAF* mutant cancers.

MEK Inhibitor Combinations

MAPK signaling is present in *RAS* and *BRAF* mutant tumors, as well as other cancer types (including almost all melanomas). MEK inhibitors have produced overall suboptimal response rates in most mutational subsets, however. The hints of activity suggest that a backbone of MEK inhibition in combination with other targeted therapy agents may be a viable treatment strategy.

One of the initial combinations proposed was MEK inhibition plus agents that block PI3K/AKT signaling. This pathway has been implicated as active in RAS mutant tumors as well as BRAF inhibitor resistance. Preclinical rationale seemed to support this approach, but preliminary studies have been disappointing. For example, selumetinib and MK-2206 (AKT inhibitor) in pretreated KRAS mutant pancreatic cancer resulted in inferior outcomes compared with FOLFOX chemotherapy; the same combination produced no responses in colorectal cancer.[66,67] Trametinib and the pan-PI3K/MTOR inhibitor GSK2126458 were also poorly tolerated and associated with low response rates in solid tumors.[68] On the other hand, trametinib in combination with buparlisib (pan-PI3K inhibitor) produced a 29% response rate in *KRAS* mutant ovarian cancer.[69] Thus, developing the most active, potent, and nontoxic combinations may prove that dual pathway inhibition is viable.

Another intriguing preclinical study suggested that combining inhibitors of MEK and CDK4/6 would produce synergistic efficacy in *NRAS* mutant melanoma.[70] In this study, MEK inhibition and *NRAS* extinction were compared in an inducible mouse model of *NRAS* mutant melanoma. MEK inhibition caused apoptosis but not cell cycle arrest, in contrast to NRAS extinction. Network modeling showed that CDK4 was a key determinant of this difference, and combining MEK and CDK4/6 inhibition induced apoptosis, cell cycle arrest, and cell death. Although dose finding and toxicities were challenging, early results from the combination of binimetinib and ribociclib demonstrated a confirmed response rate in 25% of melanoma patients and a median progression-free survival of 6.7 months, with most treated patients experiencing some degree of tumor shrinkage.[71] This approach is now being pursued in *BRAF/NRAS* wild-type melanoma and in other *RAS* mutant malignancies.

Combinations of MAPK pathway inhibitors and immunotherapy have also been explored. An initial study combining vemurafenib with ipilimumab (anti–CTLA-4) in *BRAF* mutant melanoma was halted early due to hepatotoxicity. Similarly, a trial of ipilimumab + dabrafenib + trametinib was halted early due to bowel perforations, although the doublet of ipilimumab and dabrafenib appeared tolerable.[72] More recently, combinations of anti–PD-1/PD-L1 with BRAF and/or MEK inhibitors have demonstrated promising efficacy. The triple combination of atezolizumab, cobimetinib, and vemurafenib demonstrated an 85% response rate among the first 34 patients treated.[73] Perhaps more intriguingly, the combination of atezolizumab and cobimetinib produced a 20% response rate in patients with colorectal cancer, when either drug alone would

not be expected to produce responses. Preclinical studies have suggested that MEK inhibitors promote enhanced antigen expression and effector T-cell function, suggesting that MEK inhibitors may render less immunogenic tumors sensitive to immune checkpoint inhibitors.[74,75]

Conclusions

MAPK pathway signaling is frequently dysregulated in a diverse array of deadly cancers. Targeting mutant BRAF with BRAF and MEK inhibitors in several cancers has been the primary success story in this arena to date, although overcoming acquired resistance remains the major clinical challenge. A number of promising approaches involving MEK inhibitors are poised to affect the disease course of various *RAS* mutant cancers as well.

References

1. Johnson DB, Smalley KS, Sosman JA. Molecular pathways: targeting NRAS in melanoma and acute myelogenous leukemia. *Clin Cancer Res.* 2014;20(16):4186-4192.
2. Gao J, Aksoy BA, Dogrusoz U, et al. Integrative analysis of complex cancer genomics and clinical profiles using the cBioPortal. *Sci Signal.* 2013;6:pl1.
3. Ascierto PA, Schadendorf D, Berking C, et al. MEK162 for patients with advanced melanoma harbouring NRAS or Val600 BRAF mutations: a non-randomised, open-label phase 2 study. *Lancet Oncol.* 2013;14:249-256.
4. Van Raamsdonk CD, Bezrookove V, Green G, et al. Frequent somatic mutations of GNAQ in uveal melanoma and blue naevi. *Nature.* 2009;457:599-602.
5. Johnson DB, Roszik J, Shoushtari AN, et al. Comparative analysis of the GNAQ, GNA11, SF3B1, and EIF1AX driver mutations in melanoma and across the cancer spectrum. *Pigment Cell Melanoma Res.* 2016;29(4):470-473.
6. Chen X, Wu Q, Depeille P, et al. RasGRP3 mediates MAPK pathway activation in GNAQ mutant uveal melanoma. *Cancer Cell.* 2017;31:685-696, e6.
7. Cancer Genome Atlas Network. Genomic classification of cutaneous melanoma. *Cell.* 2015;161:1681-1696.
8. Flaherty KT, Lee SJ, Zhao F, et al. Phase III trial of carboplatin and paclitaxel with or without sorafenib in metastatic melanoma. *J Clin Oncol.* 2013;31:373-379.
9. Su Y, Vilgelm AE, Kelley MC, et al. RAF265 inhibits the growth of advanced human melanoma tumors. *Clin Cancer Res.* 2012;18:2184-2198.
10. Bollag G, Hirth P, Tsai J, et al. Clinical efficacy of a RAF inhibitor needs broad target blockade in BRAF-mutant melanoma. *Nature.* 2010;467:596-599.
11. Flaherty KT, Puzanov I, Kim KB, et al. Inhibition of mutated, activated BRAF in metastatic melanoma. *N Engl J Med.* 2010;363:809-819.
12. Chapman PB, Hauschild A, Robert C, et al. Improved survival with vemurafenib in melanoma with BRAF V600E mutation. *N Engl J Med.* 2011;364:2507-2516.
13. Falchook GS, Long GV, Kurzrock R, et al. Dabrafenib in patients with melanoma, untreated brain metastases, and other solid tumours: a phase 1 dose-escalation trial. *Lancet.* 2012;379:1893-1901.
14. Long GV, Trefzer U, Davies MA, et al. Dabrafenib in patients with Val600Glu or Val600Lys BRAF-mutant melanoma metastatic to the brain (BREAK-MB): a multicentre, open-label, phase 2 trial. *Lancet Oncol.* 2012;13(11):1087-1095.
15. Hyman DM, Puzanov I, Subbiah V, et al. Vemurafenib in multiple nonmelanoma cancers with BRAF V600 mutations. *N Engl J Med.* 2015;373:726-736.
16. Corcoran RB, Atreya CE, Falchook GS, et al. Combined BRAF and MEK inhibition with dabrafenib and trametinib in BRAF V600-mutant colorectal cancer. *J Clin Oncol.* 2015;33:4023-4031.
17. Tiacci E, Park JH, De Carolis L, et al. Targeting mutant BRAF in relapsed or refractory hairy-cell leukemia. *N Engl J Med.* 2015;373:1733-1747.
18. McArthur GA, Chapman PB, Robert C, et al. Safety and efficacy of vemurafenib in BRAF(V600E) and BRAF(V600K) mutation-positive melanoma

(BRIM-3): extended follow-up of a phase 3, randomised, open-label study. *Lancet Oncol.* 2014;15:323-332.

19. Long GV, Stroyakovskiy D, Gogas H, et al. Dabrafenib and trametinib versus dabrafenib and placebo for Val600 BRAF-mutant melanoma: a multicentre, double-blind, phase 3 randomised controlled trial. *Lancet.* 2015;386:444-451.

20. Su F, Viros A, Milagre C, et al. RAS mutations in cutaneous squamous-cell carcinomas in patients treated with BRAF inhibitors. *N Engl J Med.* 2012;366:207-215.

21. Callahan MK, Rampal R, Harding JJ, et al. Progression of RAS-mutant leukemia during RAF inhibitor treatment. *N Engl J Med.* 2012;367:2316-2321.

22. Abdel-Wahab O, Klimek VM, Gaskell AA, et al. Efficacy of intermittent combined RAF and MEK inhibition in a patient with concurrent BRAF-and NRAS-mutant malignancies. *Cancer Discov.* 2014;4:538-545.

23. Infante JR, Fecher LA, Falchook GS, et al. Safety, pharmacokinetic, pharmacodynamic, and efficacy data for the oral MEK inhibitor trametinib: a phase 1 dose-escalation trial. *Lancet Oncol.* 2012;13:773-781.

24. Falchook GS, Lewis KD, Infante JR, et al. Activity of the oral MEK inhibitor trametinib in patients with advanced melanoma: a phase 1 dose-escalation trial. *Lancet Oncol.* 2012;13:782-789.

25. Flaherty KT, Robert C, Hersey P, et al. Improved survival with MEK inhibition in *BRAF*-mutated melanoma. *N Engl J Med.* 2012;367:107-114.

26. Janne PA, Shaw AT, Pereira JR, et al. Selumetinib plus docetaxel for KRAS-mutant advanced non-small-cell lung cancer: a randomised, multicentre, placebo-controlled, phase 2 study. *Lancet Oncol.* 2013;14:38-47.

27. Carvajal RD, Sosman JA, Quevedo JF, et al. Effect of selumetinib vs chemotherapy on progression-free survival in uveal melanoma: a randomized clinical trial. *JAMA.* 2014;311:2397-2405.

28. Robert C, Dummer R, Gutzmer R, et al. Selumetinib plus dacarbazine versus placebo plus dacarbazine as first-line treatment for BRAF-mutant metastatic melanoma: a phase 2 double-blind randomised study. *Lancet Oncol.* 2013;14:733-740.

29. Dombi E, Baldwin A, Marcus LJ, et al. Activity of selumetinib in neurofibromatosis type 1-related plexiform neurofibromas. *N Engl J Med.* 2016;375:2550-2560.

30. Dummer R, Schadendorf D, Ascierto PA, et al. Binimetinib versus dacarbazine in patients with advanced NRAS-mutant melanoma (NEMO): a multicentre, open-label, randomised, phase 3 trial. *Lancet Oncol.* 2017;18:435-445.

31. Dahlman KB, Xia J, Hutchinson K, et al. BRAF L597 mutations in melanoma are associated with sensitivity to MEK inhibitors. *Cancer Discov.* 2012;2(9):791-797.

32. Hutchinson KE, Lipson D, Stephens PJ, et al. BRAF fusions define a distinct molecular subset of melanomas with potential sensitivity to MEK inhibition. *Clin Cancer Res.* 2013;19:6696-6702.

33. Flaherty KT, Infante JR, Daud A, et al. Combined BRAF and MEK inhibition in melanoma with BRAF V600 mutations. *N Engl J Med.* 2012;367(18):1694-1703.

34. Johnson DB, Flaherty KT, Weber JS, et al. Combined BRAF (dabrafenib) and MEK inhibition (trametinib) in patients with BRAFV600-mutant melanoma experiencing progression with single-agent BRAF inhibitor. *J Clin Oncol.* 2014;32(33):3697-3704.

35. Johnson DB, Menzies AM, Zimmer L, et al. Acquired BRAF inhibitor resistance: A multicenter meta-analysis of the spectrum and frequencies, clinical behaviour, and phenotypic associations of resistance mechanisms. *Eur J Cancer.* 2015;51(18):2792-2799.

36. Chen G, McQuade JL, Panka DJ, et al. Clinical, molecular, and immune analysis of dabrafenib-trametinib combination treatment for BRAF inhibitor-refractory metastatic melanoma: a phase 2 clinical trial. *JAMA Oncol.* 2016;2:1056-1064.

37. Robert C, Karaszewska B, Schachter J, et al. Improved overall survival in melanoma with combined dabrafenib and trametinib. *N Engl J Med.* 2015;372(1):30-39.

38. Prahallad A, Sun C, Huang S, et al. Unresponsiveness of colon cancer to BRAF(V600E) inhibition through feedback activation of EGFR. *Nature.* 2012;483:100-103.

39. Corcoran RB, Ebi H, Turke AB, et al. EGFR-mediated re-activation of MAPK signaling contributes to insensitivity of *BRAF* mutant colorectal cancers to RAF inhibition with vemurafenib. *Cancer Discov.* 2012;2:227-235.

40. Ribas A, Gonzalez R, Pavlick A, et al. Combination of vemurafenib and cobimetinib in patients with advanced *BRAF*(V600)-mutated melanoma: a phase 1b study. *Lancet Oncol.* 2014;15:954-965.

41. Larkin J, Ascierto PA, Dreno B, et al. Combined vemurafenib and cobimetinib in *BRAF*-mutated melanoma. *N Engl J Med.* 2014;371:1867-1876.

42. Schreuer M, Jansen Y, Planken S, et al. Combination of dabrafenib plus trametinib for BRAF and MEK inhibitor pretreated patients with advanced BRAFV600-mutant melanoma: an open-label, single arm, dual-centre, phase 2 clinical trial. *Lancet Oncol.* 2017;18:464-472.

43. Konieczkowski DJ, Johannessen CM, Abudayyeh O, et al. A melanoma cell state distinction influences sensitivity to MAPK pathway inhibitors. *Cancer Discov.* 2014;4:816-827.

44. Muller J, Krijgsman O, Tsoi J, et al. Low MITF/AXL ratio predicts early resistance to multiple targeted drugs in melanoma. *Nat Commun.* 2014;5:5712.

45. Carlino MS, Fung C, Shahheydari H, et al. Preexisting MEK1P124 mutations diminish response to BRAF inhibitors in metastatic melanoma patients. *Clin Cancer Res.* 2015;21:98-105.

46. Straussman R, Morikawa T, Shee K, et al. Tumour micro-environment elicits innate resistance to RAF inhibitors through HGF secretion. *Nature.* 2012;487:500-504.

47. Wilson TR, Fridlyand J, Yan Y, et al. Widespread potential for growth-factor-driven resistance to anticancer kinase inhibitors. *Nature.* 2012;487:505-509.

48. Van Allen EM, Wagle N, Sucker A, et al. The genetic landscape of clinical resistance to RAF inhibition in metastatic melanoma. *Cancer Discov.* 2014;4:94-109.

49. Amaral T, Sinnberg T, Meier F, et al. The mitogen-activated protein kinase pathway in melanoma part I—activation and primary resistance mechanisms to BRAF inhibition. *Eur J Cancer.* 2017;73:85-92.

50. Menzies AM, Wilmott JS, Drummond M, et al. Clinicopathologic features associated with efficacy and long-term survival in metastatic melanoma patients treated with BRAF or combined BRAF and MEK inhibitors. *Cancer.* 2015;121:3826-3835.

51. Long GV, Grob JJ, Nathan P, et al. Factors predictive of response, disease progression, and overall survival after dabrafenib and trametinib combination treatment: a pooled analysis of individual patient data from randomised trials. *Lancet Oncol.* 2016;17:1743-1754.

52. Shi H, Hugo W, Kong X, et al. Acquired resistance and clonal evolution in melanoma during BRAF inhibitor therapy. *Cancer Discov.* 2014;4:80-93.

53. Rizos H, Menzies AM, Pupo GM, et al. BRAF inhibitor resistance mechanisms in metastatic melanoma: spectrum and clinical impact. *Clin Cancer Res.* 2014;20:1965-1977.

54. Haq R, Shoag J, Andreu-Perez P, et al. Oncogenic BRAF regulates oxidative metabolism via PGC1alpha and MITF. *Cancer Cell.* 2013;23:302-315.

55. Hugo W, Shi H, Sun L, et al. Non-genomic and immune evolution of melanoma acquiring MAPKi resistance. *Cell.* 2015;162:1271-1285.

56. Moriceau G, Hugo W, Hong A, et al. Tunable-combinatorial mechanisms of acquired resistance limit the efficacy of BRAF/MEK cotargeting but result in melanoma drug addiction. *Cancer Cell.* 2015;27:240-256.

57. Wagle N, Van Allen EM, Treacy DJ, et al. MAP kinase pathway alterations in BRAF-mutant melanoma patients with acquired resistance to combined RAF/MEK inhibition. *Cancer Discov.* 2014;4:61-68.

58. Long GV, Fung C, Menzies AM, et al. Increased MAPK reactivation in early resistance to dabrafenib/trametinib combination therapy of BRAF-mutant metastatic melanoma. *Nat Commun.* 2014;5:5694.

59. Das Thakur M, Salangsang F, Landman AS, et al. Modelling vemurafenib resistance in melanoma reveals a strategy to forestall drug resistance. *Nature.* 2013;494:251-255.

60. Samatar AA, Poulikakos PI. Targeting RAS-ERK signalling in cancer: promises and challenges. *Nat Rev Drug Discov.* 2014;13:928-942.

61. Morris EJ, Jha S, Restaino CR, et al. Discovery of a novel ERK inhibitor with activity in models of acquired resistance to BRAF and MEK inhibitors. *Cancer Discov.* 2013;3:742-750.

62. Li BT, Janku F, Patel MR, et al. First-in-class oral ERK1/2 inhibitor ulixertinib (BVD-523) in patients with advanced solid tumors: final results of a phase I dose escalation and expansion study. *J Clin Oncol.* 2017;35:2508-.

63. Jameson KL, Mazur PK, Zehnder AM, et al. IQGAP1 scaffold-kinase interaction blockade selectively targets RAS-MAP kinase-driven tumors. *Nat Med.* 2013;19:626-630.

64. Zhang C, Spevak W, Zhang Y, et al. RAF inhibitors that evade paradoxical MAPK pathway activation. *Nature*. 2015;526:583-586.

65. Okimoto RA, Lin L, Olivas V, et al. Preclinical efficacy of a RAF inhibitor that evades paradoxical MAPK pathway activation in protein kinase BRAF-mutant lung cancer. *Proc Natl Acad Sci U S A*. 2016;113:13456-13461.

66. Chung V, McDonough S, Philip PA, et al. Effect of selumetinib and MK-2206 vs oxaliplatin and fluorouracil in patients with metastatic pancreatic cancer after prior therapy: SWOG S1115 Study Randomized Clinical Trial. *JAMA Oncol*. 2017;3:516-522.

67. Do K, Speranza G, Bishop R, et al. Biomarker-driven phase 2 study of MK-2206 and selumetinib (AZD6244, ARRY-142886) in patients with colorectal cancer. *Invest New Drugs*. 2015;33:720-728.

68. Grilley-Olson JE, Bedard PL, Fasolo A, et al. A phase Ib dose-escalation study of the MEK inhibitor trametinib in combination with the PI3K/mTOR inhibitor GSK2126458 in patients with advanced solid tumors. *Invest New Drugs*. 2016;34:740-749.

69. Bedard PL, Tabernero J, Janku F, et al. A phase Ib dose-escalation study of the oral pan-PI3K inhibitor buparlisib (BKM120) in combination with the oral MEK1/2 inhibitor trametinib (GSK1120212) in patients with selected advanced solid tumors. *Clin Cancer Res*. 2015;21:730-738.

70. Kwong LN, Costello JC, Liu H, et al. Oncogenic NRAS signaling differentially regulates survival and proliferation in melanoma. *Nat Med*. 2012;18:1503-1510.

71. Schuler MH, Ascierto PA, Vos FYFLD, et al. Phase 1b/2 trial of ribociclib+binimetinib in metastatic NRAS-mutant melanoma: safety, efficacy, and recommended phase 2 dose (RP2D). *J Clin Oncol*. 2017;35:9519.

72. Minor DR, Puzanov I, Callahan MK, et al. Severe gastrointestinal toxicity with administration of trametinib in combination with dabrafenib and ipilimumab. *Pigment Cell Melanoma Res*. 2015;28:611-612.

73. Sullivan RJ, Gonzalez R, Lewis KD, et al. Atezolizumab (A) + cobimetinib (C) + vemurafenib (V) in BRAFV600-mutant metastatic melanoma (mel): updated safety and clinical activity. *J Clin Oncol*. 2017;35:3063.

74. Loi S, Dushyanthen S, Beavis PA, et al. RAS/MAPK activation is associated with reduced tumor-infiltrating lymphocytes in triple-negative breast cancer: therapeutic cooperation between MEK and PD-1/PD-L1 immune checkpoint inhibitors. *Clin Cancer Res*. 2016;22(6):1499-1509.

75. Ebert PJ, Cheung J, Yang Y, et al. MAP kinase inhibition promotes T cell and anti-tumor activity in combination with PD-L1 checkpoint blockade. *Immunity*. 2016;44:609-621.

CDK Inhibitors

Geoffrey I. Shapiro

Introduction

The cyclin-dependent kinases (CDKs) comprise a family of serine/threonine kinases divided into two groups based on their roles in regulating cell cycle progression (cell cycle CDKs) and transcriptional control (transcriptional CDKs). Both genetic and epigenetic events commonly lead to overactivity of the cell cycle CDKs in human cancer, such as CDKs 4 and 6, and their inhibition can lead to cell cycle arrest, senescence, and apoptosis. Recently, selective inhibitors of CDKs 4 and 6, including palbociclib, ribociclib, and abemaciclib, have transformed the treatment of estrogen receptor–positive (ER$^+$) breast cancer and have also demonstrated promise against other cancer types, both as monotherapy and in combination with inhibitors of signal transduction. Furthermore, selective CDK4/6 inhibitors display complex interactions with the immune microenvironment and have demonstrated preclinical synergy with immune checkpoint blockade.

The transcriptional CDKs phosphorylate the carboxy-terminal domain (CTD) of RNA polymerase II, facilitating efficient transcriptional initiation, elongation, and processing. Inhibition of these CDKs has been shown to disrupt expression of genes under super-enhancer control that define oncogenic states, genes with short half-life, many of which are critical for cancer cell survival, as well as genes expressed in response to cellular stresses, including those mediating DNA repair processes. This biology has propelled the continued interest in inhibition of these CDKs as an anticancer strategy. Agents targeting transcriptional CDKs frequently inhibit cell cycle CDKs as well, although recently, the targeting of cysteines remote from the ATP-binding site has resulted in the synthesis of selective compounds that have entered clinical development.

Cell Cycle CDKs and Cell Cycle Control

The cell cycle is composed of four phases: G1, S, G2, and M, during which cells undergo growth, DNA replication, and mitosis. Cell cycle regulatory CDKs, including CDKs 1, 2, 3, 4, and 6, along with their specific cyclin-binding partners, control cell growth and proliferation by tightly regulating transition through the phases of the cell cycle (Fig. 23.1).[1–3] Cyclin C-CDK3 participates in G0 exit.[4] The G1/S transition is controlled in large part by cyclin D-CDK4/6 and cyclin E-CDK2 complexes, which sequentially phosphorylate and ultimately inactivate the retinoblastoma susceptibility protein (Rb). Progression through S phase, the

G$_2$/M transition, and mitotic progression are controlled by cyclin A-CDK1/2 and cyclin B-CDK1 complexes.

Current models of G1 progression suggest that CDK phosphorylation promotes sequential intramolecular interactions that progressively modulate Rb function.[5,6] As cells exit G0, Rb is bound to E2F; this interaction not only sequesters and blocks transcriptional activation of E2F but also actively represses transcription by recruiting histone deacetylases to the promoters of genes required for S-phase entry. Following stimulation by growth factor signaling pathways, cells synthesize D-type cyclins that assemble with CDKs 4 and 6, a process that requires contribution of a Cip/Kip family member (e.g., p21$^{Waf1/Cip1}$ or p27^{Kip1}).[7] Cyclin D–dependent kinases monophosphorylate Rb at any one of 14 phosphorylation sites; monophosphorylated Rb prevents cell cycle exit and a return to G0, but is still bound to E2F transcription factors.[8] Nonetheless, CDK4/6-mediated phosphorylation displaces histone deacetylase from the Rb central pocket, thereby preventing active transcriptional repression by Rb.[6]

Although Cip/Kip family members promote activity of cyclin D–dependent kinases, they are also potent inhibitors of CDK2. Therefore, the assembly of cyclin D–dependent kinase complexes promotes the activation of cyclin E-CDK2.[7] Additionally, the displacement of histone acetylase from the central pocket facilitates a second interaction that leads to phosphorylation of the pocket by CDK2, affecting pocket structure and disrupting the binding of Rb to E2F.[6] Processive hyperphosphorylation of Rb by cyclin E-CDK2 occurs in late G1,[8] allowing E2F activation and the transcription of genes necessary for S-phase entry and progression, including cyclin E itself.[9,10] Cyclin E-CDK2 also phosphorylates p27^{Kip1}, resulting in its ubiquitination and degradation,[11,12] establishing a positive feedback loop further facilitating S-phase entry.

Cell cycle CDK activity is regulated by a number of mechanisms, including positive phosphorylation events by CDK-activating kinase (CAK; cyclin H/cdk7/MAT1),[13] negative phosphorylation events,[14] and by endogenous regulators, which not only include Cip/Kip family members but also members of the INK4 family that specifically inhibit CDKs 4 and 6.[15] INK4 family members, including p16^{INK4A} (encoded by *CDKN2A*) and p15^{INK4B} (encoded by *CDKN2B*), associate with CDK4 or CDK6 in dimeric complexes, displacing the Cip/Kip family member to CDK2 (causing its inhibition) as well as the D-cyclin, which is degraded. Therefore, as levels of p16^{INK4A} increase as cells undergo senescence,[16,17] there is potent cell cycle arrest mediated by direct CDK4/6 inhibition and indirect CDK2 inhibition.[18] Similarly, p15^{INK4B} functions as an effector of TGF-β–mediated growth arrest in concert with Cip/Kip proteins.[19,20]

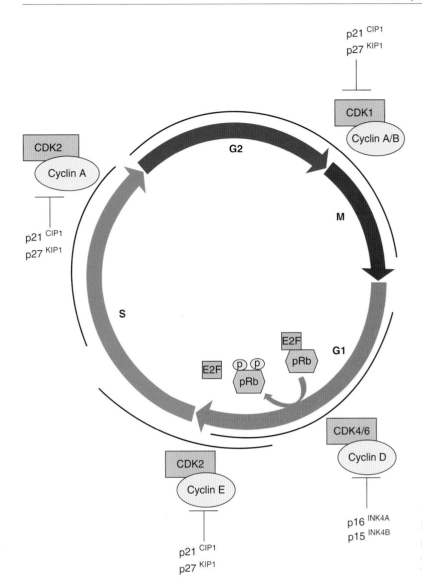

FIGURE **23.1** The mammalian cell cycle. D-cyclin–dependent kinases CDK4 and CDK6 and cyclin E-CDK2 complexes sequentially phosphorylate Rb to facilitate the G1 to S transition. Cyclin A-CDK1/2 and cyclin B-CDK1 complexes control S-phase progression, the G2/M transition, and M-phase progression.

Altered Expression of Cell Cycle CDKs and Their Regulators in Cancer

Uncontrolled cell proliferation due to dysregulation of the cell cycle is a hallmark of cancer,[21] with the growth advantage of cancer cells commonly resulting from alterations that cause elevated CDK activity (Table 23.1).

Cancer cells frequently activate CDK4/6 via increased expression of D-cyclins, often a result of gene amplification.[101] In the case of breast cancer, high levels of cyclin D1 have also been described in the absence of genomic alterations. In mantle cell lymphoma (MCL), cyclin D1 is overexpressed as a result of the hallmark $t(11;14)$ rearrangement.[102–104] Screening of primary MCLs has also revealed deletions or mutations in the 3′untranslated region that create a premature polyadenylation signal, resulting in cyclin D1 mRNAs lacking destabilization elements and contributing to the upregulation of cyclin D1 expression.[22] Additionally, mutations in cyclin D1 or cyclin D3 can directly perturb their degradation in a variety of solid tumor types or lymphomas, respectively. Such mutations directly target the T286 (cyclin D1) or T283 (cyclin D3) GSK3β

phosphorylation site or the adjacent nuclear export signal and result in nuclear retention of the cyclin, and promoting oncogenicity.[105–107] Alternative splicing of *CCND1* has also been described, resulting in the expression of cyclin D1b, which lacks the T286 phosphorylation site.[108] Hyperactivation of CDK4/6 may also directly result from amplification of the genes encoding the kinases themselves or via loss of expression of INK4 proteins; *CDKN2A*, encoding p16[INK4A], may be deleted, mutated, or silenced by promoter hypermethylation.[109] Germ-line mutations in *CDKN2A* have been described in familial cases of melanoma and pancreatic cancer.[110,111]

CCNE1, which encodes the cyclin E protein, is often amplified in cancer, and cyclin E protein is frequently overexpressed in a variety of cancer types. Notably, *CCNE1* amplification occurs in up to 20% of ovarian cancers, representing a subtype with high proliferative potential that is often resistant or refractory to standard chemotherapy[62] and that is homologous recombination (HR) repair proficient[112] and insensitive to poly(ADP-ribose) polymerase (PARP) inhibition. CDK2 activity may also be increased in cancers due to reduced or absent expression of *CDKN1B*, encoding p27[KIP1],[12,113,114] or amplification or overexpression of the genes encoding CDK2 or cyclin A. Similarly, the genes encoding CDK1 and cyclin B can also be overexpressed.

TABLE

23.1 *Representative alterations in cyclins, cell cycle CDKs, and endogenous CDK inhibitors in cancer*

Cell Cycle Gene/Protein	Alteration	Cancer Type	References
Cyclin D1	Overexpression, mutation, splice variant	Squamous cell lung cancer, squamous cell esophageal cancer, cervical cancer, gastric cancer, SCCHN, endometrial cancer, bladder cancer, mantle cell lymphoma, multiple myeloma	22–36
Cyclin D2	Overexpression, amplification	Glioma, gastric cancer, lymphoma, leukemia, testicular germ cell tumors, adrenal cancer, neuroendocrine carcinoma, squamous cell carcinoma, ovarian cancer, squamous cell carcinoma of the esophagus, other solid tumor types	37–42
Cyclin D3	Overexpression, amplification	Lymphoma, leukemia, leiomyosarcoma, GIST, bladder cancer, esophageal adenocarcinoma, anal squamous cell carcinoma, head and neck cancer, cervical cancer, breast cancer, pancreatic cancer, other solid tumor types	38,42–46
CDK4	Overexpression, amplification, mutation	Glioblastoma, osteosarcoma, rhabdomyosarcoma, melanoma, squamous cell lung cancer, squamous cell esophageal cancer, cervical cancer, pancreatic neuroendocrine cancer, adenocarcinoma of the esophagus, lung cancer	24,26,47–57
CDK6	Overexpression, amplification	Glioma, squamous cell esophageal cancer, squamous cell lung cancer, medulloblastoma, gastric cancer, pancreatic neuroendocrine cancer, adenocarcinoma of the esophagus, lymphoma	23–25,54,55,57–61
Cyclin E	Overexpression, amplification	Gastric cancer, endometrial cancer, ovarian cancer, NSCLC, breast cancer, osteosarcoma, pancreatic cancer, colorectal cancer, leukemia, lymphoma	25,58,62–81
CDK2	Overexpression	Melanoma, colorectal cancer	77,82,83
Cyclin A	Overexpression, amplification	Acute myeloid leukemia, soft tissue sarcoma, ovarian cancer, breast cancer, squamous cell carcinoma of the esophagus, hepatocellular carcinoma, thyroid carcinoma, endometrial adenocarcinoma	84–93
Cyclin B	Overexpression	Breast cancer, thyroid cancer, endometrial cancer, NSCLC, pancreatic cancer, astrocytoma, gastric cancer	90,94–100

Selective CDK4/6 Inhibitors

Overview

The universal inactivation of the Rb protein in human cancer, commonly due to excessive phosphorylation mediated by alterations that activate the D-cyclin–dependent kinases 4 and 6, has motivated the clinical development of highly selective, ATP-competitive, orally bioavailable CDK4/6 inhibitors, including palbociclib, ribociclib, and abemaciclib[115,116] (Table 23.2), all of which are FDA approved for estrogen receptor–positive (ER+) metastatic breast cancer in combination with hormonal treatment.[128] In biochemical assays, these agents demonstrate half-maximal inhibitory concentrations (IC_{50}) in the low nanomolar range, with a high degree of selectivity. In cancer cell lines, Rb phosphorylation is reduced, typically causing Rb-dependent G1 arrest. However, other biological outcomes of CDK4/6 inhibition include induction of senescence and/or apoptosis that has translated to tumor growth inhibition and/or regression against a wide variety of solid and liquid tumor xenografts.[117–120,129–131]

Early-phase trials of these agents are completed, demonstrating favorable pharmacokinetic properties and evidence of target engagement in both tumor and surrogate tissues, using immunohistochemical assays for Rb phosphorylation and antiproliferative markers indicative of G1 arrest.[121–126]

Abemaciclib is distinguished from palbociclib and ribociclib by somewhat reduced selectivity for CDK4/6 in biochemical assays, although evidence of CDK9 inhibition has not been demonstrated in cells at concentrations as high as 20 μM. Although reduced phosphorylation of Rb in skin keratinocytes was routinely observed at 4 hours post dose, based on reversibility by 24 hours, a twice-daily schedule was adopted, whereas palbociclib and ribociclib are administered once daily. Abemaciclib has also been shown to cross the blood-brain barrier in preclinical studies.[132] In the phase 1 study, concentrations in the cerebrospinal fluid of glioblastoma patients approximated those achieved in plasma. Abemaciclib produces less profound neutropenia affording continuous daily dosing[124]; in contrast, palbociclib and ribociclib require intermittent schedules, typically three weeks of every four (3/1 dosing).[121,123] For palbociclib, doses have also been established for a two-of-every-three-week schedule (2/1 dosing).[122] The reason for the reduced hematologic toxicity following abemaciclib treatment is not well understood, but may be related to greater selectivity for CDK4 over CDK6, since cyclin D3-CDK6 activity is integral to hematopoietic stem cell differentiation.[133,134] It is possible that continuous dosing contributes to a greater degree of single-agent efficacy in ER+ breast cancer than the other agents, and abemaciclib is also approved as monotherapy in this breast cancer subtype.[135]

Two other CDK4/6 inhibitors in development include G1T28 (trilaciclib),[136] formulated intravenously, and G1T38, a highly potent orally bioavailable CDK inhibitor selective for

TABLE

23.2   *Properties of FDA-approved selective CDK4/6 inhibitors*

Drug	Palbociclib PD0332991 Ibrance®	Ribociclib LEE011 Kisqali®	Abemaciclib LY2835219 Verzenio®
Activity (IC$_{50}$)			
CDK4	9 to 11 nmol/L	10 nmol/L	0.6 to 2 nmol/L
CDK6	15 nmol/L	39 nmol/L	2.4 to 5 nmol/L
CDK1	>10 μmol/L	>100 μmol/L	>1 μmol/L
CDK2	>10 μmol/L	>50 μmol/L	>500 nmol/L
CDK9	[115–118]	[115,116,119]	57 nmol/L[115,116,120]
PK parameters			
T_{max}	4.2 to 5.5 h	4 h	4 to 6 h
$t_{1/2}$	25.9 to 26.7 h[121,122]	24 to 36 h[123]	17 to 38 h[124]
PD markers	Reduced pRb and FLT-PET uptake in paired tumor biopsies (mantle cell lymphoma)[125]	Reduced pRb and Ki-67 expression in paired tumor biopsies[123]	Reduced pRb and topoisomerase IIα expression in paired tumor and skin biopsies[124]
Dosing	125 mg daily (3/1 schedule) or 200 mg daily (2/1 schedule)[121,122]	600 mg daily (3/1 schedule)[123]	200 mg twice daily (continuous dosing)[124]
Adverse events			
Major dose-limiting toxicities	Neutropenia, thrombocytopenia	Neutropenia, thrombocytopenia	Fatigue
Other reported adverse events	Anemia, nausea, anorexia, fatigue, diarrhea[121,122]	Mucositis, prolonged EKG QTc interval, nausea, elevated creatinine[123]	Diarrhea, neutropenia[124]
Early evidence of activity	Phase 1 studies: SD in 19/74 patients with advanced solid tumors; 9 patients received ≥10 cycles on 3/1 or 2/1 schedule. CRs and PR in mantle cell lymphoma; PR in a patient with growing teratoma syndrome (confirmed in phase 2 trial)[121,122,125–127]	SD lasting >6 cycles observed in 14% of treated patients. PRs in patients with *PIK3CA*-mutated, *CCND1*-amplified, and ER$^+$ breast cancer and in WT *BRAF/NRAS*, *CCND1*-amplified melanoma[123]	Clinical benefit rate of 61% among 36 patients with ER$^+$ breast cancer; responses also observed in NSCLC and melanoma[124]

CDK4/cyclin D1 and CDK6/cyclin D3, with IC$_{50}$ values of 1 and 2 nm, respectively,[137] that demonstrates activity in ER$^+$ breast cancer xenografts comparable to palbociclib. Importantly, this compound accumulated in xenografts as opposed to plasma, indicating that the possibility of less neutropenia and a continuous dosing schedule. Another preclinical study of G1T38 in castration-resistant prostate cancer (CRPC) demonstrated that in animal models, G1T38 treatment resulted in comparable efficacy to docetaxel, but exhibited significantly less toxicity.[138] Currently, G1T38 in combination with fulvestrant is being tested in a phase 1/2 clinical trial in HR$^+$/HER$^-$ locally advanced or metastatic breast cancer (NCT02983071).

Breast Cancer Monotherapy

Preclinical data with palbociclib in ER$^+$ breast cancer cell lines showed sensitivity compared to ER$^-$ cell lines, due in part to the higher incidence of Rb negativity in ER$^-$ disease,[139] but also due to the dependence of ER$^+$ breast cancer cells on cyclin D1-CDK4 for proliferation, as well as the integral relationship between cyclin D1 and estrogen receptor–mediated transcriptional events.[140]

In a phase 2 study of the 3/1 palbociclib dosing schedule in Rb$^+$ ER$^+$/HER2$^-$ and Rb$^+$ ER$^-$/HER2$^-$ advanced breast cancer patients, 1 patient achieved partial response and 5 had stable disease (SD) for ≥ 6 months among ER$^+$/HER2$^-$ patients. The median progression-free survival (PFS) was 3.8 and 1.5 months for the ER$^+$ and ER$^-$ groups ($P = 0.03$), respectively.[141] When patients were stratified by the number of prior treatments, longer PFS was seen in patients with ER$^+$ tumors who had received more than two lines of antiestrogen therapy as compared to those who received fewer therapeutic cycles (5 versus 2 months, $P = 0.023$), suggesting substantial activity in the setting of acquired endocrine resistance. Of note, cytopenia resulted in treatment interruption in 24% of patients and dose reductions in 51% of patients.

In a breast cancer expansion cohort of the initial phase 1 study, 47 patients were treated who had received a median of 7 prior systemic therapies.[124] The disease control rate was higher for ER$^+$ (29/36, 81%) versus ER$^-$ tumors (3/9, 33%), with radiographic responses exclusively in the ER$^+$ population. Among ER$^+$ patients, the clinical benefit rate was 61%; 11/36 patients (31%) achieved partial response (four of whom had continued prior endocrine therapy) and 18/36 (50%) patients had SD, including 11/36 (31%) with SD ≥24 weeks. In the overall ER⁺ patient population, the median duration of response was 13.4 months (95% CI, 3.7 to 13.4) and median PFS was 8.8 months (95% CI, 4.2 to 16.0). In some breast cancer patients in this study, fatigue and diarrhea led to dose reductions from 200 to 150 mg twice daily; however, pharmacodynamic inhibition of CDK4/6 was still demonstrated in patients treated at the reduced dose.

This expansion cohort was followed by a phase 2 study of abemaciclib initiated to evaluate its activity and toxicity profile as monotherapy in heavily pretreated patients with ER⁺/HER2⁻ metastatic breast cancer (MONARCH 1).[135] Patients received abemaciclib 200 mg, twice daily continuously with objective response rate (ORR) as the primary endpoint. Secondary endpoints included clinical benefit rate, PFS, and overall survival (OS). The confirmed ORR at the 12-month final analysis was 19.7%. The clinical benefit rate, defined as CR + PR + SD ≥ 6 months, was 42.4%. Median PFS was 6.0 months, and median OS was 17.7 months. Overall, treatment was well tolerated, with diarrhea, fatigue, and nausea being the most common side effects; adverse events led to treatment discontinuation in 7.6% of patients. This study formed the basis of the approval of abemaciclib as monotherapy in metastatic ER⁺ breast cancer.

Combined Hormonal and CDK4/6 Inhibitor–Based Treatment in ER⁺ Breast Cancer

In early studies, palbociclib and the estrogen antagonist tamoxifen were demonstrated to have synergistic effects on cell growth in breast cancer cell lines, including cells with acquired tamoxifen resistance,[139] prompting the evaluation of hormonal combinations, initially in patients with metastatic disease. Palbociclib and ribociclib have been combined with letrozole-mediated aromatase inhibition in the first-line metastatic setting. Additionally, palbociclib has been combined with the selective estrogen receptor degrader fulvestrant in patients who had progressed on prior endocrine therapy, and abemaciclib has been combined with fulvestrant in patients who had progressed on prior neoadjuvant or adjuvant hormonal therapy. Results with the three agents are remarkably similar, and all substantially increase progression-free survival compared to hormonal therapy alone (Table 23.3). Combination treatment is generally well tolerated[139–144]; although the percentage of patients experiencing grade 3 or 4 neutropenia is significantly higher with the addition of a CDK4/6 inhibitor, the incidence of febrile neutropenia remains low. Nonetheless, neutropenia can lead to treatment interruptions and dose reductions, so that additional studies may be warranted to confirm the pharmacodynamic effects of reduced doses. One such study for palbociclib is underway (NCT02384239).

TABLE 23.3 *Representative studies of combined hormonal and CDK4/6 inhibitor–based treatment in ER⁺/HER2⁻ breast cancer*

Study	Phase	Randomization	Efficacy (PFS)	Toxicity
PALOMA-1/TRIO-18[142]	2	Letrozole versus letrozole/palbociclib No prior systemic therapy for advanced disease	*Cohort 1* (*n* = 66) (ER⁺/HER2⁻) Letrozole: 5.7 mos Letrozole/palbociclib: 26.1 mos (HR 0.299) *Cohort 2* (*n* = 99) ER⁺/HER2⁻ w/ *CCND1* amplification and/or *CDKN2A* loss Letrozole: 11.1 mos Letrozole/palbociclib: 18.1 mos (HR 0.508) *Combined* (*n* = 165) Letrozole: 10.2 mos Letrozole/palbociclib: 20.2 mos	Grade 3/4 events *Neutropenia* Letrozole: 1% Letrozole/palbociclib: 54% *Febrile neutropenia* Letrozole: 0% Letrozole/palbociclib: 0% *Anemia* Letrozole: 1% Letrozole/palbociclib: 5% *Fatigue* Letrozole: 1% Letrozole/palbociclib: 4%
PALOMA-2[143]	3	2:1 Randomization of letrozole/palbociclib versus letrozole/placebo No prior systemic therapy for advanced disease	*n* = 666 Letrozole/placebo: 14.5 mos Letrozole/palbociclib: 24.8 mos (HR 0.58; *P* < 0.001)	Grade 3/4 events *neutropenia* Letrozole/placebo: 1.4% Letrozole/palbociclib: 66.4% *Febrile neutropenia* Letrozole/placebo: 0% Letrozole/palbociclib: 1.8% *Anemia* Letrozole/placebo: 1.8% Letrozole/palbociclib: 5.4%

TABLE

23.3   *Representative studies of combined hormonal and CDK4/6 inhibitor–based treatment in ER⁺/HER2⁻ breast cancer (Continued)*

Study	Phase	Randomization	Efficacy (PFS)	Toxicity
PALOMA-3[144,145]	3	Fulvestrant/palbociclib versus fulvestrant/ placebo Progression through prior endocrine therapy One previous line of chemotherapy allowed Included premenopausal patients	$n = 521$ Fulvestrant/placebo: 4.6 mos Fulvestrant/palbociclib: 9.5 mos (HR 0.46, $P < 0.0001$) *PIK3CA* mutational status had no effect on outcome	Grade 3/4 events *Neutropenia* Fulvestrant/placebo: 1% Fulvestrant/palbociclib: 65% *febrile neutropenia* Fulvestrant/placebo: 1% Fulvestrant/palbociclib: 1% *Anemia* Fulvestrant/placebo: 2% Fulvestrant/palbociclib: 3%
MONALEESA-2[146]	3	Letrozole/placebo versus letrozole/ribociclib No prior systemic therapy for advanced disease	$n = 668$ At 18 mos, PFS rate Letrozole/placebo: 42.2% Letrozole/ribociclib: 63% (HR, 0.56; $P = 3.29 \times 10^{-6}$) Response rate: Letrozole/placebo: 37.1% Letrozole/ribociclib: 52.7% ($P < 0.001$)	Grade 3/4 events *Neutropenia* Letrozole/placebo: 0.9% Letrozole/ribociclib: 59.3% *Febrile neutropenia* Letrozole/placebo: 0% Letrozole/ribociclib: 1.5% *Leukopenia* Letrozole/placebo: 0.6% Letrozole/ribociclib: 21.0%
MONARCH 2[147]	3	Fulvestrant versus fulvestrant/abemaciclib (150 mg BID) Progression on prior neoadjuvant or adjuvant endocrine therapy No prior chemotherapy allowed Included premenopausal patients Abemaciclib used at 150 mg continuously	$n = 669$ Fulvestrant: 9.3 mos Fulvestrant/abemaciclib: 16.4 mos HR 0.553, $P < 0.001$ Response rate: Fulvestrant: 21.3% Fulvestrant/abemaciclib: 48.1%	All events *Diarrhea* Fulvestrant: 24.7% Fulvestrant/abemaciclib: 86.4% *Neutropenia* Fulvestrant: 4% Fulvestrant/abemaciclib: 46.0% *Nausea* Fulvestrant: 22.9% Fulvestrant/abemaciclib: 45.1% *Fatigue* Fulvestrant: 26.9% Fulvestrant/abemaciclib: 39.9%
MONARCH 3[148]	3	Anastrozole or letrozole/ placebo versus anastrozole or letrozole/abemaciclib (150 mg BID) No prior systemic therapy for advanced disease	$n = 493$ Median PFS in AI alone arm 14.7 mo and not reached in the abemaciclib arm (HR 0.54, $P = 0.00021$) Response rate: AI alone: 44% AI/abemaciclib: 59%	Grade 3/4 events *Neutropenia* AI/placebo: 1.2% AI/abemaciclib: 21.1% *Diarrhea* AI/placebo: 1.2% AI/abemaciclib: 9.5%

Similarly, although the incidence of diarrhea is significantly higher with the addition of abemaciclib to hormonal therapy, this has been readily managed with loperamide prophylaxis.[143,144]

Neoadjuvant trials have also been conducted in patients with clinical stage II/III ER⁺/HER2⁻ disease, as a prelude to adjuvant trials and for further pharmacodynamic assessment of CDK4/6 inhibition. In the NeoPalAna study, 50 patients received anastrozole alone during cycle 0, followed by combination treatment for four 28-day cycles unless a cycle 1, day 15 biopsy demonstrated Ki-67 greater than 10% (in which case patients were discontinued due to inadequate response).[149] Anastrozole was continued until surgery, which occurred 3 to 5 weeks after palbociclib exposure ended; later, patients received an additional 10 to 12 days of palbociclib (cycle 5) immediately before surgery. In this study, serial biopsies at baseline, C1D1, C1D15, and surgery were analyzed for Ki-67, gene expression, and mutation profiles. The primary endpoint was complete cell cycle arrest (CCCA: central Ki-67 ≤2.7%). The CCCA rate was significantly higher after adding palbociclib to anastrozole (C1D15 87% versus C1D1 26%, $P < 0.001$). Palbociclib enhanced cell cycle control over anastrozole monotherapy regardless of luminal subtype (A versus B) and *PIK3CA* status with activity observed across a broad range of clinicopathologic and mutation profiles. Ki-67 recovery at surgery following palbociclib washout was suppressed by cycle 5 palbociclib. Resistance to combined treatment was associated with nonluminal subtypes and persistent E2F-target gene expression. These data indicate that palbociclib is an active antiproliferative agent for early-stage breast cancer resistant to anastrozole, although prolonged administration may be necessary to maintain its effect.[149]

Additionally, this trial employed a novel pharmacodynamic biomarker of CDK4/6 inhibition, namely, serum thymidine kinase 1 (TK1) activity. TK1 is an E2F-dependent cell cycle–regulated enzyme with peak expression in S phase and secreted by tumor cells into serum and therefore an attractive noninvasive assessment of CDK4/6 inhibition in tumor cells.

In this neoadjuvant study, despite a significant drop in tumor Ki-67 with anastrozole monotherapy, there was no statistically significant change in TK1 activity. However, a significant reduction in TK1 activity was observed 2 weeks after initiation of palbociclib (C1D15), which then rose significantly with palbociclib washout. At C1D15, TK1 activity was below the detection limit in 92% of patients, indicating a profound effect of palbociclib. There was high concordance between changes in serum TK1 and tumor Ki-67 in the same direction from C1D1 to C1D15 and from C1D15 to surgery time points, demonstrating that serum TK1 activity is a promising biomarker of CDK4/6 inhibition in ER⁺ breast cancer.[150] Further studies will be required to determine its value in predicting response or eventual resistance to CDK4/6 inhibitors.

Similarly, abemaciclib has been combined with anastrozole in the neoMONARCH study, a randomized phase 2 study in postmenopausal women with early-stage ER⁺/HER2⁻ breast cancer, in which the biological activity of combined abemaciclib and anastrozole was compared to abemaciclib and anastrozole as monotherapy.[151] Each treatment regimen was administered for 2 weeks, after which all patients received the abemaciclib and anastrozole combination for 14 weeks. Activity was assessed in tumor biopsies by determining the percentage change from baseline in Ki-67 expression following the first 2 weeks of therapy. An interim analysis at 9 months has been reported and indicated that patients receiving abemaciclib, either as monotherapy or in combination with anastrozole, showed significantly greater suppression of Ki-67 staining after 14 days of dosing than anastrozole alone. Secondary endpoints including response rates, safety, and pharmacokinetics of the abemaciclib and anastrozole combination with up to 22 additional weeks of neoadjuvant therapy have not yet been reported.

Combinations with HER2-targeted Treatment

Early preclinical data in genetically engineered mouse models have supported evaluation of CDK4/6 inhibitor–based treatment in *HER2 (ERBB2)*-amplified breast cancer.[152–154] In mice engineered to express ERBB2 under control of the MMTV promoter, breast cancer does not arise in a CCND1−/− or CDK4−/− background, demonstrating the requirement of cyclin D1-cdk4 for ERBB2-driven disease. Pharmacologic inhibition of CDK4/6 is also effective in this model. In the monotherapy breast cancer expansion cohort of abemaciclib, 4 of the 11 responses were in patients with tumors harboring *HER2* amplification, although these patients also had ER⁺ disease.[124] Further work will be required to fully define the activity in HER2⁺/ER⁻ disease. Several clinical trials are exploring the use of CDK4/6 inhibitors with therapies targeting HER2, including trastuzumab (NCT02448420), neratinib (NCT03065387), and the drug antibody conjugate trastuzumab emtansine (NCT01976169), the latter based on data suggesting that CDK4/6 inhibitors can be combined with antimitotic therapy if properly sequenced.

Mantle Cell Lymphoma

In the majority of cases, MCL is characterized by the $t(11;14)$ (q13;q32) translocation, juxtaposing the *CCND1* promoter with the B-cell IgH enhancer, driving cyclin D1 expression in B cells that normally express cyclins D2 and D3, leading to increased activity of CDK4/6.[102–104] An initial pilot study was carried out with the aim of demonstrating the pharmacodynamic effects of palbociclib-mediated CDK4/6 inhibition in MCL.[125] Seventeen heavily pretreated patients with high mantle cell international prognostic index (MIPI) scores received palbociclib on the 3/1 schedule. To directly demonstrate CDK4/6 inhibition by palbociclib, paired biopsies were performed prior to treatment and during the last few days of dosing of the first cycle and were assessed for levels of Rb phosphorylation, as well as for markers of proliferation and apoptosis. In concert with tumor biopsies, patients underwent 2-deoxy-2-[¹⁸F]fluoro-D-glucose (FDG) and 3-deoxy-3[¹⁸F]fluorothymidine (FLT) PET imaging to examine tumor metabolism and proliferation, respectively. Substantial reductions were seen in levels of Rb phosphorylation, Ki-67 expression and in the summed FLT-PET maximal standard uptake value (SUV_{max}) after 3 weeks in most patients. These pharmacologic endpoints established target engagement by palbociclib and correlated with the biological outcome of G1 arrest in patients' MCL cells (Fig. 23.2). Within the first 3 weeks of study treatment, there was no evidence of induction of apoptosis, determined by TUNEL staining.

Five of 17 heavily pretreated patients achieved PFS of greater than 1 year (range, 15 to 30 months), including one complete and two partial responses, with responses occurring later in the treatment course, after 4 to 8 cycles. Although patients with prolonged clinical benefit demonstrated marked first-cycle reductions in Rb phosphorylation (>90%), Ki-67 expression (>90%), and summed FLT SUV_{max} (>70%), these decreases also occurred in patients who did not have prolonged treatment benefit. These data suggest that initial G1 arrest may occur in the majority of MCLs exposed to palbociclib; in some cases, this outcome is reversible after a few months, while in others, effects are prolonged, leading to a substantial progression-free interval that may be associated with tumor regression over time. Of note, palbociclib was well tolerated in this population; two patients required dose reduction for hematological toxicities, but there were no treatment discontinuations.

Abemaciclib has similarly been evaluated in MCL, with similar results. Among 22 patients with relapsed or refractory disease,

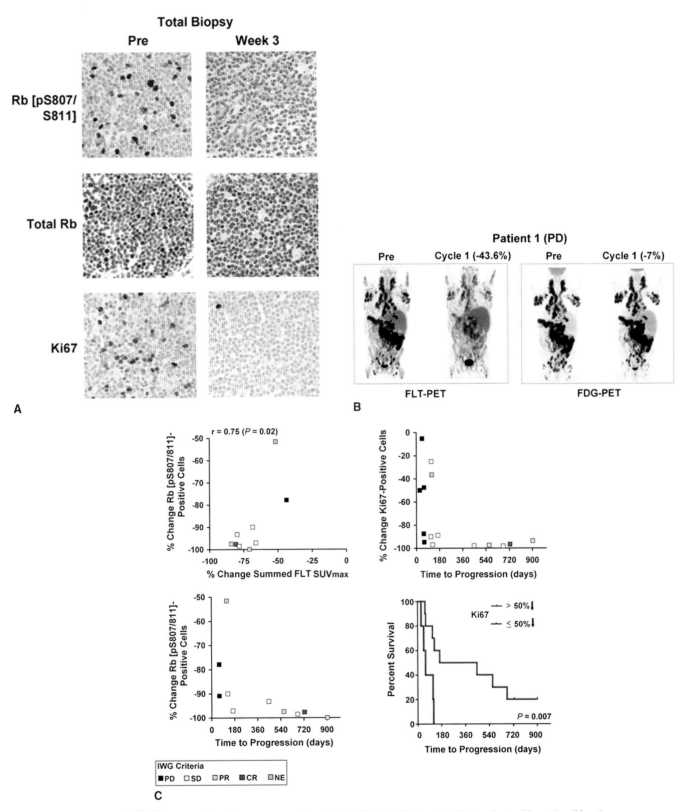

FIGURE **23.2** Pharmacodynamic assessments of the selective CDK4/6 inhibitor palbociclib in patients with mantle cell lymphoma. **A.** Paired tumor biopsies procured pretreatment and after 21 days of continuous dosing demonstrate reduced Rb phosphorylation and Ki-67 expression, consistent with CDK4/6 inhibition. **B.** FLT-PET scans demonstrate reduced SUV uptake, consistent with G1 arrest. **C.** Patients with complete response, partial response, or a prolonged progression-free interval greater than 1 year all demonstrate substantial reductions in phospho-Rb and Ki-67 expression on biopsies, as well as reduced SUV uptake on FLT-PET. However, these parameters are not sufficient to predict long-term outcome, as similar pharmacodynamic effects occurred in patients with shorter progression-free intervals. (Republished with permission of American Society of Hematology from Leonard JP, LaCasce AS, Smith MR, et al. Selective CDK4/6 inhibition with tumor responses by PD0332991 in patients with mantle cell lymphoma. *Blood.* 2012; 119(20):4597-4607; permission conveyed through Copyright Clearance Center, Inc.)

abemaciclib was associated with partial response or SD in 5 and 9 patients, respectively; of these 14 patients, eight achieved durable disease control lasting at least 6 cycles.[155]

MCL is an NF-κB–dependent disease, characterized by constitutive activation of the B-cell receptor signaling pathway.[156] Bruton's tyrosine kinase (BTK) is a critical component of this pathway, which is essential for B-cell survival[157] and is overexpressed in MCL.[158] Ibrutinib is an orally available BTK inhibitor with substantial activity in MCL; however, there is a high relapse rate.[159] Acquired ibrutinib resistance is associated with BTK C481S mutation in some patients and enhanced BTK and AKT activation without mutation in other patients. Resistant cells remain driven by enhanced CDK4 activation,[160] providing rationale for combination therapy using CDK4/6 inhibitors and ibrutinib in MCL. Additionally, prolonged early G1 arrest mediated by palbociclib has been shown to reprogram MCL cells via induction of PIK3IP1, resulting in attenuated PI3K-AKT activation, further sensitizing cells to ibrutinib when BTK is wild-type and to PI3Kδ inhibitors independent of C481S mutation.[160,161] A phase 1 dose escalation study of ibrutinib in combination with palbociclib was carried out in previously treated MCL patients who were ibrutinib and CDK4/6 inhibitor naïve.[162] Patients were treated with ibrutinib daily and palbociclib on days 1 to 21 of a 28-day cycle. The combination was well tolerated; adverse effects were primarily grade 1/2 myelosuppression, with grade 3 rash observed at the highest dose level. The combination was active at all dose levels, with a complete response (CR) rate of 44% and a median time to CR of 3 months.

Liposarcoma

CDK4 gene amplification has been identified in liposarcoma and is associated with poor prognosis.[163,164] CDK4/6 inhibition in *CDK4*-amplified liposarcoma cell line and xenograft models has been demonstrated to have antiproliferative effects,[129] prompting evaluation of palbociclib monotherapy in patients with Rb+, *CDK4*-amplified well-differentiated, or dedifferentiated liposarcoma, who had progressed on prior therapy.[165] Patients were treated at 200 mg palbociclib dose on the 2/1 schedule. Of the 30 patients enrolled in the trial, 66% were progression-free at 12 weeks, surpassing the protocol predefined endpoint of 40% PFS at 12 weeks. Eight patients remained on study for more than 40 weeks, including three with well-differentiated and five with dedifferentiated disease. Tumor regressions were seen in four patients; one patient with a dedifferentiated tumor achieved a partial response at 74 weeks, followed by a CR. Another patient experienced a reduction of a dedifferentiated component within a well-differentiated lesion, resulting in a 30% tumor decrease over a 1-year period. These two responses late in the treatment course are in line with the delayed responses observed in the MCL study, suggesting that gradual tumor regression can occur after initial CDK4/6 inhibitor–mediated tumor growth inhibition.

Following on from this study, 60 patients were enrolled in a phase 2 study of palbociclib in patients with well-differentiated/dedifferentiated liposarcomas[166] using 125 mg daily on the 3/1 schedule. At 12 weeks, the overall PFS was 57.2%, with a median PFS of 17.9 weeks and one CR lasting 2 years. In both of these studies, the most common grade 3/4 events were hematological, although they were more common on the 2/1 schedule. These events included

neutropenia (50% versus 36% on the 2/1 versus 3/1 schedules), thrombocytopenia (30% versus7%), and anemia (17% versus 3%). One incidence of febrile neutropenia occurred on the 2/1 schedule that resolved without complications.

Similar to MCL, it is critical to understand the biology underlying patients who achieve long-term clinical benefit from CDK4/6 inhibition. In this regard, studies in liposarcoma cell lines harboring coamplification of *CDK4* and *MDM2* (i.e., the 12q14 locus) have been instructive.[167] Among seven cell lines, all underwent G1 arrest in response to palbociclib within 48 hours. However, only three of the cell lines expressed markers associated with senescence, including β-galactosidase expression and formation of HPγ1 senescence–associated heterochromatic foci, and did not resume proliferation following palbociclib withdrawal. Interestingly, the senescence response (termed geroconversion) was p53 independent and required proteolytic turnover of MDM2, which occurred via CDK4/6 inhibitor–mediated dissociation of the ubiquitin-specific protease USP7/HAUSP from MDM2, priming it for autoubiquitination. The degradation of MDM2 also required the expression of the chromatin remodeling protein ATRX. It is likely that MDM2 ubiquitinates a senescence-activating protein other than p53, so that its removal promotes senescence. In addition to a role in MDM2 turnover, ATRX also promotes conversion of quiescent cells to a state of senescence after CDK4/6 inhibitor treatment by stabilizing heterochromatic foci and by repressing expression of *HRAS*, the latter mechanism with implications for combined inhibition of CDK4/6 and MAP kinase signaling.[168]

Importantly, paired tumor biopsies were procured from seven patients enrolled to the phase 2 liposarcoma study conducted with the 2/1 schedule. In all patients, there was a reduction of phosphorylated Rb following treatment. Among three patients who did not achieve clinical benefit from palbociclib, there was no evidence of reduced MDM2 in the on-treatment biopsy. In contrast, reduced MDM2 was seen in on-treatment biopsies from patients who derived benefit from palbociclib and were progression-free for an extended duration (168, 376, 500+, and 800+ days, including the patient with CR).[167] These results suggest that, as with MCL, reduced Rb phosphorylation is necessary for, but not sufficient to achieve clinical benefit with sustained disease control. Further studies will be required to determine whether the presence of ATRX or early changes in MDM2 expression may predict long-term outcome after CDK4/6 inhibition in liposarcoma or other cancer types.

Of note, while not clearly in play in liposarcoma models, the Forkhead Box M1 (FOXM1) transcription factor has been identified as a CDK4/6 phosphorylation target; this event stabilizes and activates FOXM1, maintains levels of G1/S genes, and protects cancer cells from senescence. In melanoma models, CDK4/6 inhibitor–mediated senescence is associated with reduced levels of FOXM1.[169]

Lung Cancer

Among lung cancer subsets, there has been particular interest in use of CDK4/6 inhibitors in tumors harboring *KRAS* mutation. Genetic ablation of *CDK4* in mouse models of *KRAS*-mutant non–small cell lung cancer (NSCLC) caused induction of senescence and tumor growth inhibition.[170] *KRAS*-mutant NSCLC xenografts were also demonstrated to be significantly more sensitive to abemaciclib than those harboring wild-type *KRAS*.[124]

Evaluation of CDK4/6 inhibition in advanced NSCLC was prompted by the high rate of loss of p16[INK4A] expression, due to *CDKN2A* deletion, mutation, or promoter hypermethylation. Palbociclib on the 3/1 schedule was studied in a phase 2 single-arm trial of 19 previously treated patients with recurrent or metastatic disease.[171] Eight patients achieved SD lasting 16 weeks or longer, with an overall median PFS time of 12.5 weeks. Genomic analyses were not reported to determine whether the clinical outcome was superior among patients with *KRAS*-mutant tumors.

In an expansion cohort of the phase 1 clinical trial of abemaciclib, 68 patients with advanced NSCLC were enrolled.[124] For all patients, the disease control rate (CR + PR + SD) was 49%, with 46% achieving stable disease and 22% having SD ≥24 weeks. At 6 months, the PFS rate was 26%, with four patients progression-free for longer than 12 months. In comparing patients with mutant and wild-type *KRAS*, the disease control rate was 55% in the *KRAS*-mutant population (*n* = 29) and 39% in the *KRAS* wild-type patient population (*n* = 33). SD lasting ≥24 weeks was achieved for 9/29 (31%) of those patients with *KRAS*-mutant disease compared with 4/33 patients with *KRAS* wild-type disease (12%). Median PFS in the *KRAS*-mutant and *KRAS* wild-type patient cohorts was 2.8 and 1.9 months, respectively. Partial responses were observed in two patients, one with *KRAS*-mutant NSCLC and one with *KRAS* wild-type squamous NSCLC with copy number loss of *CDKN2A*.

The activity of abemaciclib in NCSLC has been further evaluated in a phase 3 clinical trial of previously treatment *KRAS*-mutated lung cancer (JUNIPER[172]). This study randomized abemaciclib (200 mg every 12 hours) to erlotinib (150 mg orally every 24 hours), each arm with best supportive care, in patients with stage IV disease that had progressed after platinum-based chemotherapy and one other previous therapy. The trial was conceived prior to the restriction of the approval of erlotinib to *EGFR*-mutant disease. Nevertheless, the primary endpoint of improved OS was not met. In addition, the control arm showed a higher OS rate than expected based on historical data in this setting, possibly because of subsequent therapies available to patients. However, an analysis of the secondary study endpoints PFS and ORR showed evidence of monotherapy activity in the abemaciclib arm.

Predictive Genomic Biomarker for Cytotoxic Response

Despite the promise of CDK4/6 inhibition in multiple solid tumor types, ORRs have remained low and other than preserved expression of the Rb protein, biomarkers predicting activity have been slow to emerge. Additionally, as shown in Table 23.2, in the PALOMA-1 study, the improvement afforded by combined palbociclib and letrozole compared to letrozole alone was similar in unselected patients and in those whose tumors harbored *CCND1* amplification or *CDKN2A* loss.[142] Because genomic determinants of response or prolonged clinical benefit have not been elucidated, it has been difficult to incorporate patient selection strategies.

To identify cancers predicted to be most sensitive to selective CDK4/6 inhibition, a recent study conducted a systematic survey of 560 cancer cell lines and determined the absolute IC_{50} to abemaciclib derived from CellTiterGlo™ (CTG), an ATP-based measure of cell viability performed over two doubling times, which sums drug effects on cell growth, survival, and number, distinguishing cytotoxic

and cytostatic responses while normalizing for growth rate.[173] Fifteen percent of cell lines were considered highly sensitive, with IC_{50} <1 μM, the steady-state concentration achieved of abemaciclib and its active metabolites in patients. Furthermore, Rb depletion rendered highly sensitive cells resistant to abemaciclib, and results were similar when palbociclib was surveyed across 492 of the lines.

Characterization of the highly sensitive cell lines identified cancer cells with genomic alterations constituting "D-cyclin–activating features," or "DCAF," as highly sensitive to abemaciclib. These alterations included *CCND1* translocation, *CCND1-3* 3′UTR loss (resulting in mRNAs lacking destabilizing elements), *CCND2* or *CCND3* amplification, *CCNK* (encoding Kaposi's sarcoma virus D-type cyclin), and *FBXO31* loss (encoding a ubiquitin ligase controlling cyclin D1 stability). For *CCND1*, the most ubiquitously expressed of the three D-cyclin genes, mRNA and protein levels were high in both DCAF cells and less sensitive cells, which could not explain sensitivity of the former. Nonetheless, DCAF tumor cells were dependent on expression of D-cyclin, and highly sensitive cells were generally ranked in the top 10% in the Project Achilles shRNA dropout screen for dependence on a D-cyclin gene. Additionally, xenografts of DCAF cells underwent regression in response to abemaciclib, rather than the variable degree of tumor growth inhibition demonstrated by less sensitive cells. These results also explain the initial regressions observed when palbociclib was used to treat Colo-205 colon cancer xenografts, where marked regression occurred,[128] since these cells are *CCND3* amplified and therefore expected to be highly sensitive. Of note, although these tumors regrew several weeks after withdrawing palbociclib, recurrent tumors remained sensitive to palbociclib rechallenge, suggesting that they did not readily acquire therapeutic resistance.

The mechanism by which DCAF cells undergo cytotoxicity in vitro or regression in vivo remains to be determined.[174] Cyclin D–dependent kinase activity likely participates in both proliferation and prosurvival pathways, exemplified by NF-*κ*B, for which CDK6 is a cofactor, and therefore relevant for a variety of cancer types.[175] DCAF cells may be more prone to senescence, which may precede apoptosis that occurs after protracted exposure.

DCAF cells also scored as highly sensitive in a second DNA content-based assay. In contrast, most ER+ breast cancer cells scored as highly sensitive in this second assay, but were less sensitive in the CTG assay, suggesting that despite the antiproliferative effects of abemaciclib, metabolism was not completely suppressed. In fact, CDK4/6 inhibition has been linked to metabolic reprogramming in pancreatic cancer,[176] breast cancer,[177] and T-cell acute lymphoblastic leukemia (T-cell ALL) models.[178] Cyclin D3-CDK6 has been shown to phosphorylate and inhibit 6-phosphofructokinase and pyruvate kinase M2, shunting glycolytic intermediates into the pentose phosphate and serine pathways. CDK4/6 inhibition therefore results in increased aerobic glycolysis, with reduced shunting, depleted levels of the antioxidants NADPH and glutathione, and increased reactive oxygen species (ROS).[178] In DCAF cells with *CCND3* amplification or with high cyclin D3-CDK6 activity, as in T-cell ALL, this may be adequate to induce apoptosis.[179] Similar events may be occurring in other DCAF cells. In less vulnerable cells, suppression of ROS scavenging or reversal of events associated with metabolic reprogramming on which CDK4/6 inhibitor–treated cells may come to depend, including mTORC1 activation,[176] may convert partial sensitivity to efficacy similar to that observed in DCAF cells. Notably, among ER⁺ breast cancer cell lines, combined fulvestrant and abemaciclib yielded CTG curves similar to those of monotherapy-treated DCAF cells, perhaps explaining the increased response and PFS rates and profound clinical benefit of combined hormonal and CDK4/6 inhibitor treatment.

CCND1 amplification was not included in the DCAF definition. While some *CCND1*-amplified ER⁺ breast or thyroid cancer cells were highly sensitive, association of improved clinical outcome of patients with *CCND1*-amplified breast cancers to CDK4/6 inhibitor monotherapy has been inconsistent. Additionally, across histologies, this amplicon was associated with relative insensitivity, possibly because neighboring oncogenes drive growth and proliferation.

However, the DCAF alterations were borne out by the sensitivity of MCL cell lines, characterized by *CCND1* translocation, often with concomitant deletion or point mutation of the *CCND1* 3'UTR, giving rise to mRNAs lacking most of the 3'UTR, resulting in mRNA stabilization. Indeed, in the evaluations of palbociclib and abemaciclib in MCL, complete and partial responses to CDK4/6 inhibition in MCL have been described,[125,155] and it will be of interest to determine whether response correlates with the presence of 3'UTR alterations in addition to canonical D-cyclin translocation.

Importantly, DCAF alterations were shown to occur commonly in cancers in which CDK4/6 inhibitors have not been extensively evaluated (Table 23.4).[174]

Combined Inhibition of CDK4/6 and PI3k Pathway Signaling

The phosphatidylinositol 3-kinase (PI3K) pathway is a regulator of cell growth and survival, and constitutive activation of the pathway can lead to uncontrolled cell proliferation. Cyclin D1 subcellular localization and degradation are controlled by glycogen synthase kinase 3β (GSK3β), which phosphorylates cyclin D1 on Thr286, leading to nuclear export and subsequent targeting for ubiquitin-mediated proteasomal degradation. Inhibition of GSK3β by PI3K signaling causes the inhibition of Thr286 phosphorylation, leading to nuclear retention of CDK-cyclin D1 complexes, inhibition of proteasomal degradation, persistent nuclear cyclin D1

expression,[105,106] and continuous CDK4 activation. Given the crosstalk between these two pathways and their importance in various tumor types, combined inhibition of both CDK4/6 and PI3K is an attractive treatment strategy.

The PI3K pathway is frequently activated in breast cancer cells, often via *PIK3CA* mutation,[180] so that preclinical studies of combined inhibition of CDK4/6 and PI3K signaling have primarily been in breast cancer models. It has been demonstrated that Rb phosphorylation is repressed in both breast cancer cell lines sensitive to PI3K inhibition and in breast tumors from patients responsive to PI3K inhibition; in contrast, Rb phosphorylation is sustained in cells less sensitive to PI3K inhibition and in tumors that did not respond to PI3K inhibitors.[181] A combinatorial drug screen performed on multiple *PIK3CA*-mutant breast cancer cell lines with either acquired or intrinsic PI3K inhibitor resistance revealed that combined CDK4/6-PI3K inhibition synergistically reduces cell viability, translating to regression in xenograft models. These data have justified current clinical trials evaluating the addition of a PI3K inhibitor to combined CDK4/6 inhibitor and hormonal treatment, including the PI3K alpha isoform–selective agent alpelisib, in combination with ribociclib/letrozole (NCT NCT01872260) or the pan-PI3K inhibitor gedatolisib in combination with palbociclib/letrozole or palbociclib/fulvestrant (NCT02684032).

Amplification of both *CCND1* and *PIK3CA* is common in squamous cell NSCLC and head and neck cancers,[23,182] and therefore, combined CDK4/6 and PI3K inhibition may also be an effective treatment strategy in these tumor types. There is also potential for this combination in pancreatic cancer; genetically engineered mouse models of pancreatic cancer have suggested the importance of the PI3K pathway downstream from activated KRAS,[183] and synergism has been demonstrated between CDK4/6 and PI3K inhibition on proliferation and viability in p16INK4A-deficient pancreatic cancer cell lines.[184]

Combined CDK4/6 and MEK Inhibition

MEK is a critical protein in the MAPK pathway and represents a potential therapeutic target in *RAS* mutant tumors, with several MEK inhibitors, including selumetinib, trametinib, and

TABLE **23.4**	*New opportunities for evaluation of CDK4/6 inhibitors in DCAF tumors*	
DCAF Alteration	**Biological Consequence**	**Representative Tumor Types**
KSHV cyclin (K-cyclin)	Expression of D-type cyclin	Kaposi's sarcoma
FBX031 loss	Loss of ubiquitin ligase controlling D-cyclin stability	Neuroblastoma
D-cyclin gene 3'UTR loss (deletion or point mutation)	Loss of mRNA destabilizing elements; mutation causes a premature polyadenylation signal resulting in truncated mRNA lacking most of the 3'UTR	Endometrial cancer,ᵃ gastric cancer, diffuse large B-cell lymphoma
CCND2 amplification	High cyclin D2 expression	Germ cell tumor, small bowel cancer, colorectal cancer, uterine sarcoma, ovarian cancer
CCND3 amplification	High cyclin D3 expression	Ampullary carcinoma, esophagogastric cancer

ᵃTherefore, this comprehensive analysis presents clinically testable hypotheses to be evaluated in a basket study of abemaciclib that will enroll patients with tumors harboring DCAF alterations (NCT03310879), in addition to those with tumors carrying *CDK4* or *CDK6* amplification.

binimetinib, in clinical development. In patients with previously treated *KRAS*-mutant NSCLC, single-agent trametinib performed comparably to docetaxel in a randomized phase 2 trial.[185] Despite the initial promise of a randomized phase 2 trial comparing docetaxel to docetaxel combined with selumetinib in this population, a subsequent phase 3 trial did not reach a primary endpoint of improved PFS for the combination.[186] Similarly, a modestly improved PFS with binimetinib compared to dacarbazine in patients with *NRAS*-mutant melanoma was not considered sufficient to support FDA registration.[187] Overall, these findings suggest MEK inhibition, either alone or in combination with chemotherapy, may be insufficient to improve outcomes in *RAS*-mutant cancers.

Multiple preclinical models support the potential efficacy of combined CDK4/6 and MEK inhibition in *RAS*-mutant cancers. In an inducible model of *NRAS*-mutant melanoma, NRAS extinction was shown to trigger both cell cycle arrest and apoptosis, with tumor regressions. Although MEK inhibition activated apoptosis in this model, cell cycle arrest did not occur, so that cell death was balanced by continued proliferation, leading to a cytostatic response.[188] Network modeling identified CDK4 activity as the primary driver of this differential phenotype. Consequently, there was substantial in vivo synergy between MEK and CDK4/6 inhibition in this model, with similar results found in models of *KRAS*-mutant colorectal cancer[189,190] and *KRAS*-mutant NSCLC[191] treated with palbociclib and trametinib. Additional mechanisms for the synergism have also been proposed, including a MAP kinase–dependent state established in cells treated with a CDK4/6 inhibitor,[192] as well as a synergistic senescence response induced by combined CDK4/6 and MEK inhibition.

The melanoma findings were recently translated in a phase 1 trial of the MEK inhibitor binimetinib and the CDK4 inhibitor ribociclib in *NRAS*-mutant melanoma.[193,194] After assessment of 21-day (both drugs administered for 14 days) and 28-day schedules (ribociclib administered 21 of 28 days and binimetinib administered continuously), an RP2D was established with the 28-day schedule (200 mg QD ribociclib and 45 mg twice-daily binimetinib). Among 16 patients treated at the RP2D, 4 patients achieved partial response and an additional 7 patients achieved a best response of SD. Median PFS was 6.4 months, prompting initiation of a phase 2 evaluation of the combination.

In a recent phase 1 study of palbociclib and the MEK inhibitor PD-0325901, the combination was tolerable at doses of palbociclib demonstrating target engagement. Across dose levels, 32 patients with *KRAS*-mutant NSCLC were treated, with seven patients achieving partial response of SD lasting >6 months, including those with concomitant *TP53* or *CDKN2A* loss.[192]

Combined inhibition of MAP kinase signaling and CDK4/6 inhibition may also be useful in *BRAF*-mutant cancers. For example, melanoma cell lines with acquired vemurafenib resistance that exhibited reactivated MAPK signaling and cyclin D1 upregulation were sensitive to abemaciclib; CDK4/6 inhibition induced apoptosis in resistant cells, in contrast to G1 arrest in parental cells. This has led to the testing of both sequential and concomitant schedules of vemurafenib and abemaciclib in preclinical models, achieving both substantial tumor growth inhibition and regression compared to monotherapies.[195]

Intrinsic Resistance, Adaptation, and Acquired Resistance to CDK4/6 Inhibition

Loss of Rb is a primary determinant of intrinsic resistance to CDK4/6 inhibition.[196] Because the vast majority of ER+ breast cancers retain wild-type Rb expression, selection of patients based on Rb status has not been routinely incorporated into clinical trials in this population. However, in prostate cancer, loss of Rb may be a prominent feature of progression of the disease to the castrate-resistant state,[197–199] such that Rb status may ultimately define interventions such as enzalutamide/ribociclib in tumors that retain Rb expression (NCT02555189) and enzalutamide/docetaxel in tumors that lose Rb expression.[200]

Additionally, recent preclinical modeling in ER+ breast cancer patient-derived xenograft (PDX) models has shown that loss of Rb may also be a mechanism of acquired resistance.[201] During expansion of a ribociclib-sensitive PDX model, 5/8 tumors underwent regression over the first 40 days of treatment, after which 7 tumors began to regrow under drug pressure. Compared to the initially sensitive tumor, four of the seven resistant tumors had decreased levels of Rb with sustained expression of cyclin E. Genomic characterization showed the acquisition of a *RB1* frameshift mutation, *RB1 pM695fs*26*. Of note, when transplanted, these tumors remained partially sensitive to ribociclib. Digital PCR demonstrated that the mutant allele fraction increased from 0.25 in control tumors to 0.55 in ribociclib-treated tumors, indicating that the mutation was subclonal in the resistant tumor and that CDK4/6 inhibition resulted in the selection of an *RB1* mutant population of cells.

In addition to Rb loss, amplification of *CDK6* has also been described in ER+ breast cancer cells with acquired resistance to abemaciclib.[202] It is of interest that CDK6 has been linked not only to cell cycle progression but also to survival pathways, including NF-κB, for which it is a p65-bound cofactor, suggesting that elevated expression of CDK6 in resistant cells may afford the ability to overcome G1 arrest and also provide a prosurvival signal.[175] Increased expression of CDK6 in abemaciclib-resistant cells was also linked to reduced ER and PR expression and a reduced response to ER antagonists.[202]

Elevated cyclin D1 has been noted in response to ribociclib in liposarcoma cells. Of note, this appears to be an adaptive response that is reversible upon drug withdrawal.[129] Such results suggest that in some cases, intermittent schedules of CDK4/6 inhibitors may be preferable and may avoid more rapid emergence of frank resistance.

Another mechanism of rapid adaptation and resistance emerging from preclinical models is the activation of CDK2 in response to CDK4/6 inhibition. This phenomenon was first described in acute myelogenous leukemia cells; upon palbociclib exposure, an initial reduction in Rb phosphorylation was followed by a rapid decrease in p27[Kip1] expression, resulting in CDK2 activation and phosphorylation of Rb that overcame the initial G1 arrest.[203] Similarly, in the recent survey of 560 cell lines for abemaciclib sensitivity, cells with loss of *CDKN2A* (or loss of p16[INK4A] expression) were shown only to have modest sensitivity (between those of DCAF and Rb-negative cells). *CDKN2A*-mutant cells also displayed a rapid adaptation to abemaciclib, with suppression of Rb phosphorylation at 24 hours that was reversed by 72 hours with concomitant activation of CDK2, whereas DCAF cells treated with abemaciclib demonstrated continued suppression of Rb phosphorylation and CDK2 activity over time, associated with evidence of senescence and apoptosis.[173] Depletion of CDK2 from *CDKN2A*-mutant cells converted them to a DCAF phenotype. Consistent with these findings, *CDKN2A* loss was associated with a less than 8-week PFS in the phase 1 study of ribociclib.[123] Of note, in glioblastoma models, codeletion of *CDKN2A* and *CDKN2C* was required to dictate CDK4/6 inhibitor sensitivity,[204] so that it is possible that in some systems, loss of more than one INK4 protein may afford more potent G1 arrest and/or senescence that is not easily overcome.

In addition to $p27^{Kip1}$ loss, other mechanisms of CDK2 activation that may occur during early adaptation or acquired resistance in ER$^+$ breast cancer cell lines include the formation of cyclin D2-CDK2 complexes or amplification of *CCNE1*, respectively.[201] Of note, in the comprehensive cell line screen for abemaciclib sensitivity, *CCNE1* amplification was entirely absent among highly sensitive cell lines.[173] In these studies, the addition of a PI3K inhibitor was able to prevent the emergence of resistance, especially the formation of cyclin D-CDK2 complexes, via reduced expression of G1 cyclins, complete suppression of Rb phosphorylation, and inhibited activation of S-phase transcriptional programs. However, PI3K inhibition was unable to reverse acquired resistance; rather, *CCNE1*-amplified cells could be resensitized by the targeting of CDK2.[201] These results have reinvigorated interest in CDK2 inhibitors, which could be applied either concomitantly at outset, or sequentially, once CDK4/6 inhibitor resistance has emerged.

Recently, in addition to Rb loss, another mechanism of intrinsic resistance has been suggested in breast cancer, mediated by breast tumor–related kinase (BRK), a nonreceptor protein kinase that has been shown to be overexpressed in 60% of breast cancers.[205] Tyrosine phosphorylation of $p27^{Kip1}$ on residues 74, 88, and 89 facilitates activation of the CDK4-cyclin D1-$p27^{Kip1}$ complex to phosphorylate substrates such as Rb.[206–209] In breast cancer cell lines with high BRK expression, there is high affinity for $p27^{Kip1}$, with robust phosphorylation of Tyr88, conferring palbociclib resistance. These data suggest that assessment of BRK levels may be of clinical utility in breast cancer studies utilizing CDK4/6 inhibitors.[210]

Finally, in a study designed to identify novel CDK4/6 drug combinations, a kinome-wide siRNA screen was carried out to identify kinases that when inhibited may sensitize cells to ribociclib.[211] PDK (3-phosphoinositide-dependent protein kinase) upregulation was identified as a potential mechanism of resistance. PDK1 is downstream of PI3K and is required for the full activation of AKT[212] and other AGC kinases.[213,214] PDK also has been identified as being overexpressed in breast tumors, with higher expression correlated to higher tumor grade,[215] indicating a possible role in oncogenesis. Taken together, these results provide further rationale for combining PI3K and CDK4/6 inhibitors as a therapeutic strategy. Of note, elevated PDK1 was also noted in cells selected for resistance after chronic ribociclib exposure, along with higher levels of expression of cyclins D1, A, and E, as well as activated CDK2 and AKT. Treatment with a PDK1 or CDK2 inhibitor was sufficient to reverse these events and restore CDK4/6 inhibitor sensitivity.[211]

CDK4/6 Inhibition and Cytotoxic Chemotherapy

In general, the G1 arrest afforded by CDK4/6 inhibition has suggested that it will be challenging to combine these agents with standard chemotherapy, especially with agents that are cytotoxic

during the S and M phases of the cell cycle. However, recently, a novel approach has used intravenously administered trilaciclib contemporaneously with chemotherapy to transiently and reversibly block the proliferation of murine and canine bone marrow hematopoietic stem and progenitor cells and thereby provide multilineage protection from the hematologic toxicity of chemotherapy.[136] Additionally, this agent has been shown to protect murine hematopoietic stem cells from chemotherapy-induced exhaustion in a serial 5-fluorouracil treatment model.[216] When cancer cells are Rb negative, there is little risk of decreasing the antitumor efficacy of cytotoxic chemotherapy with concomitant trilaciclib. For this reason, trilaciclib is currently in development for the reduction of chemotherapy-induced myelosuppression after cisplatin/etoposide or topotecan-based treatment of small cell lung cancer (NCT03041311; NCT02514447).

There may be other advantages of combining CDK4/6 inhibition with cisplatin. It has recently been reported that silencing or palbociclib-mediated pharmacological inhibition of CDK6 increases sensitivity of epithelial ovarian cancer cells to platinum.[217] In response to platinum treatment, CDK6 phosphorylates and stabilizes the transcription factor FOXO3, eventually inducing ATR transcription. Blocking this pathway resulted in ovarian cancer cell death, due to an altered DNA damage response accompanied by increased apoptosis. These results were recapitulated in xenografts and in primary tumor cells derived from platinum-treated patients. Additionally, high CDK6 and FOXO3 expression levels in primary epithelial ovarian cancer predict poor patient survival, further suggesting that CDK6 inhibition could be exploited to improve platinum efficacy in these patients.

Nonetheless, the interaction with cisplatin may be highly dependent on cellular background. In a study of Calu-6 NSCLC cells rendered cisplatin resistant, there was upregulation of the microRNA miR-145. A predicted target of miR-145 is CDK6, and its expression was found to be down-regulated in the resistant sublines. In this model, inhibition of CDK6 inhibition antagonized cisplatin-induced NSCLC cell cytotoxicity.[218]

Additional work has attempted to combine CDK4/6 inhibitor–mediated cell cycle synchronization with paclitaxel, utilizing an alternating schedule in which 3 to 5 days of palbociclib are used before each dose of weekly taxane. Among heavily treated breast cancer patients, the approach has produced instances of partial response and prolonged SD.[219] A similar approach has been used to synchronize AML cells in order to enrich the S-phase population and augment cytarabine-induced cytotoxicity. Moreover, palbociclib inhibited expression of the homeobox (HOX)A9 oncogene, reducing the transcription of its target PIM1. Reduced PIM1 synthesis attenuated PIM1-mediated phosphorylation of the proapoptotic BAD and activated BAD-dependent apoptosis.[220]

Effects of CDK4/6 Inhibitors on Immune Microenvironment

Recent clinical successes with drugs targeting the immune checkpoints, including anti-PD-1/PD-L1 and anti-CTLA4 antibodies, have highlighted the importance of immunotherapy in treating cancer. It is therefore increasingly important to understand the effects of other cancer treatments on the immune microenvironment. Several recent studies have revealed that CDK4/6 inhibition

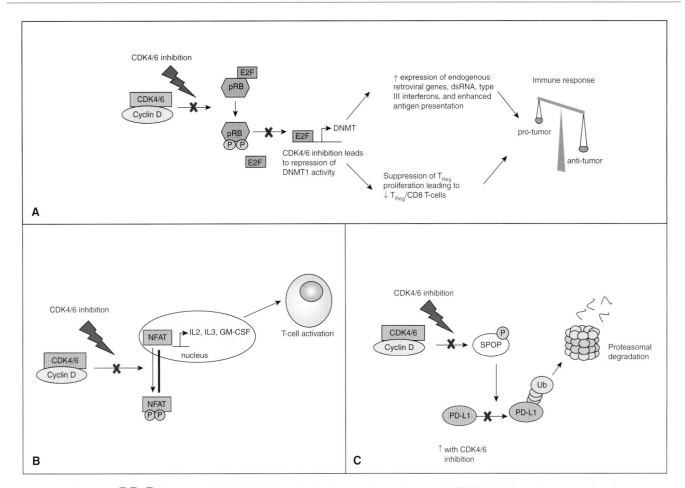

Figure **23.3** Interaction of CDK4/6 inhibition with the immune microenvironment. **A.** CDK4/6 inhibition reduces expression of DNMT1, allowing expression of endogenous retroviruses that invoke and interferon response, augmenting antigen processing and presentation. Additionally, CDK4/6 inhibition preferentially reduces the proliferation of T_{Regs}. **B.** CDK4/6 inhibition derepresses NFAT activity, allowing expression of target genes required for regulation of T-cell function. **C.** CDK4/6 inhibition blocks cyclin D-CDK4-mediated phosphorylation of the Cullin 3 adaptor SPOP, promoting its degradation and preventing the ubiquitin-mediated degradation of PD-L1. These mechanisms explain the enhanced antitumor efficacy of combined CDK4/6 inhibition and PD1/PD-L1 blockade seen in in vivo models.

promotes antitumor immunity in models of breast and other cancers[221] (Fig. 23.3). In HER2-driven genetically engineered mouse model, CDK4/6 inhibition resulted in reduced expression of DNA methyltransferase 1, a known E2F-1 transcriptional target.[222] This was associated with increased expression of endogenous retroviruses, with an increased double-strand RNA response involving type III interferon production and ultimate expression of interferon-sensitive genes that promote antigen processing and presentation via MHC1. These findings were confirmed in gene expression profiling of samples procured in the NeoPalAna study of ER+ breast cancer patients undergoing serial biopsies after neoadjuvant combined hormonal and palbociclib treatment, which showed reduced expression of E2F target genes and genes associated with the G2 and mitotic checkpoints, with concomitant enrichment of gene sets associated with the immune response, including the interferon-γ response. In addition, CDK4/6 inhibition was shown to lead to a preferential inhibition in the proliferation in regulatory T (T_{Reg}) cells, leading to a decrease in the ratio of T_{Reg} cells to CD8+ cytotoxic T cells in the tumor microenvironment, tipping the balance in favor of antitumor immunity and CD8+ T-cell–dependent clearance that is further enhanced by immune checkpoint blockade.

The selective suppression of T_{Reg} proliferation (and not that of CD8+ or conventional CD4+ T cells) might relate to the fact that T_{Reg} cells express greater than threefold higher levels of *Rb1* compared to CD8+ T cells.

In a second study, a small-molecule screen was conducted in vitro to identify agents capable of increasing the activity of T cells suppressed by PD-1 signaling, measured by IL-2 production. Short-term exposure to CDK4/6 inhibitors enhanced T-cell activation, due in part to inhibition of CDK6-mediated phosphorylation and cytoplasmic sequestration of nuclear factor of activated T-cell (NFAT) family proteins, resulting in increased nuclear accumulation of NFAT proteins, their derepression, and increased expression of target genes that are critical regulators of T-cell function.[223] In models of KRAS-driven NSCLC, such as those with activated KRAS and deleted Tp53 (*Kras^{LSL-G12D}/Tp53^{fl/fl}*), exposure to CDK4/6 inhibition increased effector T-cell infiltration and activation, coupled with greater effects on T_{Reg} compared to CD8+ T-cell proliferation. Additionally, CDK4/6 inhibition was found to augment the response to PD-1 blockade in a novel ex vivo organotypic tumor spheroid culture system and in multiple in vivo murine syngeneic models, thereby providing a rationale for combining CDK4/6 inhibitors and immunotherapies.

Finally, it has recently been reported that PD-L1 protein abundance is regulated by cyclin D-CDK4 and the Cullin 3^{SPOP} E3 ligase via proteasome-mediated degradation.[224] Inhibition of CDK4/6 in vivo elevates PD-L1 protein levels, largely by inhibiting cyclin D-CDK4-mediated phosphorylation of the Cullin 3 adaptor SPOP, thereby promoting SPOP degradation by APC/C^{Cdh1}. In mouse tumor models and in primary human prostate cancer specimens, loss-of-function mutations in SPOP compromise ubiquitination-mediated PD-L1 degradation, leading to increased PD-L1 levels and reduced numbers of tumor-infiltrating lymphocytes (TILs). As was shown in the other studies, combining CDK4/6 inhibitor treatment with anti-PD-1 immunotherapy enhances tumor regression and dramatically improves OS rates in mouse tumor models, so that PD-1 blockade overcomes the negative effects of PD-L1 expression.

Recently, the results of the first combination of a CDK4/6 inhibitor with immune checkpoint blockade were reported among 28 heavily pretreated ER$^+$ breast cancer patients who received a combination of abemaciclib and pembrolizumab.[225] At 16 weeks, a response rate of 14% was observed; although this response rate was overall lower than that reported in the single agent abemaciclib MONARCH-1 study, in the latter study, the time to response to abemaciclib was approximately 3.7 months, and at 16 weeks, the response rate was only 6.8%. These results suggest that efficacy of the abemaciclib/pembrolizumab combination may improve with longer follow-up, which will be needed to determine whether the combination appears to produce a response rate superior to that of the monotherapies. Abemaciclib combined with pembrolizumab is also being evaluated in patients with NSCLC, in both adenocarcinoma and squamous cell carcinoma cohorts. Importantly, to date, the combination has not produced any unexpected toxicities, with incidence of diarrhea similar to that seen with abemaciclib alone.

Inhibitors of Other Cell Cycle CDKs

In addition to use of a CDK2 inhibitor to counteract adaptation and acquired resistance to CDK4/6 inhibition, a CDK2 inhibitor will likely be of benefit in *CCNE1*-amplified disease, illustrated by a subgroup of patients with ovarian cancer,[62,226] where cancer cells are likely CDK2 dependent.[227] To date, inhibitors of CDK2, including dinaciclib,[228,229] seliciclib,[230] or CYC-065,[231] typically also inhibit CDK1 and/or the transcriptional CDK, CDK9, with relative equipotency. These associated activities may have advantages but may also introduce toxicity. Because CDK2 may compensate for CDK2 depletion,[232,233] combined CDK2/CDK1 inhibition may be critical to achieve S/G2 arrest in transformed cells; nonetheless, CDK1 has been shown to be highly essential for nontransformed cells in mouse knockout models,[234] so that combined CDK2/1 inhibition may lower the therapeutic index compared to selective reduction of CDK2 activity, especially in a highly CDK2-dependent cellular background. Concomitant CDK9 inhibition reduces the expression of antiapoptotic proteins, including MCL1 and XIAP, which may help convert cytostatic cell cycle inhibition to a cytotoxic response[233]; however, MCL1 is critical for neutrophil survival,[235] so that CDK9 inhibition has been associated with severe neutropenia, complicating the development of such compounds in solid tumors.

Inhibition of Transcriptional CDKs

CDK9. RNA polymerase II is the RNA polymerase responsible for the transcription of DNA to RNA, and the main mechanism of transcriptional control by CDKs 7, 8, 9, 12, and 13 is through posttranslational modification of its C-terminal domain (CTD). The CTD consists of 52 heptapeptide repeats (*N*-Tyr-Ser-Pro-Thr-Ser-Pro-Ser-C), and phosphorylation of these repeats controls its enzymatic activity.[236–238] The CDK9-cyclin T complex preferentially phosphorylates Ser5 sites of the CTD, promoting transcriptional elongation,[236,239] and affects the expression of proteins encoded by RNAs with short half-lives, including those encoding antiapoptotic proteins such as MCL1, BCL-xL, and XIAP. Thus CDK9 inhibition may be important for survival of cells addicted to these proteins, including CLL and other malignant hematopoietic cells.[240,241] This biology may in part explain the impressive response rates to drugs such as flavopiridol and dinaciclib in CLL trials, where dose-limiting toxicity has been tumor lysis syndrome.[242,243] CDK9 has been shown to be elevated in a number of cancers, including esophageal cancer[244]; pancreatic cancer, where it is a negative prognostic factor[245]; and T-and B-cell lymphomas.[246] Furthermore, in a MYC-driven model of hepatocellular carcinoma, CDK9 was shown to be required for tumor maintenance; pharmacological or shRNA-mediated CDK9 inhibition led to robust antitumor effects that correlated with MYC expression levels and depended on the role that both CDK9 and MYC play in transcription elongation.[247] Finally, another consequence of CDK9 inhibition is reduced transcription of *hDM2*, providing a mechanism for the activation of wild-type TP53.[248–250]

Dinaciclib

Currently, a few inhibitors of CDK9 remain in active development, including dinaciclib, seliciclib, and CYC-065.[228–231] These agents also inhibit cell cycle CDKs; for example, dinaciclib is a potent inhibitor of CDK1, CDK2, and CDK5 as well. In addition to its activity in CLL and other hematologic malignancies, dinaciclib has been evaluated in solid tumors on low-dose once-weekly and high-dose every-3-week schedules, with instances of partial response and prolonged SD observed.[251–253] Dinaciclib is administered intravenously and has short plasma half-life, which may be a liability as a reversible ATP-competitive inhibitor that can only be administered intermittently. Importantly, in both proliferating keratinocytes and in paired tumor biopsies, CDK2 inhibition has been demonstrated, as evidenced by reduced Rb phosphorylation at the T356 site, as well as increased expression of p27^{Kip1} in some samples,[253] stability of which is controlled by CDK2.[11,12] Additionally, increased expression of TP53 has also been demonstrated, consistent with CDK9 inhibition (Fig. 23.4). Dinaciclib has also been demonstrated to promote antitumor immunity, possibly related to its ability to relieve MYC-induced immune suppression.[254–256]

CDK12

CDK12, in concert with cyclin K, is also a regulator of transcription and RNA processing[257–259] through its ability to phosphorylate Ser2 of the RNA polymerase II CTD. It is believed to have gene specific,[260] rather than global, effects on transcription as it regulates the expression of transcription factors such as *Fos*, as well as genes associated with the DNA damage response and DNA repair,[261,262]

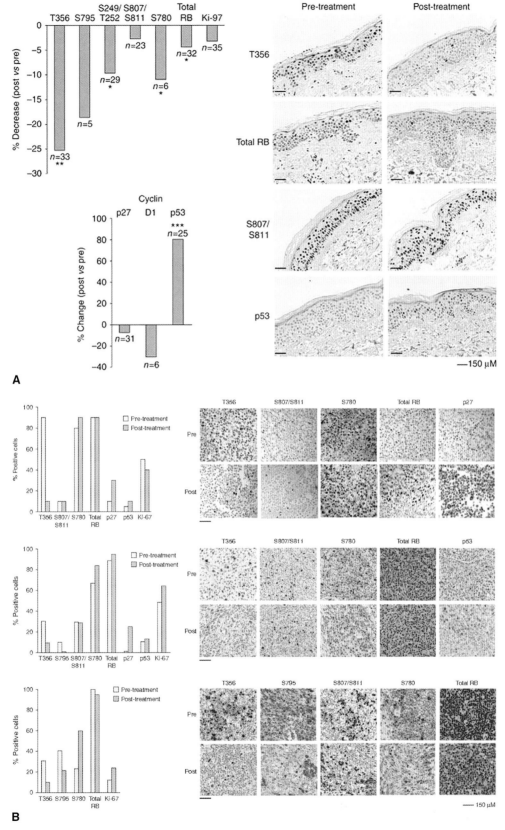

Figure 23.4 Pharmacodynamic assessments of the cell cycle/transcriptional CDK inhibitor dinaciclib. **A.** Paired skin biopsies obtained pretreatment and shortly after completion of a dinaciclib infusion demonstrate reduced phosphorylation of Rb [pT356] and increased expression of TP53, consistent with inhibition of CDK2 and CDK9, respectively. **B.** Similar data are observed in paired biopsies from melanoma patients who received dinaciclib, with reduced phosphorylation of Rb [T356] and increased p27[Kip1] as evidence of CDK2 inhibition and increased expression of TP53 as evidence of CDK9 inhibition in tumor cells. (Reprinted by permission from Nature: Mita MM, Mita AC, Moseley JL, et al. Phase 1 safety, pharmacokinetic and pharmacodynamic study of the cyclin-dependent kinase inhibitor dinaciclib administered every three weeks in patients with advanced malignancies. *Br J Cancer.* 2017;117(9):1258-1268. Copyright © 2017 Springer Nature.)

and therefore may play an important role in cancer development and treatment. Genetic alterations in the *CDK12* gene have been demonstrated in a wide variety of tumor types and include point mutations, copy number variation, and both upregulation and down-regulation of gene expression.[263] Inactivating mutations in the *CDK12* gene leading to loss of function have been characterized in ovarian carcinomas and likely promote genomic instability and tumorigenesis, primarily through their ability to impair HR repair;

these results suggest that *CDK12* mutation may be used as a marker for sensitivity to PARP inhibitors.[264,265]

Interestingly, despite the structural similarity of CDK9 and CDK12, nearly all known inhibitors of CDK9 do not inhibit CDK12[266] with the exception of dinaciclib. Dinaciclib is unique among known CDK inhibitor compounds to potently inhibit CDKs 9 and 12 (Fig. 23.5).[267] CDKs that regulate transcriptional elongation have a unique extension helix that lies the C-terminal to the

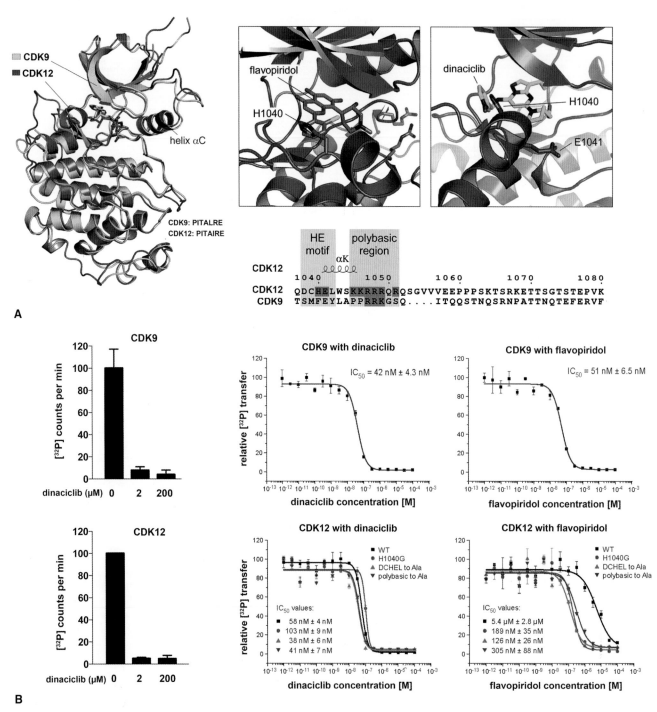

FIGURE **23.5** Dinaciclib is unique among ATP-competitive CDK inhibitor compounds for its ability to inhibit CDK12. **A.** Most CDK inhibitor compounds, such as flavopiridol, demonstrate steric hindrance with the CDK12 ATP-binding site at the H1040 site, while dinaciclib does not demonstrate this interaction. **B.** Dinaciclib inhibits CDK12 with nanomolar potency. Mutation of the H1040 site or surrounding residues of CDK12 lowers the IC50 of flavopiridol from the micromolar to nanomolar range. (Reprinted from Johnson SF, Cruz C, Greifenberg AK, et al. CDK12 Inhibition Reverses De Novo and Acquired PARP Inhibitor Resistance in BRCA Wild-Type and Mutated Models of Triple-Negative Breast Cancer. *Cell Rep.* 2016;17(9):2367-2381. Copyright © 2016 Elsevier. With permission.)

canonical CDK kinase domain. In CDK12, this extension helix interacts with the ATP-binding site and is initiated by a DCHEL motif beginning at amino acid 1038. The interaction of the C-terminal extension helix with the nucleotide-binding site of CDK12 is mediated by the H1040 and E1041 residues, and loss of the helix severely disrupts activity of the kinase.[266] CDK9 shares a similar C-terminal extension helix, but does not share the initiating 1038 DCHEL motif. Because this structural variation occurs in close proximity to the site of binding for small-molecule inhibitors of CDK9, it was considered likely responsible for the lack of shared specificity with CDK12. In silico modeling of flavopiridol, a highly potent CDK9 inhibitor, into the ATP-binding site of CDK12 revealed a significant steric clash between the benzene ring of bound flavopiridol and the H1040 residue of the DCHEL motif of CDK12. However, modeling of dinaciclib into the CDK12 ATP-binding site, in contrast with flavopiridol, did not demonstrate the same steric hindrance between the CDK12 H1040 aromatic ring and the pyridine-N-oxide ring of dinaciclib.

In triple-negative breast cancer (TNBC) cells, dinaciclib demonstrated a CDK12 inhibitory phenotype with only modest effects on cell cycle progression and profound reduction in expression of genes involved in HR repair. Consequently, dinaciclib sensitized HR repair-proficient TNBC cells to PARP inhibition and reversed de novo and acquired resistance to PARP inhibition in BRCA-mutated models, related to residual or restored HR, respectively.[267]

To ameliorate the liabilities associated with the short plasma half-life of dinaciclib, a covalent inhibitor of CDK12, THZ531, has recently been described.[268] Co-crystallization of THZ531 with CDK12-cyclin K indicates that THZ531 irreversibly targets a cysteine located outside the kinase domain (Cys-1039). THZ531 causes a loss of gene expression with concurrent loss of elongating and hyperphosphorylated RNA polymerase II. In particular, THZ531 substantially decreases the expression of DNA damage response genes and key super-enhancer–associated transcription factor genes.

CDK7

CDK7 has roles in both cell cycle control and cellular transcription, as the CDK-activating kinase (CAK) and as a component of transcription factor complex TFIIH, respectively.[269] As a transcriptional CDK, CDK7 phosphorylates the CTD of RNA polymerase II on Ser5 and Ser7, allowing for promoter clearance and transcriptional initiation.[236-238] CDK7 and cyclin H have been shown to be elevated in breast tumor tissue at the mRNA and protein level, with higher protein expression seen in ER+ tumors and associated with better prognosis[270]; in contrast, elevated expression of CDK7 mRNA and protein were found to be associated with poor prognosis of TNBC.[271] Similarly, CDK7 was found to be overexpressed in gastric cancer, where it associated with advanced stage and poor survival.[272,273]

Selective, covalent inhibitors of CDK7 targeting a cysteine outside of the kinase domain (Cys-312); the first of these, THZ1, primarily inhibits CDK7 but also has CDK12 inhibitory activity (and its chemical modification was the basis of the discovery of THZ531, the more selective CDK12 inhibitor).[274] SY-1365 is another covalent inhibitor that has recently entered phase 1 clinical trial.[275,276] CDK7 has emerged as an attractive anticancer target, since its

inhibition reduces the levels of expression of genes defining oncogenic states, especially those driven by super-enhancers.[277-279] As opposed to typical enhancers composed of transcriptional factor-binding sites located at a distance from the transcriptional start site that act via chromosomal looping events to enhance transcription, super-enhancers consist of very large clusters of enhancers that are densely occupied by transcription factors, cofactors, and chromatin regulators, typically including CDK7 and BRD4. They arise via gene amplification, translocation, or transcription factor overexpression and facilitate high level of expression of genes involved in cell identity, growth, proliferation, and survival; often, the genes and encoded proteins have short half-life, so that high-level transcription is critical to maintenance of their expression. Super-enhancers are complex structures that are highly sensitive to perturbation and therefore selectively targeted when a small-molecule CDK7 inhibitor is applied. CDK7 inhibition has been shown to have preclinical activity against *RUNX1*-dependent T-cell ALL[274] and *NMYC*-amplified neuroblastoma.[280] Small cell lung cancer,[281] ovarian cancer,[282,283] and TNBC[284] have similarly been defined as transcriptionally addicted; in the case of TNBC, there appears to be dependence on an "Achilles gene cluster," with decreased expression correlating with preclinical efficacy. CDK7 inhibition may be synergistic with MDM2 inhibitor–mediated TP53 activation[285] as well as with inhibition of antiapoptotic proteins[286] and may also reverse adaptive responses to targeted cancer therapy.[287]

Conclusions

The CDK inhibitor field has evolved rapidly over the past several years and has been invigorated by potent agents that have produced clinical benefit. For selective CDK4/6 inhibitors, future work will involve the testing of predictive biomarkers for cytotoxicity and induction of senescence, development of strategies to overcome adaptation and resistance, and continued development of combinatorial approaches with inhibitors of signal transduction and immunotherapy. Transcriptional CDK inhibition is likely to be further developed in the hematologic malignancies. Effects on expression of genes in DNA repair pathways and of genes defining oncogenic states will likely be exploitable, with novel covalent compounds overcoming the liability of short half-life that has plagued the development of ATP-competitive compounds to date. Current approvals are limited to the selective CDK4/6 inhibitor drugs in breast cancer, but these agents, as well as transcriptional CDK inhibitors, will likely enter the armamentarium of multiple cancer types over the next several years.

Acknowledgments

I thank Suzanne Hector-Barry for research and writing assistance. G.I.S. is funded by R01 CA090687, P50 CA168504 (Dana-Farber/Harvard Cancer Center Specialized Program of Research Excellence in Breast Cancer), UM1 CA186709 (Dana-Farber/Harvard Cancer Center Experimental Therapeutics Clinical Trials Network), Susan Komen Investigator-Initiated Research

Grant IIR12223953, a Basser Center for BRCA Innovation Award (University of Pennsylvania), and the Stand Up To Cancer OCRFA-NOCC Ovarian Cancer Dream Team Translational Cancer Research Grant SU2C-AACR-DT16-15.

Conflict of Interest Statement

G.I.S. has received research funding from Lilly, Pfizer, and Merck/EMD Serono. He has served on advisory boards for Lilly, Pfizer, Merck/EMD Serono, Roche, and G1 Therapeutics.

References

1. Meyerson M, Enders GH, Wu CL, et al. A family of human cdc2-related protein kinases. *EMBO J.* 1992;11:2909-2917.
2. Meyerson M, Harlow E. Identification of G1 kinase activity for cdk6, a novel cyclin D partner. *Mol Cell Biol.* 1994;14:2077-2086.
3. Shapiro GI. Cyclin-dependent kinase pathways as targets for cancer treatment. *J Clin Oncol.* 2006;24:1770-1783.
4. Ren S, Rollins BJ. Cyclin C/cdk3 promotes Rb-dependent G0 exit. *Cell.* 2004;117:239-251.
5. Lundberg AS, Weinberg RA. Functional inactivation of the retinoblastoma protein requires sequential modification by at least two distinct cyclin-cdk complexes. *Mol Cell Biol.* 1998;18:753-761.
6. Harbour JW, Luo RX, Dei Santi A, Postigo AA, Dean DC. Cdk phosphorylation triggers sequential intramolecular interactions that progressively block Rb functions as cells move through G1. *Cell.* 1999;98:859-869.
7. Sherr CJ, Roberts JM. CDK inhibitors: positive and negative regulators of G1-phase progression. *Genes Dev.* 1999;13:1501-1512.
8. Narasimha AM, Kaulich M, Shapiro GS, Choi YJ, Sicinski P, Dowdy SF. Cyclin D activates the Rb tumor suppressor by mono-phosphorylation. *Elife.* 2014;3:02872.
9. Geng Y, Eaton EN, Picon M, et al. Regulation of cyclin E transcription by E2Fs and retinoblastoma protein. *Oncogene.* 1996;12:1173-1180.
10. Hwang HC, Clurman BE. Cyclin E in normal and neoplastic cell cycles. *Oncogene.* 2005;24:2776-2786.
11. Sheaff RJ, Groudine M, Gordon M, Roberts JM, Clurman BE. Cyclin E-CDK2 is a regulator of p27Kip1. *Genes Dev.* 1997;11:1464-1478.
12. Vlach J, Hennecke S, Amati B. Phosphorylation-dependent degradation of the cyclin-dependent kinase inhibitor p27Kip1. *EMBO J.* 1997;16:5334-5344.
13. Harper JW, Elledge SJ. The role of Cdk7 in CAK function, a retro-retrospective. *Genes Dev.* 1998;12:285-289.
14. Morgan DO. Principles of CDK regulation. *Nature.* 1995;374:131-134.
15. Sherr CJ, Roberts JM. Inhibitors of mammalian G1 cyclin-dependent kinases. *Genes Dev.* 1995;9:1149-1163.
16. Alcorta DA, Xiong Y, Phelps D, Hannon G, Beach D, Barrett JC. Involvement of the cyclin-dependent kinase inhibitor p16ink4a in replicative senescence of normal human fibroblasts. *Proc Natl Acad Sci U S A.* 1996;93:13742-13747.
17. Reznikoff CA, Yeager TR, Belair CD, Savelieva E, Puthenveettil JA, Stadler WM. Elevated p16 at senescence and loss of p16 at immortalization in human papillomavirus 16 E6, but not E7 transformed human uroepithelial cells. *Cancer Res.* 1996;56:2886-2890.
18. Mitra J, Dai CY, Somasundaram K, et al. Induction of p21(WAF1/CIP1) and inhibition of Cdk2 mediated by the tumor suppressor p16(INK4a). *Mol Cell Biol.* 1999;19:3916-3928.
19. Hannon GJ, Beach D. p15ink4B Is a potential effector of TGF-beta-induced cell cycle arrest. *Nature.* 1994;371:257-261.
20. Reynisdottir I, Polyak K, Iavarone A, Massaguke J. Kip/Cip and Ink4 cdks inhibitors cooperate to induce cell cycle arrest in response to TGF-beta. *Genes Dev.* 1995;9:1831-1845.
21. Hanahan D, Weinberg RA. Hallmarks of cancer: the next generation. *Cell.* 2011;144:646-674.
22. Wiestner A, Tehrani M, Chiorazzi M, et al. Point mutations and genomic deletions in *CCND1* create stable truncated cyclin D1 mRNAs that are associated with increased proliferation rate and shorter survival. *Blood.* 2007;109:4599-4606.
23. Network CGAR. Comprehensive genomic characterization of squamous cell lung cancers. *Nature.* 2012;489:519-525.
24. Song Y, Li L, Ou Y, et al. Identification of genomic alterations in oesophageal squamous cell cancer. *Nature.* 2014;509:91-95.
25. Ooi A, Oyama T, Nakamura R, et al. Gene amplification of *CCNE1*, *CCND1*, and CDK6 in gastric cancers detected by multiplex ligation-dependent probe amplification and fluorescence in situ hybridization. *Hum Pathol.* 2017;61:58-67.
26. Cheung TH, Yu MMY, Lo KWK, Yim SF, Chung TKH, Wong YF. Alteration of cyclin D1 and CDK4 gene in carcinoma of uterine cervix. *Cancer Lett.* 2001;166:199-206.
27. Arnold A, Papanikolaou A. Cyclin D1 in breast cancer pathogenesis. *J Clin Oncol.* 2005;23:4215-4224.
28. Buckley MF, Sweeney KJ, Hamilton JA, Sini RL, Manning DL, Nicholson RI, Expression and amplification of cyclin genes in human breast cancer. *Oncogene.* 1993;8:2127-2133.
29. Gillett C, Fantl V, Smith R, et al. Amplification and overexpression of cyclin D1 in breast cancer detected by immunohistochemical staining. *Cancer Res.* 1994;54:1812-1817.
30. Wang X, Pavelic ZP, Li YQ, et al. Amplification and overexpression of the cyclin D1 gene in head and neck squamous cell carcinoma. *Clin Mol Pathol.* 1995;48:M256-M259.
31. Namazie A, Alavi S, Olopade OI, et al. Cyclin D1 amplification and p16(MTS1/CDK4I) deletion correlate with poor prognosis in head and neck tumors. *Laryngoscope.* 2002;112:472-481.
32. Ikeda Y, Oda K, Hiraike-Wada O, et al. Cyclin D1 harboring the T286I mutation promotes oncogenic activation in endometrial cancer. *Oncol Rep.* 2013;30:584-588.
33. Moreno-Bueno G, Rodriguez-Perales S, Sanchez-Estevez C, et al. Cyclin D1 gene (*CCND1*) mutations in endometrial cancer. *Oncogene.* 2003;22:6115-6118.
34. Kim CJ, Nishi K, Isono T, et al. Cyclin D1b variant promotes cell invasiveness independent of binding to CDK4 in human bladder cancer cells. *Mol Carcinog.* 2009;48:953-964.
35. Abramson VG, Troxel AB, Feldman M, et al. Cyclin D1b in human breast carcinoma and coexpression with cyclin D1a is associated with poor outcome. *Anticancer Res.* 2010;30:1279-1285.
36. Krieger S, Gauduchon J, Roussel M, Troussard X, Sola B. Relevance of cyclin D1b expression and *CCND1* polymorphism in the pathogenesis of multiple myeloma and mantle cell lymphoma. *BMC Cancer.* 2006;6:238.
37. Büschges R, Weber RG, Actor B, Lichter P, Collins VP, Reifenberger G. Amplification and expression of cyclin D genes (*CCND1 CCND2* and *CCND3*) in human malignant gliomas. *Brain Pathol.* 1999;9:435-442.
38. Helsten T, Kato S, Schwaederle M, et al. Cell-cycle gene alterations in 4,864 tumors analyzed by next-generation sequencing: implications for targeted therapeutics. *Mol Cancer Ther.* 2016;15:1682-1690.
39. Takano Y, Kato Y, van Diest PJ, Masuda M, Mitomi H, Okayasu I. Cyclin D2 Overexpression and lack of p27 correlate positively and cyclin E inversely with a poor prognosis in gastric cancer cases. *Am J Pathol.* 2000;156:585-594.
40. Hoglund M, Johansson B, Pedersen-Bjergaard J, Marynen P, Mitelman F. Molecular characterization of 12p abnormalities in hematologic malignancies: deletion of KIP1, rearrangement of TEL, and amplification of *CCND2*. *Blood.* 1996;87:324-330.
41. Rodriguez S, Jafer O, Goker H, Summersgill BM, Zafarana G, Gillis AJM. Expression profile of genes from 12p in testicular germ cell tumors of adolescents and adults associated with i(12p) and amplification at 12p11.2-p12.1. *Oncogene.* 2003;22:1880-1891.
42. Teramoto N, Pokrovskaja K, Szekely L, et al. Expression of cyclin D2 and D3 in lymphoid lesions. *Int J Cancer.* 1999;81:543-550.
43. Beltran AL, Ordonez JL, Otero AP, et al. Fluorescence in situ hybridization analysis of CCND3 gene as marker of progression in bladder carcinoma. *J Biol Regul Homeost Agents.* 2013;27:559-567.
44. Pruneri G, Mazzarol G, Fabris S, et al. Cyclin D3 immunoreactivity in gastrointestinal stromal tumors is independent of cyclin D3 gene amplification and is associated with nuclear p27 accumulation. *Mod Pathol.* 2003;16:886-892.

45. Filipits M, Jaeger U, Pohl G, et al. Cyclin D3 is a predictive and prognostic factor in diffuse large B-cell lymphoma. *Clin Cancer Res.* 2002;8:729-733.

46. Dei Tos AP, Maestro R, Doglioni C, et al. Tumor suppressor genes and related molecules in leiomyosarcoma. *Am J Pathol.* 1996;148:1037-1045.

47. Network CGAR. Comprehensive genomic characterization defines human glioblastoma genes and core pathways. *Nature.* 2008;455:1061-1068.

48. Schmidt EE, Ichimura K, Reifenberger G, Collins VP. *CDKN2* (p16/MTS1) Gene deletion or CDK4 amplification occurs in the majority of glioblastomas. *Cancer Res.* 1994;54:6321-6324.

49. Wei G, Lonardo F, Ueda T, et al. CDK4 gene amplification in osteosarcoma: reciprocal relationship with INK4A gene alterations and mapping of 12q13 amplicons. *Int J Cancer.* 1999;80:199-204.

50. Park S, Lee J, Do I-G, et al. Aberrant CDK4 amplification in refractory rhabdomyosarcoma as identified by genomic profiling. *Sci Rep.* 2014;4:3623.

51. Wölfel T, Hauer M, Schneider J, et al. A p16INK4a-insensitive *CDK4* mutant targeted by cytolytic T lymphocytes in a human melanoma. *Science.* 1995;269:1281.

52. Zuo L, Weger J, Yang Q, et al. Germline mutations in the p16INK4a binding domain of CDK4 in familial melanoma. *Nat Genet.* 1996;12:97-99.

53. Smalley KSM, Contractor R, Nguyen TK, et al. Identification of a novel subgroup of melanomas with KIT/cyclin dependent kinase-4 overexpression. *Cancer Res.* 2008;68:5743-5752.

54. Ismail A, Bandla S, Reveiller M, et al. Early G1 cyclin-dependent kinases as prognostic markers and potential therapeutic targets in esophageal adenocarcinoma. *Clin Cancer Res.* 2011;17:4513-4522.

55. Tang LH, Contractor T, Clausen R, et al. Attenuation of the retinoblastoma pathway in pancreatic neuroendocrine tumors due to increased Cdk4/Cdk6. *Clin Cancer Res.* 2012;18:4612.

56. Dobashi Y, Goto A, Fukayama M, Abe A, Ooi A. Overexpression of cdk4/cyclin D1, a possible mediator of apoptosis and an indicator of prognosis in human primary lung carcinoma. *Int J Cancer.* 2004;110:532-541.

57. Costello JF, Plass C, Arap W, et al. Cyclin-dependent kinase 6 (CDK6) amplification in human gliomas identified using two-dimensional separation of genomic DNA. *Cancer Res.* 1997;57:1250.

58. Ren W, Li W, Wang D, Hu S, Suo J, Ying X. Combining multi-dimensional data to identify key genes and pathways in gastric cancer. *PeerJ.* 2017;5:e3385.

59. Mendrzyk F, Radlwimmer B, Joos S, et al. Genomic and protein expression profiling identifies CDK6 as novel independent prognostic marker in medulloblastoma. *J Clin Oncol.* 2005;23:8853-8862.

60. Corcoran MM, Mould SJ, Orchard JA, et al. Dysregulation of cyclin dependent kinase 6 expression in splenic marginal zone lymphoma through chromosome 7q translocations. *Oncogene.* 1999;18:6271-6277.

61. Bandla S, Pennathur A, Luketich JD, et al. Comparative genomics of esophageal adenocarcinoma and squamous cell carcinoma. *Ann Thorac Surg.* 2012;93:1101-1106.

62. Patch AM, Christie EL, Etemadmoghadam D, et al. Whole-genome characterization of chemoresistant ovarian cancer. *Nature.* 2015;521:489-494.

63. Sakaguchi T, Watanabe A, Sawada H, et al. Prognostic value of cyclin E and p53 expression in gastric carcinoma. *Cancer.* 1998; 82:1238-1243.

64. Cassia R, Moreno-Bueno G, Rodríguez-Perales S, Hardisson D, Cigudosa JC, Palacios J. Cyclin E gene (CCNE) amplification and hCDC4 mutations in endometrial carcinoma. *J Pathol.* 2003;201:589-595.

65. Nakayama K, Rahman MT, Rahman M, et al. *CCNE1* amplification is associated with aggressive potential in endometrioid endometrial carcinomas. *Int J Oncol.* 2016;48:506-516.

66. Nakayama N, Nakayama K, Shamima Y, et al. Gene amplification *CCNE1* is related to poor survival and potential therapeutic target in ovarian cancer. *Cancer.* 2010;116:2621-2634.

67. Kato N, Watanabe J, Jobo T, et al. Immunohistochemical expression of cyclin E in endometrial adenocarcinoma (endometrioid type) and its clinicopathological significance. *J Cancer Res Clin Oncol.* 2003;129:222-226.

68. Karst AM, Jones PM, Vena N, et al. Cyclin E1 deregulation occurs early in secretory cell transformation to promote formation of fallopian tube derived high-grade serous ovarian cancers. *Cancer Res.* 2014;74:1141-1152.

69. Sawasaki T, Shigemasa K, Shiroyama Y, et al. Cyclin E mRNA overexpression in epithelial ovarian cancers: inverse correlation with p53 protein accumulation. *J Soc Gyn Invest.* 2001;8:179-185.

70. Erlanson M, Portin C, Linderholm B, Lindh J, Roos G, Landberg G. Expression of cyclin E and the cyclin-dependent kinase inhibitor p27 in malignant lymphomas—prognostic implications. *Blood.* 1998;92:770-777.

71. Rosen DG, Yang G, Deavers MT, et al. Cyclin E expression is correlated with tumor progression and predicts a poor prognosis in patients with ovarian carcinoma. *Cancer.* 2006;106:1925-1932.

72. Dosaka-Akita H, Hommura F, Mishina T, et al. A risk-stratification model of non-small cell lung cancers using cyclin E, Ki-67, and p21. *Cancer Res.* 2001;61:2500-2504.

73. Koutsami MK, Tsantoulis PK, Kouloukoussa M, et al. Centrosome abnormalities are frequently observed in non-small-cell lung cancer and are associated with aneuploidy and cyclin E overexpression. *J Pathol.* 2006;209:512-521.

74. Keyomarsi K, Leary N, Molnar G, Lees E, Fingert HJ, Pardee AB. Cyclin E, a potential prognostic marker for breast cancer. *Cancer Res.* 1994;54:380-385.

75. Keyomarsi K, Tucker SL, Buchholz TA, et al. Cyclin E and survival in patients with breast cancer. *N Engl J Med.* 2002;347:1566-1575.

76. Li W, Zhang G, Wang HL, Wang L. Analysis of expression of cyclin E, p27^{kip1} and Ki67 protein in colorectal cancer tissues and its value for diagnosis, treatment and prognosis of disease. *Eur Rev Med Pharmacol Sci.* 2016;20:4874-4879.

77. Kitahara K, Yasui W, Kuniyasu H, et al. Concurrent amplification of cyclin E and CDK2 genes in colorectal carcinomas. *Int J Cancer.* 1995;62:25-28.

78. Wang A, Yoshimi N, Suzui M, Yamauchi A, Tarao M, Mori H. Different expression patterns of cyclins A, D1 and E in human colorectal cancer. *J Cancer Res Clin Oncol.* 1996;122:122-126.

79. Yue H, Jiang H-Y. Expression of cell cycle regulator p57(kip2), cyclin E protein and proliferating cell nuclear antigen in human pancreatic cancer: an immunohistochemical study. *World J Gastroenterol.* 2005;11:5057-5060.

80. Lockwood WW, Stack D, Morris T, et al. Cyclin E1 is amplified and overexpressed in osteosarcoma. *J Mol Diagn.* 2011;13:289-296.

81. Wolowiec D, Benchaib M, Pernas P, et al. Expression of cell cycle regulatory proteins in chronic lymphocytic leukemias. Comparison with non-Hodgkin's lymphomas and non-neoplastic lymphoid tissue. *Leukemia.* 1995;9:1382-1388.

82. Georgieva J, Sinha P, Schadendorf D. Expression of cyclins and cyclin dependent kinases in human benign and malignant melanocytic lesions. *J Clin Pathol.* 2001;54:229-235.

83. Abdullah C, Wang X, Becker D. Expression analysis and molecular targeting of cyclin-dependent kinases in advanced melanoma: Functional analysis and molecular targeting of cyclin-dependent kinase family members in advanced melanoma. *Cell Cycle.* 2011;10:977-988.

84. Cybulski M, Jarosz B, Nowakowski A, et al. Cyclin A correlates with YB1, progression and resistance to chemotherapy in human epithelial ovarian cancer. *Anticancer Res.* 2015;35:1715-1721.

85. Gao T, Han Y, Yu L, Ao S, Li Z, Ji J. CCNA2 is a prognostic biomarker for ER+ breast cancer and tamoxifen resistance. *PLoS One.* 2014;9:e91771.

86. Klintman M, Strand C, Ahlin C, et al. The prognostic value of mitotic activity index (MAI), phosphohistone H3 (PPH3), cyclin B1, cyclin A, and Ki67, alone and in combinations, in node-negative premenopausal breast cancer. *PLoS One.* 2013;8:e81902.

87. Santala S, Talvensaari-Mattila A, Soini Y, Honkavuori-Toivola M, Santala M. High expression of cyclin A is associated with poor prognosis in endometrial endometrioid adenocarcinoma. *Tumor Biol.* 2014;35:5395-5399.

88. Furihata M, Ishikawa T, Inoue A, et al. Determination of the prognostic significance of unscheduled cyclin A overexpression in patients with esophageal squamous cell carcinoma. *Clin Cancer Res.* 1996;2:1781-1785.

89. Huuhtanen RL, Blomqvist CP, Böhling TO, et al. Expression of cyclin A in soft tissue sarcomas correlates with tumor aggressiveness. *Cancer Res.* 1999;59:2885-2890.

90. Nar A, Ozen O, Tutuncu NB, Demirhan B. Cyclin A and cyclin B1 overexpression in differentiated thyroid carcinoma. *Med Oncol.* 2012;29:294-300.

91. Ekberg J, Holm C, Jalili S, et al. Expression of cyclin A1 and cell cycle proteins in hematopoietic cells and acute myeloid leukemia and links to patient outcome. *Eur J Hematol.* 2005;75:106-115.

92. Chao Y, Shih Y-L, Chiu J-H, et al. Overexpression of cyclin A but not Skp 2 correlates with the tumor relapse of human hepatocellular carcinoma. *Cancer Res.* 1998;58:985-990.

93. Husdal A, Bukholm G, Bukholm IRK. The prognostic value and overexpression of cyclin A is correlated with gene amplification of both cyclin A and cyclin E in breast cancer patient. *Cell Oncol.* 2006;28:107-116.

94. Allan K, Jordan RC, Ang LC, Taylor M, Young B. Overexpression of cyclin A and cyclin B1 proteins in astrocytomas. *Arch Pathol Lab Med.* 2000;124:216-220.

95. Takashima S, Saito H, Takahashi N, et al. Strong expression of cyclin B2 mRNA correlates with a poor prognosis in patients with non-small cell lung cancer. *Tumor Biol.* 2014;35:4257-4265.

96. Zhou L, Li J, Zhao Y-P, et al. The prognostic value of Cyclin B1 in pancreatic cancer. *Med Oncol.* 2014; 31:107.

97. Santala S, Talvensaari-Mattila A, Soini Y, Santala M. Prognostic value of cyclin B in endometrial endometrioid adenocarcinoma. *Tumor Biol.* 2015;36:953-957.

98. Chae SW, Sohn JH, Kim D-H, et al. Overexpressions of cyclin B1, cdc2, p16 and p53 in human breast cancer: the clinicopathologic correlations and prognostic implications. *Yonsei Med J.* 2011;52:445-453.

99. Aaltonen K, Amini RM, Heikkilä P, et al. High cyclin B1 expression is associated with poor survival in breast cancer. *Br J Cancer.* 2009;100: 1055-1060.

100. Begnami MD, Fregnani JHTG, Nonogaki S, Soares FA. Evaluation of cell cycle protein expression in gastric cancer: cyclin B1 expression and its prognostic implication. *Hum Pathol.* 2010;41:1120-1127.

101. Santarius T, Shipley J, Brewer D, Stratton MR, Cooper CS. A census of amplified and overexpressed human cancer genes. *Nat Rev Cancer.* 2010;10:59-64.

102. Jares P, Colomer D, Campo E. Genetic and molecular pathogenesis of mantle cell lymphoma: perspectives for new targeted therapeutics. *Nat Rev Cancer.* 2007;7:750-762.

103. Perez-Galan P, Dreyling M, Wiestner A. Mantle cell lymphoma: biology, pathogenesis, and the molecular basis of treatment in the genomic era. *Blood.* 2011;117:26-38.

104. Bertoni F, Rinaldi A, Zucca E, Cavalli F. Update on the molecular biology of mantle cell lymphoma. *Hematol Oncol.* 2006;24:22-27.

105. Diehl JA, Cheng M, Roussel MF, Sherr CJ. Glycogen synthase kinase-3beta regulates cyclin D1 proteolysis and subcellular localization. *Genes Dev.* 1998;12:3499-3511.

106. Alt JR, Cleveland JL, Hannink M, Diehl JA. Phosphorylation-dependent regulation of cyclin D1 nuclear export and cyclin D1-dependent cellular transformation. *Genes Dev.* 2000;14:3102-3114.

107. Schmitz R, Young RM, Ceribelli M, et al. Burkitt lymphoma pathogenesis and therapeutic targets from structural and functional genomics. *Nature.* 2012;490:116-120.

108. Lu F, Gladden AB, Diehl JA. An alternatively spliced cyclin D1 isoform, cyclin D1b, is a nuclear oncogene. *Cancer Res.* 2003;63:7056-7061.

109. Shapiro GI, Park JE, Edwards CD, et al. Multiple mechanisms of p16INK4A inactivation in non-small cell lung cancer cell lines. *Cancer Res.* 1995;55:6200-6209.

110. Hansson J. Familial cutaneous melanoma. *Adv Exp Med Biol.* 2010;685: 134-145.

111. Lynch HT, Brand RE, Deters CA, Shaw TG, Lynch JF. Hereditary pancreatic cancer. *Pancreatology.* 2001; 1:466-471.

112. Etemadmoghadam D, Weir BA, Au-Yeung G, et al. Synthetic lethality between CCNE1 amplification and loss of BRCA1. *Proc Natl Acad Sci U S A.* 2013;110:19489-19494.

113. Slingerland J, Pagano M. Regulation of the cdk inhibitor p27 and its deregulation in cancer. *J Cell Physiol.* 2000;183:10-17.

114. Lloyd RV, Erickson LA, Jin L, et al. p27(kip1): a multifunctional cyclin-dependent kinase inhibitor with prognostic significance in human cancers. *Am J Pathol.* 1999;154:313-323.

115. Asghar U, Witkiewicz AK, Turner NC, Knudsen ES. The history and future of targeting cyclin-dependent kinases in cancer therapy. *Nat Rev Drug Discov.* 2015;14:130-146.

116. Sherr CJ, Beach D, Shapiro GI. Targeting CDK4 and CDK6: from discovery to therapy. *Cancer Discov.* 2016;6:353-367.

117. Fry DW, Harvey PJ, Keller PR, et al. Specific inhibition of cyclin-dependent kinase 4/6 by PD 0332991 and associated antitumor activity in human tumor xenografts. *Mol Cancer Ther.* 2004;3:1427-1438.

118. Toogood PL, Harvey PJ, Repine JT, et al. Discovery of a potent and selective inhibitor of cyclin-dependent kinase 4/6. *J Med Chem.* 2005;48:2388-2406.

119. Kim S, Loo A, Chopra R, et al. Abstract PR02: LEE011: An orally bioavailable, selective small molecule inhibitor of CDK4/6—Reactivating Rb in cancer. *Mol Cancer Ther.* 2014;12:PR02, [abstract].

120. Gelbert LM, Cai S, Lin X, et al. Preclinical characterization of the CDK4/6 inhibitor LY2835219: in-vivo cell cycle-dependent/independent antitumor activities alone/in combination with gemcitabine. *Invest New Drugs.* 2014;32:825-837.

121. Flaherty KT, Lorusso PM, Demichele A, et al. Phase I, dose-escalation trial of the oral cyclin-dependent kinase 4/6 inhibitor PD 0332991, administered using a 21-day schedule in patients with advanced cancer. *Clin Cancer Res.* 2012;18:568-576.

122. Schwartz GK, Lorusso PM, Dickson MA, et al. Phase I study of PD 0332991, a cyclin-dependent kinase inhibitor, administered in 3-week cycles (Schedule 2/1). *Br J Cancer.* 2011;104:1862-1868.

123. Infante JR, Cassier PA, Gerecitano JF, et al. A phase I study of the cyclin-dependent kinase 4/6 inhibitor ribociclib (LEE011) in patients with advanced solid tumors and lymphomas. *Clin Cancer Res.* 2016;22:5696-5705.

124. Patnaik A, Rosen LS, Tolaney SM, et al. Efficacy and safety of abemaciclib, an inhibitor of CDK4 and CDK6, for patients with breast cancer, non-small cell lung cancer, and other solid tumors. *Cancer Discov.* 2016;6:740-753.

125. Leonard JP, LaCasce AS, Smith MR, et al. Selective CDK4/6 inhibition with tumor responses by PD0332991 in patients with mantle cell lymphoma. *Blood.* 2012;119:4597-4607.

126. Vaughn DJ, Flaherty K, Lal P, et al. Treatment of growing teratoma syndrome. *N Engl J Med.* 2009;360:423-424.

127. Vaughn DJ, Hwang WT, Lal P, Rosen MA, Gallagher M, O'Dwyer PJ. Phase 2 trial of the cyclin-dependent kinase 4/6 inhibitor palbociclib in patients with retinoblastoma protein-expressing germ cell tumors. *Cancer.* 2015;121:1463-1468.

128. O'Leary B, Finn RS, Turner NC. Treating cancer with selective CDK4/6 inhibitors. *Nat Rev Clin Oncol.* 2016;13:417-430.

129. Zhang Y-X, Sicinska E, Czaplinski JT, et al. Antiproliferative effects of CDK4/6 inhibition in CDK4-amplified human liposarcoma in vitro and in vivo. *Mol Cancer Ther.* 2014;13:2184-2193.

130. Rader J, Russell MR, Hart LS, et al. Dual CDK4/CDK6 inhibition induces cell-cycle arrest and senescence in neuroblastoma. *Clin Cancer Res.* 2013;19:6173-6182.

131. Tate SC, Cai S, Ajamie RT, et al. Semi-mechanistic pharmacokinetic/pharmacodynamic modeling of the antitumor activity of LY2835219, a new cyclin-dependent kinase 4/6 inhibitor, in mice bearing human tumor xenografts. *Clin Cancer Res.* 2014; 20:3763-3774.

132. Raub TJ, Wishart GN, Kulanthaivel P, et al. Brain exposure of two selective dual CDK4 and CDK6 inhibitors and the antitumor activity of CDK4 and CDK6 inhibition in combination with temozolomide in an intracranial glioblastoma xenograft. *Drug Metab Dispos.* 2015;43:1360-1371.

133. Scheicher R, Hoelbl-Kovacic A, Bellutti F, et al. CDK6 as a key regulator of hematopoietic and leukemic stem cell activation. *Blood.* 2015;125:90-101.

134. Laurenti E, Frelin C, Xie S, et al. CDK6 Levels Regulate quiescence exit in human hematopoietic stem cells. *Cell Stem Cell.* 2015;16:302-313.

135. Dickler MN, Tolaney SM, Rugo HS, et al. MONARCH 1, A phase II study of abemaciclib, a CDK4 and CDK6 inhibitor, as a single agent, in patients with refractory HR$^+$/HER2$^-$ metastatic breast cancer. *Clin Cancer Res.* 2017;23:5218-5224.

136. Bisi JE, Sorrentino JA, Roberts PJ, Tavares FX, Strum JC. Preclinical characterization of G1T28: a novel CDK4/6 inhibitor for reduction of chemotherapy-induced myelosuppression. *Mol Cancer Ther.* 2016;15:783-793.

137. Bisi JE, Sorrentino JA, Jordan JL, et al. Preclinical development of G1T38: a novel, potent and selective inhibitor of cyclin dependent kinases 4/6 for use as an oral antineoplastic in patients with CDK4/6 sensitive tumors. *Oncotarget.* 2017;8:42343-42358.

138. Stice JP, Wardell SE, Norris JD, et al. CDK4/6 Therapeutic intervention and viable alternative to taxanes in CRPC. *Mol Cancer Res.* 2017;15:660-669.

139. Finn RS, Dering J, Conklin D, et al. PD 0332991, a selective cyclin D kinase 4/6 inhibitor, preferentially inhibits proliferation of luminal estrogen receptor-positive human breast cancer cell lines in vitro. *Breast Cancer Res.* 2009;1:R77.

140. Doisneau-Sixou SF, Sergio CM, Carroll JS, Hui R, Musgrove EA, Sutherland RL. Estrogen and antiestrogen regulation of cell cycle progression in breast cancer cells. *Endocr Relat Cancer.* 2003;10:179-186.

141. DeMichele A, Clark AS, Tan KS, et al. CDK 4/6 inhibitor palbociclib (PD0332991) in Rb+ advanced breast cancer: phase II activity, safety, and predictive biomarker assessment. *Clin Cancer Res.* 2015;21:995-1001.

142. Finn RS, Crown JP, Lang I, et al. The cyclin-dependent kinase 4/6 inhibitor palbociclib in combination with letrozole versus letrozole alone as first-line treatment of oestrogen receptor-positive, HER2-negative, advanced breast cancer (PALOMA-1/TRIO-18): a randomised phase 2 study. *Lancet Oncol.* 2015;16:25-35.

143. Finn RS, Martin M, Rugo HS, et al. Palbociclib and letrozole in advanced breast cancer. *N Engl J Med.* 2016;375:1925-1936.

144. Turner NC, Ro J, Andre F, et al. Palbociclib in hormone-receptor-positive advanced breast cancer. *N Engl J Med.* 2015;373:209-219.

145. Cristofanilli M, Turner NC, Bondarenko I, et al. Fulvestrant plus palbociclib versus fulvestrant plus placebo for treatment of hormone-receptor-positive, HER2-negative metastatic breast cancer that progressed on previous endocrine therapy (PALOMA-3): final analysis of the multicentre, double-blind, phase 3 randomised controlled trial. *Lancet Oncol.* 17:425-439.

146. Hortobagyi GN, Stemmer SM, Burris HA, et al. Ribociclib as first-line therapy for HR-positive, advanced breast cancer. *N Engl J Med.* 2016;375:1738-1748.

147. Sledge GW, Toi M, Neven P, et al. MONARCH 2: abemaciclib in combination with fulvestrant in women with HR+/HER2− advanced breast cancer who had progressed while receiving endocrine therapy. *J Clin Oncol.* 2017;35:2875-2884.

148. Goetz MP, Toi M, Campone M, et al. MONARCH 3: abemaciclib as initial therapy for advanced breast cancer. *J Clin Oncol.* 2017;35:3638-3646.

149. Ma CX, Gao F, Luo J, et al. NeoPalAna: neoadjuvant palbociclib, a cyclin-dependent kinase 4/6 inhibitor, and anastrozole for clinical stage 2 or 3 estrogen receptor-positive breast cancer. *Clin Cancer Res.* 2017;23:4055-4065.

150. Bagegni N, Thomas S, Liu N, et al. Serum TK 1 activity as a pharmacodynamic marker of cyclin-dependent kinase 4/6 inhibition in patients with early-stage breast cancer receiving neoadjuvant palbociclib. *Breast Cancer Res.* 2017;19:123.

151. Hurvitz S, Martin M, Fernández Abad M, et al. Abstract S4-06: Biological effects of abemaciclib in a phase 2 neoadjuvant study for postmenopausal patients with HR+, HER2− breast cancer. *Cancer Res.* 2017;77:S4-06, [abstract].

152. Reddy HK, Mettus RV, Rane SG, Grana X, Litvin J, Reddy EP. Cyclin-dependent kinase 4 expression is essential for neu-induced breast tumorigenesis. *Cancer Res.* 2005;65:10174-10178.

153. Yu Q, Geng Y, Sicinski P. Specific protection against breast cancers by cyclin D1 ablation. *Nature.* 2001;411:1017-1021.

154. Yu Q, Sicinska E, Geng Y, et al. Requirement for CDK4 kinase function in breast cancer. *Cancer Cell.* 2006;9:23-32.

155. Morschhauser F, Bouabdallah K, Stilgenbauer S, et al. Clinical activity of abemaciclib (LY2835219), a cell cycle inhibitor selective for CDK4 and CDK6, in patients with relapsed or refractory mantle cell lymphoma. *Blood.* 2014;124:3067, [abstract].

156. Rahal R, Frick M, Romero R, et al. Pharmacological and genomic profiling identifies NF-kappaB-targeted treatment strategies for mantle cell lymphoma. *Nat Med.* 2014;20:87-92.

157. Buggy JJ, Elias L. Bruton tyrosine kinase (BTK) and its role in B-cell malignancy. *Int Rev Immunol.* 2012;31:119-132.

158. Cinar M, Hamedani F, Mo Z, Cinar B, Amin HM, Alkan S. Bruton tyrosine kinase is commonly overexpressed in mantle cell lymphoma and its attenuation by Ibrutinib induces apoptosis. *Leuk Res.* 2013;37:1271-1277.

159. Stephens DM, Spurgeon SE. Ibrutinib in mantle cell lymphoma patients: glass half full? Evidence and opinion. *Ther Adv Hematol.* 2015;6:242-252.

160. Chiron D, Di Liberto M, Martin P, et al. Cell-cycle reprogramming for PI3K inhibition overrides a relapse-specific C481S BTK mutation revealed by longitudinal functional genomics in mantle cell lymphoma. *Cancer Discov.* 2014;4:1022-1035.

161. Chiron D, Martin P, Di Liberto M, et al. Induction of prolonged early G1 arrest by CDK4/CDK6 inhibition reprograms lymphoma cells for durable PI3Kdelta inhibition through PIK3IP1. *Cell Cycle.* 2013;12:1892-1900.

162. Martin P, Blum K, Bartlett NL, et al. A phase I trial of ibrutinib plus palbociclib in patients with previously treated mantle cell lymphoma. *Proc Am Soc Hematol.* 2016;128(22), [abstract].

163. Lee SE, Kim YJ, Kwon MJ, et al. High level of CDK4 amplification is a poor prognostic factor in well-differentiated and dedifferentiated liposarcoma. *Histol Histopathol.* 2014;29:127-138.

164. Lee S, Park H, Ha SY, et al. CDK4 amplification predicts recurrence of well-differentiated liposarcoma of the abdomen. *PLoS One.* 2014;9:e99452.

165. Dickson MA, Tap WD, Keohan ML, et al. Phase II trial of the CDK4 inhibitor PD0332991 in patients with advanced CDK4-amplified well-differentiated or dedifferentiated liposarcoma. *J Clin Oncol.* 2013;31:2024-2028.

166. Dickson MA, Schwartz GK, Keohan ML, et al. Phase 2 trial of the CDK4 inhibitor palbociclib (PD0332991) at 125 mg dose in well-differentiated or dedifferentiated liposarcoma. *JAMA Oncol.* 2016;2:937-940.

167. Kovatcheva M, Liu DD, Dickson MA, et al. MDM2 turnover and expression of ATRX determine the choice between quiescence and senescence in response to CDK4 inhibition. *Oncotarget.* 2015;6:8226-8243.

168. Kovatcheva M, Liao W, Klein ME, et al. ATRX is a regulator of therapy induced senescence in human cells. *Nat Commun.* 2017;8:386.

169. Anders L, Ke N, Hydbring P, et al. A systematic screen for CDK4/6 substrates links FOXM1 phosphorylation to senescence suppression in cancer cells. *Cancer Cell.* 2011;20:620-634.

170. Puyol M, Martín A, Dubus P, et al. A synthetic lethal interaction between K-Ras oncogenes and Cdk4 unveils a therapeutic strategy for non-small cell lung carcinoma. *Cancer Cell.* 2010;18:63-73.

171. Gopalan PK, Pinder MC, Chiappori A, Ivey AM, Gordillo Villegas A, Kaye FJ. A phase II clinical trial of the CDK 4/6 inhibitor palbociclib (PD 0332991) in previously treated, advanced non-small cell lung cancer (NSCLC) patients with inactivated *CDKN2A. J Clin Oncol.* 2014;32:8077, [abstract].

172. Goldman JW, Shi P, Reck M, Paz-Ares L, Koustenis A, Hurt KC. Treatment rationale and study design for the JUNIPER study: a randomized phase III study of abemaciclib with best supportive care versus erlotinib with best supportive care in patients with stage IV non–small-cell lung cancer with a detectable KRAS mutation whose disease has progressed after platinum-based chemotherapy. *Clin Lung Cancer.* 2016;17:80-84.

173. Gong X, Litchfield LM, Webster Y, et al. Genomic aberrations that activate D-type cyclins are associated with enhanced sensitivity to the CDK4 and CDK6 inhibitor abemaciclib. *Cancer Cell.* 2017;32:761-776.

174. Shapiro GI. Genomic biomarkers predicting response to selective CDK4/6 inhibition: progress in an elusive search. *Cancer Cell.* 2017;32:721-723.

175. Handschick K, Beuerlein K, Jurida L, et al. Cyclin-dependent kinase 6 is a chromatin-bound cofactor for NF-kappaB-dependent gene expression. *Mol Cell.* 2014;53:193-208.

176. Franco J, Balaji U, Freinkman E, Witkiewicz AK, Knudsen ES. Metabolic reprogramming of pancreatic cancer mediated by CDK4/6 inhibition elicits unique vulnerabilities. *Cell Rep.* 2016;14:979-990.

177. Torres-Guzman R, Calsina B, Hermoso A, et al. Preclinical characterization of abemaciclib in hormone receptor positive breast cancer. *Oncotarget.* 2017;8:69493-69507.

178. Wang H, Nicolay BN, Chick JM, et al. The metabolic function of cyclin D3-CDK6 kinase in cancer cell survival. *Nature.* 2017;546:426-430.

179. Choi YJ, Li X, Hydbring P, et al. The requirement for cyclin D function in tumor maintenance. *Cancer Cell.* 2012;22:438-451.

180. Miller TW, Hennessy BT, González-Angulo AM, et al. Hyperactivation of phosphatidylinositol-3 kinase promotes escape from hormone dependence in estrogen receptor–positive human breast cancer. *J Clin Invest.* 2010;120:2406-2413.

181. Vora Sadhna R, Juric D, Kim N, et al. CDK 4/6 Inhibitors sensitize *PIK3CA* mutant breast cancer to PI3K inhibitors. *Cancer Cell.* 2014;26:136-149.

182. Schwaederle M, Elkin SK, Tomson BN, Carter JL, Kurzrock R. Squamousness: next-generation sequencing reveals shared molecular features across squamous tumor types. *Cell Cycle.* 2015;14:2355-2361.

183. Eser S, Reiff N, Messer M, et al. Selective requirement of PI3K/PDK1 signaling for Kras oncogene-driven pancreatic cell plasticity and cancer. *Cancer Cell.* 23:406-420.

184. Franco J, Witkiewicz AK, Knudsen ES. CDK4/6 inhibitors have potent activity in combination with pathway selective therapeutic agents in models of pancreatic cancer. *Oncotarget.* 2014;5:6512-6525.

185. Blumenschein GR, Smit EF, Planchard D, et al. MEK114653: a randomized, multicenter, phase II study to assess efficacy and safety of trametinib compared to docetaxel in *KRAS*-mutant advanced non-small cell lung cancer. *J Clin Oncol.* 2013;31:A8029, [abstract].

186. Jänne PA, Shaw AT, Pereira JR, et al. Selumetinib plus docetaxel for *KRAS*-mutant advanced non-small-cell lung cancer: a randomised, multicentre, placebo-controlled, phase 2 study. *Lancet Oncol.* 2013;14:38-47.

187. Dummer R, Schadendorf D, Ascierto PA, et al. Binimetinib versus dacarbazine in patients with advanced *NRAS*-mutant melanoma (NEMO): a multicentre, open-label, randomised, phase 3 trial. *Lancet Oncol.* 2017;18: 435-445.

188. Kwong LN, Costello JC, Liu H, et al. Oncogenic NRAS signaling differentially regulates survival and proliferation in melanoma. *Nat Med.* 2012;18:1503-1510.

189. Lee MS, Helms TL, Feng N, et al. Efficacy of the combination of MEK and CDK4/6 inhibitors in vitro and in vivo in *KRAS* mutant colorectal cancer models. *Oncotarget.* 2016;7:39595-39608.

190. Ziemke EK, Dosch JS, Maust JD, et al. Sensitivity of *KRAS*-mutant colorectal cancers to combination therapy that cotargets MEK and CDK4/6. *Clin Cancer Res.* 2016;22:405-414.

191. Tao Z, Le Blanc JM, Wang C, et al. Coadministration of trametinib and palbociclib radiosensitizes *KRAS*-mutant non–small cell lung cancers. *Clin Cancer Res.* 2016;22:122-133.

192. Shapiro GI, Hilton J, Gandi L, et al. Abstract CT046: Phase I dose escalation study of the CDK4/6 inhibitor palbociclib in combination with the MEK inhibitor PD-0325901 in patients with *RAS*-mutant solid tumors. *Cancer Res.* 2017;77:CT046, [abstract].

193. Van Herpen C, Postow MA, Carlino MS, et al. 3300 A phase 1b/2 study of ribociclib (LEE011; CDK4/6 inhibitor) in combination with binimetinib (MEK162; MEK inhibitor) in patients with *NRAS*-mutant melanoma. *Eur J Cancer.* 51:S663, [abstract].

194. Schuler MH, Ascierto PA, De Vos FY, et al. Phase 1/b/2 trial of ribociclib and binimetinib in metastatic *NRAS*-mutant melanoma: safety, efficacy, and recommended phase 2 dose (RP2D). *J Clin Oncol.* 2017;35(suppl):9519, [abstract].

195. Yadav V, Burke TF, Huber L, et al. The CDK4/6 inhibitor LY2835219 overcomes vemurafenib resistance resulting from MAPK reactivation and cyclin D1 upregulation. *Mol Cancer Ther.* 2014;13:2253-2263.

196. Dean JL, Thangavel C, McClendon AK, Reed CA, Knudsen ES. Therapeutic CDK4/6 inhibition in breast cancer: key mechanisms of response and failure. *Oncogene.* 2010;29(28):4018-4032.

197. McNair C, Xu K, Mandigo AC, et al. Differential impact of RB status on E2F1 reprogramming in human cancer. *J Clin Invest.* 2018;128(1):341-358.

198. Sharma A, Yeow WS, Ertel A, et al. The retinoblastoma tumor suppressor controls androgen signaling and human prostate cancer progression. *J Clin Invest.* 2010;120:4478-4492.

199. Thangavel C, Boopathi E, Liu Y, et al. RB Loss promotes prostate cancer metastasis. *Cancer Res.* 2017;77:982-995.

200. Aparicio A, Den RB, Knudsen KE. Time to stratify? The retinoblastoma protein in castrate-resistant prostate cancer. *Nat Rev Urol.* 2011;8:562-568.

201. Herrera-Abreu MT, Palafox M, Asghar U, et al. Early adaptation and acquired resistance to CDK4/6 inhibition in estrogen receptor–positive breast cancer. *Cancer Res.* 2016;76:2301-2313.

202. Yang C, Li Z, Bhatt T, et al. Acquired CDK6 amplification promotes breast cancer resistance to CDK4/6 inhibitors and loss of ER signaling and dependence. *Oncogene.* 2017;36:2255-2264.

203. Wang L, Wang J, Blaser BW, et al. Pharmacologic inhibition of CDK4/6: mechanistic evidence for selective activity or acquired resistance in acute myeloid leukemia. *Blood.* 2007;110:2075-2083.

204. Wiedemeyer WR, Dunn IF, Quayle SN, et al. Pattern of retinoblastoma pathway inactivation dictates response to CDK4/6 inhibition in GBM. *Proc Natl Acad Sci U S A.* 2010;107:11501-11506.

205. Barker KT, Jackson LE, Crompton MR. BRK tyrosine kinase expression in a high proportion of human breast carcinomas. *Oncogene.* 1997;15: 799-805.

206. Kardinal C, Dangers M, Kardinal A, et al. Tyrosine phosphorylation modulates binding preference to cyclin-dependent kinases and subcellular localization of p27 in the acute promyelocytic leukemia cell line NB4. *Blood.* 2006;107:1133-1140.

207. Jäkel H, Peschel I, Kunze C, Weinl C, Hengst L. Regulation of p27^{Kip1} by mitogen-induced tyrosine phosphorylation. *Cell Cycle.* 2012;11:1910-1917.

208. Ray A, James MK, Larochelle S, Fisher RP, Blain SW. p27^{Kip1} inhibits cyclin D-cyclin-dependent kinase 4 by two independent modes. *Mol Cell Biol.* 2009;29:986-999.

209. James MK, Ray A, Leznova D, Blain SW. Differential modification of p27^{Kip1} controls its cyclin D-cdk4 inhibitory activity. *Mol Cell Biol.* 2008;28:498-510.

210. Patel P, Asbach B, Shteyn E, et al. Brk/protein tyrosine kinase 6 phosphorylates p27^{KIP1}, regulating the activity of cyclin D–cyclin-dependent kinase 4. *Mol Cell Biol.* 2015;35:1506-1522.

211. Jansen VM, Bhola NE, Bauer JA, et al. Kinome-wide RNA interference screen reveals a role for PDK1 in acquired resistance to CDK4/6 inhibition in ER-positive breast cancer. *Cancer Res.* 2017;77:2488-2499.

212. Alessi DR, James SR, Downes CP, et al. Characterization of a 3-phosphoinositide-dependent protein kinase which phosphorylates and activates protein kinase Balpha. *Curr Biol.* 1997;7:261-269.

213. Mora A, Komander D, van Aalten DMF, Alessi DR. PDK1, the master regulator of AGC kinase signal transduction. *Semin Cell Devl Biol.* 2004;15:161-170.

214. Tan J, Li Z, Lee PL, et al. PDK1 Signaling toward PLK1—MYC activation confers oncogenic transformation, tumor-initiating cell activation, and resistance to mTOR-targeted therapy. *Cancer Discov.* 2013;3:1156-1171.

215. Lin HJ, Hsieh FC, Song H, Lin J. Elevated phosphorylation and activation of PDK-1/AKT pathway in human breast cancer. *Br J Cancer.* 2005;93:1372-1381.

216. He S, Roberts PJ, Sorrentino JA, et al. Transient CDK4/6 inhibition protects hematopoietic stem cells from chemotherapy-induced exhaustion. *Sci Transl Med.* 2017;9:3986.

217. Dall'Acqua A, Sonego M, Pellizzari I, et al. CDK6 protects epithelial ovarian cancer from platinum-induced death via FOXO3 regulation. *EMBO Mol Med.* 2017;9:1415-1433.

218. Bar J, Gorn-Hondermann I, Moretto P, et al. miR profiling identifies cyclin-dependent kinase 6 downregulation as a potential mechanism of acquired cisplatin resistance in non-small-cell lung carcinoma. *Clin Lung Cancer.* 2015;16:e121-e129.

219. Clark AS, O'Dwyer P, Troxel A, et al. Palbociclib and paclitaxel on an alternating schedule for advanced breast cancer: results of a phase Ib trial [abstract]. In: *Proceedings of the Thirty-Eighth Annual CTRC-AACR San Antonio Breast Cancer Symposium*: 2015 Dec 8-12; San Antonio, TX. Philadelphia (PA): AACR; Cancer Res 2016;76(suppl 4):Abstract nr P6-13-08.

220. Yang C, Boyson CA, Di Liberto M, et al. CDK4/6 inhibitor PD 0332991 sensitizes acute myeloid leukemia to cytarabine-mediated cytotoxicity. *Cancer Res.* 2015;75:1838-1845.

221. Goel S, DeCristo MJ, Watt AC, et al. CDK4/6 inhibition triggers antitumour immunity. *Nature.* 2017;548:471-475.

222. Kimura H, Nakamura T, Ogawa T, Tanaka S, Shiota K. Transcription of mouse DNA methyltransferase 1 (Dnmt1) is regulated by both E2F-Rb-HDAC-dependent and -independent pathways. *Nucleic Acids Res.* 2003;31: 3101-3113.

223. Deng J, Wang ES, Jenkins RW, et al. CDK4/6 inhibition augments anti-tumor immunity by enhancing T cell activation. *Cancer Discov.* 2018;8(2):216-233.

224. Zhang J, Bu X, Wang H, et al. Cyclin D-CDK4 kinase destabilizes PD-L1 via Cul3(SPOP) to control cancer immune surveillance. *Nature.* 2018;553(7686):91-95.

225. Rugo HS, Kabos P, Dickler MN, et al. A phase 1b study of abemaciclib plus pembrolizumab for patients with hormone receptor-positive (HR+), human epidermal growth factor receptor 2-negative (HER2⁻) metastatic breast cancer (MBC) [abstract]. In: Proceedings of the 2017 San Antonio Breast Cancer Symposium; 2017 Dec 5-9; San Antonio, TX. Philadelphia (PA): AACR; Cancer Res 2018;78(suppl 4):Abstract nr P1-09-01.

226. Etemadmoghadam D, deFazio A, Beroukhim R, et al. Integrated genome-wide DNA copy number and expression analysis identifies distinct mechanisms of primary chemoresistance in ovarian carcinomas. *Clin Cancer Res.* 2009;15:1417-1427.

227. Etemadmoghadam D, George J, Cowin PA, Amplicon-dependent *CCNE1* expression is critical for clonogenic survival after cisplatin treatment and is correlated with 20q11 gain in ovarian cancer. *PLoS One.* 2010;5:e15498.

228. Parry D, Guzi T, Shanahan F, et al. Dinaciclib (SCH 727965), a novel and potent cyclin-dependent kinase inhibitor. *Mol Cancer Ther.* 2010;9:2344-2353.

229. Paruch K, Dwyer MP, Alvarez C, et al. Discovery of dinaciclib (SCH 727965): a potent and selective inhibitor of cyclin-dependent kinases. *ACS Med Chem Lett.* 2010;1:204-208.

230. Aldoss IT, Tashi T, Ganti AK. Seliciclib in malignancies. *Expert Opin Investig Drugs.* 2009;18:1957-1965.

231. Kawakami M, Mustachio LM, Rodriguez-Canales J, et al. Next-generation CDK2/9 inhibitors and anaphase catastrophe in lung cancer. *J Natl Cancer Inst.* 2017;109:1093.

232. L'Italien L, Tanudji M, Russell L, Schebye XM. Unmasking the redundancy between Cdk1 and Cdk2 at G2 phase in human cancer cell lines. *Cell Cycle.* 2006;5:984-993.

233. Cai D, Latham VM, Jr, Zhang X, Shapiro GI. Combined depletion of cell cycle and transcriptional cyclin-dependent kinase activities induces apoptosis in cancer cells. *Cancer Res.* 2006;66:9270-9280.

234. Santamaria D, Barriere C, Cerqueira A, et al. Cdk1 is sufficient to drive the mammalian cell cycle. *Nature.* 2007;448:811-815.

235. Dzhagalov I, St John A, He YW. The antiapoptotic protein Mcl-1 is essential for the survival of neutrophils but not macrophages. *Blood.* 2007;109:1620-1626.

236. Jeronimo C, Collin P, Robert F. The RNA polymerase II CTD: the increasing complexity of a low-complexity protein domain. *J Mol Biol.* 2016;428:2607-2622.

237. Meinhart A, Kamenski T, Hoeppner S, Baumli S, Cramer P. A structural perspective of CTD function. *Genes Dev.* 2005;19:1401-1415.

238. Loyer P, Trembley JH, Katona R, Kidd VJ, Lahti JM. Role of CDK/cyclin complexes in transcription and RNA splicing. *Cell Signal.* 2005;17:1033-1051.

239. Eick D, Geyer M. The RNA polymerase II carboxy-terminal domain (CTD) code. *Chem Rev.* 2013;113:8456-8490.

240. Chen R, Keating MJ, Gandhi V, Plunkett W. Transcription inhibition by flavopiridol: mechanism of chronic lymphocytic leukemia cell death. *Blood.* 2005;106:2513-2519.

241. Gregory GP, Hogg SJ, Kats LM, et al. CDK9 inhibition by dinaciclib potently suppresses Mcl-1 to induce durable apoptotic responses in aggressive MYC-driven B-cell lymphoma in vivo. *Leukemia.* 2015;29:1437-1441.

242. Christian BA, Grever MR, Byrd JC, Lin TS. Flavopiridol in chronic lymphocytic leukemia: a concise review. *Clin Lymphoma Myeloma.* 2009;9 (suppl 3):S179-S185.

243. Flynn J, Jones J, Johnson AJ, et al. Dinaciclib is a novel cyclin-dependent kinase inhibitor with significant clinical activity in relapsed and refractory chronic lymphocytic leukemia. *Leukemia.* 2015;29:1524-1529.

244. Tong Z, Chatterjee D, Deng D, et al. Antitumor effects of cyclin dependent kinase 9 inhibition in esophageal adenocarcinoma. *Oncotarget.* 2017;8:28696-28710.

245. Kretz A-L, Schaum M, Richter J, et al. CDK9 is a prognostic marker and therapeutic target in pancreatic cancer. *Tumor Biol.* 2017;39:1010428317694304.

246. Bellan C, De Falco G, Lazzi S, et al. CDK9/CYCLIN T1 expression during normal lymphoid differentiation and malignant transformation. *J Pathol.* 2004;203:946-952.

247. Huang CH, Lujambio A, Zuber J, et al. CDK9-mediated transcription elongation is required for MYC addiction in hepatocellular carcinoma. *Genes Dev.* 2014;28:1800-1814.

248. Alonso M, Tamasdan C, Miller DC, Newcomb EW. Flavopiridol induces apoptosis in glioma cell lines independent of retinoblastoma and p53 tumor suppressor pathway alterations by a caspase-independent pathway. *Mol Cancer Ther.* 2003;2:139-150.

249. Demidenko ZN, Blagosklonny MV. Flavopiridol induces p53 via initial inhibition of Mdm2 and p21 and, independently of p53, sensitizes apoptosis-reluctant cells to tumor necrosis factor. *Cancer Res.* 2004;64:3653-3660.

250. Desai BM, Villanueva J, Nguyen TT, et al. The anti-melanoma activity of dinaciclib, a cyclin-dependent kinase inhibitor, is dependent on p53 signaling. *PLoS One.* 2013;8:e59588.

251. Nemunaitis JJ, Small KA, Kirschmeier P, et al. A first-in-human, phase 1, dose-escalation study of dinaciclib, a novel cyclin-dependent kinase inhibitor, administered weekly in subjects with advanced malignancies. *J Transl Med.* 2013;11:259.

252. Mita MM, Joy AA, Mita A, et al. Randomized phase II trial of the cyclin-dependent kinase inhibitor dinaciclib (MK-7965) versus capecitabine in patients with advanced breast cancer. *Clin Breast Cancer.* 2014;14:169-176.

253. Mita MM, Mita AC, Moseley JL, et al. Phase 1 safety, pharmacokinetic and pharmacodynamic study of the cyclin-dependent kinase inhibitor dinaciclib administered every three weeks in patients with advanced malignancies. *Br J Cancer.* 2017;177:1258-1268.

254. Hossain DMS, Ugarte F, Sawant A, et al. Dinaciclib induces immunogenic cell death and enhances anti-PD-1-mediated tumor suppression [abstract]. In: Proceedings of the 107th Annual Meeting of the American Association for Cancer Research; 2016 Apr 16-20; New Orleans, LA. Philadelphia (PA): AACR; Cancer Res 2016;76(suppl 14):Abstract nr 562.

255. Casey SC, Baylot V, Felsher DW. MYC: master regulator of immune privilege. *Trends Immunol.* 2017;38:298-305.

256. Casey SC, Tong L, Li Y, et al. MYC regulates the antitumor immune response through CD47 and PD-L1. *Science.* 2016;352:227-231.

257. Bartkowiak B, Greenleaf AL. Expression, purification, and identification of associated proteins of the full-length hCDK12/CyclinK complex. *J Biol Chem.* 2015;290:1786-1795.

258. Davidson L, Muniz L, West S. 3' End formation of pre-mRNA and phosphorylation of Ser2 on the RNA polymerase II CTD are reciprocally coupled in human cells. *Genes Dev.* 2014;28:342-356.

259. Liang K, Gao X, Gilmore JM, et al. Characterization of human cyclin-dependent kinase 12 (CDK12) and CDK13 complexes in C-terminal domain phosphorylation, gene transcription, and RNA processing. *Mol Cell Biol.* 2015;35:928-938.

260. Juan HC, Lin Y, Chen HR, Fann MJ. Cdk12 is essential for embryonic development and the maintenance of genomic stability. *Cell Death Differ.* 2016;23:1038-1048.

261. Blazek D, Kohoutek J, Bartholomeeusen K, et al. The Cyclin K/Cdk12 complex maintains genomic stability via regulation of expression of DNA damage response genes. *Genes Dev.* 2011;25:2158-2172.

262. Eifler TT, Shao W, Bartholomeeusen K, et al. Cyclin-dependent kinase 12 increases 3' end processing of growth factor-induced c-FOS transcripts. *Mol Cell Biol.* 2015;35:468-478.

263. Chilà R, Guffanti F, Damia G. Role and therapeutic potential of CDK12 in human cancers. *Cancer Treat Rev.* 2016;50:83-88.

264. Bajrami I, Frankum JR, Konde A, et al. Genome-wide profiling of genetic synthetic lethality identifies CDK12 as a novel determinant of PARP1/2 inhibitor sensitivity. *Cancer Res.* 2014;74:287-297.

265. Joshi PM, Sutor SL, Huntoon CJ, Karnitz LM. Ovarian cancer-associated mutations disable catalytic activity of CDK12, a kinase that promotes homologous recombination repair and resistance to cisplatin and poly(ADP-ribose) polymerase inhibitors. *J Biol Chem.* 2014;289:9247-9253.

266. Bosken CA, Farnung L, Hintermair C, et al. The structure and substrate specificity of human Cdk12/Cyclin K. *Nat Commun.* 2014;5:3505.

267. Johnson SF, Cruz C, Greifenberg AK, et al. CDK12 inhibition reverses de novo and acquired PARP inhibitor resistance in BRCA wild-type and mutated models of triple-negative breast cancer. *Cell Rep.* 2016;17:2367-2381.

268. Zhang T, Kwiatkowski N, Olson CM, et al. Covalent targeting of remote cystein residues to develop CDK12 and 13 inhibitors. *Nat Chem Biol.* 2016;12:876-884.

269. Fisher RP. Secrets of a double agent: CDK7 in cell-cycle control and transcription. *J Cell Sci.* 2005;118:5171-5180.

270. Patel H, Abduljabbar R, Lai C-F, et al. Expression of CDK7, Cyclin H, and MAT1 is elevated in breast cancer and is prognostic in estrogen receptor–positive breast cancer. *Clin Cancer Res.* 2016;22:5929-5938.

271. Li B, Ni Chonghaile T, Fan Y, et al. Therapeutic rationale to target highly expressed CDK7 conferring poor outcomes in triple-negative breast cancer. *Cancer Res.* 2017;77:3834-3845.

272. Nasch G, Mohammadifard M, Mohammadifard M. Upregulation of cyclin-dependent kinase 7 and matrix metalloproteinase-14 expression contribute to metastatic properties of gastric cancer. *IUBMB Life.* 2016;68:799-805.

273. Wang Q, Li M, Zhang X, et al. Upregulation of CDK7 in gastric cancer cell promotes tumor cell proliferation and predicts poor prognosis. *Exp Mol Pathol.* 2016;100:514-521.

274. Kwiatkowski N, Zhang T, Rahl PB, et al. Targeting transcription regulation in cancer with a covalent CDK7 inhibitor. *Nature*. 2014;511:616-620.

275. Hu S, Ke N, Ren Y, et al. SY-1365, a potent and selective CDK7 inhibitor, exhibits promising anti-tumor activity in multiple preclinical models of aggressive solid tumors. *Proc Am Assoc Cancer Res*. 2017;A1151, [abstract].

276. Tolcher A, Do KT, D'i Tomaso E, et al. A phase 1 study of SY-1365, a selective CDK7 inhibitor, in adult patients with advanced solid tumors. *Proc ESMO Congress*. 2017;A425 (TiP), [abstract].

277. Dowen JM, Fan ZP, Hnisz D, et al. Control of cell identity genes occurs in insulated neighborhoods in mammalian chromosomes. *Cell*. 2014;159:374-387.

278. Whyte WA, Orlando DA, Hnisz D, et al. Master transcription factors and mediator establish super-enhancers at key cell identity genes. *Cell*. 2013;153:307-319.

279. Hnisz D, Shrinivas K, Young RA, Chakraborty AK, Sharp PA. A phase separation model for transcriptional control. *Cell*. 2017;169:13-23.

280. Chipumuro E, Marco E, Christensen CL, et al. CDK7 inhibition suppresses super-enhancer-linked oncogenic transcription in MYCN-driven cancer. *Cell*. 2014;159:1126-1139.

281. Christensen CL, Kwiatkowski N, Abraham BJ, et al. Targeting transcriptional addictions in small cell lung cancer with a covalent CDK7 inhibitor. *Cancer Cell*. 2014;26:909-922.

282. Zhang Z, Peng H, Wang X, et al. Preclinical efficacy and molecular mechanism of targeting CDK7-dependent transcriptional addiction in ovarian cancer. *Mol Cancer Ther*. 2017;16:1739-1750.

283. Francavilla C, Lupia M, Tsafou K, et al. Phosphoproteomics of primary cells reveals druggable kinase signatures in ovarian cancer. *Cell Rep*. 2017;18:3242-3256.

284. Wang Y, Zhang T, Kwiatkowski N, et al. CDK7-Dependent transcriptional addiction in triple-negative breast cancer. *Cell*. 2015;163:174-186.

285. Kalan S, Amat R, Schachter MM, et al. Activation of the p53 transcriptional program sensitizes cancer cells to Cdk7 inhibitors. *Cell Rep*. 2017;21:467-481.

286. Cayrol F, Praditsuktavorn P, Fernando TM, et al. THZ1 targeting CDK7 suppresses STAT transcriptional activity and sensitizes T-cell lymphomas to BCL2 inhibitors. *Nat Commun*. 2017;8:14290.

287. Rusan M, Li K, Li Y, et al. Suppression of adaptive responses to targeted cancer therapy by transcriptional repression. *Cancer Discov*. 2018;8(1):59-73.

Drugs Targeting the ABL and JAK Kinases

James A. Kennedy, Samantha O. Luk, and Gabriela Hobbs

Chronic Myeloid Leukemia

Chronic myeloid leukemia (CML) is a clonal stem cell neoplasm characterized by the universal presence of the BCR-ABL fusion protein.[1] This fusion results from a reciprocal translocation that juxtaposes the c-ABL1 oncogene at 9q34 and the housekeeping gene BCR on chromosome 22q11, generating the Philadelphia chromosome.[2] This resulting fusion protein has dysregulated tyrosine kinase activity and is both necessary and sufficient for the development of CML.[3]

In CML, BCR-ABL drives the uncontrolled production of mature and maturing granulocytes, predominantly neutrophils. In the absence of treatment, CML classically has a triphasic clinical course as it progresses from an indolent chronic phase, characterized by leukocytosis and splenomegaly, to an accelerated phase, where blood counts are more difficult to control, and ultimately onto a terminal blast crisis, where myeloid or lymphoid blasts proliferate uncontrollably, similar to acute leukemia.[4]

In the late 1990s, the standard of care in the pharmacologic treatment of chronic phase CML was interferon-α (IFN-α). Either alone or in combination with low-dose cytarabine (ARA-C), this immunomodulatory cytokine could normalize hematologic parameters and, in a subset of patients, decrease the numbers of Philadelphia-positive (Ph+) cells.[5-7] However, the modest disease-modifying activity of IFN-α came at the cost of significant side effects including flu-like symptoms, cytopenias, depression, and autoimmune disease. The only curative therapy for CML was allogeneic bone marrow transplantation.

CML is a unique malignancy in that a single genetic event drives the disease, making it uniquely susceptible to agents that target BCR-ABL. This understanding of disease pathophysiology underpinned the development of tyrosine kinase inhibitors (TKIs), small molecules designed to specifically inhibit BCR-ABL. The approval of the first such agent, imatinib, in 2001 was a historic watershed moment in clinical oncology. It not only transformed the treatment of CML and the outlook of patients with this disease, but it also ushered in the era of molecularly targeted cancer therapeutics, fundamentally altering the manner in which oncologists treat disease.

The following will provide an overview of the basic pharmacology and clinical use of imatinib as well as the second- and third-generation TKIs.

Imatinib

Mechanism of Action

Imatinib mesylate (Gleevec, formerly STI571; Fig. 24.1A) is a member of the 2-phenylaminopyrimidine class of TKIs and acts as a potent inhibitor of c-ABL and consequently BCR-ABL, as well as the PDGFR (platelet-derived growth factor receptor) and c-KIT kinases. Imatinib has minimal activity against other tyrosine and serine/threonine kinases.[8] Its key pharmacologic features are provided in Table 24.1.

Imatinib targets the ATP-binding site of its target kinases, acting as a competitive inhibitor. It binds to the inactive conformation of ABL and prevents the enzyme from phosphorylating its downstream signaling substrates that drive cellular proliferation and survival. Imatinib contacts 21 amino acids within the ABL kinase domain and fits into a tight-binding pocket stabilized by hydrophobic interactions and hydrogen bonds (Fig. 24.2A).[9]

Resistance to imatinib emerges by a number of mechanisms, most commonly via point mutations within the kinase domain that reduce its binding affinity for the drug.[10-12] Changes to amino acids in the vicinity of the drug's binding pocket can directly reduce binding by altering required hydrophobic and hydrogen-bonding interactions and/or by causing topographical changes that result in steric hindrance (e.g., T315I; Fig. 24.2B). Binding can also be affected indirectly, as certain point mutants promote the kinase to remain in an active conformation, as opposed to the inactive form, which is required for imatinib binding (e.g., Y253F/H).[13,14] Other less well-characterized mechanisms of drug resistance include BCR-ABL overexpression, achieved via gene amplification,[15] the increased cellular expression of drug exporters (e.g., ABCB1/MRD-1),[16] and the activation of compensatory signaling pathways, which can be achieved by overexpressing SRC family kinases.[17]

Clinical Pharmacology and Metabolism

Imatinib is 98% orally bioavailable and rapidly absorbed following ingestion, reaching a maximum concentration (C_{max}) in the serum between two to four hours after administration in healthy individuals.[18] Based on case reports, it appears that imatinib is absorbed in the upper gastrointestinal (GI) tract, as patients who have undergone surgical procedures that bypass or limit transit time through the upper GI tract have lower serum drug levels postoperatively, in some instances necessitating increased drug dosing to maintain clinical response.[19-21] A proportional increase in the mean imatinib area under the curve (AUC) is seen with increasing drug doses. Imatinib is approximately 95% protein bound at clinically relevant concentrations, predominantly to albumin and α1-acid glycoprotein.[22]

Imatinib is primarily metabolized by the cytochrome P450 (CYP) 3A4 enzyme and to a lesser extent by CYP 1A2, CYP 2D6, CYP 2C9, and CYP 2C19. Its major active metabolite is an N-demethylated piperazine derivative (N-desmethyl-imatinib), which comprises

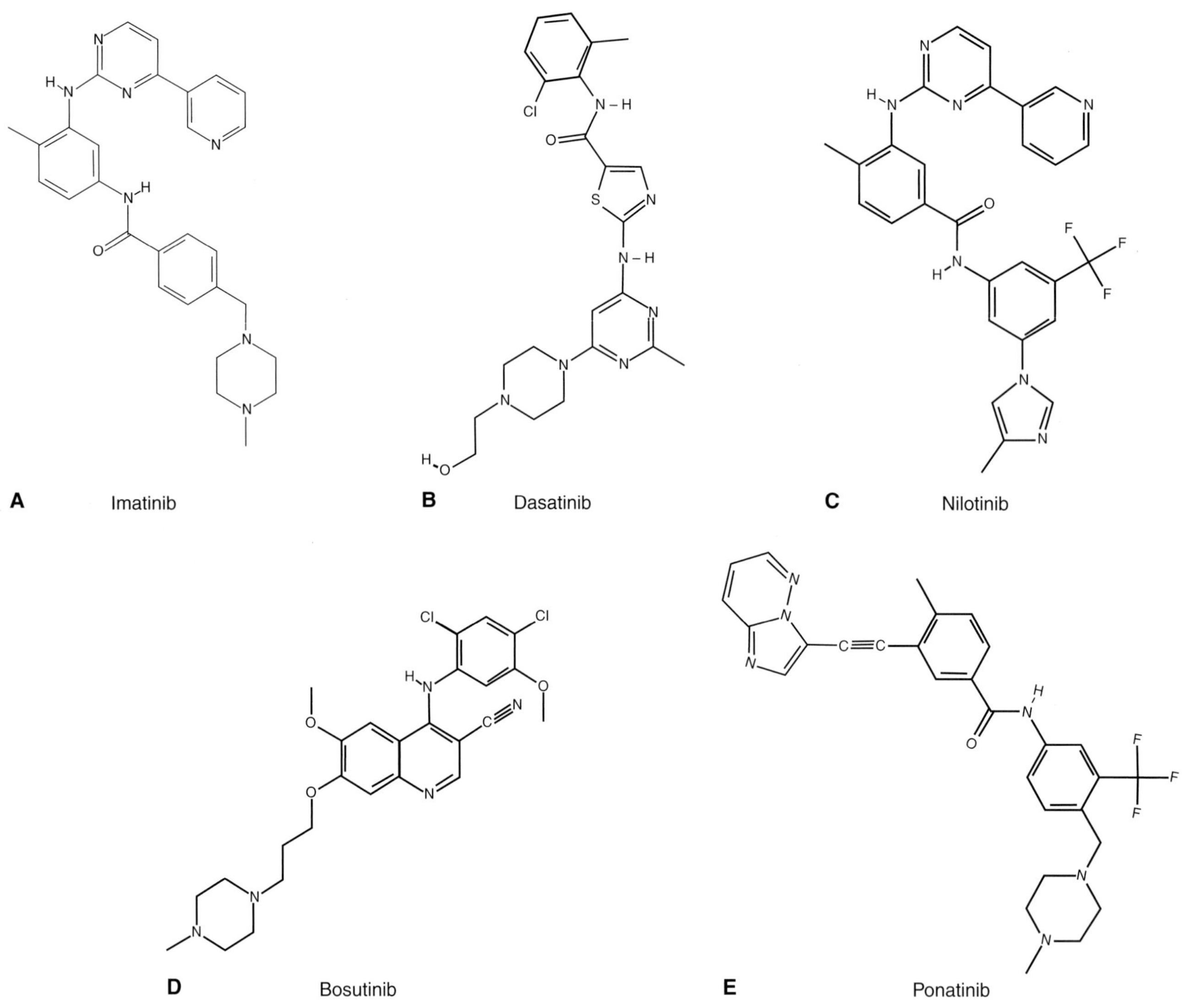

FIGURE **24.1** Chemical structures of the small molecule tyrosine kinase inhibitors of BCR-ABL. **(A)** Imatinib, **(B)** dasatinib, **(C)** nilotinib, **(D)** bosutinib, and **(E)** ponatinib.

TABLE

24.1 *Key features of imatinib*

Mechanism of action	Competitive inhibitor of ATP-binding site of c-ABL as well as c-KIT and PDGF receptor tyrosine kinases
Metabolism	CYP 3A4
Pharmacokinetics	t_{max}: 2 to 4 hours Bioavailability: 98% Protein binding: 95% $t_{1/2}$: 18 to 20 hours
Elimination	Fecal (85% to 90%) and urinary (10% to 15%)
Drug interactions	Concomitant strong CYP 3A4 inhibitors and inducers: closely monitor, potentially dose adjust
	Concomitant CYP 3A4 substrates: closely monitor substrate if narrow therapeutic index and consider alternative agents
Toxicity	Myelosuppression, rash, fatigue, fluid retention, muscle cramps, GI upset, liver toxicity, and electrolyte abnormalities. Bone mineral loss with long-term use. Rarely associated with cardiotoxicity/congestive heart failure
Precautions	Elderly patients are at higher risk of cardiotoxicity/congestive heart failure and severe fluid retention

$t_{1/2}$, half-life; t_{max}, time to maximum concentration.

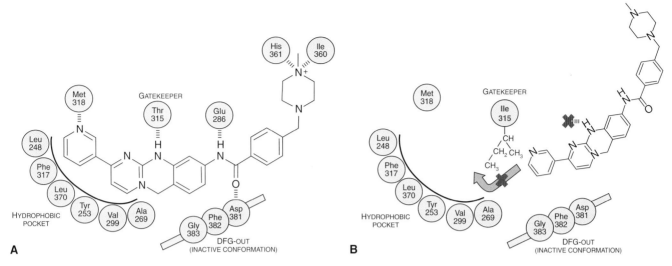

FIGURE 24.2 A. Schematic of the key intermolecular interactions that occur between imatinib and its binding site in BCR-ABL. Imatinib forms six hydrogen bonds with BCR-ABL (depicted with dashed lines) as well as numerous van der Waals interactions, in particular between the pyridine/pyrimidine groups of imatinib and a hydrophobic pocket beyond the T315 gatekeeper residue. Imatinib binds to the inactive DFG (aspartate-phenylalanine-glycine)-out conformation of BCR-ABL, forming a hydrogen bond with D381. **B.** Disruption of imatinib binding by the T315I mutation. The bulky isoleucine side chain causes steric hindrance, preventing drug access to the hydrophobic pocket, and also disrupts a key hydrogen bond interaction with the pyrimidine amino group of imatinib.

approximately 15% of the total AUC of imatinib.[22,23] The elimination half-life is 18 to 20 hours for imatinib and 40 hours for N-desmethyl-imatinib.[22] Steady-state levels are typically reached by seven days for imatinib and by two weeks for N-desmethyl-imatinib.[23] Elimination of imatinib and its metabolites occurs primarily via the feces (85% to 90%) with the remainder in the urine. The majority of a single dose of drug is excreted within 7 days.

Summary of Literature/Efficacy

In preclinical studies, imatinib was shown to reduce the proliferation of BCR-ABL–expressing cell lines and inhibit hematopoietic colony formation by mononuclear cells from chronic phase CML patients, but not healthy individuals.[24] Based on these encouraging results in the laboratory, imatinib was then evaluated in a phase 1 trial of CP-CML patients who had lost response to IFN-*α*.[25] Remarkable clinical activity was seen in this population; complete hematologic responses were observed in 98% of patients, and complete cytogenetic responses (CCyR) were seen in 53.7% (see Table 24.2 for definitions of response types in CML). As such, imatinib moved forward in larger clinical studies, culminating in the phase III International Randomized Study of Interferon and STI571 (IRIS).[26] This trial enrolled patients with newly diagnosed chronic phase CML and randomized them to receive imatinib 400 mg once daily or combination therapy with IFN-*α* and low-dose ARA-C.[26] In IRIS, imatinib was superior for all efficacy and toxicity endpoints. At 18 months, 95% of imatinib patients had achieved a complete hematologic response and 85% had a major cytogenetic response (MCyR), compared to 55% and 22%, respectively, in the IFN-*α*/ARA-C arm. Imatinib also resulted in significantly improved disease control; the rate of freedom from progression to accelerated phase and blast crisis was 97% in the imatinib arm compared to 91.5% with combination therapy.[26] Long-term follow-up of patients enrolled in the IRIS study has continued to show evidence of this drug's efficacy. At 10 years, imatinib-treated

patients had an overall survival (OS) of 83% and an estimated rate of freedom from progression of 92%.[27]

Ultimately, the IRIS study established imatinib as a new standard of care for the upfront treatment of chronic phase CML. However, small numbers of individuals progress on therapy, largely due to compliance issues or the development of resistance, either by mutations in the ABL kinase domain or by increased expression of BCR-ABL (see *Mechanism of Action* section).[10,11,28] Given that both of these resistance mechanisms could potentially be overcome by higher drug concentrations, several clinical trials were performed

TABLE 24.2	*Response definitions for CML therapy*
Response Type	**Clinical/Lab Criteria[76]**
Complete hematological response (CHR)	Platelet count < 450 × 10⁹/L WBC count < 10 × 10⁹/L Differential: no immature granulocytes, basophils < 5% Nonpalpable spleen
Major cytogenetic response (MCyR)	Conventional cytogenetics: ≤35% Ph+ metaphases[a]
Complete cytogenetic response (CCyR)	Conventional cytogenetics: no Ph+ metaphases[a]
Major molecular response (MMR)	Peripheral blood *BCR-ABL1* transcript level ≤ 0.1% (3-log reduction) according to the International Scale (IS)[b]

[a]Requires evaluation of at least 20 metaphases from a bone marrow sample.
[b]Requires detection of >10,000 *ABL1* (control) transcripts.

comparing the standard imatinib dose of 400 mg daily to 800 mg daily. Across these studies, there were no consistent differences in remission rates or survival, but high-dose imatinib was associated with increased toxicity.[29-32] Interestingly, in some studies, major molecular response (MMR, corresponding to a >3-log reduction in *BCR-ABL1* transcript levels) did occur earlier in patients taking higher doses of drug[31,32]; however, the impact of this finding on long-term clinical outcomes remains unknown.

Toxicity

In newly diagnosed CML patients starting imatinib, the most common side effect is cytopenias, which can pose a significant challenge, particularly among patients with advanced disease. In the IRIS study, 60.8% of patients experienced neutropenia (14.3% with grade 3/4), 44.6% of patients experienced anemia (3.1% with grade 3/4), and 56.6% experienced thrombocytopenia (16.5% with grade 3/4).[26] Another common side effect is fluid retention, as 62% to 72% of patients experiencing some form of edema, predominantly occurring in the periorbital region or lower limbs. Typically, this can be managed with diuretics and supportive care; however, severe grade 3/4 fluid retention occurred in about 2.5% to 11% of subjects in the initial clinical trials of imatinib, necessitating dose reduction. These events occur more frequently in the elderly, in patients presenting in accelerated phase or blast crisis, and in individuals taking higher imatinib doses.[22,26] Hepatotoxicity can also be a challenging side effect of imatinib, which often necessitates close monitoring. About 43.2% of patients in the IRIS study experienced elevations in serum alanine or aspartate aminotransferase with 6.8% of patients experiencing grade 3/4 transaminase elevations.[26] In a phase II study in GI stromal tumor (GIST) patients, 2.7% of patients had bilirubin elevations while on imatinib.[33] Transaminase and bilirubin elevations were usually managed with dose reduction or interruption for a median time of 1 week.[22]

Other common nonhematologic adverse events related to imatinib include fatigue (30% to 39%), nausea (49.5% to 73%), vomiting (22.5% to 58%), diarrhea (43% to 57%), muscle cramps (28% to 62%), musculoskeletal pain (38% to 49%), and rash (36% to 47%).[22] Congestive heart failure and cardiotoxicity have been noted in rare instances.[22,34-36]

Overall, only a minority of imatinib-treated patients discontinue drug due to intolerance. Many of the initial toxicities of imatinib, such as cytopenias, resolve with long-term use. However, certain side effects, specifically fatigue and edema, remain particularly troublesome in some individuals. In addition, long-term imatinib treatment may be associated with bone mineral loss, suggesting that bone health should be monitored in these patients.[37,38]

Drug Interactions

As mentioned above, imatinib is predominantly metabolized by CYP 3A4; consequently, it is subject to numerous drug interactions. Strong CYP 3A4 inhibitors such as the azoles, amiodarone, and grapefruit juice can increase imatinib levels[22]; for example, when imatinib was coadministered with ketoconazole, the mean imatinib C_{max} increased by 26% and AUC increased by 40%.[39] A similar increase, both at the plasma and cellular level, is seen with coadministration of medications that inhibit the efflux pump P-glycoprotein (PGP), such as fluconazole, cyclosporine, verapamil, erythromycin, and clarithromycin. On the other hand,

strong CYP 3A4 inducers can drive more rapid imatinib clearance and thereby decrease exposure. For example, when coadministered with rifampin, imatinib clearance increased by 3.8-fold, resulting in significantly lower mean C_{max} (decreased by 54%) and AUC (decreased by 74%).[40] As such, close monitoring of clinical effects and potential dose adjustment is required when imatinib is given with strong CYP 3A4 inducers/inhibitors and PGP inhibitors.

Conversely, the levels of other medications metabolized by CYP 3A4 can be affected by concomitant imatinib administration. For example, when simvastatin, a CYP 3A4 substrate, was coadministered with imatinib, there was a twofold increase in its C_{max} and a threefold increase in its AUC. Consequently, when CYP 3A4 substrates with narrow therapeutic windows are administered alongside imatinib, either careful monitoring of drug levels is required (as would be the case with tacrolimus, sirolimus, and cyclosporine) or alternative agents should be utilized (as would be the case with warfarin).[22]

Lastly, in vitro studies have demonstrated that imatinib can inhibit the O-glucuronidation of acetaminophen; this effect, together with inhibition of CYP 2D6, is postulated to increase systemic exposure to acetaminophen. Though this has not been evaluated in detail in humans, caution is suggested when imatinib and acetaminophen are coadministered.[41]

Dasatinib

Mechanism of Action

Dasatinib (Sprycel, formerly BMS-354825) is a second-generation TKI that was first synthesized in an effort to develop small molecules able to inhibit both ABL and SRC kinases.[42] It is a thiazolylamino-pyrimidine, structurally unrelated to imatinib (Fig. 24.1B), and is 325-fold more potent at inhibiting BCR-ABL while additionally targeting c-KIT, PDGFR-α/β, and ephrin receptor tyrosine kinases, as well as SRC family kinases (including SRC, LYN, FGR, FYN, HCK, LCK, and YES), which have been implicated in imatinib resistance.[17,42] The key pharmacological features of dasatinib are provided in Table 24.3.

Dasatinib is active against a wide variety of *BCR-ABL* point mutants, a benefit conferred by the manner in which it binds to the fusion kinase.[43-45] Like imatinib, it associates with the ATP-binding domain of ABL; however, it relies less on P-loop interactions and thereby is less affected by point mutations in this region. Second, dasatinib can bind to both the inactive and active conformations of BCR-ABL, likely contributing not only to its increased potency, but also conferring resistance to those point mutants that stabilize the active kinase conformation. However, dasatinib does form a critical interaction with T315, resulting in a lack of activity against the mutations affecting this residue.[43]

Clinical Pharmacology and Metabolism

Dasatinib has a rapid onset after oral ingestion; it is detectable in the body within 30 minutes of ingestion and reaches its C_{max} between 30 minutes and 6 hours.[46,47] Given this time frame, it is likely absorbed in the upper GI tract, similar to imatinib. Dasatinib has pH-dependent solubility, which significantly decreases at pH values >4. Consequently, gastric pH–modifying agents, such as proton pump inhibitors (PPIs) and H2-receptor antagonists have been shown to reduce its bioavailability.[48-51] Therefore, their coadministration with dasatinib is not recommended.[47]

TABLE

24.3   *Key features of dasatinib*

Mechanism of action	Competitive inhibitor of c-ABL ATP-binding site, also inhibits c-KIT, PDGFR-α/β, ephrin, and SRC family kinases
Metabolism	CYP 3A4 with minor contribution from FMO-3 and UGT
Pharmacokinetics	t_{max}: 0.5 to 6 hours Protein binding: 96% V_d: 2,505 L $t_{1/2}$: 3 to 5 hours
Elimination	Fecal (85%) and urinary (4%)
Drug interactions	Avoid concomitant strong CYP 3A4 inducers/inhibitors, PPIs, and H2 receptor antagonists
Toxicity	Myelosuppression, fluid retention, pleural effusions, PAH, bleeding, diarrhea, rash, musculoskeletal pain, headache, fatigue, nausea, myalgia, vomiting
Precautions	Monitor for PAH; drug discontinuation is required upon diagnosis
	Monitor for fluid retention (including pleural effusion); might require dose interruption, adjustment, and/or discontinuation

V_d, volume of distribution; $t_{1/2}$, half-life; FMO, flavin-containing monooxygenase; UGT, uridine diphosphate-glucuronosyltransferase; PAH, pulmonary arterial hypertension.

Dasatinib is 96% protein bound, with an estimated volume of distribution of 2,505 L suggesting extensive distribution in the extravascular space. Dasatinib is metabolized primarily by hepatic CYP 3A4 and to a lesser extent by flavin-containing monooxygenase 3 (FMO-3) and uridine diphospho-glucuronosyltransferase (UGT).[52] Dasatinib's primary metabolite is equipotent to the parent drug and constitutes approximately 5% of the total AUC suggesting that it has a limited clinical role.[46,47] Interestingly, dasatinib appears to have time-dependent antileukemic activity as higher rates of MMR at 3 months were observed in patients with a prolonged time spent above the half maximal inhibitory concentration (IC$_{50}$, calculated based on the phosphorylation of CrkL [CT10 regulator of kinase like] in bone marrow CD34+ cells).[53] Dasatinib is primarily eliminated in the feces (85%) with the remainder via the urine, with 19% and 0.1%, respectively, in an unmetabolized form. The overall terminal half-life ranges from 3 to 5 hours.[47]

Summary of Literature/Efficacy

Early-phase studies evaluated the efficacy of dasatinib in patients from all CML disease phases that were imatinib resistant/intolerant.[54–56] Dasatinib had significant clinical activity in these individuals; specifically, in the chronic phase setting, dasatinib at a dose of 70 mg twice daily led to complete hematologic response in 91% and CCyR in 49%, with a progression-free survival (PFS) of 90% at a median follow-up of 15 months.[54] Dasatinib was subsequently studied in the frontline setting. In the phase III multicenter **Das**atinib versus **I**matinib **S**tudy in treatment-**N**aïve CML Patients (DASISION) trial, dasatinib 100 mg once daily was compared to imatinib once 400 mg daily in patients with newly diagnosed chronic phase CML.[57] At 12 months, dasatinib was superior to imatinib with respect to CCyR (77% versus 66%, the trial's primary endpoint) as well as MMR (46% versus 28%). Dasatinib achieved these molecular milestones more rapidly than imatinib and was not highly toxic. At 5 years of follow-up, dasatinib maintained its advantage with respect to CCyR and MMR, but this did not translate into improved PFS or OS (Table 24.4).[58]

Toxicity

Cytopenias are the most common toxicity associated with dasatinib. Myelosuppression is dose-related but generally reversible and can be managed with either dose interruption or reduction.[47] In the DASISION study, 65% of patients experienced neutropenia (21% with grade 3/4), 70% of patients experienced thrombocytopenia (19% with grade 3/4), and 90% of patients experienced anemia (10% with grade 3/4).[47,57] The next most common side effect associated with dasatinib is fluid retention; 19% of patients in the DASISION study experienced this in some form, most commonly pleural effusion (10%) or superficial edema (9%).[57] Fluid retention

TABLE

24.4   *Clinical responses at 5-years of follow-up in the frontline phase 3 trials of chronic phase CML*

Trial	Drug	Dose	5-y MMR	5-y PFS	5-y OS
DASISION[58]	Imatinib	400 mg once daily	64%	86%	90%
	Dasatinib	100 mg once daily	76%	85%	91%
ENESTnd[75]	Imatinib	400 mg once daily	60%	91%	92%
	Nilotinib	300 mg twice daily	77%	92%	94%
	Nilotinib	400 mg twice daily	77%	96%	96%

typically can be managed with diuretics and/or dose modifications.[47] Other common nonhematologic drug-related adverse events associated with dasatinib include diarrhea (17%), rash (11%), musculoskeletal pain (11%), fatigue (8%), nausea (8%), myalgia (6%), and vomiting (5%).[57] Of note, headache is common with therapy initiation (seen in 12% of DASISION patients) but tends to improve with time.

While the aforementioned side effects are similar to those seen with imatinib, dasatinib does have some distinct toxicities. In the 5-year follow-up of the DASISION trial, pleural effusion was reported in 28% of patients receiving dasatinib versus 0.8% of those receiving imatinib.[58] The rate of pleural effusions increases by approximately 4% to 5% with each year of therapy.[57–60] The development of an effusion does not necessitate permanent discontinuation of dasatinib. Often, effusions resolve with temporary dose interruptions, diuretics, and/or short courses of glucocorticoids.[61]

Pulmonary arterial hypertension (PAH) is a rare but serious late complication of dasatinib therapy; at the 5-year follow-up of DASISION, PAH was diagnosed in 5% of patients in the dasatinib arm compared to 0.4% in the imatinib arm.[58] In the French pulmonary hypertension registry, nine patients were documented to have moderate to severe PAH attributable to dasatinib between November 2006 and September 2010. The median time between drug initiation and the diagnosis of PAH was 34 months (range: 8 to 48 months). Dasatinib was discontinued in each instance, and all but one patient showed clinical, functional, and/or hemodynamic improvements afterward.[62] Although there are no clear guidelines for screening or monitoring for PAH, providers should be aware of this complication and permanently discontinue therapy upon diagnosis.

Bleeding episodes have also been reported in up to 20% to 25% of patients on dasatinib, with 10% having grade III to IV severity. These typically involve the GI tract and mucosal surfaces (uterus, gingiva) and can be managed with supportive medical care and dose interruption or reduction. Dasatinib causes reversible inhibition of platelet aggregation, which is thought to contribute to bleeding, which usually, but not always, occurs in the setting of thrombocytopenia.[63] In a detailed analysis of phase I/II patients receiving dasatinib, bleeding events most commonly occurred in the GI tract (81% of cases); drug discontinuation was required in 47% of these instances, with a median interruption of 17 days.[64]

Drug Interactions

Like imatinib, dasatinib is primarily metabolized by CYP 3A4; consequently, its levels can be affected by coadministration of strong CYP 3A4 inhibitors, which can increase its levels, and strong CYP 3A4 inducers, which can decrease its levels. It also can influence the metabolism of other CYP 3A4 substrates, and careful monitoring is required if these medications have a narrow therapeutic index.[47]

As discussed above, the solubility of dasatinib is pH dependent; therefore, concomitant H2 receptor antagonists and PPIs should be avoided.[47] For patients requiring gastric acid suppression, over-the-counter magnesium or aluminum hydroxide-based antacids may be used as an alternative, as their administration either 2 hours before or after dasatinib was not shown to influence the AUC in a small phase I trial.[47,51]

Nilotinib

Mechanism of Action

Nilotinib (Tasigna, formerly AMN107; Fig. 24.1C) is a second-generation TKI that was rationally designed in an effort to optimize drug binding to BCR-ABL. Its key pharmacologic features are provided in Table 24.5. Like imatinib, it binds to the inactive conformation of BCR-ABL at the ATP-binding site. However, by replacing imatinib's polar N-methylpiperazine heterocycle with a lipophilic trifluoromethyl/imidazole phenyl group, the topological fit of nilotinib is enhanced, resulting in approximately 30-fold greater potency ($IC_{50} < 30$ nM) and enhanced selectivity. Nilotinib lacks activity against SRC family kinases and inhibits the KIT and PDGF receptor tyrosine kinases less potently than imatinib.[65,66]

TABLE 24.5	*Key features of nilotinib*		
Mechanism of action	Competitive inhibitor of ATP-binding site of c-ABL as well as the KIT and PDGFR-α/β tyrosine kinases		
Metabolism	CYP 3A4		
Pharmacokinetics	t_{max}: 2.2 to 3 hours	Protein binding: 98%	$t_{1/2}$: 15 to 17 hours
Elimination	Fecal (93%)		
Drug interactions	Avoid concomitant strong CYP 3A4 inhibitors/inducers, medications that prolong the QT interval and PPIs		
Toxicity	Myelosuppression, rash, pruritus, headache, fatigue, nausea, myalgia, alopecia, diarrhea; elevation of serum glucose, cholesterol, transaminases, and lipase		
	Rare, but serious side effects: pancreatitis, cardiovascular events (including peripheral artery occlusion), and QT prolongation/sudden cardiac death		
Precautions	Take on an empty stomach		
	Can prolong QT interval—assess at baseline and 7 days after initiation; avoid medications that can also prolong QT; monitor if concomitant CYP 3A4 inhibitors are initiated		
	Monitor serum lipase with dose adjustment/interruption as necessary		
	Contains lactose		

$t_{1/2}$, half-life; t_{max}, time to maximum concentration.

Despite its structural similarity to imatinib, nilotinib exhibits activity against a wide variety of *BCR-ABL* point mutants.[44,65] This is likely a consequence of both its increased potency as well as the nature of its binding interactions, which rely heavily upon the lipophilic moiety that is absent from imatinib.[66] However, like imatinib and dasatinib, nilotinib does form a crucial hydrogen-bonding interaction with threonine-315; consequently, it too lacks activity against T315I point mutants.[44,65]

Clinical Pharmacology and Metabolism

The absolute oral bioavailability of nilotinib has not been determined.[67] It reaches its C_{max} approximately 3 hours after ingestion of an oral dose when given once daily and 2.2 hours when given twice daily.[67] Importantly, the bioavailability of nilotinib is increased with food; in healthy volunteers, when nilotinib was administered with a high-fat meal, its AUC was increased by 82% as compared to an empty stomach.[68] Given that the type and quantity of food intake can variably affect the systemic exposure of nilotinib, it is recommended that it is taken on an empty stomach.[67,68]

Like the other TKIs, the upper GI tract is thought to play a key role in nilotinib absorption. Patients who have undergone total gastrectomy have 53% lower median steady-state trough nilotinib concentrations as compared to those who have not undergone the procedure.[69] Nilotinib has pH-dependent solubility, which decreases at higher pH. Consequently, like dasatinib, nilotinib AUC is decreased by coadministration of PPIs.[67,70]

In vitro studies have found that nilotinib is 98% protein bound. It is primarily metabolized via CYP 3A4, generating metabolites that lack significant pharmacological activity.[67] Its elimination half-life is approximately 15 to 17 hours.[67,71] Of note, coadministration with food, which affects nilotinib absorption, does not alter its $t_{1/2}$.[68] About 93% of nilotinib is eliminated in the feces, with 69% in the parent form.

Summary of Literature/Efficacy

Following demonstration of its activity in preclinical models of CML,[65] nilotinib was evaluated in early-phase clinical trials in patients with imatinib-intolerant/imatinib-resistant CML.[71–73] Hematologic and cytogenetic responses were observed in all disease phases, with the exception of patients harboring the T315I mutation. Specifically, in the chronic phase CML setting, nilotinib at a dose of 400 mg twice daily led to CCyR rates as high as 31% and an OS between 79% and 95% at 12 months.[72,73] These favorable results in the imatinib-intolerant/-resistant population led to a phase III study, **E**valuating **N**ilotinib **E**fficacy and **S**afety in Clinical **T**rials-**n**ewly **d**iagnosed patients (ENESTnd) that compared imatinib to nilotinib in newly diagnosed chronic phase CML patients.[74] This study randomized patients to receive nilotinib 300 mg twice daily (BID), nilotinib 400 mg BID or imatinib 400 mg once daily. At 12 months, the rates of MMR, the trial's primary endpoint, were significantly higher for both nilotinib arms (44% for 300 mg BID, 43% for 400 mg BID, 22% for imatinib). Regardless of dose, patients receiving nilotinib also had an improvement in the time to progression compared to those receiving imatinib. At 5 years of follow-up, nilotinib maintained its advantage with respect to CCyR and MMR, with 52% to 54% of patients in the nilotinib groups achieving an MMR 4.5 (BCR-ABL ≤ 00032%) compared to 31% in the imatinib arm.[75] However,

similar to the DASISION trial with dasatinib, this did not translate into substantially improved PFS or OS (Table 24.4).

Toxicity

Like imatinib and dasatinib, the most common side effect associated with nilotinib is myelosuppression, typically during the first 2 months of therapy. In the ENESTnd study, anemia, neutropenia, and thrombocytopenia occurred at rates similar to those seen in patients receiving imatinib.[74] Nonhematologic adverse events associated with nilotinib at a dose of 300 mg twice daily included rash (31%), pruritus (15%), headache (14%), fatigue (11%), nausea (11%), myalgia (10%), alopecia (8%), and diarrhea (8%), the majority of which were grade 1/2.[74] Fluid retention occurs in patients receiving nilotinib, albeit at lower rates than those receiving imatinib.

Nilotinib does have certain toxicities distinct from dasatinib and imatinib; in particular, it significantly increases cardiovascular (CV) risk. In the 5-year follow-up of the ENESTnd trial, new or worsening elevations of blood glucose and total cholesterol occurred in 51% and 27% of nilotinib-treated patients, respectively.[75] CV events, including ischemic heart disease, stroke, and peripheral artery occlusive disease, occurred in 10.4% of nilotinib-treated patients versus 2.1% of imatinib-treated patients. Peripheral artery occlusion was exclusively seen with nilotinib, affecting 2.5% of patients.[75] Consequently, NCCN guidelines suggest that CV risk factors and pre-existing peripheral artery disease should be considered prior to initiating nilotinib, and if an arterial block develops during therapy, the drug should be discontinued.[76]

Nilotinib can also lead to transaminitis, increased total bilirubin levels, and elevations in serum lipase levels, the latter which may be associated with overt pancreatitis. This risk appears to be highest in patients with a previous history of pancreatitis. Consequently, serum lipase levels should be checked periodically, with dose reduction for significant elevations, and prompt discontinuation if associated with abdominal symptoms.[67]

Nilotinib has a black box warning for QT prolongation, and rare reports of sudden cardiac death have been noted among patients receiving this drug.[67] Consequently, ECGs should be obtained at baseline, 7 days after therapy initiation, and periodically thereafter, including after all dose adjustments. Electrolyte levels should be obtained at baseline and hypokalemia and hypomagnesemia should be corrected before nilotinib initiation.[76] Dose adjustment is required in the face of QT prolongation.[67]

Five-year follow-up of the ENESTnd trial showed that nilotinib at a starting dose of 400 mg twice daily results in higher rates of many adverse events, in particular CV disease (13.4% [400 mg BID] versus 7.5% [300 mg BID] versus 2.1% [imatinib]).[75] Overall, serious adverse events occurred in 33% of patients at the higher nilotinib dose compared to 26% at the lower dose and led to drug discontinuation in 20% and 12% of patients, respectively. This toxicity profile, taken together with the efficacy findings described above (Table 24.4), suggests that nilotinib 300 mg twice daily provides a better balance of benefit and risk in the frontline treatment of chronic phase CML patients compared to higher doses.

Drug Interactions

Nilotinib, like imatinib and dasatinib, is predominantly metabolized by CYP 3A4; therefore, it is associated with a similar set of drug interactions. Concomitant administration of strong CYP 3A4 inhibitors or inducers should be avoided. Moreover, nilotinib can potentially interfere with the metabolism of other CYP 3A4 substrates; for example, the C_{max} of midazolam increases by 20% when coadministered with nilotinib.[77] As such, caution should be used when nilotinib is given alongside CYP 3A4 substrates that have a narrow therapeutic index.

In vitro studies have suggested that nilotinib can inhibit other drug metabolizing enzymes including CYP 2C8, CYP 2C9, CYP 2D6, UGT 1A1, and PGP while inducing others, such as CYP 2B6, CYP 2C8, and CYP 2C9.[67] However, the in vivo significance of these findings remains unclear; for example, when coadministered with warfarin (a CYP 2C9 substrate), there was no significant change in warfarin's C_{max} or AUC.[78]

As discussed above, nilotinib has increased solubility at acidic pH; consequently, medications that alter gastric pH have the potential to interfere with its bioavailability. This has been confirmed for PPIs, as concomitant use of nilotinib and esomeprazole reduced the nilotinib C_{max} by 27% and AUC by 34%[70]; as such, coadministration with PPIs is not recommended. Interestingly, H2 receptor antagonists and antacid suspensions do not appear to alter drug levels when taken 2 hours after nilotinib and may serve as treatment alternatives.[79]

Lastly, as nilotinib can increase the QT interval, the simultaneous usage of medications that likewise prolong the QT should be avoided.[67] Moreover, the QT interval should be carefully monitored if a medication capable of inhibiting CYP 3A4 (and thereby increasing nilotinib levels) is initiated.

Bosutinib

Mechanism of Action

Bosutinib (Bosulif, formerly SKI-606) is a dual ABL1 and SRC kinase inhibitor. This 4-anilino-3-quinolinecarbonitrile molecule is structurally unrelated to imatinib (Fig. 24.1D), as it was originally synthesized as a SRC inhibitor.[80] Bosutinib inhibits BCR-ABL activity at an IC_{50} of less than 10 nM, exhibiting significantly higher potency than imatinib; however, it exhibits no activity against PDGFR-α/β or c-KIT.[66]

Bosutinib binds to both the active and inactive conformations of the ABL kinase domain. Compared to the other TKIs, its physical interaction with ABL is most similar to that of dasatinib, with some notable differences. First, it forms a hydrogen-bond network with residues in the kinase domain, not directly, but instead by engaging a pair of structured water molecules.[81] Second, as opposed to forming a hydrogen bond with T315I, it makes a van der Waals interaction via its nitrile group.[82] Nevertheless, this interaction is critical for bosutinib to gain access to the structured water molecules within its binding site.[81] Consequently, though bosutinib displays activity against a range of BCR-ABL1 kinase domain mutants, it is not effective against T315I.[83]

Clinical Pharmacology and Metabolism

Compared to the other first-and second-generation TKIs, bosutinib has lower oral bioavailability (34% with food) and is absorbed more slowly, reaching C_{max} approximately 4 to 6 hours after administration.[84–86] Its absorption is affected by both food intake and gastric pH. Bosutinib's C_{max} and AUC increase with food, with less accompanying diarrhea and nausea compared to the fasting state.[87] Consequently, bosutinib is recommended to be taken with food.[85] The solubility of bosutinib is pH dependent; coadministration of PPIs decreases bosutinib's C_{max} and AUC by 46% and 26%, respectively.[88]

Bosutinib has a very large volume of distribution of 6,080 L and is 94% to 96% protein bound.[85] Bosutinib is converted by CYP 3A4 to two major inactive metabolites: oxydechlorinated (M2) bosutinib and N-desmethylated (M5) bosutinib. These contribute 19% and 25% to the AUC, respectively. Bosutinib's mean terminal elimination half-life is 22.5 hours, enabling steady-state concentrations to be reached in approximately 7 days.[85,86] The majority of bosutinib, both parent drug and metabolites, is excreted in the feces (91%) and minor component in the urine (3%).[85,87]

Summary of Literature/Efficacy

Bosutinib was first studied as a second-line agent in the treatment of CML in a large phase I/II open-label clinical trial that included patients in all disease phases with documented resistance or intolerance to one or more TKIs.[86,89] In each of these populations, bosutinib showed evidence of clinical activity as a second-line agent, and importantly, responses were seen in individuals with BCR-ABL1 resistance mutations, with the notable exception of T315I. In chronic phase patients with imatinib resistance/intolerance, 53% had a major cytogenetic response at a median follow-up of 24.2 months, and 41% achieved CCyR.[86] At 2 years, the PFS and OS rates in this population were 81% and 91%, respectively.[89]

Based on these findings, bosutinib was next studied in the upfront setting in chronic phase CML. In the phase III BELA trial, bosutinib 500 mg once daily was compared to imatinib 400 mg once daily.[90] In terms of the trial's primary endpoint, CCyR at 12 months, bosutinib did not exhibit superiority (70% for bosutinib versus 68% for imatinib). In secondary analyses, bosutinib had significantly higher rates of MMR, as well as a shorter times to CCyR/MMR and lower rates of transformation to accelerated/blast phase; however, this did not translate into increased EFS or OS, at either 12 or 24 months of follow-up.[90,91] Of note, in BELA, the treatment discontinuation rates were higher with bosutinib than imatinib, largely due to early GI and hepatic toxicity (see *Toxicity* section below), which likely affected efficacy outcomes in this trial. A follow-up phase III trial (BFORE) compared a lower dose of bosutinib (400 mg once daily) to imatinib in the upfront treatment of CML. Results from this study, first presented at the American Society of Clinical Oncology (ASCO) meeting in 2017, showed that bosutinib achieved higher rates of MMR at 12 months than imatinib (47.2% versus 36.9%), achieving its primary endpoint. Additionally, bosutinib showed higher rates of CCyR and shorter times to CCyR/MMR.[92] Together, these findings suggest that the lower starting dose of bosutinib used in BFORE may offer a more ideal balance between efficacy and toxicity in the first-line treatment of chronic phase CML.

Toxicity

Bosutinib shares many side effects with the other TKIs, including early myelosuppression, which can be managed with dose adjustment, as well as hepatotoxicity, fluid retention, kidney dysfunction, diarrhea, nausea/vomiting, fatigue, myalgia, rash, and headache.[85,91] However, it has some key differences in its toxicity profile. In the BELA trial, bosutinib caused less neutropenia, musculoskeletal events, and edema compared to imatinib. Moreover, there was no signal for a higher incidence of peripheral artery occlusion, PAH, or pleural effusion.[91] On the other hand, bosutinib causes significant GI side effects—in BELA, 70% of patients experienced diarrhea (12% with grade 3/4), compared to 25% of patients taking imatinib (1% grade 3/4). This typically occurred during the first month of treatment, was short-lived, and could be effectively managed with antidiarrheal medications and/or dose interruption/reduction.[91,93] Compared to imatinib, bosutinib also results in more frequent increases in ALT (23% versus 4%) and AST (12% versus 4%).[91] Transaminitis usually arises within the first few months of treatment and can be managed via dose reduction/interruption without risk of progression to permanent hepatic injury. Consequently, liver enzymes should be monitored for the first 3 months of treatment.[85]

Drug interactions

Similar to the other TKIs, bosutinib is metabolized primarily by CYP 3A4; thus, its levels can be influenced by strong CYP 3A4 inhibitors and inducers, and it can interfere with the metabolism of other CYP 3A4 substrates. Also, given that bosutinib is a substrate of the PGP drug efflux pump, coadministration of PGP inhibitors can increase its plasma concentrations.

As discussed above, bosutinib's solubility is pH dependent, and the concomitant administration of PPIs can decrease its absorption.[88] Consequently, their coadministration is not recommended. If gastric protection is required, H2 receptor antagonists or antacids, separated from bosutinib by at least 2 hours, can be considered, though their effects on its pharmacokinetics have not been studied in detail.[85]

Ponatinib

Mechanism of Action

Ponatinib (Iclusig, formerly AP24534; Fig. 24.1E) is a third-generation TKI, specifically designed to overcome the T315I point mutation, which confers resistance to imatinib, dasatinib, nilotinib, and bosutinib. Its key pharmacologic features are provided in Table 24.6.

The T315 residue acts as a gatekeeper to the ATP-binding site of the ABL kinase domain, and mutation to isoleucine eliminates molecular interactions critical for the binding of the aforementioned TKIs (Fig. 24.2B).[43] Ponatinib includes a carbon-carbon triple bond that can form a hydrophobic interaction with the isoleucine side chain, enabling it to productively bind to the ATP-binding site of the inactive conformation of T315I BCR-ABL and inhibit its kinase activity with an IC_{50} of 2.0 nM.[94] Moreover, in addition to T315I, ponatinib can inhibit all documented BCR-ABL kinase domain mutants, as well as native ABL, SRC, and members of the VEGF, FGFR, and PDGFR families of receptor tyrosine kinases.[94]

Clinical Pharmacology and Metabolism

Ponatinib is slowly absorbed and takes approximately 6 hours to reach C_{max} after oral administration.[95] There is a proportional relationship between drug dose and both the C_{max} and AUC.[96] In contrast to bosutinib, ponatinib's absorption, AUC, and C_{max} are not affected by ingestion with food.[97] Like many of the other TKIs, ponatinib requires an acidic environment to enter solution, and coadministration with PPIs decreases its C_{max} and AUC while also increasing the time to C_{max}.[95,98]

After absorption, ponatinib distributes extensively throughout the body, with a volume of distribution of approximately 1,223 L. Ponatinib is 99% protein bound and, in in vitro studies, is not displaced by other highly bound medications.[95] Ponatinib is metabolized via cytochrome P450 enzymes, esterases, and amidases into inactive metabolites. CYP 3A4 is the major CYP isoform involved, with minor contributions from CYP 2C8, CYP 2D6, and CYP 3A5.[99] Ponatinib's mean terminal half-life is approximately 24 hours; consequently, steady-state concentrations should be established in about 7 days.[95,96] Ponatinib and its metabolites are mainly excreted in the feces (87%) with a minor component in the urine (5%).[95,99]

Summary of Literature/Efficacy

Ponatinib was first evaluated in a phase I clinical trial that included 60 CML patients at various disease phases, the majority whom had received two or more prior TKI therapies. Of patients in chronic

---

TABLE 24.6	Key features of ponatinib
Mechanism of action	Competitive inhibitor of c-ABL ATP-binding site, designed to overcome the T315I mutation. Also inhibits SRC, VEGF, FGFR, and PDGFR receptor tyrosine kinases
Metabolism	CYP 3A4, esterases, and amidases with minor contribution from CYP 2C8, CYP 2D6, and CYP 3A5
Pharmacokinetics	t_{max}: <6 hours Protein binding: >99% V_d: 1,223 L $t_{1/2}$: 24 hours
Elimination	Fecal (87%) and urinary (5%)
Drug interactions	Avoid concomitant strong CYP 3A4 inhibitors/inducers and PPIs
Toxicity	Myelosuppression, arterial occlusion, heart failure, hypertension, cardiac arrhythmias, hepatotoxicity, serum lipase elevation/pancreatitis, ocular toxicity, neuropathy, venous thromboembolism, fluid retention, rash, myalgia, fatigue, and GI upset
Precautions	Black box warning for arterial occlusion, venous thromboembolism, heart failure, and hepatotoxicity
	Monitor blood pressure, serum lipase, liver enzymes. Eye examination recommended at baseline then periodically
	Contains lactose

t_{max}, time to maximum concentration; V_d, volume of distribution; $t_{1/2}$, half-life.

phase, 98% achieved complete hematologic response and 72% reached MCyR; of note, all 12 patients with a documented T315I mutation responded, with 92% achieving MCyR.[96] The follow-up phase II **P**onatinib Ph+ **A**LL and **C**ML **E**valuation (PACE) trial enrolled CML patients in all disease phases with either documented resistance/intolerance of second-generation TKIs (dasatinib or nilotinib) or T315I mutations.[100] All patients received ponatinib at a dose of 45 mg once daily, and at a median follow-up of 15 months, 56% of chronic phase patients achieved MCyR, 46% reached CCyR, and 34% had an MMR. Responses were seen in both those patients with intolerance/resistance to second-generation TKIs, as well as the subgroup with *BCR-ABL* T315I mutations; in fact, no single *BCR-ABL* mutation was found to be associated with ponatinib resistance. Among patients with accelerated or blast phase disease, ponatinib also resulted in clinically significant responses as MCyR was obtained in 39% and 23% of patients, respectively.[100]

Ponatinib was studied in the frontline setting in the EPIC (**E**valuation of **P**onatinib versus **I**matinib in **C**ML) trial, a phase III study of treatment-naïve chronic phase CML patients who were randomized to receive imatinib 400 mg once daily or ponatinib 45 mg once daily.[101] This trial was terminated prematurely due to a concern over high rates of vascular adverse events in ongoing follow-up of the aforementioned phase I and II trials of ponatinib. At the time of termination, only 23 patients had completed their 12-month follow-up, limiting analysis of the study's primary endpoint, MMR at 12 months. MMR was achieved in 8/10 patients in the ponatinib group versus 5/13 patients in the imatinib group, but patient numbers were not sufficient to establish the statistically superiority of ponatinib.[101]

The initial analysis of the PACE trial was done at a median follow-up of 15 months and reported that CV, cerebrovascular, and peripheral vascular events occurred in 7%, 4%, and 5% of patients, respectively.[100] At the time, it was not clear how many of these events could be directly attributed to the study drug, in part due to the single-arm design of this trial. However, with longer periods of follow-up, a significantly higher proportion of patients in the PACE cohort were shown to be affected by vascular events; at 5-years of follow-up, 29% of patients had experienced arterial occlusion events.[102] A pooled analysis across the three major ponatinib clinical trials has suggested an association between dose intensity and risk of peripheral arterial occlusive disease, with the risk being highest among the elderly as well as individuals with a history of ischemic CV disease.[103]

As such, prospective studies aiming to evaluate the efficacy and risk profile of ponatinib at a lower dose intensity, achieved either by starting at a lower dose or by decreasing the dose after achieving response, are currently underway. OPTIC is a phase II trial of patients with TKI-refractory CML where patients will be started on one of three doses of ponatinib (15, 30 and 45 mg/day) and, upon achievement of MCyR, the dose will be reduced to 15 mg/day. The OPTIC-2L phase III trial will compare nilotinib 400 mg twice daily against two starting doses of ponatinib (15 and 30 mg/day) in patients with imatinib-resistant CP-CML.

Toxicity

As discussed above, ponatinib significantly increases the risk of CV disease, most notably arterial thrombotic events, including myocardial infarction, stroke, and peripheral vascular disease. It can also lead to congestive heart failure, symptomatic arrhythmias, and

treatment-emergent hypertension. At 4-years of follow-up of the PACE trial, fatal or serious heart failure occurred in 6% of ponatinib-treated patients.[95] Hypertension occurred in 68% of patients in the PACE trial, including individuals with and without pre-existing hypertension. Symptomatic elevations of blood pressure necessitating urgent clinical intervention occurred in 12% of patients, and there have been rare reports of posterior reversible encephalopathy syndrome (PRES).[95]

As a result of these CV risks, before ponatinib initiation, risk factors for CV disease, such as pre-existing hypertension, hyperlipidemia, smoking, and estrogen-based hormonal replacement, should be identified and managed. Many practitioners initiate low-dose aspirin in the absence of contraindications. While on therapy, all patients should be monitored for evidence of arterial thrombotic events and heart failure; if these events arise, ponatinib should be stopped immediately.[76] Patients should have regular assessment of their blood pressure, and treatment-emergent hypertension should be medically managed.[95]

Ponatinib has a number of other notable side effects, including several shared with the other TKIs. It causes myelosuppression, usually early in the course of therapy, which can be managed with dose interruption/reduction. In terms of nonhematologic adverse events, ponatinib causes fluid retention (most commonly peripheral edema, rarely pleural or pericardial effusions), arthralgia/myalgia, rash, and GI symptomatology. Though many TKIs cause transaminitis, ponatinib appears to be particularly hepatotoxic. In the PACE trial, transaminase elevations occurred in 56% of patients (8% grade 3/4), with rare cases of fulminant hepatic failure. Consequently, ponatinib carries a black box warning for hepatotoxicity, and it is recommended that liver function tests be monitored at baseline and then at least monthly. Dose modification is required for significant elevations of AST and ALT, and a lower starting dose of 30 mg daily is recommended for patients with baseline hepatic impairment.[95]

Aside from CV-related side effects, ponatinib also has a number of other toxicities that are relatively unique compared to the other TKIs. Peripheral neuropathy occurred in 20% of patients in PACE, was typically mild (only 2% had grade 3/4 toxicity), and arose during the first month of treatment.[95] Ponatinib also carries a black box warning for venous thromboembolism, which occurred in 6% of patients in the PACE trial at 4-years follow-up. Ponatinib frequently causes elevation in serum lipase and occasional overt pancreatitis; in the PACE trial, these complications arose in 42% and 7% of ponatinib-treated patients, respectively.[95] Consequently, patients on ponatinib should have lipase checked every 2 weeks for the first 2 months of therapy and then monthly afterward or as clinically indicated. More frequent monitoring should be considered in individuals with a history of pancreatitis or risk factors such as alcohol abuse. Dose reduction/interruption is required in the setting of lipase elevations and overt pancreatitis.[95] Lastly, long-term follow-up of ponatinib patients has found that it can lead to ocular toxicity ranging from conjunctival symptoms (14% of patients in PACE) to visual blurring (6%) and retinal toxicity (2%). Consequently, comprehensive eye exams are recommended at baseline and periodically during treatment.

Drug interactions

Ponatinib's drug interactions are similar to the other TKIs. It is primarily metabolized by CYP 3A4, so strong inhibitors and inducers of this enzyme can affect its concentration and should be avoided if possible. When coadministered with ketoconazole, a strong CYP 3A4 inhibitor, ponatinib's C_{max} and AUC increased by 47% and 78%, respectively.[104] As this has the potential to result in increased rates of adverse events, when strong CYP 3A4 inhibitors must be used concurrently with ponatinib, a lower starting dose (30 mg daily) is recommended.[95]

As described above, ponatinib's solubility is pH dependent; as such, its absorption can be affected by medications that alter gastric pH. In a phase I study of 20 healthy subjects, concomitant use of ponatinib and lansoprazole resulted in a 25% decrease in C_{max}, a longer time to C_{max}, and a 6% decrease in AUC.[98] Coadministration of PPIs should be avoided, but if necessary, patients should be monitored for evidence of reduced efficacy.[95]

Omacetaxine

Mechanism of Action

Omacetaxine mepesuccinate (Synribo, formerly CGX-653; Fig. 24.3) is semisynthetic derivative of the plant alkaloid homoharringtonine, originally isolated from *Cephalotaxus harringtonii*, an evergreen tree found in China, India, and Japan.[105] It is not a TKI, but instead a cell cycle–dependent inhibitor of protein synthesis that acts by blocking the binding of aminoacyl transfer RNAs to the A-site of the ribosome, preventing the elongation step of translation, and leading to a global decrease in mRNA translation efficacy.[106,107] In particular, omacetaxine inhibits the synthesis of antiapoptotic proteins of the Bcl-2 family, including Mcl-1 (myeloid cell leukemia 1), leading to apoptosis of stem/progenitor cells in CML patients.[108]

Clinical Pharmacology and Metabolism

Omacetaxine is injected subcutaneously and rapidly absorbed, reaching C_{max} in approximately 30 minutes. Its volume of distribution

Omacetaxine

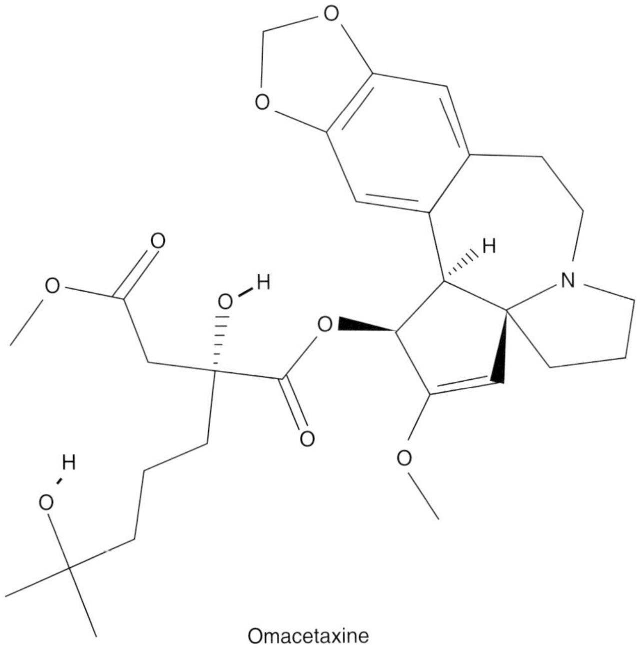

FIGURE **24.3** Chemical structure of the protein synthesis inhibitor omacetaxine.

is 141 L, and the drug is less than 50% protein bound. Omacetaxine is metabolized through esterases to its inactive metabolites 4′-desmethylhomoharringtonine (4′-DMHHT) and cephalotaxine.[109] In a pharmacokinetic analysis, the concentration of 4′-DMHHT was 10% that of the parent compound, while cephalotaxine was usually undetectable.[110] Omacetaxine has a half-life of approximately 6 hours, and its excretion is nearly equally split between the urine and feces, with the latter occurring more slowly.[109,111]

Summary of Literature/Efficacy

Omacetaxine was initially studied in chronic phase CML in a series of small trials in the pre-TKI era, either as monotherapy or in combination with other agents such as low-dose cytarabine or IFN-α.[112–114] These studies established the clinical efficacy of subcutaneous omacetaxine in CML, but its development slowed as oral TKIs came to dominate the treatment of chronic phase patients. However, a role for omacetaxine in the treatment of patients with resistance/intolerance to multiple TKIs has emerged in recent years. In an early case report, an imatinib-resistant patient with a T315I mutation was treated with omacetaxine, resulting in a complete hematologic response and selective disappearance of the T315I mutant clone.[115] Further case reports and case series replicated this finding, eventually leading to two single-arm open-label phase II trials: CML-202, which enrolled patients with imatinib intolerance/resistance and a documented T315I mutation, and CML-203, which enrolled patients with intolerance to imatinib and at least one other TKI. In both of these studies, omacetaxine was administered as a subcutaneous injection at a dose of 1.25 mg/m² twice daily. During the initial induction phase, the drug was dosed twice daily for 14 consecutive days, every 28 days, until hematologic response was achieved, to a maximum of six cycles. Once response was achieved, a maintenance phase of treatment commenced, where omacetaxine was dosed twice daily for 7 consecutive days of a 28-day cycle.

In a pooled analysis of chronic phase patients from both trials, hematologic responses were achieved in 56 of 81 patients (69%), and the trials' primary endpoint, MCyR, was obtained in 16 of 81 patients (20%), with a median duration of 17.7 months.[116] Among patients with accelerated phase CML, responses were also seen, as 14% achieved a major hematologic response, with a median duration of 4.7 months, but no MCyR were documented.[117] Together, these trials established that omacetaxine can result in clinically meaningful responses in heavily pretreated chronic and accelerated phase CML patients, leading to its approval by the FDA for this indication in 2012. To date, omacetaxine has not been evaluated head to head versus TKIs in the upfront treatment of chronic phase CML, so its role in this setting remains unknown.

Toxicity

Omacetaxine causes significant hematologic toxicity. While on omacetaxine, 76% of patients developed thrombocytopenia (68% grade 3/4), 61% developed anemia (36% grade 3/4), and 53% developed neutropenia (47% grade 3/4), frequently complicated by fever.[109] Median time to resolution of grade 3/4 thrombocytopenia was 31 days, whereas the median time to resolution of grade 3/4 neutropenia was 19 days.[116] Consequently, complete blood counts should be performed weekly during the induction phase of treatment and biweekly during the early stages of maintenance with dose adjustments for significant cytopenias. Severe neutropenia (ANC $< 0.5 \times 10^9$/L) or thrombocytopenia (platelet count $< 50 \times 10^9$/L) should prompt delay of the next cycle of treatment until counts recover above these thresholds. Moreover, the number of dosing days in the next cycle should be reduced by 2 (i.e., 12 days during induction; 5 days during maintenance).[109]

Omacetaxine also causes a number of nonhematologic toxicities, most notably bacterial, viral, and fungal infections (seen in 48% of chronic phase patients, with 11% grade 3/4) and diarrhea (seen in 41%, with 1% grade 3/4). Other less common side effects associated with omacetaxine include nausea/vomiting, fatigue, pyrexia, asthenia, musculoskeletal pain, headache, anorexia, hyperglycemia, and local injection site reactions.[109,116]

Drug Interactions

Omacetaxine is not a substrate, inhibitor, or inducer of cytochrome P450 enzymes; thus, there is limited potential for CYP-related drug interactions. It was found to be a PGP substrate in vitro, but concomitant use of omacetaxine and loperamide, another substrate, did not affect the efflux of either drug, suggesting that this interaction is of limited clinical consequence.[109]

Clinical Use of Targeted CML Therapeutics

At present, three TKIs are approved for the frontline therapy of CML (imatinib, dasatinib, and nilotinib), while all of the TKIs and omacetaxine can be used as second-line therapies or beyond. Details regarding their approved CML indications and dosing are provided in Table 24.7.

With this range of available agents, deciding which drug to use in a given clinical scenario poses a challenge for health care providers. The following will briefly cover this and other practical aspects of TKI use, including the molecular monitoring of therapy and drug interruption.

Frontline Therapy of Chronic Phase CML

As discussed above, in trials comparing imatinib to second-generation TKIs, dasatinib and nilotinib were not associated with significantly improved survival (Table 24.4). As such, clinical guidelines state that any of these three TKIs are an appropriate choice for frontline therapy in chronic phase CML.[76,118] However, in these same studies, both second-generation agents were associated with higher rates of molecular response and lower disease progression rates, particularly among intermediate-and high-risk patients as defined by the

---

TABLE 24.7   *Approved indications for TKIs and omacetaxine in CML*

Indication	Dose	Details
Chronic Phase CML		
Frontline therapy		
Imatinib	400 mg once daily	
Dasatinib	100 mg once daily	
Nilotinib	300 mg twice daily	
Second-line therapy		
Imatinib	600 to 800 mg once daily	Only use after a 2nd-generation TKI if issue is tolerability, not efficacy
Dasatinib	100 mg once daily	
Nilotinib	400 mg twice daily	
Bosutinib	500 mg once daily	
Ponatinib	45 mg once daily	If T315I-positive disease or no other TKI is indicated
Omacetaxine	1.25 mg/m² SC twice daily	If resistance/intolerance to 2 or more TKIs

Indication	Dose	AP	BC	Details
Advanced phase (AP/BC) CML				
Imatinib	600 mg once daily	✓	✓	
Dasatinib	140 mg once daily	✓	✓	
Nilotinib	400 mg twice daily	✓		
Bosutinib	500 mg twice daily	✓	✓	If resistant/intolerant to a prior TKI
Ponatinib	45 mg once daily	✓	✓	If T315I-positive disease or no other TKI is indicated
Omacetaxine	1.25 mg/m² SC twice daily	✓		If resistance/intolerance to 2 or more TKIs

AP, accelerated phase; BC, blast crisis.

Sokal et al. [119] or Hasford et al. [120] scoring systems. As such, NCCN guidelines suggest that dasatinib and nilotinib may be preferable alternatives to imatinib as first-line therapy in these patient populations. [76]

In addition to disease risk, other important considerations in the selection of first-line TKI therapy include patient comorbidities, the toxicity profiles of each drug, and the ease of administration. The TKIs share numerous side effects, such as cytopenias, rash, myalgia, electrolyte abnormalities, and liver toxicity; however, differences do exist in their toxicity profiles. In general, imatinib has the most favorable side effect profile of the TKIs approved for first-line therapy in chronic phase CML. Due to its association with pleural effusions and pulmonary hypertension, dasatinib should be used with caution in patients with pre-existing lung disease. Similarly, nilotinib should be avoided in patients with a history of CV disease, as it can result in elevated blood glucose and lipids and is associated with higher rates of CV events and progression of peripheral vascular disease. [76] Notably, given that concurrent food intake can variably affect nilotinib absorption, it is recommended that the drug be taken on an empty stomach, with no food for 2 hours before and 1 hour after each dose. [67] This can prove to be a challenge for patients, as the medication is taken twice daily. Ultimately, a thorough, personalized assessment of the risk-benefit balance is crucial for guiding TKI selection in the frontline setting.

Following their initiation, response to the TKIs is monitored by performing complete blood counts (initially on a weekly basis and then spaced out periodically) and by quantitative assessment of BCR-ABL1 transcript levels via RT-PCR every 3 months. This molecular testing is reported according to the international scale (IS)—for a given patient, the ratio of BCR-ABL1 transcripts to ABL1 transcripts (an internal control) is calculated and then normalized to a reference baseline, common across all laboratories. Values are reported as the number of log reductions in the BCR-ABL1/ABL1 transcript levels between the patient and the standardized reference, with a 3-log reduction corresponding to an MMR. [121] For chronic phase CML, guidelines provide molecular response milestones at various times after the initiation of therapy (Table 24.8). [76,118] If patients fail to reach these benchmarks, patient compliance and drug interactions must be evaluated, and testing for BCR-ABL1 resistance mutations is warranted.

Traditionally, TKIs have been dosed indefinitely in CML patients, but the feasibility of discontinuing therapy in individuals who have maintained deep molecular responses for extended periods is an area of ongoing investigation. In the **Stop Im**atinib (STIM) trial, patients with a 5-log reduction in BCR-ABL1 transcript levels and undetectable minimal residual disease discontinued drug with close molecular monitoring. [122] At 12 months after imatinib discontinuation, molecular remissions were maintained in 41% of patients, with the majority of recurrences occurring within the first 6 months of treatment cessation. Importantly, resumption of imatinib post-relapse resulted in the re-establishment of undetectable MRD in the majority of patients. Similar results have been obtained in other prospective clinical trials, suggesting that, with close monitoring, TKIs can be safely discontinued in select subset of patients, with the hope of obtaining extended treatment-free remissions. This is reflected in the 2016 NCCN CML guidelines, which outline strict criteria for both the selection of patients to attempt treatment discontinuation (most notably CP patients, with 4-log reduction in BCR-ABL1 transcript levels for >2 years) and for molecular monitoring post discontinuation. [76] TKI discontinuation has the potential to greatly improve patient quality of life by enabling drug holidays and will prove particularly useful in patients contemplating pregnancy, as all TKIs are contraindicated in this setting.

Second-Line Treatment and Beyond

While the introduction of TKIs into the frontline treatment of chronic phase CML has revolutionized care of this disease, with survival approaching that of age-matched controls, small numbers of individuals either do not tolerate these drugs, or progress on therapy, often secondary to the development of tyrosine kinase domain mutations. Failure to reach response milestones (Table 24.8) should prompt evaluation of patient compliance, as well as BCR-ABL mutational analysis.

If drug intolerance is the issue, the next-line TKI should be chosen on the basis of a potentially more favorable side effect profile. For example, in patients having significant fluid retention and/or GI side effects due imatinib, nilotinib may prove to be more tolerable, as it is associated with lower rates of these complications. [74]

Lack or loss of efficacy should also prompt a change in therapy. In the case of first-line imatinib, dose escalation to 600 or 800 mg daily was traditionally used in this scenario. However, given that multiple other TKIs are readily available, this approach should only be used in patients with no BCR-ABL1 mutations and good tolerance of the standard dose, or for individuals where no other TKIs can be used due to lack of availability or potential side effects. The decision regarding which TKI should be used in the second-line setting should take into account each drug's unique toxicity profile (and how this aligns with patient comorbidities), as well as each drug's activity against the various BCR-ABL1 mutations (Table 24.9). Of note, imatinib is not recommended for disease that is resistant to primary treatment with nilotinib and dasatinib. Moreover, the emergence of a T315I mutation, which confers resistance to all TKIs except ponatinib, limits treatment options to ponatinib, omacetaxine, or allogeneic stem cell transplant. [76]

Other Clinical Uses of TKIs

Aside from CML, TKIs are also used in the treatment of a number of other malignancies. The Philadelphia chromosome is present in a subset of acute lymphoblastic leukemia (ALL) patients and is associated with particularly poor prognosis. A number of studies have shown that the incorporation of TKIs into induction chemotherapy

TABLE **24.8**	*Response milestones for TKI therapy*	
Time after Therapy Initiation	Optimal Goal	Failure
3 months	IS ≤ 10%	CHR not achieved
6 months	IS ≤ 1%	IS > 10%
12 months	IS ≤ 0.1% (MMR)	IS > 1%
Beyond 12 months	IS ≤ 0.1% (MMR)	Loss of best response

Adapted from ELN guidelines: Baccarani M, Deininger MW, Rosti G, et al. European LeukemiaNet recommendations for the management of chronic myeloid leukemia: 2013. *Blood.* 2013;122:872-884.

24.9 *TKI options for BCR-ABL1 TKD mutations*

Recommended Treatment	*BCR-ABL1* Mutation
Dasatinib	Y253H
	E255K/V
	F359V/C/I
Nilotinib	F317L/V/I/C
	T315A
	V299L
Bosutinib	Y253H
	E255K/V
	F317L/V/I/C
	F359V/C/I
	T315A
Ponatinib	T315I

Adapted with permission from the NCCN Clinical Practice Guidelines in Oncology (NCCN Guidelines®) for Chronic Myeloid Leukemia V.1.2017. © 2018 National Comprehensive Cancer Network, Inc. All rights reserved. The NCCN Guidelines® and illustrations herein may not be reproduced in any form for any purpose without the express written permission of NCCN. To view the most recent and complete version of the NCCN Guidelines, go online to NCCN.org. The NCCN Guidelines are a work in progress that may be refined as often as new significant data becomes available. NCCN makes no warranties of any kind whatsoever regarding their content, use or application and disclaims any responsibility for their application or use in any way.

regimens results in complete remission (CR) in greater than 90% of Ph+ ALL cases, significantly higher than historical controls.[123,124] In practice, second-generation TKIs are typically used in this setting, with ponatinib reserved for patients with T315I mutations. Once CR is attained, it is recommended that eligible patients proceed with allogeneic stem cell transplant, but in the nontransplant population, TKIs are included in the consolidation and maintenance phases of treatment, an approach that can result in lasting remissions.[125,126]

Due to its ability to inhibit kinases other than BCR-ABL, imatinib has also been approved for clinical use in malignancies other than CML and Ph+ ALL. Chromosomal rearrangements involving the *PDGFRA* and *PDGFRB* genes, which result in the constitutive activation of these kinases, are well documented in patients with hypereosinophilic syndrome (HES) as well as myelodysplastic syndrome/myeloproliferative neoplasm (MDS/MPN) overlap conditions. Imatinib has emerged as a treatment option in these patient populations; in particular, in HES expressing the constitutively active FIP1L1-PDGFR-α fusion kinase, imatinib at a starting dose of 100 mg daily can result in molecular remissions.[127] Systemic mastocytosis is another myeloproliferative disorder, characterized by the accumulation of mast cells in the skin, bone marrow, and other tissues. These cells express the receptor tyrosine kinase KIT on their surface, and their development relies on signaling via the stem cell factor-KIT axis. Imatinib is used for cytoreduction in patients with advanced systemic mastocytosis in order to mitigate organ dysfunction; specifically, it is active in patients who lack the KIT D816V mutation, as this change confers drug resistance.[128,129] Lastly, outside of the

realm of hematologic malignancies, imatinib is used in the treatment of GIST, which is associated with activating mutations in KIT or PDGFR-α,[130,131] as well as dermatofibrosarcoma protuberans, which is associated with chromosomal rearrangements that lead to the overexpression of PDGFB and constitutive PDGFR-β signaling.[132]

Philadelphia-Negative Myeloproliferative Neoplasms

The Philadelphia-negative myeloproliferative neoplasms (Ph− MPNs) are a group of phenotypically related clonal hematopoietic diseases, namely, polycythemia vera (PV), essential thrombocythemia (ET), and primary myelofibrosis (MF). These stem cell disorders are characterized by the overproduction of mature myeloid cells, a prolonged clinical course, and the risk of transformation into acute myeloid leukemia (AML). The underlying molecular pathogenesis of Ph− MPNs involves constitutive activation of JAK-STAT signaling, achieved in the vast majority of cases by acquired mutations in one of *JAK2*, *MPL*, or *CALR* (Fig. 24.4).[133]

Both ET, which is characterized by isolated thrombocytosis, and PV, which features panmyelosis with a predominant erythrocytosis, carry a significant risk of thrombohemorrhagic complications. Accordingly, treatment approaches aim to reduce this risk, using one or more of low-dose aspirin, phlebotomy (for PV only), and cytoreduction with agents such as hydroxyurea (HU) or IFN-α. Compared to ET and PV, MF is a more clinically aggressive entity, as it is associated with progressive bone marrow fibrosis, peripheral blood cytopenias, splenomegaly, and constitutional symptoms, such as pruritus, fatigue, night sweats, and bone pain. Historically, treatment approaches for MF were largely unsatisfactory; however, since the discovery of the JAK2V617F mutation in 2005,[134–137] a major change in the therapeutic landscape of MF has occurred, with the development of targeted inhibitors of the JAK kinases. JAK inhibitors significantly relieve constitutional symptoms and reduce splenomegaly, but do not modify underlying disease biology. The following will discuss the emerging role of inhibitors of JAK-STAT signaling in the treatment of the Ph− MPNs, focusing on the FDA-approved agent ruxolitinib, as well as agents that are currently in clinical development.

Ruxolitinib

Mechanism of Action

Ruxolitinib (Jakafi, formerly INCB018424) is an oral inhibitor of the Janus kinase (JAK) family of protein tyrosine kinases. A summary of its key pharmacologic features is provided in Table 24.10. Ruxolitinib is a cyclopentylpropionitrile derivative (Fig. 24.5A) that acts as a potent and selective inhibitor of JAK1 ($IC_{50} = 3.3 \pm 1.2$ nM) and JAK2 ($IC_{50} = 2.8 \pm 1.2$ nM) with modest activity against TYK2 ($IC_{50} = 19 \pm 3.2$ nM) and JAK3 ($IC_{50} = 428 \pm 243$ nM).[138] Ruxolitinib acts as a type I kinase inhibitor by competitively binding to the ATP-binding pocket of its targets, locking them in an active conformation and inhibiting activity. The crystal structure of ruxolitinib bound to either JAK1 or JAK2 has not yet been solved.[139]

Importantly, response to ruxolitinib occurs in MF patients regardless of their *JAK2* mutational status, suggesting that it acts via generalized inhibition of JAK-STAT signaling and not by specifically targeting the JAK2V617F kinase. In keeping with this notion, treatment with

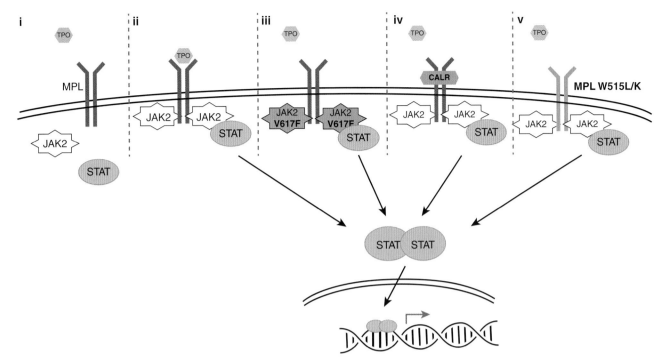

FIGURE **24.4** Mechanisms driving constitutive JAK-STAT signaling in the myeloproliferative neoplasms. In the normal state, activation of JAK-STAT signaling requires binding of a cytokine to its cognate receptor, illustrated here as thrombopoietin (TPO) binding to myeloproliferative leukemia protein (MPL) in panels **(i)** and **(ii)**. In MPNs, JAK-STAT signaling is constitutively activated in the absence of cytokine binding by **(iii)** activating mutations in JAK2, most commonly JAK2 V617F, **(iv)** mutations causing truncation of CALR that drive MPL signaling via interaction with its extracellular domain, and **(v)** activating point mutations in MPL, such as W515L and W515K.

ruxolitinib does not significantly decrease the *JAK2V617F* allelic burden in patients.[140] Instead, it is thought that this drug's clinical efficacy in MF may be due in part to its ability to attenuate proinflammatory cytokine signaling. Patients with MF are known to have significantly elevated circulating levels of proinflammatory cytokines, and it has been hypothesized that this cytokine-driven inflammatory state may contribute to the constitutional symptoms, bone marrow fibrosis, and extramedullary hematopoiesis characteristic of this disease.[141,142] Consistent with this model, levels of proinflammatory cytokines, such as tumor necrosis factor-α and interleukin-6 are significantly decreased in MF patients treated with ruxolitinib.[143]

The finding that the MF disease clone does not significantly decrease upon treatment with ruxolitinib has raised the question as to how these cells are able to maintain JAK-STAT signaling in the presence of this inhibitor. In contrast to imatinib, kinase domain mutations do not appear to play a significant role in conferring resistance to JAK inhibitors. Instead, JAK-STAT signaling persists in the presence of ruxolitinib via heterodimerization of JAK kinases. In this scenario, instead of JAK2 being activated by homodimerization, it is activated *in trans* by JAK1 or TYK2. Heterodimerization has been observed not only in experimental models of myeloproliferative neoplasms but also in patients treated with ruxolitinib and other type I JAK kinase inhibitors.[144]

TABLE

24.10 *Key features of ruxolitinib*

Mechanism of action	ATP-competitive inhibitor of JAK1/2 with minor inhibition of TYK2/JAK3			
Metabolism	CYP 3A4, CYP 2C9			
Pharmacokinetics	t_{max}: 1 to 2 h Bioavailability: 95% Protein binding: 97% V_d: 72 to 75 L $t_{1/2}$: 2 to 3 h			
Elimination	Renal (74%) and fecal (22%)			
Drug interactions	Dose adjustment required when given with CYP 3A4 inhibitors			
	Avoid use with fluconazole doses >200 mg			
Toxicity	Myelosuppression, infections (including latent tuberculosis/viral reactivation), bruising, dizziness, headache, weight gain, flatulence, elevated transaminases and lipids			
Precautions	Serious infections should be resolved prior to initiation			
	Abrupt discontinuation can result in MF symptom exacerbation			
	Increases risk of nonmelanoma skin cancer			

t_{max}, time to maximum concentration; V_d, volume of distribution; $t_{1/2}$, half-life.

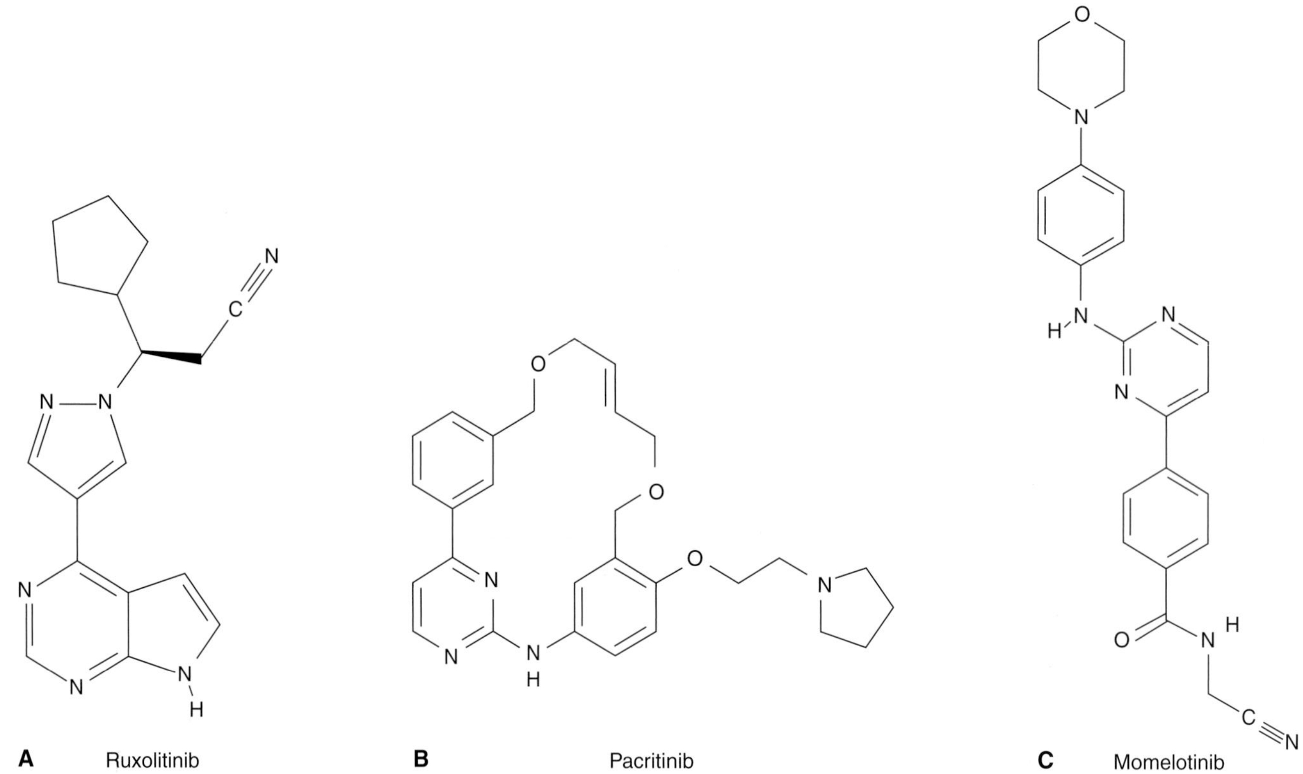

FIGURE 24.5 Chemical structures of the JAK inhibitors. **(A)** Ruxolitinib, **(B)** pacritinib, and **(C)** momelotinib.

Clinical Pharmacology and Metabolism

Ruxolitinib is rapidly absorbed after oral administration, with C_{max} achieved within one to two hours. Its bioavailability is at least 95%, and there is no effect of food on absorption. Ruxolitinib has a volume of distribution of 72 to 75 L, and it is approximately 97% protein bound, mainly to albumin. Ruxolitinib is primarily metabolized by CYP 3A4, and to a lesser extent by CYP 2C9, generating active metabolites. Its mean elimination half-life is 2 to 3 hours, and when taken together with its metabolites, the mean $t_{1/2}$ is 5.8 hours.[145–147] Ruxolitinib is 74% excreted in the urine and 22% via the feces, with less than 1% in an unmetabolized form.[145,146] Given the involvement of both the liver and kidney its excretion, dose adjustments are recommended for patients with hepatic and/or renal impairment.[146]

Summary of Literature/Efficacy

In preclinical studies, ruxolitinib was found to inhibit the proliferation of JAK2V617-dependent cell lines, suppress erythroid colony formation in PV patients, and, in a mouse model of JAK2V617F+ myeloproliferative disease, reduce splenomegaly and prolong survival.[138] Following promising results in early-phase clinical trials, where ruxolitinib caused sustained reductions in splenomegaly and improvements in MF-related symptoms,[147] it proceeded to two randomized controlled phase III studies: COMFORT-I, which compared ruxolitinib to placebo,[143] and COMFORT-II, which compared it to the best available alternative therapy.[148] In both, all patients had intermediate-2 or high-risk disease, according to the International Prognostic Scoring System (IPSS),[149] and had platelet counts of greater than $100 \times 10^9/L$. The primary endpoint in these studies was a splenic volume reduction of 35% at 24 and 48 weeks.

Secondary endpoints included durability of response, symptomatic improvement as measured by the MF symptom assessment form, and OS. In both trials, ruxolitinib resulted in a significant reduction in spleen size and symptom scores[143,148]; moreover, a pooled followup analysis has demonstrated a statistically significant improvement in OS.[150] However, ruxolitinib did not appear to fundamentally alter the disease biology in these patients as it led only to small reductions in both the *JAK2* mutant allele burden and bone marrow fibrosis while not reducing the risk of disease progression to AML.[140]

In addition to its use in MF, ruxolitinib is now FDA approved for PV. The RESPONSE trial compared the efficacy and safety of ruxolitinib to best available therapy in phlebotomy-dependent PV patients with splenomegaly who were resistant to or intolerant of HU.[151] In this study, ruxolitinib resulted in a significant increase in the proportion of patients achieving hematocrit control, as well as improvement in both spleen size and PV-associated symptomatology. Subsequently, a similar patient population without splenomegaly was assessed in the RESPONSE-2 trial, where ruxolitinib similarly improved hematocrit control and symptomatology.[152]

Toxicity

The most common toxicities associated with ruxolitinib are new or worsening cytopenias, a consequence of the drug's on-target activity. In COMFORT-I, 96% of ruxolitinib-treated patient experienced anemia (45% grade 3/4), compared to 87% (19% grade 3/4) in the placebo arm. Sixty percent of ruxolitinib patients required red cell transfusions, compared to 38% in the placebo group. Neutropenia also occurred more frequently with ruxolitinib-treated patients, affecting 19% of individuals (7% grade 3/4). Thrombocytopenia was particularly common with ruxolitinib treatment (70% versus

31%, with 13% grade 3/4) especially among patients with lower baseline platelet counts. The median time to onset was 8 weeks, and it was typically reversible with dose reduction/interruption.[143] As a result of this toxicity, ruxolitinib dosing is adjusted according to the platelet count.[146]

Importantly, ruxolitinib causes immunosuppression, leading to an increased susceptibility to infections. The urinary tract is most commonly affected, but more serious infections include reactivation of tuberculosis, hepatitis B, herpes zoster, and JC virus (leading to progressive multifocal leukoencephalopathy). It is also associated with an increased risk of nonmelanoma skin cancers; consequently, periodic skin examinations are recommended.[146]

Common nonhematological side effects associated with ruxolitinib include bruising (23% of COMFORT-1 patients), dizziness (18%), headache (15%), weight gain (7%), and flatulence (5%), all of which are typically mild.[143] Ruxolitinib can also cause mild abnormalities in AST and ALT as well as increased blood cholesterol levels. Lipid parameters should be checked 8 to 12 weeks after ruxolitinib initiation.[146]

Lastly, the discontinuation of ruxolitinib can lead to the rapid return of MF-related symptoms. In order to avoid this rebound phenomenon, with the exception of dose interruption for cytopenias, ruxolitinib should be tapered as opposed to abruptly stopped.

Drug Interactions

As ruxolitinib is extensively metabolized by CYP 3A4, drugs that inhibit or induce this enzyme can significantly influence its levels. For example, when ruxolitinib was coadministered with ketoconazole, a strong CYP 3A4 inhibitor, its C_{max} increased by 33%, AUC increased by 91%, and half-life nearly doubled.[153] Consequently, when strong CYP 3A4 inhibitors, such as boceprevir, clarithromycin, conivaptan, grapefruit juice, itraconazole, ketoconazole, posaconazole, and voriconazole, are administered with ruxolitinib, dose adjustment is required to minimize the potential for toxicity. For MF patients with a platelet count greater than or equal to 100×10^9/L, the starting dose of ruxolitinib should be reduced to 10 mg twice daily; however, if the platelet count falls below this threshold, coadministration with a strong CYP 3A4 inhibitor, regardless of ruxolitinib dose, is not recommended.[146] Fluconazole, a strong inhibitor of not only CYP 3A4 but also CYP 2C9, the other main contributor to ruxolitinib metabolism, should be used with particular caution; in addition to the aforementioned dose adjustments, fluconazole at amounts greater than 200 mg daily should be avoided.[146]

On the other hand, the coadministration of ruxolitinib with strong CYP 3A4 inducers has the potential to decrease drug exposure. For example, when given with rifampin, the C_{max} and AUC decreased by 32% and 61%, respectively. However, this resulted in only a 10% decrease in ruxolitinib activity, as measured by the inhibition of IL-6 stimulated STAT3 phosphorylation in whole blood, a discrepancy potentially explained by the activity of ruxolitinib's metabolites.[153] No dose adjustment is recommended when ruxolitinib is coadministered with CYP 3A4 inducers, but drug efficacy should be monitored.[146]

Clinical Use of Ruxolitinib

Ruxolitinib is currently the only JAK inhibitor approved for clinical use. Its original indication was for MF patients with intermediate-2 or high-risk disease, defined by the presence of two or more IPSS risk factors (age >65 years, hemoglobin of <10 g/dL, leukocyte count of $>25 \times 10^9$/L, ≥1% circulating myeloblasts, and/or the presence of constitutional symptoms). More recently, with the results from the RESPONSE trials, it has been approved for use in PV for HU-resistant patients, who require ongoing phlebotomy or have elevated WBC and PLT counts despite the maximum-tolerated HU dose, and HU-intolerant patients, who have significant cytopenias or unacceptable nonhematologic toxicities due to HU. The starting dose is 10 mg twice daily for PV and 20 mg twice daily for MF, with adjustments based on the platelet count, hepatic/renal dysfunction, and the concomitant usage of strong CYP 3A4 inhibitors, as discussed above.

Ruxolitinib represents a major treatment advance for patients with Ph− MPNs, in particular MF, where treatment options before its introduction were highly unsatisfactory. However, despite the benefits it confers with respect to splenomegaly and symptomatology, ruxolitinib is associated with a high rate of discontinuation mainly due to loss of efficacy and cytopenias, and importantly, it does not appear to significantly alter underlying disease biology.[140]

In order to address these limitations, multiple lines of investigation are actively ongoing. First, in attempts to more effectively target the MF disease clone, multiple clinical trials using ruxolitinib in combination with other agents are currently underway. Second, in order to mitigate ruxolitinib's significant on-target side effects of anemia and thrombocytopenia, there is significant interest in the development of novel JAK inhibitors that are less myelosuppressive. Here, we will briefly discuss two of these agents, pacritinib and momelotinib, that have shown promise in this area.

Pacritinib

Basic Pharmacology

Pacritinib (Fig. 24.5B) is a selective inhibitor of JAK2 with additional activity against *fms*-like tyrosine kinase 3 (FLT3), colony-stimulating factor 1 receptor (CSF1R), and interleukin-1 receptor–associated kinase 1 (IRAK1).[154] In early-phase clinical trials, pacritinib was less myelosuppressive than ruxolitinib,[155] a property that likely stems from its kinase profile, as it inhibits IRAK1, which is known to suppress hematopoiesis, and has no activity against JAK1.[154]

Pacritinib reaches C_{max} between 4 to 8 hours after oral administration, and its absorption is not affected by food.[156–158] It has moderately bioavailability (58.6%), with a volume of distribution of 112 L, and is greater than 99% protein bound.[158,159] Pacritinib is predominantly metabolized by CYP 3A4, and consequently, the concomitant administration of strong inhibitors or inducers of this enzyme can influence its levels. Pacritinib has a mean elimination half-life of 2 to 3 days, and it is primarily excreted in the feces (85%) with a minor component in the urine (3%).[157,159,160]

Results from Clinical Trials

In phase I/II trials of MF patients, pacritinib induced splenic responses with limited myelosuppression.[155,156] These findings led to the phase III PERSIST-1 trial, which enrolled patients with intermediate and high-risk MF, with no exclusions for baseline anemia or thrombocytopenia, and randomized them to received either pacritinib 400 mg once daily or best available therapy (excluding other

JAK inhibitors).[161] Pacritinib resulted in significant spleen volume reduction, the trial's primary endpoint, as well as a decrease in MF-related symptoms. Importantly, pacritinib showed consistent benefits across subgroups, including those patients with baseline anemia and thrombocytopenia. In the PERSIST-2 trial, pacritinib, dosed either at 400 mg once daily or 200 mg twice daily, was compared to best available therapy in patients with MF and platelets less than 100×10^9/L. Prior JAK2 inhibitor use was allowed, and best available therapy could include ruxolitinib. As reported at the 2016 American Society of Hematology Annual Meeting, pacritinib achieved significantly higher rates of splenic response compared to best available therapy and showed a nonsignificant trend toward decreased MF-related symptoms.[162]

In these clinical trials, the most common side effects associated with pacritinib were cytopenias (in particular anemia and thrombocytopenia), diarrhea, nausea, and vomiting. Of note, pacritinib was associated with cardiac complications, including QT prolongation (5% of patients in PERSIST-1) and heart failure (4%).[161] In February of 2016, the FDA placed a full clinical hold on pacritinib due to concerns over excess mortality from cardiac and bleeding events in patients from both PERSIST trials. However, upon further review of safety data, the hold was lifted in February 2017, with plans for a dose exploration trial, targeting patients who have failed prior ruxolitinib.

Looking forward, a JAK inhibitor that can be safely administered to MF patients with significant thrombocytopenia would fill an important niche, and the results from the PERSIST trials suggest that pacritinib may yet prove to be a valuable option in this patient population.

Momelotinib

Basic Pharmacology

Momelotinib (Fig. 24.5C) is a potent and selective ATP-competitive inhibitor of JAK1, JAK2, and TYK2. In early-phase clinical trials, momelotinib was unexpectedly noted to improve anemia.[163,164] This finding, which is unique among the JAK inhibitors studied to date, appears to be mediated by momelotinib targeting the inflammation-driven component of anemia in MF patients. In an experimental model using rats, momelotinib has been shown to inhibit the type 1 bone morphogenic protein receptor kinase activin A receptor (ACVR1) leading to a reduction of hepcidin production by the liver, thereby improving the mobilization of iron from cellular stores.[165]

Momelotinib achieves C_{max} approximately 2 hours after oral ingestion.[166] When taken with a high-fat meal, its C_{max} and AUC are both increased by 28%, whereas coadministration with a PPI reduces these values by 36% and 33%, respectively; in both scenarios, these differences are not expected to be of clinical relevance.[167] At steady state, momelotinib has an elimination half-life between 3.9 and 6.1 hours, but little else has been reported to date regarding its metabolism and excretion.[163]

Results from Clinical Trials

The therapeutic efficacy of momelotinib in MF was established by phase I/II trials showing that it could induce splenic responses as well as improvements in disease-related symptoms and red cell transfusion requirements.[163,164] These prompted the evaluation of momelotinib in two phase 3 clinical trials, whose results have only

been presented in abstract form to date. SIMPLIFY-1 compared momelotinib to ruxolitinib in JAK inhibitor–naive patients with intermediate-and high-risk MF. Momelotinib was noninferior to ruxolitinib with respect to the primary endpoint of splenic volume reduction of ≥35% at 24 weeks; however, statistical noninferiority was not achieved for the key secondary endpoint of total symptom score improvement (28.4% for momelotinib versus 42.2% for ruxolitinib). Exploratory analyses of anemia-related outcomes showed that momelotinib resulted in significantly higher rates of transfusion independence as well as reduced transfusion requirements.[168] The SIMPLIFY-2 trial studied MF patients who had previously received ruxolitinib and required either transfusional support or dose reduction. Patients were randomized to receive momelotinib or best available therapy, where 88% of patients continued on ruxolitinib. There was no significant difference in splenic response rates between the two groups (6.7% for momelotinib versus 5.8% for best available therapy). However, in exploratory analyses, momelotinib did demonstrate superior rates of symptomatic improvement and transfusion independence.[169]

Common side effects associated with momelotinib include diarrhea, which is typically mild and self-limiting, and dizziness, which is primarily associated with the first dose of drug. The latter is often associated with low-grade hypotension, light-headedness, and flushing and usually resolves in less than an hour without any interventions.[164] The main hematologic toxicity of momelotinib is thrombocytopenia, and as predicted by early-phase clinical trials, it caused less anemia than ruxolitinib in SIMPLIFY-1.[168] Peripheral sensory neuropathy is a toxicity specifically associated with momelotinib. In early-phase clinical trials, this occurred in 44% of subjects with a median onset of 32 weeks. While momelotinib-associated neuropathy tends to be mild, severe episodes have been documented, and dose reduction and/or discontinuation improves symptoms in only a minority of individuals.[170]

Due to the failure of momelotinib to show noninferiority to ruxolitinib in the upfront setting in SIMPLIFY-1, and superiority as a potential second-line agent in patients on ruxolitinib in SIMPLIFY-2, its role in the clinical landscape of MF patients remains unclear at this time. Encouragingly, across studies, it has consistently resulted in improvement in anemia-related outcomes, unlike all other JAK inhibitors studied to date. As such, momelotinib may find its eventual niche as an agent specifically utilized in the treatment of MF patients with significant red cell transfusion requirements. Moreover, given its effects on hepcidin, whose elevation is central to the pathophysiology of anemia of chronic disease, momelotinib may also prove to have a role in the treatment of this distinct patient population.

References

1. Arber DA, Orazi A, Hasserjian R, et al. The 2016 revision to the World Health Organization classification of myeloid neoplasms and acute leukemia. *Blood.* 2016;127:2391-2405.
2. Rowley JD. Letter: A new consistent chromosomal abnormality in chronic myelogenous leukaemia identified by quinacrine fluorescence and Giemsa staining. *Nature.* 1973;243:290-293.
3. Konopka JB, Watanabe SM, Witte ON. An alteration of the human c-abl protein in K562 leukemia cells unmasks associated tyrosine kinase activity. *Cell.* 1984;37:1035-1042.

4. Faderl S, Talpaz M, Estrov Z, O'Brien S, Kurzrock R, Kantarjian HM. The biology of chronic myeloid leukemia. *N Engl J Med.* 1999;341:164-172.

5. Italian Cooperative Study Group on Chronic Myeloid Leukemia; Tura S, Baccarani M, et al. Interferon alfa-2a as compared with conventional chemotherapy for the treatment of chronic myeloid leukemia. *N Engl J Med.* 1994;330:820-825.

6. Allan NC, Richards SM, Shepherd PC. UK Medical Research Council randomised, multicentre trial of interferon-alpha n1 for chronic myeloid leukaemia: improved survival irrespective of cytogenetic response. The UK Medical Research Council's Working Parties for Therapeutic Trials in Adult Leukaemia. *Lancet.* 1995;345:1392-1397.

7. Guilhot F, Chastang C, Michallet M, et al. Interferon alfa-2b combined with cytarabine versus interferon alone in chronic myelogenous leukemia. French Chronic Myeloid Leukemia Study Group. *N Engl J Med.* 1997;337:223-229.

8. Buchdunger E, Zimmermann J, Mett H, et al. Inhibition of the Abl protein-tyrosine kinase in vitro and in vivo by a 2-phenylaminopyrimidine derivative. *Cancer Res.* 1996;56:100-104.

9. Nagar B, Bornmann WG, Pellicena P, et al. Crystal structures of the kinase domain of c-Abl in complex with the small molecule inhibitors PD173955 and imatinib (STI-571). *Cancer Res.* 2002;62:4236-4243.

10. Gorre ME, Mohammed M, Ellwood K, et al. Clinical resistance to STI-571 cancer therapy caused by BCR-ABL gene mutation or amplification. *Science.* 2001;293:876-880.

11. von Bubnoff N, Schneller F, Peschel C, Duyster J. BCR-ABL gene mutations in relation to clinical resistance of Philadelphia-chromosome-positive leukaemia to STI571: a prospective study. *Lancet.* 2002;359:487-491.

12. Balabanov S, Braig M, Brümmendorf TH. Current aspects in resistance against tyrosine kinase inhibitors in chronic myelogenous leukemia. *Drug Discov Today Technol.* 2014;11:89-99.

13. Weisberg E, Manley PW, Cowan-Jacob SW, Hochhaus A, Griffin JD. Second generation inhibitors of BCR-ABL for the treatment of imatinib-resistant chronic myeloid leukaemia. *Nat Rev Cancer.* 2007;7:345-356.

14. Roumiantsev S, Shah NP, Gorre ME, et al. Clinical resistance to the kinase inhibitor STI-571 in chronic myeloid leukemia by mutation of Tyr-253 in the Abl kinase domain P-loop. *Proc Natl Acad Sci U S A.* 2002;99:10700-10705.

15. le Coutre P, Tassi E, Varella-Garcia M, et al. Induction of resistance to the Abelson inhibitor STI571 in human leukemic cells through gene amplification. *Blood.* 2000;95:1758-1766.

16. Eechoute K, Sparreboom A, Burger H, et al. Drug transporters and imatinib treatment: implications for clinical practice. *Clin Cancer Res.* 2011;17:406-415.

17. Donato NJ, Wu JY, Stapley J, et al. BCR-ABL independence and LYN kinase overexpression in chronic myelogenous leukemia cells selected for resistance to STI571. *Blood.* 2003;101:690-698.

18. Malcovati L, Karimi M, Papaemmanuil E, et al. SF3B1 mutation identifies a distinct subset of myelodysplastic syndrome with ring sideroblasts. *Blood.* 2015;126:233-241.

19. Liu H, Artz AS. Reduction of imatinib absorption after gastric bypass surgery. *Leuk Lymphoma.* 2011;52:310-313.

20. Pavlovsky C, Egorin MJ, Shah DD, Beumer JH, Rogel S, Pavlovsky S. Imatinib mesylate pharmacokinetics before and after sleeve gastrectomy in a morbidly obese patient with chronic myeloid leukemia. *Pharmacotherapy.* 2009;29:1152-1156.

21. Yoo C, Ryu MH, Kang BW, et al. Cross-sectional study of imatinib plasma trough levels in patients with advanced gastrointestinal stromal tumors: impact of gastrointestinal resection on exposure to imatinib. *J Clin Oncol.* 2010;28:1554-1559.

22. Imatinib [package insert]. East Hanover, NJ: Novartis Pharmaceutical Corporation; 2016.

23. Larson RA, Druker BJ, Guilhot F, et al. Imatinib pharmacokinetics and its correlation with response and safety in chronic-phase chronic myeloid leukemia: a subanalysis of the IRIS study. *Blood.* 2008;111:4022-4028.

24. Druker BJ, Tamura S, Buchdunger E, et al. Effects of a selective inhibitor of the Abl tyrosine kinase on the growth of Bcr-Abl positive cells. *Nat Med.* 1996;2:561-566.

25. Druker BJ, Talpaz M, Resta DJ, et al. Efficacy and safety of a specific inhibitor of the BCR-ABL tyrosine kinase in chronic myeloid leukemia. *N Engl J Med.* 2001;344:1031-1037.

26. O'Brien SG, Guilhot F, Larson RA, et al. Imatinib compared with interferon and low-dose cytarabine for newly diagnosed chronic-phase chronic myeloid leukemia. *N Engl J Med.* 2003;348:994-1004.

27. Hochhaus A, Larson RA, Guilhot F, et al. Long-term outcomes of imatinib treatment for chronic myeloid leukemia. *N Engl J Med.* 2017;376:917-927.

28. Corbin AS, Rosée PL, Stoffregen EP, Druker BJ, Deininger MW. Several Bcr-Abl kinase domain mutants associated with imatinib mesylate resistance remain sensitive to imatinib. *Blood.* 2003;101:4611-4614.

29. Baccarani M, Rosti G, Castagnetti F, et al. Comparison of imatinib 400 mg and 800 mg daily in the front-line treatment of high-risk, Philadelphia-positive chronic myeloid leukemia: a European LeukemiaNet Study. *Blood.* 2009;113:4497-4504.

30. Deininger MW, Kopecky KJ, Radich JP, et al. Imatinib 800 mg daily induces deeper molecular responses than imatinib 400 mg daily: results of SWOG S0325, an intergroup randomized PHASE II trial in newly diagnosed chronic phase chronic myeloid leukaemia. *Br J Haematol.* 2014;164:223-232.

31. Kalmanti L, Saussele S, Lauseker M, et al. Safety and efficacy of imatinib in CML over a period of 10 years: data from the randomized CML-study IV. *Leukemia.* 2015;29:1123-1132.

32. Cortes JE, Baccarani M, Guilhot F, et al. Phase III, randomized, open-label study of daily imatinib mesylate 400 mg versus 800 mg in patients with newly diagnosed, previously untreated chronic myeloid leukemia in chronic phase using molecular end points: tyrosine kinase inhibitor optimization and selectivity study. *J Clin Oncol.* 2010;28:424-430.

33. Verweij J, Casali PG, Zalcberg J, et al. Progression-free survival in gastrointestinal stromal tumours with high-dose imatinib: randomised trial. *Lancet.* 2004;364:1127-1134.

34. Pulido EG, Riquelme A, Ballesteros J, Vaz MA. Congestive heart failure in a 77-year-old woman receiving adjuvant treatment with imatinib for a large gastric gastrointestinal stromal tumour. *Anticancer Drugs.* 2012;23(Suppl):S15-S17.

35. Ran HH, Zhang R, Lu XC, Yang B, Fan H, Zhu HL. Imatinib-induced decompensated heart failure in an elderly patient with chronic myeloid leukemia: case report and literature review. *J Geriatr Cardiol.* 2012;9:411-414.

36. Turrisi G, Montagnani F, Grotti S, Marinozzi C, Bolognese L, Fiorentini G. Congestive heart failure during imatinib mesylate treatment. *Int J Cardiol.* 2010;145:148-150.

37. Berman E, Girotra M, Cheng C, et al. Effect of long term imatinib on bone in adults with chronic myelogenous leukemia and gastrointestinal stromal tumors. *Leuk Res.* 2013;37:790-794.

38. Berman E, Nicolaides M, Maki RG, et al. Altered bone and mineral metabolism in patients receiving imatinib mesylate. *N Engl J Med.* 2006;354:2006-2013.

39. Dutreix C, Peng B, Mehring G, et al. Pharmacokinetic interaction between ketoconazole and imatinib mesylate (Glivec) in healthy subjects. *Cancer Chemother Pharmacol.* 2004;54:290-294.

40. Bolton AE, Peng B, Hubert M, et al. Effect of rifampicin on the pharmacokinetics of imatinib mesylate (Gleevec, STI571) in healthy subjects. *Cancer Chemother Pharmacol.* 2004;53:102-106.

41. Haouala A, Widmer N, Duchosal MA, Montemurro M, Buclin T, Decosterd LA. Drug interactions with the tyrosine kinase inhibitors imatinib, dasatinib, and nilotinib. *Blood.* 2011;117:e75-e87.

42. Lombardo LJ, Lee FY, Chen P, et al. Discovery of N-(2-chloro-6-methyl-phenyl)-2-(6-(4-(2-hydroxyethyl)-piperazin-1-yl)-2-methylpyrimidin-4-ylamino)thiazole-5-carboxamide (BMS-354825), a dual Src/Abl kinase inhibitor with potent antitumor activity in preclinical assays. *J Med Chem.* 2004;47:6658-6661.

43. Tokarski JS, Newitt JA, Chang CYJ, et al. The structure of Dasatinib (BMS-354825) bound to activated ABL kinase domain elucidates its inhibitory activity against imatinib-resistant ABL mutants. *Cancer Res.* 2006;66:5790-5797.

44. O'Hare T, Walters DK, Stoffregen EP, et al. In vitro activity of Bcr-Abl inhibitors AMN107 and BMS-354825 against clinically relevant imatinib-resistant Abl kinase domain mutants. *Cancer Res.* 2005;65:4500-4505.

45. Shah NP, Tran C, Lee FY, Chen P, Norris D, Sawyers CL. Overriding imatinib resistance with a novel ABL kinase inhibitor. *Science.* 2004;305:399-401.

46. Demetri GD, Lo Russo P, MacPherson IR, et al. Phase I dose-escalation and pharmacokinetic study of dasatinib in patients with advanced solid tumors. *Clin Cancer Res.* 2009;15:6232-6240.

47. *Dasatinib [package insert].* Princeton, NJ: Bristol-Myers Squibb Company; 2017.

48. Matsuoka A, Takahashi N, Miura M, et al. H2-receptor antagonist influences dasatinib pharmacokinetics in a patient with Philadelphia-positive acute lymphoblastic leukemia. *Cancer Chemother Pharmacol.* 2012;70:351-352.

49. Takahashi N, Miura M, Niioka T, Sawada K. Influence of H2-receptor antagonists and proton pump inhibitors on dasatinib pharmacokinetics in Japanese leukemia patients. *Cancer Chemother Pharmacol.* 2012;69:999-1004.

50. Pape E, Michel D, Scala-Bertola J, et al. Effect of esomeprazole on the oral absorption of dasatinib in a patient with Philadelphia-positive acute lymphoblastic leukemia. *Br J Clin Pharmacol.* 2016;81:1195-1196.

51. Eley T, Luo FR, Agrawal S, et al. Phase I study of the effect of gastric acid pH modulators on the bioavailability of oral dasatinib in healthy subjects. *J Clin Pharmacol.* 2009;49:700-709.

52. Christopher LJ, Cui D, Wu C, et al. Metabolism and disposition of dasatinib after oral administration to humans. *Drug Metab Dispos.* 2008;36:1357-1364.

53. Ishida Y, Murai K, Yamaguchi K, et al. Pharmacokinetics and pharmacodynamics of dasatinib in the chronic phase of newly diagnosed chronic myeloid leukemia. *Eur J Clin Pharmacol.* 2016;72:185-193.

54. Hochhaus A, Baccarani M, Deininger M, et al. Dasatinib induces durable cytogenetic responses in patients with chronic myelogenous leukemia in chronic phase with resistance or intolerance to imatinib. *Leukemia.* 2008;22:1200-1206.

55. Apperley JF, Cortes JE, Kim D-W, et al. Dasatinib in the treatment of chronic myeloid leukemia in accelerated phase after imatinib failure: the START a trial. *J Clin Oncol.* 2009;27:3472-3479.

56. Cortes J, Rousselot P, Kim D-W, et al. Dasatinib induces complete hematologic and cytogenetic responses in patients with imatinib-resistant or -intolerant chronic myeloid leukemia in blast crisis. *Blood.* 2007;109:3207-3213.

57. Kantarjian H, Shah NP, Hochhaus A, et al. Dasatinib versus imatinib in newly diagnosed chronic-phase chronic myeloid leukemia. *N Engl J Med.* 2010;362:2260-2270.

58. Cortes JE, Saglio G, Kantarjian HM, et al. Final 5-year study results of DASISION: the dasatinib versus imatinib study in treatment-naive chronic myeloid leukemia patients trial. *J Clin Oncol.* 2016;34:2333-2340.

59. Jabbour E, Kantarjian HM, Saglio G, et al. Early response with dasatinib or imatinib in chronic myeloid leukemia: 3-year follow-up from a randomized phase 3 trial (DASISION). *Blood.* 2014;123:494-500.

60. Kantarjian HM, Shah NP, Cortes JE, et al. Dasatinib or imatinib in newly diagnosed chronic-phase chronic myeloid leukemia: 2-year follow-up from a randomized phase 3 trial (DASISION). *Blood.* 2012;119:1123-1129.

61. Shah NP, Kantarjian HM, Kim DW, et al. Intermittent target inhibition with dasatinib 100 mg once daily preserves efficacy and improves tolerability in imatinib-resistant and -intolerant chronic-phase chronic myeloid leukemia. *J Clin Oncol.* 2008;26:3204-3212.

62. Montani D, Bergot E, Gunther S, et al. Pulmonary arterial hypertension in patients treated by dasatinib. *Circulation.* 2012;125:2128-2137.

63. Quintás-Cardama A, Han X, Kantarjian H, Cortes J. Tyrosine kinase inhibitor-induced platelet dysfunction in patients with chronic myeloid leukemia. *Blood.* 2009;114:261-263.

64. Quintas-Cardama A, Kantarjian H, Ravandi F, et al. Bleeding diathesis in patients with chronic myelogenous leukemia receiving dasatinib therapy. *Cancer.* 2009;115:2482-2490.

65. Weisberg E, Manley PW, Breitenstein W, et al. Characterization of AMN107, a selective inhibitor of native and mutant Bcr-Abl. *Cancer Cell.* 2005;7:129-141.

66. Manley PW, Cowan-Jacob SW, Mestan J. Advances in the structural biology, design and clinical development of Bcr-Abl kinase inhibitors for the treatment of chronic myeloid leukaemia. *Biochim Biophys Acta.* 2005;1754:3-13.

67. Nilotinib [package insert]. Novartis Pharmaceuticals Corporation; 2012.

68. Tanaka C, Yin OQ, Sethuraman V, et al. Clinical pharmacokinetics of the BCR-ABL tyrosine kinase inhibitor nilotinib. *Clin Pharmacol Ther.* 2010;87:197-203.

69. Kim KP, Ryu MH, Yoo C, et al. Nilotinib in patients with GIST who failed imatinib and sunitinib: importance of prior surgery on drug bioavailability. *Cancer Chemother Pharmacol.* 2011;68:285-291.

70. Yin OQ, Gallagher N, Fischer D, et al. Effect of the proton pump inhibitor esomeprazole on the oral absorption and pharmacokinetics of nilotinib. *J Clin Pharmacol.* 2010;50:960-967.

71. Kantarjian H, Giles F, Wunderle L, et al. Nilotinib in imatinib-resistant CML and Philadelphia chromosome-positive ALL. *N Engl J Med.* 2006;354:2542-2551.

72. Kantarjian HM, Giles F, Gattermann N, et al. Nilotinib (formerly AMN107), a highly selective BCR-ABL tyrosine kinase inhibitor, is effective in patients with Philadelphia chromosome–positive chronic myelogenous leukemia in chronic phase following imatinib resistance and intolerance. *Blood.* 2007;110:3540-3546.

73. le Coutre P, Ottmann OG, Giles F, et al. Nilotinib (formerly AMN107), a highly selective BCR-ABL tyrosine kinase inhibitor, is active in patients with imatinib-resistant or -intolerant accelerated-phase chronic myelogenous leukemia. *Blood.* 2008;111:1834-1839.

74. Saglio G, Kim DW, Issaragrisil S, et al. Nilotinib versus imatinib for newly diagnosed chronic myeloid leukemia. *N Engl J Med.* 2010;362:2251-2259.

75. Hochhaus A, Saglio G, Hughes TP, et al. Long-term benefits and risks of front-line nilotinib vs imatinib for chronic myeloid leukemia in chronic phase: 5-year update of the randomized ENESTnd trial. *Leukemia.* 2016;30:1044-1054.

76. Pallera A, Altman JK, Berman E, et al. NCCN guidelines insights: chronic myeloid leukemia, version 1.2017. *J Natl Compr Canc Netw.* 2016;14:1505-1512.

77. Zhang H, Sheng J, Ko JH, et al. Inhibitory effect of single and repeated doses of nilotinib on the pharmacokinetics of CYP3A substrate midazolam. *J Clin Pharmacol.* 2015;55:401-408.

78. Yin OQ, Gallagher N, Fischer D, et al. Effects of nilotinib on single-dose warfarin pharmacokinetics and pharmacodynamics: a randomized, single-blind, two-period crossover study in healthy subjects. *Clin Drug Investig.* 2011;31:169-179.

79. Yin OQ, Bedoucha V, McCulloch T, et al. Effects of famotidine or an antacid preparation on the pharmacokinetics of nilotinib in healthy volunteers. *Cancer Chemother Pharmacol.* 2013;71:219-226.

80. Boschelli DH, Ye F, Wang YD, et al. Optimization of 4-phenylamino-3-quinolinecarbonitriles as potent inhibitors of Src kinase activity. *J Med Chem.* 2001;44:3965-3977.

81. Levinson NM, Boxer SG. A conserved water-mediated hydrogen bond network defines bosutinib's kinase selectivity. *Nat Chem Biol.* 2014;10:127-132.

82. Levinson NM, Boxer SG. Structural and spectroscopic analysis of the kinase inhibitor bosutinib and an isomer of bosutinib binding to the Abl tyrosine kinase domain. *PLoS One.* 2012;7:e29828.

83. Puttini M, Coluccia AML, Boschelli F, et al. In vitro and in vivo activity of SKI-606, a novel Src-Abl inhibitor, against imatinib-resistant Bcr-Abl+ neoplastic cells. *Cancer Res.* 2006;66:11314-11322.

84. Hsyu PH, Mould DR, Abbas R, Amantea M. Population pharmacokinetic and pharmacodynamic analysis of bosutinib. *Drug Metab Pharmacokinet.* 2014;29:441-448.

85. Bosutinib [package insert]. New York, NY: Pfizer Labs; 2012.

86. Cortes JE, Kantarjian HM, Brummendorf TH, et al. Safety and efficacy of bosutinib (SKI-606) in chronic phase Philadelphia chromosome-positive chronic myeloid leukemia patients with resistance or intolerance to imatinib. *Blood.* 2011;118:4567-4576.

87. Abbas R, Hug BA, Leister C, Gaaloul ME, Chalon S, Sonnichsen D. A phase I ascending single-dose study of the safety, tolerability, and pharmacokinetics of bosutinib (SKI-606) in healthy adult subjects. *Cancer Chemother Pharmacol.* 2012;69:221-227.

88. Abbas R, Leister C, Sonnichsen D. A clinical study to examine the potential effect of lansoprazole on the pharmacokinetics of bosutinib when administered concomitantly to healthy subjects. *Clin Drug Investig.* 2013;33:589-595.

89. Gambacorti-Passerini C, Kantarjian HM, Kim D-W, et al. Long-term efficacy and safety of bosutinib in patients with advanced leukemia following resistance/intolerance to imatinib and other tyrosine kinase inhibitors. *Am J Hematol.* 2015;90:755-768.

90. Cortes JE, Kim D-W, Kantarjian HM, et al. Bosutinib versus imatinib in newly diagnosed chronic-phase chronic myeloid leukemia: results from the BELA trial. *J Clin Oncol.* 2012;30:3486-3492.

91. Brummendorf TH, Cortes JE, de Souza CA, et al. Bosutinib versus imatinib in newly diagnosed chronic-phase chronic myeloid leukaemia: results from the 24-month follow-up of the BELA trial. *Br J Haematol.* 2015;168:69-81.

92. Cortes JE, Gambacorti-Passerini C, Deininger MWN, et al. Bosutinib (BOS) versus imatinib (IM) for newly diagnosed chronic myeloid leukemia (CML): Initial results from the BFORE trial. *J Clin Oncol.* 2017;35:7002.

93. Gambacorti-Passerini C, Brummendorf TH, Kim DW, et al. Bosutinib efficacy and safety in chronic phase chronic myeloid leukemia after imatinib resistance or intolerance: minimum 24-month follow-up. *Am J Hematol.* 2014;89:732-742.

94. O'Hare T, Shakespeare WC, Zhu X, et al. AP24534, a pan-BCR-ABL inhibitor for chronic myeloid leukemia, potently inhibits the T315I mutant and overcomes mutation-based resistance. *Cancer Cell.* 2009;16:401-412.

95. *Ponatinib [package insert].* Cambridge, MA: ARIAD Pharmaceuticals, Inc.; 2017.

96. Cortes JE, Kantarjian H, Shah NP, et al. Ponatinib in refractory Philadelphia chromosome-positive leukemias. *N Engl J Med.* 2012;367:2075-2088.

97. Narasimhan NI, Dorer DJ, Niland K, Haluska F, Sonnichsen D. Effects of food on the pharmacokinetics of ponatinib in healthy subjects. *J Clin Pharm Ther.* 2013;38:440-444.

98. Narasimhan NI, Dorer DJ, Davis J, Turner CD, Sonnichsen D. Evaluation of the effect of multiple doses of lansoprazole on the pharmacokinetics and safety of ponatinib in healthy subjects. *Clin Drug Investig.* 2014;34:723-729.

99. Ye YE, Woodward CN, Narasimhan NI. Absorption, metabolism, and excretion of [14C]ponatinib after a single oral dose in humans. *Cancer Chemother Pharmacol.* 2017;79:507-518.

100. Cortes JE, Kim DW, Pinilla-Ibarz J, et al. A phase 2 trial of ponatinib in Philadelphia chromosome-positive leukemias. *N Engl J Med.* 2013;369:1783-1796.

101. Lipton JH, Chuah C, Guerci-Bresler A, et al. Ponatinib versus imatinib for newly diagnosed chronic myeloid leukaemia: an international, randomised, open-label, phase 3 trial. *Lancet Oncol.* 2016;17:612-621.

102. Kantarjian HM, Pinilla-Ibarz J, Coutre PD, et al. Five-year results of the ponatinib phase II PACE trial in heavily pretreated CP-CML patients (pts). *J Clin Oncol.* 2017;35:7012.

103. Dorer DJ, Knickerbocker RK, Baccarani M, et al. Impact of dose intensity of ponatinib on selected adverse events: Multivariate analyses from a pooled population of clinical trial patients. *Leuk Res.* 2016;48:84-91.

104. Narasimhan NI, Dorer DJ, Niland K, Haluska F, Sonnichsen D. Effects of ketoconazole on the pharmacokinetics of ponatinib in healthy subjects. *J Clin Pharmacol.* 2013;53:974-981.

105. Kantarjian HM, Talpaz M, Santini V, Murgo A, Cheson B, O'Brien SM. Homoharringtonine: history, current research, and future direction. *Cancer.* 2001;92:1591-1605.

106. Tujebajeva RM, Graifer DM, Karpova GG, Ajtkhozhina NA. Alkaloid homoharringtonine inhibits polypeptide chain elongation on human ribosomes on the step of peptide bond formation. *FEBS Lett.* 1989;257:254-256.

107. Gürel G, Blaha G, Moore PB, Steitz TA. U2504 determines the species specificity of the A-site cleft antibiotics: the structures of tiamulin, homoharringtonine, and bruceantin bound to the ribosome. *J Mol Biol.* 2009;389:146-156.

108. Allan EK, Holyoake TL, Craig AR, Jørgensen HG. Omacetaxine may have a role in chronic myeloid leukaemia eradication through downregulation of Mcl-1 and induction of apoptosis in stem/progenitor cells. *Leukemia.* 2011;25:985-994.

109. *Omacetaxine [package insert].* North Wales, PA: Teva Pharmaceuticals USA, Inc.; 2012.

110. Nemunaitis J, Mita A, Stephenson J, et al. Pharmacokinetic study of omacetaxine mepesuccinate administered subcutaneously to patients with advanced solid and hematologic tumors. *Cancer Chemother Pharmacol.* 2013;71:35-41.

111. Nijenhuis CM, Hellriegel E, Beijnen JH, et al. Pharmacokinetics and excretion of (14)C-omacetaxine in patients with advanced solid tumors. *Invest New Drugs.* 2016;34:565-574.

112. Kantarjian HM, Talpaz M, Smith TL, et al. Homoharringtonine and low-dose cytarabine in the management of late chronic-phase chronic myelogenous leukemia. *J Clin Oncol.* 2000;18:3513-3521.

113. O'Brien S, Kantarjian H, Keating M, et al. Homoharringtonine therapy induces responses in patients with chronic myelogenous leukemia in late chronic phase. *Blood.* 1995;86:3322-3326.

114. O'Brien S, Kantarjian H, Koller C, et al. Sequential homoharringtonine and interferon-alpha in the treatment of early chronic phase chronic myelogenous leukemia. *Blood.* 1999;93:4149-4153.

115. Legros L, Hayette S, Nicolini FE, et al. BCR-ABL(T315I) transcript disappearance in an imatinib-resistant CML patient treated with homoharringtonine: a new therapeutic challenge? *Leukemia.* 2007;21:2204-2206.

116. Cortes JE, Nicolini FE, Wetzler M, et al. Subcutaneous omacetaxine mepesuccinate in patients with chronic-phase chronic myeloid leukemia previously treated with 2 or more tyrosine kinase inhibitors including imatinib. *Clin Lymphoma Myeloma Leuk.* 2013;13:584-591.

117. Cortes JE, Kantarjian HM, Rea D, et al. Final analysis of the efficacy and safety of omacetaxine mepesuccinate in patients with chronic- or accelerated-phase chronic myeloid leukemia: Results with 24 months of follow-up. *Cancer.* 2015;121:1637-1644.

118. Baccarani M, Deininger MW, Rosti G, et al. European LeukemiaNet recommendations for the management of chronic myeloid leukemia: 2013. *Blood.* 2013;122:872-884.

119. Sokal JE, Cox EB, Baccarani M, et al. Prognostic discrimination in "good-risk" chronic granulocytic leukemia. *Blood.* 1984;63:789-799.

120. Hasford J, Pfirrmann M, Hehlmann R, et al. A new prognostic score for survival of patients with chronic myeloid leukemia treated with interferon alfa. Writing Committee for the Collaborative CML Prognostic Factors Project Group. *J Natl Cancer Inst.* 1998;90:850-858.

121. Hughes T, Deininger M, Hochhaus A, et al. Monitoring CML patients responding to treatment with tyrosine kinase inhibitors: review and recommendations for harmonizing current methodology for detecting BCR-ABL transcripts and kinase domain mutations and for expressing results. *Blood.* 2006;108:28-37.

122. Mahon F-X, Réa D, Guilhot J, et al. Discontinuation of imatinib in patients with chronic myeloid leukaemia who have maintained complete molecular remission for at least 2 years: the prospective, multicentre Stop Imatinib (STIM) trial. *Lancet Oncol.* 2010;11:1029-1035.

123. Yanada M, Takeuchi J, Sugiura I, et al. High complete remission rate and promising outcome by combination of imatinib and chemotherapy for newly diagnosed BCR-ABL-positive acute lymphoblastic leukemia: a phase II study by the Japan Adult Leukemia Study Group. *J Clin Oncol.* 2006;24:460-466.

124. Fielding AK, Rowe JM, Buck G, et al. UKALLXII/ECOG2993: addition of imatinib to a standard treatment regimen enhances long-term outcomes in Philadelphia positive acute lymphoblastic leukemia. *Blood.* 2014;123:843-850.

125. Schultz KR, Bowman WP, Aledo A, et al. Improved early event-free survival with imatinib in Philadelphia chromosome-positive acute lymphoblastic leukemia: a children's oncology group study. *J Clin Oncol.* 2009;27:5175-5181.

126. Alvarnas JC, Brown PA, Aoun P, et al. Acute lymphoblastic leukemia, version 2.2015. *J Natl Compr Canc Netw.* 2015;13:1240-1279.

127. Baccarani M, Cilloni D, Rondoni M, et al. The efficacy of imatinib mesylate in patients with FIP1L1-PDGFRalpha-positive hypereosinophilic syndrome. Results of a multicenter prospective study. *Haematologica.* 2007;92:1173-1179.

128. Pardanani A, Elliott M, Reeder T, et al. Imatinib for systemic mast-cell disease. *Lancet.* 2003;362:535-536.

129. Vega-Ruiz A, Cortes JE, Sever M, et al. Phase II study of imatinib mesylate as therapy for patients with systemic mastocytosis. *Leuk Res.* 2009;33:1481-1484.

130. Hirota S, Isozaki K, Moriyama Y, et al. Gain-of-function mutations of c-kit in human gastrointestinal stromal tumors. *Science.* 1998;279:577-580.

131. Heinrich MC, Corless CL, Duensing A, et al. PDGFRA activating mutations in gastrointestinal stromal tumors. *Science.* 2003;299:708-710.

132. Sjöblom T, Shimizu A, O'Brien KP, et al. Growth inhibition of dermatofibrosarcoma protuberans tumors by the platelet-derived growth factor receptor antagonist STI571 through induction of apoptosis. *Cancer Res.* 2001;61:5778-5783.

133. Spivak JL. Myeloproliferative neoplasms. *N Engl J Med.* 2017;376: 2168-2181.

134. James C, Ugo V, Le Couédic J-P, et al. A unique clonal JAK2 mutation leading to constitutive signalling causes polycythaemia vera. *Nature.* 2005;434:1144 1148.

135. Levine RL, Wadleigh M, Cools J, et al. Activating mutation in the tyrosine kinase JAK2 in polycythemia vera, essential thrombocythemia, and myeloid metaplasia with myelofibrosis. *Cancer Cell.* 2005;7:387-397.

136. Baxter EJ, Scott LM, Campbell PJ, et al. Acquired mutation of the tyrosine kinase JAK2 in human myeloproliferative disorders. *Lancet.* 2005;365:1054-1061.

137. Kralovics R, Passamonti F, Buser AS, et al. A gain-of-function mutation of JAK2 in myeloproliferative disorders. *N Engl J Med.* 2005;352:1779-1790.

138. Quintás-Cardama A, Vaddi K, Liu P, et al. Preclinical characterization of the selective JAK1/2 inhibitor INCB018424: therapeutic implications for the treatment of myeloproliferative neoplasms. *Blood.* 2010;115:3109-3117.

139. Zhou T, Georgeon S, Moser R, Moore DJ, Caflisch A, Hantschel O. Specificity and mechanism-of-action of the JAK2 tyrosine kinase inhibitors ruxolitinib and SAR302503 (TG101348). *Leukemia.* 2014;28:404-407.

140. Deininger M, Radich J, Burn TC, Huber R, Paranagama D, Verstovsek S. The effect of long-term ruxolitinib treatment on JAK2p.V617F allele burden in patients with myelofibrosis. *Blood.* 2015;126:1551-1554.

141. Tefferi A, Vaidya R, Caramazza D, Finke C, Lasho T, Pardanani A. Circulating interleukin (IL)-8, IL-2R, IL-12, and IL-15 levels are independently prognostic in primary myelofibrosis: a comprehensive cytokine profiling study. *J Clin Oncol.* 2011;29:1356-1363.

142. Kleppe M, Kwak M, Koppikar P, et al. JAK-STAT pathway activation in malignant and nonmalignant cells contributes to MPN pathogenesis and therapeutic response. *Cancer Discov.* 2015;5:316-331.

143. Verstovsek S, Mesa RA, Gotlib J, et al. A double-blind, placebo-controlled trial of ruxolitinib for myelofibrosis. *N Engl J Med.* 2012;366:799-807.

144. Koppikar P, Bhagwat N, Kilpivaara O, et al. Heterodimeric JAK-STAT activation as a mechanism of persistence to JAK2 inhibitor therapy. *Nature.* 2012;489:155-159.

145. Shilling AD, Nedza FM, Emm T, et al. Metabolism, excretion, and pharmacokinetics of [14C]INCB018424, a selective Janus tyrosine kinase 1/2 inhibitor, in humans. *Drug Metab Dispos.* 2010;38:2023-2031.

146. Ruxolitinib [package insert]. Wimington, DE: Incyte Pharmaceuticals, Inc.; 2016.

147. Verstovsek S, Kantarjian H, Mesa RA, et al. Safety and efficacy of INCB018424, a JAK1 and JAK2 inhibitor, in myelofibrosis. *N Engl J Med.* 2010;363:1117-1127.

148. Harrison C, Kiladjian J-J, Al-Ali HK, et al. JAK inhibition with ruxolitinib versus best available therapy for myelofibrosis. *N Engl J Med.* 2012;366:787-798.

149. Cervantes F, Dupriez B, Pereira A, et al. New prognostic scoring system for primary myelofibrosis based on a study of the International Working Group for Myelofibrosis Research and Treatment. *Blood.* 2009;113:2895-2901.

150. Vannucchi AM, Kantarjian HM, Kiladjian J-J, et al. A pooled analysis of overall survival in COMFORT-I and COMFORT-II, 2 randomized phase III trials of ruxolitinib for the treatment of myelofibrosis. *Haematologica.* 2015;100:1139-1145.

151. Vannucchi AM. Ruxolitinib versus standard therapy for the treatment of polycythemia vera. *N Engl J Med.* 2015;372:1670-1671.

152. Passamonti F, Griesshammer M, Palandri F, et al. Ruxolitinib for the treatment of inadequately controlled polycythaemia vera without splenomegaly (RESPONSE-2): a randomised, open-label, phase 3b study. *Lancet Oncol.* 2017;18:88-99.

153. Shi JG, Chen X, Emm T, et al. The effect of CYP3A4 inhibition or induction on the pharmacokinetics and pharmacodynamics of orally administered ruxolitinib (INCB018424 phosphate) in healthy volunteers. *J Clin Pharmacol.* 2012;52:809-818.

154. Singer JW, Al-Fayoumi S, Ma H, Komrokji RS, Mesa R, Verstovsek S. Comprehensive kinase profile of pacritinib, a nonmyelosuppressive Janus kinase 2 inhibitor. *J Exp Pharmacol.* 2016;8:11-19.

155. Komrokji RS, Seymour JF, Roberts AW, et al. Results of a phase 2 study of pacritinib (SB1518), a JAK2/JAK2(V617F) inhibitor, in patients with myelofibrosis. *Blood.* 2015;125:2649-2655.

156. Verstovsek S, Odenike O, Singer JW, Granston T, Al-Fayoumi S, Deeg HJ. Phase 1/2 study of pacritinib, a next generation JAK2/FLT3 inhibitor, in myelofibrosis or other myeloid malignancies. *J Hematol Oncol.* 2016;9:137.

157. Verstovsek S, Odenike O, Scott B, et al. Phase I dose-escalation trial of SB1518, a novel JAK2/FLT3 inhibitor, in acute and chronic myeloid diseases, including primary or post-essential thrombocythemia/polycythemia vera myelofibrosis. *Blood* 2009;114(22),3905.

158. Verstovsek S, Machida C, Dean J, Myint H. PACRITINIB Inhibitor of tyrosine-protein kinase JAK2 inhibitor of FLT-3 treatment of myelofibrosis. *Drugs Future.* 2013;38:375-386.

159. Al-Fayoumi S, Campbell MS, Amberg S, Zhou H, Millard L, Dean JP. Clinical pharmacology profile of pacritinib (PAC), a novel JAK2/FLT3 inhibitor. *Blood* 2015;126(23), 5178.

160. Jayaraman R, Pasha MK, Williams A, Goh KC, Ethirajulu K. Metabolism and disposition of pacritinib (SB1518), an orally active janus kinase 2 inhibitor in preclinical species and humans. *Drug Metab Lett.* 2015;9: 28-47.

161. Mesa RA, Vannucchi AM, Mead A, et al. Pacritinib versus best available therapy for the treatment of myelofibrosis irrespective of baseline cytopenias (PERSIST-1): an international, randomised, phase 3 trial. *Lancet Haematol.* 2017;4:e225-e236.

162. Mascarenhas J, Hoffman R, Talpaz M, et al. Results of the persist-2 phase 3 study of pacritinib (PAC) versus best available therapy (BAT), including ruxolitinib (RUX), in patients (pts) with myelofibrosis (MF) and platelet counts ≤100,000/μl. *Blood.* 2016;128:LBA-5.

163. Pardanani A, Laborde RR, Lasho TL, et al. Safety and efficacy of CYT387, a JAK1 and JAK2 inhibitor, in myelofibrosis. *Leukemia.* 2013;27: 1322-1327.

164. Gupta V, Mesa RA, Deininger MWN, et al. A phase 1/2, open-label study evaluating twice-daily administration of momelotinib in myelofibrosis. *Haematologica.* 2017;102:94-102.

165. Asshoff M, Petzer V, Warr MR, et al. Momelotinib inhibits ACVR1/ALK2, decreases hepcidin production, and ameliorates anemia of chronic disease in rodents. *Blood.* 2017;129:1823-1830.

166. Gupta V, Baer MR, Oh ST, et al. Phase III randomized, open-label, active-controlled study of momelotinib versus best available therapy in ruxolitinib-treated patients with myelofibrosis. *Journal of Clinical Oncology* 2015;33(suppl 15).

167. Xin Y, Shao L, Deng W, et al. The relative bioavailability, food effect and drug interaction with omeprazole of momelotinib tablet formulation. *Blood* 2013;122(21):5239.

168. Mesa RA, Kiladjian J-J, Catalano JV, et al. Phase 3 trial of momelotinib (MMB) vs ruxolitinib (RUX) in JAK inhibitor (JAKi) naive patients with myelofibrosis (MF). *Journal of Clinical Oncology* 2017;35(suppl 15):7000.

169. Harrison CN, Vannucchi AM, Platzbecker U, et al. Phase 3 randomized trial of momelotinib (MMB) versus best available therapy (BAT) in patients with myelofibrosis (MF) previously treated with ruxolitinib (RUX). *Journal of Clinical Oncology* 2017;35(suppl 15):7001.

170. Abdelrahman RA, Begna KH, Al-Kali A, et al. Momelotinib treatment-emergent neuropathy: prevalence, risk factors and outcome in 100 patients with myelofibrosis. *Br J Haematol.* 2015;169:77-80.

The PI3K/AKT/mTOR Signaling System

Bruce A. Chabner

Overview

The PI3K/AKT/mTOR pathway is a key regulator of cellular growth and survival and is mutated and/or activated in many different human cancers (Table 25.1). As a critical pathway for monitoring and responding to the nutritional status, stress, and growth opportunities of cells, it has become a target of great interest in cancer therapeutics. Unfortunately, despite its central role in tumor

TABLE 25.1	Components of the mTOR pathway with evidence of involvement in human cancers
Mutated/Overexpressed Protein	**Types of Cancer**
PTEN	• Lung • Breast cancer • Prostate cancer • H&N cancer • Glioblastoma
AKT	• Breast cancer • Thyroid
PI3K	• Breast cancer • Endometrium • Colon • Liver
eIF4E	• H&N squamous carcinoma • Renal cancer • Lymphoma
TSC1/2	Benign tumor syndrome (hamartoma syndromes, including tuberous sclerosis complex, PTEN-related hamartoma syndromes, and Peutz-Jeghers syndrome)
S6K1	Breast cancer
RICTOR	• Amplified in many tumors, associated with poor prognosis and drug resistance • Squamous and small cell lung • Gastroesophageal cancers • Melanoma • Neuroendocrine tumors

cell survival, attempts to develop new therapies that block this pathway have met with limited success, the most useful being the drugs that inhibit mTOR function.

The extended pathway headed by PI3K is shown in Figure 25.1. Depending on cell type and its mutational status, the four multiple isoforms of PI3K (α, β, δ, and γ) are variably activated by phosphorylation through signals generated from tyrosine kinase growth factor receptors such as the insulin growth factor receptor (IGFR), epidermal growth factor receptor family, ALK, ROS, KIT, and others; from integrins and other cell adhesion molecules; from G-protein–coupled receptors; and from intermediary proteins such as RAS.[1] In addition PI3K is activated by cross talk with other basic signaling pathways, including MAP kinase, JAK-STAT, cyclin-dependent kinases, and hormonal pathways.[2] The signaling activates the several PI3K isoforms expressed in various tissues. Thus, while breast cancers are heavily dependent on signaling from PI3Kα, lymphoid tissues respond primarily to PI3Kδ. Cross talk from the MAP kinase pathway predominates in solid tumors, while JAK-STAT is a particularly important source of input for hematological malignancies. In general, phosphorylation events flow through PI3K to AKT and thence to mTOR.

The mechanism of activation of PI3K by a receptor tyrosine kinase begins with recruitment of PI3K through binding of its Src homology 2 (SH2) domain of the p85 regulatory subunit of PI3K to specific phosphotyrosine (YxxM) components of the primary signaling complex.[3] In action mediated by its p110 catalytic subunit, PI3K phosphorylates the D3 position of phosphoinositides to generate phosphatidylinositol-3,4,5-triphosphate (PIP$_3$). PIP$_3$ in turn binds to the pleckstrin homology (PH) domain of the PH domain–containing kinase (PDK1) and the serine/threonine kinase AKT, anchoring both proteins to the cell membrane, leading to their activation. AKT1 is activated at two critical amino acids: by phosphorylation of T308, in its catalytic domain, by PDK1, and then by subsequent phosphorylation of S473 by several other kinases (including mTOR when bound to the *rapamycin-insensitive* companion of mTOR [RICTOR] in the target of rapamycin complex 2 [TORC2]).[4] AKT is expressed in three different isoforms: AKT1, AKT2, and AKT3, which are variably expressed in most tissues and mutated in various tumors.[5]

The membrane translocation and activation of AKT are opposed by the tumor suppressor phosphatase and tensin homologue on chromosome 10 (PTEN). PTEN is a phosphatase that antagonizes PI3K by dephosphorylating PIP$_3$, preventing activation of AKT and PDK1.[6] Once activated, AKT phosphorylates the consensus sequence RXRXX(S/T) in many downstream targets,[7] leading to alterations in the expression of proteins important in cell cycle

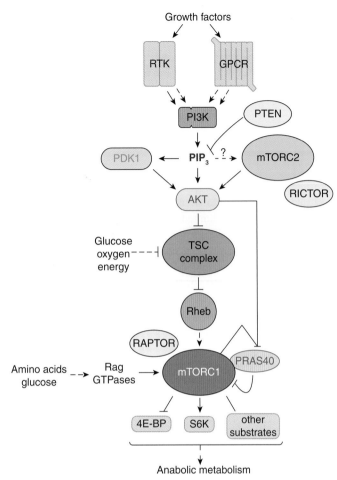

FIGURE 25.1 Activated integrin receptors, growth factor receptors (RTKs), G-protein–coupled receptors (GPCRs), and cytokine receptors stimulate sequential phosphorylations through the PI3K/AKT signaling pathway, leading to the activation of the mTORC1 complex. Activation of mTORC1 leads to the phosphorylation of S6K1 and 4E-BP1. S6K1 phosphorylates rpS6, while phosphorylated 4E-BP1 dissociates from eIF4E, enhancing mRNA translation and stimulating proliferation, angiogenesis, and the suppression of apoptosis. Shown also in the active mTORC1 complex are the regulatory protein, RAPTOR, which complexes with and promotes mTORC1 activity, and Rheb, a second essential component. TSC (tuberous sclerosis complex) proteins 1 and 2 inactivate Rheb by phosphorylation, thus inhibiting mTORC1 activity, while AKT, when activated by a second mTOR complex, mTORC2, inactivates the TSC complex and restores mTORC1 function. mTOR inhibitors, such as temsirolimus, bind to FK506-binding protein (FKBP12) and displace RAPTOR, inhibiting the kinase activity of the mTORC1 complex. A second cofactor, RICTOR, activates mTORC2, is amplified in many tumors, and is associated with rapalog resistance. (Figure modified from Dibble CC, Cantley LC. Regulations of mTORC1 by PI3K signaling. *Trends Cell Biol.* 2015;25:545-555, with permission.)

progression, apoptosis, angiogenesis, cytoskeletal arrangement, and the regulation of ribonucleic acid (RNA) transcription and protein translation.

While AKT is undoubtedly a critical substrate of activated PI3K, the inhibition of PI3K also diminishes Rac activation and other important downstream targets. Phosphoprotein profiling and functional genomic studies demonstrate that many cancer cell lines and human breast tumors with mutations of the catalytic (p110α) subunit of PI3K (PI3KCA) have only minimal AKT activation and

little requirement of AKT for anchorage-independent growth.[8] These cells, instead, are characterized by robust PDK1 activation and have dependency on the PDK1 substrate serum/glucocorticoid regulated kinase 3 (SGK3). SGK3 undergoes PI3K- and PDK1-dependent activation in PIK3CA-mutant cancer cells. Therefore, PI3K activation may promote cancer through both AKT-dependent and AKT-independent mechanisms, with important implications for the treatment of patients with these tumors.

Cell cycle progression is promoted by AKT through inhibitory phosphorylation of the cyclin-dependent kinase inhibitors p21 and p27 and by the inhibition of glycogen synthase kinase 3β (GSK3β), which stabilizes cyclin D1.[9,10] AKT also regulates apoptosis by inactivating the proapoptotic protein BAD, which controls the release of cytochrome c from mitochondria.[11] AKT phosphorylation of the FoxO family of transcription factors inhibits transcription of the proapoptotic genes Bim, Fas-L, and IGFBP-1.[12] AKT also phosphorylates IκB kinase (IKK), which increases the activity of nuclear factor-κB (NF-κB) and the transcription of prosurvival genes.[13] AKT phosphorylation of the human homologue of mouse double-minute 2 (MDM2) leads to inhibition of p53, with further effects on cell cycle progression, apoptosis, and DNA repair.[14]

Role of mTOR

mTOR, a serine/threonine kinase, is a highly conserved 250-kD phosphoprotein and serves as a critical convergence point in cellular signaling pathways for cell growth, metabolism, proliferation, and angiogenesis[15] (Fig. 25.1). It controls protein translation in response to nutrients, hypoxia, energy levels, hormones, and growth factors. AKT can directly activate mTOR through phosphorylation. AKT also causes indirect activation of mTOR by inhibitory phosphorylation of tuberous sclerosis complex (TSC), which in its unphosphorylated state binds to and inhibits Rheb, a necessary cofactor in the mTORC1 complex.

mTOR exerts its metabolic effects through two catalytic complexes: (a) target of rapamycin complex 1 (TORC1), which, in its active state, is bound to regulatory-associated protein of mTOR (RAPTOR) and to Rheb, and (b) the TORC2 complex, in which mTOR is bound to and activated by RICTOR (the rapamycin-insensitive companion of mTOR).

Activation of mTORC1 regulates cellular growth and proliferation through control of protein synthesis. The function of the mTORC1 complex is to initiate messenger RNA (mRNA) translation. mTORC1 phosphorylates S6 kinase 1 (S6K1) at threonine 389, which in turn phosphorylates the ribosomal protein S6, eukaryotic initiation factor (eIF4B), and eukaryotic elongation factor (eEF) 2 protein kinase, all critical to cellular protein synthesis.[16] The mTORC1 complex also phosphorylates 4E-binding protein 1 (4E-BP1), a translational repressor, causing 4E-BP1 to dissociate from eIF4E, the mRNA cap-binding protein.[17] After dissociation from 4E-BP1, eIF4E can then promote the translation of 5'-cap mRNA species and the synthesis of cyclin D1, c-Myc, HIF-1α, and VEGF. pS6 levels have become an important biomarker for the activity of the mTORC1 complex in clinical studies of PI3K pathway inhibitors.[18]

The TORC2 complex has become an increasingly important focus of drug development because of its insensitivity to rapalogs and the growing appreciation of its role in cancer progression. It phosphorylates AKT at serine 473 in a positive feedback mechanism[4]; pAKT in turn activates mTORC1, as described above (Fig. 25.1), and promotes many of the key properties of the cancer cell, including proliferation, survival, angiogenesis, and migration. This activation of AKT responds to and is believed to overcome mTORC1 inhibition. The activity of mTORC1 is also regulated through a cellular energy–sensing pathway, responsive to cellular levels of amino acids and adenosine triphosphate (ATP), and is inhibited through multiple steps by the tumor suppressor protein LKB1, which is inactivated in Peutz-Jeghers syndrome.[19] LKB1 activates adenosine monophosphate (AMP)–activated kinase, which subsequently activates TSC1/2, thereby leading to mTOR inhibition.

Deregulation of the AKT Pathway in Human Cancer

The PI3k/AKT/mTOR pathway can be activated in cancer by loss of the tumor suppressor PTEN function, amplification or activating mutation of PI3K, amplification or mutation of AKT, or activation of upstream growth factor receptors (Table 25.1). Recent studies also demonstrate that mTOR signaling is inhibited by the p53 tumor suppressor gene and that loss of p53 function, the most common molecular defect in human cancers, results in mTOR activation.[15] Both PTEN phospholipase and PI3K3CA, the catalytic subunit of PIK3α, are frequently mutated across many human cancers.[8] PTEN mutations occur commonly in prostate cancer, renal cell cancer (RCC), hepatocellular carcinoma (HCC), melanoma, breast and endometrial cancer, and glioblastoma. Activating mutations in the PI3KCA gene, the catalytic subunit of PI3K, have been discovered in large numbers of human tumors, including 27% of breast and 19% of colon cancers, according to the Catalogue of Somatic Mutations in Cancer database. Three recurrent oncogenic "hotspot" mutations comprise the majority of somatic PI3KCA mutations.[21] Gene mutation in the p85 regulatory domain of PI3K has also been noted in colon and ovarian cancers.[22] Amplification of AKT1 has been described in human gastric carcinoma, and amplification of AKT2 has been reported in pancreatic, ovarian, gastric, head and neck, and breast carcinomas.[23]

The importance of mTOR in the genesis of human cancer is illustrated by its dysregulation in many forms of inherited cancer.[19-26] Abnormal activation of the PI3K/mTOR pathway through loss of tumor suppressor gene function is the cause of several tumor predisposition syndromes, including tuberous sclerosis (TSC1/2), Cowden's syndrome (PTEN), and the Peutz-Jeghers syndrome (LKB1).[19] Loss of function mutations of TSC1 in bladder cancer leads to activation of mTOR and may be a biomarker for sensitivity to everolimus (see below) in bladder cancer.[24] Many different point mutations that activate mTOR, either by increasing catalytic activity, by decreasing the binding affinity of suppressive cofactors, or by preventing the inhibitory binding of FKBP12-rapalog complex, have been found pre- and post treatment with rapalogs in renal clear-cell carcinoma samples.[25,26]

Deregulation of the PI3K/AKT/mTOR pathway is associated with high-risk or poor prognosis human cancers. PTEN genomic deletion is associated with pAKT expression and androgen receptor signaling in poorer outcome, hormone-refractory prostate cancer.[27] PI3K mutations and loss of PTEN are associated with resistance to hormonal therapy of breast cancer[18] and with resistance to anti-HER2–directed therapies in breast cancer.[28]

Further reports implicate mTOR activation in the regulation of estrogen receptor activation and in resistance to antiestrogen therapies in breast cancer and have led to successful trials of rapalogs with hormone antagonists, as described below. mTORC1 stimulates estrogen receptor alpha (ERα) transcriptional activity by mediating the phosphorylation of ERα at S167 (through S6K activation) and directly at S104/106.[29] mTOR also increases ERα translation through phosphorylation of the elongation factor, eIF4E, a marker for tamoxifen resistance.[30]

There is growing evidence that mutations in mTOR or its cofactors may play at least an accessory role in human carcinogenesis. mTOR is overexpressed in many cancers, and activating mutations, as described above, are found in *VHL*-mutated clear-cell renal cancers and other tumors. RICTOR, which is a necessary component for the function of the mTORC2 complex, is amplified in many human cancers, including squamous cell and small cell carcinoma of the lung (14% to 18%), neuroendocrine prostate cancer (18%), gastroesophageal cancers (10%), and melanoma (44% of cell lines), and is frequently coamplified with receptor tyrosine kinases, including HER2.[31] Amplification of RICTOR is associated with more rapid tumor progression, a poor prognosis, and, in breast cancer, resistance to HER2 therapy.[32]

mTOR Inhibitors

Rapamycin (Sirolimus, Rapamune)

Rapamycin is a macrolide antibiotic derived from the bacteria *Streptomyces hygroscopicus* isolated from a soil sample from Easter Island (Rapa Nui).[33] Rapamycin has immunosuppressive properties and is most useful for maintenance of immunosuppression in organ transplantation. Rapamycin was subsequently found to induce p53-independent apoptosis of rhabdomyosarcoma cell lines and decrease cyclin D1 expression and proliferation in pancreatic cancer cell lines,[34,35] leading to the exploration of anticancer effects of this and closely related molecules.

Rapamycin's pharmacologic action is mediated through its binding to the binding protein FKBP12; the rapamycin-FKBP12 complex in turn binds to a site near the catalytic phosphorylating domain of mTORC1, prevents RAPTOR activation, and inhibits mTOR-induced phosphorylation of downstream targets, S6K and 4E-BP1; this finding suggested that rapalog antitumor effects are due to suppression of RNA translation and protein synthesis dependent on these targets (Fig. 25.1). Rapamycin also inhibits cell cycling at the G1/S-phase transition point through the loss of mTOR stimulation of cyclin-dependent kinase, cyclin D1 turnover, and an increased association of p27^{kip1} with cyclin E/cdk2.[36] Prolonged exposure to rapamycin or its analogues may also lead to tissue-specific AKT inhibition, through depletion of mTORC2, which normally activates AKT.

Poor aqueous solubility and chemical instability limited the development of rapamycin as an intravenous (IV) anticancer drug. Two analogues have emerged as effective anticancer medications.

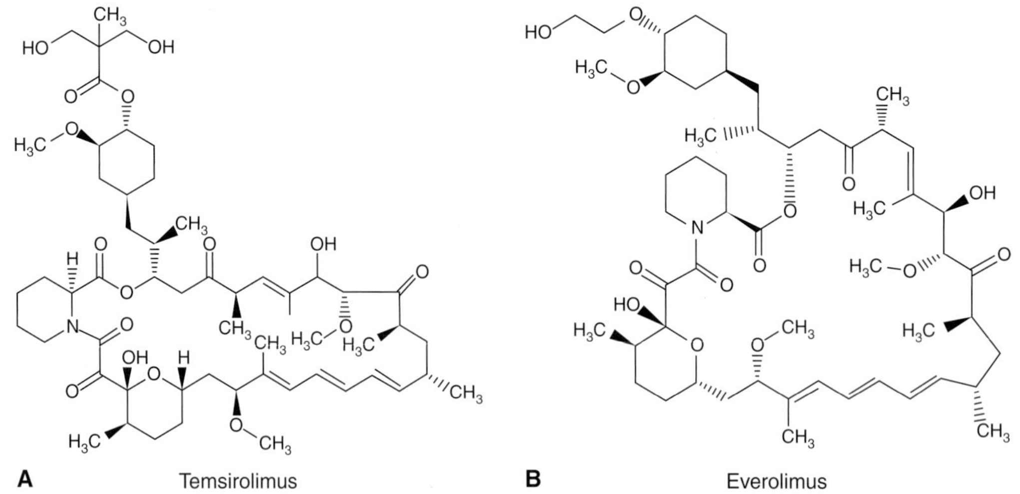

FIGURE **25.2** Structures of temsirolimus (**A**) and everolimus (**B**), both esterified analogs of rapamycin (sirolimus).

Temsirolimus (CCI-779, Torisel)

Temsirolimus (Fig. 25.2A) is an ester analog of rapamycin. Temsirolimus itself has in vitro activity,[37] but when administered in vivo, is rapidly hydrolyzed to sirolimus, which, because of its long half-life in plasma, becomes the predominant mTOR inhibitor. The efficacy of intermittent intravenous dosing with temsirolimus is of interest since the immunosuppressive effects of the drug resolve within 24 hours after dosing, while its inhibition of S6K and other downstream targets persists for days.

Early-phase clinical trials with temsirolimus demonstrated prolonged stable disease and occasional tumor responses, particularly in RCC. Its toxicity included rash, mucositis, thrombocytopenia, hypertriglyceridemia, nausea, anorexia, edema, fatigue, hypercholesterolemia, and a worrisome pneumonitis.[38] Temsirolimus is approved as initial therapy for poor-risk renal cell carcinomas, where it produced a three-month improvement in survival as compared to IFN-α. Its key pharmacological properties are presented in Table 25.2. Note its dependence on hepatic CYP metabolism and therefore interaction with inducers or inhibitors of CYP3A4; the longer, 54-hour plasma half-life of its primary metabolite, sirolimus; and the need to decrease doses to 10 mg/wk in patients with severe hepatic dysfunction.[39]

Approval was based on a phase 3 study of 626 RCC patients who received either temsirolimus alone (25 mg IV weekly), interferon alpha alone, or a combination of the two agents.[40] Patients treated with temsirolimus had an improved median survival of 10.9 months compared to patients treated with interferon alpha, who had a median survival of 7.3 months ($P = 0.008$). Patients treated with the combination of agents survived a median of 8.4 months; therefore, combination therapy is not recommended.

Temsirolimus is also approved as second-line therapy in mantle cell lymphoma,[41] although it is infrequently used as the result of multiple new agents being developed in the past 5 years.

TABLE

25.2 *Key features of rapalogs*

	Everolimus (oral, 10 mg/d)	Temsirolimus (IV, 25 mg/wk)
C_{max}	13 mg/mL	600 ng/mL
Area under C × T curve	Approximately 1,000 µg·h/L	1580 µg·h/L
Clearance	CYP3A4 > 3A5 > 2C8	CYP3A4
$t_{1/2}$	30 h	17 h (metabolite, sirolimus, 54 h)
Dose-limiting toxicity	Stomatitis, rash, fatigue, hyperglycemia Anemia, thrombocytopenia, pneumonitis	Same
Drug interactions	CYP inducers decrease drug levels and decrease toxicity. CYP inhibitors increase drug levels and toxicity. Chemotherapy increases side effects	Same
Dose adjustment	50% decrease for mild to moderate liver dysfunction; do not use for patients with severe liver dysfunction	10 mg/wk for patients with severe liver dysfunction. Do not use in patients with severe renal dysfunction or dialysis

Dose escalation of IV weekly temsirolimus to levels as high as 250 mg led to new and significantly more profound toxicities, including altered mental states, and has not been associated with improved clinical benefit. Temsirolimus in combination with cytotoxic chemotherapy such as paclitaxel and platinum analogues is associated with dose-limiting mucositis, increased myelosuppression, and other toxicity.[42]

Everolimus (RAD001, Afinitor)

Everolimus (Fig. 25.2B) is a hydroxyethyl ester of rapamycin and was initially developed as an oral therapy for transplant and, subsequently, for anticancer applications. As shown in Table 25.2, everolimus is rapidly absorbed after oral administration (bioavailability of 30%, decreased by fatty meals) and, with a $t_{1/2}$ of approximately 30 hours, can be given on a daily schedule.[18] Following ingestion of an oral dose of 10 mg/d, plasma levels reach steady state within 1 week, and trough levels average 13 ng/mL. Like temsirolimus, it is primarily cleared by CYP3A4 and also by CYP3A5 and CYP2C8. Drug interactions with CYP inducers and inhibitors are prominent, and everolimus dosage should be reduced to 5 mg/d in patients with moderate liver dysfunction.

The FDA approved everolimus for relapsed advanced renal cell carcinoma based on results from the phase 3 RECORD-1 trial, in which treatment with everolimus more than doubled the time to progression relative to placebo (4.0 versus 1.9 months) and reduced the risk of disease progression by 70%.[44] Patients in the control arm were allowed to cross over to the everolimus arm upon disease progression.

Everolimus is also approved in patients with advanced neuroendocrine cancer.[45] The partial response rate was only 17%, but an additional 75% of patients have stable disease for greater than 3 months.

A search for biomarkers predictive of response to mTOR inhibition identified an inactivating mutation in the TSC1 gene, a negative regulator of mTOR C1 activity. Eight percent of bladder cancer tumors exhibit this mutation, and Iyer et al., in their heralded "N of 1" study, reported a dramatic, multiyear response to everolimus in such a patient.[46] There have been no subsequent comprehensive trials of everolimus in TSC1 mutant patients.

Because of evidence that PI3K pathway activation may underlie resistance to hormonal therapy in breast cancer, a series of trials were initiated with the combination of everolimus and tamoxifen and with exemestane, a steroid aromatase inhibitor, in breast cancer patients refractory to nonsteroidal aromatase antagonists.[18,47] Everolimus plus exemestane produced a strikingly positive 4.5-month improvement in progression-free survival (PFS) versus exemestane alone in BOLERO-2, but with no improvement in survival.[48] Everolimus was generally well tolerated, but oral mucositis (56%), rash (36%), weakness (33%), and the less common occurrence of grade 3 or 4 drug-related toxicities, such as pneumonitis (12%), led to drug discontinuation in 29% of patients. Hypercholesterolemia, hyperglycemia, and anemia and thrombocytopenia are often noted in patients receiving rapalog treatment. PIK3CA mutation was not predictive of response, although a low PI3K activity signature, associated with high mTOR activation, may be useful, as evidenced in other trials of everolimus with tamoxifen

or letrazole.[18] There were no pharmacokinetic interactions with the hormonal agents.

Similar trials have been pursued with a combination of everolimus, trastuzumab, and vinorelbine in patients with HER2-amplified, trastuzumab/taxane-resistant metastatic breast cancer (BOLERO-3), based on the prominence of PI3K3 pathway mutations in resistant patients.[49] Everolimus added to trastuzumab and chemotherapy improved progression-free survival by less than 2 months. A post hoc subset analysis indicated a positive outcome in the 47% of patients with tumors that had a PIK3CA, PTEN, or AKT mutation and therefore PI3K pathway activation, while patients without these mutations experienced no benefit.[50] Further trials are underway.

Resistance to mTORC1 Inhibitors

As discussed previously, resistance to rapalogs arises through several mechanisms: (a) activating point mutations in the mTORC1 catalytic domain and (b) mutations that prevent inhibitory binding of the FKBP12-rapalog complex. Shokat's laboratory has described a new set of mTORC1 inhibitors that contain elements, joined by a linker, that inhibit the adjoining catalytic and FKB12 binding sites.[25] An additional factor in resistance to rapalogs is their modest inhibitory effect on mTORC2, which provides positive feedback to PI3K and AKT through phosphorylation at S473, overcoming mTORC1 inhibition. Amplification of RAPTOR[32] may also play a role in stimulating mTORC2 and overcoming rapalog inhibition. Compounds that inhibit both mTOR complexes are now in clinical evaluation but have not yielded definitive results.

TORC1/TORC2 Inhibitors

Inhibition of mTORC1 by rapamycin analogues inhibits S6K and prevents an inhibitory phosphorylation of IRS1. This mechanism leads to increased PI3K activation and activating phosphorylation of AKT, which may allow survival of cancer cells treated with an mTOR inhibitor. Several agents inhibit both mTORC1 and mTORC2, preventing the second activating phosphorylation of AKT at Ser473 and countering the stimulatory effects of mTORC1 inhibition on AKT activation. A series of ATP-competitive inhibitors of TORC1/TORC2 kinases are in early clinical development but at this point have not shown striking activity.[51]

PI3K Inhibitors

The frequency of PI3K mutations in many human solid tumors and hematological malignancies and their association with drug resistance in breast cancer have spurred interest in developing inhibitors of PI3K. It is unclear whether pan- versus isoform-specific inhibition of PI3K would have the greatest clinical utility in oncology, although current studies favor isoform-specific inhibitors, based on the higher response rates and lower toxicity associated with early trials of α-specific inhibitors in breast cancer.[52]

A number of inhibitors of the α, β, δ, and γ class I PI3K isoforms, including pan inhibitors and isoform-specific drugs, have entered clinical trials,[52,53] with limited success in solid tumors. The δ inhibitors, which have been uniquely active in follicular lymphomas, and chronic lymphocytic leukemia (CLL) will be considered separately below. In general, the trials in solid tumors, despite the presence of activating PI3K pathway mutations, have been hampered by low response rates and minimal evidence of enhancement of either hormonal therapy or HER2-directed regimens. The trials in breast cancer and other solid tumors have included pan-PI3K inhibitors such as buparlisib (Novartis),[54] as well as PIK3CA-specific inhibitors such as alpelisib (Novartis),[55] and combined PI3K/mTORC1 inhibitors such as gedatolisib (Pfizer).[56] The drugs have been compromised by frequent toxicities such as rash, altered mood and mental status, hypertension, and hyperglycemia.[52,57] In breast cancer trials, responses appeared to be more common, and PFS is longer in patients with tumors that had underlying PI3K pathway activating mutations.[52,53,58] Mayer et al. found numerous different loss of function mutations in PTEN at different metastatic sites in a patient at autopsy after progression on a PI3KCA inhibitor BYL719,[59] suggesting the potential of unique clonal development of drug resistance through multiple different mutations in a single protein.

PI3K𝛿 Inhibitors in Lymphoid Malignancy

The PI3K𝛿 isoform plays a significant physiological role in mediating intracellular signaling through the B-cell lymphocyte receptor and is highly expressed in most B-cell tumors.[60] It has thus become a high-interest target for inhibitors of B-cell tumor proliferation and survival. Two primary compounds, idelalisib, an oral selective PI3K𝛿 inhibitor,[61] and copanlisib, an intravenously administered, combined PI3K𝛼 and PI3K𝛿 inhibitor,[62] have achieved FDA approval: idelalisib for treatment of relapsed/refractory CLL in combination with rituximab and for relapsed/refractory follicular or small cell lymphoma as a single agent, and copanlisib for relapsed follicular lymphoma (Fig. 25.3).

Their key features are shown in Table 25.3. This class of drugs has promising activity in other lymphoid malignancies (mantle cell lymphoma, marginal zone lymphoma, and large cell lymphoma). However, toxicity seems increased in treatment-naïve patients, particularly in the case of idelalisib, and drug combinations of

Idelalisib

Copanlisib

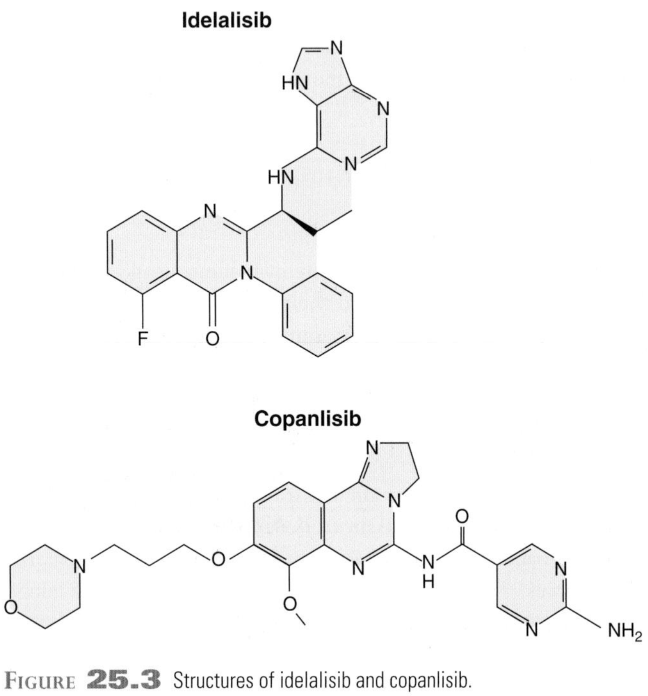

FIGURE **25.3** Structures of idelalisib and copanlisib.

idelalisib with lenalidomide and venetoclax and with bendamustine have also been poorly tolerated, with serious intervening infections, hampering further development of combination first-line therapies.

Idelalisib

The B-cell receptor engages antigen and, in response, activates intracellular pathways that promote expansion of the B-cell population and prevent apoptosis.[63] Key components of this pathway, downstream from the B-cell receptor, are the Bruton tyrosine kinase (BTK) (see Chapter 24) and spleen kinase (SIK), as well the p110 catalytic unit of PI3K𝛿. B-cell lymphoid tumor cells require the same active pathway for proliferation and survival. There is evidence for activation of the PI3K pathway in all histological categories of lymphoma. In the aggressive diffuse large B-cell lymphomas, activating mutations in PIK3CA and PTEN loss are found in a significant subset of tumors, while in mantle cell lymphomas, PTEN loss and PIK3CA mutation are frequent findings.[63] In the low-grade lymphomas, p110𝛿 is highly expressed and, with BTK, has become a favored target for drug development.

Idelalisib has direct inhibitory effects on B-cell proliferation and survival. It also decreases T-cell and NK cytokine production and alters microenvironmental support of lymphoma survival[64] and induces exit of both normal and malignant B cells from the bone marrow compartment. Idelalisib selectively blocks the activity of the PI3k𝛿 activity, with an in vitro IC_{50} of 2.5 nM.[64] It has 100- to 450-fold less efficacy against the other PI3K isoforms. It induces apoptosis in normal and malignant B cells in culture and in early clinical trials showed significant activity in heavily pretreated CLL and follicular and small cell lymphoma.

Initial clinical trials established an acceptable toxicity profile at a dose of 150 mg bid and demonstrated response rates of 48% in a heterogeneous group of heavily pretreated lymphoid malignancies.[65] Further studies confirmed this level of activity for follicular and small lymphocytic lymphoma, leading to FDA approval.[64] A second key trial found a 77% response rate with rituximab in refractory CLL, after progression on first line drugs, including a 54% response rate in the high-risk category of del 17p/p53 mutated subgroup,[61] leading to FDA approval for CLL. The drug also has important activity in relapsed/refractory mantle cell lymphoma and marginal zone lymphoma.[64]

Clinical Pharmacology and Toxicity

Idelalisib is administered as a fixed dose of 150 mg bid and is cleared through aldehyde oxidase, CYP3A4, and glucuronidation metabolism.[66] Its plasma $t_{1/2}$ is 8 to 9 hours. A small (15%) proportion of administered drug is excreted unchanged in the urine. CYP3A4 inducers reduce drug level, while inhibitors and renal or hepatic dysfunction increase exposure (CxT). Inducers/inhibitors should be used with caution in conjunction with idelalisib. While clearance is delayed modestly in patients with severe hepatic or renal dysfunction, with a 50% to 65% increase in AUC, no dose adjustment is necessary in such patients.

As a monotherapy, idelalisib's primary grade 3 or greater toxicities are diarrhea (14%) and pneumonitis (3%), the latter on occasion a fatal event. Transaminase elevations occur in 25% of patients, prompting the recommendation to monitor liver enzymes during

TABLE

25.3   *Key features of idelalisib and copanlisib[66,71]*

Drug	Idelalisib (150 mg PO)[a]	Copanlisib (60 mg IV)
Mechanism of action	Inhibition of PI3Kδ	Inhibition of PI3Kα and PI3Kδ
Clearance	Aldehyde oxidase, CYP3A; 15% renal excretion	CYP3A4
C_{max}	447 ng/mL	318 ng/mL (dose 0.8 mg/kg)
AUC	100 h µg/mL	1,400 h µg/mL (dose 0.8 mg/kg)
$t_{1/2}$	8.2 to 9.5 h	32 to 38 h
Drug interactions	CYP3A inducers/inhibitors	CYP3A4 inducers/inhibitors
	Increased autoimmune reactions in treatment-naïve patients and in combination therapies	
Dose adjustment	None for mild or moderate hepatic for renal dysfunction. Do not use in severe hepatic dysfunction[a]	None
Toxicity	Diarrhea, pneumonitis, neutropenia, transaminitis, infection, autoimmunity	Hypertension, hyperglycemia, neutropenia, transaminitis

[a]Jin F, Robeson M, Zhou H, et al. The pharmacokinetics and safety of idelalisib in subjects with moderate or severe hepatic impairment. *J Clin Pharmacol.* 2015;55:944-952.

therapy; in the majority of patients, elevated enzyme levels return toward normal with continued therapy. Neutropenia, fatigue, and fever have also been noted. However, attempts to use the drug in first-line combinations have been hampered by evidence of opportunistic infection and autoimmunity. Increased neutropenia, transaminitis, and colitis were reported in combination with rituximab, as compared to monotherapy.[61] In combination with lenalidomide and rituximab for CLL, idelalisib caused unacceptable toxicity, with a sepsis-like syndrome (culture negative) of fever and hypotension, as well as severe liver toxicity, pneumonitis, and colitis. These findings, together with evidence of T_{reg} suppression, suggest an autoimmune basis for its organ toxicities.[64,67] When studied in combination with rituximab and bendamustine, idelalisib led to a high rate of neutropenia and bacterial infections and reactivation of cytomegalovirus.[68] With ofatumumab, idelalisib caused a similar spectrum of toxicity, along with *Pneumocystis jirovecii* pneumonia.[69] *P. jirovecii* prophylaxis is now mandated for all patients receiving idelalisib.

Copanlisib

In contrast to the highly specific inhibition of p110δ by idelalisib, copanlisib inhibits both PIK3CA and PI3Kδ at subnanomolar concentrations, with lesser activity against the β and γ isoforms. Preclinical activity against lymphoma and myeloma cell lines prompted its testing in lymphoid tumors in the clinic, where it proved to have a response rate of 59% in relapsed/refractory follicular lymphoma, leading to its FDA approval in 2017.[70] The recommended dose is fixed at 60 mg, given as a 1-hour IV infusion on days 1, 8, and 15 of a 28-day cycle.

The drug is slowly metabolized by CYP3A4, and its clearance is potentially affected by interaction with inducers or inhibitors of this enzyme. A significant portion of unchanged drug is eliminated in stool (30%) and urine (15%). It has a terminal $t_{1/2}$ of 32 to 38 hours in plasma.[71] No dose adjustment is indicated for hepatic

dysfunction. Its primary toxicities are hyperglycemia and hypertension, likely related to its inhibition of p110α, as well as neutropenia, modest gastrointestinal symptoms, and, rarely, pneumonitis (5%).[63]

Acknowledgments

The author has extensively revised Chapter 30 from the fifth edition and wishes to acknowledge the fine contribution of those authors, Helen Chen, Austin Doyle, Naoko Takebe, William Timmer, and Percy Ivy, all from the National Cancer Institute, to the current manuscript.

References

1. Wymann MP, Pirola L. Structure and function of phosphoinositide 3-kinases. *Biochim Biophys Acta.* 1998;1436(1-2):127-150.
2. Tolcher AW, Peng W, Calvo E. Rational approaches for combination therapy strategies targeting the MAP Kinase pathway in solid tumors. *Mol Cancer Ther.* 2018;17:3-16.
3. Maira SM, Voliva C, Garcia-Echeverria C. Class IA phosphatidylinositol 3-kinase: from their biologic implication in human cancers to drug discovery. *Expert Opin Ther Targets.* 2008;12(2):223-238.
4. Sarbassov DD, Guertin DA, Ali SM, et al. Phosphorylation and regulation of Akt/PKB by the rictor-mTOR complex. *Science.* 2005;307(5712):1098-1101.
5. Zinda MJ, Johnson MA, Paul JD, et al. AKT-1, -2, and -3 are expressed in both normal and tumor tissues of the lung, breast, prostate, and colon. *Clin Cancer Res.* 2001;7(8):2475-2479.
6. Cantley LC, Neel BG. New insights into tumor suppression: PTEN suppresses tumor formation by restraining the phosphoinositide 3-kinase/AKT pathway. *Proc Natl Acad Sci U S A.* 1999;96(8):4240-4245.
7. Obata T, Yaffe MB, Leparc GG, et al. Peptide and protein library screening defines optimal substrate motifs for AKT/PKB. *J Biol Chem.* 2000;275(46):36108-36115.
8. Vasudevan KM, Barbie DA, Davies MA, et al. AKT-independent signaling downstream of oncogenic PIK3CA mutations in human cancer. *Cancer Cell.* 2009;16(1):21-32.

9. Diehl JA, Cheng M, Roussel MF, et al. Glycogen synthase kinase-3beta regulates cyclin D1 proteolysis and subcellular localization. *Genes Dev.* 1998;12(22):3499-3511.

10. Zhou BP, Liao Y, Xia W, et al. Cytoplasmic localization of p21Cip1/WAF1 by Akt-induced phosphorylation in HER-2/neu-overexpressing cells. *Nat Cell Biol.* 2001;3(3):245-252.

11. Datta SR, Dudek H, Tao X, et al. Akt phosphorylation of BAD couples survival signals to the cell-intrinsic death machinery. *Cell.* 1997;91(2):231-241.

12. Greer EL, Brunet A. FOXO transcription factors at the interface between longevity and tumor suppression. *Oncogene.* 2005;24(50):7410-7425.

13. Plas DR, Thompson CB. Akt-dependent transformation: there is more to growth than just surviving. *Oncogene.* 2005;24(50):7435-7442.

14. Zhou BP, Liao Y, Xia W, et al. HER-2/neu induces p53 ubiquitination via Akt-mediated MDM2 phosphorylation. *Nat Cell Biol.* 2001;3(11):973-982.

15. Guertin DA, Sabatini DM. Defining the role of mTOR in cancer. *Cancer Cell.* 2007;12(1):9-22.

16. Holz MK, Ballif BA, Gygi SP, et al. mTOR and S6K1 mediate assembly of the translation preinitiation complex through dynamic protein interchange and ordered phosphorylation events. *Cell.* 2005;123(4):569-580.

17. Martin DE, Hall MN. The expanding TOR signaling network. *Curr Opin Cell Biol.* 2005;17(2):158-166.

18. Gambos A, Barthelemy P, Awada A. Evaluating the pharmacokinetics and pharmacodynamics of everolimus for treating breast cancer. *Expert Opin Drug Metab Toxicol.* 2015;11:823-834.

19. Inoki K, Corradetti MN, Guan KL. Dysregulation of the TSC-mTOR pathway in human disease. *Nat Genet.* 2005;37(1):19-24.

20. Feng Z, Zhang H, Levine AJ, et al. The coordinate regulation of the p53 and mTOR pathways in cells. *Proc Natl Acad Sci U S A.* 2005;102(23): 8204-8209.

21. Samuels Y, Wang Z, Bardelli A, et al. High frequency of mutations of the PIK3CA gene in human cancers. *Science.* 2004;304(5670):554.

22. Philp AJ, Campbell IG, Leet C, et al. The phosphatidylinositol 3′-kinase p85{alpha} gene is an oncogene in human ovarian and colon tumors. *Cancer Res.* 2001;61(20):7426-7429.

23. Mayer IA, Arteaga CL. The PI3K/AKT pathway as a target for cancer treatment. *Annu Rev Med.* 2016;67:11-28.

24. Shaw RJ, Bardeesy N, Manning BD, et al. The LKB1 tumor suppressor negatively regulates mTOR signaling. *Cancer Cell.* 2004;6(1):91-99.

25. Rodrik-Outmezquine VS, Okaniwa M, Yao Z, et al. Overcoming mTOR resistance mutations with a new-generation mTOR inhibitor. *Nature.* 2016;534:272-277.

26. Xu J, Pham CG, Albanese SK, et al. Mechanistically distinct cancer-associated mTOR activation clusters predict sensitivity to rapamycin. *J Clin Invest.* 2016;126:3526-3540.

27. Sircar K, Yoshimoto M, Monzon FA, et al. PTEN genomic deletion is associated with p-Akt and AR signalling in poorer outcome, hormone refractory prostate cancer. *J Pathol.* 2009;218(4):505-513.

28. Rimawi MF, De Angelis C, Contreras A, et al. Low PTEN levels and PIK3CAA mutations predicts resistanced to neoadjuvant lapatinib and trastuzumab without chemotherapy in patients with HER2 over-expressing breast cancer. *Breast Cancer Res Treat.* 2018;167:731-740.

29. Aleyev A, Salamon RS, Berger SM, et al. mTORC1 directly phosphorylates and activates ERα upon estrogen stimulation. *Oncogene.* 2016;35:3535-3543.

30. Geter PA, Ernlund AW, Bakogianni S, et al. Hyperactive mTOR and MNK1 phosphorylation of eIF4E confer tamoxifen resistance and estrogen independence through selective mRNA translation reprogramming. *Genes Dev.* 2017;31:2235-2249.

31. Jeboli A, Dumaz N. The role of RICTOR downstream of receptor tyrosine kinase in cancers. *Mol Cancer.* 2018;17:39-48.

32. Morrison MJ, Hicks DJ, Jones B, et al. Rictor/mTOR2 drives progression and therapeutic resistance of Her-2-amplified breast cancers. *Cancer Res.* 2016;76:4752-4764.

33. Vezina C, Kudelski A, Sehgal S. Rapamycin (AY-22, 989), a new antifungal antibiotic. I. Taxonomy of the producing streptomycete and isolation of the active principle. *J Antibiot (Tokyo).* 1975;28(10):721-726.

34. Grewe M, Gansauge F, Schmid RM, et al. Regulation of cell growth and cyclin D1 expression by the constitutively active FRAP-p70s6K pathway in human pancreatic cancer cells. *Cancer Res.* 1999;59(15):3581-3587.

35. Hosoi H, Dilling MB, Shikata T, et al. Rapamycin causes poorly reversible inhibition of mTOR and induces p53-independent apoptosis in human rhabdomyosarcoma cells. *Cancer Res.* 1999;59(4):886-894.

36. Kato JY, Matsuoka M, Polyak K, et al. Cyclic AMP-induced G1 phase arrest mediated by an inhibitor (p27Kip1) of cyclin-dependent kinase 4 activation. *Cell.* 1994;79(3):487-496.

37. Gibbons J, Discafani C, Peterson R, et al. The effect of CCI-779, a novel macrolide anti-tumor agent, on the growth of human tumor cells in vitro and in nude mouse xenografts in vivo. *Proc Am Assoc Cancer Res.* 1999;40:A2000.

38. Raymond E, Alexandre J, Faivre S, et al. Safety and pharmacokinetics of escalated doses of weekly intravenous infusion of CCI-779, a novel mTOR inhibitor, in patients with cancer. *J Clin Oncol.* 2004;22(12):2336-2347.

39. Danesi, R, Boni J, Ravaud A. Oral and intravenously administered mTOR inhibitors for metastatic renal cell carcinoma: Pharmacokinetic consideration and clinical implications. *Cancer Treat Rev.* 2013;39:784-792.

40. Hudes G, Carducci M, Tomczak P, et al. Temsirolimus, interferon alfa, or both for advanced renal-cell carcinoma. *N Engl J Med.* 2007;356(22):2271-2281.

41. Fakhri B, Kahl B. Current and emerging treatment options for mantle cell lymphoma. *Ther Adv Hemat.* 2017;8:223-234.

42. Oza AM, Kollmannsberger C, Group NCT, et al. Phase I study of temsirolimus (CCI-779), carboplatin, and paclitaxel in patients (pts) with advanced solid tumors: NCIC CTG IND 179. *ASCO Meeting Abstracts.* 2009;27(15S):3558.

43. Schuler W, Sedrani R, Cottens S, et al. SZD-RAD, a new rapamycin derivative: pharmacological properties in vitro and in vivo. *Transplantation.* 1997;61(1):36-42.

44. Motzer RJ, Escudier B, Oudard S, et al. Efficacy of everolimus in advanced renal cell carcinoma: a double-blind, randomised, placebo-controlled phase III trial. *Lancet.* 2008;372(9637):449-456.

45. Yao JC, Phan A, Chang DZ, et al. Phase II study of RAD001 (everolimus) and depot octreotide (sandostatin LAR) in advanced low grade neuroendocrine carcinoma (LGNET). *J Clin Oncol (Meeting Abstracts).* 2007;25(18 suppl):4503.

46. Iyer G, Hanrahan AJ, Milowsky MI, et al. Genome sequencing identifies a basis for everolimus sensitivity. *Science.* 2012;338:221-226.

47. Fagan DH, Fettig LM, Avdulov S, et al. Acquired Tamoxifen resistance in MCF-7 breast cancer cells requires hyperactivation of eIF4F-Mediated translation. *Horm Cancer.* 2017;8:219-229.

48. Piccart M, Hortobagyi GN, Campone M, et al. Everolimus plus exemestane for hone-receptor-positive human epidermal growth factor-2-negative advanced breast cancer: overall survival results from BOLERO-2. *Ann Oncol.* 2014;25:2357-2362.

49. Andre F, O'Regan R, Ozguroglu M, et al. Everolimus for women with trastuzumab-resistant, HER2-positive, advanced breast cancer (BOLERO-3): a randomized double-blind, placebo-controlled phase 3 trial. *Lancet Oncol.* 2014;15:580-591.

50. Andre F, Hurvitz S, Fasolo A, et al. Molecular alterations and everolimus efficacy in human epidermal growth factor receptor 2-overexpressing metastatic breast cancers; Combined exploratory biomarker analysis from BOLERO-1 and BOLERO-3. *J Clin Oncol.* 2016;34(18):2115-2124.

51. Bendell JC, Kelley RK, Shin KC, et al. A phase 1 dose-escalation study to assess safety, tolerability, pharmacokinetics, and preliminary efficacy of the dual mTORC1/mmTORC2 inhibitor CC-223 in patients with advanced solid tumors or multiple myeloma. *Cancer.* 2015;121:3481-3490.

52. Janku F. Phosphoinositide-3-Kinase (PI3K) pathway inhibitors in solid tumors: from laboratory to patients. *Cancer Treat Rev.* 2017;59:93-101.

53. Raphael J, Desautels D, Pritchard KI, Petkova E, Shah PS. Phosphoinositide 3-kinase inhibitors in advanced breast cancer: a systematic review and meta-analysis. *Eur J Cancer.* 2018;91:36-46.

54. Criscitiello C, Viale G, Curigliano G, et al. Profile of buparlisib and its potential in the treatment of breast cancer: evidence to date. *Breast Cancer.* 2018;10:23-29.

55. Rodon JD, Tabernero J, Janku F, et al. Phosphatidylinositol 3-Kinase α-Selective inhibition with alpelisib (BYL7619) in PIK3CA-altered solid tumors: results from the first-in-human study. *J Clin Oncol.* 2018;36(13):1291-1299. doi: 1200/JCO.2017.72.7107.

56. Shapiro GI, Bell-McGuinn KM, Molina JR, et al. First-in-human study of PF 05212384 (PKI-587), a small-molecule, intravenous, dual inhibitor of PI3K and mTOR in patients with advanced cancer. *Clin Cancer Res.* 2015;21:1888-1895.

57. Greenwell IB, Ip A, Cohen JB. PI3K Inhibitors: understanding toxicity mechanisms and management. *Oncology*. 2017;31:821-828.

58. Juric D, Castel P, Griffith M, et al. Convergent loss of PTEN leads to clinical resistance to a PI(3)Kα inhibitor. *Nature*. 2015;516:240-244.

59. Mayer IA, Abramson VG, Formisano L, et al. A Phase 1b study of alpelisib (BYL19), a PI3Kα-specific inhibitor, with letrozole in ER+/Her2- metastatic breast Cancer. *Clin Cancer Res*. 2017;23(1):26-34.

60. Clayton E, Bardi G, Bell SF, et al. A crucial role for the p110delta subunit of phosphatidylinositol 3-kinase in B cell development and activation. *J Exp Med*. 2002;196:753-763.

61. Furman RR, Sharman JP, Coutre SE Idelalisib and rituximab in relapsed chronic lymphocytic leukemia. *N Engl J Med*. 2014;370(11):997-1007.

62. Markham A. Copanlisib: first global approval. *Drugs*. 2017;77:2057-2062.

63. Lampson BL, Brown JR. PI3Kδ-selective and PI3Kα/δ-combinatorial inhibitors in clinical development for B-cell non-Hodgkin Lymphoma. *Expert Opin Investig Drugs*. 2017;26:1267-1279.

64. Cheah CY, Fowler NH. Idelalisib in the management of lymphoma. *Blood*. 2016;128:331-336.

65. Gopal AK, Kahl BS, de Vos S, et al. PI3Kδ inhibition by idelalisib in patients with relapsed indolent lymphoma. *N Engl J Med*. 2014;370:1008-1018.

66. Jin F, Gao Y, Fang L, Li X. Population pharmacokinetic modeling of idelalisib, a novel PI3Kδ inhibitor, in healthy subjects and patients with hematologic malignancies. *Cancer Chemother Pharmacol*. 2016;77:89-98.

67. Zelenetz AD, Barrientos JC, Brown JR, et al. Idelalisib or placebo in combination with bendamustine and rituximab in patients with relapsed or refractory chronic lymphocytic leukaemia: interim results from a phase 3, randomized, double-blind, placebo-controlled trial. *Lancet Oncol*. 2017;18:297-311.

68. Lampson BL, Kasar SN, Matos TR, et al. Idelalisib give front-line for treatment of chronic lymphocytic leukemia causes frequent immune-mediated hepatotoxicity. *Blood*. 2016;128:195-203.

69. Jones JA, Robak T, Brown, JR, et al. Efficacy and safety of idelalisib in combination with ofatumumab for previously treated chronic lymphocytic leukemia: an open-label, randomised phase 3 trial. *Lancet Haematol*. 2017;4:e114-e126.

70. Dreyling M, Santoro A, Luigina M, et al. Phosphatidylinositol 3-kinase inhibition by copanlisib in relapsed or refractory indolent lymphoma. *J Clin Oncol*. 2017;35:3898-3905.

71. Patnaik A, Appleman LJ, Tolcher AW, et al. First-in-human phase I study of copanlisib (BAY 80-6946), an intravenous pan-class 1 phosphatidylinositol 3-kinase inhibitor, in patients with advanced solid tumors and non-Hodgkin's lymphomas. *Ann Oncol*. 2016;27:1928-1940.

Inhibitors of Tumor Angiogenesis

Ami N. Shah and William J. Gradishar

Neoplasms occur when a normal cell acquires molecular changes that allow the cell to divide and metastasize in an unsupervised manner. This process requires a supply of nutrients, which is provided by the vasculature. In the early 1970s, Judah Folkman first proposed the theory of tumor angiogenesis, which he defined as the process of recruitment of new vessels to a tumor as it grows.[1] His hypothesis was that tumors are unable to grow beyond a certain size in the absence of a new vascular supply. Subsequent data have supported this hypothesis, indicating that angiogenesis is a critical step in tumor growth and metastases.[2,3] A concentrated effort over the last 2 decades had led to the development of antiangiogenic cancer therapies as a component of cancer therapy.

The growth and maturation of new vasculature is a highly complex process involving interactions of multiple cellular pathways and communication between cells and the extracellular matrix. Many of the key molecules have been identified and have become potential therapeutic targets. As one of the first steps in this process, tumors produce signaling molecules that activate angiogenesis or downregulate the expression of inhibitors of angiogenesis. This step alters the microenvironment to favor an "angiogenic switch."[4,5] In the normal microenvironment, endothelial cells are usually quiescent. In contrast, once the "angiogenic switch" occurs, proliferating endothelial cells form new blood vessels. These blood vessels are structurally abnormal with a leaky basement membrane, which allows tumor cells to become integrated into the vessel wall. This neovasculature is then responsible for the supply of nutrients to the tumor. Angiogenesis was once considered the ideal target for antineoplastic therapy, since it is a unique process that occurs only at tumor sites and not in normal human organs, potentially limiting the toxicities related to these agents. Unfortunately, the reality has been a more tempered effect of antiangiogenic therapies that help improve progression-free survival (PFS) and overall survival (OS) in some tumors but are associated with toxicities and eventual disease progression.

Our arsenal of Food and Drug Association (FDA)-approved drugs targeting angiogenesis has grown immensely over the last decade to include monoclonal antibodies targeting vascular endothelial growth factor (VEGF) and its receptor VEGFR, a soluble VEGF binding protein, and receptor tyrosine kinase inhibitors (TKIs) that target VEGFR along with numerous other receptor tyrosine kinases. This chapter reviews the process of angiogenesis and the rationale for the development of angiogenesis inhibitors as antineoplastic therapies. The chemistry, pharmacology, indications

for use, common toxicities, mechanisms of resistance, and clinical studies leading to approval for the current FDA-approved angiogenesis inhibitors will be covered. Finally, we will discuss and highlight some important areas in need of ongoing research.

Tumor Angiogenesis

Since Judah Folkman initially proposed the concept of tumor angiogenesis in 1971, much work has been done to elucidate the key players in this critical process. Initiation of tumor angiogenesis leads to a cascade of events that must occur in concert in order for successful tumor angiogenesis to occur. Without angiogenesis, tumors cannot exceed a few cubic millimeters in size.[2]

Angiogenic Switch

The normal microenvironment has an antiangiogenic disposition. As tumors grow, they are initially dependent on the normal microenvironment for oxygen and other nutrients. However, since the diffusion limit of oxygen is around 100 μm, as tumors expand, those cells that are no longer within the oxygen diffusion perimeter become hypoxic.[6] In the setting of hypoxia, multiple intracellular molecules are activated. One well-characterized result of hypoxia is the activation of the hypoxia inducible factor-1 (HIF-1) transcriptional complex.[7] Activation of this complex leads to upregulation of proangiogenic factors, such as VEGF, platelet-derived growth factor (PDGF), and nitric oxide synthase (NOS), which are released into the microenvironment. Consistent with this finding, HIF-1 is upregulated in many cancers.[7] However, like most pathways in oncogenesis, redundancy is present and the HIF system is also influenced by many oncogenic pathways, including the insulin-like growth factor-1, epidermal growth factor (EGF), mutant Ras, and Src kinase pathways, as well as tumor suppressor mutations, including PTEN, p53, p14ARF, and pVHL (von Hippel-Lindau).[7] The activation of HIF-1 is a critical step in initiation of the "angiogenic switch" in which the normal microenvironment changes from antiangiogenic to proangiogenic and new blood vessel formation is started. The neovasculature supplies the tumor with oxygen and nutrients and produces growth factors that directly promote tumor growth.[8] Although there are antineoplastic therapies that in addition to their primary target affect HIF-1α, there are no selective HIF-1α inhibitors that have been successfully developed.[9]

The Vascular Endothelial Growth Factor and VEGF Receptor Family

Activation of the VEGF pathway is critical in both physiologic and pathologic angiogenesis. The complexities of this system are beyond the scope of this chapter; therefore, only a brief overview is provided. Detailed reviews are available elsewhere.[10-12] The VEGF receptor family is made up of three tyrosine kinase receptors. Of these, only VEGFR-1 and VEGFR-2 bind the main ligand important in tumor angiogenesis, VEGF-A.[10,12] VEGF-A, usually referred to as VEGF, belongs to a family of genes including placenta growth factor (PLGF), VEGF-B, VEGF-C, and VEGF-D. The biology of VEGF and its primary receptors, VEGFR-1 and VEGFR-2, will be discussed in this chapter (Table 26.1).

The two circulating isoforms of VEGF, $VEGF_{121}$ and $VEGF_{165}$, are the major mediators of tumor angiogenesis.[11] One of the main inducers of VEGF expression is tumor hypoxia.[13] This is mediated in part by HIF-1.[14] Interestingly, loss of the *vHL* tumor suppressor gene in renal cell carcinomas (RCC) results in constitutive overexpression of HIF-1 leading to elevated VEGF expression in these tumors.[15] Several other major growth factors, including EGF, transforming growth factors alpha (TGF-α) and beta (TGF-β), keratinocyte growth factor, insulin-like growth factor-1, fibroblast growth factor (FGF), and PDGF, have also been shown to upregulate VEGF mRNA expression.[10] In addition, oncogenic mutations or amplifications of the Ras oncogene and inflammatory cytokines (IL-1α and IL-6) are associated with VEGF gene induction.[16] VEGF production can also originate from tumor-associated stromal cells suggesting that paracrine or autocrine release of these factors cooperates with hypoxia to induce tumor angiogenesis via VEGF upregulation.[11] Vascular permeability is also mediated by VEGF, which forms fenestrations in blood vessels.[12] Therefore, agents targeting VEGF are also thought to exert antitumorigenic effects by allowing improved delivery of other agents, such as chemotherapy, to tumors.[17]

The VEGF-1 and VEGF-2 receptors are expressed normally on vascular endothelial cells engaged in angiogenesis as well as on bone marrow-derived cells. In addition, many solid and hematologic tumors also express the VEGF receptors, primarily VEGFR-1.[11] These receptors have a similar protein structure with seven immunoglobulin-like domains in the extracellular region, a single transmembrane region, and a consensus tyrosine kinase sequence that is interrupted by a kinase-insert domain. Interestingly, the VEGF receptors can also be expressed inside the cell, where they can promote cell survival by an "intracrine" mechanism.[11]

The role of VEGFR-1 (also known as Flt-1) in angiogenesis remains controversial (Table 26.1). The data suggest that the function of VEGFR-1 differs depending on the developmental stage of the animal, the cell type on which it is being expressed, and the ligand to which it is binding (VEGF-A, VEGF-B, or PLGF).[10,11] Studies linking VEGFR-1 to angiogenesis have found that expression of VEGFR-1 is upregulated by hypoxia. Similar to the VEGF, this is mediated by HIF-1. However, VEGFR-1 has also been identified as a negative regulator of VEGF, especially in embryonic development. In addition, its signal transduction properties are very weak. In general, VEGFR-1 is thought to have little role in tumor angiogenesis.

VEGFR-2 (also known as KDR or Flk-1) is the main regulator of endothelial cell proliferation and survival, as well as vascular permeability (Table 26.1).[12] Upon VEGF ligand binding, the receptor undergoes dimerization and tyrosine phosphorylation. In endothelial cells, this VEGFR-2 activation leads to initiation of several signaling cascades.[11] This includes activation of the mitogen-activating protein kinase (MAPK) pathway, which involves phospholipase C-γ (PLC γ), protein kinase C (PKC), Raf kinase, and MEK. Activation of this pathway results in DNA synthesis and cell growth. Other pathways initiated by VEGFR-2 are the phosphatidylinositol 3′-kinase (PI3K)/Akt pathway that leads to increased endothelial cell survival and the Src family pathway that results in cell migration. Many of these pathways are abnormally expressed in tumors and have been targeted with specific inhibitors. In addition, the neuropilin (NRP) receptors also bind to VEGF and can act as coreceptors with VEGFR-2 to regulate angiogenesis; therefore, these receptors may be targeted by novel agents in the future.[11]

Other Molecular Pathways Important in Tumor Angiogenesis

Matrix metalloproteinases (MMPs) are a family of structurally related endopeptidases that are involved in the degradation of extracellular matrix components (ECM) and mediate remodeling and invasion of the ECM by new vessels by regulating endothelial cell attachment, proliferation, and migration.[18] These observations suggest that MMP inhibitors (MMPIs) could inhibit tumor progression at both the primary tumor site and sites of metastases. Several MMPIs have been developed with promising preclinical data. However, clinical trials in numerous cancers were disappointing, potentially due to the lack of specificity for a particular MMP.[19]

TABLE 26.1	The VEGF signaling family	
Receptor	**Ligands**	**Role of Receptor in Angiogenesis**
VEGFR-1 (Flt-1)	VEGF-A VEGF-B PLGF	Varies by developmental stage, cell-type, and ligand binding Little role in tumor angiogenesis
VEGFR-2 (KDR/Flk-1)	VEGF-A VEGF-C VEGF-D	Main mediator of endothelial cell survival and proliferation as well as vascular permeability Tumor angiogenesis primarily induced via VEGF-A
VEGFR-3 (Flt-4)	VEGF-C VEGF-D	Little role in tumor angiogenesis Important for lymphangiogenesis

Interaction between endothelial cells and the ECM is critical to tumor angiogenesis. The integrins are transmembrane receptors that bind to ECM proteins and play a significant role in this interaction. Studies have implicated a number of endothelial cell integrins in the regulation of endothelial cell growth, survival, and migration during angiogenesis.[20] In addition, integrin signaling is dysfunctional in cancer cells and their expression may correlate with prognosis. Several inhibitors of these endothelial cell integrins have been developed and tested in early phase clinical trials with signs of potential benefit.[20]

Another receptor tyrosine kinase pathway involved in tumor angiogenesis involves the tie-2 receptor.[11] This receptor is expressed principally on the vascular endothelium. Its major ligands are angiopoietin-1 (ang-1) and angiopoietin-2 (ang-2). In concert with VEGF, this pathway stabilizes and matures new capillaries. Ang-1, ang-2, and tie-2 expressions have been correlated with prognosis in several cancers. Peptibodies against ang-2 have been developed and have been shown to prolong PFS in recurrent ovarian cancer without side effects typically associated with VEGF inhibition.[21]

Another pathway that also appears to play an important role in tumor angiogenesis is the notch receptor pathway. The notch receptors are cell surface receptors implicated in cell fate, differentiation, and proliferation.[11,22] The ligands for these receptors are the transmembrane proteins, jagged and delta-like ligand (Dll), which are expressed on adjacent cells. Vascular endothelial cells express notch 1 and 4, as well as jagged 1, Dll-1, and Dll4. Notch-Dll4 signaling is essential for vascular development in the embryo and Dll4 is upregulated in tumor vasculature. This is thought to be in part VEGF-mediated. Novel agents targeting this pathway are also currently in early phase clinical development.[23]

Preclinical Development of VEGF Inhibitors

VEGF and its receptors are overexpressed in a number of malignancies, including colorectal, lung, breast, renal cell, endometrial carcinomas, and acute myelogenous leukemia.[10,11] The majority of retrospective studies correlating VEGF or VEGFR expression to prognosis suggest that high levels are associated with a worse prognosis.[24–26]

In vitro and in vivo studies indicate the importance of VEGF signaling in enhancing proliferation and inhibiting apoptosis of endothelial cells. In addition to tumor angiogenesis, VEGF signaling is critical in developmental endothelial cell growth and in endothelial cell growth after normal tissue injury. However, established blood vessels are not VEGF-dependent. Therefore, agents targeting this pathway should have effects on the peritumoral vasculature and not on the established vasculature critical for normal human physiology. Based on the data indicating the importance of VEGF signaling in tumor angiogenesis, animal studies were done and demonstrated that inhibition of VEGF signaling interrupts tumor growth and invasion.[27–30] Limitations of these preclinical observations experimental tumors maybe more VEGF-dependent because they were rapidly grown and models may not represent

VEGF activity in the metastatic setting. Nevertheless, the abundance of preclinical data supporting the antineoplastic potential of these agents led to the development of multiple drugs targeting the VEGF pathway.

VEGF Activity in Malignancy

Different tumors have variable VEGF dependency and sensitivity to pathway inhibition. Clear cell RCC can be exquisitely sensitive to antiangiogenic therapies because a significant portion have mutations in the VHL gene leading to HIF-1 induction and subsequent VEGF and PDGF upregulation.[8] Hepatocellular carcinoma (HCC) and neuroendocrine tumors are highly vascular tumors, suggesting dependency on angiogenesis. Ovarian, cervical, gastroesophageal, colorectal (CRC), non–small cell lung (NSCLC), and thyroid cancer have also demonstrated sensitivity to VEGF inhibition.[31] Interestingly, prostate cancer and pancreatic cancer have not shown benefit from VEGF-inhibition, potentially related to redundant angiogenic pathways and poor vasculature.[32,33] Numerous drugs have successfully targeted the VEGF pathway to improve outcomes in these disease types. Their pharmacologic properties (Table 26.2) and studies leading to their FDA approvals (Table 26.3) are summarized with more details in this chapter.

Toxicities of VEGF Pathway Inhibitors

All currently approved antiangiogenic therapies inhibit VEGFR-2 activation and downstream activity. Accordingly, recurring pathway-related toxicities are seen with all anti-angiogenic drugs currently in practice. The most frequent and/or severe toxicities are hypertension, proteinuria, thrombosis, hemorrhage, gastrointestinal fistula or perforation, poor wound healing, and reversible posterior leukoencephalopathy (RPLS). Some severe toxicities are rare, making large studies or meta-analyses helpful in determining whether the risk is increased with antiangiogenic medications. If severe, the drug should be interrupted. Dose reduction or drug discontinuation may be needed.

Of these toxicities, hypertension occurs most frequently. VEGF helps maintain blood pressure by mediating nitric oxide production and creating new vasculature that reduces resistance. Study population variations make direct comparisons difficult, but hypertension incidence ranged from 8% with ramucirumab, around 25% with bevacizumab, around 20% to 40% with sorafenib, sunitinib, and pazopanib, and 68% with lenvatinib.[34] A meta-analysis of over 30,000 patients treated with VEGF-targeted TKIs noted that 23% developed hypertension of all grades and 4.4% developed >grade 3 hypertension.[35] Patients with a history of hypertension, age >60, or BMI >25 kg/m^2 are at increased risk.[36] The degree of elevation is dose dependent. Some studies suggest that developing hypertension is associated with efficacy, although this is not consistently observed.[37–39] While hypertension is primarily low grade, up to one in four patients may need treatment for hypertension.[8]

TABLE
26.2 Pharmacology/pharmacokinetics of small molecular inhibitors

Drug	Target/Mechanism	FDA-Approved Indications, year	Recommended Dosing	Plasma Half-Life	Primary Metabolism	Drug Interactions	Food Interaction
Bevacizumab	Monoclonal antibody, VEGF	mCRC 2004 (1st line), 2006 (2nd line) NSCLC 2006 RCC 2009 Ovarian cancer 2016 Breast cancer 2009 (withdrawn)	5 to 15 mg/kg IV q 2 to 3 wks	20 d	—	Increased HFSR with sorafenib. Microangiopathic hemolytic anemia with sunitinib.	None expected
Ziv-Aflibercept	Fusion protein, VEGF	mCRC 2012	4 mg/kg IV q 2 wks	6 d	—	No formal studies	None expected
Ramucirumab	Monoclonal antibody, VEGFR2	NSCLC 2014 Gastric/GE junction 2014 mCRC 2015	8 mg/kg IV q 2 wks; except NSCLC with docetaxel 10 mg/g q 3 wks	14 d	—	No formal studies	None expected
Sorafenib	TKI, VEGFR2, FLT3, PDGFR, FGFR-1	RCC 2005 HCC 2007 DTC 2013	400 mg PO bid	1 to 2 d	CYP3A4, UGT1A9	P450 inhibitors & inducers, inhibits P450	Take on empty stomach, high-fat decreases absorption
Sunitinib	c-kit, VEGFR1-3, PDGFR, FLT3, CSF-1R, RET	RCC 2006 GIST 2006 PNET 2011	RCC & GIST: 50mg PO QD week 1 to 4 of 6 wk cycle PNET: 37.5 mg PO QD continuous	40 to 60 h	CYP3A4	P450 inhibitors & inducers	None expected
Pazopanib	VEGFR1-3, PDGFR, FGFR1, FGFR3, c-kit, and others	RCC 2009 STS 2012	800 mg PO daily	31 h	CYP3A4, 1A2, 2C8	P450 inhibitors & inducers, inhibits P450	Take on empty stomach, food increased absorption
Axitinib	VEGFR1-3	RCC 2nd line 2012	5mg PO bid	2.6 to 6.1 h	CYP3A4, 2C19, A2	P450 inhibitors & inducers	No dose adjustment
Cabozantinib	VEGFR1-3, MET, AXL, RET, KIT, FLT3	MTC 2012 RCC 2016	140 mg PO daily MTC 60 mg PO daily RCC	55 to 99 h	CYP3A4, 2C9	P450 inhibitors & inducers, inhibits P450	Take on empty stomach, food increased absorption
Lenvatinib	VEGFR1-3, RET, FGFR, KIT, PDGFR	Thyroid cancer 2015 RCC (+ everolimus) 2016	24 mg PO daily DTC 18 mg PO daily + everolimus 5 mg PO daily RCC	28 h	CYP3A4	P450 inhibitors & inducers	No dose adjustment
Regorafenib	VEGFR1-3, RET, c-kit, PDGFR, FGFR1 FGFR2, and more	mCRC 2013 HCC 2017	160 mg daily days 1 to 21, 28-day cycle	25 to 51 h	CYP3A4	P450 inhibitors & inducers	Take with food, food increased absorption

TABLE
26.3 *Important phase II/III trials leading to drug approvals for anti-angiogenic medications*

	Study	Phase	Patient Population/study	Experimental Arm	Control	PFS	OS
Bevacizumab	AVOREN	III	649 patients, metastatic RCC, first line	Bevacizumab + IFNα	Placebo + IFNα	10.2 versus 5.5 mo*	23.3 versus 21.3 mo ~
	CALBG 90206	III	732 patients, metastatic RCC, first line	Bevacizumab + IFNα	Placebo + IFNα	8.5 versus 5.3 mo*	18.3 versus 17.4 mo ~
	Hurwitz et al.[68]	III	813 patients, metastatic CRC, first line	Bevacizumab + irinotecan-based CT	Irinotecan-based CT	10.6 versus 6.2 mo*	20.3 versus 15.6 mo *~
	NO16966	III	1401 patients metastatic CRC, previously untreated	Bevacizumab + oxaliplatin-based CT	Oxaliplatin-based CT	9.4 versus 8.0 mo*	21.2 versus 19.9 mo ~
	E3200	III	830 patients metastatic CRC, 2nd line after 5-FU and irinotecan	Bevacizumab and FOLFOX or bevacizumab	FOLFOX	7.3 versus 2.7 versus 4.7 mo*	13.0 versus 10.8 *~
	ML18147	III	829 patients, metastatic CRC, 2nd line after bevacizumab + CT	Bevacizumab + 2nd line CT	2nd line CT	5.7 versus 4.1 mo*	11.2 versus 9.8 mo *~
	E4599	III	878 patients, advanced nonsquamous NSCLC, first line	Carboplatin/paclitaxel + bevacizumab → bevacizumab maintenance	Carboplatin/paclitaxel	6.2 versus 4.5 mo*	12.3 versus 10.3 mo *~
	BRAIN	II	167 patients, GBM, prior temozolomide and radiation	Bevacizumab, bevacizumab + irinotecan	Historic controls	4.2, 5.6 mo	9.2, 8.7 mo
	GOG 420	III	452 patients persistent, recurrent, or metastatic cervical cancer	Chemotherapy doublet + bevacizumab	Chemotherapy doublet	7.6 versus 5.7 mo *	17.0 versus 13.3 mo *~
	AURELIA	III	361 patients, platinum resistance epithelial ovarian, fallopian tube, primary peritoneal cancer	Chemotherapy + bevacizumab	Bevacizumab	6.7 versus 3.4 mo ~	16.6 versus 13.3 mo
Aflibercept	VELOUR	III	1226 patients, second line after oxaliplatin for mCRC	FOLFIRI + aflibercept	FOLFIRI + placebo	6.9 versus 4.8 mo*	13.5 versus 12.6 mo *~
Ramucirumab	RAISE	III	1072 patients, second line after oxaliplatin and bevacizumab for mCRC	FOLFIRI + ramucirumab	FOLFIRI + placebo	5.7 versus 4.5 mo*	13.3 versus 11.7 mo *~
	REVEL	III	1253 patients, second line after platinum-based CT for advanced NSCLC	Docetaxel + ramucirumab	Docetaxel + placebo	4.5 versus 3.0 mo*	10.5 versus 9.1 mo *~
	REGARD	III	355 patients, second line after CT for gastric or gastroesophageal adenocarcinoma	Ramucirumab	Placebo	2.1 versus 1.3 mo *	5.2 versus 3.8 mo *~
	RAINBOW	III	665 patients, second line after CT for gastro-esophageal adenocarcinoma	Paclitaxel + ramucirumab	Paclitaxel + placebo	4.4 versus 2.9 mo*	9.6 versus 7.4 mo~
Sorafenib	TARGET	III	903 patients, second line after cytokine therapy for clear cell RCC	Sorafenib	Placebo	5.5 versus 2.8 mo*	17.8 versus 15.2 mo~
	SHARP	III	602 patients, first-line advanced HCC	Sorafenib	Placebo	5.5 versus 2.8 mo*	10.7 versus 7.9 mo *~
	DECISION	III	417 patients, progressive radioiodine refractory DTC	Sorafenib	Placebo	10.8 versus 5.8 mo*~	–

TABLE

26.3 Important phase II/III trials leading to drug approvals for anti-angiogenic medications (Continued)

	Study	Phase	Patient Population/study	Experimental Arm	Control	PFS	OS
Sunitinib	Motzer et al.[132]	III	750 patients, first-line clear cell metastatic RCC	Sunitinib	IFN-α	11 versus 5 mo*~	26.4 versus 21.8 mo
	Demetri et al.[135]	III	312 patients, second line after imatinib metastatic GIST	Sunitinib	Placebo	27.3 versus 6.4 wks *~	73 versus 65 mo
	Raymond et al.[136]	III	171 patients, progressive, metastatic pancreatic neuroendocrine tumor	Sunitinib	Placebo	11.4 versus 5.5 mo*~	38.6 versus 29.1 mo
Pazopanib	Sternberg et al.[48]	III	435 patients, first line or after cytokine therapy, advanced RCC	Pazopanib	Placebo	9.2 versus 4.2*~	23 versus 21 mo
	COMPARZ	III	1110 patients, first-line metastatic clear cell RCC	Pazopanib	Sunitinib	8.4 versus 9.5 mo~	28.3 versus 29.1 mo
	PALETTE	III	369 patients, progressive after chemotherapy, STS	Pazopanib	Placebo	4.6 versus 1.6 mo*~	12.5 versus 10.7 mo
Axitinib	AXIS	III	723 patients, second-line advanced RCC	Axitinib	Sorafenib	6.7 versus 4.7 mo*~	20.1 versus 19.2
Cabozantinib	METEOR	III	658 patients, second line after at least one anti-VEGF TKI advanced clear cell RCC	Cabozantinib	Everolimus	7.4 versus 3.8 mo*~	21.4 versus 16.5*
	EXAM	III	330 patients, progressive metastatic medullary thyroid cancer	Cabozantinib	Placebo	11.2 versus 4.0 mo*~	26.6 versus 21.1 mo
Lenvatinib	Motzer et al. Lancet Oncol 2015.[164]	II	153 patients, second line after one anti-VEGF TKI, advanced clear cell RCC	Lenvatinib 18 mg daily + everolimus 5 mg daily	Lenvatinib 24 mg daily versus everolimus 10 mg daily	14.6 versus 7.4 versus 5.5 mo*~	25.5 versus 18.4 versus 17.5
	SELECT	III	392 patients, progressive radioiodine refractory DTC	Lenvatinib	Placebo	18.3 versus 3.6*~	—
Regorafenib	CORRECT	III	760 patients refractory to fluoropyrimidine, oxaliplatin, irinotecan, anti-VEGF, and anti-EGFR if KRAS wild-type, metastatic CRC	Regorafenib	Placebo	1.9 versus 1.7 mo*	6.4 versus 5.0 mo*~
	CONCUR	III	204 patients refractory to standard chemotherapy for metastatic CRC	Regorafenib	Placebo	3.2 versus 1.7 mo*	8.8 versus 6.3 mo*~
	GRID	III	199 patients refractory to imatinib and sunitinib, advanced GIST	Regorafenib	Placebo	4.8 versus 0.9 mo*~	—
	RESOURCE	III	573 patients, prior sorafenib advanced HCC	Regorafenib	Placebo	3.1 versus 1.5*	10.6 versus 7.8*~

Legend: (*) = statistically significant results; (~) = primary endpoint.

Prior to initiation of antiangiogenic therapy, patients should have baseline cardiac risk factors assessed and optimized, including control of blood pressure. Blood pressure should be closely monitored, particularly when therapy is beginning. Although the optimal strategy has not been determined, drug-induced hypertension can be managed with calcium channel blockers and angiotensin-converting enzyme inhibitors.[40]

Proteinuria of any grade is common with bevacizumab, but >grade 3 proteinuria occurs in only 2.2% of patients.[41] With anti-VEGF TKIs, a meta-analysis of 6882 patients found proteinuria of any grade occurred in 18.7% and >grade 3 occurred in 2.4% of patients. RCC is associated with higher rates of proteinuria in bevacizumab-treated patient, although this difference was not seen with anti-VEGF TKIs.[42] Proteinuria often does not prompt a change in treatment as short-term clinical consequences of proteinuria are limited in patients with advanced disease.

As a class, VEGF inhibitors have shown increased rates of arterial thromboembolism. However, whether they increase the rate of venous thromboembolism is not clear. While the pathophysiology associated with increased risk is uncertain, one possible mechanism for these toxicities is VEGF inhibition that causes endothelial cell dysfunction and/or apoptosis. The resulting exposed basement membrane is prothrombotic but the loss of integrity of endothelial vessel lining can increase risk for hemorrhage. VEGF is also involved in the production of prostaglandins and nitric oxide, so its inhibition promotes a prothrombotic state.[43]

A meta-analysis using individual patient data from five trials evaluating bevacizumab with chemotherapy found the relative risk for arterial thromboembolism was 2.0 (95% CI 1.05 to 3.75) in patients treated with chemotherapy and bevacizumab compared to chemotherapy alone. The risk was higher in patients >65 years and with a prior history of arterial thromboembolism.[44] Data analyzing the addition of bevacizumab to chemotherapy have not consistently shown an increased risk for venous thromboembolism when compared to chemotherapy alone.[45,46] In placebo-controlled trial of ramucirumab monotherapy, an increased rate of arterial thromboembolism was seen (1.7% versus 0%) but not venous thromboembolism (3% versus 5%) with ramucirumab therapy compared to placebo.[47] Increased rates of arterial thromboembolism are also seen with anti-VEGF TKIs. A meta-analysis of over 10,000 patients who received sorafenib or sunitinib found a RR for arterial thromboembolism of 3.0 (95% CI 1.25 to 7.37) when compared to control. An increase in rates of arterial thromboembolism was also seen with pazopanib and lenvatinib.[48,49] The risk for venous thromboembolism with anti-angiogenic TKIs therapy was not increased (RR 1.10, 95% CI 0.73 to 1.66) in a meta-analysis of 7441 patients who received sorafenib, sunitinib, pazopanib, vandetanib, or axitinib.[50]

Bevacizumab has been shown to have increased bleeding risks in multiple meta-analyses. One included over 12,000 patients and found all-grade, severe, and fatal bleeding occurred in 30.4%, 3.5%, and 0.8% of patients, respectively. When compared to controls, the RR for bleeding was 2.48 (95% CI 1.93 to 3.18). A higher dose was associated with increased risk.[51] Similarly, a meta-analysis of 27 studies with patients treated with anti-VEGF TKIs found an incidence of 9.1% all-grade bleeding and 1.3% severe bleeding. The risk of all-grade bleeding events was elevated (RR 1.67, 95%

CI 1.19 to 2.33), but the risk for severe bleeding was not significantly increased (RR 1.23, 95% CI 0.86 to 1.77). The most common high-grade events were hemoptysis and CNS hemorrhage.[52]

If anticoagulation is warranted in patients on anti-VEGF therapy, an individual assessment of the risks and benefits of anticoagulation should be considered and caution should be used given the risk for hemorrhage associated with this class of drugs. Retrospective data indicate that the combination of bevacizumab and therapeutic anticoagulation is not associated with an increased rate of severe bleeding episodes (<1%).[53]

Gastrointestinal perforation and fistula formation is another class-associated complication. Hypotheses for its mechanism include ulceration from tumor necrosis and impaired healing, thrombosis, and mesenteric ischemia.[54] A meta-analysis of various tumor types found a 1% rate of perforation. One in five of those perforations were fatal. The rate varies based on tumor type, with CRC and RCC having increased risk compared to lung cancer.[55] Early studies of heavily pretreated epithelial ovarian cancer patients showed high rates (~10%) of gastrointestinal perforation or fistula.[56] However, more recent studies evaluating bevacizumab with chemotherapy as part of first-line systemic therapy suggest much lower rates.[57,58] Ramucirumab is associated with low rates of severe gastrointestinal complications (0.7% perforation).[47] However, fatal events have occurred. Studies with antiangiogenic TKIs report a rate of 1.3% for gastrointestinal perforation, which was not increased compared to placebo (HR 2.99, 95% 0.85 to 10.53).[59]

Angiogenesis is important for early wound healing. VEGF inhibition can impair wound healing, as is seen with bevacizumab and anti-VEGF TKIs.[60-62] This is especially relevant with bevacizumab given its long half-life.

While rare (<1%), RPLS can occur in the setting of anti-VEGF therapy. Adequate management of hypertension is important as uncontrolled hypertension increases the risk of RPLS.[8]

Fatigue and dysphonia are common but typically not severe toxicities seen with many antiangiogenic agents. Off-target toxicities are more common with anti-VEGF TKIs as they act by competitive ATP inhibition, affecting other tyrosine kinases. These include thyroid dysfunction, stomatitis, gastrointestinal symptoms (diarrhea, nausea, and weight loss), hand-foot skin reaction (HFSR), decreased left ventricle ejection fraction, prolonged QTC, and hepatic toxicity.[8]

Antibodies and Proteins Targeting the Vascular Endothelial Growth Factor Pathway

Bevacizumab (Avastin)

Chemistry

Bevacizumab is a recombinant humanized monoclonal immunoglobulin G (IgG) antibody generated by engineering VEGF-binding residues of a murine neutralizing antibody into the framework of a normal human IgG.[27] It consists of approximately 93% human and 7% murine protein sequences.[63] Bevacizumab has a molecular weight of approximately 149 kDa (kilodaltons). It comes in a clear to slightly opalescent, colorless to pale brown, sterile, pH 6.2 solution for intravenous infusion.

Mechanism of Action

Bevacizumab binds and neutralizes the biologically active forms of VEGF by recognizing the binding sites for the VEGF receptors. This prevents the interaction of VEGF with its receptors on the surface of endothelial cells. Bevacizumab neutralizes all isoforms of human VEGF with a dissociation constant (K_d) of 1.1.[63] Inhibition of VEGF-induced proliferation of endothelial cells as well as tumor angiogenesis in vitro has been noted with bevacizumab. Preclinical studies showed that the administration of bevacizumab to mice with various tumor xenografts caused growth inhibition and decreased metastatic progression. Given that VEGF is produced and acts locally in a tumor site, the capacity of an antibody to interfere with its effects is somewhat surprising. Unlike antibodies targeting receptors, ligands can be difficult to sop up.

Pharmacokinetics, interactions, and special populations

Bevacizumab is administered as an intravenous formulation. The predicted time to reach steady state was 100 days and its half-life is 20 days.[64] The clearance of bevacizumab varied with body weight, sex, and tumor burden. Bevacizumab has been tested at doses from 3 to 20 mg/kg, but a clear dose-response relationship has not been identified. In CRC, a dose of 5 mg/kg was more effective than 10 mg/kg.[65] On the other hand, in renal cell cancer and non–small cell lung cancer, higher doses up to 15 mg/kg are more effective than lower doses.[66,67] Although there are no dedicated studies, no dose adjustments are recommended for renal or hepatic dysfunction. There is increased toxicity in elderly patients, but no dose adjustment is recommended. In pediatrics, there are limited clinical data with osteonecrosis of the jaw as an additional observed toxicity. Fetal harm is expected with bevacizumab exposure during pregnancy based on its mechanism of action and animal studies.

Toxicities

The most common adverse events seen with bevacizumab (occurred in >10% of patients and at least twice as frequent as the control arm) were epistaxis, headache, hypertension, rhinitis, proteinuria, taste alteration, dry skin, rectal hemorrhage, lacrimation disorder, and exfoliative dermatitis. The combination of bevacizumab and chemotherapy compared to chemotherapy alone had higher rates of grade 3 or 4 neutropenia (21% versus 14% in metastatic CRC). Adverse events led to discontinuation of bevacizumab in 8.4% to 20.3% of patients. Rates of toxicities vary depending on the treatment population (tumor type and setting of therapy). As an example, in a study of chemotherapy plus bevacizumab 5 mg/kg every 2 weeks versus placebo in patients with metastatic CRC, 85 versus 74% experienced grade 3 or 4 events and 45% versus 40% experience an adverse event requiring hospitalization. Hypertension occurred in 22.4% versus 8.3% of patients, grade 3 or 4 diarrhea in 32 versus 25% of patients, and grade 3 or 4 leukopenia in 37% versus 31% of patients.[68] Anti-VEGF class adverse events as described earlier are seen with bevacizumab. It carries black box warnings for gastrointestinal perforation, impaired wound healing, and hemorrhage. The package insert recommends to holding the drug 28 days prior to and after surgery and until there is complete wound healing. It also recommends avoidance of the drug in severe hemorrhage or recent hemoptysis.

Therapeutic Uses

Renal Cell Cancer

A randomized phase II trial evaluated low-dose bevacizumab (3 mg/kg every 2 weeks), high-dose bevacizumab (10 mg/kg every 2 weeks), and placebo in patients with metastatic clear cell RCC whose disease progressed after or could not receive interleukin-2. There was a difference between PFS in the high-dose group compared with the placebo group (4.8 versus 2.5 months; $P < 0.001$), but no improvement in OS occurred in any of the cohorts.[69] The higher dose was used in future studies. The AVOREN trial was a multicenter, randomized, double-blind, placebo-controlled phase III study of 649 patients with previously untreated metastatic RCC. Patients received interferon alpha-2a (IFNα) and bevacizumab or placebo. PFS was significantly longer in the combination group (10.2 versus 5.4 months, HR 0.63, 95% CI 0.45 to 0.72) as was response rate (31% versus 13%).[66] A second phase III study, CALGB 90206, included 732 untreated metastatic RCC patients with the same treatment arms. It showed a similar improvement in PFS.[70] Both studies had a trend toward improved OS but the difference was not statistically significant. However, the majority of patients received poststudy treatments that may obscure a survival benefit.[71,72] No trials evaluated bevacizumab and IFNα compared to bevacizumab alone. Bevacizumab with IFNα was granted FDA approval for treating metastatic RCC in 2009. Trials evaluating other combinations including bevacizumab with sorafenib and temsirolimus have shown increased toxicity and/or no significant improvement.[73]

Colorectal Cancer

Bevacizumab was approved by the FDA in 2004 for use with 5-fluorouracil (5-FU)–based chemotherapy as first-line therapy for patients with metastatic CRC. This approval was based on two clinical trials in patients with previously untreated metastatic disease.[65,68] In the initial phase II trial, patients were assigned to one of the three treatment regimens: 5-FU/leucovorin (LV), 5-FU/LV plus bevacizumab 5 mg/kg every 2 weeks, or 5FU/LV plus bevacizumab 10 mg/kg every 2 weeks.[65] The time to progression was improved in the 5 mg/kg bevacizumab group when compared with the control group (9.0 versus 5.2 months; $P = 0.005$), as was the overall response rate (40% versus 17%; $P = 0.029$). However, this improvement was not seen in the cohort that received the higher-dose bevacizumab. The phase III trial randomly assigned 413 patients to IFL (irinotecan, bolus 5-FU, and LV) and 402 patients to IFL plus bevacizumab 5 mg/kg every 2 weeks.[68] The group that received bevacizumab had a better overall response rate (44.8 versus 34.8; $P = 0.004$) and improved PFS. The study met its primary endpoint with improvement in median survival from 15.6 months in the IFL cohort to 20.3 months in the IFL plus bevacizumab group ($P < 0.001$). Grade 3 or 4 adverse events were significantly increased with bevacizumab when compared to placebo.

Another study evaluated the addition of bevacizumab to oxaliplatin-based chemotherapy regimens.[74] The phase III NO16966 study randomly assigned 1,401 patients to FOLFOX (5-FU, LV, and oxaliplatin every 2 weeks) or XELOX (capecitabine and oxaliplatin every 3 weeks) plus bevacizumab (5 mg/kg with FOLFOX, 7.5 mg/kg with XELOX) versus placebo. Median PFS for the bevacizumab-containing arms was significantly better than the placebo-containing arms (9.3 versus 8.0 months; $P = 0.0023$). No statistically significant difference in median OS or response rate was seen between the two arms. Interestingly, although the protocol specified treatment until disease progression, 50% of patients discontinued the treatment for reasons unrelated to progressive disease. The most common reasons for treatment discontinuation were related to chemotherapy and included neurotoxicity, gastrointestinal events, general disorders, and hematologic events. Theories for the smaller clinical benefit noted in this study when compared to the previously discussed study using IFL include early treatment discontinuation and a smaller incremental benefit when bevacizumab is combined with more active regimens. The toxicities associated with bevacizumab in metastatic CRC were similar in all the large phase III studies.

Subsequent studies with bevacizumab in CRC have focused on several clinical questions regarding its use as second-line therapy, the efficacy of novel combinations with bevacizumab, and its use in the adjuvant setting.

A phase III open-label randomized multicenter three-arm trial compared FOLFOX every 2 weeks, FOLFOX plus bevacizumab, and bevacizumab monotherapy in patients who had previously received a 5-FU–based and irinotecan-based regimen. The bevacizumab monotherapy arm was closed early based on lack of efficacy. Median OS was longer in the FOLFOX plus bevacizumab arm than in the FOLFOX only arm (13.0 versus 10.8 months; $P = 0.0012$).[75] This study led to FDA approval of bevacizumab with 5-FU–based chemotherapy for second-line therapy in metastatic CRC. Another study investigated the continuation of bevacizumab with second-line chemotherapy in 829 patients who had previously received chemotherapy with bevacizumab. A modest benefit in OS was found with continuation of bevacizumab (11.2 versus 9.8 months, HR 0.81, 95% CI 0.69 to 0.94). Patients in the bevacizumab arm also experienced an increase in toxicity as has been observed with bevacizumab and chemotherapy combinations.[31]

Two trials evaluated the addition of an EGFR-targeting monoclonal antibody in addition to chemotherapy and bevacizumab. The combination of bevacizumab with capecitabine and oxaliplatin-based chemotherapy with or without cetuximab was studied in a phase III open-label randomized study of 755 subjects with previously untreated metastatic CRC. PFS was significantly shorter in the cetuximab-containing arm; however, a subset analysis showed that those patients whose tumors had wild-type KRAS had improved PFS from the addition of cetuximab.[76] Similar results of worse toxicity and decreased PFS were also noted in a first-line phase III study using oxaliplatin- or irinotecan-based chemotherapy with bevacizumab with or without panitumumab.[77] NSABP C-08 evaluated if the addition of bevacizumab to adjuvant FOLFOX improved outcomes in patients with stage II or III CRC that had been resected. No difference was found in the 3-year DFS (77.4% versus 75.5%) or OS and more toxicity was seen.[78] These negative findings were confirmed by the AVANT BO17920 and QUASAR2 trial.[79,80]

Non–Small Cell Lung Cancer

The addition of bevacizumab to standard chemotherapy has also been beneficial in advanced nonsquamous, NSCLC. The E4599 trial was a phase III randomized study of 878 patients with stage IIIB or IV NCSCL.[81] This trial evaluated carboplatin/paclitaxel versus carboplatin/paclitaxel plus bevacizumab 15 mg/kg. Bevacizumab was continued after completion of chemotherapy. Notably, patients needed to have adequate organ function, an ECOG performance status of 0 to 1, and could not have hemoptysis, brain metastases, or squamous cell cancer histology. The median OS was 12.3 months in the group assigned to chemotherapy plus bevacizumab, as compared with 10.3 months in the chemotherapy-alone group (HR 0.79; $P = 0.003$). The median PFS and tumor response rates were also significantly better in the bevacizumab arm. Important toxicities included a statistically significant increase in rates of grade 4 neutropenia (25.5% versus 16.8%) and grade 3 febrile neutropenia (4.0% versus 1.8%). Grade 3 or higher bleeding events were noted in 4.4% of bevacizumab-treated patients and in only 0.7% of control patients. Fifteen subjects had grade 5 events in the bevacizumab arm: five subjects with febrile neutropenia, five with hemoptysis, two with hematemesis, two with cerebrovascular events, and one with pulmonary embolism. This study led to the FDA approval of bevacizumab in combination with carboplatin and paclitaxel for the first-line therapy of advanced NSCLC with nonsquamous histology in 2006. Another first-line study and a meta-analysis of trials evaluating bevacizumab with standard chemotherapy in advanced nonsquamous NSCLC confirmed the modest benefit of bevacizumab.[82,83]

Glioblastoma multiforme

The FDA granted accelerated approval of bevacizumab for the treatment of advanced glioblastoma multiforme in May 2009. This was based on a noncomparative phase II study (the BRAIN study) of 167 patients with recurrent glioblastoma multiforme after prior treatment with temozolomide and radiation. Patients were randomly assigned to either bevacizumab alone at 10 mg/m^2 every 2 weeks or bevacizumab with irinotecan. Patients with active intracranial hemorrhage were excluded. Patients were stratified by Karnofsky performance status and relapse (first or second). Six-month PFS and objective response rates were the co-primary endpoints. These were compared to expected results from historical controls. The 6-month PFS was 50.2% in the combination therapy arm and 35.1% in the bevacizumab-alone arm, both of which were much higher than the expected rate of 15%. In addition, response rates were 33% in the combination arm and 20% in the bevacizumab-alone arm. Median OS was equivalent in both arms, 8.9 months in the single-agent arm and 9.7 months in the combination arm. Grade 3 or worse adverse events were higher in the combination arm (67.1% versus 47.6%).[84] A second phase II study in glioblastoma with prior temozolomide and radiation therapy evaluated lomustine, bevacizumab, or the combination of bevacizumab and lomustine. The primary outcome, 9-month OS, was 43%, 38%, and 63% in the three treatment arms, respectively.[85] However, a phase III trial evaluating lomustine compared to lomustine plus bevacizumab did not show a benefit in OS.[86] Notably, these studies have shown that intracranial hemorrhage with bevacizumab in glioblastoma occurs but rates are low (2% to 3%). Although bevacizumab has not clearly shown a benefit in OS as second-line treatment, it has demonstrated radiographic responses and a steroid-sparing effect.[84,85] Two studies evaluated adding bevacizumab to temozolomide and radiation as part of the initial treatment for glioblastoma. Despite improvements in PFS, bevacizumab did not improve OS and was associated with increased toxicities.[87,88]

Cervical Cancer

The FDA expanded bevacizumab's approval to include persistent, recurrent, or metastatic cervical cancer in 2014. This was based on results from the GOG 240, which randomized 452 patients to chemotherapy with or without bevacizumab 15 mg/kg every 3 weeks. Patients had a good performance status (ECOG PS 0 or 1) and about three fourths of the patients had received prior therapy with a platinum and chemotherapy. The trial was a 2×2 design with patients receiving either paclitaxel and topotecan or paclitaxel and cisplatin for chemotherapy. No difference was seen between the chemotherapy regimens, so the bevacizumab analysis was done combining both chemotherapy regimens. The addition of bevacizumab was associated with improved ORR, PFS, and OS. The OS was 17.0 versus 13.3 mo (HR 0.71, 98% CI 0.54 to 0.95) and response rate was 48% versus 35% (P = 0.008). Toxicities were increased with bevacizumab and were in line with previously described toxicities. Notably, the rate of gastrointestinal-vaginal fistulas was significantly higher with bevacizumab (8.2% versus 0.9%). All fistulas occurred in patients who had received prior radiation. The addition of bevacizumab was associated with higher toxicity.[89]

Ovarian Cancer

In a phase II study of single-agent bevacizumab at 15 mg/kg every 3 weeks in 62 patients with persistent or recurrent epithelial ovarian cancer or primary peritoneal cancer, 13 patients (21.0%) experienced clinical responses (two complete, 11 partial) with a median response duration of 10 months.[90] Activity was seen in other phase II trials with and without concurrent chemotherapy. These led to a phase III study, the AURELIA study, that included 361 patients with platinum-resistant ovarian cancer. These patients had an initial benefit with platinum therapy, received no more than two lines of prior therapy, and did not have a history of bowel obstruction. Patients were randomized to investigator's choice chemotherapy (paclitaxel, topotecan, or pegylated liposomal doxorubicin) alone or with bevacizumab 10 mg/kg. Crossover to single-agent bevacizumab at disease progression was permitted in the chemotherapy-alone arm and 40% of this group received bevacizumab monotherapy. The addition of bevacizumab resulted in an improved ORR (31% versus 13%) and PFS (6.7 versus 3.4 months, HR 0.48, 95% CI 0.38 to 0.60). However, the impact on OS was not statistically significant (16.6 versus 13.3 months, HR 0.85, 95% CI 0.66 to 1.08), which maybe at least partially related to crossover. Although toxicities increased with bevacizumab (i.e., hypertension, proteinuria), the rates of severe complications remained low. This includes a perforation rate of 2.2% (lower than in previous ovarian cancer and bevacizumab trials.[91] Data from the AURELIA study led to the FDA approval of bevacizumab for platinum-resistant recurrent epithelial ovarian, fallopian tube, or primary peritoneal cancer.

Two additional studies evaluated bevacizumab for first-line therapy in newly diagnosed epithelial ovarian cancer. GOG 218 treated 1873 woman with stage III or IV disease to standard chemotherapy (carboplatin and paclitaxel), chemotherapy and bevacizumab, or chemotherapy and bevacizumab with bevacizumab maintenance. The median PFS was 10.3, 11.2, and 14.1 months, respectively. Only the maintenance group had a significant improvement in PFS, and none of the groups showed improvement in OS.[58] The second study, ICON7, included over 1500 patients to chemotherapy or chemotherapy with concurrent bevacizumab followed by bevacizumab maintenance. It also showed a modest improvement in PFS without an OS benefit.[92] Unplanned subgroup analyses in both studies of high-risk patients (ascites, residual disease, inoperable, or metastatic) showed a survival benefit but has not been validated prospectively.[58,92] Given the limited benefit in PFS, without improvement in OS and with increased toxicity, bevacizumab has not been approved for first-line therapy in ovarian cancer.

Bevacizumab in other histologies

With the important role angiogenesis plays in cancer biology, bevacizumab has been evaluated in many tumor types. It has demonstrated activity in endometrial cancer, angiosarcoma, and mesothelioma, although its use in these settings is off-label.[93-95] In gastric cancer although improved response rates and PFS were seen, it did not prolong survival.[96] Similarly, there was initial promise for its use in breast cancer, but ultimately no benefit in survival was seen. In pancreatic cancer, a well-designed phase III study failed to show benefit with bevacizumab.[97]

Bevacizumab's accelerated approval in 2008 for first-line treatment of human epidermal receptor-2 (Her2)–negative metastatic breast cancer was revoked in 2011. The initial accelerated approval was based on the ECOG 2100 trial of paclitaxel with or without bevacizumab in first-line treatment for metastatic breast cancer. The study showed an impressive improvement in PFS of 6 months from 5.9 to 11.8 months and an improved response rate (21.2% versus 36.9%) with the addition of bevacizumab. However, the OS was unchanged (25.2 versus 26.7 months, HR 0.88, P = 0.16).[98] Subsequent studies and a meta-analysis of these data failed to show improvement in survival or quality of life. The addition of bevacizumab was also associated with increased toxicity.[99] After review of these findings, the FDA decided to withdraw its approval of bevacizumab for breast cancer.

Clinical Summary: Bevacizumab

Bevacizumab has demonstrated modest activity with improvements in PFS and OS as monotherapy or in combination with chemotherapy in multiple different tumors. This monoclonal antibody is only available as an intravenous infusion. The dose of bevacizumab varies with disease state and coadministered chemotherapy. There are no known drug-drug interactions. However, its use in combination with other chemotherapy has increased toxicities. Toxicities associated with bevacizumab are those described for VEGF pathway inhibition. The prolongation of survival from bevacizumab is quite modest. The toxicities of bevacizumab must be balanced against the degree of expected benefit in deciding upon its use.

Ziv-Aflibercept (VEGF-trap, Zaltrap)

Chemistry

Ziv-Aflibercept is a fusion protein of human VEGF receptor extracellular domain and the Fc portion of human immunoglobulin G1.[100] It is a dimeric glycoprotein with a molecular weight of 115 kDa with glycosylation. It is a clear, colorless to pale yellow solution at a pH of 6.2 that should be diluted with sodium chloride or dextrose solution for infusion.

Mechanism of action

Aflibercept serves as a soluble decoy receptor that binds VEGF-A, VEGF-B, and placental growth factor (PlGF). Aflibercept was developed to provide more effective antiangiogenic action given its inhibition of VEGF-B and PlGF in addition to the VEGF-A inhibition shared with bevacizumab. PlGF levels increase in the setting of VEGF inhibition. Aflibercept's inhibition of PlGF pathways may help address a potential mechanism of bevacizumab resistance. Animal xenograft models suggested increased antitumor activity when compared to bevacizumab.[101]

Pharmacokinetics, Interactions, and Special Populations

The recommended dosing is 4 mg/kg as an IV infusion over 2 hours every 2 weeks. It has an elimination half-life of 6 days (range 4 to 7 days).[102] Based on population pharmacokinetic analysis, aflibercept exposure in patients with mild to moderate hepatic impairment and mild, moderate, or severe renal dysfunction was similar to patients with normal liver and kidney function, respectively. While no formal drug interaction studies have been conducted, there are no contraindicated drugs or predicted interactions. It has not been adequately studied in pediatric patients. In elderly patients, it is associated with increased toxicity, especially diarrhea and dehydration. However, no dose adjustment is recommended for age. Based on its mechanism of action and animal studies demonstrating embryotoxicity and teratogenicity, fetal harm is expected if there is exposure during pregnancy.

Toxicity

When the combination of aflibercept with FOLFIRI is compared to placebo with FOLFIRI in patients with refractory metastatic CRC, there was an increase in many common side effects including diarrhea (69.2% versus 56.5%), fatigue (60.4% versus 50.2%), stomatitis (54.8% versus 34.9%), infection (46.2% versus 32.7%), hypertension (41.4% versus 10.7%), hemorrhage (37.8% versus 19%), anorexia (31.9% versus 23.8%), weight loss (31.9% versus 14.4%), dysphonia (25.4% versus 3.3%), HFSR% (11% versus 4.3%), and neutropenia (67.8% versus 56.3%).[103] The most common > grade 3 toxicities were hypertension, diarrhea, fatigue, and stomatitis. Grade 3 or greater adverse events were more frequent in the aflibercept arm than placebo (83.5 versus 62.5%). Toxicities including hypertension, vascular events, proteinuria, and risk for gastrointestinal perforation or fistula were consistent with those seen with other anti-VEGF therapies.

Therapeutic Uses

Colorectal Cancer

A phase I study of aflibercept demonstrated safety and preliminary efficacy in combination with FOLFIRI in advanced solid malignancies.[104] A following phase II study demonstrated very limited single-agent activity with expected toxicities evaluated in refractory metastatic CRC patients with and without prior bevacizumab exposure. For bevacizumab-naïve patients, the median PFS was 2.0 months, the median OS was 10.4 months, and partial response rate was 21%. For patients with prior bevacizumab, the median PFS was 2.4 months, median OS was 8.5 months, partial response rate was 2%, and stable disease rate was 12%.[105] The phase III VELOUR trial

evaluated the efficacy of aflibercept versus placebo in combination with 5-fluorouracil, leucovorin, and irinotecan (FOLFIRI) in patients with metastatic CRC who had progressed on prior oxaliplatin-based chemotherapy.[103] The study included 1226 patients of which 69.5% had not received prior bevacizumab therapy. There was a statistically significant improvement in the primary endpoint of median OS (13.5 versus 12.6 months, HR 0.817, 95% CI 0.71 to 0.93) as well as median PFS (6.9 versus 4.8 months, HR 0.76, 95% CI 0.66 to 0.87) and response rate 19.8 versus 11.1%. Even in patients with prior bevacizumab, there was a trend towards improved OS (HR 0.86, 95% 0.67 to 1.10) and a statistically significant prolongation of median PFS (HR 0.66, 95% CI 0.51 to 0.85). Based on this study, the FDA approved the drug in 2012 for oxaliplatin-resistant metastatic CRC. The AFFIRM trial, a phase II trial evaluating the benefit of aflibercept in the first-line setting for metastatic CRC in combination with FOLFOX, demonstrated no difference in the median PFS or response rate.[106]

Clinical Summary

Aflibercept is a fusion protein that behaves as a decoy receptor, binding to VEGF-A, VEGF-B, and PlGF. The added inhibition of VEGF-B and PlGF was hypothesized to provide benefit over bevacizumab in circumventing a potential resistance pathway. However, its role is clinical practice thus far is limited. It showed only modest benefit in second-line treatment with irinotecan-based chemotherapy for mCRC. The role of aflibercept is still poorly defined with the lack of data directly comparing it with bevacizumab, the benefit of continuation of bevacizumab after progression, costs and toxicities associated with aflibercept, and much more extensive clinical experience with bevacizumab.[5] Studies in other histologies have helped define toxicities, but survival benefit was not seen in phase III studies in pancreatic and NSCLC.[107,108]

Ramucirumab (Cyramza)

Chemistry

Ramucirumab is a recombinant IgG1 monoclonal antibody that binds to the VEGFR-2 receptor.

Mechanism of Action

Ramucirumab has specific binding to VEGFR-2, thus inhibiting its ligand-associated activity. By blocking binding of VEGFA ligand to VEGFR-2, phosphorylation of VEGFR2 and downstream signaling is inhibited. Its increased specificity for VEGFR-2 when compared to bevacizumab leaves VEGFR-1 unbound and able to serve as a decoy receptor for VEGFA, increasing the degree of inhibition.[109]

Pharmacokinetics, Interactions, and Special Populations

The recommended dose is 8 mg/kg every 2 weeks as monotherapy, with paclitaxel for gastric and gastroesophageal junction (GEJ) carcinoma or with FOLFIRI for CRC. In NSCLC, ramucirumab 10 mg/kg is given every 3 weeks with docetaxel. The terminal half-life is 14 days. Based on pharmacokinetic data, there is no dose adjustment recommended for renal dysfunction or mild to moderate hepatic dysfunction. Of note, clinical deterioration was seen with single-agent ramucirumab in patients with Childs-Pugh B or C. There are no known drug interactions. No difference in efficacy was observed in older patients treated with ramucirumab and no dose adjustment is recommended for age. It has not been studied adequately in pediatric patients. Based on its mechanism of action, there is concern for fetal harm.

Toxicity

When given as a single agent, for a median duration of 8 weeks in gastric or GEJ adenocarcinoma patients, the most common toxicities that were increased with ramucirumab compared to placebo were hypertension (16% versus 8%) and diarrhea (14% versus 9%). Other relevant toxicities included neutropenia (4.7% versus 0.9%), epistaxis (4.7% versus 0.9%), and rash (4.2% versus 1.7%).[47] In the RAINBOW trial, gastric and GEJ cancer patients were randomized to receive paclitaxel and ramucirumab or paclitaxel and placebo with a median duration of exposure of 18 weeks. The most common toxicities likely associated ramucirumab (based on increased incidence when compared with the placebo arm) were fatigue (57% versus 44%), neutropenia (54% versus 41%), diarrhea (32% versus 23%), epistaxis (31% versus 7%), stomatitis (20% versus 7%), hypertension (25% versus 6%), and thrombocytopenia (13% versus 6%). Severe adverse events (>grade 3) occurred in 47% of patients compared with 42% in the placebo and paclitaxel arm. Despite the higher rate of neutropenia, neutropenic fever was rare and similar between both groups (3% versus 2%). The rate of discontinuation due to adverse events was also similar between the two groups (12% versus 11%).[110] The combination with docetaxel had a similar adverse event profile as with paclitaxel. In this study, the rate of grade 3 or 4 adverse events increased from 72% to 79% with the addition of ramucirumab to docetaxel.[111] When combined with FOLFIRI, toxicities were as expected with each individual drug, with an increased rate of discontinuation most frequently due to neutropenia and thrombocytopenia.[112] Toxicities expected with antiangiogenic medications including bleeding and clotting events, gastrointestinal perforation, hypertension, and impaired wound healing were seen.

Therapeutic Uses

Colorectal Cancer

The double-blind, phase III RAISE study included 1072 patients with metastatic CRC who had progressed after first-line treatment with fluoropyrimidine, oxaliplatin, and bevacizumab.[112] Patients were randomized to receive FOLFIRI with ramucirumab or placebo. There was a modest improvement in the primary endpoint of median OS (13.3 versus 11.7 months, HR 0.84, 95% CI 0.73 to 0.98) and improved median PFS (5.7 versus 4.5, HR 0.79, 95% CI 0.70 to 0.90). There was an accompanying increase in toxicity as described above. The hazard ratio for improved survival is similar to that seen in studies evaluating other antiangiogenic agents (bevacizumab and aflibercept) in the second-line setting for patients with metastatic CRC.[31,103]

Gastroesophageal Junction and Gastric Cancer

Based on safety and activity demonstrated in earlier phase trials, the REGARD trial investigated ramucirumab monotherapy compared to placebo as second-line therapy for gastric or GEJ

adenocarcinoma. This phase III international trial of 355 patients showed improvement in OS that just met statistical significance (HR 0.78, 95% CI 0.60, 0.998).[47] The RAINBOW trial evaluated combination therapy in a similar patient population. It was a large double-blinded international trial of patients with advanced gastric or GEJ adenocarcinoma with disease progression on or within 4 months of first-line chemotherapy. The study randomized 665 patients with a good performance status (ECOG 0 or 1) to ramucirumab with paclitaxel or placebo with paclitaxel. There was improvement in the primary endpoint of median OS (9.6 versus 7.3 months, HR 0.81, 95% CI 0.68 to 0.96). There was concordant improvement in median PFS (4.4 versus 2.9 months, HR 0.64, 95% CI 0.54 to 0.75) and response rate (28% versus 16%). Patients who received ramucirumab were more likely to have stable or improved quality of life scores and delayed symptom deterioration when compared to those treated with placebo. This suggests the increased toxicity with ramucirumab may be outweighed by improved disease control.[113] Data from the REGARD and RAINBOW studies led to ramucirumab's 2012 FDA approval as monotherapy or with paclitaxel for second-line treatment of advanced or metastatic gastric or GEJ cancer.

A subsequent randomized phase II trial evaluated ramucirumab with FOLFOX versus placebo with FOLFOX in the first-line setting in 168 patients with advanced GEJ cancer. No benefit in the primary endpoint of median PFS (6.4 versus 6.7 months, HR 0.98) or median OS (11.7 versus 11.5 months) was seen.[114] This is consistent with the lack of benefit in the AVAGAST clinical trial of bevacizumab with chemotherapy in the front-line setting for advanced gastric cancer.[96]

Non–Small Cell Lung Cancer

The REVEL trial evaluated 1253 patients with NSCLC who progressed after initial platinum-based chemotherapy. The study population consisted of patients with ECOG performance status 0 or 1, 26% of patients had squamous histology, and 14% of patients had received prior bevacizumab. Patients were randomized to docetaxel with or without ramucirumab. The study met its primary endpoint with improved median OS (10.5 versus 9.1 months HR 0.86, 95% CI 0.75 to 0.98). The median PFS was superior with ramucirumab plus docetaxel compared with the docetaxel plus placebo (4.5 versus 3.0 months, HR 0.76, 95% CI 0.68 to 0.86). This modest improvement in survival and outcomes was associated with an increase in toxicity.[111] Quality of life data from the REVEL study have similar quality of life, symptoms, and time to deterioration in both arms.[115] Ramucirumab was approved for metastatic NSCLC in 2014.

Clinical Summary

Ramucirumab is a monoclonal antibody with specific VEGFR-2–binding activity. Toxicities are consistent with those expected with VEGF inhibition. Clinical trials have led to its approval in gastric cancer, NSCLC, and mCRC. However, with its modest impact on survival, cost, and toxicities, careful evaluation of risks and benefits should be undertaken. Further studies to evaluate its use in earlier lines of therapy, other tumor types, and in novel combinations are underway.

Oral Tyrosine Kinase Inhibitors of the Vascular Endothelial Growth Factor Receptor

There are a rapidly growing number of VEGFR-targeting TKIs. As a class, these drugs offer the advantage of oral dosing, a shorter half-life, and targeting of other tyrosine kinases that maybe involved with tumor pathogenesis or resistance. Unfortunately, disadvantages include lower target affinity and more promiscuous activity with increased off-target side effects and a dependence on an oral route for administration.

Sorafenib (Nexavar)

Chemistry

Sorafenib tosylate is also known by the chemical name, 4-(4{3-[4-chloro-3(trifluoromethyl)phenyl]ureidophenoxy)-N-methylpyridine-2-carboxamide-4-methylbenzenesulfonate. Its molecular formula is $C_{21}H_{16}ClF_3N_4O_3 \times C_7H_8O_3S$ and it has a molecular weight of 637.0 g/mole.[116,117]

Mechanism of Action

Sorafenib targets the adenosine triphosphate (ATP)-binding site of multiple receptor tyrosine kinases including VEGFR-1, -2, and -3. In addition, sorafenib is known to target Raf kinase, PDGFR β; FMS-like tyrosine kinase 3 (Flt-3); c-Kit protein (KIT); and RET receptor tyrosine kinases.[116] These receptor tyrosine kinases are important for tumor angiogenesis, proliferation, and metastatic progression.

Pharmacokinetics, Interactions, and Special Populations

Sorafenib is an orally bioavailable drug that reaches peak plasma levels approximately 3 hours after administration.[116] With a high-fat meal, sorafenib bioavailability is reduced 29% compared with fasting bioavailability. Therefore, it is recommended that it be taken on an empty stomach. In vitro binding of sorafenib to human plasma proteins is 99.5%. The mean elimination half-life is between 25 and 48 hours. Sorafenib is metabolized primarily in the liver.[116] Oxidative metabolism of sorafenib is mediated by CYP3A4, and glucuronidation is mediated by UGT1A9. The parent drug accounts for approximately 70% to 85% of the circulating analytes in plasma at steady state. After oral administration, the majority of the dose is excreted in feces, with only 19% excreted in urine as glucuronidated metabolites. In patients with mild (Child-Pugh A) or moderate (Child-Pugh B) hepatic impairment, drug exposure values were within the range observed in patients with no hepatic impairment with no dose adjustments needed.[116] A phase I study of sorafenib did demonstrate that patients with a baseline bilirubin 3 to 10× upper limit normally did not tolerate sorafenib even at 200 mg dosed every 3rd day and those with a baseline albumin of less than 2.5 g/dL could only tolerate 200 mg once daily. In patients with moderate renal dysfunction, no relationship was observed between renal function and steady-state sorafenib area under the curve (AUC) at doses of 400 mg twice daily.[116] A phase I study showed that 400 mg twice daily is tolerated in those patients with CrCl of 40 to 59 mL/min and the maximum tolerated dose was 200 mg once daily with a CrCl 20 to 39.[116]

Cytochrome P450 3A4 (CYP3A4) inhibition did not alter the mean AUC of an oral dose of sorafenib.[116] Although not clinically reported, inducers of CYP3A4 activity are expected to increase metabolism of sorafenib and thus decrease sorafenib concentrations. Administration of sorafenib tablets did not alter the exposure of concomitantly given midazolam (CYP3A4 substrate), dextromethorphan (CYP2D6 substrate), omeprazole (CYP2C19 substrate), or warfarin (CYP2C9 substrate). However, exposure to CYP2B6 and CYP2C8 substrates is expected to increase when given with sorafenib. The pharmacokinetic parameters of several chemotherapeutic agents are affected by sorafenib. The AUC of irinotecan (and other UGT1A1 and UGT1A9 substrates), docetaxel, and doxorubicin increases with coadministration of sorafenib. In addition, the AUC of 5-FU changes with sorafenib.

The safety, efficacy, and pharmacokinetic profile of sorafenib in pediatric patients have not been established, although a phase I study in children with solid tumors suggested that the maximum tolerated dose was 200 mg/m² twice daily.[118] Toxicities were more frequent in the elderly.[119] Nevertheless, its use was associated with an improved quality of life in the elderly. If used during pregnancy, fetal harm is expected because of its mechanism of action and animal studies.

Toxicity

The most common any-grade side effects with sorafenib when compared to placebo in RCC were diarrhea (43% versus 13%), hypertension (17% versus 2%), rash or desquamation (40% versus 16%), and HFSR (30% versus 7%), Cardiac ischemia or infarction occurred in 12 patients in the sorafenib group (3%) and 2 patients in the placebo group (<1%) (P = 0.01).[120] In patients with HCC, predominant side effects included grade 1 or 2 diarrhea, weight loss, HFSR, alopecia, anorexia, and voice changes. Grade 3 adverse events that were significantly increased in the sorafenib group included diarrhea (8% versus 2%), HFSR (8% versus 4%), weight loss (2% versus 1%), hypophosphatemia (11% versus 2%), and grade 3 or 4 thrombocytopenia (4% versus <1%).[121]

Therapeutic Uses

Renal Cell Cancer

Sorafenib was the first VEGF TKI approved for RCC based on results of the TARGET trial. This was a phase III randomized double-blind placebo-controlled trial of sorafenib in 903 patients with clear cell RCC that was resistant to cytokine therapy.[120] Patients had good performance status (ECOG 0 and 1), low or intermediate prognostic risk RCC, and no prior antiangiogenic therapy. Sorafenib was dosed at 400 mg twice daily. A preplanned interim analysis of PFS showed a statistically significant benefit of sorafenib over placebo (5.5 versus 2.8 months; P < 0.01). Consequently, crossover was permitted. There was a nonsignificant improvement in median OS (17.8 versus 15.2 mo, HR = 0.88; P = 0.146).[122] Interestingly, a secondary analysis censoring those placebo patients who crossed over showed a survival benefit for sorafenib, suggesting that the survival endpoint had likely been affected by the crossover. Based on this study, the FDA has approved sorafenib for advanced RCC in 2005.

Since that time, two studies compared sorafenib with axitinib in the first- and second-line setting in metastatic RCC.[123,124] These demonstrated an improved PFS with axitinib, although this was also associated with increased toxicity. A phase III study evaluating its adjuvant use in high-risk RCC failed to show improved survival.[125] As a result of these studies and rapidly increasing options for treatment in RCC, sorafenib's use in RCC is decreasing.

Hepatocellular Carcinoma

The investigation of sorafenib for HCC stemmed from literature implicating the Raf-1 and VEGF pathways in the molecular pathogenesis of HCC.[121] Preclinical studies in hepatocellular cell lines showed that sorafenib had antiproliferative activity. It also reduced tumor angiogenesis and tumor cell signaling and increased tumor apoptosis in a mouse xenograft model of human HCC. A subsequent single-arm phase II study involving 137 patients with advanced HCC showed that sorafenib treatment resulted in a median OS of 9.2 months and a median time to progression of 5.5 months, an improvement over historical data.[126] This was followed by the SHARP trial, a randomized placebo-controlled multicenter phase III study of 602 previously untreated patients with Child-Pugh liver function class A cirrhosis and advanced HCC.[121] Patients received either sorafenib 400 mg twice daily or placebo. The primary endpoint, median OS, was significantly improved in the sorafenib group (10.7 versus 7.9 months, HR 0.69; $P < 0.001$). No significant difference was noted between the two groups in the median time to symptomatic progression (4.1 versus 4.9 mo, $P = 0.77$). Only 2% of patients in the sorafenib group had a partial response. This study was the basis of the FDA's approval of sorafenib for advanced HCC in 2007. Since then, sorafenib failed to show benefit as adjuvant treatment for HCC.[127]

Thyroid

In 2013, the FDA-approved indications for sorafenib were expanded to include progressive differentiated thyroid cancer (DTC) that is radioiodine refractory. The approval was based on a phase III study of 417 patients with progressive radioiodine refractory DTC who were randomized to sorafenib or placebo. The primary endpoint of mPFS improved from 5.8 to 10.8 months with sorafenib (HR 0.59, 95% CI 0.45 to 0.76). Toxicity was common and required dose adjustment in 64.3% and discontinuation of drug in 18.8% of patients.[128] Analysis after a third of the patients had died did not show a benefit in survival.

Clinical Summary: Sorafenib

Sorafenib is a multiple receptor TKI that is approved for the treatment of advanced RCC, HCC, and DTC. With its broad spectrum of activity, it has also demonstrated activity in various other tumor types. It is an oral agent, metabolized in the liver, with a number of drug interactions. Side effects include class effects of VEGF inhibitors and TKIs. Rash, skin reactions, and gastrointestinal side effects are frequently seen. Despite its modest benefit in metastatic disease, adjuvant studies have not shown a survival benefit.

Sunitinib Malate (Sutent)

Chemistry

Sunitinib malate is described chemically as butanedioic acid, hydroxy-, (2S)-, compound with N-[2-(diethylamino)ethyl]-5-[(Z)-(5-fluoro-1,2-dihydro-2-oxo-3H-indol-3-ylidene)methyl]-2,4-dimethyl-1H-pyrrole-3-carboxamide (1:1).[129] The molecular formula is $C_{22}H_{27}FN_4O_2 \cdot C_4H_6O_5$ and the molecular weight is 532.6 daltons. It is a yellow to orange powder with a pK_a of 8.95.

Mechanism of Action

Sunitinib is an oral inhibitor of multiple receptor tyrosine kinases. Some of its known receptor targets include VEGFR, PDGFR, KIT, Flt-3, colony-stimulating factor receptor type 1 (CSF-1R), and the glial cell line–derived neurotrophic factor receptor (RET).[129] These receptor tyrosine kinases play a key role in tumor growth, angiogenesis, and metastatic progression.

Both the VEGF and PDGF pathways are thought to play a role in the pathogenesis of renal clear cell carcinoma, as noted above. Sunitinib's activity in gastrointestinal stromal tumors (GIST) likely primarily relates to its targeting of KIT, which can be constitutively active.

Pharmacokinetics, Interactions, and Special Populations

Sunitinib is an oral agent. It reaches its peak plasma concentrations between 6 and 12 hours after dosing and levels are unaffected by concomitant food intake.[129] Binding of sunitinib and its primary metabolite to human plasma proteins in vitro were 95% and 90%, respectively. Metabolism of sunitinib to its primary active metabolite occurs predominantly by the hepatic cytochrome P450 enzyme CYP3A4. The terminal half-lives of sunitinib and its active metabolite are approximately 40 to 60 hours and 80 to 110 hours, respectively. Steady-state conditions of sunitinib and its active metabolite are reached in about 2 weeks. The majority of sunitinib is eliminated in the feces. No clinically relevant effects of age, body weight, creatinine clearance, race, sex, or ECOG performance score on sunitinib's pharmacokinetics have been identified. Cotreatment with the potent CYP3A4 inhibitor ketoconazole doubled the sunitinib AUC, whereas cotreatment with the potent CYP3A4 inducer rifampin reduced the AUC by half. Therefore, caution should be used with drugs known to be inducers or inhibitors of CYP3A4. In addition, when administered with bevacizumab in a phase I trial, microangiopathic hemolytic anemia was observed. Its recommended dosing for RCC and GIST is 50 mg daily with 4 weeks on treatment, 2 weeks off. For pancreatic neuroendocrine tumor (PNET), sunitinib is given continuously at 37.5 mg daily. Mild and moderate hepatic dysfunction and mild, moderate, or severe renal dysfunction do not require dose adjustment. However, it is metabolized by the liver and has not been studied in Child-Pugh Class C hepatic dysfunction.

Sunitinib is likely to have fetal harm if taken during pregnancy based on its mechanism of action and animal studies. Breastfeeding is not recommended while taking sunitinib due to the potential secretion into breast milk. The safety, efficacy, and pharmacokinetic profile of sunitinib in pediatric patients have not been established, although a phase I trial suggests similar pharmacokinetics.[130] Elderly patients achieve clinical benefit with increase in some toxicities (i.e., fatigue, decreased appetite).[131]

Toxicities

Toxicities with sunitinib are consistent with those expected from VEGF TKIs. In a large phase III trial, the most frequent toxicities with sunitinib compared to IFN-α included gastrointestinal side effects (diarrhea 66%, nausea 58%, stomatitis 47%), HFSR (29%), hypertension (34%), rash (29%), and fatigue (62%).[132] A decline in left ventricular ejection fraction was seen in 10% of patients, but only 2% of these were severe. Dose-dependent QT interval prolongation is also seen. An increase in bleeding was seen compared to IFN-α (37% versus 10%). Abnormalities of liver enzymes, neutropenia, and thrombocytopenia were also seen. Dose interruptions and reductions were seen in over half of sunitinib-treated patients. Although severe hepatotoxicity is uncommon, rare cases of liver failure and death were observed.

Therapeutic Uses

Renal Cell Cancer

After promising phase II studies in RCC, sunitinib was evaluated with a phase III trial comparing sunitinib to the standard first-line therapy of interferon alpha (IFN-α).[132] In this study, 750 patients with previously untreated, metastatic RCC with a clear cell histologic component were treated with either sunitinib 50 mg once daily for 4 weeks, followed by a 2-week break, or IFN-α at a dose of 9 million units subcutaneously three times weekly. Over 90% of patients had favorable or intermediate risk disease. The primary endpoint of median PFS was longer in the sunitinib group than in the IFN-α group (11 versus 5 months, HR 0.42; $P < 0.001$). A higher response rate was noted with sunitinib than IFN-α (47% versus 12%; $P < 0.001$). Despite subsequent anti-VEGF therapy in the majority of patients in both treatment arms, an advantage in OS was seen in the sunitinib arm (26.4 versus 21.8 months, HR 0.82, 95% CI 0.67 to 1.00).[133] Notably, patients in the sunitinib group reported a significantly better quality of life than did patients in the IFN-α group ($P < 0.001$). In 2006, the FDA approved sunitinib for advanced RCC. Studies evaluating it as adjuvant therapy in high-risk RCC showed a prolongation in disease-free survival but no benefit in OS and added toxicity leading to frequent discontinuation.[125,134]

Gastrointestinal Stromal tumor

Sunitinib targets GIST primarily through the KIT receptor tyrosine kinase, not via VEGF-mediated antiangiogenic effects. An international, randomized, double-blind, placebo-controlled trial in patients having advanced GISTs and imatinib intolerance or resistance led to its FDA approval in GIST after imatinib therapy in 2006. The study compared sunitinib 50 mg/d 4 weeks on/2 weeks off ($n = 207$) to placebo ($n = 105$).[135] The primary endpoint of time to tumor progression showed significant benefit with sunitinib (27.3 versus 6.4 weeks, HR, 0.33; $P < 0.0001$). This led to unblinding of the study and crossover of all placebo patients to open-label sunitinib. Objective response rates were low (6.8% with partial response and 17.4% with stable disease >22 weeks). An initial advantage in OS was diminished with subsequent follow-up, in the context of crossover and subsequent therapies.

Pancreatic Neuroendocrine Tumor

In a phase III study of 171 patients with progressive metastatic PNET, sunitinib 37.5 mg daily was compared to placebo.[136] Efficacy noted at an interim analysis resulted in early termination of accrual. The primary endpoint of median PFS showed improvement with sunitinib versus placebo of 11.4 versus 5.5 months. Response rates

were low (9.3%) and an initial benefit in OS was not statistically significant in subsequent analysis, potentially due to crossover to sunitinib in 69% of patients in the placebo arm. This led to its 2011 FDA approval for well-differentiated PNET that is unresectable, advanced, or metastatic.

Clinical Summary: Sunitinib

Sunitinib is used to treat advanced RCC, PNET, and GISTs. Standard dosing is 50 mg daily with 4 weeks on/2 weeks off in RCC and GIST and 37.5 mg daily in PNET. Alternative schedule to improve tolerability has also been studied. It is metabolized through the liver and inducers or inhibitors of CYP3A4 may affect sunitinib concentrations. Side effects include those typically described with VEGF inhibition and TKI use. Although not approved for these indications, studies have shown activity in other malignancies including soft tissue sarcomas (STS) and refractory thyroid cancer. It has not been shown to offer benefit in the adjuvant setting in RCC.

Pazopanib Hydrochloride (Votrient)

Chemistry

Pazopanib hydrochloride is a synthetic imidazolylpyrimidine known chemically as 5-[[4-[(2,3-dimethylindazol-6-yl)-methylamino]pyrimidin-2-yl]amino]-2-methylbenzenesulfonamide.[137] The molecular formula is $C_{21}H_{23}N_7O_2S$ and the molecular weight is 437.522 g/mol.[117]

Mechanism of Action

Pazopanib is a small molecule multi-TKI that competitively binds to the ATP-binding pocket of multiple intracellular tyrosine kinase domains. This results in the inhibition of VEGF-1, -2, -3, PDGFR-α and -β, and c-kit with more modest inhibition of FGFR-1 and -3, interleukin receptor-2 receptor-inducible T cell kinase (ItK), leukocyte-specific protein tyrosine kinase (Lck), and transmembrane glycoprotein receptor tyrosine kinase (c-Fms). Its antioncogenic action is thought to be primarily antiangiogenic via inhibition of VEGFR-2. Pazopanib's prevention of ATP binding to the intracellular tyrosine kinase domain inhibits VEGF-induced VEGFR-2 phosphorylation and downstream signal transduction.[137]

Pharmacokinetics, Drug Interactions, and Special Populations

Pazopanib is manufactured as 200 mg tablet that is gray and capsule shaped. Administration results in a peak concentration at 2 to 4 hours. It reached a plateau in steady-state concentration at a dose of >800 mg daily.[138] At 800 mg daily, patients achieved a mean C_{max} of 132 μM and a steady-state concentration of >15 μg/mL in 93% of patients (a level that correlated with clinical activity). Accordingly, 800 mg daily was the recommended phase II dose and is the currently recommended initial dose.

The tablet should not be crushed as doing so increased the AUC by 46% and C_{max} by twofold, while decreasing the time to maximum concentration. Administration with food caused a twofold increase in bioavailability. Therefore, pazopanib should be taken at least 2 hours after and 1 hour before a meal. Its half-life is for elimination is 31.1 hours (range 20.3 to 52.3 hours). Pazopanib has >99%

binding to human plasma protein. It is metabolized by CYP3A4 with a minor contribution from CYP1A2 and CYP2C8. Pazopanib is primarily eliminated in the feces, with renal clearance accounting for <4%. For patients with mild hepatic dysfunction, the standard dose of 800 mg daily was tolerated; moderate hepatic dysfunction, the maximum tolerated dose was 200 mg daily; and severe hepatic dysfunction, pazopanib is not recommended. There are no recommended dose adjustments for renal dysfunction.

Given its primary metabolism by CYP3A4, coadministration with strong enzyme inhibitors should be avoided, and if needed, the pazopanib starting dose should be reduced to 400 mg daily. Concomitant use with ketoconazole (a potent inhibitor of CYP3A4) resulted in an increase of the 24-hour AUC of 66%. Pazopanib's solubility is pH dependent, and concomitant use with a proton pump inhibitor resulted in a 40% reduction of drug exposure. Accordingly, drugs increasing gastric pH should be avoided or if needed should be changed to short-acting medications that are separated by several hours from pazopanib. Pazopanib inhibits multiple CYP enzymes, UGT1A1, and OATP1B1, thus potentially increasing concentrations of drugs metabolized by these enzymes. However, in clinic studies, it was shown to not change exposure to caffeine (CYP1A2 substrate), warfarin (CYP2C9 substrate), or omeprazole (CYP2C19 substrate). It did increase exposure to midazolam (CYP3A4 substrate) by 30% and dextromethorphan (CYP2D6 substrate) by 33% to 64%. Additionally, concurrent use with paclitaxel (a CYP3A4 and CYP2C8 substrate) caused a 26% to 31% increase in paclitaxel levels.

There is only limited phase I data of pazopanib in pediatric patients. Based on its mechanism of action, pazopanib is not recommended during pregnancy or with breastfeeding. Pazopanib may affect fertility based on male and female rats.

Toxicity

In a phase III clinical trial evaluating pazopanib in patients with advanced RCC, the most common clinical toxicities of any grade when compared to placebo were diarrhea (52% versus 9%), hypertension (40% versus 10%), hair color changes (38% versus 3%), nausea (26% versus 9%), anorexia (22% versus 10%), vomiting (21% versus 8%), and fatigue (19% versus 8%). Abnormalities of transaminases (ALT, 53% versus 22%), bilirubin (36% versus 10%), and electrolytes (hypophosphatemia, 34% versus 11%) were seen. Mild neutropenia and thrombocytopenia were seen in about one third of patients. The most common grade 3 or higher adverse reactions include hypertension (4%) and diarrhea (4%). Arterial thrombotic events occurred in 3% of patients (myocardial ischemia in 2%, cerebrovascular event in <1%, and TIA in <1%). Hemorrhagic events were also more common in pazopanib-treated patients (13% versus 5%), with about 1% having a serious hemorrhagic event.[48,139] QTc prolongation >500 ms was seen in 2% of patients and torsades de pointes occurred in 2 of 977 patients on pazopanib monotherapy clinical trials. Cardiac dysfunction (although primarily asymptomatic) was noted in 13% of patients with advanced RCC and 11% of patients with STS receiving pazopanib monotherapy.[140,141] Other rare but severe adverse events observed in with pazopanib monotherapy in a phase III clinic trial include gastrointestinal perforation or fistula, interstitial lung disease, thrombotic microangiopathy, and RPLS syndrome. Pazopanib

carries a black box warning for hepatotoxicity given severe and fatal reported cases of hepatotoxicity. Patients should have regular monitoring of liver tests with drug interruptions, dose reductions, or drug discontinuation as necessary based on degree or recurrence of abnormality. Baseline and periodic electrocardiogram and electrolytes are recommended given concern for QTc prolongation.

In a phase III studies, 14% to 24% of patients discontinued pazopanib due to adverse events.[140,142] Health-related quality of life (HRQoL) outcomes for pazopanib-treated patients support its tolerability. Rates of HRQoL deterioration was similar to placebo-treated RCC and STS patients, and patients who had a treatment response to pazopanib had less HRQoL worsening.[143,144] When compared with sunitinib, pazopanib was associated with more transaminase abnormalities, but less fatigue, HFSR, and thrombocytopenia.[140] In an early crossover study, 70% (95% CI 60.9–78.4%) of mRCC patients reported a preference for pazopanib over sunitinib.[145]

Therapeutic Uses

Renal Cell Cancer

After showing single-agent activity in phase I and II trials in RCC, pazopanib was approved by the FDA for the treatment of advanced RCC in 2009 based on results of a phase III randomized, double-blind, placebo-controlled clinical trial.[48,139] Of the 435 patients with locally advanced or metastatic RCC who were randomized to pazopanib or placebo in a 2:1 fashion, 54% were treatment-naïve and the rest had received prior cytokine therapy. Patients had clear cell (91%) or predominantly clear cell histology (9%). The study showed that pazopanib prolonged the primary endpoint of PFS from 4.2 to 9.2 months. The hazard ratio for recurrence was 0.46 (95% CI 0.34 to 0.62). The response rate was 30% (95% CI, 25.1% to 35.6%) versus 3% with placebo and the median duration of response was over a year. Although no OS benefit was observed, this was thought to be related to a high crossover rate. Over half of patients originally in the placebo arm received pazopanib in an open-label extension arm.[139] An additional phase III trials evaluating pazopanib in mRCC with clear cell histology demonstrated pazopanib's noninferiority to sunitinib with a PFS of 8.4 months and OS of 28.3 months.[140,146] Accordingly, pazopanib carries a category 1 designation for the first-line treatment of predominantly clear cell histology mRCC in the NCCN guidelines and is also indicated for subsequent lines of therapy. Although it has not been well studied in non–clear cell mRCC, it is FDA-approved for this indication and is considered an acceptable treatment option with supportive phase II data.[147]

Soft Tissue Sarcoma

A phase II trial of pazopanib demonstrated activity in pazopanib in three of four STS subcategories including leiomyosarcoma, synovial sarcoma, and other STS but not liposarcoma.[148] A subsequent phase III, international trial randomized 369 STS patients 2:1 to pazopanib 800 mg daily or placebo.[141] Liposarcoma and GIST were excluded and patients must have had progressive disease during or after standard chemotherapy (including an anthracycline). Pazopanib demonstrated improved PFS (4.6 versus 1.6 months) with a hazard ratio of 0.31 (95% CI 0.24 to 0.40; $P < 0.0001$). The difference in OS (12.5 versus 10.7 months) was not statistically significant (HR 0.86, 0.67–1.11; $P = 0.25$). These studies led to pazopanib's approval in 2012 by the FDA for the treatment of advanced STS (except liposarcoma and GIST) who has received prior chemotherapy. Ongoing studies are evaluating pazopanib's efficacy in liposarcoma and phase II data suggest some efficacy in refractory GIST with significant associated toxicities.[149]

Clinical Summary

Pazopanib has actions at multiple receptor tyrosine kinases and is approved for the treatment of advanced clear cell RCC and STS (except liposarcoma and GIST). It carries typical toxicities associated with VEGF inhibition and anti-VEGF TKIs. It is recommended to monitor liver tests during therapy. Additionally, gastrointestinal side effects and fatigue are common. Loss of hair pigmentation is a unique side effect. Pazopanib is associated with less HFSR than sorafenib or sunitinib. Although not approved by the FDA for other indications, pazopanib has demonstrated activity in other malignancies including differentiated advanced thyroid cancer, where the NCCN guidelines endorse its use in an appropriate patient who does not have options for clinical trials based on data from a single-arm phase II trial of 39 patients demonstrating a response rate of 49% (95% CI 35 to 68).[150] Its role in combination therapy and activity in other malignancies is under further investigation. A randomized phase III trial of adjuvant pazopanib did not show improvement in disease-free survival.

Axitinib (Inlyta)

Chemistry

Axitinib is a substituted indazole inhibitor, with the chemical name N-methyl-2-[[3-[(E)-2-pyridin-2-ylethenyl]-1H-indazol-6-yl]sulfanyl]benzamide and molecular formula $C_{22}H_{18}N_4OS$. It has a molecular weight of 386.5 g/mol.[151]

Mechanism of Action

Axitinib is a potent small molecule receptor TKI of VEGFR-1, -2, -3 at subnanomolar concentrations.[151] It causes more potent and selective VEGFR inhibition, with limited PDGFR-β and c-Kit inhibition at low nanomolar concentrations. It binds to the intracellular tyrosine kinase domain of VEGFR and prevents VEGF-mediated VEGFR autophosphorylation, inhibiting endothelial cell proliferation and survival.

Pharmacokinetics, Drug Interactions, and Special Populations

Axitinib is produced as 1 and 5 mg tablets that have a red film coat. The recommended starting dose is 5 mg twice daily. If this dose is tolerated without adverse events greater than grade 2, normal blood pressure, and no antihypertensive use for at least 2 consecutive weeks, the dose can be increased to 7 mg twice daily, then again to 10 mg twice daily. For adverse events, the dose can also be decreased to 3 mg twice daily followed by 2 mg twice daily.

Axitinib has greater and faster absorption when a patient is fasting, but given the limited impact on overall AUC, it can be taken with or without food. Its median T_{max} is 2.8 to 4.1 hours and its oral bioavailability is 58%.[151] The drug is >99% plasma protein bound, preferentially to albumin. It has a plasma half-life of 4.1 hours and is primarily metabolized hepatically by CYP3A4/5, with some activity via CYP1A2, CYP2C19, and UGT1A1.

Ketoconazole increased and rifampin decreased axitinib concentrations. Accordingly, concomitant use of strong CYP3A4/5 inhibitors should be avoided, or if needed, the dose of axitinib should be reduced to 50% with further titration based on tolerance. Strong and moderate inducers of CYP3A4/5 should be avoided. Axitinib can be administered with antiacid medication, as studies with proton pump inhibition caused increased absorption time but not change overall drug exposure.

Mild hepatic dysfunction did not affect drug exposure, but the dose should be reduced by about half for patients with moderate hepatic impairment and titrated further based on tolerability. It has not been studies in severe hepatic dysfunction. Although no studies specifically aimed at evaluating the impact of renal dysfunction have been conducted, drug clearance is not significantly impacted by renal dysfunction. No dose adjustment is recommended for mild to severe renal dysfunction, but caution is recommended for axitinib use in end-stage renal disease. Analysis of covariates in multiple pharmacokinetic studies for axitinib suggests decreased clearance in patients over the age of 60 years when compared with those younger. However, this difference was not considered clinically significant and no dose adjustments are recommended based on age.[151] Its use in pediatric patients has not been studied. Embryo-fetal toxicities were noted in mice, but there are not adequate studies in pregnant women.

Toxicity

The toxicity profile of axitinib has been demonstrated in multiple tumor types in phase I and II clinical trials. The AXIS trial was a large phase III trial evaluating axitinib in refractory metastatic RCC patients.[124] Common toxicities of any grade included gastrointestinal (diarrhea 55%, decreased appetite 34%, nausea 32%, weight loss 25%, vomiting 24%), hypertension (40%), fatigue (39%), dysphonia (31%), and HFSR (27%). Anemia and creatinine elevation of any grade were seen in 35% and 55% of patients, respectively. With the standard dosing strategy, the most commonly experienced >grade 3 side effects were gastrointestinal (diarrhea 11%), hypertension (16%), and fatigue (11%). In the AXIS trial, 34% of patients experienced a serious adverse event, but only 4% of patients stopped the medication due to side effects (compared to 8% in the sorafenib arm). Despite these side effects, patient-reported outcomes were similar to sorafenib and relatively stable until near the end of treatment when they worsened, presumably from progression of disease.[152] Other rare or severe side effects include arterial and venous thromboembolic events, hemorrhage, gastrointestinal perforation or fistula, and RPLS syndrome. Patients should have monitoring of standard blood work, thyroid function, and blood pressure.

Therapeutic Use
RCC

Axitinib produces more potent and selective VEGFR inhibition than first-generation oral antiangiogenic medications. After demonstrating safety and activity in phase I and II trials, axitinib was evaluated compared to sorafenib in the first- and second-line setting for RCC with the hope it would have less off-target effects and an improved therapeutic index.[153] The AXIS trial was a large international randomized phase III trial evaluating 723 patients with advanced RCC (clear cell histology) who had progressed despite standard first-line therapy (sunitinib, bevacizumab and interferon-alpha, temsirolimus, or cytokines). Patients were randomized to receive sorafenib 400 mg twice daily or axitinib 5 mg twice daily with titration up to 10 mg twice daily as tolerated. An objective response was seen in 19% of patients and stable disease >20 months was seen in 27% of patients treated with axitinib. AXIS showed an improvement in median PFS with axitinib to 6.7 months from 4.7 months with sorafenib arm (HR 0.665, 95% CI 0.544 to 0.812).[124] This led to axitinib's FDA approval for second-line treatment of advanced RCC in 2012. However, no benefit was shown in OS (axitinib 20.1 versus sorafenib 19.2 months, HR 0.969, 95% CI 0.800 to 1.174).[154] Interestingly, a post hoc exploratory analysis showed that patients who developed hypertension on axitinib therapy with a diastolic blood pressure >90 mm Hg had improved OS and PFS. Axitinib was also compared to sorafenib in 288 treatment-naïve patients with metastatic renal clear cell carcinoma. There was no statistically significant difference in median PFS between the two groups (mPFS axitinib 10.1 versus sorafenib 6.5 mo, HR 0.77, 95% CI 0.56 to 1.05).[123] Although axitinib was tolerated, serious adverse events were higher in the axitinib group (34% versus 25%). Thus, axitinib's use in advanced RCC is limited to patients with clear cell histology and progression on prior therapy.

Clinical Summary

Compared with other anti-VEGF TKIs, axitinib offers more potent and selective VEGFR targeting. Nevertheless, its toxicity profile is similar to other anti-VEGF TKIs. It is approved for use in the second-line setting for advanced RCC. Interestingly, an exploratory analysis suggested that there is a correlation between hypertension on axitinib therapy and disease response. Further studies evaluating its use in other malignancies and in the adjuvant setting are ongoing.

Cabozantinib (Cometriq, Cabometyx)

Chemistry

Cabozantinib's chemical name is 1-N-[4-(6,7-dimethoxyquinolin-4-yl)oxyphenyl]-1-N'-(4-fluorophenyl)cyclopropane-1,1-dicarboxamide, a molecular formula is $C_{28}H_{24}FN_3O_5$, and a molecular weight is 501.5 g/mol.[117]

Mechanism of Action

Cabozantinib is a small molecule inhibitor of multiple receptor tyrosine kinases that acts by reversible competitive inhibition of ATP. It is a potent inhibitor of VEGFR-1, -2, -3, and MET. It also has activity at RET, KIT, AXL, and FLT3.[155]

Pharmacokinetics (Absorption, Distribution, and Elimination)

Cabozantinib is manufactured under the brand name Cometriq in medullary thyroid cancer as 20 and 80 mg capsules. For RCC, it is also known as Cabometyx and produced as 20, 40, and 60 mg tablets. The recommended dose is 140 mg daily for medullary thyroid

cancer. Although 140 mg was the maximum tolerated dose, a subsequent study showed efficacy with improved tolerability at lower doses. Accordingly, 60 mg daily was studied and approved for RCC. The T_{max} is 2 to 5 hours after an oral dose.[156] The tablet has a 19% higher C_{max}; nevertheless, there is less than a 10% difference in AUC between the formulations. Food increases oral absorption by 41% to 57%, thus food should be avoided 2 hours before and 1 hour after administration. In human plasma, it is >99.7% protein bound and has a half-life of 55 to 99 hours with steady state achieved at day 15. It is metabolized by CYP3A4.

Mild and moderate hepatic impairments increase the AUC by 81% and 63%, respectively. Cabozantinib has not been studied in severe hepatic impairment. Mild to moderate renal impairment did not significantly change drug exposure, and exposure has not been studied in severe renal impairment. CYP3A4 inhibitors increased and inducers decreased cabozantinib concentrations. Accordingly, these drugs should be avoided or the dose of cabozantinib should be adjusted. Change in gastric pH with proton pump inhibition does not result in a clinically meaningful change in drug exposure.

Cabozantinib has not been studied in pediatric populations. Age did not make a statistically significant difference in drug exposure in clinical trials with adult patients, although there were limited patients enrolled >65 years. The drug has not been studied in pregnant or nursing women, but embryo-fetal abnormalities were noted in animal studies.

Toxicity

When given as a second-line therapy in the METEOR trial of advanced RCC patients, the most common toxicities of any grade included gastrointestinal side effects (diarrhea 74%, nausea 56%, decreased appetite 46%, emesis 32%, and weight loss 31%), fatigue (56%), HFSR (42%), hypertension (37%), dysgeusia (24%), and hypothyroidism (20%).[157] The most common severe toxicities (> grade 3) were hypertension (15%), diarrhea (11%), fatigue (9%), and HFSR (8%). Toxicities were more common and more severe at higher doses studied in the medullary thyroid carcinoma population. As with other VEGF pathway inhibitors, severe adverse events included hypertension, RPLS, venous or arterial thrombosis, gastrointestinal perforation or fistula, proteinuria, and hemorrhage. Diarrhea, hypertension, and hypothyroidism are managed with standard medical therapies and if needed interruption and/or reduction in dose.

Therapeutic Uses

Medullary Thyroid Cancer

Given its inhibitory effect of the RET, MET, and VEGFR2 pathways, cabozantinib is of interest in medullary thyroid cancers. A phase I clinical trial showed activity with a 29% partial response rate in patients with medullary thyroid cancer.[158] These results were followed by further investigation in the EXAM trial, a phase III, double-blind, placebo-controlled trial involving 330 patients with progressive metastatic medullary thyroid cancer. This showed an improvement in PFS from 4.0 months in the placebo arm to 11.2 months in the cabozantinib arm, leading to its approval by the FDA in 2012 for progressive medullary thyroid cancer.[159] A response rate of 28% was observed cabozantinib and responses occurred in patients with hereditary and sporadic medullary thyroid cancer.

There was no statistically significant difference in OS. However, the subgroup of patients harboring RET mutations had a more pronounced improvement in PFS and a statically significant 25-month improvement in OS. A subsequent analysis showed that subgroups without RET or RAS mutations did not demonstrate improved PFS but cabozantinib still had activity, with a response rate of 21%.[160] VEGF pathway activity in medullary thyroid cancer and responses in patients without RET and RAS mutations suggest that cabozantinib's VEGFR-2 inhibition has relevance, but it is not likely the dominant mechanism of action.

Renal Cell Cancer

Preclinical RCC models demonstrated that chronic antiangiogenic treatment with sunitinib is associated with an increase in MET and AXL signaling and suggest that these are potential resistance mechanisms.[161] VHL tumor suppressor gene is associated with upregulation of VEGFR as well as MET and AXL signaling. High expression of MET and AXL is associated with a poor prognosis. Its inhibitory effect at MET and AXL in addition to VEGFR-2 provides rationale for cabozantinib as first and second line after initial antiangiogenic therapy in advanced RCC.

A phase 1 study of heavily pretreated RCC patients demonstrated a 28% response rate. This was followed by a phase III study, the METEOR trial, 658 patients with advanced clear cell RCC who had received at least one prior VEGFR TKI.[157] Patients were randomized to cabozantinib 60 mg daily or everolimus 10 mg daily. The trial demonstrated improvement in the primary endpoint of median PFS from 3.8 months with everolimus to 7.4 months with cabozantinib (HR 0.58, 95% CI 0.45 to 0.75). Additionally, the cabozantinib arm had an improved ORR (24 versus 4%) and OS (21.4 versus 16.5 months) (HR 0.66, 95% CI 0.53 to 0.83). These findings resulted in cabozantinib's approval for advanced RCC in patients who have received prior anti-angiogenic therapy.

Cabozantinib's efficacy as a second-line anti-VEGF TKI in clear cell RCC and its MET and AXL inhibitory action led to a phase II randomized trial, CABOSUN, evaluating its efficacy in the frontline setting.[162] The study randomized 157 patients with poor-risk untreated advanced clear cell RCC to cabozantinib or sunitinib. Patients treated with cabozantinib had an improved mPFS of 8.2 months compared with 5.6 months in the sunitinib group. Cabozantinib also showed benefit in rate of progression or death with a HR of 0.66 (95% CI 0.46 to 0.95) and ORR (46% versus 18%). Whether cabozantinib moves to the front-line setting in poor-risk RCC patients is still to be determined given limitations of this phase II study and the changing landscape of RCC therapy.

Clinical Summary

Cabozantinib is produced under different trade names and doses for medullary thyroid cancer and RCC. It offers inhibition of MET and AXL signaling, which are increased with VHL loss and sunitinib-resistant RCC. Cabozantinib improved PFS, OS, and response rate when compared to everolimus in the second-line setting. Furthermore, cabozantinib demonstrated an impressive response rate of 46% in the first-line setting along with the improvement in rate of progression and death and PFS in a phase II study when compared to sunitinib. However, the study has notable limitations, and with the rapidly changing treatment landscape in RCC, the ideal sequencing of cabozantinib in treatment of advanced RCC is still to be determined. In medullary thyroid cancer, its action is likely primarily related to RET inhibition; however, VEGFR may offer additional antitumor benefit. Further studies are evaluating its efficacy in non–clear cell RCC, in combination with immune checkpoint inhibition in RCC, and various other tumor histologies.

Lenvatinib (Lenvima)

Chemistry

The chemical name for lenvatinib is 4-[3-Chloro-4-(cyclopropylaminocarbonyl)aminophenoxy]-7-methoxy-6-quinolinecarboxamide. Its molecular formula is $C_{21}H_{19}ClN_4O_4$ and molecular weight is 426.8g/mol.[117]

Mechanism of Action

Lenvatinib is a multiple receptor TKI with action at VEGFR-1, -2, -3; FGFR1, 2, 3, 4; PDGFR-α; KIT; and RET. Its action is by competitive inhibition of ATP at its binding site.[49]

Pharmacokinetics, Drug Interactions, and Special Populations

Lenvatinib is produced as 4 mg and 10 mg capsules. The recommended dose is 24 mg daily for DTC and 18 mg daily when given in combination with everolimus 5 mg daily in RCC. It reaches its T_{max} at 1 to 4 hours after oral administration.[163] Food delayed rate of absorption but did not affect drug absorption. The drug is highly protein bound and has an elimination half-life of 28 hours. It is metabolized by CYP3A4. Drug exposure was not significantly changed with renal impairment and increased with increasing degree of hepatic dysfunction. For severe renal or hepatic dysfunction, the recommended dose is 14 mg and 10 mg daily for DTC and RCC, respectively.

CYP3A inhibition with ketoconazole increased lenvatinib C_{max} by 19% and its induction with rifampicin did not significantly change C_{max}. Lenvatinib's effects on CYP substrates are unlikely to cause a clinically meaningful change in lenvatinib exposure.

In elderly patients, lenvatinib continues to demonstrate improvements in PFS and OS but is associated with higher rates of toxicities. It has not been studied adequately in children, but growth retardation and other toxicities in juvenile animal studies. Additionally, animal studies demonstrated fetal and embryo toxicity, teratogenicity, and excretion in breast milk. Adequate contraception with use is advised and women should not breastfeed while taking lenvatinib.

Toxicity

In the phase III SELECT trial of patients with progressive radioiodine refractory DTC, patients received lenvatinib 24 mg daily.[49] The median duration of therapy was 13.8 months. Frequent toxicities of any grade with lenvatinib compared to placebo were hypertension (68% versus 9%), diarrhea (59% versus 8%), fatigue (59% versus 28%), decreased appetite (50% versus 11%), nausea (41% versus 13%), stomatitis (36% versus 6%), HFSR (32% versus 1%), and proteinuria (31% versus 2%). Grade 3 or higher treatment-related toxicities occurred in 76% of patients compared with 10% in the placebo arm. Dose reductions were required in 67% of patients, but only 14% discontinued therapy compared with 3% in the placebo arm. The most common >grade 3 toxicities with lenvatinib versus placebo arm were hypertension (42% versus 2%), proteinuria (10% versus 0%), decreased weight (9% versus 0%), fatigue (9% versus 2%), and diarrhea (8% versus 0%). Diarrhea and anorexia were the most frequent causes of dose reductions. Of note, there were six reported treatment-related deaths in the lenvatinib group, including one from pulmonary embolism and another from hemorrhagic stroke.

The combination of lenvatinib 18 mg with everolimus 5 mg as approved for advanced RCC is associated with described side effects expected with each individual drug.[164] There was a higher rate of adverse events in the combination arm than each single agent; however, the treatment duration was also significantly longer in the combination arm. Diarrhea was significantly more frequent with the combination, grade 1 to 2 occurring in 65% and grade 3 in 20% of patients.

Therapeutic Uses

Renal Cell Cancer

Studies demonstrate activity of the FGF pathway as a resistance pathway to anti-VEGF therapies. With lenvatinib's inhibitory action at VEGFR and FGF pathways, there was interest in evaluating its efficacy in RCC with progression after prior antiangiogenic therapy. Additionally, the MTOR pathway has been implicated in the pathogenesis of RCC and everolimus has demonstrated efficacy in the second-line setting in RCC. A phase Ib study demonstrated safety of the combination of lenvatinib 18 mg daily with everolimus 5 mg daily. This was followed by a phase II clinical trial comparing lenvatinib 24 mg daily, everolimus 10 mg daily, and the combination of lenvatinib 18 mg daily with everolimus 5 mg daily.[164] The study included 153 patients with advanced clear cell RCC who had progressed after prior therapy with VEGF-targeted therapy. Patients were randomized 1:1:1 in an open-label design. The median PFS was 14.6 months for the combination, 7.4 months for lenvatinib, and 5.5 months for everolimus. The combination had a superior PFS when compared to everolimus with a HR of 0.4 (95% CI 0.24 to 0.68). Compared to lenvatinib single agent, the HR was 0.66 (95% CI 0.39 to 1.10). The objective response rate was 43% with the combination compared with 27% with lenvatinib and 6% with everolimus alone. The median OS 25.5 months for the combination, 18.4 months for lenvatinib, and 17.5 months for everolimus. The HR of the combination versus everolimus was 0.55 (95% CI 0.30 to 1.01) and versus lenvatinib was 0.75 (95% CI 0.43 to 1.3). As a result of these data, the combination of lenvatinib and everolimus was granted FDA approval in 2016 for advanced RCC that has progressed despite one prior antiangiogenic therapy. Given these promising findings, the phase III CLEAR trial is underway, evaluating lenvatinib with everolimus versus lenvatinib with pembrolizumab versus sunitinib at first-line treatment in patients with advanced RCC (NCT 02811861).

Differentiated Thyroid Cancer

VEGF pathway signaling in DTC is associated with more aggressive disease and increased risk for metastases. Additionally, BRAF, RAS, RET, and PDGFR-α are active pathways. Accordingly, receptor TKIs with multiple sites of action are of interest. A phase II trial of lenvatinib in radioiodine refractory DTC showed an objective response rate of 50% and median PFS of 12.6 months.[165] Even in patients with prior antiangiogenic therapy, an ORR of 59% was seen. A follow-up phase III study, the SELECT trial, was a double blind study comparing lenvatinib 24 mg daily to placebo in 392 patients with progressive radioiodine refractory DTC.[49] One in four patients had received prior therapy with a TKI. The primary endpoint of mPFS was impressively improved from 3.6 months in the placebo group to 18.3 months in lenvatinib-treated patients. The ORR was 65% and the HR for disease progression or death was 0.21 (99% confidence interval 0.14 to 0.31, P < 0.001). At an interim analysis, median OS in the lenvatinib group had not been reached and a median OS benefit was not yet demonstrated. However, the study had allowed crossover at progression in the placebo group. After adjusting for crossover, OS was improved in the lenvatinib group with a rank-preserving structural failure time-adjusted HR of 0.53 (95% CI 0.34 to 0.82, P = 0.005). This study led to the FDA approval of the drug in 2015.

Clinical Summary

Lenvatinib is a multiple receptor TKI. While most toxicities are in line with those seen with anti-VEGF TKIs, lenvatinib has higher rates of hypertension but less QT prolongation. Lenvatinib in combination with everolimus as first-line advanced RCC therapy compared to everolimus showed improvement in PFS, OS, and response rate (although OS did not meet statistical significance). However, this was a phase II trial, the combination has not been compared directly to other important first-line agents, and the combination comes with added toxicity and cost. Accordingly, when and if to use, the combination needs to be further studied. However, these data may lead to a change in paradigm with evaluation of combination treatment approaches in RCC. Additionally, lenvatinib showed the most impressive extension of PFS seen thus far in radioiodine refractory DTC.

Regorafenib (Stivarga)

Chemistry

Regorafenib is a biaryl compound with the chemical name for regorafenib is 4-(4-(((4-chloro-3-(trifluoromethyl)phenyl)carbamoyl)amino)-3-fluorophenoxy)-n-methylpyridine-2-carboxamide. Its molecular formula is $C_{21}H_{15}ClF_4N_4O_3$ and molecular weight is 482.8 g/mol. Its structure differs only slightly from sorafenib with the addition of fluorine in its central phenyl ring.[166]

Mechanism of Action

Regorafenib is an ATP-competitive inhibitor of multiple receptor tyrosine kinases. At levels achieved with clinical use, it has action at receptors involved with angiogenesis, tumor growth, and tumor microenvironment. It inhibits VEGFR-1, -2, -3, TIE2, RET, KIT, BRAF, PDGFR, and FGFR.[166] In CRC and HCC, its activity is thought to be through its inhibition of angiogenesis, its inhibition of tumor growth, and its impact on the microenvironment. In GIST, its activity may be primarily based on its KIT inhibition rather than antiangiogenic properties.[167]

Pharmacokinetics, Drug Interactions, and Special Populations

Regorafenib is available as a 40 mg tablet with an FDA-approved dose of 160 mg daily on days 1 to 21 in a 28-day cycle. It has a 69% bioavailability with a T_{max} of 4 hours. It is highly plasma bound (99.5%) and metabolized by CYP3A4 and UGT1A9. Its metabolites (M-2 ad M-5) have similar activity. The half-life for regorafenib, M-2, and M5 are 28, 25, and 51 hours, respectively. Mild and moderate hepatic impairment did not change exposure to regorafenib or its active metabolites. Its use in the setting of severe hepatic impairment has not been studied. Mild renal impairment did not affect drug exposure. The effect of more severe renal dysfunction has not been well studied. Strong inducers of CYP3A4 resulted in a decrease in regorafenib, no change in M-2, and increase in M-5. Accordingly, avoidance of strong CYP3A4 inducers or inhibitors is recommended.

No differences in safety or efficacy were seen in the relatively smaller subgroup of elderly patients enrolled in regorafenib clinical trials. It has not been studied in pediatric patients. Animal studies demonstrated embryolethality and teratogenicity. Pregnancy and nursing should be avoided when taking regorafenib.

Toxicity

In refractory metastatic CRC patients evaluated in the CORRECT trial, the most frequent toxicities with regorafenib (mean duration of therapy 2.8 months) compared to placebo were fatigue (47% versus 28%), HFSR (47% versus 8%), gastrointestinal side effects (diarrhea 34% versus 7%, anorexia 30% versus 15%, oral mucositis 27% versus 4%), dysphonia (29% versus 4%), hypertension (28% versus 6%), and rash (26% versus 4%).[168] Adverse events > grade 3 occurred in 54% versus 14% of patients. The most common serious adverse reactions were HFSR (17% versus <1%), fatigue (9% versus 5%), diarrhea (7% versus 1%), hypertension (7% versus 1%), and rash (6% versus 0%). When compared to placebo, 70% required drug interruption and 20% of patients required dose reductions. This profile was consistent with that seen in the CONCUR trial.[169]

Therapeutic Uses

Colorectal Cancer

A phase 1b study of regorafenib 160 mg daily on days 1 to 21 in a 28-day cycle showed a promising disease control rate in refractory metastatic CRC. The CORRECT trial was a placebo-controlled phase III evaluating regorafenib in refractory metastatic CRC. It enrolled 760 patients who had progressed despite prior fluoropyrimidine, oxaliplatin, irinotecan, an anti-VEGF agent, and if KRAS wild-type, an anti-EGFR therapy, and showed only a modest benefit.[168] In this heavily pretreated setting when regorafenib was compared to placebo, the primary endpoint of median OS was improved from 6.4 versus 5 months (HR 0.77, 95% CI 0.64 to 0.94). Although statistically significant, the difference in median PFS was only 1.9 versus 1.7 months (HR 0.49, 95% CI 0.42 to 0.58). While only five patients (1%) demonstrated an objective response, disease control rate (partial response or stable disease >6 weeks) was improved in the regorafenib group (41% versus 15%). These data led to regorafenib's approval by the FDA in 2012 for refractory metastatic CRC. A second placebo-controlled, randomized phase III

trial (the CONCUR trial) confirmed benefit with regorafenib.[169] This study included 204 Asian patients with metastatic CRC who progressed after standard chemotherapy. Prior anti-VEGF or anti-EGFR targeted therapy was not required, and 40% of patients had not received prior targeted therapy. Regorafenib-treated patients had improved OS (8.8 versus 6.3 months, HR 0.55, 95% CI 0.40 to 0.77), median PFS (3.2 versus 1.7 months, HR 0.31, 95% CI 0.22 to 0.44), and disease control (51% versus 7%). An exploratory analysis showed a statistically significant benefit only in the patients who had not received prior targeted therapy. However, this analysis was limited by a small sample size and differences in subsequent therapies between the groups.

Gastrointestinal Stromal Tumor

The GRID trial evaluated regorafenib compared to placebo in 199 patients with metastatic or unresectable GIST refractory to prior therapy with sunitinib and imatinib.[167] Overall, the tolerability was similar to those described in CRC. Median PFS was improved from 0.9 months with placebo to 4.8 months with regorafenib. The lack of benefit in OS was thought to be a result of crossover at progression in the placebo arm. The FDA approved regorafenib for GIST refractory to imatinib and sunitinib in 2013. Regorafenib's activity in GIST is thought to be primarily an antitumor effect from KIT inhibition rather than an antiangiogenic effect.

Hepatocellular Carcinoma

Since the approval of sorafenib for unresectable HCC, multiple clinical trials of combinations with sorafenib or in the second-line after sorafenib failure have failed to demonstrate improved outcomes. The RESOURCE trial evaluated regorafenib compared to placebo in 573 sorafenib-treated HCC patients who had progression of disease.[170] Patients had a preserved performance status (ECOG 0 to 1) and liver function (Childs-Pugh A). Regorafenib demonstrated an improved median OS (10.6 versus 7.8 months, HR 0.63, 95% CI 0.50 to 0.79). Regorafenib received FDA approval for HCC patients previously treated with sorafenib in 2017.

Clinical Summary

Regorafenib is a multiple TKI with modest activity in a number of different malignancies. It is currently approved for use in refractory CRC, HCC, and GIST. It causes a range of toxicities typically seen in this class of medications, with fatigue, rash, and gastrointestinal symptoms being particularly common. With its current indications, it is important to weight the modest improvement in outcomes with associated side effects and impact on quality of life in patients with refractory disease.

VEGF Inhibitors in Clinical Development

There are many candidate oral anti-VEGF TKIs in various stages of development. Tivozanib has potent and selective VEGF-1, -2, and -3 inhibition and a longer half-life. It is being developed with the hope that its selectivity will reduce off-target side effects. A phase III study in the first-line setting of tivozanib compared to sorafenib and allowed crossover at progression.[171] It showed improved PFS without improved OS and was not approved by the FDA with these findings. Studies in breast and CRC have been negative and a second phase III RCC study is ongoing. Cediranib also inhibits all three VEGFRs and is being studied for use in ovarian cancer, STS, and other malignancies. One phase III study in recurrent platinum-sensitive ovarian cancer found the addition of cediranib to platinum chemotherapy followed by cediranib maintenance improved PFS but added toxicity that led to its frequent discontinuation in the maintenance phase.[172] Nintedanib inhibits VEGFR, FGFR, and PDGFR. It demonstrated a very modest PFS benefit as second-line therapy with docetaxel in NSCLC that was more pronounced in patients with adenocarcinoma.[173] It is approved in the EU for this indication. A number of other VEGF TKIs, including brivanib and motesanib, have been evaluated in numerous clinical trials but failed to show improvement over current therapies, are associated with more toxicities, or require further data.

Mechanisms of Resistance to VEGF Inhibition

Despite the growing number and indications for antiangiogenic agents, their impact on disease progression is temporary. Elucidating mechanisms of resistance and strategies to overcome this is of great interest. Unlike resistance to other therapies targeting tyrosine kinases on the tumor, antiangiogenic resistance is not reliant on mutations in the target tyrosine kinase (on endothelial cells). Our understanding of resistance pathways is incomplete, but proposed mechanisms of acquired resistance include upregulation of VEGF signaling pathways, VEGF-independent angiogenesis, and selection of tumor cells than can survival in hypoxic conditions.

Resistance may be reversible and resistant tumors may still be VEGF-dependent. Preclinical models demonstrate similar gene expression profiles between treat-naïve tumors and sorafenib-resistant tumors implanted into treatment naïve mice and given a treatment holiday. These were distinct from gene expression of resistant tumors, suggesting reversal of changes associated with resistance.[174] Clinically, this principle was seen in case series of sunitinib-resistant RCC that responded to reintroduction of sunitinib after a treatment break.[175] Persistent VEGF-dependence despite progression is evidenced by continued benefit of bevacizumab after progression on therapy in CRC and efficacy of second-line anti-VEGF TKIs despite first-line antiangiogenic agents.[31,124,157,176]

After decreased blood flow with antiangiogenic therapy, perfusion scanning shows restored perfusion of tumors prior to disease progression. This suggests restoration of angiogenesis instead of simply adaption to grow in hypoxic conditions. One mechanism postulated to achieve this is that antiangiogenic agents cause tumor tissue hypoxia and a resultant increase in HIF1A. This causes induction of proangiogenic pathways including VEGF, FGFR, MET, and AXL. An increase in MET and AXL expression is seen in preclinical models and supported by cabozantinib's activity despite resistance to front-line anti-VEGF therapy.[161,177,178] Other VEGF-independent angiogenic pathways include expression of alternate proangiogenic signals and recruitment of bone marrow vascular progenitor cells and proangiogenic monocytes. Resistance may also result from decreased dependency on angiogenesis by selection of tumor cells that can survive in hypoxic conditions or cooption of existing vessels to abrogate the need for VEGF. More details regarding these resistance mechanisms can be found in a number of detailed reviews.[8,75,179]

Biomarkers

Although our armamentarium of angiogenesis inhibitors is growing, their impact on PFS and OS is modest (particularly in non-RCC tumors). Furthermore, they are associated with frequent low-grade toxicities, rare but severe high-grade toxicities, and significant increases in cost. Consequently, there is interest in identifying biomarkers that may help predict patients more likely to respond to VEGF inhibition or to develop severe toxicities. Unfortunately, clinically validated, predictive biomarkers have not been identified. Plasma levels and tissue expression of VEGF and VEGFR-2 and microvessel density are prognostic, but not predictive. Permeability imaging and protein signatures have been studied, but not validated clinically.[8] Further research is needed to identify strategies that optimize the use of angiogenesis inhibitors.

Conclusion

We have a growing arsenal of agents targeting tumor angiogenesis induced by the VEGF pathway that have shown clinical utility in the treatment of a variety of malignancies. There are currently 10 drugs approved by the FDA that target angiogenesis as their primary mechanism of action. Numerous others are in development that target the VEGF pathway or other mechanisms of angiogenesis. However, significant challenges remain with the development and clinical use of angiogenesis inhibitors.

The antiangiogenesis monoclonal antibodies (bevacizumab and ramucirumab) and decoy receptor (aflibercept) have limited single-agent activity and provide modest benefit in combination with chemotherapy. Therefore, the toxicities of chemotherapy are difficult to avoid with these medications. The oral TKIs have single-agent activity in several malignancies but come with toxicities associated with VEGF pathway and receptor tyrosine kinase inhibition. Resistance eventually develops to each of these agents. Interestingly, a number of studies have shown additional benefit of subsequent antiangiogenic therapy after initial anti-VEGF resistance. So far, studies evaluating their use in the adjuvant setting have been uniformly disappointing.

Despite the hypothesis that targeting tumor angiogenesis would have minimal toxicities given the lack of angiogenesis in normal tissues, significant side effects and serious complications have been noted with each of these agents. This includes life-threatening toxicities such as arterial thrombotic events, gastrointestinal perforations, and bleeding. These toxicities may limit the utility of these agents, especially in the adjuvant treatment setting, when many patients may already be cured of their disease.

With the development of novel targeted agents for malignancies, one of the main challenges facing researchers is identifying predictive markers to help classify which patients are likely to benefit from each individual agent. Despite over 30 years of research on angiogenesis with successful identification of many of the key players in this process, no biomarker has been identified that predicts response to the angiogenesis inhibitors. Future studies will evaluate new antiangiogenic agents, novel combinations that target angiogenesis, and their use in other malignancies.

References

1. Folkman J, Tumor angiogenesis: therapeutic implications. *N Engl J Med.* 1971;285(21):1182-1186.

2. Folkman J, Angiogenesis in cancer, vascular, rheumatoid and other disease. *Nat Med.* 1995;1(1):27-31.

3. Hanahan D, Weinberg RA. The hallmarks of cancer. *Cell.* 2000;100(1):57-70.

4. Folkman J, et al. Induction of angiogenesis during the transition from hyperplasia to neoplasia. *Nature.* 1989;339(6219):58-61.

5. Bergers G, Benjamin LE, Tumorigenesis and the angiogenic switch. *Nat Rev Cancer.* 2003;3(6):401-410.

6. Torres Filho IP, et al. Noninvasive measurement of microvascular and interstitial oxygen profiles in a human tumor in SCID mice. *Proc Natl Acad Sci U S A.* 1994;91(6):2081-2085.

7. Semenza GL. Targeting HIF-1 for cancer therapy. *Nat Rev Cancer,* 2003;3(10):721-732.

8. Jayson GC, et al. Antiangiogenic therapy in oncology: current status and future directions. *Lancet.* 2016;388(10043):518-529.

9. Masoud GN, Li W. HIF-1α pathway: role, regulation and intervention for cancer therapy. *Acta Pharm Sin B.* 2015;5(5):378-389.

10. Ferrara N, Gerber HP, LeCouter J, The biology of VEGF and its receptors. *Nat Med.* 2003;9(6):669-676.

11. Kerbel RS. Tumor angiogenesis. *N Engl J Med.* 2008;358(19):2039-2049.

12. Neufeld G, et al. Vascular endothelial growth factor (VEGF) and its receptors. *Faseb J.* 1999;13(1):9-22.

13. Dor Y, Porat R, Keshet E. Vascular endothelial growth factor and vascular adjustments to perturbations in oxygen homeostasis. *Am J Physiol Cell Physiol.* 2001;280(6):C1367.

14. Carmeliet P, et al. Role of HIF-1alpha in hypoxia-mediated apoptosis, cell proliferation and tumour angiogenesis. *Nature.* 1998;394(6692):485-490.

15. Maxwell PH, et al. The tumour suppressor protein VHL targets hypoxia-inducible factors for oxygen-dependent proteolysis. *Nature.* 1999;399(6733):271-275.

16. Okada F, et al. Impact of oncogenes in tumor angiogenesis: mutant K-ras up-regulation of vascular endothelial growth factor/vascular permeability factor is necessary, but not sufficient for tumorigenicity of human colorectal carcinoma cells. *Proc Natl Acad Sci U S A.* 1998;95(7):3609-3614.

17. Tong RT, et al. Vascular normalization by vascular endothelial growth factor receptor 2 blockade induces a pressure gradient across the vasculature and improves drug penetration in tumors. *Cancer Res.* 2004;64(11):3731-3736.

18. Hidalgo M, Eckhardt SG, Development of matrix metalloproteinase inhibitors in cancer therapy. *J Natl Cancer Inst.* 2001;93(3):178-193.

19. Cathcart J, Pulkoski-Gross A, Cao J. Targeting matrix metalloproteinases in cancer: Bringing new life to old ideas. *Genes Dis.* 2015;2(1):26-34.

20. Avraamides CJ, Garmy-Susini B, Varner JA. Integrins in angiogenesis and lymphangiogenesis. *Nat Rev Cancer.* 2008;8(8):604-617.

21. Monk BJ, et al. Anti-angiopoietin therapy with trebananib for recurrent ovarian cancer (TRINOVA-1): a randomised, multicentre, double-blind, placebo-controlled phase 3 trial. *Lancet Oncol.* 2014;15(8):799-808.

22. Shih I-M, Wang T.L. Notch signaling, γ-secretase inhibitors, and cancer therapy. *Cancer Res.* 2007;67(5):1879.

23. Kangsamaksin T, et al. NOTCH decoys that selectively block DLL/NOTCH or JAG/NOTCH disrupt angiogenesis by unique mechanisms to inhibit tumor growth. *Cancer Discov.* 2015;5(2):182-197.

24. Harada Y, Ogata Y, Shirouzu K. Expression of vascular endothelial growth factor and its receptor KDR (kinase domain-containing receptor)/Flk-1 (fetal liver kinase-1) as prognostic factors in human colorectal cancer. *Int J Clin Oncol.* 2001;6(5):221-228.

25. Herbst RS, Onn A, Sandler A, Angiogenesis and lung cancer: prognostic and therapeutic implications. *J Clin Oncol.* 2005;23(14):3243-3256.

26. Linderholm BK, et al. The expression of vascular endothelial growth factor correlates with mutant p53 and poor prognosis in human breast cancer. *Cancer Res,* 2001;61(5):2256-2260.

27. Kim KJ, et al. Inhibition of vascular endothelial growth factor-induced angiogenesis suppresses tumour growth in vivo. *Nature.* 1993;362(6423):841-844.

28. Millauer B, et al. Dominant-negative inhibition of Flk-1 suppresses the growth of many tumor types in vivo. *Cancer Res.* 1996;56(7):1615-1620.

29. Prewett M, et al. Antivascular endothelial growth factor receptor (fetal liver kinase 1) monoclonal antibody inhibits tumor angiogenesis and growth of several mouse and human tumors. *Cancer Res.* 1999;59(20):5209-5218.

30. Skobe M, et al. Halting angiogenesis suppresses carcinoma cell invasion. *Nat Med.* 1997;3(11):1222-1227.

31. Bennouna J, et al. Continuation of bevacizumab after first progression in metastatic colorectal cancer (ML18147): a randomised phase 3 trial. *Lancet Oncol.* 2013;14(1):29-37.

32. Kindler HL, et al. Gemcitabine plus bevacizumab compared with gemcitabine plus placebo in patients with advanced pancreatic cancer: phase III trial of the Cancer and Leukemia Group B (CALGB 80303). *J Clin Oncol.* 2010;28(22):3617-3622.

33. Michaelson MD, et al. Randomized, placebo-controlled, phase III trial of sunitinib plus prednisone versus prednisone alone in progressive, metastatic, castration-resistant prostate cancer. *J Clin Oncol.* 2014;32(2):76-82.

34. An MM, et al. Incidence and risk of significantly raised blood pressure in cancer patients treated with bevacizumab: an updated meta-analysis. *Eur J Clin Pharmacol.* 2010;66(8):813-821.

35. Liu B, et al. Incidence and risk of hypertension associated with vascular endothelial growth factor receptor tyrosine kinase inhibitors in cancer patients: a comprehensive network meta-analysis of 72 randomized controlled trials involving 30013 patients. *Oncotarget.* 2016;7(41):67661-67673.

36. Hamnvik OP, et al. Clinical risk factors for the development of hypertension in patients treated with inhibitors of the VEGF signaling pathway. *Cancer.* 2015;121(2):311-319.

37. Rini BI, et al. Hypertension as a biomarker of efficacy in patients with metastatic renal cell carcinoma treated with sunitinib. *J Natl Cancer Inst.* 2011;103(9):763-773.

38. Mir O, et al. An observational study of bevacizumab-induced hypertension as a clinical biomarker of antitumor activity. *Oncologist.* 2011;16(9):1325-1332.

39. Hurwitz HI, et al. Analysis of early hypertension and clinical outcome with bevacizumab: results from seven phase III studies. *Oncologist.* 2013;18(3):273-280.

40. Maitland ML, et al. Initial assessment, surveillance, and management of blood pressure in patients receiving vascular endothelial growth factor signaling pathway inhibitors. *J Natl Cancer Inst.* 2010;102(9):596-604.

41. Wu S, et al., Bevacizumab increases risk for severe proteinuria in cancer patients. *J Am Soc Nephrol.* 2010;21(8):1381-1389.

42. Zhang Z-F, et al. Risks of proteinuria associated with vascular endothelial growth factor receptor tyrosine kinase inhibitors in cancer patients: A systematic review and meta-analysis. *PLoS One.* 2014;9(3):e90135.

43. Zangari M, et al. Thrombotic events in patients with cancer receiving antiangiogenesis agents. *J Clin Oncol.* 2009;27(29):4865-4873.

44. Scappaticci FA, et al. Arterial thromboembolic events in patients with metastatic carcinoma treated with chemotherapy and bevacizumab. *J Natl Cancer Inst.* 2007;99(16):1232-1239.

45. Hurwitz HI, et al. Venous thromboembolic events with chemotherapy plus bevacizumab: a pooled analysis of patients in randomized phase II and III studies. *J Clin Oncol.* 2011;29(13):1757-1764.

46. Nalluri SR, et al. Risk of venous thromboembolism with the angiogenesis inhibitor bevacizumab in cancer patients: a meta-analysis. *JAMA.* 2008;300(19):2277-2285.

47. Fuchs CS, et al. Ramucirumab monotherapy for previously treated advanced gastric or gastro-oesophageal junction adenocarcinoma (REGARD): an international, randomised, multicentre, placebo-controlled, phase 3 trial. *Lancet.* 2014;383(9911):31-39.

48. Sternberg CN, et al. Pazopanib in locally advanced or metastatic renal cell carcinoma: results of a randomized phase III trial. *J Clin Oncol.* 2010;28(6):1061-1068.

49. Schlumberger M, et al. Lenvatinib versus placebo in radioiodine-refractory thyroid cancer. *N Engl J Med.* 2015;372(7):621-630.

50. Sonpavde G, et al. Venous thromboembolic events with vascular endothelial growth factor receptor tyrosine kinase inhibitors: a systematic review and meta-analysis of randomized clinical trials. *Crit Rev Oncol Hematol.* 2013;87(1):80-89.

51. Hapani S, et al. Increased risk of serious hemorrhage with bevacizumab in cancer patients: a meta-analysis. *Oncology.* 2010;79(1-2):27-38.

52. Qi WX, et al. Incidence and risk of hemorrhagic events with vascular endothelial growth factor receptor tyrosine-kinase inhibitors: an up-to-date meta-analysis of 27 randomized controlled trials. *Ann Oncol.* 2013;24(12):2943-2952.

53. Leighl NB, et al. Bleeding events in bevacizumab-treated cancer patients who received full-dose anticoagulation and remained on study. *Br J Cancer.* 2011;104(3):413-418.

54. Verheul HM, Pinedo HM, Possible molecular mechanisms involved in the toxicity of angiogenesis inhibition. *Nat Rev Cancer.* 2007;7(6):475-485.

55. Hapani S, Chu D, Wu S, Risk of gastrointestinal perforation in patients with cancer treated with bevacizumab: a meta-analysis. *Lancet Oncol.* 2009;10(6):559-568.

56. Richardson DL, et al. Which factors predict bowel complications in patients with recurrent epithelial ovarian cancer being treated with bevacizumab? *Gynecol Oncol.* 2010;118(1):47-51.

57. Perren TJ, et al. A phase 3 trial of bevacizumab in ovarian cancer. *N Engl J Med.* 2011;365(26):2484-2496.

58. Burger RA, et al. Incorporation of bevacizumab in the primary treatment of ovarian cancer. *N Engl J Med.* 2011;365(26):2473-2483.

59. Qi WX, et al. Risk of gastrointestinal perforation in cancer patients treated with vascular endothelial growth factor receptor tyrosine kinase inhibitors: a systematic review and meta-analysis. *Crit Rev Oncol Hematol.* 2014;89(3):394-403.

60. Scappaticci FA, et al. Surgical wound healing complications in metastatic colorectal cancer patients treated with bevacizumab. *J Surg Oncol.* 2005;91(3):173-180.

61. Kozloff M, et al. Clinical outcomes associated with bevacizumab-containing treatment of metastatic colorectal cancer: the BRiTE observational cohort study. *Oncologist.* 2009;14(9):862-870.

62. Chapin BF, et al. Safety of presurgical targeted therapy in the setting of metastatic renal cell carcinoma. *Eur Urol.* 2011;60(5):964-971.

63. Gerber HP, Ferrara N, Pharmacology and pharmacodynamics of bevacizumab as monotherapy or in combination with cytotoxic therapy in preclinical studies. *Cancer Res.* 2005;65(3):671-680.

64. Han K, et al. Population pharmacokinetics of bevacizumab in cancer patients with external validation. *Cancer Chemother Pharmacol.* 2016;78(2):341-351.

65. Kabbinavar F, et al. Phase II, randomized trial comparing bevacizumab plus fluorouracil (FU)/leucovorin (LV) with FU/LV alone in patients with metastatic colorectal cancer. *J Clin Oncol.* 2003;21(1):60-65.

66. Escudier B, et al. Bevacizumab plus interferon alfa-2a for treatment of metastatic renal cell carcinoma: a randomised, double-blind phase III trial. *Lancet.* 2007;370(9605):2103-2111.

67. Johnson DH, et al. Randomized phase II trial comparing bevacizumab plus carboplatin and paclitaxel with carboplatin and paclitaxel alone in previously untreated locally advanced or metastatic non-small-cell lung cancer. *J Clin Oncol.* 2004;22(11):2184-2191.

68. Hurwitz H, et al. Bevacizumab plus irinotecan, fluorouracil, and leucovorin for metastatic colorectal cancer. *N Engl J Med.* 2004;350(23):2335-2342.

69. Yang JC, et al. A randomized trial of bevacizumab, an anti-vascular endothelial growth factor antibody, for metastatic renal cancer. *N Engl J Med.* 2003;349(5):427-434.

70. Rini BI, et al. Bevacizumab plus interferon alfa compared with interferon alfa monotherapy in patients with metastatic renal cell carcinoma: CALGB 90206. *J Clin Oncol.* 2008;26(33):5422-5428.

71. Escudier B, et al. Phase III trial of bevacizumab plus interferon alfa-2a in patients with metastatic renal cell carcinoma (AVOREN): final analysis of overall survival. *J Clin Oncol.* 2010;28(13):2144-2150.

72. Rini BI, et al. Phase III trial of bevacizumab plus interferon alfa versus interferon alfa monotherapy in patients with metastatic renal cell carcinoma: final results of CALGB 90206. *J Clin Oncol.* 2010;28(13):2137-2143.

73. Flaherty KT, et al. BEST: a randomized phase II study of vascular endothelial growth factor, RAF kinase, and mammalian target of rapamycin combination targeted therapy with bevacizumab, sorafenib, and temsirolimus in advanced renal cell carcinoma—A trial of the ECOG-ACRIN Cancer Research Group (E2804). *J Clin Oncol* 2015. 33(21):2384-2391.

74. Saltz LB, et al. Bevacizumab in combination with oxaliplatin-based chemotherapy as first-line therapy in metastatic colorectal cancer: a randomized phase III study. *J Clin Oncol.* 2008;26(12):2013-2019.

75. Giantonio BJ, et al. Bevacizumab in combination with oxaliplatin, fluorouracil, and leucovorin (FOLFOX4) for previously treated metastatic colorectal cancer: results from the Eastern Cooperative Oncology Group Study E3200. *J Clin Oncol.* 2007;25(12):1539-1544.

76. Tol J, et al. Chemotherapy, bevacizumab, and cetuximab in metastatic colorectal cancer. *N Engl J Med.* 2009;360(6):563-572.

77. Hecht JR, et al. A randomized phase IIIB trial of chemotherapy, bevacizumab, and panitumumab compared with chemotherapy and bevacizumab alone for metastatic colorectal cancer. *J Clin Oncol.* 2009;27(5):672-680.

78. Allegra CJ, et al. Initial safety report of NSABP C-08: A randomized phase III study of modified FOLFOX6 with or without bevacizumab for the adjuvant treatment of patients with stage II or III colon cancer. *J Clin Oncol.* 2009;27(20):3385-3390.

79. de Gramont A, et al. Bevacizumab plus oxaliplatin-based chemotherapy as adjuvant treatment for colon cancer (AVANT): a phase 3 randomised controlled trial. *Lancet Oncol.* 2012;13(12):1225-1233.

80. Kerr RS, et al. Adjuvant capecitabine plus bevacizumab versus capecitabine alone in patients with colorectal cancer (QUASAR 2): an open-label, randomised phase 3 trial. *Lancet Oncol.* 2016;17(11):1543-1557.

81. Sandler A, et al. Paclitaxel-carboplatin alone or with bevacizumab for non-small-cell lung cancer. *N Engl J Med.* 2006;355(24):2542-2550.

82. Reck M, et al. Phase III trial of cisplatin plus gemcitabine with either placebo or bevacizumab as first-line therapy for nonsquamous non-small-cell lung cancer: AVAiL. *J Clin Oncol.* 2009;27(8):1227-1234.

83. Soria JC, et al. Systematic review and meta-analysis of randomised, phase II/III trials adding bevacizumab to platinum-based chemotherapy as first-line treatment in patients with advanced non-small-cell lung cancer. *Ann Oncol.* 2013;24(1):20-30.

84. Friedman HS, et al. Bevacizumab alone and in combination with irinotecan in recurrent glioblastoma. *J Clin Oncol.* 2009;27(28):4733-4740.

85. Taal W, et al. Single-agent bevacizumab or lomustine versus a combination of bevacizumab plus lomustine in patients with recurrent glioblastoma (BELOB trial): a randomised controlled phase 2 trial. *Lancet Oncol.* 2014;15(9):943-953.

86. Wick W, et al. EORTC 26101 phase III trial exploring the combination of bevacizumab and lomustine in patients with first progression of a glioblastoma. *J Clin Oncol.* 2016;34(15 suppl):2001-2001.

87. Gilbert MR, et al. A randomized trial of bevacizumab for newly diagnosed glioblastoma. *N Engl J Med.* 2014;370(8):699-708.

88. Chinot OL, et al. Bevacizumab plus radiotherapy-temozolomide for newly diagnosed glioblastoma. *N Engl J Med.* 2014;370(8):709-722.

89. Tewari KS, et al. Improved survival with bevacizumab in advanced cervical cancer. *N Engl J Med.* 2014;370(8):734-743.

90. Burger RA, et al. Phase II trial of bevacizumab in persistent or recurrent epithelial ovarian cancer or primary peritoneal cancer: a Gynecologic Oncology Group Study. *J Clin Oncol.* 2007;25(33):5165-5171.

91. Pujade-Lauraine E, et al. Bevacizumab combined with chemotherapy for platinum-resistant recurrent ovarian cancer: The AURELIA open-label randomized phase III trial. *J Clin Oncol.* 2014;32(13):1302-1308.

92. Oza AM, et al. Standard chemotherapy with or without bevacizumab for women with newly diagnosed ovarian cancer (ICON7): overall survival results of a phase 3 randomised trial. *Lancet Oncol.* 2015;16(8):928-936.

93. Agulnik M, et al. An open-label, multicenter, phase II study of bevacizumab for the treatment of angiosarcoma and epithelioid hemangioendotheliomas. *Ann Oncol.* 2013;24(1):257-263.

94. Lorusso D, et al. Randomized phase II trial of carboplatin-paclitaxel (CP) compared to carboplatin-paclitaxel-bevacizumab (CP-B) in advanced (stage III-IV) or recurrent endometrial cancer: The MITO END-2 trial. *J Clin Oncol.* 2015;33(15_suppl):5502.

95. Zalcman G, et al. Bevacizumab for newly diagnosed pleural mesothelioma in the Mesothelioma Avastin Cisplatin Pemetrexed Study (MAPS): a randomised, controlled, open-label, phase 3 trial. *Lancet.* 2016;387(10026):1405-1414.

96. Ohtsu A, et al. Bevacizumab in combination with chemotherapy as first-line therapy in advanced gastric cancer: a randomized, double-blind, placebo-controlled phase III study. *J Clin Oncol.* 2011;29(30):3968-3976.

97. Kindler HL, et al. A double-blind, placebo-controlled, randomized phase III trial of gemcitabine (G) plus bevacizumab (B) versus gemcitabine plus placebo (P) in patients (pts) with advanced pancreatic cancer (PC): A preliminary analysis of Cancer and Leukemia Group B (CALGB. *J Clin Oncol.* 2007;25(18_suppl):4508.

98. Miller K, et al. Paclitaxel plus bevacizumab versus paclitaxel alone for metastatic breast cancer. *N Engl J Med.* 2007;357(26):2666-2676.

99. Miles DW, et al. First-line bevacizumab in combination with chemotherapy for HER2-negative metastatic breast cancer: pooled and subgroup analyses of data from 2447 patients. *Ann Oncol.* 2013;24(11):2773-2780.

100. Ricci V, M Ronzoni, T Fabozzi, Aflibercept a new target therapy in cancer treatment: a review. *Crit Rev Oncol Hematol.* 2015;96(3):569-576.

101. Chiron M, et al. Differential antitumor activity of aflibercept and bevacizumab in patient-derived xenograft models of colorectal cancer. *Mol Cancer Ther.* 2014;13(6):1636.

102. Lockhart AC, et al. Phase I study of intravenous vascular endothelial growth factor Trap, aflibercept, in patients with advanced solid tumors. *J Clin Oncol.* 2010;28(2):207-214.

103. Van Cutsem E, et al. Addition of aflibercept to fluorouracil, leucovorin, and irinotecan improves survival in a phase III randomized trial in patients with metastatic colorectal cancer previously treated with an oxaliplatin-based regimen. *J Clin Oncol.* 2012;30(28):3499-3506.

104. Van Cutsem E, et al. Phase I dose-escalation study of intravenous aflibercept administered in combination with irinotecan, 5-fluorouracil and leucovorin in patients with advanced solid tumours. *Eur J Cancer.* 2013;49(1):17-24.

105. Tang PA, et al. Phase II clinical and pharmacokinetic study of aflibercept in patients with previously treated metastatic colorectal cancer. *Clin Cancer Res.* 2012;18(21):6023-6031.

106. Folprecht G., et al. Oxaliplatin and 5-FU/folinic acid (modified FOLFOX6) with or without aflibercept in first-line treatment of patients with metastatic colorectal cancer: the AFFIRM study. *Ann Oncol* 2016;27(7):1273-1279.

107. Rougier P, et al. Randomised, placebo-controlled, double-blind, parallel-group phase III study evaluating aflibercept in patients receiving first-line treatment with gemcitabine for metastatic pancreatic cancer. *Eur J Cancer.* 2013;49(12):2633-2642.

108. Ramlau R, et al. Aflibercept and Docetaxel versus Docetaxel alone after platinum failure in patients with advanced or metastatic non-small-cell lung cancer: a randomized, controlled phase III trial. *J Clin Oncol.* 2012;30(29):3640-3647.

109. Javle M, Smyth EC, Chau I, Ramucirumab: Successfully targeting angiogenesis in gastric cancer. *Clin Cancer Res.* 2014;20(23):5875-5881.

110. Wilke H, et al. Ramucirumab plus paclitaxel versus placebo plus paclitaxel in patients with previously treated advanced gastric or gastro-oesophageal junction adenocarcinoma (RAINBOW): a double-blind, randomised phase 3 trial. *Lancet Oncol.* 2014;15(11):1224-1235.

111. Garon EB, et al. Ramucirumab plus docetaxel versus placebo plus docetaxel for second-line treatment of stage IV non-small-cell lung cancer after disease progression on platinum-based therapy (REVEL): a multicentre, double-blind, randomised phase 3 trial. *Lancet.* 2014;384(9944):665-673.

112. Tabernero J, et al. Ramucirumab versus placebo in combination with second-line FOLFIRI in patients with metastatic colorectal carcinoma that progressed during or after first-line therapy with bevacizumab, oxaliplatin, and a fluoropyrimidine (RAISE): a randomised, double-blind, multicentre, phase 3 study. *Lancet Oncol.* 2015;16(5):499-508.

113. Al-Batran SE, et al. Quality-of-life and performance status results from the phase III RAINBOW study of ramucirumab plus paclitaxel versus placebo plus paclitaxel in patients with previously treated gastric or gastroesophageal junction adenocarcinoma. *Ann Oncol.* 2016;27(4):673-679.

114. Yoon HH, et al. Ramucirumab combined with FOLFOX as front-line therapy for advanced esophageal, gastroesophageal junction, or gastric adenocarcinoma: a randomized, double-blind, multicenter Phase II trial. *Ann Oncol.* 2016;27(12):2196-2203.

115. Perol M, et al. Quality of life results from the phase 3 REVEL randomized clinical trial of ramucirumab-plus-docetaxel versus placebo-plus-docetaxel in advanced/metastatic non-small cell lung cancer patients with progression after platinum-based chemotherapy. *Lung Cancer.* 2016;93:95-103.

116. Kane RC, et al. Sorafenib for the treatment of advanced renal cell carcinoma. *Clin Cancer Res.* 2006;12(24):7271-7278.

117. National Center for Biotechnology Information. PubChem Compound Database;CID=216239,https://pubchem.ncbi.nlm.nih.gov/compound/216239.

118. Widemann BC, et al. A phase I trial and pharmacokinetic study of sorafenib in children with refractory solid tumors or leukemias: A children's oncology group phase I consortium report. *Clin Cancer Res,* 2012;18(21):6011-6022.

119. Eisen T, et al. Sorafenib for older patients with renal cell carcinoma: subset analysis from a randomized trial. *J Natl Cancer Inst.* 2008;100(20):1454-1463.

120. Escudier B, et al. Sorafenib in advanced clear-cell renal-cell carcinoma. *N Engl J Med.* 2007;356(2):125-134.

121. Llovet JM, et al. Sorafenib in advanced hepatocellular carcinoma. *N Engl J Med.* 2008;359(4):378-390.

122. Bukowski RM et al. Final results of the randomized phase III trial of sorafenib in advanced renal cell carcinoma: Survival and biomarker analysis. *J Clin Oncol.* 2007;25(18_suppl):5023.

123. Hutson TE, et al. Axitinib versus sorafenib as first-line therapy in patients with metastatic renal-cell carcinoma: a randomised open-label phase 3 trial. *Lancet Oncol.* 2013;14(13):1287-1294.

124. Rini BI, et al. Comparative effectiveness of axitinib versus sorafenib in advanced renal cell carcinoma (AXIS): a randomised phase 3 trial. *Lancet.* 2011;378(9807):1931-1939.

125. Haas NB, et al. Adjuvant sunitinib or sorafenib for high-risk, non-metastatic renal-cell carcinoma (ECOG-ACRIN E2805): a double-blind, placebo-controlled, randomised, phase 3 trial. *Lancet.* 2016;387(10032):2008-2016.

126. Abou-Alfa GK, et al. Phase II study of sorafenib in patients with advanced hepatocellular carcinoma. *J Clin Oncol.* 2006;24(26):4293-4300.

127. Bruix J, et al. Adjuvant sorafenib for hepatocellular carcinoma after resection or ablation (STORM): a phase 3, randomised, double-blind, placebo-controlled trial. *Lancet Oncol.* 2015;16(13):1344-1354.

128. Brose MS, et al. Sorafenib in radioactive iodine-refractory, locally advanced or metastatic differentiated thyroid cancer: a randomised, double-blind, phase 3 trial. *Lancet.* 2014;384(9940):319-328.

129. Goodman VL, et al. Approval summary: sunitinib for the treatment of imatinib refractory or intolerant gastrointestinal stromal tumors and advanced renal cell carcinoma. *Clin Cancer Res.* 2007;13(5):1367-1373.

130. Dubois SG, et al. Phase I and pharmacokinetic study of sunitinib in pediatric patients with refractory solid tumors: a children's oncology group study. *Clin Cancer Res.* 2011;17(15):5113-5122.

131. Hutson TE, et al. Efficacy and safety of sunitinib in elderly patients with metastatic renal cell carcinoma. *Br J Cancer.* 2014;110(5):1125-1132.

132. Motzer RJ, et al. Sunitinib versus interferon alfa in metastatic renal-cell carcinoma. *N Engl J Med.* 2007;356(2):115-124.

133. Motzer RJ et al., Overall survival and updated results for sunitinib compared with interferon alfa in patients with metastatic renal cell carcinoma. *J Clin Oncol.* 2009;27(22):3584-3590.

134. Ravaud A, et al. Adjuvant sunitinib in high-risk renal-cell carcinoma after nephrectomy. *N Engl J Med.* 2016;375(23):2246-2254.

135. Demetri GD, et al. Efficacy and safety of sunitinib in patients with advanced gastrointestinal stromal tumour after failure of imatinib: a randomised controlled trial. *Lancet.* 2006;368(9544):1329-1338.

136. Raymond E, et al. Sunitinib malate for the treatment of pancreatic neuroendocrine tumors. *N Engl J Med.* 2011;364(6):501-513.

137. Hamberg P, J Verweij, S Sleijfer, (Pre-)clinical pharmacology and activity of pazopanib, a novel multikinase angiogenesis inhibitor. *Oncologist.* 2010;15(6):539-547.

138. Verheijen RB, et al. Clinical pharmacokinetics and pharmacodynamics of pazopanib: Towards optimized dosing. *Clin Pharmacokinet.* 2017;56(9):987-997

139. Sternberg CN, et al. A randomised, double-blind phase III study of pazopanib in patients with advanced and/or metastatic renal cell carcinoma: final overall survival results and safety update. *Eur J Cancer.* 2013;49(6):1287-1296.

140. Motzer RJ, et al. Pazopanib versus sunitinib in metastatic renal-cell carcinoma. *N Engl J Med.* 2013;369(8):722-731.

141. van der Graaf, WT, et al. Pazopanib for metastatic soft-tissue sarcoma (PALETTE): a randomised, double-blind, placebo-controlled phase 3 trial. *Lancet.* 2012;379(9829):1879-1886.

142. Sternberg CN, et al. An open-label extension study to evaluate safety and efficacy of pazopanib in patients with advanced renal cell carcinoma. *Oncology.* 2014;87(6):342-350.

143. Cella D, et al. Health-related quality of life in patients with advanced renal cell carcinoma receiving pazopanib or placebo in a randomised phase III trial. *Eur J Cancer.* 2012;48(3):311-323.

144. Coens C, et al. Health-related quality-of-life results from PALETTE: a randomized, double-blind, phase 3 trial of pazopanib versus placebo in patients with soft tissue sarcoma whose disease has progressed during or after prior chemotherapy—a European Organization for research and treatment of cancer soft tissue and bone sarcoma group global network study (EORTC 62072). *Cancer.* 2015;121(17):2933-2941.

145. Escudier B, et al. Randomized, controlled, double-blind, cross-over trial assessing treatment preference for pazopanib versus sunitinib in patients with metastatic renal cell carcinoma: PISCES study. *J Clin Oncol.* 2014;32(14):1412-1418.

146. Motzer RJ, et al. Overall survival in renal-cell carcinoma with pazopanib versus sunitinib. *N Engl J Med.* 2014;370(18):1769-1770.

147. Jung KS, et al. Pazopanib for the treatment of non-clear cell renal cell carcinoma: A single-arm, open-label, multicenter, phase II study. *Cancer Res Treat.* 2018;50(2):488-494.

148. Sleijfer S, et al. Pazopanib, a multikinase angiogenesis inhibitor, in patients with relapsed or refractory advanced soft tissue sarcoma: A phase II study from the european organisation for research and treatment of cancer—soft tissue and bone sarcoma group (EORTC Study 62043). *J Clin Oncol.* 2009;27(19):3126-3132.

149. Mir O, et al. Pazopanib plus best supportive care versus best supportive care alone in advanced gastrointestinal stromal tumours resistant to imatinib and sunitinib (PAZOGIST): a randomised, multicentre, open-label phase 2 trial. *Lancet Oncol.* 2016;17(5):632-641.

150. Bible KC, et al. Efficacy of pazopanib in progressive, radioiodine-refractory, metastatic differentiated thyroid cancers: results of a phase 2 consortium study. *Lancet Oncol.* 2010;11(10):962-972.

151. Chen Y, et al. Clinical pharmacology of axitinib. *Clin Pharmacokinet.* 2013;52(9):713-725.

152. Cella D, et al. Patient-reported outcomes for axitinib vs sorafenib in metastatic renal cell carcinoma: phase III (AXIS) trial. *Br J Cancer.* 2013;108(8):1571-1578.

153. Rixe O, et al. Axitinib treatment in patients with cytokine-refractory metastatic renal-cell cancer: a phase II study. *Lancet Oncol.* 2007;8(11):975-984.

154. Motzer RJ, et al. Axitinib versus sorafenib as second-line treatment for advanced renal cell carcinoma: overall survival analysis and updated results from a randomised phase 3 trial. *Lancet Oncol.* 2013;14(6):552-562.

155. Yakes FM, et al. Cabozantinib (XL184), a novel MET and VEGFR2 inhibitor, simultaneously suppresses metastasis, angiogenesis, and tumor growth. *Mol Cancer Ther.* 2011;10(12):2298-2308.

156. Lacy SA, DR Miles, LT Nguyen, Clinical pharmacokinetics and pharmacodynamics of cabozantinib. *Clin Pharmacokinet.* 2017;56(5):477-491.

157. Choueiri TK, et al. Cabozantinib versus everolimus in advanced renal cell carcinoma (METEOR): final results from a randomised, open-label, phase 3 trial. *Lancet Oncol.* 2016;17(7):917-927.

158. Kurzrock R, et al. Activity of XL184 (cabozantinib), an oral tyrosine kinase inhibitor, in patients with medullary thyroid cancer. *J Clin Oncol.* 2011;29(19):2660-2666.

159. Elisei R, et al. Cabozantinib in progressive medullary thyroid cancer. *J Clin Oncol.* 2013;31(29):3639-3646.

160. Sherman SI, et al. Correlative analyses of RET and RAS mutations in a phase 3 trial of cabozantinib in patients with progressive, metastatic medullary thyroid cancer. *Cancer.* 2016;122(24):3856-3864.

161. Zhou L, et al. Targeting MET and AXL overcomes resistance to sunitinib therapy in renal cell carcinoma. *Oncogene.* 2016;35(21):2687-2697.

162. Choueiri TK, et al. Cabozantinib versus sunitinib as initial targeted therapy for patients with metastatic renal cell carcinoma of poor or intermediate risk: the alliance A031203 CABOSUN trial. *J Clin Oncol.* 2016;35(6):591-597.

163. Hussein Z, et al. Clinical pharmacokinetic and pharmacodynamic profile of lenvatinib, an orally active, small-molecule, multitargeted tyrosine kinase inhibitor. *Eur J Drug Metab Pharmacokinet.* 2017;42(6):903-914

164. Motzer RJ, et al. Lenvatinib, everolimus, and the combination in patients with metastatic renal cell carcinoma: a randomised, phase 2, open-label, multicentre trial. *Lancet Oncol.* 2015;16(15):1473-1482.

165. Sherman SI, et al. A phase II trial of the multitargeted kinase inhibitor E7080 in advanced radioiodine (RAI)-refractory differentiated thyroid cancer (DTC). *J Clin Oncol.* 2011;9(15_suppl):5503-5503.

166. Wilhelm SM, et al. Regorafenib (BAY 73-4506): a new oral multikinase inhibitor of angiogenic, stromal and oncogenic receptor tyrosine kinases with potent preclinical antitumor activity. *Int J Cancer.* 2011;129(1):245-255.

167. Demetri GD, et al. Efficacy and safety of regorafenib for advanced gastrointestinal stromal tumours after failure of imatinib and sunitinib (GRID): an international, multicentre, randomised, placebo-controlled, phase 3 trial. *Lancet.* 381(9863):295-302.

168. Grothey A, et al. Regorafenib monotherapy for previously treated metastatic colorectal cancer (CORRECT): an international, multicentre, randomised, placebo-controlled, phase 3 trial. *Lancet.* 2013;381(9863):303-312.

169. Li J., et al. Regorafenib plus best supportive care versus placebo plus best supportive care in Asian patients with previously treated metastatic colorectal cancer (CONCUR): a randomised, double-blind, placebo-controlled, phase 3 trial. *Lancet Oncol.* 2015;16(6):619-629.

170. Bruix J, et al. Regorafenib for patients with hepatocellular carcinoma who progressed on sorafenib treatment (RESORCE): a randomised, double-blind, placebo-controlled, phase 3 trial. *Lancet.* 2017;389(10064):56-66.

171. Motzer RJ, et al. Tivozanib versus sorafenib as initial targeted therapy for patients with metastatic renal cell carcinoma: results from a phase III trial. *J Clin Oncol.* 2013;31(30):3791-3799.

172. Ledermann JA, et al. Cediranib in patients with relapsed platinum-sensitive ovarian cancer (ICON6): a randomised, double-blind, placebo-controlled phase 3 trial. *Lancet.* 2016;387(10023):1066-1074.

173. Reck M, et al. Docetaxel plus nintedanib versus docetaxel plus placebo in patients with previously treated non-small-cell lung cancer (LUME-Lung 1): a phase 3, double-blind, randomised controlled trial. *Lancet Oncol.* 2014;15(2):143-155.

174. Zhang L, et al. Resistance of renal cell carcinoma to sorafenib is mediated by potentially reversible gene expression. *PLoS One.* 2011. 6(4):e19144.

175. Porta C, Paglino C, Grünwald V, Sunitinib re-challenge in advanced renal-cell carcinoma. *Br J Cancer.* 2014. 111(6):1047-1053.

176. Izar B, et al. Pharmacokinetics, clinical indications, and resistance mechanisms in molecular targeted therapies in cancer. *Pharmacol Rev.* 2013. 65(4):1351-1395.

177. Rini, BI, Atkins MB, Resistance to targeted therapy in renal-cell carcinoma. *Lancet Oncol.* 2009;10(10):992-1000.

178. Choueiri TK, Motzer RJ, Systemic therapy for metastatic renal-cell carcinoma. *N Engl J Med.* 2017;376(4):354-366.

179. Bergers G, D. Hanahan, Modes of resistance to anti-angiogenic therapy. *Nat Rev Cancer.* 2008;8(8):592-603.

Hormone Antagonists

Section 13.4

Hormone

Antagonists

Endocrine Therapy of Breast Cancer

Laura M. Spring and Beverly Moy

Endocrine therapy plays a critical role in the prevention and treatment of breast cancer at all stages of its pathogenesis.[1] This chapter provides an understanding of (a) estrogen synthesis and metabolism, (b) the endocrine regulation of these processes, (c) the molecular basis of estrogen signaling through the estrogen receptor (ER), (d) the response of breast cancer cells to the modulation of ER signaling, (e) the pharmacology of antiestrogen therapeutics, and (f) endocrine therapy resistance.

Estrogen Structure, Biosynthesis, Transport, and Metabolism

Structure of Estrogen

Estrogens are steroids containing a hydrated four-ring structure (cyclopentane-perhydro-phenanthrene), in which a five-sided cyclopentane ring (designated the D ring) is attached to three six-sided phenanthrene rings (designated the A, B, and C rings) (Figs. 27.1 [35.1 from the last edition] and 27.2 [35.2]).

The three endogenous estrogens are estradiol, estrone, and estriol. Estradiol and estrone can be formed directly by aromatization of testosterone and androstenedione, respectively. Estradiol can also be readily formed from estrone and is the principally active estrogen (Fig. 27.3).[2-5] The common and systematic names of selected steroidal hormones and their structures are shown in Figure 27.2.[2-5] The physiologic effects of estrogens are summarized in Table 27.1.

Estrogen Biosynthesis

Estrogen biosynthesis begins from cholesterol. Cytochrome P-450 enzymes convert cholesterol to different steroid hormones via alteration of side chains on the molecule.[6] The final step in estrogen synthesis is aromatization, which is catalyzed by the P-450 aromatase monooxygenase enzyme complex.[6,7] The endocrine regulation of the CYP19 gene on chromosome 15, which spans 120 kb, is intricate, primarily due to a complex and tissue-specific promoter structure, with regulatory elements targeted by gonadotropins, glucocorticoids, growth factors, cytokines, and the intracellular signaling molecule cAMP.[8-11]

In premenopausal women, estrogens are predominantly produced by the ovaries. By contrast, in postmenopausal women, estrogens are formed from the extragonadal conversion of androgens to estrogens via aromatase. Androgens from the ovaries and adrenal glands are released into circulation and converted to estrogens in tissues with aromatase activity, including adipose tissue and muscle.[12]

Estrogen Transport

Estrogens circulate in the bloodstream predominantly bound to albumin and steroid-binding globulins. The estrogens and androgens are transported via testosterone and estradiol-binding globulin or sex steroid–binding globulin.[13] The unbound, or free, hormone, which makes up only 2% to 3% of total circulating estrogens, enters the cell by diffusion through the cell membrane.[6] Once inside the cell, estrogens bind to the ER, thereby starting a complex series of signaling events in the target cell. Local estrogen synthesis within tissues such as the breast may also act as a paracrine factor.[14]

The Estrogen Receptor

ER Structure

The ER is a member of the nuclear hormone receptor superfamily that includes the progesterone receptor (PgR), androgen receptor (AR), glucocorticoid receptor (GR), and mineralocorticoid receptor. This receptor family also includes receptors for nonsteroidal nuclear hormones such as the retinoids, vitamin D or deltanoids, and thyroid hormones.

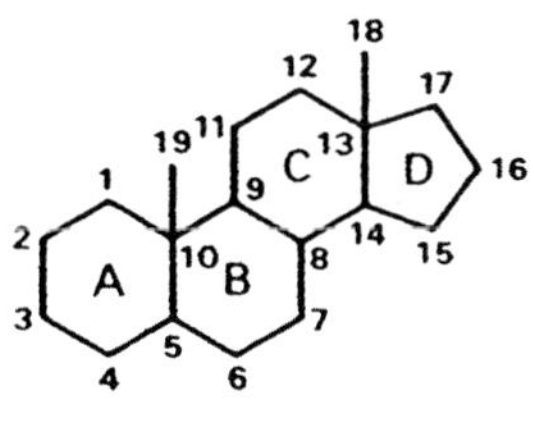

FIGURE **27.1** The structure and numbering of the cyclopentane-perhydrophenanthrene nucleus.

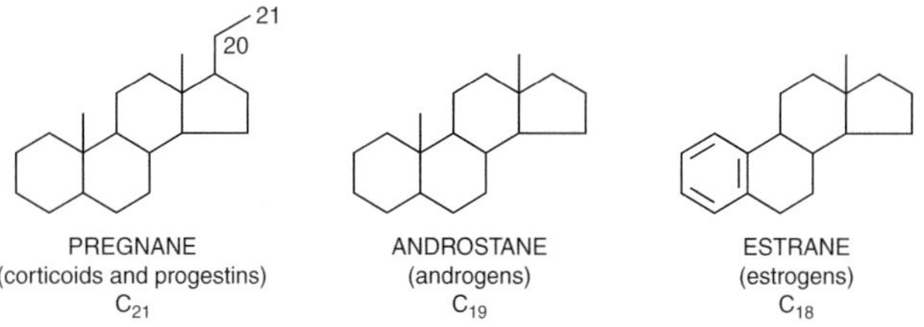

FIGURE **27.2** The structure and names of the five major steroid hormones. (Trivial name is followed by systematic.) Cortisol, 4-pregnen-11β, 17α, 21-triol-3,20-dione; aldosterone, 4-pregnen-11β,21-diol-18-al-3,20-dione; progesterone, 4-pregnen-3,20-dione; testosterone, 4-androsten-17β-ol-3-one; estradiol, 1,3,5(10)-estratrien-3,17β-diol.

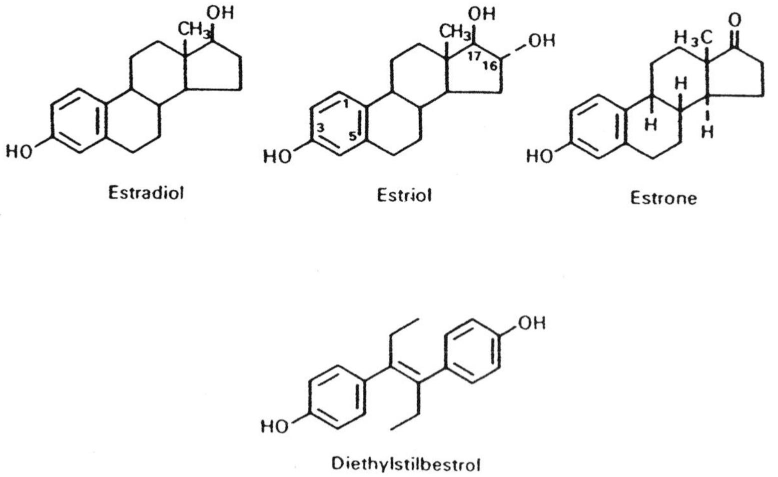

FIGURE **27.3** Endogenous and synthetic estrogens.

The ER, like most nuclear hormone receptors, operates as a ligand-dependent transcription factor that binds to DNA at estrogen response elements (EREs) to direct changes in gene expression in response to hormone binding.[6,15] The ER protein structure includes six domains, designated A to E (Fig. 27.4). Estradiol binds to the ligand-binding site in the E domain. The E domain also mediates ER dimerization, with assistance from residues in domain C. The sequence-specific DNA-binding function resides in domain C. Domain D contains a nuclear localization signal required for transfer of the ER from the cytoplasm to the nucleus. Sequences that promote transcription, or activation functions (AFs), are present in domains A and B (AF1) and domain E (AF2). The basic structure and functional components of steroid hormones follow the same pattern, with a hormone-binding site, a dimerization domain, transactivation domain(s), and a nuclear localization signal.[16]

ER Subtypes: ERα and ERβ

The first identified ER, now known as "ERα," was discovered in the late 1960s, and the gene was cloned in 1986. The second ER, named "ERβ," was first reported in 1996 and has provided a further layer of complexity to our understanding of estrogen-regulated gene expression.[17,18] Furthermore, each subtype of ER exists in several isoforms. At the amino acid level, ERα and ERβ are highly homologous in the DNA-binding domain, but less so in the ligand-binding domain. This structural comparison suggests that the two subtypes would recognize and bind to similar DNA sites. However, the differences in the ligand-binding domain suggest that responses to different ligands may be more distinct than anticipated from primary sequence analysis.[19] There is no consensus on the clinical significance of ERβ since many different studies have conflicting findings. However, breast cancers that coexpress ERα and ERβ tend to be node positive and of a higher grade than tumors that express ERα alone.[20] ERβ-expressing tumors tend to be PgR negative.[21]

Classical ER Signal Transduction

Ligand-Dependent ER Signaling

The well-described classical ER signaling pathway is illustrated in Figure 27.5. Estrogens bind to the ligand-binding domain of the ER, leading to the release of the receptor from heat shock protein 90. This ligand binding is then followed by phosphorylation of the receptor at specific serine residues, ER dimerization, and then sequence-specific DNA binding to a sequence referred to as an ERE. In the presence of estrogen, messenger RNA (mRNA) transcription is promoted through AF2. Residues in AF1 also promote transcription, although the function of AF1 does not require the presence of estrogen.[22] The consensus DNA-binding sites for each of the nuclear hormones are illustrated in Figure 27.6. While the ER binds most strongly to the ERE consensus sequence, it is also capable of promoting transcription through sequences that have only partial homology to a classic ERE. In these cases, nearby response elements for other transcription factors (e.g., SP-1) contribute to ER activity.[22–24] The characteristics of the target gene promoter are critical to the specific nuclear actions of the activated ER. Other factors that are critical are the structure of the bound ligand and the balance of coactivators and corepressors associated with the ER-ligand complex. In addition, ERα and ERβ can either homodimerize or heterodimerize, and this has an impact on their activity at the DNA-binding site.[25]

ER Coactivators and Corepressors

Ligand-bound receptors interact with a family of coactivator and corepressor proteins that are sensitive to the conformational changes that occur in the ligand-binding domain of each receptor. These coregulatory proteins interact with the ER to either increase

TABLE

27.1 *Physiologic effects of estrogens*

Growth and maintenance of female genitalia
Pubertal expression of female secondary sex characteristics
Breast enlargement
Increase in size and pigmentation of nipple and areolae
Molding of body contour with alteration of subcutaneous fat deposition
Promotion of female psyche formation
Alteration in skin texture
Maintenance of pregnancy (in concert with progestins)
Sodium retention

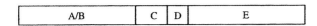

A/B   AF-1 transactivation domain
C   DNA Binding and homodimerization domain
D   NLS and HSP90 binding domain
E   AF-2 transactivation domain

% amino acid homology in relation to GR

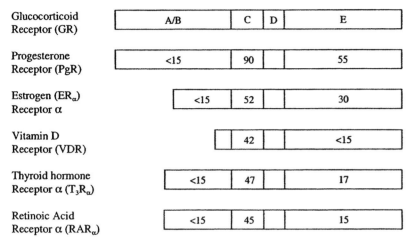

FIGURE **27.4** Examples of amino acid homology between nuclear hormone receptors. A/B, activation function 1 transactivation domain; C, DNA-binding and homodimerization domain; D, nuclear localization signal and heat shock protein 90-binding domain; E, activation function 2 transaction domain.

or decrease transcriptional activity at a promoter site. One key mechanism for the coactivator and corepressor modulation of ER transcription likely involves histone acetylation and methylation.[26] In addition to alteration of chromatin structure and histone acetylation, coactivators may also promote interactions between the nuclear hormone receptor and the basal transcriptional machinery to activate gene transcription.[16] Corepressors have the opposite

function and negatively regulate transcription via recruitment of histone deacetylases.[27]

In general, coactivators and corepressors appear to be expressed at similar levels in many different tissues, suggesting that the responses to estrogen agonists and antagonists are not determined simply by the relative abundance of these cofactors. Instead, differential regulation of coactivator activity appears to occur through other signal transduction pathways.[26]

Nonclassical ER Signal Transduction

ER Activation by Other Signal Transduction Pathways

In addition to classical ER signaling, other ER signaling pathways have been described (Fig. 27.7). Nuclear hormones are not simply receptors for lipid-soluble hormones, but are also critical signaling targets for protein phosphorylation–dependent second messenger pathways.[28] These nuclear hormone receptors cross-talk with growth factor pathways that determine the ultimate cellular responses to a complex set of extracellular signals.

ER expression and function are strongly influenced by growth factor signaling (Fig. 27.7B). As a result, ER expression levels correlate with distinct patterns of growth factor receptor overexpression. For example, when ErbB2 or EGFR is activated in experimental systems, ER expression is suppressed. This suggests that EGFR and ErbB2 signaling can bypass the requirement for estrogen for breast cancer cell growth and drive breast cancer cells into an ER-negative, endocrine therapy–resistant state.[29] In other circumstances, EGFR and ErbB2 signaling can activate the ER in an estrogen-independent manner. Signaling of these growth factors through the mitogen-activated protein kinase (MAPK) cascade leads to phosphorylation of the Ser118 residue in the ERα AF1 domain.[30,31] This, in turn,

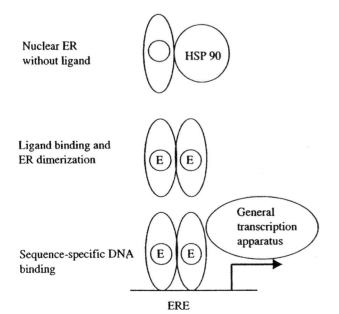

FIGURE **27.5** Simplified operational details of nuclear hormone action, using the estrogen receptor as an example. E, estrogen-occupied ligand-binding site; ER, estrogen receptor; ERE, estrogen response element; HSP, heat shock protein.

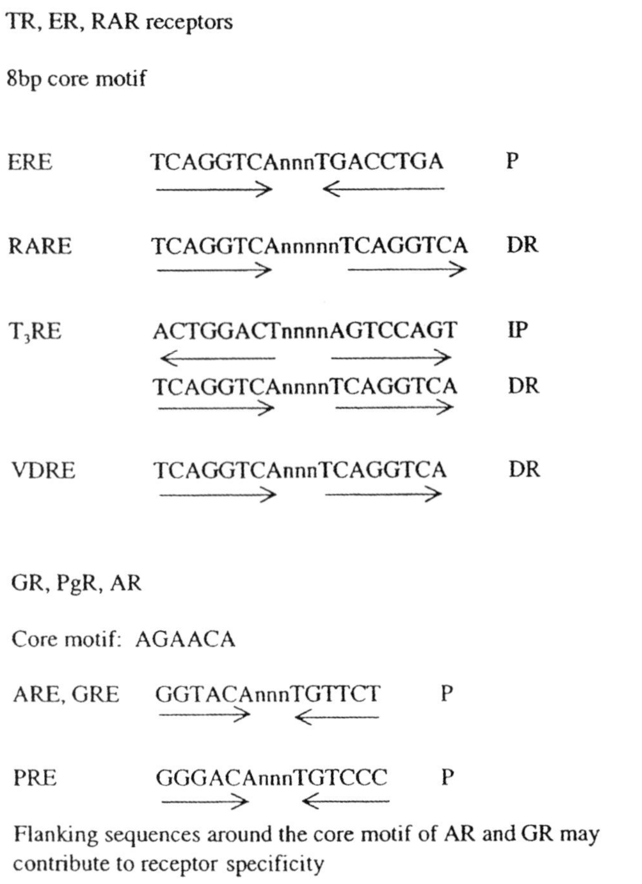

TR, ER, RAR receptors

8bp core motif

ERE	TCAGGTCAnnnTGACCTGA	P
	→ ←	
RARE	TCAGGTCAnnnnnTCAGGTCA	DR
	→ →	
T₃RE	ACTGGACTnnnnAGTCCAGT	IP
	← ←	
	TCAGGTCAnnnnTCAGGTCA	DR
	→ →	
VDRE	TCAGGTCAnnnTCAGGTCA	DR
	→ →	

GR, PgR, AR

Core motif: AGAACA

ARE, GRE	GGTACAnnnTGTTCT	P
	→ ←	
PRE	GGGACAnnnTGTCCC	P
	→ ←	

Flanking sequences around the core motif of AR and GR may contribute to receptor specificity

FIGURE 27.6 Consensus core response element motifs for nuclear hormone receptors. AR, androgen receptor; ARE, androgen receptor response element; DR, direct repeat; ER, estrogen receptor; ERE, estrogen response element; GR, glucocorticoid receptor; GRE, glucocorticoid response element; IP, inverted palindrome; n, any nucleotide; P, palindrome; PgR, progesterone receptor; PRE, progesterone receptor response element; RAR, retinoic acid receptor; RARE, retinoic acid receptor response element; T₃RE, triiodothyronine receptor response element; VDRE, vitamin D receptor response element.

leads to recruitment of coactivators, allowing ligand-independent gene transcription by the ER.[29,32] As discussed in the "Endocrine Resistance" section, insights into the cross talk between the ER and other signal transduction pathways provide a potential strategy for novel therapeutic combinations as well as an approach to novel predictive tests for endocrine therapy sensitivity.

Tamoxifen: The First Selective Estrogen Receptor Modulator

High doses of estrogen had long been recognized as effective treatment for estrogen receptor–positive (ER+) breast cancer, but serious side effects such as thromboembolism prompted the development of alternative strategies.[33] The antiestrogen tamoxifen, a nonsteroidal triphenylethylene synthesized in 1966, was first developed as an oral contraceptive but paradoxically was found to induce ovulation. Activity in metastatic breast cancer was first described in the early 1970s.[34] Since then, tamoxifen has become a prototype drug for the endocrine treatment of ER+ breast cancer, with use in prevention and treatment of all stages of the disease.

Tamoxifen rapidly became the drug of choice for advanced disease, with response rates ranging from 16% to 56% in early studies.[35-37] It became the preferred drug in large part due to its safety and tolerability. Tamoxifen's tolerability was one of the chief reasons for its success in adjuvant and prevention trials, as patients are able to take it for prolonged periods of time with acceptable levels of toxicity.[34,38-40] Widespread use of tamoxifen has likely contributed to the decline in breast cancer mortality observed in high-incidence Western countries.[41]

In addition to its generally antagonist effects on the breast, tamoxifen has estrogen agonist effects on other organs including the endometrium,[42-44] the coagulation system,[45,46] bone,[47,48] and liver.[49,50] Therefore, tamoxifen is correctly described as a selective estrogen receptor modulator (SERM) with organ-specific mixed agonist and antagonist effects. The agonist properties of tamoxifen are illustrated occasionally in advanced breast cancer (ABC) when "flare reactions" and withdrawal responses are seen.

Clinical Use

Tamoxifen is used for the treatment of ER+ invasive breast cancer in the neoadjuvant, adjuvant, and metastatic settings. Tamoxifen is also used in the treatment of ductal carcinoma in situ and for breast cancer prevention in high-risk patients. It is also capable of reducing the incidence of breast cancer in women at high risk by 49% if taken prophylactically (see below).

Tamoxifen Metabolism and Pharmacokinetics

The metabolism of tamoxifen is complex.[51] Ten major metabolites have been identified in patient's sera.[52-54] The most abundant plasma metabolite of tamoxifen is N-desmethyltamoxifen.[55] Metabolism of tamoxifen is mediated in the liver by cytochrome P450–dependent oxidases. The metabolites are excreted largely in the bile as conjugates.[56] Endoxifen (4-hydroxy-N-desmethyltamoxifen), a second metabolite of tamoxifen, appears to be most responsible for tamoxifen activity.

The initial plasma half-life of tamoxifen ranges from 4 to 14 hours, with a secondary half-life of approximately 7 days.[51,56-58] Steady-state concentrations of tamoxifen are achieved after 4 to 16 weeks of treatment due to the long plasma half-life of the agent.[58] The biologic half-life of the metabolite N-desmethyltamoxifen is 14 days, with a steady-state concentration reached at 8 weeks. These long half-lives reflect the high level of plasma binding to protein (>99%) and enterohepatic recirculation.[58] Only free tamoxifen or metabolites can bind to ERs. Tamoxifen persists in the plasma of patients for at least 6 weeks after discontinuation of treatment.[59] A thorough analysis indicated that a single dose of 20 mg a day is the most appropriate approach to tamoxifen administration.[59] Because most tamoxifen is bound to serum proteins, tamoxifen is present in low concentrations in the cerebrospinal fluid, suggesting that the response to tamoxifen is likely to be poor in leptomeningeal disease and central nervous system metastasis.[60]

Drug Interactions

The CYP3A family is responsible for N-demethylation of tamoxifen (Fig. 27.8). Many other drugs are substrates for this enzyme family, such as erythromycin, nifedipine, cyclosporine, testosterone, diltiazem, and cortisol. The combination of tamoxifen with these types of drugs could potentially interfere with tamoxifen metabolism.[61]

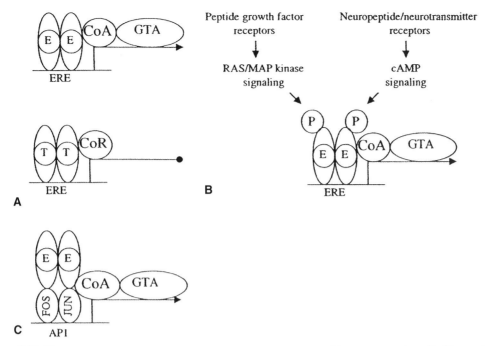

FIGURE **27.7** More complex models of estrogen receptor (ER) models. **A.** Estrogen (E) promotes coactivator (CoA) interactions that activate the general transcription apparatus (GTA). Tamoxifen (T) promotes corepressor (CoR) interactions that prevent activation of the general transcription apparatus. **B.** Estrogen receptor is phosphorylated by protein kinases activated by growth factors and neurotransmitters. **C.** ER interacts with other DNA-binding transcription factors to modulate the transcription of genes that do not possess an ERE. cAMP, cyclic adenosine monophosphate; ERE, estrogen response element; MAPK, mitogen-activated protein kinase; P, phosphate.

CYP2D6, which is commonly involved in drug hydroxylation, is the major CYP isoform responsible for the generation of the metabolites 4-hydroxytamoxifen and endoxifen from tamoxifen.[62] A pilot clinical trial of 12 breast cancer patients on adjuvant tamoxifen observed that plasma concentrations of endoxifen appeared to be influenced by the patient's CYP2D6 genotype.[63] The plasma concentrations of endoxifen were significantly lower in patients who were carriers of nonfunctional CYP2D6 allelic variants compared with those who had two functional wild-type alleles.[63] While a retrospective study of 1,325 patients reported time to breast

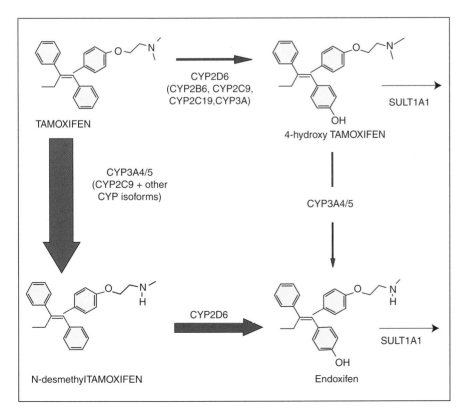

FIGURE **27.8** Selected transformation pathways of tamoxifen and the main CYP enzymes involved. The relative contribution of each pathway to the overall oxidation of tamoxifen is shown by the thickness of the *arrow*.

cancer recurrence was significantly shortened in poor metabolizers of tamoxifen, the BIG 1-98 study found no correlation between CYP2D6 allelic status and disease outcome.[64,65] Furthermore, no association between CYP2D6 genotype and clinical outcomes was seen in the ATAC trial.[66] Current NCCN and ASCO guidelines do not recommend CYP2D6 testing.[67]

The activity of CYP2D6 is also reduced by serotonin selective reuptake inhibitor (SSRI) antidepressants.[63,68] In view of the widespread use of SSRIs in patients with a history of breast cancer, a detailed study was done to determine their effects on tamoxifen metabolites.[69] Levels of 4-hydroxy-N-desmethyltamoxifen, a metabolite generated via CYP3A4 and CYP2D6 activity, were 64% lower in women taking SSRIs. Other studies also showed that plasma endoxifen concentrations were lower in patients who were also taking the SSRI paroxetine.[69] It is therefore reasonable to avoid potent and intermediate CYP2D6 inhibiting agents, especially paroxetine and fluoxetine, when there are appropriate alternative options. For example, several mild inhibitors of CYP2D6, such as citalopram, escitalopram, sertraline, and venlafaxine, have been shown to have little to no effect on tamoxifen metabolism.[70,71]

Medroxyprogesterone acetate has also been found to alter the metabolism of tamoxifen.[72] Reports of an interaction between warfarin and tamoxifen have prompted the manufacturer to list concurrent warfarin use as a contraindication.[73] Supratherapeutic effects of warfarin have been reported in patients also receiving tamoxifen; however, the number of cases studied is small. The mechanism of this interaction is likely inhibition of hepatic metabolism of warfarin by tamoxifen. Therefore, close monitoring of coagulation indices is warranted when warfarin and tamoxifen are prescribed together.[73]

Tamoxifen Side Effects

Although tamoxifen remains a standard endocrine therapy for early-stage breast cancer and ABC, important side effects should be considered. The tamoxifen chemoprevention trial, National Surgical Adjuvant Breast Project (NSABP) P1, established one of the most comprehensive sources of information on tamoxifen toxicity because the true incidence of tamoxifen side effects was not obscured by tumor-related medical problems.[74] In NSABP P1, the excess incidence of serious adverse events (pulmonary embolus, deep venous thrombosis, cerebrovascular accident, cataract, and endometrial cancer) for patients receiving tamoxifen therapy was five to six events per 1,000 patient-years of treatment. Other side effects of tamoxifen included hot flashes, nausea, and vaginal discharge. Depression is also considered a side effect of tamoxifen, although there was no clear evidence of this association for women who received tamoxifen or placebo in NSABP P1. In summary, tamoxifen is usually well tolerated and safe, and serious side effects occur in no more than 1 in 200 patients annually.

Ophthalmologic Side Effects

Tamoxifen retinopathy, with macular edema and loss of visual acuity, was first reported in patients receiving 120 to 160 mg/d. Three

of the four originally reported patients also had corneal opacities.[75] The retinal lesions are superficial, white, refractile bodies 3 to 10 µm in diameter in the macula and 30 to 35 µm in diameter in the paramacular tissues, and they occur in the nerve fiber layer, suggesting that they are products of axonal degeneration.[76] Additional cases have been described among patients receiving 30 to 180 mg/d.[77] Other ophthalmologic findings reported include optic neuritis, macular edema, crystalline macular deposits with reduced visual acuity, intraretinal crystals with noncystoid macular edema, refractile deposits in the paramacular areas with progressive retinal pigment atrophy, bilateral optic disc edema with visual impairment and retinal hemorrhages, tapetoretinal degeneration, and two cases of superior ophthalmic vein thrombosis.[77–80] It is worth emphasizing that, in the NSABP P1 chemoprevention study in which standard tamoxifen dosing was utilized, the only significant optic toxicity at increased incidence compared with placebo was cataract formation.[74]

Thrombosis

The increased risk of thrombosis associated with tamoxifen therapy may be initiated by decreased levels of antithrombin III levels. Enck and Rios found a decreased functional activity of antithrombin III in 42% of tamoxifen-treated patients.[45] Others found reduced antithrombin III and protein C levels in women taking tamoxifen.[81] The incidence of venous thrombosis in this study was 5.62%, compared with 0% in controls. In the P1 prevention trial, the average annual rates of stroke, pulmonary embolism, and deep venous thrombosis per 1,000 women were increased by 0.53, 0.46, and 0.50 cases, respectively.[74] The NSABP B-14 study reported thromboembolic events in 12 patients (0.9%), with one fatal pulmonary embolus, compared with two thromboemboli (0.2%) in controls,[82] a rate similar to that occurring in the P1 prevention trial.[74] In the P1 trial, tamoxifen-related thrombotic events were more likely to occur in patients with higher body mass index but not with factor V Leiden or prothrombin gene mutations.[83]

Hematologic Side Effects

Thrombocytopenia occurs in 5% of patients and is usually transient, resolving after the first week of treatment. Leukopenia is less frequent and is also transient.[84] The mechanism of these side effects is unclear.

Lipoprotein Effects

Changes in serum lipoproteins in patients taking tamoxifen are indicative of an estrogenic agonist effect: an increase in total triglycerides, a decrease in total cholesterol, an increase in low-density lipoprotein (LDL) triglycerides, and a decrease in LDL cholesterol. Many studies substantiate the effect of tamoxifen on lowering total cholesterol and, in most cases, LDL cholesterol and apolipoprotein B.[84–86] Despite these potentially favorable effects, there was no evidence of an improvement in the rate of cardiovascular mortality in either the Oxford meta-analysis of tamoxifen trials or the P1 prevention trial.[38,74] It is possible that beneficial effects of improved lipoprotein levels induced by tamoxifen are counteracted in part by increased incidence of thromboembolism.

Hepatic Toxicity

Tamoxifen has been associated with various hepatic abnormalities, including cholestasis, jaundice, peliosis hepatitis, and hepatitis. Carcinogenicity studies in rats reveal hepatocellular carcinoma in dosages ranging from 5 to 35 mg/kg/d.[87] A dose of 20 to 40 mg given to humans is 5-to 10-fold lower than the rat dose range of 5 mg/kg, and an increase in hepatocellular carcinoma in humans taking tamoxifen has not been reported. This is significant because tamoxifen metabolites form adducts with DNA and could be mutagenic and carcinogenic.[87]

Bone Side Effects

The positive effect of tamoxifen on bone mineral content in postmenopausal women can be considered an advantageous side effect due to its estrogen agonistic activity.[88,89] In the P1 study, a nonsignificant decrease in fracture rate was documented.[90] In premenopausal women, bone mineral density is decreased, possibly because in a high-estrogen environment, tamoxifen may operate predominantly as an antagonist.[88,91]

Gynecologic Side Effects

A change in the duration of menses or heaviness of flow and an increased incidence of ovarian cysts may occur. A small increase in endometrial cancer occurs, but screening for endometrial cancer is complicated by tamoxifen-induced benign endometrial hyperplasia and polyp formation. The risk of endometrial cancer relates to age and duration of tamoxifen treatment. In the original Swedish report, the highest frequency occurred among those treated for 5 years and the Swedish patients received the high dose of 40 mg daily.[92] Of 17 tamoxifen-related endometrial cancers, 16 were grade 1 or 2, although three patients died from their endometrial cancer.[92] A case-control study found that exposure to tamoxifen interacts with other risk factors for endometrial cancer such as a history of hormone replacement therapy and higher body mass index.[93] In addition to endometrial cancer, the risk of uterine sarcoma, a very rare malignancy, is also increased by tamoxifen. Data from six NSABP trials in which over 17,000 women were randomized to tamoxifen or placebo shows that the rate of uterine sarcoma was increased to 0.17 per 1,000 years in women taking tamoxifen versus 0 per 1,000 years in those taking placebo.[94]

Recommendations for gynecologic follow-up of patients taking tamoxifen have varied from observation to yearly vaginal ultrasound to yearly endometrial biopsy, with no solid data supporting any of these approaches. Yearly pelvic examinations and rapid investigation of postmenopausal bleeding, but not radiologic or biopsy screening, are currently recommended.

Pregnancy

Given the possible teratogenicity of tamoxifen, women should use contraception while on the drug. Of a series of 50 pregnancies on file at AstraZeneca Pharmaceuticals in women taking tamoxifen, there were 19 normal births, 8 terminated pregnancies, 13 unknown outcomes, and 10 infants with a fetal and neonatal disorder, 2 of whom had craniofacial defects. Yet in another report, 85 women taking tamoxifen for prevention of breast cancer became pregnant; none of these pregnancies resulted in fetal abnormalities.[95] Another case of an infant born with ambiguous genitalia after in utero exposure through 20 weeks has also been reported.[96] The evidence for the teratogenicity of tamoxifen is primarily derived from animal studies, in which reproductive organ abnormalities and increased susceptibility to carcinogens were found.[97] Nevertheless, tamoxifen is contraindicated in women who are pregnant or planning pregnancy.

Male Breast Cancer

Among men taking tamoxifen, one series reported a decrease in libido in 29.2%.[98] Impotence has been studied in men treated with tamoxifen for male infertility. One paper reports a loss of libido in four cases (9%), whereas studies that reported an increase in testosterone levels with tamoxifen did not report an increase in impotence.[99,100] These data suggest that tamoxifen has minimal effect on sexual function and is probably not the cause of impotence.

Flare Reactions and Withdrawal Responses

Tamoxifen has been characterized as having both estrogen agonist and antagonist actions. These functions are also tissue and perhaps tumor specific. Tamoxifen's agonist effects on the endometrium, bones, and clotting profile have been described. On the breast its antagonist actions are manifest by anti–breast cancer effects. In patients with ABC tamoxifen's occasional paradoxical effects are manifest by the phenomena of a clinical flare and a drug withdrawal response. A clinical flare reaction is characterized by a dramatic increase in bone pain and an increase in the size and number of metastatic skin nodules with erythema if present.[101] Typically, symptoms occur from 2 days to 3 weeks after starting treatment and can be accompanied by hypercalcemia, which occurs in approximately 5% of patients.[102] Tumor regression may occur as the reaction subsides.[103]

Other SERMs

Background

The structures of other SERMs and antiestrogens are provided in Figure 27.9. Alternative antiestrogens with a modified mixed agonist and antagonist profile have been evaluated with an eye toward developing drugs that are antiestrogenic in the breast and endometrium but retain beneficial effects on bone mineralization. However, although ideal SERMs may represent a small advance in terms of safety, they are not necessarily more efficacious. In general, antiestrogens that exhibit a mixed agonist and antagonist profile, even if modified in a way that improves tissue-specific toxicities, are likely to exhibit resistance and toxicity profiles that overlap those of tamoxifen.[104] This may be because any antiestrogen that triggers ER dimerization and DNA binding is prone to the same coactivator-based resistance mechanisms that may limit the activity of tamoxifen.

Raloxifene

Raloxifene [6-hydroxy-2-(4-hydroxyphenyl)-benzo[b]thien-3-yl]–[4-[2-(1-piperidinyl) ethoxy] phenyl] is the first approved drug to exhibit a "modified" SERM profile; however, the first approved indication for raloxifene was osteoporosis, not breast cancer.[105] An early evaluation of activity in tamoxifen-resistant breast cancer was disappointing.[106] Consequently, raloxifene is not used for the treatment of either early-stage breast cancer or ABC. However,

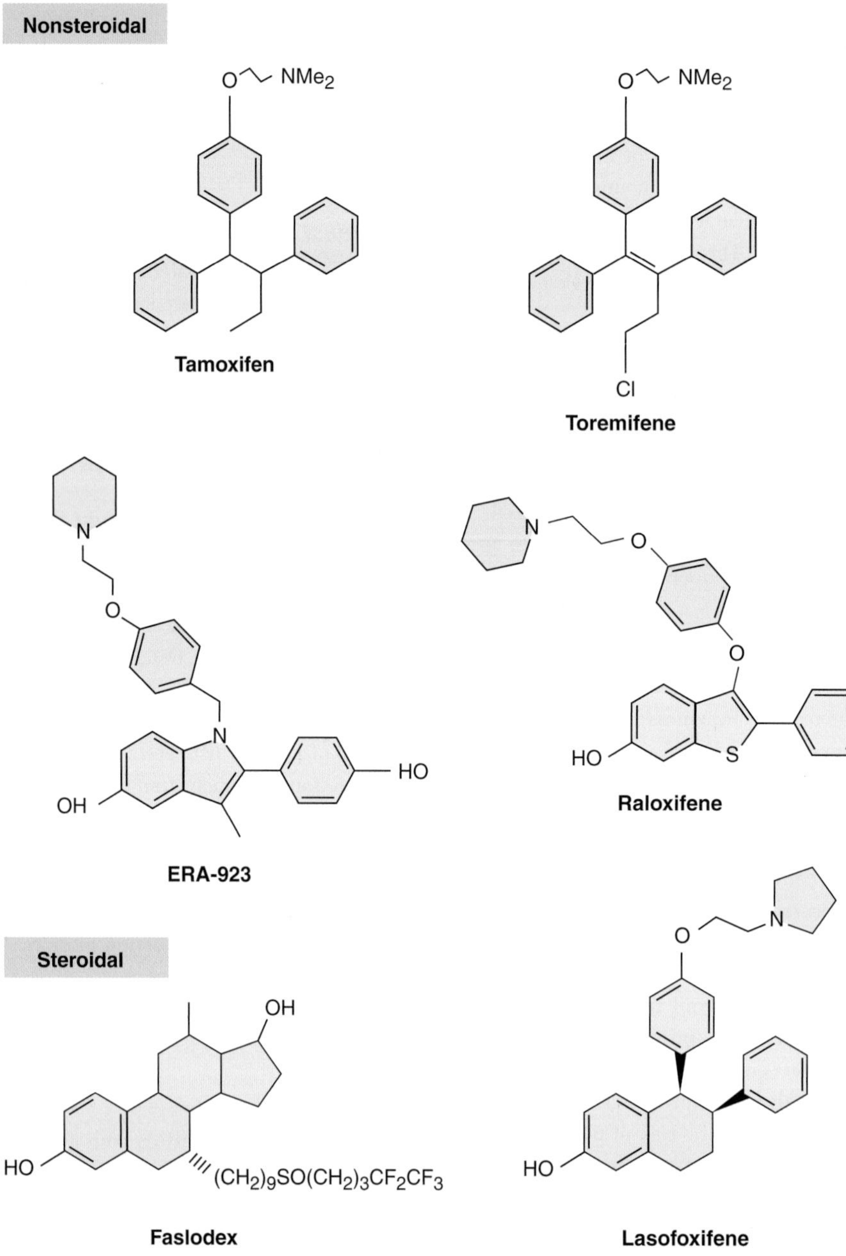

FIGURE **27.9** Antiestrogens. SERM, selective estrogen receptor modulator.

raloxifene has been approved in the breast cancer prevention setting.[107] The NSABP-P2 prevention trial demonstrated that in women at high risk for developing breast cancer, raloxifene is as effective as tamoxifen in reducing the risk of invasive breast cancer and has a lower risk of thromboembolic events, endometrial cancer, and cataracts.[108] It is important to note that raloxifene has a nonstatistically significant higher risk of noninvasive (in situ) breast cancer compared to tamoxifen, raising the possibility that it may not be as effective in long-term prevention of invasive cancer.

Mechanism of Action

While raloxifene has agonist and antagonist activity similar to tamoxifen in breast tissue and bones, its nil or only very mild agonist effect on the endometrium results in no or very mild increase in endometrial cancer risk, a distinct advantage over tamoxifen. Raloxifene is a benzothiophene with a structure that includes

a flexible "hinge" region. This modification results in a nearly orthogonal orientation of its side chains. This is markedly different from tamoxifen, which has a rigid triphenylethylene structure.[109] Although both drugs bind to the ER, their structural differences lead to dissimilar conformations of the ER-ligand complex.[110] In the Ishikawa endometrial carcinoma cell line, tamoxifen, but not raloxifene, induces recruitment of coactivators SRC-1, AIB1, and CBP to the c-Myc and IGF-1 promoters.[111] This recruitment of coactivators is critical to tamoxifen's transactivating ability and agonist activity in the endometrium. The comparative inability of raloxifene to assemble this coactivator complex may account for its lower agonist activity in the endometrium.

Clinical Use

Raloxifene is indicated for breast cancer prevention in postmenopausal women at high risk for developing breast cancer.

Pharmacology and Metabolism

Raloxifene binds to the ER with a K_d of about 50 pmol/L, which is comparable to the value for estradiol.[112] The drug is given at 60 mg/d, and after oral administration, it is rapidly absorbed, reaching its maximal concentration in about 30 minutes.[112] While absorption is 60%, first-pass metabolism limits the drug's bioavailability to 2%. After absorption, raloxifene is distributed widely throughout the body and is bound to plasma proteins, including albumin. The half-life of the drug is 27.7 hours.[113]

Metabolism of raloxifene, as mentioned, is primarily via first-pass glucuronidation. The agent does not appear to be metabolized by the CYP enzyme systems, and there are no other known metabolites.[113] Elimination occurs primarily through bile and feces, with just a small amount found in the urine.

Drug Interactions

Cholestyramine causes a 60% reduction in raloxifene absorption and enterohepatic circulation.[113] Unlike tamoxifen, raloxifene has a minor interaction with warfarin, with just a 10% decrease in prothrombin time. Concomitant therapy with ampicillin reduced the raloxifene peak concentration by 28%, which was felt to be clinically insignificant.[113]

Skeletal Effects

Raloxifene has been demonstrated to have estrogen agonist activity in bone in both animal models and in clinical trials. The multiple outcomes of raloxifene evaluation (MORE) study enrolled 7,705 women with osteoporosis to determine if the drug could decrease the rate of fractures.[114] While vertebral fractures were reduced by 30%, nonvertebral fractures were not significantly different. However, bone mineral density was increased in both the spine and femoral neck.

Endometrial Effects

Unlike estrogen and tamoxifen, raloxifene does not have stimulatory activity in the uterus. In the mature rats, uterine weight and endothelial height were unchanged with raloxifene exposure.[115] However, in the more sensitive immature rat uterine assay, raloxifene is agonistic but less so than tamoxifen. Clinically, raloxifene does not promote uterine proliferation.[115] The 4-year update of the MORE trial confirmed that the rates of vaginal bleeding and endometrial cancer in patients taking raloxifene are the same as that in those on placebo.[116]

Cardiovascular Effects

Raloxifene has estrogen agonist effects on lipid metabolism, with reduction of serum cholesterol levels by 70% in postmenopausal rat models.[115] In clinical trials, raloxifene reduces serum LDL, fibrinogen, lipoprotein (a), homocysteine, and C-reactive protein. Unlike tamoxifen, however, raloxifene does not affect triglycerides or high-density lipoprotein (HDL). While these findings could argue for a possible cardiovascular protective effect, this has not been demonstrated in clinical study.[115] In the MORE trial, there was no difference between arms in cardiovascular events or cerebrovascular events in the overall cohort; however, subgroup analysis with multiple comparisons revealed that women with increased cardiovascular risk had a relative risk reduction in cardiac events of 40% when taking raloxifene.[113] The randomized placebo-controlled RUTH (Raloxifene Use for the Heart) trial failed to show any benefit of raloxifene in the prevention of coronary heart disease but, in fact, increased the incidence of blood clots and death from stroke, possibly related to its hypercoagulable effects.[117,118]

Other Side Effects

Other major symptoms provoked by raloxifene compared to placebo in the MORE trial included hot flashes (9.7% versus 6.4%), leg cramps (5.5% versus 1.9%), and thromboembolic events (1.4% versus 0.47%).[114] Some reports suggest that the increased risk of thromboembolic events is similar to that seen with tamoxifen and is perhaps the side effect of most concern when the drug is used in clinical practice. However, in the NSABP P2 prevention trial, thromboembolic events occurred significantly less often in patients treated with raloxifene compared with tamoxifen.[108] Raloxifene has been demonstrated to be teratogenic in animal studies.[109]

Toremifene

Toremifene is approved in the United States for treatment of advanced ER+ breast cancer, though its use has decreased.[119] Toremifene has antiestrogenic activity similar to that of tamoxifen.[120] The drug acts as almost a pure antiestrogen in rats and is partially agonistic in mice. Unlike tamoxifen, however, this drug has no hepatocarcinogenicity or DNA adduct-forming ability in rats.[120] It was hoped, therefore, that toremifene would provide a safer SERM for long-term use, such as in the adjuvant setting, although studies comparing the two drugs have shown no clear advantage over tamoxifen. As a result, toremifene's use in the clinic has been somewhat limited. The major CYP-mediated metabolites of toremifene are N-demethyl-toremifene and 4-hydroxytoremifene. The mean terminal half-life of toremifene and these metabolites is from 5 to 6 days.[121] The side effects are similar to those of tamoxifen, with hot flashes being the most common. Toremifene is cross-resistant with tamoxifen and should not be used in tamoxifen-resistant disease.[120]

Fulvestrant: A Pure Antiestrogen

Background

Given the finding that resistance to tamoxifen may sometimes be due to its partial agonist effects, pure antiestrogens without agonist activity were developed as endocrine agents. Fulvestrant, a pure antiestrogen, is a 7 α-alkylamide analog of 17 β-estradiol (Fig. 27.9). This drug is also often called a "selective estrogen receptor down-regulator"(SERD), because it has been demonstrated to decrease the level of ER protein in the cell.[121]

Mechanism of Action

Fulvestrant is a steroidal antiestrogen that acts in a distinctly different manner than the SERMs. The drug binds the ER, like SERMs, but its long, bulky alkylamide side chain at the 7 α position interferes with ER function. Crystallographic and fluorescence energy transfer studies of the drug indicate that it binds to ERα and promotes receptor dimerization (but less potently than SERMs), suggesting that its downstream effects may lie at the level of interaction of the drug-ER complex with coactivators and/or corepressors.[122] The result is that the ER cannot bind DNA and is eliminated more rapidly via proteosome degradation, leading to a marked reduction in ER protein levels.[122,123] In this way, fulvestrant completely blocks ER-mediated gene transcription completely. In vitro, this results in inhibition of tamoxifen-resistant breast cancer cell lines by fulvestrant. In addition, the drug has no growth stimulatory effect in a tamoxifen-stimulated MCF-7 breast cancer xenograft model.[122] In primate studies, fulvestrant also acts as a pure antiestrogen outside of the breast, with complete inhibition of estrogen stimulation of uterine tissue.[124]

The antiproliferative effects of fulvestrant may be augmented by its ability to suppress insulin-like growth factor receptor signaling. This appears to occur both in vitro and in animal models. Finally, fulvestrant also has activity as an aromatase inhibitor, although it is not known how much this property contributes to the clinical activity of the drug.[125]

The effects of fulvestrant on ER, PgR, proliferation, and apoptosis have been examined in benign endometrial tissue and malignant breast tissue. When fulvestrant was given for a week before hysterectomy, it was found to decrease a Ki-67–based proliferation assay; however, ER and PgR levels were not affected. By contrast, short-term exposure to fulvestrant before breast surgery decreased ER and PgR expression, proliferation, and increased apoptosis.[126,127] These data suggest that, as in the case of other antiestrogens, there may be differences in the action of fulvestrant at different organ sites.

While current experience with fulvestrant in breast cancer is limited to postmenopausal women, there have been trials with benign gynecologic conditions that demonstrate its antiestrogenic properties in premenopausal women.[128]

Clinical Use

Fulvestrant is used in the treatment of postmenopausal women with ER+ metastatic breast cancer, following progression on tamoxifen or an aromatase inhibitor. However, recent phase III data from the FALCON trial comparing fulvestrant 500 mg versus anastrozole 1 mg for endocrine therapy-naïve hormone receptor–positive (HR+) ABC demonstrated progression-free survival (PFS) was significantly longer in the fulvestrant group, 16.6 months, versus 13.8 months in the anastrozole group (HR 0.797, $P = 0.0486$).[129] Fulvestrant is also approved in combination with the cyclin-dependent kinase (CDK) 4/6 inhibitor palbociclib in pre-or postmenopausal HR+, HER2-negative ABC patients with disease progression on prior endocrine therapy based on the phase III PALOMA-3 trial.[130] A number of ongoing clinical trials are exploring novel oral SERDs.

Pharmacology

In vitro, fulvestrant has an ER-binding affinity 100-fold greater than that of tamoxifen.[123] Because the drug is not reliably absorbed orally, it is formulated as a monthly depot intramuscular injection. With this preparation, peak levels of fulvestrant occur at a median of 8 to 9 days after dosing and decline thereafter, but the levels remain above the projected therapeutic threshold at day 28. In pharmacokinetic studies, the area under the curve (AUC) was 140 μg × day/Liter in the first month and 208 μg × day/Liter after 6 months, suggesting drug accumulation.[131] Because a single injection of the 5-mL volume can be difficult in some patients, the drug is often given as two 2.5-mL injections (250 mg each); this

alternative method of delivery has no effect on the pharmacokinetics of the drug.[132] Based on studies exploring the key issue of whether fulvestrant would be more effective with a loading dose, patients now receive an additional 500 mg at day 14 of cycle 1 and begin monthly dosing with cycle 2.[133]

Metabolism

Fulvestrant is known to undergo oxidation, hydroxylation, and conjugation with glucuronic acid and/or sulfate in the liver, with negligible renal excretion. The half-life of the drug is approximately 40 days.[134]

Side Effects

In preclinical studies, fulvestrant has been reported to cause decreased bone mineral density in adult female rats, suggesting that osteoporosis might be a side effect.[132]

The frequency of hot flashes with fulvestrant in clinical trials has been similar to the frequency with aromatase inhibitors, with the exception of one trial that compared fulvestrant and tamoxifen in the metastatic setting and found decreased hot flashes with fulvestrant.[135] No other side effects in this trial were statistically different between the two drugs.

In early clinical studies, fulvestrant did not cause a change in sex hormone–binding globulin, prolactin, or serum lipids. In addition, there was no increase in endometrial thickness in patients undergoing hysterectomy.[131] In more recent clinical trials for metastatic breast cancer, fulvestrant has been well tolerated, with hot flashes and gastrointestinal disturbances as the most common adverse events. Tolerability was similar between fulvestrant and anastrozole in two phase III trials with a treatment-related withdrawal rate of 2.5%.[123]

Aromatase Inhibitors

Aromatase Background

Postmenopausal Estrogen

The therapeutic effect of reducing estrogen levels for patients with breast cancer was originally restricted to patients with functioning ovaries. However, postmenopausal women produce significant amounts of estrogen through aromatization of circulating adrenal androgens in peripheral normal tissues, such as fat, muscle, liver, and the epithelial and stromal components of the breast.[136,137] Peripheral aromatization is increased in certain medical conditions, including obesity, hepatic disease, and hyperthyroidism, but is independent of pituitary hormone secretion. The relative proportion of estrogens synthesized in extragonadal sites increases with age, and eventually, nonovarian estrogens predominate in the circulation.[138]

Intratumoral Aromatase

Aromatase is a key enzyme responsible for the biosynthesis of estrogens. It catalyzes the conversion of testosterone to estradiol. Expression of aromatase in the breast led to the hypothesis that local synthesis of estrogens contributes to breast cancer growth in postmenopausal women.[139,140] In support of this theory, the decline in estrogen concentrations after menopause is less marked in breast tissue than in plasma due to a combination of aromatase activity and to a lesser extent preferential estrogen uptake from the circulation.[52] Furthermore, aromatase activity has been shown to correlate with a marker of breast cancer cell proliferation, and quadrants of the breast bearing a breast cancer have more aromatase expression than those not bearing tumors.[141]

Development of Aromatase Inhibitors

Steroidal Versus Nonsteroidal

Two distinct solutions evolved to the problem of designing potent, specific, and safe aromatase inhibitors.[142] One strategy was to develop "steroidal" aromatase inhibitors that are resistant to aromatase action and that bind aromatase and block conversion of androgenic substrates (type 1 inhibitors). An alternative was to develop a family of "nonsteroidal" inhibitors that disrupt the aromatase active site by coordinating within the heme complex without affecting the steroid binding sites of other steroidogenic enzymes (type 2 inhibitors). Both approaches led to the successful introduction of potent and specific aromatase inhibitors into clinical practice.

Early Aromatase Inhibitors

In 1973, Griffiths et al. first demonstrated the activity of aminoglutethimide, an inhibitor of cholesterol conversion to pregnenolone in the treatment of metastatic breast cancer.[143] Subsequently, it was appreciated that inhibition of aromatase, rather than suppression of general steroidogenesis, was key to the therapeutic action of aminoglutethimide.[144,145] Although the drug has well-documented efficacy in the metastatic setting, its side effect profile is concerning. Aminoglutethimide inhibits the formation of glucocorticoids by blocking P-450 enzymes involved in cholesterol side chain cleavage.[146] This lack of specificity exposes patients to the risk of glucocorticoid deficiency. Furthermore, other concerning side effects include rash, nausea, somnolence, and blood dyscrasias.[146,147]

These observations provided a strong rationale for the development of more potent and selective aromatase inhibitors. While second-generation aromatase inhibitors, such as fadrozole and formestane, had improved potency and selectivity, the third-generation aromatase inhibitors provided superior clinical results and rendered both aminoglutethimide and the second-generation drugs obsolete in breast cancer therapeutics.

Exemestane: Steroidal Aromatase Inhibitor

Background

Exemestane, an androstenedione derivative, exhibits tight or even irreversible binding to the aromatase active site.[148] The compound is therefore considered a "mechanism-based" or "suicide" inhibitor because it permanently inactivates aromatase.

Clinical Use

Exemestane is used in the adjuvant setting for postmenopausal women with ER+ breast cancer and for premenopausal women in combination with ovarian suppression. It is also used in the metastatic setting as monotherapy, in combination with CDK 4/6 inhibitors, and in combination with the mTOR inhibitor everolimus based on BOLERO-2.[149]

Pharmacology

Exemestane (Fig. 27.10) has potent aromatase activity with a K^i of 26 nM and no cholesterol side chain cleavage (desmolase) or 5-reductase activity. An oral dose is rapidly absorbed, and peak plasma concentrations are reached within 2 hours of administration. The absorption of exemestane is enhanced by high-fat foods, and it is recommended that the drug be taken after eating.[150] Plasma concentrations fall below the limit of detection 4 hours later (for the approved 25-mg dose), although inhibition of the enzyme persists for at least 5 days.[150] Steady-state levels are achieved within 7 days with daily dosing, and the time to maximal estradiol suppression is 3 to 7 days.[151] The smallest that maximally suppressed of plasma estrone, estradiol, and estrone sulfate and urinary estrone and estradiol was 25 mg, now the recommended daily dosage. This dosage inactivates peripheral aromatase by 98% and reduces basal plasma estrone, estradiol, and estrone sulfate levels by 85% to 95% in postmenopausal women.[152] Other endocrine parameters, such as cortisol, aldosterone, dehydroepiandrosterones, 17-OH-progesterone, follicle-stimulating hormone (FSH), and LH, are not significantly affected by 25 mg of exemestane.[153]

Metabolism

Exemestane is extensively metabolized, with rapid oxidation of the methylene group at position 6 and reduction of the 17-keto group, along with subsequent formation of many secondary metabolites. The drug is excreted in both the urine and feces. As a consequence, clearance is affected by both renal and hepatic insufficiency, with threefold elevations in the AUC under either condition. Metabolism occurs through CYP3A4 and aldoketoreductases.[151,154] While exemestane does not bind to the ER and only weakly binds to the AR, with an affinity of 0.28% relative to DHT, the binding affinity of the 17-dihydrometabolite for AR is 100 times that of the parent compound.[155] As a result, there is slight androgenic activity in the rat with this drug. A screen of potential metabolites for aromatase activity did not reveal any compounds with inhibitory activity greater than exemestane.[156]

Toxicities

In clinical studies, exemestane has been well tolerated and has had a treatment-related discontinuation rate of less than 3%.[154] At high doses in rat studies, exemestane has been observed to have androgenic effects. Similarly, at high doses in clinical trials, androgenic side effects, including hypertrichosis, hair loss, hoarseness, and acne, have been reported in 4% of patients.[154] Other reported side effects include hot flashes, increased sweating, and nausea.

With all aromatase inhibitors, bone loss is a significant concern. However, there was some thought that the androgenic properties of exemestane metabolites might mitigate this effect. Initial studies in postmenopausal women using bone turnover biomarkers suggest that exemestane has a significantly smaller negative impact on bone formation and bone resorption than letrozole.[157] Despite these findings, results of the Intergroup Exemestane Study (IES) showed that postmenopausal patients on exemestane experience more osteoporosis than those on tamoxifen.[158] This may be in part due to improvement in BMD with tamoxifen rather than loss with exemestane. BMD profiles suggest an early mild decrease in exemestane-treated women with stabilization thereafter. Cessation

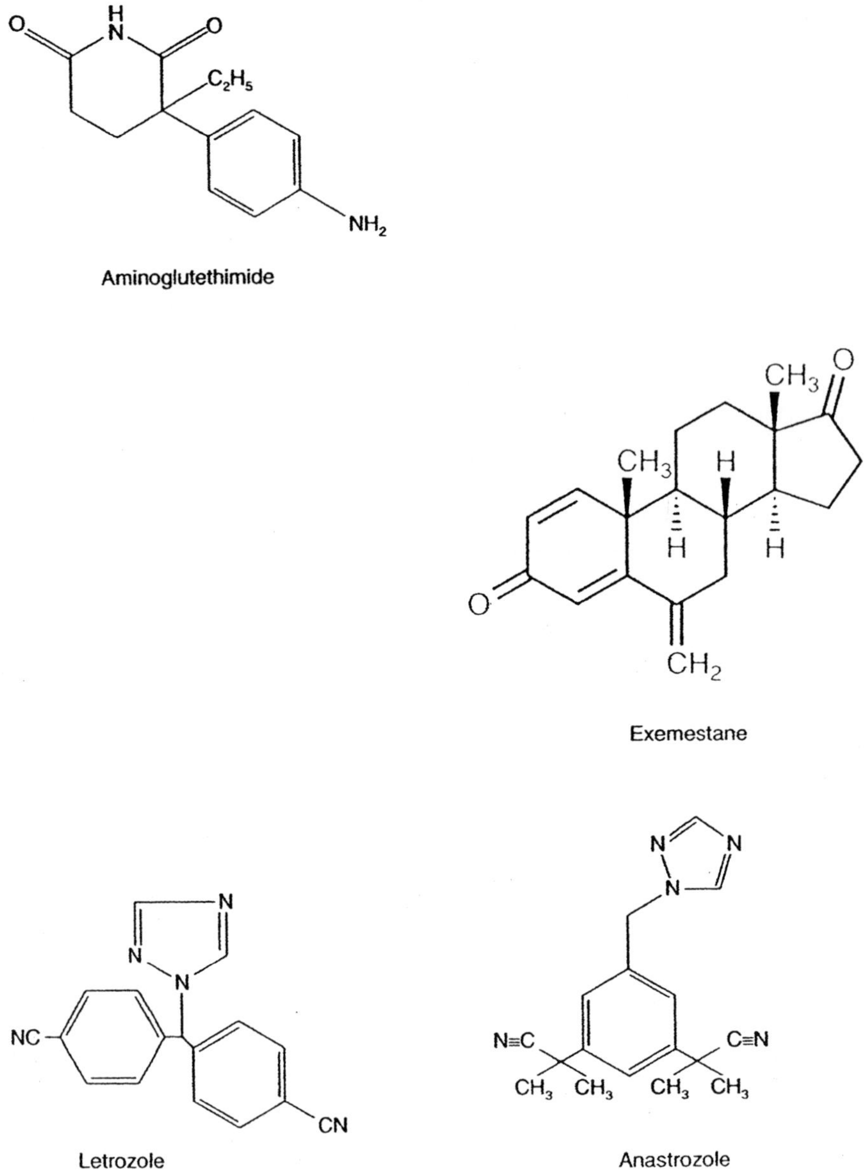

Aminoglutethimide

Exemestane

Letrozole

Anastrozole

FIGURE **27.10** Aromatase inhibitors.

of exemestane with recovery of estrogen levels results in approximate return to placebo-controlled levels within 12 to 24 months after stopping treatment.[159]

Other side effects that were increased in the exemestane group in the IES trial included visual disturbances, arthralgia, and diarrhea. Conversely, patients on tamoxifen experienced more gynecologic symptoms, vaginal bleeding, thromboembolic disease, and cramps.[158]

Drug Interactions

Given that exemestane is extensively metabolized by CYP3A4, interference with other drugs that induce or inhibit this P-450 enzyme may occur. Interestingly, however, ketoconazole does not significantly influence the pharmacokinetics of exemestane, suggesting that with CYP3A4 inhibition exemestane may be metabolized via a different route or that renal excretion may compensate.[151]

Exemestane has mild androgenic activity, which may exert antitumor effects independent of its aromatase inhibitory action. Other advantages are its irreversible inhibition of aromatase, its better toxicity profile, and improved quality of life.

Nonsteroidal Aromatase Inhibitors

The nonsteroidal approach to aromatase inhibition has yielded two compounds widely applied in the clinic today, anastrozole and letrozole (Fig. 27.10).[160]

Anastrozole

Clinical Use

Anastrozole is used to treat postmenopausal women with ER+ breast cancer in the neoadjuvant, adjuvant, and metastatic settings. It is also approved in combination with a CDK 4/6 inhibitor, palbociclib or ribociclib, for the first-line treatment of ABC.[161,162]

Pharmacokinetics

Anastrozole [2,2′-[5-(1H-1,2,4-triazol-1-ylmethyl)-1,3-phenylene]bis (2-methyl-propiononitrile)] is a competitive aromatase inhibitor with high potency and was the first selective aromatase inhibitor approved in North America and Europe. It inhibits human placental aromatase and has an IC50 of 15 nM.[163] Anastrozole is rapidly absorbed, with the C_{max} occurring within 2 hours after administration, and it is 40% bound to plasma proteins. The mean C_{max} at the 1-mg dose was 13.1 ng/mL.[163] Pharmacodynamic studies reveal that subjects receiving 1 mg/d orally achieved 96.7% aromatase inhibition, with maximal estradiol suppression and a decrease of estradiol ranging from 78% to 86% from baseline. Suppression is maintained long term, and there is no compensatory rise in androstenedione levels. The drug has a half-life of 38 to 61 hours and reaches steady-state levels in 7 days, with maximal estrogen suppression within 3 to 4 hours.[154,163] There is no effect on glucocorticoid or mineralocorticoid secretion as tested by ACTH stimulation.[163] In addition, anastrozole at a dosage of 1 mg daily does not have an effect on gonadotropins or FSH. Importantly, even at higher doses (5 to 10 mg), anastrozole administration does not affect basal or ACTH-stimulated cortisol and aldosterone levels.[154]

Metabolism

Elimination of anastrozole is primarily by metabolic degradation, and less than 10% of the drug is cleared as unchanged drug. Degradation occurs through *N*-dealkylation, hydroxylation, and glucuronidation, and metabolites are excreted predominantly in the urine.[163]

Anastrozole has no effect on CYP2A6 but does inhibit CYP1A2 and CYP2C8, with an IC50 of 30 and 48 μmol/L, respectively. In clinical use, the drug is present at much lower levels than required to inhibit these enzymes.[154]

Toxicity

Anastrozole is well tolerated overall. In the ATAC (Arimidex, Tamoxifen Alone, or in Combination) trial, a large adjuvant trial comparing anastrozole versus tamoxifen versus their combination, anastrozole demonstrated a favorable toxicity profile with prolonged use.[164] Compared with patients taking tamoxifen, patients in the anastrozole arm of the study experienced less vaginal bleeding (4.8% versus 8.7%), vaginal discharge (3.0% versus 12.2%), endometrial malignancy (0.1% versus 0.7%), ischemic cerebrovascular events (1.1% versus 2.3%), and venous thromboembolic events (2.2% versus 3.8%). Anastrozole, however, did result in an increase in fractures (7.1% versus 4.4%) and in musculoskeletal complaints (30.3% versus 23.7%). Given that there was no placebo control in this trial, part of the increased incidence of fractures is likely due to protective effects of tamoxifen in addition to the deleterious effects of anastrozole.

Drug Interactions

To date, clinically significant drug interactions with anastrozole have been minimal. Coadministration with tamoxifen has been shown to lead to a 27% decrease in steady-state levels of anastrozole.[164] However, given the ATAC trial findings that combining tamoxifen and anastrozole provides inferior clinical outcomes compared with anastrozole alone, the combination of these drugs will not be used clinically in the future. It is unclear whether this pharmacokinetic interaction might contribute to the inferiority of the combination arm in ATAC.

Letrozole

Clinical Use

Letrozole is used to treat postmenopausal women with ER+ breast cancer in the neoadjuvant, adjuvant, and metastatic settings. It is also approved in combination with a CDK 4/6 inhibitor, palbociclib

or ribociclib. Letrozole was the aromatase inhibitor used in the pivotal trials that led to the approval of palbociclib (PALOMA-1, PALOMA-2) and ribociclib (MONALEESA-2) for the first-line treatment of HR+ ABC.[165–167]

Pharmacokinetics

Letrozole (4,4′-[(1H-1,2,4-triazol-1-yl)methylene]bisbenzonitrile) was the second nonsteroidal selective aromatase inhibitor approved for the treatment of ABC. The drug has a profile similar to anastrozole, combining high potency, selectivity, and good clinical activity against breast cancer.[160] The IC50 for placental aromatase is 11.5 nM, so it is marginally more potent than anastrozole or exemestane, but this did not translate to greater clinical benefit in the randomized phase III study MA.27 comparing exemestane to anastrozole.[168] For comparison, the IC50 for aminoglutethimide is 1,900 nM. Oral absorption is rapid, with high bioavailability that is only minimally affected by food.[151] Aromatase inhibition at the recommended 2.5-mg dose of letrozole reaches 98.9%,[151] and both letrozole doses examined in phase III trials, 0.5 and 2.5 mg, suppress estrogen levels over 90% (<0.5 pmol/L).[169] Letrozole reaches peak concentration within 2 hours, and steady-state levels are achieved within 14 to 40 days.[151] Maximal estrogen suppression occurs within 2 to 3 days, and the half-life of the drug is 2 to 4 days.[151]

Although letrozole has high specificity for aromatase, two studies have shown effects on either cortisol levels or aldosterone levels; however, these two studies had conflicting results.[170,171] In addition, changes in glucocorticoid and mineralocorticoid levels were small and not clinically meaningful. In these studies, no changes were found in 11-deoxycortisol, 17-hydroxyprogesterone, ACTH, or plasma renin levels. In addition, plasma androgens, thyroid function, LH, and FSH remained unchanged.

Comparison with Anastrozole

While letrozole appears to have characteristics similar to those of anastrozole, comparison of the drugs at the recommended doses has revealed minor differences in potency. In a preclinical model of aromatase-dependent breast cancer growth, letrozole had greater antitumor activity than did anastrozole and tamoxifen.[172] In a double-blind, cross-over study, letrozole was found to suppress aromatization by greater than 99.1% versus 97.3% for anastrozole ($P = 0.0022$). In addition, suppression of plasma estrone sulfate was greater with letrozole treatment.[173] However, data from a study in metastatic disease revealed no difference between the two drugs.[174] A clinical trial in early-stage breast cancer (the FACE trial) directly comparing efficacy and toxicity of these two nonsteroidal inhibitors also did not find any differences in clinical outcomes.[175]

Metabolism

As with anastrozole, metabolic clearance of letrozole is mainly through the liver, and the half-life of 50 hours allows a once-a-day dosing schedule. CYP3A4 and CYP2A6 convert letrozole to its major metabolite, 4,4′-methanol-bisbenzonitrile, which is then subjected to glucuronidation. Letrozole can be safely prescribed for patients with renal insufficiency, because only 5% of the drug is cleared in the urine. However, the drug should be used with caution in treating patients with severe liver impairment.[151] There are no known drug interactions with erythromycin, warfarin, or cimetidine. As with anastrozole, coadministration of tamoxifen reduces letrozole levels by 37%; in the case of letrozole, this is likely due to the induction of CYP3A4.[176]

Toxicity

Like anastrozole, letrozole is well tolerated overall, with 2% of patients discontinuing the drug due to adverse events in one study.[177] A large adjuvant trial using letrozole versus placebo in patients who had completed 5 years of tamoxifen treatment has provided data on toxicities associated with long-term letrozole use.[178] After a median follow-up of 2.4 years, patients on letrozole experienced an increased incidence of hot flashes (47.2% versus 40.5%), arthritis (5.6% versus 3.5%), arthralgias (21.3% versus 16.6%), and myalgias (11.8% versus 9.5%). In addition, there was a trend toward increased osteoporosis (5.8% versus 4.5%). Compared with placebo, patients on letrozole had less vaginal bleeding (4.3% versus 6.0%). Discontinuations rates were nearly identical for placebo and letrozole in this population selected for having tolerated 5 years of prior antiestrogen therapy with tamoxifen.

Aromatase Inhibitors in Premenopausal Women

Hereditary aromatase deficiency, due to inherited loss-of-function mutations in the aromatase gene, is associated with a syndrome of hypergonadotropic hypogonadism, multicystic ovaries, virilism, and bone demineralization in childhood. These problems are reversible with low-dose estrogens.[179,180] Polycystic ovary syndrome in adult women has a less well-defined etiology, although low aromatase activity is believed to play a part.[181] Treatment of premenopausal women with aromatase inhibitors may therefore be complicated by polycystic ovaries and virilization and can result in higher levels of estradiol. To circumvent these problems, the treatment of premenopausal women with ABC with a luteinizing hormone–releasing hormone (LHRH) analog and selective aromatase inhibitor combination is utilized. In the adjuvant setting, the IBCSG Tamoxifen and Exemestane Trial (TEXT) and the IBCSG Suppression of Ovarian Function Trial (SOFT) explored the use of triptorelin in combination with either exemestane or tamoxifen and demonstrated benefit with the addition of ovarian suppression among higher-risk patients.[182,183]

Progestins

Historically, megestrol acetate was a favored second-line therapy for patients with tamoxifen-resistant disease. However, the use of megestrol acetate has been superceded by third-generation aromatase inhibitors and fulvestrant, which both have better side effect and efficacy profiles.[184]

Luteinizing Hormone–Releasing Hormone Agonists

Background

Oophorectomy has been a standard therapy option for breast cancer for more than 100 years. As adjuvant therapy for premenopausal women, oophorectomy is associated with a marked reduction in relapse and death from breast cancer.[185] The development of LHRH agonists has provided the option of reversible medical ovarian ablation. The only randomized comparison between ovariectomy and LHRH agonist therapy was underpowered, but it did not reveal significant differences between these two approaches to estrogen deprivation.[186] Because premenopausal women treated with LHRH agonists have plasma estradiol concentrations typical for postmenopausal women, surgical oophorectomy and treatment with LHRH agonists are generally held to be equivalent.[186–188] Premenopausal women with breast cancer treated with LHRH agonists have objective response rates of between 36% and 44%.[188] Treatment with LHRH agonists is currently used in premenopausal women in both the adjuvant and metastatic setting, with or without tamoxifen or an aromatase inhibitor. Despite the fact that a number of LHRH agonists have been tested in breast cancer, goserelin acetate is the only one approved for this disease. The general characteristics of different LHRH agonists are detailed in Table 27.2 and Figure 27.11.

Mechanism of Action

LHRH agonists reduce circulating concentrations of estrogens in premenopausal women via an inhibitory effect on the hypothalamic-pituitary-gonadal axis. The drugs bind to the LHRH receptors on the pituitary gland, leading to an initial stimulation of FSH and LH production during the first few days of treatment.[187] After this initial stimulation, the ligand-receptor complexes cluster and become sequestered inside the cell; this leads to a reduction in the number of active receptors on the surface. This mechanism accounts for the paradoxical inhibition of pituitary gonadotropic cells with continuous instead of pulsatile LHRH agonism.[189] As a result, after a few days of stimulation, FSH and LH levels fall and remain persistently suppressed, reaching levels comparable to the postmenopausal state within 21 days.[189] Plasma progesterone, estrone, estrone sulfate, and estradiol levels decrease to postmenopausal levels after 6 weeks of treatment. There is no change in androstenedione, prolactin, or cortisol levels.

Goserelin: Pharmacology and Metabolism

Goserelin is a synthetic decapeptide analog of LHRH that is administered as a subcutaneous depot, providing gradual release of the drug. A 3.6-mg depot formulation is given once a month. In addition, a 10.8-mg depot can be given once every 3 months, although this formulation is approved only for prostate cancer, not breast cancer.

When administered as a solution subcutaneously, goserelin has been observed to have a half-life of about 4 hours.[190] After administration of the 3.6-mg depot, there is an initial, short-duration peak of goserelin in the serum at 8 hours. A more prolonged peak then occurs at about 14 days. There is no accumulation of the drug with multiple administration of the depots. After administration of the 10.8-mg depot, the serum concentration profile is notably different than for the 3.6-mg depot. After an initial release over a few days, the profile shows a downward trend, with a shallow second peak at 5 weeks.

Elimination of goserelin is primarily in the urine (93%), with only 2% found in the feces. Excretion occurs fairly rapidly, with greater than 75% of a dose being excreted within 12 hours.[190] In the urine, approximately 20% of the drug is excreted unchanged, and the remaining products are fragments of the decapeptide. With renal impairment, goserelin clearance decreases, and there

TABLE
27.2 *Pharmacology of luteinizing hormone–releasing hormone agonists*

Mechanisms of action	Inhibition of gonadotropin secretion with resultant castration levels of testosterone in men and estrogens in women	
	Direct inhibitory effects on steroidogenesis through blockade of 17,20-desmolase and 17α-hydroxylase enzymes	
	Direct antitumor effect on human mammary cancer in vitro	
Pharmacokinetics	Gonadotropin-releasing hormone	$t_{1/2a}$, 2–8 min
		$t_{1/2b}$, 15–60 min
	Goserelin s.c.	4.9 h
	Triptorelin s.c.	2.8 h
Elimination	Enzymatic degradation by pyroglutamate aminopeptidase, endopeptidase, and postproline-cleaving enzymes and renal excretion	
Drug interactions	None known	
Toxicity	Hot flashes	
	Reduced libido	
	Impotence	
	Local irritation at the injection site	
	Polyuria and polydipsia	
	Gastrointestinal problems, such as indigestion, nausea and vomiting, and constipation	
	Taste sensations	
	Peripheral edema	
	Rash	
	Gynecomastia and mastodynia	
	Disease flare	
	General allergic reaction	
Precautions	Because there is an initial surge of luteinizing hormone, FSH, and testosterone, an acute exacerbation of disease may be seen	

$t_{1/2}$, half-life.

is a corresponding increase in half-life. With hepatic impairment, differences in the pharmacokinetic parameters of goserelin were minimal, with a small increase in C_{max} but not in AUC as compared with controls.[190] Given the wide therapeutic window of goserelin, it is not considered necessary to alter dosing in patients with either renal or hepatic insufficiency.

Following an initial dose of the 3.6-mg depot, LH and FSH levels rise to a peak at about 48 hours.[190] In women with benign gynecologic conditions, the levels then rapidly decline to below baseline

GnRH

pyro Glu-His-Trp-Ser-Tyr-Gly-Leu-Arg-Pro-Gly-NH2

Goserelin

pyro Glu-His-Trp-Ser-Tyr-D-Ser (tert Butyl)-Leu-Arg-Pro-Azgly

Tripterelin

pyro Glu-His-Trp-Ser-Tyr-D-Trp-Leu-Arg-Pro-Gly-NH2

FIGURE **27.11** Gonadotropin-releasing hormone (GnRH) and analogs. Arg, arginine; Glu, glucose; Gly, glycerol; His, histidine; Leu, leucine; Pro, proline; Ser, serine; Trp, tryptophan; Tyr, tyrosine.

by day 3. The levels are greatly reduced after day 8. Estradiol levels rise transiently at 3 days, followed by a decrease of estradiol; similar results are seen with progesterone. Estradiol levels return to normal within 3 months of stopping goserelin. With the 10.8-mg depot, there is an initial increase in LH and FSH in the first week, and castrate range is achieved within 21 days.

While ovarian ablation is achieved in most patients treated with LHRH agonists, there are reports of failure with normal treatment doses.[191] In a study with three different LHRH analogs, residual ovarian estrogen production was detected in 5 of 40 patients at 3 months despite profound suppression of LH in all patients.[192] In addition, up to 9% of patients treated for endometriosis had persistence of uterine bleeding episodes at 6 months.[193]

Triptorelin: Pharmacology and Metabolism

Triptorelin is a synthetic decapeptide analog of LHRH that is not approved for use in breast cancer treatment (approved for advanced prostate cancer), but it was the agent used in the TEXT and SOFT studies.[194] The drug can be administered as an intramuscular injection of a suspension of microspheres at a dose of 3.75 mg once a month or 11.25 mg every 3 months.[195] With the monthly formulation, peak serum levels of the drug occur during the first week and then remain at a detectable plateau level for about 4 weeks.

As with goserelin, initially, levels of LH and FSH increase but fall to low levels after 1 to 2 weeks,[196] and estradiol levels reach nadir levels by 21 days.[195] Studies in patients with hepatic and renal insufficiency show that clearance of the drug decreases by about half under both conditions. Given the generous therapeutic window of triptorelin, however, dose modification does not appear to be necessary.[197]

LHRH Agonist Toxicity

Potential side effects in women include hot flashes, nausea and vomiting, headache, dizziness, vaginitis, sweating, emotional lability, breast atrophy, tumor flare, diarrhea, local reaction, irritability, hives, loss of bone density, and severe polydipsia and polyuria in one patient.[187,198,199] Also, amenorrhea is induced in all women. Measurement of antithrombin III concentrations after treatment with goserelin revealed no change. This suggests there may be no increased or decreased risk of thromboembolic episodes with this therapy. There are limited data available on known drug-drug interactions.

Endocrine Resistance

Despite the proven clinical efficacy of endocrine therapy in all stages of breast cancer, hormone-refractory breast cancer remains a formidable challenge. Some ER-positive tumors are intrinsically resistant, and all patients with ER-positive metastatic disease ultimately become refractory to endocrine treatments.[200] From a clinical standpoint, hormone-refractory breast cancer can be considered to exhibit either primary resistance (no response to endocrine therapy) or acquired resistance (progression after disease regression or stability). The molecular mechanisms of resistance can be divided into three groups: (a) ER mutation, splice variants, and isoform ratio; (b) coactivator and corepressor effects; and (c) activation of other signaling pathways.

ER Mutation, Splice Variants, and Isoform Ratio

One hypothesis to explain the variable clinical response to endocrine therapy in ER-positive breast cancer invokes ER gene mutation or splice variants.[201–203] ER mutations that allow ligand-independent activity have been described in human tumors. Early work demonstrated a missense mutation substituting tyrosine 537 for asparagine in the LBD was equally active in the absence of ligand, with tamoxifen or with estradiol.[204] In recent years, there has been broader recognition of gain-of-function mutations in *ESR1*, the gene encoding the ER, with an estimated 20% of patients with ER+ ABC exhibiting such mutations.[205] *ESR1* mutations are associated with resistance to aromatase inhibitor therapy, and therefore, one therapeutic strategy is to consider SERDs.[206] These mutations can be detected through both metastatic tissue genotyping and through analysis of circulating tumor DNA (ctDNA), and the presence of *ESR1* mutations is associated with shorter PFS on subsequent AI-based therapy.[207] However, evaluation of primary breast tumors has established that such somatic mutations in ER are rare, occurring in fewer than 1% of either ER-positive or ER-negative breast cancers[208] and do not explain the majority of instances of primary endocrine resistance.[201,209]

Another potential alteration of ER function may occur through changes in the ERα-ERβ ratio.[210] Steroidal antiestrogens have been shown to activate ERβ-mediated transcription while they repress ERα activity.[211] Although the biologic significance of this remains unclear, this observation suggests that increased ERβ might counter inhibitory effects of antiestrogens, but there is conflicting data regarding this issue. In support of this hypothesis, a relatively small study demonstrated that ERβ mRNA levels were twice as high as ERα mRNA levels in tamoxifen-resistant tumors compared with tamoxifen-responsive tumors.[212]

ERα and ERβ splice variants may also play a role in endocrine resistance. Alternatively spliced ER mRNA variants have also been commonly identified in normal and malignant breast tissues.[18] An ERα transcript that has received particular attention lacks exon 5; exon 4 directly splices into exon 6, with preservation of the reading frame.[213] The exon 5–deleted variant binds to DNA but not to estrogen, and it activates transcription in an estrogen-independent manner (a dominant positive receptor). These properties imply a role in estrogen-independent growth. However, coexpression of the exon 5–deleted variant with an intact ER did not alter the transcriptional response to estrogen, arguing against a critical role in breast cancer pathogenesis.[214]

At least five isoforms and one tyrosine mutant of ERβ have been identified; however, their role in hormone-resistance is not clear.[18] The most interesting ERβ variant is ERβcx, which lacks amino acid residues important for ligand binding. Although ERβcx does not bind estrogen, it does heterodimerize with ERα and inhibits DNA binding. This, in turn, results in a dominant negative effect on ligand-dependent transcription of the ER.[22] Higher levels of ERβcx in tumors have been correlated with resistance to tamoxifen; however, confirmatory studies are required.[18]

Coactivators and Corepressors

Given the role of coactivators and corepressors in regulating ER activity, it is not surprising that they might also contribute to endocrine response. NCoA3 (AIB1) was initially identified based on its amplification in breast cancer.[209] When expressed in cultured cells, AIB1 promotes tamoxifen's agonist activity, suggesting a role in endocrine resistance.[215] Overexpression of another coactivator, NCoA1, similarly increases tamoxifen's agonist activity, indicating a role in tamoxifen resistance.[216]

Conversely, decreased activity of corepressors has also been implicated as a mechanism of resistance. In a mouse model of tamoxifen resistance, NCoR1 levels were decreased.[210] Together, these findings suggest that alteration of the coactivator-corepressor balance can result in conversion of tamoxifen from an antagonist to an agonist.

Growth Factor Signaling Pathways

As previously discussed, ER function is strongly influenced by peptide growth factor signaling, including EGFR, ErbB2, and IGF-1-R, that leads to stimulation of ER activity in the absence of estrogen. These mitogenic pathways are often elevated in non-responsive tumors that exhibit either primary or acquired resistance, which may lead to downstream activation of kinases that phosphorylate the ER and/or ER coregulators.[217–219] In this way, these growth factor pathways can allow the ER to function in the absence of ligand.

EGF has been shown to mimic the effect of estrogens on uterine cell proliferation in ovariectomized mice, and tumors overexpressing EGFR are less likely to be sensitive to endocrine therapy.[217] Similar results have been demonstrated with overexpression of ErbB2.[217] Several groups have evaluated response to endocrine therapy with respect to ErbB2 tumor status or circulating ErbB2 levels.[220-222] These studies have found a markedly decreased response to hormones in patients with ErbB2-overexpressing tumors.

Recently, the paired box 2 gene product (PAX2) has been identified as a crucial mediator of ER cross talk with ErbB2.[223] PAX2 and the ER coactivator AIB1/SRC-3 compete for binding and regulation of ErbB2 transcription. This suggests an intrinsic transcriptional link between tumors driven by ER and those driven by ErbB2. PAX2 may be a primary determinant of tamoxifen response in breast cancer cells.

Additionally, the expression and activation of the Ras/Raf-1/MAPK pathway play an important role in the development and progression of cancer. An analysis of breast tumors showed that expression and activation of the Ras pathway were associated with loss of benefit from treatment with tamoxifen but not chemotherapy.[224] This finding is consistent with other studies of the Ras pathway in lung and colon cancer. Patients with a polymorphism of TC21, a member of the Ras superfamily, had higher recurrence rates on tamoxifen.[225]

Strategies to Combat Endocrine Resistance

There has been remarkable growth in the number of endocrine therapies available for the treatment of breast cancer. With more options, the clinical efficacy of endocrine therapy has improved; however, the improvement has been incremental in nature. Our increasing understanding of the molecular basis of endocrine resistance has led to the use of combinations of endocrine agents with newer signal transduction inhibitors for the treatment of breast cancer, such as combinations of endocrine therapy with agents such as CDK4/6 inhibitors, such as palbociclib and ribociclib, and mTOR inhibitors, such as everolimus (Fig. 27.12). A number of other targeted agents, particularly PI3K inhibitors and Akt inhibitors, are being extensively evaluated in clinical trials in combination with endocrine therapy (Fig. 27.12). The inhibition of multiple growth pathways simultaneously could potentially combat the redundancy and cross talk of growth signals, thereby providing effective, well-tolerated therapy.

Future Directions

With the advent of advanced techniques, such as DNA microarrays and proteomic technologies, the characterization of different types of tumors will continue to make major strides. With regard to endocrine therapy, significant achievements have already been

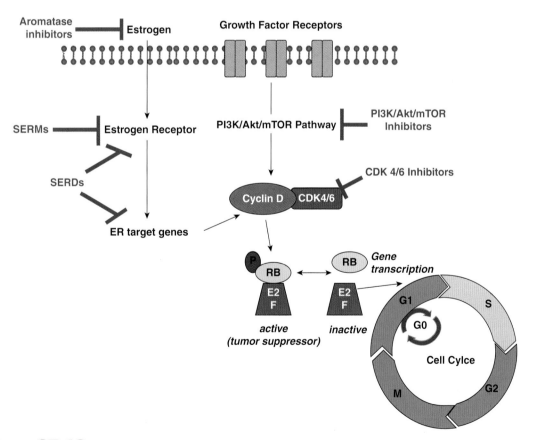

FIGURE 27.12 Endocrine-based combination therapy. Summary of the interaction of endocrine therapies and targeted therapies to halt cell growth. SERMs, selective estrogen receptor modulators; SERDs, selective estrogen receptor degraders; PI3K, phosphoinositide 3-kinase; Akt, protein kinase B; mTOR, mechanistic target of rapamycin; CDK 4/6, cyclin-dependent kinase 4/6; P, phosphate; RB, retinoblastoma.

made. Several groups have demonstrated that supervised cluster analysis of DNA microarray data allows identification of a set of genes that can distinguish between ER-positive and ER-negative breast tumors.[226,227] The marked difference in the gene expression profile of these breast cancer subtypes suggests the possibility of distinct precursor cells. Interestingly, only a small number of genes that discriminate between ER-positive and ER-negative tumors are involved in ER signaling.[228]

Further subclassification of breast tumors will continue. Given that resistance to endocrine agents does not entirely overlap, further work with other agents will likely show different resistance and sensitivity patterns associated with various endocrine therapies. This will undoubtedly help define how to use different endocrine agents as well as rationale combinations with targeted therapies. Furthermore, as signal transduction inhibitors are tested in combination with endocrine therapy, DNA microarrays will be critical in determining which targeted drug cocktail to use against a specific tumor.

In addition to predicting the ER status of tumors and their response to therapy, gene expression profiling has the potential to help elucidate which signaling pathways are critical in tumors and thus provide strategies to improve treatment. It is important to note that, with DNA microarray analysis, the delineation of differences in signaling pathways between tumors is only inferential. While these advanced analytic procedures can help generate hypotheses, the findings from these studies still require testing with more traditional laboratory techniques. A number of laboratories have identified and characterized changes in gene expression that occur with various endocrine agents.[229,230] Proteomic technologies, which are beginning to allow large-scale interrogation of signaling pathways, will be critical in achieving this goal. Integration of these technologies into clinical trial design is essential.

The determination of predictive biomarkers for targeted therapy is currently a major goal in the oncology community. Interestingly, the use of endocrine therapy for ER/PR-positive breast cancer provides the oldest paradigm for this approach. In addition, this history gives a glimpse of the promise and limitations of targeted therapy. Endocrine resistance remains a problem that we are only beginning to address in the clinic. Finally, classical endocrine therapy continues to evolve with ongoing clinical investigation into the optimal endocrine agent, duration of therapy, and scheduling of therapy. However, with the development of new technologies and new drugs, endocrine therapy can be a foundation on which to build more effectively tailored and targeted treatments.

References

1. Love RR, Philips J. Oophorectomy for breast cancer: history revisited. *J Natl Cancer Inst.* 2002;94:1433-1434.
2. IUPAC Commission on the Nomenclature of Organic Chemistry (CNOC) and IUPAC-IUB Commission on Biochemical Nomenclature (CBN). The nomenclature of steroids. Revised tentative rules. *Eur J Biochem.* 1969;10:1-19.
3. Briggs MJ. *Steroid Biochemistry and Pharmacology.* London: Academic Press; 1970.
4. Brotherton J. *Sex Hormone Pharmacology.* London: Academic Press; 1976.
5. Briggs MH, Christie GA. *Advances in Steroid Biochemistry and Pharmacology.* London: Academic Press; 1977.
6. Gruber CJ, Tschugguel W, Schneeberger C, et al. Production and actions of estrogens. *N Engl J Med.* 2002;346:340-352.
7. Brodie A. Aromatase inhibitors in breast cancer. *Trends Endocrinol Metab.* 2002;13:61-65.
8. Chen SA, Besman MJ, Sparkes RS, et al. Human aromatase: cDNA cloning, Southern blot analysis, and assignment of the gene to chromosome 15. *DNA.* 1988;7:27-38.
9. Agarwal VR, Bulun SE, Leitch M, et al. Use of alternative promoters to express the aromatase cytochrome P450 (CYP19) gene in breast adipose tissues of cancer-free and breast cancer patients. *J Clin Endocrinol Metab.* 1996;81:3843-3849.
10. Santner SJ, Pauley RJ, Tait L, et al. Aromatase activity and expression in breast cancer and benign breast tissue stromal cells. *J Clin Endocrinol Metab.* 1997;82:200-208.
11. Zhou D, Clarke P, Wang J, et al. Identification of a promoter that controls aromatase expression in human breast cancer and adipose stromal cells. *J Biol Chem.* 1996;271:15194-15202.
12. Grodin JM, Siiteri PK, MacDonald PC. Source of estrogen production in postmenopausal women. *J Clin Endocrinol Metab.* 1973;36:207-214.
13. Simpson ER. Sources of estrogen and their importance. *J Steroid Biochem Mol Biol.* 2003;86:225-230.
14. Kutsky RJ. *Handbook of Vitamins, Minerals, and Hormones.* 2nd ed. New York: Van Nostrand Reinhold; 1981:1-492.
15. Evans RM. The steroid and thyroid hormone receptor superfamily. *Science.* 1988;240:889-895.
16. Shao W, Brown M. Advances in estrogen receptor biology: prospects for improvements in targeted breast cancer therapy. *Breast Cancer Res.* 2004;6:39-52.
17. Yang NN, Venugopalan M, Hardikar S, et al. Identification of an estrogen response element activated by metabolites of 17beta-estradiol and raloxifene. *Science.* 1996;273:1222-1225.
18. Speirs V, Carder PJ, Lane S, et al. Oestrogen receptor beta: what it means for patients with breast cancer. *Lancet Oncol.* 2004;5:174-181.
19. Barkhem T, Carlsson B, Nilsson Y, et al. Differential response of estrogen receptor alpha and estrogen receptor beta to partial estrogen agonists/antagonists. *Mol Pharmacol.* 1998;54:105-112.
20. Saunders FJ. Effects of norethynodrel combined with mestranol on the offspring when administered during pregnancy and lactation in rats. *Endocrinology.* 1967;80:447-452.
21. Williams MT, Clark MR, Ling WY. Role of cyclic AMP in the action of luteinizing hormone on steroidogenesis in the corpus luteum. In: George WJ, Ignarro LJ, eds. *Adv Cyclic Nucleotide Res.* New York: Raven Press; 1978:573.
22. Weihua Z, Andersson S, Cheng G, et al. Update on estrogen signaling. *FEBS Lett.* 2003;546:17-24.
23. Krege JH, Hodgin JB, Couse JF, et al. Generation and reproductive phenotypes of mice lacking estrogen receptor beta. *Proc Natl Acad Sci U S A.* 1998;95:15677-15682.
24. Porter W, Wang F, Wang W, et al. Role of estrogen receptor/Sp1 complexes in estrogen-induced heat shock protein 27 gene expression. *Mol Endocrinol.* 1996;10:1371-1378.
25. Pace P, Taylor J, Suntharalingam S, et al. Human estrogen receptor beta binds DNA in a manner similar to and dimerizes with estrogen receptor alpha. *J Biol Chem.* 1997;272:25832-25838.
26. McDonnell DP, Norris JD. Connections and regulation of the human estrogen receptor. *Science.* 2002;296:1642-1644.
27. Beato M, Candau R, Chavez S, et al. Interaction of steroid hormone receptors with transcription factors involves chromatin remodelling. *J Steroid Biochem Mol Biol.* 1996;56:47-59.
28. Lannigan DA. Estrogen receptor phosphorylation. *Steroids.* 2003;68:1-9.
29. El-Ashry D, Miller DL, Kharbanda S, et al. Constitutive Raf-1 kinase activity in breast cancer cells induces both estrogen-independent growth and apoptosis. *Oncogene.* 1997;15:423-435.
30. Kato S, Masuhiro Y, Watanabe M, et al. Molecular mechanism of a crosstalk between oestrogen and growth factor signalling pathways. *Genes Cells.* 2000;5:593-601.
31. Kato S, Endoh H, Masuhiro Y, et al. Activation of the estrogen receptor through phosphorylation by mitogen-activated protein kinase. *Science.* 1995;270:1491-1494.

32. Mueller H, Kueng W, Schoumacher F, et al. Selective regulation of steroid receptor expression in MCF-7 breast cancer cells by a novel member of the heregulin family. *Biochem Biophys Res Commun.* 1995;217:1271-1278.

33. Ingle JN, Ahmann DL, Green SJ, et al. Randomized clinical trial of diethylstilbestrol versus tamoxifen in postmenopausal women with advanced breast cancer. *N Engl J Med.* 1981;304:16-21.

34. Furr BJ, Jordan VC. The pharmacology and clinical uses of tamoxifen. *Pharmacol Ther.* 1984;25:127-205.

35. Osborne CK. Tamoxifen in the treatment of breast cancer. *N Engl J Med.* 1998;339:1609-1618.

36. Morgan LR, Schein PS, Woolley PV, et al. Therapeutic use of tamoxifen in advanced breast cancer: correlation with biochemical parameters. *Cancer Treat Rep.* 1976;60:1437-1443.

37. Rose C, Mouridsen HT. Treatment of advanced breast cancer with tamoxifen. *Recent Results Cancer Res.* 1984;91:230-242.

38. Early Breast Cancer Trialists' Collaborative Group. Tamoxifen for early breast cancer: an overview of the randomised trials. *Lancet.* 1998;351:1451-1467.

39. Ingle JN, Krook JE, Green SJ, et al. Randomized trial of bilateral oophorectomy versus tamoxifen in premenopausal women with metastatic breast cancer. *J Clin Oncol.* 1986;4:178-185.

40. Muss HB, Case LD, Atkins JN, et al. Tamoxifen versus high-dose oral medroxyprogesterone acetate as initial endocrine therapy for patients with metastatic breast cancer: a Piedmont Oncology Association study. *J Clin Oncol.* 1994;12:1630-1638.

41. Hermon C, Beral V. Breast cancer mortality rates are levelling off or beginning to decline in many western countries: analysis of time trends, age-cohort and age-period models of breast cancer mortality in 20 countries. *Br J Cancer.* 1996;73:955-960.

42. Jordan VC, Assikis VJ. Endometrial carcinoma and tamoxifen: clearing up a controversy. *Clin Cancer Res.* 1995;1:467-472.

43. Uziely B, Lewin A, Brufman G, et al. The effect of tamoxifen on the endometrium. *Breast Cancer Res Treat.* 1993;26:101-105.

44. Kavak ZN, Binöz S, Ceyhan N, et al. The effect of tamoxifen on the endometrium, serum lipids and hypothalamus pituitary axis in the postmenopausal breast cancer patients. *Acta Obstet Gynecol Scand.* 2000;79:604-607.

45. Enck RE, Rios CN. Tamoxifen treatment of metastatic breast cancer and antithrombin III levels. *Cancer.* 1984;53:2607-2609.

46. Love RR, Surawicz TS, Williams EC. Antithrombin III level, fibrinogen level, and platelet count changes with adjuvant tamoxifen therapy. *Arch Intern Med.* 1992;152:317-320.

47. Barakat RR. The effect of tamoxifen on the endometrium. *Oncology (Williston Park).* 1995;9:129-134; discussion 139-140, 142.

48. Barni S, Lissoni P, Tancini G, et al. Effects of one-year adjuvant treatment with tamoxifen on bone mineral density in postmenopausal breast cancer women. *Tumori.* 1996;82:65-67.

49. Schapira DV, Kumar NB, Lyman GH. Serum cholesterol reduction with tamoxifen. *Breast Cancer Res Treat.* 1990;17:3-7.

50. Love RR, Newcomb PA, Wiebe DA, et al. Effects of tamoxifen therapy on lipid and lipoprotein levels in postmenopausal patients with node-negative breast cancer. *J Natl Cancer Inst.* 1990;82:1327-1332.

51. Fromson JM, Pearson S, Bramah S. The metabolism of tamoxifen (I.C.I. 46,474). I. In laboratory animals. *Xenobiotica.* 1973;3:693-709.

52. Lyman SD, Jordan VC. Metabolism of nonsteroidal antiestrogens. In: Craig Jordan V, ed. *Estrogen/Antiestrogen Action and Breast Cancer Therapy.* Madison, Wisconsin: University of Wisconsin Press; 1986.

53. Bain RR, Jordan VC. Identification of a new metabolite of tamoxifen in patient serum during breast cancer therapy. *Biochem Pharmacol.* 1983;32:373-375.

54. Robinson SP, Jordan VC. Metabolism of antihormonal anticancer agents. In: Powlis C, ed. *Anticancer Drugs: Antimetabolite Metabolism and Natural Anticancer Agents*, pp. 279-289 (section 5.2). Pergamon Press: Oxford; 1994.

55. Adam HK, Douglas EJ, Kemp JV. The metabolism of tamoxifen in human. *Biochem Pharmacol.* 1979;28:145-147.

56. Fromson JM, Pearson S, Bramah S. The metabolism of tamoxifen (I.C.I. 46,474). II. In female patients. *Xenobiotica.* 1973;3:711-714.

57. Fabian C, Tilzer L, Sternson L. Comparative binding affinities of tamoxifen, 4-hydroxytamoxifen, and desmethyltamoxifen for estrogen receptors isolated from human breast carcinoma: correlation with blood levels in patients with metastatic breast cancer. *Biopharm Drug Dispos.* 1981;2:381-390.

58. Fabian C, Sternson L, El-Serafi M, et al. Clinical pharmacology of tamoxifen in patients with breast cancer: correlation with clinical data. *Cancer.* 1981;48:876-882.

59. Fabian C, Sternson L, Barnett M. Clinical pharmacology of tamoxifen in patients with breast cancer: comparison of traditional and loading dose schedules. *Cancer Treat Rep.* 1980;64:765-773.

60. Noguchi S, Miyauchi K, Imaoka S, et al. Inability of tamoxifen to penetrate into cerebrospinal fluid. *Breast Cancer Res Treat.* 1988;12:317-318.

61. Jacolot F, Simon I, Dreano Y, et al. Identification of the cytochrome P450 IIIA family as the enzymes involved in the N-demethylation of tamoxifen in human liver microsomes. *Biochem Pharmacol.* 1991;41:1911-1919.

62. Desta Z, Ward BA, Soukhova NV, et al. Comprehensive evaluation of tamoxifen sequential biotransformation by the human cytochrome P450 system in vitro: prominent roles for CYP3A and CYP2D6. *J Pharmacol Exp Ther.* 2004;310:1062-1075.

63. Stearns V, Johnson MD, Rae JM, et al. Active tamoxifen metabolite plasma concentrations after coadministration of tamoxifen and the selective serotonin reuptake inhibitor paroxetine. *J Natl Cancer Inst.* 2003;95:1758-1764.

64. Schroth W, Goetz MP, Hamann U, et al. Association between CYP2D6 polymorphisms and outcomes among women with early stage breast cancer treated with tamoxifen. *JAMA.* 2009;302:1429-1436.

65. Regan MM, Leyland-Jones B, Bouzyk M, et al. CYP2D6 genotype and tamoxifen response in postmenopausal women with endocrine-responsive breast cancer: the breast international group 1-98 trial. *J Natl Cancer Inst.* 2012;104:441-451.

66. Rae JM, Drury S, Hayes DF, et al. Abstract S1-7: lack of correlation between gene variants in tamoxifen metabolizing enzymes with primary endpoints in the ATAC trial. *Cancer Res.* 2010;70:S1-S7.

67. Gradishar WJ, Anderson BO, Balassanian R, et al. Invasive breast cancer version 1.2016, NCCN clinical practice guidelines in oncology. *J Natl Compr Can Netw.* 2016;14:324-354.

68. Crewe HK, Lennard MS, Tucker GT, et al. The effect of selective serotonin re-uptake inhibitors on cytochrome P4502D6 (CYP2D6) activity in human liver microsomes. *Br J Clin Pharmacol.* 1992;34:262-265.

69. Jin Y, Desta Z, Stearns V, et al. CYP2D6 genotype, antidepressant use, and tamoxifen metabolism during adjuvant breast cancer treatment. *J Natl Cancer Inst.* 2005;97:30-39.

70. Henry NL, Stearns V, Flockhart DA, et al. Drug interactions and pharmacogenomics in the treatment of breast cancer and depression. *Am J Psychiatry.* 2008;165:1251-1255.

71. Ahern TP, Pedersen L, Cronin-Fenton DP, et al. No increase in breast cancer recurrence with concurrent use of tamoxifen and some CYP2D6-inhibiting medications. *Cancer Epidemiol Biomarkers Prev.* 2009;18:2562-2564.

72. Reid AD, Horobin JM, Newman EL, et al. Tamoxifen metabolism is altered by simultaneous administration of medroxyprogesterone acetate in breast cancer patients. *Breast Cancer Res Treat.* 1992;22:153-156.

73. Fogarty PF, Rick ME, Swain SM. Tamoxifen and thrombosis: current clinical observations and treatment guidelines. In: Devita VT, Hellman S, Rosenberg SA, eds. *Cancer: Principles and Practice of Oncology.* 6th ed. Philadelphia, PA: Lippincott Williams & Wilkins; 2002.

74. Fisher B, Costantino JP, Wickerham DL, et al. Tamoxifen for prevention of breast cancer: report of the National Surgical Adjuvant Breast and Bowel Project P-1 Study. *J Natl Cancer Inst.* 1998;90:1371-1388.

75. Kaiser-Kupfer MI, Lippman ME. Tamoxifen retinopathy. *Cancer Treat Rep.* 1978;62:315-320.

76. Kaiser-Kupfer MI, Kupfer C, Rodrigues MM. Tamoxifen retinopathy. A clinicopathologic report. *Ophthalmology.* 1981;88:89-93.

77. McKeown CA, Swartz M, Blom J, et al. Tamoxifen retinopathy. *Br J Ophthalmol.* 1981;65:177-179.

78. Gerner EW. Low-dose tamoxifen retinopathy. *Can J Ophthalmol.* 1992;27:358.

79. Griffiths MF. Tamoxifen retinopathy at low dosage. *Am J Ophthalmol.* 1987;104:185-186.

80. Bentley CR, Davies G, Aclimandos WA. Tamoxifen retinopathy: a rare but serious complication. *BMJ.* 1992;304:495-496.

81. Pemberton KD, Melissari E, Kakkar VV. The influence of tamoxifen in vivo on the main natural anticoagulants and fibrinolysis. *Blood Coagul Fibrinolysis.* 1993;4:935-942.

82. Fisher B, Costantino J, Redmond C, et al. A randomized clinical trial evaluating tamoxifen in the treatment of patients with node-negative breast cancer who have estrogen-receptor-positive tumors. *N Engl J Med.* 1989;320:479-484.

83. Abramson N, Costantino JP, Garber JE, et al. Effect of Factor V Leiden and prothrombin G20210—>A mutations on thromboembolic risk in the national surgical adjuvant breast and bowel project breast cancer prevention trial. *J Natl Cancer Inst.* 2006;98:904-910.

84. Jones AL, Powles TJ, Treleaven JG, et al. Haemostatic changes and thromboembolic risk during tamoxifen therapy in normal women. *Br J Cancer.* 1992;66:744-747.

85. Bruning PF, Bonfrer JM, Hart AA, et al. Tamoxifen, serum lipoproteins and cardiovascular risk. *Br J Cancer.* 1988;58:497-499.

86. Ingram D. Tamoxifen use, oestrogen binding and serum lipids in postmenopausal women with breast cancer. *ANZ J Surg.* 1990;60:673-675.

87. Pathak DN, Bodell WJ. DNA adduct formation by tamoxifen with rat and human liver microsomal activation systems. *Carcinogenesis.* 1994;15:529-532.

88. Turken S, Siris E, Seldin D, et al. Effects of tamoxifen on spinal bone density in women with breast cancer. *J Natl Cancer Inst.* 1989;81:1086-1088.

89. Fornander T, Rutqvist LE, Sjöberg HE, et al. Long-term adjuvant tamoxifen in early breast cancer: effect on bone mineral density in postmenopausal women. *J Clin Oncol.* 1990;8:1019-1024.

90. Fisher B, Costantino JP, Wickerham DL, et al. Tamoxifen for the prevention of breast cancer: current status of the National Surgical Adjuvant Breast and Bowel Project P-1 Study. *J Natl Cancer Inst.* 2005;97:1652-1662.

91. Gotfredsen A, Christiansen C, Palshof T. The effect of tamoxifen on bone mineral content in premenopausal women with breast cancer. *Cancer.* 1984;53:853-857.

92. Kedar RP, Bourne TH, Powles TJ, et al. Effects of tamoxifen on uterus and ovaries of postmenopausal women in a randomised breast cancer prevention trial. *Lancet.* 1994;343:1318-1321.

93. Bernstein L, Deapen D, Cerhan JR, et al. Tamoxifen therapy for breast cancer and endometrial cancer risk. *J Natl Cancer Inst.* 1999;91:1654-1662.

94. Wysowski DK, Honig SF, Beitz J. Uterine sarcoma associated with tamoxifen use. *N Engl J Med.* 2002;346:1832-1833.

95. Cullins SL, Pridjian G, Sutherland CM. Goldenhar's syndrome associated with tamoxifen given to the mother during gestation. *JAMA.* 1994;271:1905-1906.

96. Woo JC, Yu T, Hurd TC. Breast cancer in pregnancy: a literature review. *Arch Surg.* 1960;138:91-98; discussion 99.

97. Halakivi-Clarke L, Cho E, Onojafe I, et al. Maternal exposure to tamoxifen during pregnancy increases carcinogen-induced mammary tumorigenesis among female rat offspring. *Clin Cancer Res.* 2000;6:305-308.

98. Anelli TF, Anelli A, Tran KN, et al. Tamoxifen administration is associated with a high rate of treatment-limiting symptoms in male breast cancer patients. *Cancer.* 1994;74:74-77.

99. Traub AI, Thompson W. The effect of tamoxifen on spermatogenesis in subfertile men. *Andrologia.* 1981;13:486-490.

100. Gooren LJ. Androgen levels and sex functions in testosterone-treated hypogonadal men. *Arch Sex Behav.* 1987;16:463-473.

101. Plotkin D, Lechner JJ, Jung WE, et al. Tamoxifen flare in advanced breast cancer. *JAMA.* 1978;240:2644-2646.

102. Beex L, Pieters G, Smals A, et al. Tamoxifen versus ethinyl estradiol in the treatment of postmenopausal women with advanced breast cancer. *Cancer Treat Rep.* 1981;65:179-185.

103. Howell A, Dodwell DJ, Anderson H, et al. Response after withdrawal of tamoxifen and progestogens in advanced breast cancer. *Ann Oncol.* 1992;3:611-617.

104. O'Regan RM, Cisneros A, England GM, et al. Effects of the antiestrogens tamoxifen, toremifene, and ICI 182,780 on endometrial cancer growth. *J Natl Cancer Inst.* 1998;90:1552-1558.

105. Lufkin EG, Whitaker MD, Nickelsen T, et al. Treatment of established postmenopausal osteoporosis with raloxifene: a randomized trial. *J Bone Miner Res.* 1998;13:1747-1754.

106. Buzdar AU, Marcus C, Holmes F, et al. Phase II evaluation of Ly156758 in metastatic breast cancer. *Oncology.* 1988;45:344-345.

107. Ettinger B, Black DM, Mitlak BH, et al. Reduction of vertebral fracture risk in postmenopausal women with osteoporosis treated with raloxifene:

results from a 3-year randomized clinical trial. Multiple Outcomes of Raloxifene Evaluation (MORE) Investigators. *JAMA.* 1999;282:637-645.

108. Vogel VG, Costantino JP, Wickerham DL, et al. Effects of tamoxifen vs raloxifene on the risk of developing invasive breast cancer and other disease outcomes: the NSABP Study of Tamoxifen and Raloxifene (STAR) P-2 trial. *JAMA.* 2006;295:2727-2741.

109. Goldstein SR, Siddhanti S, Ciaccia AV, et al. A pharmacological review of selective oestrogen receptor modulators. *Hum Reprod Update.* 2000;6:212-224.

110. Wijayaratne AL, Nagel SC, Paige LA, et al. Comparative analyses of mechanistic differences among antiestrogens. *Endocrinology.* 1999;140:5828-5840.

111. Shang Y, Brown M. Molecular determinants for the tissue specificity of SERMs. *Science.* 2002;295:2465-2468.

112. Morello KC, Wurz GT, DeGregorio MW. Pharmacokinetics of selective estrogen receptor modulators. *Clin Pharmacokinet.* 2003;42:361-372.

113. Snyder KR, Sparano N, Malinowski JM. Raloxifene hydrochloride. *Am J Health Syst Pharm.* 2000;57:1669-1675; quiz 1676-1678.

114. Cummings SR, Eckert S, Krueger KA, et al. The effect of raloxifene on risk of breast cancer in postmenopausal women: results from the MORE randomized trial. Multiple Outcomes of Raloxifene Evaluation. *JAMA.* 1999;281:2189-2197.

115. Hochner-Celnikier D. Pharmacokinetics of raloxifene and its clinical application. *Eur J Obstet Gynecol Reprod Biol.* 1999;85:23-29.

116. Cauley JA, Norton L, Lippman ME, et al. Continued breast cancer risk reduction in postmenopausal women treated with raloxifene: 4-year results from the MORE trial. Multiple outcomes of raloxifene evaluation. *Breast Cancer Res Treat.* 2001;65:125-134.

117. Barrett-Connor E, Mosca L, Collins P, et al. Effects of raloxifene on cardiovascular events and breast cancer in postmenopausal women. *N Engl J Med.* 2006;355:125-137.

118. Grady D, Cauley JA, Geiger MJ, et al. Reduced incidence of invasive breast cancer with raloxifene among women at increased coronary risk. *J Natl Cancer Inst.* 2008;100:854-861.

119. Vogel CL. Phase II and III clinical trials of toremifene for metastatic breast cancer. *Oncology (Williston Park).* 1998;12:9-13.

120. Wiseman LR, Goa KL. Toremifene. A review of its pharmacological properties and clinical efficacy in the management of advanced breast cancer. *Drugs.* 1997;54:141-160.

121. Wiebe VJ, Benz CC, Shemano I, et al. Pharmacokinetics of toremifene and its metabolites in patients with advanced breast cancer. *Cancer Chemother Pharmacol.* 1990;25:247-251.

122. Tamrazi A, Carlson KE, Daniels JR, et al. Estrogen receptor dimerization: ligand binding regulates dimer affinity and dimer dissociation rate. *Mol Endocrinol.* 2002;16:2706-2719.

123. Johnston SRD. Fulvestrant (AstraZeneca). *Curr Opin Investig Drugs.* 2002;3:305-312.

124. Dauvois S, Danielian PS, White R, et al. Antiestrogen ICI 164,384 reduces cellular estrogen receptor content by increasing its turnover. *Proc Natl Acad Sci U S A.* 1992;89:4037-4041.

125. Dukes M, Miller D, Wakeling AE, et al. Antiuterotrophic effects of a pure antioestrogen, ICI 182,780: magnetic resonance imaging of the uterus in ovariectomized monkeys. *J Endocrinol.* 1992;135:239-247.

126. Long BJ, Tilghman SL, Yue W, et al. The steroidal antiestrogen ICI 182,780 is an inhibitor of cellular aromatase activity. *J Steroid Biochem Mol Biol.* 1998;67:293-304.

127. DeFriend DJ, Howell A, Nicholson RI, et al. Investigation of a new pure antiestrogen (ICI 182780) in women with primary breast cancer. *Cancer Res.* 1994;54:408-414.

128. Ellis PA, Saccani-Jotti G, Clarke R, et al. Induction of apoptosis by tamoxifen and ICI 182780 in primary breast cancer. *Int J Cancer.* 1997;72:608-613.

129. Robertson JFR, Bondarenko IM, Trishkina E, et al. Fulvestrant 500 mg versus anastrozole 1 mg for hormone receptor-positive advanced breast cancer (FALCON): an international, randomised, double-blind, phase 3 trial. *Lancet.* 2017;388:2997-3005.

130. Turner NC, Ro J, André F, et al. Palbociclib in Hormone-Receptor–Positive advanced breast cancer. *N Engl J Med.* 2015;373:209-219.

131. Thomas EJ, Walton PL, Thomas NM, et al. The effects of ICI 182,780, a pure anti-oestrogen, on the hypothalamic-pituitary-gonadal axis and on endometrial proliferation in pre-menopausal women. *Hum Reprod.* 1994;9:1991-1996.

132. Howell A, DeFriend DJ, Robertson JF, et al. Pharmacokinetics, pharmacological and anti-tumour effects of the specific anti-oestrogen ICI 182780 in women with advanced breast cancer. *Br J Cancer.* 1996;74:300-308.

133. Leo AD, Jerusalem G, Petruzelka L, et al. Final overall survival: fulvestrant 500mg vs 250mg in the randomized CONFIRM trial. *J Natl Cancer Inst.* 2013;106:djt337. doi:10.1093/jnci/djt337.

134. Robertson JFR, Harrison MP. Equivalent single-dose pharmacokinetics of two different dosing methods of prolonged-release fulvestrant ("Faslodex") in postmenopausal women with advanced breast cancer. *Cancer Chemother Pharmacol.* 2003;52:346-348.

135. Howell A, Robertson JFR, Abram P, et al. Comparison of fulvestrant versus tamoxifen for the treatment of advanced breast cancer in postmenopausal women previously untreated with endocrine therapy: a multinational, double-blind, randomized trial. *J Clin Oncol.* 2004;22:1605-1613.

136. Labrie F, Labrie C, Bélanger A, et al. EM-652 (SCH 57068), a third generation SERM acting as pure antiestrogen in the mammary gland and endometrium. *J Steroid Biochem Mol Biol.* 1999;69:51-84.

137. Santen RJ, Santner SJ, Pauley RJ, et al. Estrogen production via the aromatase enzyme in breast carcinoma: which cell type is responsible? *J Steroid Biochem Mol Biol.* 1997;61:267-271.

138. Longcope C. Metabolic clearance and blood production rates of estrogens in postmenopausal women. *Am J Obstet Gynecol.* 1971;111:778-781.

139. Abul-Hajj YJ, Iverson R, Kiang DT. Aromatization of androgens by human breast cancer. *Steroids.* 1979;33:205-222.

140. Dowsett M, Lee K, Macaulay VM, et al. The control and biological importance of intratumoural aromatase in breast cancer. *J Steroid Biochem Mol Biol.* 1996;56:145-150.

141. Lu Q, Nakmura J, Savinov A, et al. Expression of aromatase protein and messenger ribonucleic acid in tumor epithelial cells and evidence of functional significance of locally produced estrogen in human breast cancers. *Endocrinology.* 1996;137:3061-3068.

142. Brodie AM, Njar VC. Aromatase inhibitors and breast cancer. *Semin Oncol.* 1996;23:10-20.

143. Griffiths CT, Hall TC, Saba Z, et al. Preliminary trial of aminoglutethimide in breast cancer. *Cancer.* 1973;32:31-37.

144. Samojlik E, Santen RJ, Wells SA. Adrenal suppression with aminoglutethimide. II. Differential effects of aminoglutethimide on plasma androstenedione and estrogen levels. *J Clin Endocrinol Metab.* 1977;45:480-487.

145. Santen RJ, Santner S, Davis B, et al. Aminoglutethimide inhibits extraglandular estrogen production in postmenopausal women with breast carcinoma. *J Clin Endocrinol Metab.* 1978;47:1257-1265.

146. Goldhirsch A, Gelber RD. Endocrine therapies of breast cancer. *Semin Oncol.* 1996;23:494-505.

147. Lawrence B, Santen RJ, Lipton A, et al. Pancytopenia induced by aminoglutethimide in the treatment of breast cancer. *Cancer Treat Rep.* 1978;62:1581-1583.

148. Johnston SRD, Dowsett M. Aromatase inhibitors for breast cancer: lessons from the laboratory. *Nat Rev Cancer.* 2003;3:821-831.

149. Baselga J, Campone M, Piccart M, et al. Everolimus in postmenopausal hormone-receptor–positive advanced breast cancer. *N Engl J Med.* 2012;366:520-529.

150. Evans TR, Di Salle E, Ornati G, et al. Phase I and endocrine study of exemestane (FCE 24304), a new aromatase inhibitor, in postmenopausal women. *Cancer Res.* 1992;52:5933-5939.

151. Lønning P, Pfister C, Martoni A, et al. Pharmacokinetics of third-generation aromatase inhibitors. *Semin Oncol.* 2003;30:23-32.

152. Scott LJ, Wiseman LR. Exemestane. *Drugs.* 1999;58:675-680; discussion 681-682.

153. Zilembo N, Noberasco C, Bajetta E, et al. Endocrinological and clinical evaluation of exemestane, a new steroidal aromatase inhibitor. *Br J Cancer.* 1995;72:1007-1012.

154. Lønning PE, Paridaens R, Thürlimann B, et al. Exemestane experience in breast cancer treatment. *J Steroid Biochem Mol Biol.* 1997;61:151-155.

155. Di Salle E, Giudici D, Ornati G, et al. 4-Aminoandrostenedione derivatives: a novel class of irreversible aromatase inhibitors. Comparison with FCE 24304 and 4-hydroxyandrostenedione. *J Steroid Biochem Mol Biol.* 1990;37:369-374.

156. Buzzetti F, Di Salle E, Longo A, et al. Synthesis and aromatase inhibition by potential metabolites of exemestane (6-methylenandrosta-1,4-diene-3,17-dione). *Steroids.* 1993;58:527-532.

157. Goss PE, Strasser-Weippl K. Prevention strategies with aromatase inhibitors. *Clin Cancer Res.* 2004;10:372S-379S.

158. Coombes RC, Hall E, Gibson LJ, et al. A randomized trial of exemestane after two to three years of tamoxifen therapy in postmenopausal women with primary breast cancer. *N Engl J Med.* 2004;350:1081-1092.

159. Lønning PE, Geisler J, Krag LE, et al. Effects of exemestane administered for 2 years versus placebo on bone mineral density, bone biomarkers, and plasma lipids in patients with surgically resected early breast cancer. *J Clin Oncol.* 2005;23:5126-5137.

160. Miller WR. Aromatase inhibitors: mechanism of action and role in the treatment of breast cancer. *Semin Oncol.* 2003;30:3-11.

161. Ibrance (palbociclib) [prescribing information]. Available at http://labeling.pfizer.com/ShowLabeling.aspx?id=2191#S14

162. Kisqali (ribociclib) Prescribing Information. Available at https://www.pharma.us.novartis.com/sites/www.pharma.us.novartis.com/files/kisqali.pdf

163. Plourde PV, Dyroff M, Dukes M. Arimidex: a potent and selective fourth-generation aromatase inhibitor. *Breast Cancer Res Treat.* 1994;30:103-111.

164. Baum M, Buzdar A, Cuzick J, et al. Anastrozole alone or in combination with tamoxifen versus tamoxifen alone for adjuvant treatment of postmenopausal women with early-stage breast cancer: results of the ATAC (Arimidex, Tamoxifen Alone or in Combination) trial efficacy and safety update analyses. *Cancer.* 2003;98:1802-1810.

165. Finn RS, Crown JP, Lang I, et al. The cyclin-dependent kinase 4/6 inhibitor palbociclib in combination with letrozole versus letrozole alone as first-line treatment of oestrogen receptor-positive, HER2-negative, advanced breast cancer (PALOMA-1/TRIO-18): a randomised phase 2 study. *Lancet Oncol.* 2015;16:25-35.

166. Finn RS, Martin M, Rugo HS, et al. Palbociclib and letrozole in advanced breast cancer. *N Engl J Med.* 2016;375:1925-1936.

167. Hortobagyi GN, Stemmer SM, Burris HA, et al. Ribociclib as first-line therapy for HR-Positive, advanced breast cancer. *N Engl J Med.* 2016;375:1738-1748.

168. Goss PE, Ingle JN, Pritchard KI, et al. Exemestane versus anastrozole in postmenopausal women with early breast cancer: NCIC CTG MA.27—a randomized controlled phase III trial. *J Clin Oncol.* 2013;31:1398-1404.

169. Klein KO, Demers LM, Santner SJ, et al. Use of ultrasensitive recombinant cell bioassay to measure estrogen levels in women with breast cancer receiving the aromatase inhibitor, letrozole. *J Clin Endocrinol Metab.* 1995;80:2658-2660.

170. Bajetta E, Zilembo N, Dowsett M, et al. Double-blind, randomised, multicentre endocrine trial comparing two letrozole doses, in postmenopausal breast cancer patients. *Eur J Cancer.* 1999;35:208-213.

171. Bisagni G, Cocconi G, Scaglione F, et al. Letrozole, a new oral non-steroidal aromatase inhibitor in treating postmenopausal patients with advanced breast cancer. A pilot study. *Ann Oncol.* 1996;7:99-102.

172. Brodie A, Lu Q, Yue W, et al. Intratumoral aromatase model: the effects of letrozole (CGS 20267). *Breast Cancer Res Treat* 1998;49(Suppl 1):S23-S26; discussion S33-S37.

173. Geisler J, Haynes B, Anker G, et al. Influence of letrozole and anastrozole on total body aromatization and plasma estrogen levels in postmenopausal breast cancer patients evaluated in a randomized, cross-over study. *J Clin Oncol.* 2002;20:751-757.

174. Rose C, Vtoraya O, Pluzanska A, et al. An open randomised trial of second-line endocrine therapy in advanced breast cancer. comparison of the aromatase inhibitors letrozole and anastrozole. *Eur J Cancer.* 2003;39:2318-2327.

175. Smith I, Yardley D, Burris H, et al. Comparative efficacy and safety of adjuvant letrozole versus anastrozole in postmenopausal patients with hormone receptor–positive, node-positive early breast cancer: final results of the randomized phase III Femara Versus Anastrozole Clinical Evaluation (FACE) Trial. *J Clin Oncol.* 2017;35(10):1041-1048.

176. Dowsett M, Pfister C, Johnston SR, et al. Impact of tamoxifen on the pharmacokinetics and endocrine effects of the aromatase inhibitor letrozole in postmenopausal women with breast cancer. *Clin Cancer Res.* 1999;5:2338-2343.

177. Dombernowsky P, Smith I, Falkson G, et al. Letrozole, a new oral aromatase inhibitor for advanced breast cancer: double-blind randomized trial showing a dose effect and improved efficacy and tolerability compared with megestrol acetate. *J Clin Oncol.* 1998;16:453-461.

178. Goss PE, Ingle JN, Martino S, et al. A randomized trial of letrozole in post-menopausal women after five years of tamoxifen therapy for early-stage breast cancer. *N Engl J Med.* 2003;349:1793-1802.

179. Ito Y, Fisher CR, Conte FA, et al. Molecular basis of aromatase deficiency in an adult female with sexual infantilism and polycystic ovaries. *Proc Natl Acad Sci U S A.* 1993;90:11673-11677.

180. Conte FA, Grumbach MM, Ito Y, et al. A syndrome of female pseudo-hermaphrodism, hypergonadotropic hypogonadism, and multicystic ovaries associated with missense mutations in the gene encoding aromatase (P450arom). *J Clin Endocrinol Metab.* 1994;78:1287-1292.

181. Agarwal SK, Judd HL, Magoffin DA. A mechanism for the suppression of estrogen production in polycystic ovary syndrome. *J Clin Endocrinol Metab.* 1996;81:3686-3691.

182. Francis PA, Regan MM, Fleming GF, et al. Adjuvant ovarian suppression in premenopausal breast cancer. *N Engl J Med.* 2015;372:436-446.

183. Pagani O, Regan MM, Walley BA, et al. Adjuvant exemestane with ovarian suppression in premenopausal breast cancer. *N Engl J Med.* 2014;371:107-118.

184. Buzdar A, Jonat W, Howell A, et al. Anastrozole, a potent and selective aromatase inhibitor, versus megestrol acetate in postmenopausal women with advanced breast cancer: results of overview analysis of two phase III trials. Arimidex Study Group. *J Clin Oncol.* 1996;14:2000-2011.

185. Ovarian ablation in early breast cancer: overview of the randomised trials. Early Breast Cancer Trialists' Collaborative Group. *Lancet.* 1996;348:1189-1196.

186. Taylor CW, Green S, Dalton WS, et al. Multicenter randomized clinical trial of goserelin versus surgical ovariectomy in premenopausal patients with receptor-positive metastatic breast cancer: an intergroup study. *J Clin Oncol.* 1998;16:994-999.

187. Harvey HA, Lipton A, Max DT, et al. Medical castration produced by the GnRH analogue leuprolide to treat metastatic breast cancer. *J Clin Oncol.* 1985;3:1068-1072.

188. Klijn JG, de Jong FH, Lamberts SW, et al. LHRH-agonist treatment in clinical and experimental human breast cancer. *J Steroid Biochem.* 1985;23:867-873.

189. Chrisp P, Goa KL. Goserelin. A review of its pharmacodynamic and pharmacokinetic properties, and clinical use in sex hormone-related conditions. *Drugs.* 1991;41:254-288.

190. Cockshott ID. Clinical pharmacokinetics of goserelin. *Clin Pharmacokinet.* 2000;39:27-48.

191. Jiménez-Gordo AM, de las Heras B, Zamora P, et al. Failure of goserelin ovarian ablation in premenopausal women with breast cancer: two case reports. *Gynecol Oncol.* 2000;76:126-127.

192. Filicori M, Flamigni C, Cognigni G, et al. Comparison of the suppressive capacity of different depot gonadotropin-releasing hormone analogs in women. *J Clin Endocrinol Metab.* 1993;77:130-133.

193. Reichel RP, Schweppe KW. Goserelin (Zoladex) depot in the treatment of endometriosis. Zoladex Endometriosis Study Group. *Fertil Steril* 1992;57:1197-1202.

194. Winer EP, Hudis C, Burstein HJ, et al. American Society of Clinical Oncology technology assessment on the use of aromatase inhibitors as adjuvant therapy for women with hormone receptor-positive breast cancer: status report 2002. *J Clin Oncol.* 2002;20:3317-3327.

195. Donnez J, Dewart PJ, Hedon B, et al. Equivalence of the 3-month and 28-day formulations of triptorelin with regard to achievement and maintenance of medical castration in women with endometriosis. *Fertil Steril.* 2004;81:297-304.

196. Drieu K, Devissaguet JP, Duboistesselin R, et al. Pharmacokinetics of D-Trp6 LHRH in man: sustained release polymer microsphere study (I.M. route). *Prog Clin Biol Res.* 1987;243A:435-437.

197. Müller FO, Terblanchè J, Schall R, et al. Pharmacokinetics of triptorelin after intravenous bolus administration in healthy males and in males with renal or hepatic insufficiency. *Br J Clin Pharmacol.* 1997;44:335-341.

198. Nicholson RI, Syne JS, Daniel CP, et al. The binding of tamoxifen to oestrogen receptor proteins under equilibrium and non-equilibrium conditions. *Eur J Cancer.* 1979;15:317-329.

199. Blamey RW, Jonat W, Kaufmann M, et al. Survival data relating to the use of goserelin depot in the treatment of premenopausal advanced breast cancer. *Eur J Cancer.* 1993;29A:1498.

200. Moy B, Goss PE. Estrogen receptor pathway: resistance to endocrine therapy and new therapeutic approaches. *Clin Cancer Res.* 2006;12:4790-4793.

201. Tonetti DA, Jordan VC. The role of estrogen receptor mutations in tamoxifen-stimulated breast cancer. *J Steroid Biochem Mol Biol.* 1997;62:119-128.

202. Karnik PS, Kulkarni S, Liu XP, et al. Estrogen receptor mutations in tamoxifen-resistant breast cancer. *Cancer Res.* 1994;54:349-353.

203. Fuqua SA, Chamness GC, McGuire WL. Estrogen receptor mutations in breast cancer. *J Cell Biochem.* 1993;51:135-139.

204. Zhang QX, Borg A, Wolf DM, et al. An estrogen receptor mutant with strong hormone-independent activity from a metastatic breast cancer. *Cancer Res.* 1997;57:1244-1249.

205. Jeselsohn R, Buchwalter G, De Angelis C, et al. ESR1 mutations—a mechanism for acquired endocrine resistance in breast cancer. *Nat Rev Clin Oncol.* 2015;12:573-583.

206. Bardia A, Iafrate JA, Sundaresan T, et al. Metastatic breast cancer with ESR1 mutation: clinical management considerations from the Molecular and Precision Medicine (MAP) tumor board at Massachusetts general hospital. *Oncologist.* 2016;21:1035-1040.

207. Schiavon G, Hrebien S, Garcia-Murillas I, et al. Analysis of ESR1 mutation in circulating tumor DNA demonstrates evolution during therapy for metastatic breast cancer. *Sci Transl Med.* 2015;7:313ra182.

208. Roodi N, Bailey LR, Kao WY, et al. Estrogen receptor gene analysis in estrogen receptor-positive and receptor-negative primary breast cancer. *J Natl Cancer Inst.* 1995;87:446-451.

209. Ali S, Coombes RC. Endocrine-responsive breast cancer and strategies for combating resistance. *Nat Rev Cancer.* 2002;2:101-112.

210. Riggins RB, Schrecengost RS, Guerrero MS, et al. Pathways to tamoxifen resistance. *Cancer Lett.* 2007;256:1-24.

211. Paech K, Webb P, Kuiper GG, et al. Differential ligand activation of estrogen receptors ERalpha and ERbeta at AP1 sites. *Science.* 1997;277:1508-1510.

212. Speirs V, Malone C, Walton DS, et al. Increased expression of estrogen receptor beta mRNA in tamoxifen-resistant breast cancer patients. *Cancer Res.* 1999;59:5421-5424.

213. Zhang QX, Borg A, Fuqua SA. An exon 5 deletion variant of the estrogen receptor frequently coexpressed with wild-type estrogen receptor in human breast cancer. *Cancer Res.* 1993;53:5882-5884.

214. Rea D, Parker MG. Effects of an exon 5 variant of the estrogen receptor in MCF-7 breast cancer cells. *Cancer Res.* 1996;56:1556-1563.

215. Webb P, Nguyen P, Shinsako J, et al. Estrogen receptor activation function 1 works by binding p160 coactivator proteins. *Mol Endocrinol.* 1998;12:1605-1618.

216. Smith CL, Nawaz Z, O'Malley BW. Coactivator and corepressor regulation of the agonist/antagonist activity of the mixed antiestrogen, 4-hydroxytamoxifen. *Mol Endocrinol.* 1997;11:657-666.

217. Schiff R, Massarweh S, Shou J, et al. Breast cancer endocrine resistance: how growth factor signaling and estrogen receptor coregulators modulate response. *Clin Cancer Res.* 2003;9:447S-454S.

218. Arpino G, Green SJ, Allred DC, et al. HER-2 amplification, HER-1 expression, and tamoxifen response in estrogen receptor-positive metastatic breast cancer: a southwest oncology group study. *Clin Cancer Res.* 2004;10:5670-5676.

219. Gutierrez MC, Detre S, Johnston S, et al. Molecular changes in tamoxifen-resistant breast cancer: relationship between estrogen receptor, HER-2, and p38 mitogen-activated protein kinase. *J Clin Oncol.* 2005;23:2469-2476.

220. Wright C, Nicholson S, Angus B, et al. Relationship between c-erbB-2 protein product expression and response to endocrine therapy in advanced breast cancer. *Br J Cancer.* 1992;65:118-121.

221. Leitzel K, Teramoto Y, Konrad K, et al. Elevated serum c-erbB-2 antigen levels and decreased response to hormone therapy of breast cancer. *J Clin Oncol.* 1995;13:1129-1135.

222. Yamauchi H, O'Neill A, Gelman R, et al. Prediction of response to antiestrogen therapy in advanced breast cancer patients by pretreatment circulating levels of extracellular domain of the HER-2/c-neu protein. *J Clin Oncol.* 1997;15:2518-2525.

223. Hurtado A, Holmes KA, Geistlinger TR, et al. Regulation of ERBB2 by oestrogen receptor-PAX2 determines response to tamoxifen. *Nature.* 2008;456:663-666.

224. McGlynn LM, Kirkegaard T, Edwards J, et al. Ras/Raf-1/MAPK pathway mediates response to tamoxifen but not chemotherapy in breast cancer patients. *Clin Cancer Res.* 2009;15:1487-1495.

225. Rokavec M, Schroth W, Amaral SMC, et al. A polymorphism in the TC21 promoter associates with an unfavorable tamoxifen treatment outcome in breast cancer. *Cancer Res.* 2008;68:9799-9808.

226. van 't Veer LJ, Dai H, van de Vijver MJ, et al. Gene expression profiling predicts clinical outcome of breast cancer. *Nature.* 2002;415:530-536.

227. Gruvberger S, Ringnér M, Chen Y, et al. Estrogen receptor status in breast cancer is associated with remarkably distinct gene expression patterns. *Cancer Res.* 2001;61:5979-5984.

228. Cleator S, Ashworth A. Molecular profiling of breast cancer: clinical implications. *Br J Cancer.* 2004;90:1120-1124.

229. Frasor J, Stossi F, Danes JM, et al. Selective estrogen receptor modulators: discrimination of agonistic versus antagonistic activities by gene expression profiling in breast cancer cells. *Cancer Res.* 2004;64:1522-1533.

230. Cunliffe HE, Ringnér M, Bilke S, et al. The gene expression response of breast cancer to growth regulators: patterns and correlation with tumor expression profiles. *Cancer Res.* 2003;63:7158-7166.

Hormone Therapy for Prostate Cancer

Richard J. Lee

Introduction

Androgens stimulate the growth of normal and cancerous prostate cells. The critical role of androgens for prostate cancer growth was established in 1941 and led to the Nobel Prize in 1966 being awarded to Dr. Charles Huggins.[1,2] Importantly, these findings established androgen deprivation therapy (ADT) as the mainstay of treatment for patients with advanced prostate cancer. This chapter outlines (a) androgen synthesis and regulation, (b) the molecular basis of androgen signaling through the androgen receptor (AR), (c) mechanisms of hormone therapy resistance, (d) clinical applications, and (e) the pharmacology of therapies that manipulate androgen signaling.

Androgen Structure, Synthesis, and Signaling

Androgen Structure and Biosynthesis

In men, testosterone is the principal secreted androgen. The Leydig cells of the testes synthesize the majority of the testosterone. Like other steroids, testosterone has a hydrated four-ring structure and is ultimately derived from cholesterol. Cholesterol may be derived from the diet and resultant plasma pool or synthesized endogenously. Cholesterol is first converted to pregnenolone by side-chain cleavage involving CYP11A1 in the mitochondria. The enzymatic pathways leading to testosterone synthesis are illustrated in Figure 28.1. The steps leading to the androgen precursors dehydroepiandrosterone (DHEA) and androstenedione are shared by the adrenal glands and gonads. These steps are catalyzed by 3β-hydroxysteroid dehydrogenase and a single CYP17 enzyme that possesses both 17α-hydroxylase and 17,20-lyase activities.[3]

The final step leading to testosterone production is catalyzed by 17β-reductase in the Leydig cells. The enzyme 5α-reductase catalyzes the conversion of testosterone to dihydrotestosterone (DHT) in androgen target tissues (Fig. 28.2). Two isoenzymes of 5α-reductase exist: type 1 in the liver, nongenital skin, and bone, and type 2 in the urogenital tissue in men and genital skin in men and women.[4] Although both testosterone and DHT act via the AR, DHT binds AR with higher affinity and thereby activates gene expression more efficiently. Thus, tissues that express 5α-reductase may have more potent androgen signaling due to conversion of testosterone to DHT.

The CYP19 aromatase complex, present in liver and adipose tissue, converts testosterone to estradiol. Estradiol circulates at lower levels than do androgens in men but stimulates bone growth and increases bone mineral density in men via the estrogen receptor.[5]

Control of Androgen Levels

Testosterone levels are regulated via the hypothalamic-pituitary-testicular axis. The hypothalamus secretes gonadotropin-releasing hormone (GnRH, also termed luteinizing hormone–releasing hormone or LHRH) in a pulsatile manner. GnRH binds to GnRH receptors on pituitary gonadotropin-producing cells and causes the release of both luteinizing hormone (LH) and follicle-stimulating hormone (FSH). LH is the principal stimulus of testosterone synthesis and secretion from testicular Leydig cells in men (Fig. 28.3).

Maintenance of androgen levels occurs by negative feedback. Testosterone inhibits both hypothalamic GnRH pulse frequency and pituitary LH secretion. Estradiol, synthesized from testosterone, can also inhibit GnRH pulse frequency and diminish pituitary responsiveness to GnRH.[6]

The Androgen Receptor

AR is essential for the development of the prostate gland.[7] The *AR* gene is located on the X chromosome at q11.2-12. AR is a member of the nuclear hormone receptor superfamily and is a ligand-dependent transcription factor. AR is composed of 919 amino acids, with characteristic domains of a nuclear receptor, including ligand-and DNA-binding domains and a long *N*-terminal transactivation domain that is capable of binding to the C-terminus and autoregulating AR activity. AR signaling is regulated by negative feedback on *AR* gene transcription. Castration results in increased *AR* transcription.[8]

Two polymorphic trinucleotide repeat segments exist in the transactivation domain of AR: $(CAG)_n$ and $(GGN)_n$.[9] CAG repeat length and AR mRNA and protein expression are inversely correlated,[10] whereas GGN length and AR transcriptional activity are positively correlated.[11] Increased long-term androgen stimulation due to CAG or GGN repeat lengths is postulated to lead to increased proliferation and subsequently higher rates of somatic mutations. However, numerous large genetic association studies have reported conflicting results; therefore, there is no clear association between these *AR* polymorphisms and prostate cancer risk.[12–16]

AR Signaling

AR is sequestered in the cytoplasm by chaperone proteins such as heat shock proteins. Upon ligand binding, AR is released from the chaperone proteins and can translocate to the nucleus. AR binds in a homodimeric conformation to DNA sequences known as androgen response elements (AREs), which can vary substantially in different gene promoters [reviewed in Gelmann[8]].

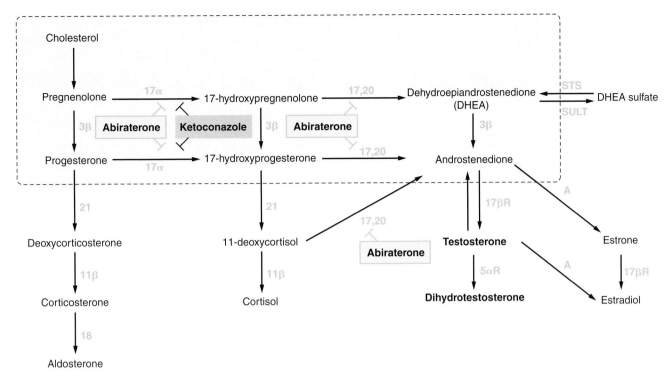

FIGURE 28.1 Steroid synthesis pathways. The enclosed area contains the pathways used by the adrenal glands and gonads. Enzymes are labeled in *red*. Steps inhibited by ketoconazole and abiraterone are indicated. Enzymes: 17*α*, 17*α*-hydroxylase (CYP17); 17,20, C-17,20-lyase (also CYP17); 3*β*, 3*β*-hydroxysteroid dehydrogenase; 21, 21-hydroxylase; 11*β*, 11*β*-hydroxylase; 18, aldosterone synthase; 17*β*R, 17*β*-reductase; 5*α*R, 5*α*-reductase; A, aromatase; SULT, sulfotransferase; STS, sulfatase.

In addition to ligand-stimulated activation of AR, increased AR signaling may occur via growth factor receptors such as HER2,[17,18] IL-6R,[19] EGFR, and IGF-1R.[20] In experimental systems, overexpression of these growth factor receptor tyrosine kinases led to enhanced AR signaling, via downstream activation of growth and survival pathways mediated by AKT, ERK, and STAT. The contribution of purported ligand-independent AR activation to disease progression in prostate cancer patients is unknown.

AR also binds to cytoplasmic proteins such as the tyrosine kinases SRC and Ack1. Ligand-bound AR binds and activates SRC and

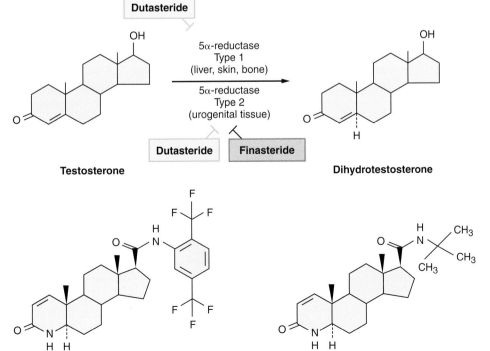

FIGURE 28.2 The action of 5*α*-reductase. Two isoforms of 5*α*-reductase convert testosterone to DHT in different tissues. The 5*α*-reductase inhibitor dutasteride can inhibit both isoforms, whereas finasteride can only inhibit type 2.

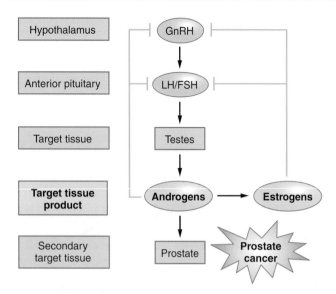

FIGURE **28.3** The hypothalamic-pituitary-testicular axis. Gonadotropin-releasing hormone (*GnRH*) is secreted from the hypothalamus and induces release of luteinizing hormone (*LH*) and follicle-stimulating hormone (*FSH*) from the pituitary gland. LH stimulates testosterone synthesis from testicular Leydig cells. Testosterone promotes prostate gland development and stimulates prostate cancer cell growth. Testosterone can be converted to estrogens. Androgens and estrogens can inhibit hypothalamic GnRH pulse frequency and pituitary LH production by negative feedback.

downstream effectors including ERK. SRC can also phosphorylate and potentiate AR activity via the AR SH3 domain.[21] In the setting of hormone therapy for prostate cancer, SRC may thereby sensitize AR to subphysiologic levels of androgens.[22] Ack1 is a kinase downstream of EGFR/HER2 signaling and also targets AR for tyrosine phosphorylation and activation.[23] The mechanisms of activation of AR via growth factor receptor and cytoplasmic tyrosine kinases may occur in the castrate state and are putative targets for therapeutic intervention.

Mechanisms of Resistance to Hormone Therapy

While response to hormone therapy is nearly universal, resistance to hormonal manipulations develops in most men. In the castrate state, AR signaling despite low circulating androgen levels supports continued prostate cancer growth. AR signaling may occur due to androgens produced from nongonadal sources, AR gene mutations, AR gene amplification, AR splice variants, or ligand-independent activation via growth factor receptor or cytoplasmic tyrosine kinases (as described above).

Nongonadal sources of androgens include the adrenal glands and the prostate cancer cells themselves. Adrenal-produced androstenedione is converted to testosterone in peripheral tissues and tumors.[24] Intratumoral de novo androgen synthesis may also provide sufficient androgen for AR-driven cell proliferation.[25]

Numerous somatic missense mutations have been detected in the *AR* gene in human prostate cancer tissues, cell lines, and xenografts. Primary prostate tumors or metastatic deposits examined prior to initiation of therapy exhibit a range in *AR* mutation frequency from 8% to 44%.[26,27] *AR* mutation frequency in metastases of patients who have progressed despite hormone therapy ranges from 18% to 50%.[28,29] Treatment with antiandrogens favors the selection of recurrent cancer with mutant AR.[29]

Most *AR* gene mutations in prostate cancer cluster in three regions, the ligand-binding domain (LBD), a region flanking the ligand-dependent transactivation function-2 domain (AF-2), and the boundary of the hinge region and the LBD.[30] Mutations in these regions may contribute to altered androgen signaling and disease progression in the context of hormone therapy in patients. Mutations in the LBD can broaden the spectrum of AR agonists to include other steroid hormones such as estrogen, progesterone, and glucocorticoids, as well as antiandrogens.[28,29,31,32] Mutations flanking the AF-2 region increase AR stability and sensitivity to very low levels of DHT[33]; the enhanced AR signaling may also result from altered p160 coactivator interaction with AF-2.[30] Mutations near the hinge region have enhanced transactivation activity, potentially due to a reduction in binding to nuclear corepressors.[34]

Amplification of *AR* may reflect a distinct adaptation of prostate cancer cells to castrate levels of circulating androgens. *AR* amplification occurs in recurrent tumors from 30% of patients with metastatic disease but is not present in the corresponding untreated primary tumors of the same patients.[35] Amplification of *AR* can also occur in patients being treated with AR antagonists; in these patients, testosterone levels are typically above normal.[29,36]

The most recently described mechanism of hormonal resistance to AR-directed therapy involves expression of AR mRNA splice variants.[37] These genes may not be mutated, but alternative splicing leads to variant protein products that have constitutively active AR function. Several AR variants (or "AR-Vs") have been characterized. AR-Vs are truncated AR proteins that lack the LBD but retain the transactivation domain and therefore may be resistant to inhibition by AR-targeted hormonal agents. The most clinically prevalent is AR-V7, which was first described in metastatic prostate cancer (Fig. 28.4).[38,39] AR-V7 expression has been associated with resistance to the newer androgen-targeted agents *abiraterone acetate* (ZYTIGA) and *enzalutamide* (XTANDI) (described later in this chapter),[40] but not taxane chemotherapy[41] in patients with metastatic castration-resistant prostate cancer (mCRPC). AR-V7 expression is thus considered a potential biomarker for selection of treatment in advanced prostate cancer.[42] The characterization and clinical significance of other AR-Vs including AR-V9[43] continue to emerge and may have future therapeutic implications.

Together, these findings reflect the critical importance of AR signaling for growth and survival of cancer cells throughout the clinical course of prostate cancer.

Clinical Applications

Chemoprevention of Prostate Cancer

Prostate cancer is the most common malignancy for men in the United States, with an estimated 161,360 new diagnoses in 2017.[44] Strategies for prostate cancer prevention in healthy men are based on evidence that androgens influence prostate cancer development. Drugs that target 5α-reductase reduce androgen levels in the prostate. *Finasteride* (PROSCAR) inhibits type 2 5α-reductase, whereas *dutasteride* (AVODART) inhibits both isoenzymes of 5α-reductase (see Fig. 28.2). Two randomized, placebo-controlled trials were designed to measure the effect of a 5α-reductase inhibitor on prostate cancer incidence. The Prostate Cancer Prevention Trial randomized

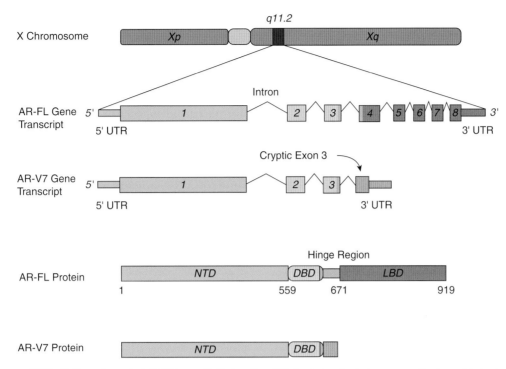

FIGURE **28.4** The splice variant AR-V7 is constitutively active. *AR* is located on the X chromosome. The transcript structures for full-length AR (AR-FL) and the splice variant AR-V7 demonstrate the alternative splicing to cryptic exon 3, which truncates the AR transcript and eliminates the ligand binding domain (compare the AR-FL and AR-V7 protein structures). Peptide positions are as indicated. AR-V7 can therefore bind DNA and cause transactivation but is resistant to therapeutic androgen manipulation.

18,882 healthy men over age 55 with a normal rectal exam and a PSA less than 3.0 mg/mL to daily finasteride or placebo.[45] Finasteride was associated with a significant 24.8% reduction in prostate cancer prevalence over the 7-year study period. However, high-grade prostate cancer was more frequently diagnosed in the finasteride group (6.4% versus 5.1%, $P = 0.005$). The uncertainty of increased high-grade cancers associated with finasteride has led to limited adoption of finasteride as a chemoprevention agent.[46] A randomized, placebo-controlled study of dutasteride in 8,200 healthy men aged 50 to 75 but with higher PSA levels (2.5 to 10 ng/mL) revealed a 22.4% reduction in prostate cancer prevalence over 4 years, with no difference in high-grade tumors.[47,48]

Localized Prostate Cancer

Localized prostate cancer is frequently curable with surgery or radiation therapy. Hormone therapy may be employed in conjunction with radiation therapy for patients with high-risk or locally advanced disease (currently defined by the pathologic Gleason sum of 8 to 10, or serum prostate-specific antigen (PSA) greater than 20, or clinical T3/4 stage defined by a palpable mass extending outside of the prostate capsule). The Radiation Therapy Oncology Group (RTOG) protocol 85-31 established that lifelong ADT combined with definitive radiotherapy is associated with better disease control and freedom from progression, compared with radiotherapy alone.[49] Subsequent studies in Europe and the United States, such as RTOG protocol 92-02,[50] further defined the standard use of prolonged (28 to 36 months) ADT for patient who opt for radiotherapy for high-risk, localized disease. While there is no benefit for the addition of ADT to radiation for good-risk, localized disease, the absolute benefit of short-course ADT along with contemporary

radiation therapy for intermediate-risk, localized prostate cancer will likely be defined by RTOG protocol 08-15.[51] This protocol has been fully accrued but not yet reported.

Recurrent Prostate Cancer

For patients who have undergone radical prostatectomy, the serum PSA should become undetectable. A detectable level of PSA indicates persistence or recurrence of prostate cancer. In the absence of distant metastasis on scans, the PSA source may be a local recurrence of prostate cancer in the pelvis. "Salvage" radiation therapy directed at the prostatic fossa is associated with long-term freedom from cancer recurrence in a subset of patients. Given the benefit of hormone therapy combined with radiation as primary treatment of prostate cancer, trials evaluated the benefit of adding hormone therapy to salvage radiation therapy. The largest study, RTOG 96-01, randomized 760 patients to salvage radiation with or without antiandrogen therapy (*bicalutamide* [CASODEX] at 150 daily; see below for discussion of antiandrogens). Patients who received hormone therapy with salvage radiation had higher rates of overall survival and lower rates of metastatic prostate cancer and death from disease.[52]

Metastatic Prostate Cancer

When distant metastases are present, hormone therapy is the primary treatment. Standard approaches either reduce the concentration of endogenous androgens or inhibit their effects. ADT is the standard first-line treatment.[53] ADT is accomplished via surgical castration (bilateral orchiectomy) or medical castration (using GnRH agonists or antagonists). Other hormone therapy approaches are used in second-line treatment and include antiandrogens, estrogens, and inhibitors of steroidogenesis (*see below*).

Nearly all patients with metastatic prostate cancer respond to ADT. ADT is considered palliative, not curative, treatment.[54] ADT can alleviate cancer-related symptoms, produce objective responses, and normalize serum PSA in over 90% of patients. ADT provides important quality of life (QOL) benefits, including reduction of bone pain and reduction of rates of pathologic fracture, spinal cord compression, and ureteral obstruction. ADT alone does not clearly prolong survival.[53]

From 2015 to 2017, four studies altered the standard of care for the initial management of metastatic prostate cancer. Two studies added six cycles of *docetaxel* (Taxotere) chemotherapy to ADT,[55,56] and two studies added continuous *abiraterone acetate* (Zytiga, an oral steroidogenesis inhibitor; described below) with prednisone to ADT.[57,58] Docetaxel or abiraterone acetate was started within 3 to 4 months of ADT initiation. All four studies demonstrated an improvement in overall survival for patients with newly diagnosed metastatic prostate cancer, and the addition of either docetaxel or abiraterone to ADT for "castration-sensitive" prostate cancer has quickly become the standard of care.

The duration of response to ADT alone for patients with metastatic disease is variable but typically lasts 14 to 20 months.[59,60] By comparison, the median time to progression was improved with the addition of docetaxel (20.2 versus 11.7 months for ADT alone)[55] or abiraterone (33.0 versus 14.8 months for ADT alone).[58] Disease progression despite ADT signifies progression to mCRPC. However, many men respond to secondary hormonal manipulations. Despite castrate levels of testosterone, low-level androgen (DHEA) synthesis from the adrenal glands or the tumor cells themselves may permit the continued androgen-driven growth of prostate cancer cells. Therefore, antiandrogens (which competitively bind the AR), inhibitors of steroidogenesis (such as ketoconazole or abiraterone), and estrogens are frequently employed as secondary hormone therapies. Unlike the nearly universal response to ADT, only the minority of patients experience symptomatic relief or tumor regression when treated with secondary hormone therapies. When prostate cancer becomes refractory to further hormonal therapies, it is considered androgen independent. Other life-prolonging, FDA-approved mCRPC treatment options include cytotoxic chemotherapy such as docetaxel[61,62] or *cabazitaxel* (Jevtana),[63] the autologous cellular immunotherapy *sipuleucel-T* (Provenge),[64] or the radionuclide therapy *radium-223* (Xofigo).[65] The median overall survival benefit of these manipulations is generally between 2 and 6 months.

Approaches to Hormone Therapy

Hormone therapy for prostate cancer includes the following options:

- Bilateral orchiectomy (surgical castration)
- GnRH agonists (medical castration, alternatively termed LHRH agonists)
- GnRH antagonists
- Antiandrogens
- Estrogens
- Inhibitors of steroidogenesis
- Combined androgen blockade (CAB)

The efficacy of each treatment approach for metastatic prostate cancer is described herein. These approaches have not been directly compared in one large trial. A systematic review of various forms of monotherapy (including orchiectomy, GnRH agonists, estrogens, antiandrogens) involving over 6,600 patients in 24 randomized controlled trials (RCTs) suggested that survival is equivalent among these therapies.[66] In addition to its use in metastatic prostate cancer, hormone therapy has an important cytoreductive role when used prior to (neoadjuvant) and concurrently with radiation therapy for locally advanced prostate cancer.[49,50,67,68]

Bilateral Orchiectomy

Bilateral orchiectomy is the standard against which other forms of hormone therapy are compared. Orchiectomy is a relatively simple, cost-effective procedure with minor surgical risks.[69] Serum testosterone levels decrease rapidly to castrate levels (<20 ng/mL) after surgery,[70] with concomitant improvements in bone pain and other symptoms such as spinal cord compression.[2] The use of orchiectomy as initial hormone therapy has largely been supplanted by medical castration (described below). However, orchiectomy remains a useful alternative for patients in whom an immediate decrease in testosterone is necessary, such as pending spinal cord compression, or in whom costs or adherence to medical therapy may be an issue. In many countries, bilateral orchiectomy remains the standard of care for initial hormone therapy of metastatic prostate cancer.

The endocrine side effects of orchiectomy include vasoactive symptoms (hot flushes), weight gain, mood lability, fatigue, gynecomastia, cognitive changes, impotence, loss of libido, osteopenia, and dyslipidemia.[69] The psychological impact of orchiectomy is an important consideration for men considering surgical versus medical castration. In a study of 159 men with metastatic prostate cancer who were provided with standard information regarding the costs, benefits, and risks of either orchiectomy or monthly GnRH agonist therapy, only 22% selected orchiectomy.[71]

Gonadotropin-Releasing Hormone Agonists

Medical castration was first reported in 1982.[72] In the United States, the most common form of ADT involves chemical suppression of the pituitary gland with GnRH agonists. Synthetic GnRH analogs have greater receptor affinity and reduced susceptibility to enzymatic degradation than the naturally occurring GnRH molecule and are 100-fold more potent (Fig. 28.5).[73] GnRH agonists bind to GnRH receptors on pituitary gonadotropin-producing cells, causing an initial release of both LH and FSH and a subsequent increase in testosterone production from testicular Leydig cells. After approximately 1 week of therapy, GnRH receptors are downregulated on the gonadotropin-producing cells, causing a decline in the pituitary response.[74] The fall in serum LH leads to a decrease in testosterone production to castrate levels, within 3 to 4 weeks of the first treatment. Subsequent treatments maintain testosterone at castrate levels.[75]

During the transient rise in LH, the resultant testosterone surge may induce an acute stimulation of prostate cancer growth and a "flare" of symptoms from metastatic deposits. Patients may experience an increase in bone pain or obstructive bladder symptoms, lasting for 2 to 3 weeks.[76] A placebo-controlled trial demonstrated that 2 to 4 weeks of antiandrogen therapy (see below) coadministered with a GnRH agonist can counteract this flare phenomenon.[77]

Agonists
GnRH:
pyroGlu-His-Trp-Ser-Tyr-Gly-Leu-Arg-Pro-Gly-NH2

Goserelin:
pyroGlu-His-Trp-Ser-Tyr-D-Ser(tBu)-Leu-Arg-Pro-Azgly-NH2

Leuprolide:
5-oxo-Pro-His-Trp-Ser-Tyr-D-Leu-Leu-Arg-N-ethyl-Prolinamide

Triptorelin:
pyroGlu-His-Trp-Ser-Tyr-D-Trp-Leu-Arg-Pro-Gly-NH2

Antagonists
Abarelix:
Ac-D-Nal-D-Cpa-D-Pal-Ser-Tyr(N-Me)-D-Asn-Leu-Lys(iPr)-Pro-D-Ala-NH2

Degarelix:
Ac-D-Nal-D-Cpa-D-Pal-Ser-Aph (L-hydroorotyl)-D-Aph (carbamoyl)-Leu-Lys(iPr)-Pro-D-Ala-NH2

FIGURE **28.5** Gonadotropin-releasing hormone (GnRH), agonists, and antagonists. GnRH agonists and antagonists are structurally modified peptides. Ac, acetyl; Aph, 4-amino phenylalanine; Arg, arginine; Azgly, azaglycyl; Cpa, chlorophenylalanyl; D-Nal, 3-(2-naphthyl)-D-alanyl; Glu, glutamate; Gly, glycine; His, histidine; Leu, leucine; Pal, 3-pyridylalanyl; Pro, proline; Ser, serine; tBu, tert-butyl; Trp, tryptophan; Tyr, tyrosine.

Current depot forms of GnRH agonists are the result of progressive improvements in drug development. GnRH agonists in common use include *leuprolide* (LUPRON), *goserelin* (ZOLADEX), *triptorelin* (TRELSTAR), and *buserelin* (SUPREFACT; not available in the United States) (Table 28.1). Long-acting preparations of both leuprolide and goserelin are available in doses that are approved for 1-, 3-, 4-, and 6-month administrations.

Common side effects of GnRH agonists include vasomotor flushing, loss of libido, impotence, gynecomastia, fatigue, anemia, weight gain, decreased insulin sensitivity, altered lipid profiles, osteoporosis and fractures, and loss of muscle mass.[78] The spectrum of side effects of GnRH agonists is distinct from the metabolic syndrome.[79] The risk of fracture is a significant contributor to morbidity associated with ADT. Observational studies of the Surveillance, Epidemiology, and End Results (SEER) program and Medicare data ($n = 50,613$) revealed a significantly increased number of fractures in men on ADT (19.4% versus 12.6% for those not receiving ADT, $P < 0.001$).[80] Skeletal-related events due to ADT, including fractures, may be significantly mitigated by bisphosphonate therapy, such as *zoledronic acid* (ZOMETA),[81] or inhibitors of osteoclast activation, such as *denosumab* (XGEVA).[82]

Importantly, large observational studies of prostate cancer patients from SEER and Medicare data ($n = 73,196$)[83] and the Veterans Health Administration data ($n = 37,443$)[84] have demonstrated associations between GnRH agonist therapy and incident diabetes and cardiovascular disease. GnRH agonist therapy was associated with statistically significantly increased risks of incident diabetes (adjusted hazard ratio [aHR] = 1.28), incident coronary heart disease (aHR = 1.19), myocardial infarction (12.8 events per 1,000 person-years for GnRH agonist therapy versus 7.3 for no ADT; aHR 1.28), sudden cardiac death (aHR = 1.35), and stroke (aHR = 1.22).[84] Despite these observations, there is no convincing evidence that ADT is associated with increased cardiovascular mortality (reviewed in Saylor and Smith[78]). Careful evaluation of risks and benefits of ADT for an individual patient is of paramount importance. Prospective studies of these issues of survivorship, as well as effective management strategies of potential complications, are important future considerations.

TABLE
28.1 *Key features of GnRH agonists*

Mechanism of action	Inhibition of luteinizing hormone (LH) secretion, with resultant decrease in testosterone to castrate levels
Onset of action	After an initial increase, testosterone falls to castrate levels in 2 to 4 weeks
Pharmacokinetics	Leuprolide, $t_{1/2}$: 3 h Goserelin, $t_{1/2}$: 4 h Triptorelin, $t_{1/2}$: 3 h
Elimination	Metabolized to smaller peptides, eliminated by the liver and kidneys
Drug interactions	None known
Toxicity	Vasomotor flushing Impotence Loss of libido Local irritation at injection site Gynecomastia and mastodynia Disease flare Weight gain Loss of lean muscle mass (sarcopenia) Anemia Osteoporosis, osteopenia, and fractures Diabetes mellitus Altered lipid profiles Coronary heart disease, myocardial infarction, sudden cardiac death Stroke
Precautions	(1) Transient increases in testosterone may cause disease flare; administer with 2 to 4 weeks of antiandrogen therapy. (2) No dose adjustments for renal impairment or moderate hepatic impairment; pharmacokinetics in severe hepatic impairment have not been determined.

GnRH Agonists Versus Orchiectomy

Medical castration compared with surgical castration offers the possibility of reversibility of hypogonadal symptoms upon cessation of therapy and improved psychological tolerance. The GnRH agonists leuprolide and goserelin have been compared with orchiectomy in randomized trials. A meta-analysis of ten randomized trials involving 1,908 patients comparing a GnRH agonist with orchiectomy found equivalence in overall survival, progression-related outcomes, and time to treatment failure.[66,85–88] The 2-year survival hazard ratio with GnRH agonists compared with orchiectomy was 1.26 (95% CI, 0.92 to 1.39).[66] Although no trials have directly compared the GnRH agonists, the meta-analysis found no evidence of a difference in efficacy among the GnRH agonists leuprolide, goserelin, or buserelin.[66]

Despite the high price of GnRH agonists versus the one-time procedure of orchiectomy, GnRH agonists are given to the majority of American prostate cancer patients for initial ADT.[71,89] The American Society of Clinical Oncology (ASCO) guidelines from 2004 and updated in 2007 maintain the recommendation of GnRH agonists or bilateral orchiectomy as first-line initial hormone therapy.[69,89]

Gonadotropin-Releasing Hormone Antagonists

GnRH antagonists have been developed to suppress testosterone while avoiding the flare phenomenon of GnRH agonists (see Fig. 28.5). Other than avoidance of the initial flare, GnRH antagonist therapy offers no apparent advantage compared with GnRH agonists. The first available GnRH antagonist, *abarelix* (Plenaxis), rapidly achieves medical castration.[90] However, local reactions and anaphylaxis have discouraged its clinical acceptance and have led to its withdrawal from the market. A second GnRH antagonist, *degarelix* (Firmagon), is not associated with systemic allergic reactions and is approved for prostate cancer in the United States.[91] Degarelix is currently available as a subcutaneous monthly injection.

Antiandrogens (AR Antagonists)

Antiandrogens bind to the AR and competitively inhibit ligand binding and consequent AR translocation from the cytoplasm to the nucleus. Unlike surgical or medical castration, antiandrogen monotherapy does not decrease LH production; therefore, testosterone levels are normal or increased. Men treated with antiandrogen monotherapy maintain some degree of potency and libido and do not have the same spectrum of side effects seen with castration.

Antiandrogens, when compared with GnRH agonists, cause more gynecomastia, mastodynia, and hepatotoxicity but less bone loss and vasomotor flushing.[92] Antiandrogens are generally well tolerated and are associated with PSA responses in 20% to 50% of previously untreated patients (median duration, 3 to 6 months).[93]

Currently, antiandrogen monotherapy is not indicated as first-line treatment for patients with advanced prostate cancer. Numerous studies have examined the effectiveness of antiandrogens compared with surgical castration, GnRH agonists, or *diethylstilbestrol* (DES) treatment. A meta-analysis of eight trials indicated that nonsteroidal antiandrogens had equivalent overall survival relative to castration, although the association between nonsteroidal antiandrogens and *decreased* survival approached statistical significance.[66]

Antiandrogens are most commonly used in clinical practice to prevent the initial flare reaction to GnRH agonists or as secondary hormone therapy when the disease progresses to mCRPC.

From a structural standpoint, antiandrogens are classified as steroidal, including *cyproterone* (Androcur) and *megestrol*, or nonsteroidal, including *flutamide* (Eulexin and others), *bicalutamide* (Casodex), *nilutamide* (Nilandron), and *enzalutamide* (Xtandi) (Fig. 28.6 and Table 28.2). The steroidal antiandrogens are rarely used. The antiandrogens are taken orally. Among these, enzalutamide has the highest activity and is the most widely used as secondary hormone therapy for mCRPC in the United States, based on overall survival benefit in phase III clinical trials.

Cyproterone is associated with liver toxicity and has inferior efficacy compared with other forms of ADT.[94,95] In a phase III study, cyproterone was inferior to medical castration with goserelin in delaying time to progression.[95] On this basis, cyproterone is not approved in the United States for treatment of men with metastatic prostate cancer, although it is used in Europe.

Flutamide has a half-life of 5 hours and is therefore given as a 250-mg dose every 8 hours. It is metabolized in the liver by CYP1A2 to the major active metabolite, hydroxyflutamide, which has a half-life of 9.5 hours, and to at least five other minor metabolites.[96,97] The common side effects include diarrhea, breast tenderness, and nipple tenderness. Less commonly, nausea, vomiting, and hepatotoxicity occur.[98,99] Hepatotoxicity is uncommon (3 per 10,000 patients) but can be fatal, and therefore flutamide administration should include close monitoring of serum aminotransferases.[98,99]

Bicalutamide has a serum half-life of 5 to 6 days and is taken once daily at a dose of 50 mg/d when given with a GnRH agonist.

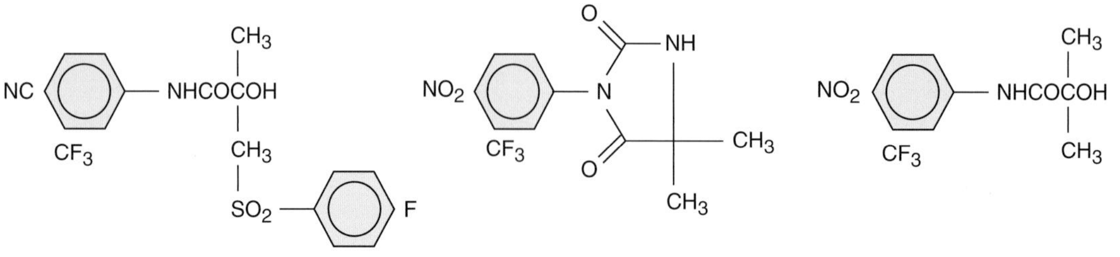

FIGURE **28.6** The nonsteroidal antiandrogens.

TABLE **28.2** Key features of nonsteroidal antiandrogens				
	Enzalutamide	**Bicalutamide**	**Flutamide**	**Nilutamide**
Typical dosing	160 mg daily	50 mg daily	250 mg every 8 h	150 mg daily
$t_{1/2}$	5.8 d	5 to 6 d	Parent drug, 5 h	45 h
			Hydroxyflutamide, 9.5 h	
Metabolism	CYP2C8	(1) CYP3A4	CYP1A2	CYP2C19
	CYP3A4	(2) Hydroxylation then glucuronidation		
Elimination	Urine	Bile and urine	Urine	Urine
Drug interactions	Precaution with strong CYP2C8 (e.g., gemfibrozil) or CYP3A4 inhibitors (e.g., itraconazole)	May displace warfarin from protein-binding sites and lead to prolonged prothrombin times	May displace warfarin from protein-binding sites and lead to prolonged prothrombin times	May increased plasma levels of phenytoin and theophylline
Toxicity	Fatigue	Vasomotor instability	Diarrhea	Nausea
	Seizure (rare)	Gynecomastia	Gynecomastia	Alcohol intolerance
	Diarrhea	Mastodynia	Mastodynia	Diminished ocular adaptation to darkness
	Hypertension		Rare fatal hepatotoxicity	Rare interstitial pneumonitis
Precautions	Contraindicated in patients with prior history of seizures	Elimination is increased in severe hepatic insufficiency	Monitor liver function	Least favorable toxicity profile

Bicalutamide is well tolerated at higher doses with rare additional side effects. Similar to flutamide, breast tenderness and gynecomastia occur in over half of treated men.[100,101] Bicalutamide is a racemate with antiandrogenic activity almost exclusive to the (R)-enantiomer. Whereas (S)-bicalutamide is rapidly metabolized by glucuronidation, (R)-bicalutamide is thought to be metabolized by both hepatic CYP3A4 activity and hydroxylation followed by glucuronidation. (R)-bicalutamide metabolites are eliminated in bile and urine. The elimination half-life of bicalutamide is increased in severe hepatic insufficiency and is unchanged in renal insufficiency.[102]

Bicalutamide is as effective as flutamide in terms of PSA response, objective response, and QOL, with less diarrhea and hepatotoxicity.[103] Daily bicalutamide (either low or high dose) is significantly inferior compared with surgical or medical castration.[104,105] Although the ease of administration and favorable toxicity are attractive, concerns about inferior survival have limited the use of bicalutamide monotherapy. Neither bicalutamide nor flutamide are approved as monotherapy at any dose for treatment of prostate cancer in the United States and are thus most commonly used in combination with GnRH agonists.

Nilutamide is a second-generation antiandrogen with an elimination half-life of 45 hours, allowing once-daily administration at 150 mg/d.[106] Common side effects include mild nausea, alcohol intolerance (5% to 20%), and diminished ocular adaptation to darkness (25% to 40%); rarely, interstitial pneumonitis occurs.[107,108] It is metabolized in the liver by CYP2C19 to at least five products that are all excreted in the urine.[109] Nilutamide appears to offer no

benefit over the first-generation drugs above and has the least favorable toxicity profile.[110]

Enzalutamide (formerly MDV3100) is the most recently developed, FDA-approved antiandrogen. It has higher affinity for AR compared with bicalutamide.[111] Enzalutamide has a half-life of 5.8 days and is primarily metabolized in the liver.[112] It is administered at 160 mg once daily. In terms of mechanism of action, enzalutamide is thought to more effectively inhibit nuclear translocation of the AR, DNA binding of the AR, and coactivator recruitment compared with the other antiandrogens.

Enzalutamide is FDA approved in the mCRPC setting as secondary hormone therapy. The AFFIRM study randomized 1,199 men with mCRPC who had previously received docetaxel chemotherapy to enzalutamide or placebo.[113] Enzalutamide was associated with improved overall survival (18.4 versus 13.6 months with placebo; HR 0.63; $P < 0.001$), PSA reduction greater than 50% (54% versus 2%; $P < 0.001$), and radiographic progression-free survival (8.3 versus 3.0 months; HR 0.40; $P < 0.001$), among other endpoints. The PREVAIL study similarly randomized 1,717 men with mCRPC but without prior docetaxel chemotherapy to enzalutamide or placebo.[114] Enzalutamide was associated with improved overall survival, radiographic progression-free survival, and PSA response rate, among other measures. The most common side effect was fatigue, though this was generally mild, and high-grade fatigue was not significantly different between enzalutamide and placebo in these studies. Importantly, although seizures were described in earlier clinical trials, these phase III trials did not demonstrate a statistically significant seizure risk. Nonetheless, enzalutamide should be used with caution (if at all) in patients with a prior history of seizures or with medical conditions or medications that might lower the seizure threshold.

Enzalutamide has been compared directly with bicalutamide in a phase II RCT of 375 mCRPC patients.[115] The TERRAIN study met its primary endpoint of improved progression-free survival with enzalutamide (15.7 versus 5.8 months with bicalutamide; HR 0.44; $P < 0.0001$). These recent trials have established enzalutamide as the most effective antiandrogen for mCRPC.

Are Antiandrogens as Effective as Castration?

The different antiandrogens have not been directly compared in a clinical trial. One meta-analysis of eight trials involving 2,717 patients examined the effectiveness of antiandrogens compared with castration, GnRH agonist, or DES.[66] Three studies examined flutamide[116–119] and five studies used bicalutamide.[120–124] One study with flutamide[118] and two studies on bicalutamide[121,124] found statistically significant longer survival in the control arms; no significant survival difference was seen in the other five studies. Overall, the nonsteroidal antiandrogens had equivalent overall survival relative to orchiectomy, although the association between nonsteroidal antiandrogens and decreased survival approached statistical significance (HR 1.22, 95% CI 0.99 to 1.40).[66] Current ASCO guidelines suggest that nonsteroidal antiandrogen monotherapy be discussed but should not be offered.[89]

Estrogens

High estrogen levels can reduce testosterone to castrate levels in 1 to 2 weeks via negative feedback on the hypothalamic-pituitary axis. Estrogen may also compete with androgens for steroid hormone receptors and may thereby exert a cytotoxic effect on prostate cancer cells.[125] Numerous estrogenic compounds have been tested in prostate cancer. Estrogens cause a hypercoagulable state and increase cardiovascular mortality (including increased myocardial infarctions, strokes, and pulmonary emboli) in prostate cancer patients and are not considered standard treatment options.[126] One benefit is that estrogens prevent bone loss.[127]

Most early studies on the use of estrogens used DES and were conducted between 1960 and 1975 by the Veterans Administration Cooperative Urological Research Group (VACURG). Two studies compared orchiectomy to different doses of DES to placebo.[126,128,129] DES was as effective as orchiectomy for metastatic prostate cancer but was associated with an increase in cardiovascular events, including myocardial infarction, cerebrovascular accident, and pulmonary embolism; men who received placebo lived longer than men receiving DES, due to higher rates of noncancer deaths in the DES groups.[128–132] The emerging availability of GnRH agonists led to the marked decline in the use of DES. Due to its cardiovascular toxicity and unacceptable mortality at any dose level, DES is not indicated for prostate cancer treatment and is not available in North America for that purpose.

Other Estrogens

Other synthetic oral estrogens have similar associated cardiovascular toxicity of DES, but without the efficacy. These compounds include conjugated estrogens (PREMARIN), *ethinyl estradiol* (ESTINYL), *medroxyprogesterone acetate* (PROVERA), and *chlorotrianisene* (TACE).

Premarin (1.25 mg three times daily) is approved for metastatic prostate cancer in the United States. In a randomized phase II study of 45 men with castration-resistant prostate cancer who received Premarin either once or three times daily along with 1 mg of daily warfarin, 25% of men on the higher dose achieved at least a 50% decrease in serum PSA. Only three patients in the entire group had a venous thromboembolic event.[133]

Oral estrogens are associated with elevated serum levels of coagulation factor VII and decreased levels of antithrombin III, which may account for their hypercoagulable complications.[134] Parenteral or transdermal estrogens avoid first-pass portal circulation, and indeed parenteral polyestradiol phosphate was associated with a decreased level of antithrombin III but no change in factor VII.[134] Transdermal estradiol was associated with castrate levels of testosterone and a biochemical response in all patients of a 20 patient study, without significant cardiovascular toxicity after a median follow-up of 15 months.[135] Intramuscular estrogen has also been attempted; a recent randomized study of parenteral estrogen versus CAB demonstrated equivalent disease control and survival but significantly more nonfatal cardiovascular events.[136]

Inhibitors of Steroidogenesis

In the castrate state, nongonadal sources of androgens may support continued prostate cancer growth (see section on "Mechanisms of resistance to hormone therapy"). Inhibitors of steroidogenesis are effective secondary hormone manipulations to further lower circulating or intratumoral androgen levels. Among these, abiraterone has supplanted ketoconazole in terms of efficacy and clinical benefit, based on phase III clinical trials that established the role of abiraterone as secondary hormone therapy in mCRPC[137,138] and with initial ADT for metastatic castration-sensitive disease.[57,58]

Ketoconazole, an oral antifungal agent, interrupts the synthesis of an essential fungal membrane sterol. Ketoconazole inhibits both testicular and adrenal steroidogenesis by blocking cytochrome P450 enzymes, primarily CYP17 (17α-hydroxylase) (*see* Fig. 28.2). Ketoconazole is typically administered as secondary hormone therapy, to reduce adrenal androgen synthesis in mCRPC.[139] Ketoconazole causes significant diarrhea and hepatic enzyme elevations, limiting its use as initial hormone therapy. Consequent poor patient adherence deters from its efficacy. Ketoconazole is given in doses of 200 or 400 mg three times daily. Hydrocortisone supplementation is coadministered to compensate for inhibition of adrenal steroidogenesis at the 400-mg dose level. High-dose ketoconazole plus corticosteroids demonstrates PSA declines for 27% to 63% of patients with CRPC. Lower doses may have comparable activity with less toxicity.[140]

Abiraterone is an irreversible inhibitor of both 17α-hydroxylase and C-17,20-lyase CYP17 activity, with greater potency and selectivity compared with ketoconazole (*see* Fig. 28.2). The parent compound, abiraterone acetate, is orally bioavailable and has been well tolerated in mCRPC patients as secondary hormone therapy in phase I and II studies.[141,142] With continuous administration, abiraterone increased adenocorticotrophic hormone (ACTH) levels, resulting in mineralocorticoid excess. Therefore, abiraterone acetate is administered with daily low-dose glucocorticoids, such as prednisone.

Abiraterone was initially FDA approved in the mCRPC setting as secondary hormone therapy. The "Cougar-301" study randomized 1,195 men with mCRPC who had previously received docetaxel chemotherapy to abiraterone acetate with prednisone or placebo.[138] Abiraterone was associated with improved overall survival (14.8 versus 10.9 months with placebo; HR 0.65; $P < 0.001$), PSA reduction greater than 50% (29% versus 6%; $P < 0.001$), and radiographic progression-free survival (5.6 versus 3.6 months; HR 0.40; $P < 0.001$), among other endpoints. The "Cougar-302" study similarly randomized 1,088 men with mCRPC but without prior docetaxel chemotherapy to abiraterone acetate with prednisone or placebo.[137] Abiraterone was associated with improved overall survival, among other measures. Notable adverse events with abiraterone included cardiac disorders, liver function test abnormalities, and hypertension.

In 2017, two phase III trials were published establishing the role for abiraterone acetate in metastatic castration-sensitive prostate cancer. The LATITUDE trial randomized 1,199 patients starting ADT to abiraterone acetate with prednisone or ADT alone.[58] The STAMPEDE trial similarly randomized 1,917 patients but included metastatic disease (1,002 subjects) and nonmetastatic disease (915 subjects).[57] In both trials, patients were randomized within 3 months of starting ADT. For patients with metastatic disease, abiraterone acetate was associated with improved overall survival in both studies with remarkably similar hazard ratios of 0.62 and 0.61 for LATITUDE[58] and STAMPEDE,[57] respectively. Thus, for many men with newly diagnosed, metastatic castration-sensitive prostate cancer, the current standard of care combines ADT with abiraterone acetate or docetaxel (as described above under "Clinical Applications").[55,56]

Combined Androgen Blockade

CAB requires administration of ADT with an antiandrogen. The theoretical advantage is that the GnRH agonist will deplete testicular androgens, while the antiandrogen component competes at the receptor with residual androgens made by the adrenal glands or by the cancer cells. CAB provides maximal relief of androgen stimulation. However, the benefit of CAB over ADT monotherapy is controversial. Numerous large trials have compared CAB with ADT monotherapy, with variable results (selected studies are summarized in Table 28.3).[59,60,143,144,146–151] Notably, the largest studies, Intergroup 0105[60] and Intergroup 0036,[59] were performed by the same group and demonstrated conflicting results. Several meta-analyses of these trials suggest a benefit for CAB in 5-year survival but not at earlier time points.[152–154] Toxicity and costs associated with CAB are higher.[155] Current ASCO guidelines suggest that CAB should be discussed, with the emphasis that there may be a gain in overall survival at the cost of higher toxicity.[89]

Future Directions

Despite decades since the 1941 discovery of the role of androgens in prostate cancer growth, optimal hormonal control of advanced prostate cancer remains an area of active investigation. Newer agents targeting steroidogenesis, such as abiraterone, and new antiandrogens, such as enzalutamide, have altered the standard approach to prostate cancer therapy since their initial FDA approvals in 2011 and 2012, respectively. Other agents in development target AR including the AR variants without the ligand binding domain, or other proteins involved in AR activation and signaling, such as the SRC cytoplasmic tyrosine kinase. The effectiveness and appropriate therapeutic use of such agents are the subject of ongoing clinical trials.

Advances in technologies including gene expression profiling, whole transcriptome sequencing, and capture of circulating tumor cells from peripheral blood may allow the development of predictive biomarkers of response to current and future therapies. Indeed, tailoring of a patient's therapy based on AR mutation, amplification, splice variant expression, or dominant signaling pathways represents a prime opportunity for improvement in the hormonal control of metastatic prostate cancer.

TABLE

28.3 *Selected larger studies examining CAB versus ADT monotherapy*

Study	Intervention (*n*)	Median Overall Survival	*P*
INT0036[59]	Leuprolide + flutamide (303)	35.6 mo	0.035
	Leuprolide + placebo (300)	28.3 mo	
International Anandron Study Group[143]	Orchiectomy + nilutamide (225)	27.3 mo	0.0326
	Orchiectomy + placebo (232)	23.6 mo	
EORTC 30853[144]	Goserelin + flutamide (149)	34.4 mo	0.02
	Orchiectomy (148)	27.1 mo	
INT0105[60]	Orchiectomy + flutamide (700)	33.5 mo	0.16
	Orchiectomy + placebo (687)	29.9 mo	
International Prostate Cancer Study Group[145]	Goserelin + flutamide (293)	3.3 y	0.172
	Goserelin (293)	3.2 y	
DAPROCA 86[146]	Goserelin + flutamide (129)	22.7 mo	0.49
	Orchiectomy (133)	27.6 mo	

References

1. Huggins C, Hodges CV. Studies on prostatic cancer: I. The effects of castration, of estrogen, and of androgen injection on serum phosphatases in metastatic carcinoma of the prostate. *Cancer Res.* 1941;1:293-297.

2. Huggins C, Stevens RE Jr, Hodges CV. Studies on prostatic cancer: II. The effects of castration on advanced carcinoma of the prostate gland. *Arch Surg.* 1941;43:209-233.

3. Miller WL. Molecular biology of steroid hormone synthesis. *Endocr Rev.* 1988;9:295-318.

4. Russell DW, Wilson JD. Steroid 5alpha-reductase: two genes/two enzymes. *Annu Rev Biochem.* 1994;63:25-61.

5. Bilezikian JP, Morishima A, Bell J, et al. Increased bone mass as a result of estrogen therapy in a man with aromatase deficiency. *N Engl J Med.* 1998;339:599-603.

6. Hayes FJ, Seminara SB, DeCruz S, et al. Aromatase inhibition in the human male reveals a hypothalamic site of estrogen feedback. *J Clin Endocrinol Metab.* 2000;85:3027-3035.

7. Yeh S, Tsai M-Y, Xu Q, et al. Generation and characterization of androgen receptor knockout (ARKO) mice: an in vivo model for the study of androgen functions in selective tissues. *Proc Natl Acad Sci U S A.* 2002;99:13498-13503.

8. Gelmann EP. Molecular biology of the androgen receptor. *J Clin Oncol.* 2002;20:3001-3015.

9. Mononen N, Schleutker J. Polymorphisms in genes involved in androgen pathways as risk factors for prostate cancer. *J Urol.* 2009;181:1541-1549.

10. Chamberlain NL, Driver ED, Miesfeld RL. The length and location of CAG trinucleotide repeats in the androgen receptor N-terminal domain affect transactivation function. *Nucl Acids Res.* 1994;22:3181-3186.

11. Brockschmidt FF, Nothen MM, Hillmer AM. The two most common alleles of the coding GGN repeat in the androgen receptor gene cause differences in protein function. *J Mol Endocrinol.* 2007;39:1-8.

12. Zeegers MP, Kiemeney LALM, Nieder AM, et al. How strong is the association between CAG and GGN repeat length polymorphisms in the androgen receptor gene and prostate cancer risk? *Cancer Epidemiol Biomarkers Prev.* 2004;13:1765-1771.

13. Lindström S, Zheng SL, Wiklund F, et al. Systematic replication study of reported genetic associations in prostate cancer: strong support for genetic variation in the androgen pathway. *Prostate.* 2006;66:1729-1743.

14. Freedman ML, Pearce CL, Penney KL, et al. Systematic evaluation of genetic variation at the androgen receptor locus and risk of prostate cancer in a Multiethnic Cohort Study. *Am J Hum Genet.* 2005;76:82-90.

15. Chang B-l, Zheng S, Hawkins G, et al. Polymorphic GGC repeats in the androgen receptor gene are associated with hereditary and sporadic prostate cancer risk. *Hum Genet.* 2002;110:122-129.

16. Miller EA, Stanford JL, Hsu L, et al. Polymorphic repeats in the androgen receptor gene in high-risk sibships. *Prostate.* 2001;48:200-205.

17. Mellinghoff IK, Vivanco I, Kwon A, et al. HER2/neu kinase-dependent modulation of androgen receptor function through effects on DNA binding and stability. *Cancer Cell.* 2004;6:517-527.

18. Craft N, Shostak Y, Carey M, et al. A mechanism for hormone-independent prostate cancer through modulation of androgen receptor signaling by the HER-2/neu tyrosine kinase. *Nat Med.* 1999;5:280-285.

19. Hobisch A, Eder IE, Putz T, et al. Interleukin-6 regulates prostate-specific protein expression in prostate carcinoma cells by activation of the androgen receptor. *Cancer Res.* 1998;58:4640-4645.

20. Culig Z, Hobisch A, Cronauer MV, et al. Androgen receptor activation in prostatic tumor cell lines by insulin-like growth factor-I, keratinocyte growth factor, and epidermal growth factor. *Cancer Res.* 1994;54:5474-5478.

21. Kousteni S, Bellido T, Plotkin LI, et al. Nongenotropic, sex-nonspecific signaling through the estrogen or androgen receptors: dissociation from transcriptional activity. *Cell.* 2001;104:719-730.

22. Guo Z, Dai B, Jiang T, et al. Regulation of androgen receptor activity by tyrosine phosphorylation. *Cancer Cell.* 2006;10:309-319.

23. Mahajan NP, Liu Y, Majumder S, et al. Activated Cdc42-associated kinase Ack1 promotes prostate cancer progression via androgen receptor tyrosine phosphorylation. *Proc Natl Acad Sci U S A.* 2007;104:8438-8443.

24. Stanbrough M, Bubley GJ, Ross K, et al. Increased expression of genes converting adrenal androgens to testosterone in androgen-independent prostate cancer. *Cancer Res.* 2006;66:2815-2825.

25. Montgomery RB, Mostaghel EA, Vessella R, et al. Maintenance of intratumoral androgens in metastatic prostate cancer: a mechanism for castration-resistant tumor growth. *Cancer Res.* 2008;68:4447-4454.

26. Marcelli M, Ittmann M, Mariani S, et al. Androgen receptor mutations in prostate cancer. *Cancer Res.* 2000;60:944-949.

27. Tilley WD, Buchanan G, Hickey TE, et al. Mutations in the androgen receptor gene are associated with progression of human prostate cancer to androgen independence. *Clin Cancer Res.* 1996;2:277-285.

28. Taplin M-E, Bubley GJ, Shuster TD, et al. Mutation of the androgen-receptor gene in metastatic androgen-independent prostate cancer. *N Engl J Med.* 1995;332:1393-1398.

29. Taplin M-E, Bubley GJ, Ko Y-J, et al. Selection for androgen receptor mutations in prostate cancers treated with androgen antagonist. *Cancer Res.* 1999;59:2511-2515.

30. Buchanan G, Greenberg NM, Scher HI, et al. Collocation of androgen receptor gene mutations in prostate cancer. *Clin Cancer Res.* 2001;7:1273-1281.

31. Veldscholte J, Ris-Stalpers C, Kuiper GGJM, et al. A mutation in the ligand binding domain of the androgen receptor of human LNCaP cells affects steroid binding characteristics and response to anti-androgens. *Biochem Biophys Res Commun.* 1990;173:534-540.

32. Zhao X-Y, Malloy PJ, Krishnan AV, et al. Glucocorticoids can promote androgen-independent growth of prostate cancer cells through a mutated androgen receptor. *Nat Med.* 2000;6:703-706.

33. Gregory CW, Johnson RT Jr, Mohler JL, et al. Androgen receptor stabilization in recurrent prostate cancer is associated with hypersensitivity to low androgen. *Cancer Res.* 2001;61:2892-2898.

34. Buchanan G, Yang M, Harris JM, et al. Mutations at the boundary of the hinge and ligand binding domain of the androgen receptor confer increased transactivation function. *Mol Endocrinol.* 2001;15:46-56.

35. Visakorpi T, Hyytinen E, Koivisto P, et al. In vivo amplification of the androgen receptor gene and progression of human prostate cancer. *Nat Genet.* 1995;9:401-406.

36. Palmberg C, Koivisto P, Hyytinen E, et al. Androgen receptor gene amplification in a recurrent prostate cancer after monotherapy with the nonsteroidal potent antiandrogen Casodex (bicalutamide) with a subsequent favorable response to maximal androgen blockade. *Eur Urol.* 1997;31:216-219.

37. Antonarakis ES, Armstrong AJ, Dehm SM, et al. Androgen receptor variant-driven prostate cancer: clinical implications and therapeutic targeting. *Prostate Cancer Prostatic Dis.* 2016;19:231-241.

38. Hu R, Dunn TA, Wei S, et al. Ligand-independent androgen receptor variants derived from splicing of cryptic exons signify hormone-refractory prostate cancer. *Cancer Res.* 2009;69:16-22.

39. Guo Z, Yang X, Sun F, et al. A novel androgen receptor splice variant is upregulated during prostate cancer progression and promotes androgen depletion–resistant growth. *Cancer Res.* 2009;69:2305-2313.

40. Antonarakis ES, Lu C, Wang H, et al. AR-V7 and resistance to enzalutamide and abiraterone in prostate cancer. *N Engl J Med.* 2014;371:1028-1038.

41. Antonarakis ES, Lu C, Luber B, et al. Androgen receptor splice variant 7 and efficacy of taxane chemotherapy in patients with metastatic castration-resistant prostate cancer. *JAMA Oncol.* 2015;1:582-591.

42. Luo J. Development of AR-V7 as a putative treatment selection marker for metastatic castration-resistant prostate cancer. *Asian J Androl.* 2016;18:580-585.

43. Kohli M, Ho Y, Hillman DW, et al. Androgen receptor variant AR-V9 is coexpressed with AR-V7 in prostate cancer metastases and predicts abiraterone resistance. *Clin Cancer Res.* 2017;23:4704-4715.

44. Siegel RL, Miller KD, Jemal A. Cancer statistics, 2017. *CA Cancer J Clin.* 2017;67:7-30.

45. Thompson IM, Goodman PJ, Tangen CM, et al. The influence of finasteride on the development of prostate cancer. *N Engl J Med.* 2003;349:215-224.

46. Kramer BS, Hagerty KL, Justman S, et al. Use of 5alpha-reductase inhibitors for prostate cancer chemoprevention: American Society of Clinical Oncology/American Urological Association 2008 Clinical Practice Guideline. *J Clin Oncol.* 2009;27:1502-1516.

47. Andriole G, Bostwick D, Brawley O, et al. Chemoprevention of prostate cancer in men at high risk: rationale and design of the reduction by dutasteride of prostate cancer events (REDUCE) trial. *J Urol.* 2004;172:1314-1317.

48. Andriole G, Bostwick D, Brawley O, et al. Further analyses from the REDUCE prostate cancer risk reduction trial. *J Urol.* 2009;181: 555-555.

49. Pilepich MV, Caplan R, Byhardt RW, et al. Phase III trial of androgen suppression using goserelin in unfavorable-prognosis carcinoma of the prostate treated with definitive radiotherapy: report of Radiation Therapy Oncology Group Protocol 85-31. *J Clin Oncol.* 1997;15:1013-1021.

50. Hanks GE, Pajak TF, Porter A, et al. Phase III trial of long-term adjuvant androgen deprivation after neoadjuvant hormonal cytoreduction and radiotherapy in locally advanced carcinoma of the prostate: the Radiation Therapy Oncology Group Protocol 92–02. *J Clin Oncol.* 2003;21:3972-3978.

51. Jones CU, Hunt D, McGowan DG, et al. Radiotherapy and short-term androgen deprivation for localized prostate cancer. *N Engl J Med.* 2011;365:107-118.

52. Shipley WU, Seiferheld W, Lukka HR, et al. Radiation with or without antiandrogen therapy in recurrent prostate cancer. *N Engl J Med.* 2017;376:417-428.

53. Sharifi N, Gulley JL, Dahut WL. Androgen deprivation therapy for prostate cancer. *JAMA.* 2005;294:238-244.

54. Walsh PC, Deweese TL, Eisenberger MA. A structured debate: immediate versus deferred androgen suppression in prostate cancer--evidence for deferred treatment. *J Urol.* 2001;166:508-516.

55. Sweeney CJ, Chen Y-H, Carducci M, et al. Chemohormonal therapy in metastatic hormone-sensitive prostate cancer. *N Engl J Med.* 2015;373:737-746.

56. James ND, Sydes MR, Clarke NW, et al. Addition of docetaxel, zoledronic acid, or both to first-line long-term hormone therapy in prostate cancer (STAMPEDE): survival results from an adaptive, multiarm, multistage, platform randomised controlled trial. *Lancet.* 2016;387:1163-1177.

57. James ND, de Bono JS, Spears MR, et al. Abiraterone for prostate cancer not previously treated with hormone therapy. *N Engl J Med.* 2017;377:338-351.

58. Fizazi K, Tran N, Fein L, et al. Abiraterone plus prednisone in metastatic, castration-sensitive prostate cancer. *N Engl J Med.* 2017;377:352-360.

59. Crawford ED, Eisenberger MA, McLeod DG, et al. A controlled trial of leuprolide with and without flutamide in prostatic carcinoma. *N Engl J Med.* 1989;321:419-424.

60. Eisenberger MA, Blumenstein BA, Crawford ED, et al. Bilateral orchiectomy with or without flutamide for metastatic prostate cancer. *N Engl J Med.* 1998;339:1036-1042.

61. Petrylak DP, Tangen CM, Hussain MHA, et al. Docetaxel and estramustine compared with mitoxantrone and prednisone for advanced refractory prostate cancer. *N Engl J Med.* 2004;351:1513-1520.

62. Tannock IF, de Wit R, Berry WR, et al: Docetaxel plus prednisone or mitoxantrone plus prednisone for advanced prostate cancer. *N Engl J Med.* 2004;351:1502-1512.

63. de Bono JS, Oudard S, Ozguroglu M, et al. Prednisone plus cabazitaxel or mitoxantrone for metastatic castration-resistant prostate cancer progressing after docetaxel treatment: a randomised open-label trial. *Lancet.* 2010;376:1147-1154.

64. Kantoff PW, Higano CS, Shore ND, et al. Sipuleucel-T immunotherapy for castration-resistant prostate cancer. *N Engl J Med.* 2010;363:411-422.

65. Parker C, Nilsson S, Heinrich D, et al. Alpha emitter radium-223 and survival in metastatic prostate cancer. *N Engl J Med.* 2013;369:213-223.

66. Seidenfeld J, Samson DJ, Hasselblad V, et al. Single-therapy androgen suppression in men with advanced prostate cancer: a systematic review and meta-analysis. *Ann Intern Med.* 2000;132:566-577.

67. Pilepich MV, Winter K, John MJ, et al. Phase III Radiation Therapy Oncology Group (RTOG) trial 86-10 of androgen deprivation adjuvant to definitive radiotherapy in locally advanced carcinoma of the prostate. *Int J Radiat Oncol Biol Phys.* 2001;50:1243-1252.

68. Roach M, III, DeSilvio M, Lawton C, et al. Phase III trial comparing whole-pelvic versus prostate-only radiotherapy and neoadjuvant versus adjuvant combined androgen suppression: Radiation Therapy Oncology Group 9413. *J Clin Oncol.* 2003;21:1904-1911.

69. Loblaw DA, Mendelson DS, Talcott JA, et al. American Society of Clinical Oncology recommendations for the initial hormonal management of androgen-sensitive metastatic, recurrent, or progressive prostate cancer. *J Clin Oncol.* 2004;22:2927-2941.

70. Oefelein MG, Feng A, Scolieri MJ, et al. Reassessment of the definition of castrate levels of testosterone: implications for clinical decision making. *Urology.* 2000;56:1021-1024.

71. Cassileth BR, Soloway MS, Vogelzang NJ, et al. Patients' choice of treatment in stage D prostate cancer. *Urology.* 1989;33:57-62.

72. Tolis G, Ackman D, Stellos A, et al. Tumor growth inhibition in patients with prostatic carcinoma treated with luteinizing hormone-releasing hormone agonists. *Proc Natl Acad Sci U S A.* 1982;79:1658-1662.

73. Schally AV, Coy DH, Arimura A. LH-RH agonists and antagonists. *Int J Gynaecol Obstet.* 1980;18:318-324.

74. Conn PM, Crowley WFJ. Gonadotropin-releasing hormone and its analogues. *N Engl J Med.* 1991;324:93-103.

75. Limonta P, Montagnani Marelli M, Moretti RM. LHRH analogues as anti-cancer agents: pituitary and extrapituitary sites of action. *Expert Opin Investig Drugs.* 2001;10:709-720.

76. Waxman J, Man A, Hendry WF, et al. Importance of early tumour exacerbation in patients treated with long acting analogues of gonadotrophin releasing hormone for advanced prostatic cancer. *Br Med J (Clin Red Ed).* 1985;291:1387-1388.

77. Kuhn JM, Billebaud T, Navratil H, et al. Prevention of the transient adverse effects of a gonadotropin-releasing hormone analogue (buserelin) in metastatic prostatic carcinoma by administration of an antiandrogen (nilutamide). *N Engl J Med.* 1989;321:413-418.

78. Saylor PJ, Smith MR. Metabolic complications of androgen deprivation therapy for prostate cancer. *J Urol.* 2009;181:1998-2008.

79. Smith MR. Treatment-related diabetes and cardiovascular disease in prostate cancer survivors. *Ann Oncol.* 2008;19:vii86-vii90.

80. Shahinian VB, Kuo Y-F, Freeman JL, et al. Risk of fracture after androgen deprivation for prostate cancer. *N Engl J Med.* 2005;352:154-164.

81. Saad F, Gleason DM, Murray R, et al. A randomized, placebo-controlled trial of zoledronic acid in patients with hormone-refractory metastatic prostate carcinoma. *J Natl Cancer Inst.* 2002;94:1458-1468.

82. Smith MR, Egerdie B, Toriz NH, et al. Denosumab in men receiving androgen-deprivation therapy for prostate cancer. *N Engl J Med.* 2009;361:745-755.

83. Keating NL, O'Malley AJ, Smith MR. Diabetes and cardiovascular disease during androgen deprivation therapy for prostate cancer. *J Clin Oncol.* 2006;24:4448-4456.

84. Keating NL, O'Malley AJ, Freedland SJ, et al. Diabetes and cardiovascular disease during androgen deprivation therapy: observational study of veterans with prostate cancer. *J Natl Cancer Inst.* 2010;102:39-46.

85. The Leuprolide Study Group. Leuprolide versus diethylstilbestrol for metastatic prostate cancer. *N Engl J Med.* 1984;311:1281-1286.

86. Vogelzang NJ, Chodak GW, Soloway MS, et al. Goserelin versus orchiectomy in the treatment of advanced prostate cancer: final results of a randomized trial. *Urology.* 1995;46:220-226.

87. Turkes AO, Peeling WB, Griffiths K. Treatment of patients with advanced cancer of the prostate: phase III trial, zoladex against castration; a study of the British Prostate Group. *J Steroid Biochem.* 1987;27:543-549.

88. Kaisary AV, Tyrrell CJ, Peeling WB, et al. Comparison of LHRH analogue (Zoladex) with orchiectomy in patients with metastatic prostatic carcinoma. *Br J Urol.* 1991;67:502-508.

89. Loblaw DA, Virgo KS, Nam R, et al. Initial hormonal management of androgen-sensitive metastatic, recurrent, or progressive prostate cancer: 2007. Update of an American Society of Clinical Oncology Practice Guideline. *J Clin Oncol.* 2007;25:1596-1605.

90. Trachtenberg J, Gittleman M, Steidle C, et al. A phase 3, multicenter, open label, randomized study of abarelix versus leuprolide plus daily antiandrogen in men with prostate cancer. *J Urol.* 2002;167:1670-1674.

91. Klotz L, Boccon-Gibod L, Shore ND, et al. The efficacy and safety of degarelix: a 12-month, comparative, randomized, open-label, parallel-group phase III study in patients with prostate cancer. *BJU Int.* 2008;102:1531-1538.

92. McLeod DG. Tolerability of nonsteroidal antiandrogens in the treatment of advanced prostate cancer. *Oncologist.* 1997;2:18-27.

93. Nakabayashi M, Regan MM, Lifsey D, et al. Efficacy of nilutamide as secondary hormonal therapy in androgen-independent prostate cancer. *BJU Int.* 2005;96:783-786.

94. Schroder FH, Collette L, de Reijke TM, et al. Prostate cancer treated by anti-androgens: is sexual function preserved? *Br J Cancer.* 1999;82:283-290.

95. Thorpe SC, Azmatullah S, Fellows GJ, et al. A prospective, randomised study to compare goserelin acetate (Zoladex) versus cyproterone acetate (Cyprostat) versus a combination of the two in the treatment of metastatic prostatic carcinoma. *Eur Urol.* 1996;29:47-54.

96. Luo S, Martel C, Chen C, et al. Daily dosing with flutamide or casodex exerts maximal antiandrogenic activity. *Urology*. 1997;50:913-919.

97. Shet MS, McPhaul M, Fisher CW, et al. Metabolism of the antian-drogenic drug (Flutamide) by human CYP1A2. *Drug Metab Dispos*. 1997;25:1298-1303.

98. Wysowski DK, Fourcroy JL. Flutamide hepatotoxicity. *J Urol*. 1996;155:209-212.

99. Wysowski DK, Freiman JP, Tourtelot JB, et al. Fatal and nonfatal hepatotoxicity associated with flutamide. *Ann Intern Med*. 1993;118:860-864.

100. Kolvenbag GJ, Furr BJ. Bicalutamide ('Casodex') development: from theory to therapy. *Cancer J Sci Am*. 1997;3:192-203.

101. Iversen P, Tyrrell CJ, Kaisary AV, et al. Bicalutamide monotherapy compared with castration in patients with nonmetastatic locally advanced prostate cancer: 6.3 years of followup. *J Urol*. 2000;164:1579-1582.

102. Cockshott ID. Bicalutamide: clinical pharmacokinetics and metabolism. *Clin Pharmacokinet*. 2004;43:855-878.

103. Schellhammer PF. Combined androgen blockade for the treatment of metastatic cancer of the prostate. *Urology*. 1996;47:622-628.

104. Bales GT, Chodak GW. A controlled trial of bicalutamide versus castration in patients with advanced prostate cancer. *Urology*. 1996;47:38-43.

105. Tyrrell CJ, Kaisary AV, Iversen P, et al. A randomised comparison of 'Casodex' (bicalutamide) 150 mg monotherapy versus castration in the treatment of metastatic and locally advanced prostate cancer. *Eur Urol*. 1998;33:447-456.

106. Mahler C, Verhelst J, Denis L. Clinical pharmacokinetics of the antiandrogens and their efficacy in prostate cancer. *Clin Pharmacokinet*. 1998;34:405-417.

107. Decensi AU, Boccardo F, Guarneri D, et al. Monotherapy with nilutamide, a pure nonsteroidal antiandrogen, in untreated patients with metastatic carcinoma of the prostate. the Italian Prostatic Cancer Project. *J Urol*. 1991;146:377-378.

108. Pfitzenmeyer P, Foucher P, Piard F, et al. Nilutamide pneumonitis: a report on eight patients. *Thorax*. 1992;47:622-627.

109. Creaven PJ, Pendyala L, Tremblay D. Pharmacokinetics and metabolism of nilutamide. *Urology*. 1991;37:13-19.

110. Dole EJ, Holdsworth MT. Nilutamide: an antiandrogen for the treatment of prostate cancer. *Ann Pharmacother*. 1997;31:65-75.

111. Tran C, Ouk S, Clegg NJ, et al. Development of a second-generation antiandrogen for treatment of advanced prostate cancer. *Science*. 2009;324:787-790.

112. Gibbons JA, Ouatas T, Krauwinkel W, et al. Clinical pharmacokinetic studies of enzalutamide. *Clin Pharmacokinet*. 2015;54:1043-1055.

113. Scher HI, Fizazi K, Saad F, et al. Increased survival with enzalutamide in prostate cancer after chemotherapy. *N Engl J Med*. 2012;367:1187-1197.

114. Beer TM, Armstrong AJ, Rathkopf DE, et al. Enzalutamide in metastatic prostate cancer before chemotherapy. *N Engl J Med*. 2014;371:424-433.

115. Shore ND, Chowdhury S, Villers A, et al. Efficacy and safety of enzalutamide versus bicalutamide for patients with metastatic prostate cancer (TERRAIN): a randomised, double-blind, phase 2 study. *Lancet Oncol*. 2016;17:153-163.

116. Lund F, Rasmussen F. Flutamide versus stilboestrol in the management of advanced prostatic cancer. A controlled prospective study. *Br J Urol*. 1988;61:140-142.

117. Koutsilieris M, Tolis G. Long-term follow-up of patients with advanced prostatic carcinoma treated with either buserelin (HOE 766) or orchiectomy: classification of variables associated with disease outcome. *Prostate*. 1985;7:31-39.

118. Chang A, Yeap B, Davis T, et al. Double-blind, randomized study of primary hormonal treatment of stage D2 prostate carcinoma: flutamide versus diethylstilbestrol. *J Clin Oncol*. 1996;14:2250-2257.

119. Boccon-Gibod L, Fournier G, Bottet P, et al. Flutamide versus orchidectomy in the treatment of metastatic prostate carcinoma. *Eur Urol*. 1997;32:391-395.

120. Iversen P, Tyrrell CJ, Kaisary AV, et al. Casodex (bicalutamide) 150-mg monotherapy compared with castration in patients with previously untreated nonmetastatic prostate cancer: results from two multicenter randomized trials at a median follow-up of 4 years. *Urology*. 1998;51:389-396.

121. Iversen P. Update of monotherapy trials with the new anti-androgen, Casodex (ICI 176,334). International Casodex Investigators. *Eur Urol*. 1994;26:5-9.

122. Chodak G, Sharifi R, Kasimis B, et al. Single-agent therapy with bicalutamide: a comparison with medical or surgical castration in the treatment of advanced prostate carcinoma. *Urology*. 1995;46:849-855.

123. Kaisary AV, Tyrrell CJ, Beacock C, et al. A randomised comparison of monotherapy with Casodex 50 mg daily and castration in the treatment of metastatic prostate carcinoma Casodex Study Group. *Eur Urol*. 1995;28:215-222.

124. Iversen P, Tveter K, Varenhorst E. Randomised study of Casodex 50 MG monotherapy vs orchidectomy in the treatment of metastatic prostate cancer. The Scandinavian Casodex Cooperative Group. *Scand J Urol Nephrol*. 1996;30:93-98.

125. Landstrom M, Damber JE, Bergh A. Estrogen treatment postpones the castration-induced dedifferentiation of Dunning R3327-PAP prostatic adenocarcinoma. *Prostate*. 1994;25:10-18.

126. Byar DP, Corle DK. Hormone therapy for prostate cancer: results of the Veterans Administration Cooperative Urological Research Group studies. *NCI Monogr*. 1988;7:165-170.

127. Scherr D, Pitts WRJ, Vaugh EDJ. Diethylstilbestrol revisited: androgen deprivation, osteoporosis and prostate cancer. *J Urol*. 2002;167:535-538.

128. Byar DP. The Veterans Administration Cooperative Urological Research Group's studies of cancer of the prostate. *Cancer*. 1973;32:1126-1130.

129. The Veterans Administration Co-operative Urological Research Group. Treatment and survival of patients with cancer of the prostate. *Surg Gynecol Obstet*. 1967;124:1011-1017.

130. Bailar JC, III, Byar DP. Estrogen treatment for cancer of the prostate. Early results with 3 doses of diethylstilbestrol and placebo. *Cancer*. 1970;26:257-261.

131. Waymont B, Lynch TH, Dunn JA, et al. Phase III randomised study of zoladex versus stilboestrol in the treatment of advanced prostate cancer. *Br J Urol*. 1992;69:614-620.

132. de Voogt HJ, Smith PH, Pavone-Macaluso M, et al. Cardiovascular side effects of diethylstilbestrol, cyproterone acetate, medroxyprogesterone acetate and estramustine phosphate used for the treatment of advanced prostatic cancer: results from European Organization for Research on Treatment of Cancer trials 30761 and 30762. *J Urol*. 1986;135:303-307.

133. Pomerantz M, Manola J, Taplin M-E, et al. Phase II study of low dose and high dose conjugated estrogen for androgen independent prostate cancer. *J Urol*. 2007;177:2146-2150.

134. Mikkola AKK, Ruutu ML, Aro JLV, et al. Parenteral polyestradiol phosphate vs orchidectomy in the treatment of advanced prostatic cancer. Efficacy and cardiovascular complications: a 2-year follow-up report of a national, prospective prostatic cancer study. *Br J Urol*. 1998;82:63-68.

135. Ockrim JL, Lalani EN, Laniado ME, et al. Transdermal estradiol therapy for advanced prostate cancer—forward to the past? *J Urol*. 2003;169:1735-1737.

136. Hedlund PO, Damber J-E, Hagerman I, et al. Parenteral estrogen versus combined androgen deprivation in the treatment of metastatic prostatic cancer: Part 2. Final evaluation of the Scandinavian Prostatic Cancer Group (SPCG) Study No. 5. *Scand J Urol Nephrol*. 2008;42:220-229.

137. Ryan CJ, Smith MR, de Bono JS, et al. Abiraterone in metastatic prostate cancer without previous chemotherapy. *N Engl J Med*. 2013;368:138-148.

138. de Bono JS, Logothetis CJ, Molina A, et al. Abiraterone and increased survival in metastatic prostate cancer. *N Engl J Med*. 2011;364:1995-2005.

139. Small EJ, Halabi S, Dawson NA, et al. Antiandrogen withdrawal alone or in combination with ketoconazole in androgen-independent prostate cancer patients: a phase III trial (CALGB 9583). *J Clin Oncol*. 2004;22:1025-1033.

140. Harris KA, Weinberg V, Bok RA, et al. Low dose ketoconazole with replacement doses of hydrocortisone in patients with progressive androgen independent prostate cancer. *J Urol*. 2002;168:542-545.

141. Attard G, Reid AHM, Yap TA, et al, Phase I clinical trial of a selective inhibitor of CYP17, abiraterone acetate, confirms that castration-resistant prostate cancer commonly remains hormone driven. *J Clin Oncol*. 2008;26:4563-4571.

142. Attard G, Reid AHM, A'Hern R, et al. Selective inhibition of CYP17 with abiraterone acetate is highly active in the treatment of castration-resistant prostate cancer. *J Clin Oncol*. 2009;27:3742-3748.

143. Dijkman GA, Janknegt RA, De Reijke TM, et al. Long-term efficacy and safety of nilutamide plus castration in advanced prostate cancer, and the significance of early prostate specific antigen normalization. *J Urol*. 1997;158:160-163.

144. Denis LJ, Carnelro de Moura JL, Bono A, et al. Goserelin acetate and flutamide versus bilateral orchiectomy: a phase III EORTC trial (30853). *Urology.* 1993;42:119-129.

145. Tyrrell CJ, Altwein JE, Klippel F, et al. Comparison of an LH-RH analogue (Goeserelin acetate, 'Zoladex') with combined androgen blockade in advanced prostate cancer: final survival results of an international multicentre randomized-trial. International Prostate Cancer Study Group. *Eur Urol.* 2000;37:205-211.

146. Iversen P, Rasmussen F, Klarskov P, et al. Long-term results of Danish Prostatic Cancer Group trial 86. Goserelin acetate plus flutamide versus orchiectomy in advanced prostate cancer. *Cancer.* 1993;72:3851-3854.

147. Denis LJ, Keuppens F, Smith PH, et al. Maximal androgen blockade: final analysis of EORTC phase III trial 30853. *Eur Urol.* 1998;33:144-151.

148. Akaza H, Yamaguchi A, Matsuda T, et al. Superior anti-tumor efficacy of bicalutamide 80 mg in combination with a luteinizing hormone-releasing hormone (LHRH) agonist versus LHRH agonist monotherapy as first-line treatment for advanced prostate cancer: interim results of a randomized study in Japanese patients. *Jpn J Clin Oncol.* 2004;34:20-28.

149. Usami M, Akaza H, Arai Y, et al. Bicalutamide 80 mg combined with a luteinizing hormone-releasing hormone agonist (LHRH-A) versus LHRH-A monotherapy in advanced prostate cancer: findings from a phase III randomized, double-blind, multicenter trial in Japanese patients. *Prostate Cancer Prostatic Dis.* 2007;10:194-201.

150. Boccardo F, Rubagotti A, Barichello M, et al. Bicalutamide monotherapy versus flutamide plus goscrelin in prostate cancer patients: results of an Italian Prostate Cancer Project Study. *J Clin Oncol.* 1999;17:2027-2038.

151. Beland G, Elhilali M, Fradet Y, et al. Total androgen ablation: Canadian experience. *Urol Clin North Am.* 1991;18:75-82.

152. Prostate Cancer Trialists' Collaborative Group. Maximum androgen blockade in advanced prostate cancer: an overview of the randomised trials. *Lancet.* 2000;355:1491-1498.

153. Schmitt B, Bennett C, Seidenfeld J, et al. Maximal androgen blockade for advanced prostate cancer. *Cochrane Database Syst Rev.* 2000;2:CD001526.

154. Samson DJ, Seidenfeld J, Schmitt B, et al. Systematic review and meta-analysis of monotherapy compared with combined androgen blockade for patients with advanced prostate carcinoma. *Cancer* 2002;95: 361-376.

155. Bayoumi AM, Brown AD, Garber AM. Cost-effectiveness of androgen suppression therapies in advanced prostate cancer. *J Natl Cancer Inst.* 2000;92:1731-1739.

Section *IV*

Immune-Based Therapies

Monoclonal Antibodies

Ramya Ramaswami and Dan L. Longo

Introduction

Monoclonal antibodies (mAbs) have advanced cancer treatment. At the turn of the 20th century, Paul Ehrlich developed the term "magic bullet" to describe chemicals that are designed to target a specific germ. Over time, this concept has been reapplied in cancer therapies directed specifically against tumor cells.[1] Before the advent of mAbs, passive administration of antibodies was used to treat malignant disease without notable success. Lack of specificity is presumed to have been the reason for the failure. Monoclonal antibody development using hybridoma technology originated in 1975.[2] Fusing a normal lymphocyte producing an antibody of defined specificity with a myeloma cell that proliferated but did not secrete an immunoglobulin molecule led to a hybridoma, a factory for producing monoclonal antibodies. It was possible to generate antibodies that were highly specific against nearly any antigen, including those associated with tumor cells. In 1980, Nadler et al. conducted the first proof of principle trial describing the use of a murine monoclonal antibody known as AB 89.[3] It was administered to a patient with non-Hodgkin's lymphoma and produced a transient decrease in the number of circulating tumor cells. Although this treatment did not result in a durable clinical response, AB 89 caused minor toxicity to the patient. The careful study of this first patient identified problems with murine monoclonal antibodies that would have to be addressed for mAbs to achieve success including down-regulation of target antigen expression, secretion of soluble antigen that distracts the antibody from its tumor target, poor activation of human immune cytotoxic mechanisms, and the development of antibodies to the treating antibody.

The first Food and Drug Administration (FDA) approval of a monoclonal antibody for administration to a person came in 1986 (an anti-CD3 antibody for autoimmune disease) and the first for a cancer indication in 1997 (rituximab anti-CD20).[4] There are now over 40 mAbs that are FDA approved for a wide variety of indications including asthma, autoimmunity, infections, macular degeneration, inflammatory diseases, osteoporosis, anticoagulant reversal, and cancer; several billions of dollars are spent on developing new mAbs.[5] A novel bifunctional antibody (emicizumab) has even been designed to replace factor VIII function in hemophilia A by doing what factor VIII does, bridging factor IXa and factor X. In cancer therapy, mAbs are used in conjunction with chemotherapy and are part of guidelines for the treatment of cancers ranging from lymphoma to colorectal cancer.[6,7]

In addition to high specificity, another advantage of mAbs is their ability to act as delivery molecules for other cytotoxic agents like drugs, toxins, and radioisotopes. There are at least five applications of mAbs in cancer therapy.[8] First, antibodies have a variety of effector mechanisms (complement fixation, activation of various effector cells, direct inhibitory effects) that act on the target to which they bind. Second, antibodies can serve as targeting moieties to specifically deliver diverse killing or inhibitory molecules or effector cells to a specific site. Third, antibodies can be directed at soluble protein or proteoglycan hormones or cytokines or their cellular receptors to antagonize a particular function such as cell growth, invasion, or migration or reverse immunosuppression. Fourth, antibodies can be used as antigens to elicit antitumor responses against immunoglobulin-expressing tumors. Fifth, antibodies can be used to alter the pharmacologic behavior of other substances to either increase or decrease their half-life or alter their distribution (e.g., antibodies to digoxin used to treat digoxin toxicity or to dabigatran to reverse anticoagulant effect).

This chapter reviews the biochemical structure, properties, and applications of mAbs. The safety issues related to this type of therapy are also addressed. The landscape of mAbs is a rapidly evolving field; therefore, this chapter will focus on pharmacologic principles developed from studies to date and will need to be supplemented by the reader in real time as new data and new agents emerge.

Antibody Structure

Antibody structure was initially elucidated by using antibodies as probes of other antibodies. Three sets of determinants were defined. *Isotypes* are determinants that distinguish among the main classes of antibodies of a particular species and are defined by antibodies made in different species. Humans have five main heavy chain isotypes (M, G, A, D, E) and two light chain isotypes (κ, λ). *Allotypes* are small sequence differences or allelic differences between immunoglobulins of the same isotype in different individuals within a species and are defined by antibodies made in the same species. *Idiotypes* are antigenic determinants formed by the antigen-combining site of an antibody that distinguish each clonal B-cell product.

Antibodies are generally composed of four chains, two identical heavy polypeptide chains (molecular weight approximately 50,000 Da) and two identical light chains (molecular weight approximately 22 to 25,000 Da). The heavy chain has four domains that are comprised of 100 amino acids each, and the light chain has two domains. The heavy chain domains are referred to as V_H, C_H1, C_H2, and C_H3, where V indicates "variable" and C denotes "constant." The light chain domains are known as V_L and C_L. Each chain has a portion with limited sequence variability called the constant region (Fc) and a portion with extensive sequence variability called the variable

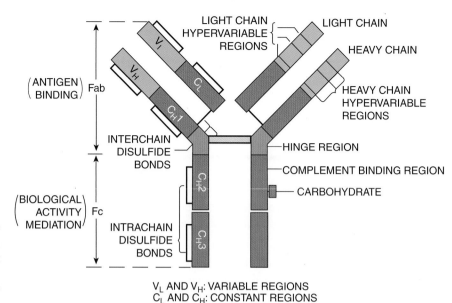

Figure 29.1 A schematic depiction of antibody structure and function relationships. (Reprinted from Wasserman RL, Capra, JD. Immunoglobulins. In: Horowitz MI, Pigman W, eds. *The Glycoconjugates*. New York: Academic Press; 1977:323. Copyright © 1977 Academic Press, Inc. With permission.)

region. The heavy and light chains are bonded and linked by disulfide bonds and aligned such that the variable regions of the light and heavy chain are adjacent to each other (Fig. 29.1). Interheavy chain bonds are located between C$_H$1 and C$_H$2, which forms a hinge region. This area determines the flexibility of the antigen-binding region relative to the Fc and how the antibody can bind to the antigen. A specific antigen is bound by the antibody in the pocket formed by the heavy and light chains (i.e., intertwined V$_H$ and V$_L$ domains)—known as the fragment of antigen binding (Fab). The contact regions between the antigen and the antibody are usually defined by two or three short stretches of peptides that are regions of hypervariability within the variable regions. These are called complementarity-determining regions (CDRs).

Antibodies are linked to immune effector functions by the Fc fragment, which is capable of initiating complement-dependent cytotoxicity (CDC) using complement fixation or targeting immune effector cells using antibody-dependent cellular cytotoxicity (ADCC). Therapeutic antibodies are usually of the IgG class. The Fc portion for IgG also contains a receptor for neonatal FcR (FcRn), which mediates vectorial transport of the antibody and provides protection from catabolism and elimination.[9] mAbs will exert an effect for a longer period of time and will be less rapidly degraded by ensuring stable complexes with FcRn.[9,10]

The development and maturity of B-cells is a highly specialized process in the human body. The expression of an antibody begins with the B-cell progenitor and V gene selection for heavy and light chain V selection that leads to surface expression and secretion by the B-cell. These heavy and light chain genes, in addition to minigene domains, are involved with structure and maturation of B-cells. For example, the minigenes—diversity (D) and joining (J) regions for heavy chain and J regions for light chain—contribute to the CDR3, a variable component of antibodies. Antibodies need to be varied to address the number and diversity of antigens present.[11] There are approximately 80 functional VH genes, 12 D regions, and 6 J regions on the heavy chain locus that can generate over 6,000 combinations. The locus of the light chain has a smaller number of distinct V genes, but this can generate 400 combinations.

Together, the combinations of heavy and light chains may lead to over 2×10^6 combinations.

Following interaction with an antigen, activated B-cells proliferate and secrete antibody. They also undergo CDR mutagenesis, affinity maturation, chain switch, and plasma cell differentiation.[12] These plasma cells remain in the spleen, tissues, or lymph nodes and secrete large quantities of antibody, which is the main function of the fully matured plasma cell.

Antibody Naming

The names of antibodies signify the origin of the product. All monoclonal antibodies and their fragments end with the suffix -mab. The next part of the name is derived from the animal source. A prefix is then added to provide a unique antibody name. The following letters are used as common animal source identifiers:

Infix 2	Infix 2 + -mab suffix
u = human	-umab
o = mouse	-omab
a = rat	-amab
zu = humanized	-zumab
xi = chimera	-ximab

Infix 1 provides a part of the name that highlights the indication for the product. Examples include:

Viral—vir-

Immune—lim-

Cardiovascular—cir-

Interleukins—kin-

Tumor—tum-

A consonant from the infix-1 may be removed to help with the pronunciation of the antibody name.

If the antibody is radiolabeled or conjugated to a chemical or toxin, the conjugate is identified with a separate word or chemical designation. For example, zolimomab aritox indicates the addition of aritox, a ricin chain. For radiolabeled antibody substances, the name of the isotope, element symbol, isotope number, and the antibody name are provided in the name: technetium Tc^{99m} biciromab. Separate words are used to describe the presence of a chelator if one is used to conjugate an antibody to a toxin or isotope, such as indium In^{111} satumomab pendetide.

Antibody Function

It is possible to generate an antibody of defined specificity that can bind to nearly any biological molecule by immunizing mice and isolating and immortalizing the B-cell that produces the desired antibody. The B-cell is then fused to an immunoglobulin non–producing B-cell line, yielding the monoclonal murine-derived antibodies first used in clinical trials. The efficacy of murine antibodies was limited by several factors. First, murine antibodies cooperate with human effector mechanisms poorly such that important mechanisms like complement fixation and ADCC were activated weakly or not at all. Second, the human host has developed sophisticated methods to remove animal proteins rapidly from the blood. Therefore, the biological half-life of murine antibodies is short, indeed, much shorter than the biological half-life of human IgG antibodies (approximately 23 days). Third, murine antibodies are themselves immunogenic. Thus, human antimouse antibodies to the therapeutic agent result in even more rapid clearance on repeat administration. Other factors that compromised efficacy of early antibody trials were tumor-related. Initially, targets were suboptimal. The target molecule could be shed into the serum and distract the antibody from reaching the cell producing the target. In some cases, target molecules were down-regulated such that resistance to the therapeutic antibody emerged.

Many of these problems were addressed in a single technical development: the recombinant production of chimeric antibodies that contained the framework and constant regions of human immunoglobulins with the murine-derived antigen-binding portion of the molecule (the variable or hypervariable regions). The first of these chimeric antibodies to gain FDA approval and to become widely used clinically was rituximab, an anti-CD20 antibody. The success of rituximab against lymphoid malignancies derived in large measure from the persistence of the company that owned the rights to it. Based on the rather minor antitumor activity of the murine anti-CD20 antibody, a peer-review process would likely have terminated its clinical development. However, the industrial sponsor took the development a step further and generated a chimeric antibody. That final step corrected nearly all of the defects of the murine antibody and pointed the way to other effective antibodies for clinical use.

At the cellular level, mAbs act on various components to cause tumor cell death. It is the noncovalent interaction between antibody and antigen that initiates these effects. The strength and association of an antibody to one antigen is known as affinity, which is a measure of the concentration of antibody required to bind a given proportion of the antigen pool. Therefore, it provides information on therapeutic doses. The antibody-antigen dissociation constant K_D, expressed in molar units, is a measure of affinity. Higher affinity is related to smaller values of K_D. The site that the antibody attaches to is known as the epitope, which can also influence the effects that the antibody has on exerting CDC, ADCC, or other changes in target cells.

Pharmacokinetics

Several pharmacokinetic properties make mAbs a useful cancer therapy. First, half-life can equate to days in many cases; thus, convenient dosing schedules can be employed to accommodate other agents. Second, compared to many other cancer therapies such as small-molecule inhibitors, mAbs are not substrates of multidrug resistance efflux pumps.[13] Third, in many cases, concomitant medications generally do not interfere with the pharmacokinetics of mAbs.[14]

The majority of mAbs for cancer therapy are administered via the intravenous or subcutaneous routes. In cases where subcutaneous routes or intramuscular routes are used, the lymphatic system facilitates absorption. The bioavailability following subcutaneous administration may be low compared with small-molecule drugs due to effects on proteolytic degradation in the lymphatic system.[15] Furthermore, subcutaneous administration may also mean that it takes a few days to reach a peak plasma concentration due to slow absorption into the systemic circulation. Despite these differences, in cases such as trastuzumab (anti-HER2), intravenous and subcutaneous administration has been shown to exert the same effects and outcomes.[16,17]

mAbs are designed to bind to the antigen with high affinity and this interaction can affect drug distribution. mAbs have a limited ability to distribute from the blood compartment to the peripheral tissue using diffusion due to their size.[18] The effect of mAb distribution may be subject to heterogeneous characteristics of tumor tissues. Elevated interstitial pressure within tumor tissue may also reduce diffusion and delivery of mAbs to the tumor.[19] Factors such as the presence of a "binding-site barrier" may mean that the penetration of the mAb is limited to the periphery of the tumor tissue.[20,21] This can be overcome with the use of antibody fragments that consist of the antigen-binding parts (Fab).[22] These fragments may move past the blood-tissue barrier easily compared with intact mAbs. However, fragments may be compromised in their ability to activate immune mechanisms. Other factors that impede the effects of mAbs include the heterogeneity of antigen expression on tumor surface, the immunosuppressive tumor microenvironment, and the disordered vasculature in tumors.[23]

mAbs are metabolized to peptides and amino acids that are excreted by the kidney or can be reused in the body for de novo synthesis of proteins. Several routes may be used to excrete mAbs such as proteolysis by the liver, reticuloendothelial system (RES), target-mediated elimination, and nonspecific endocytosis.[15] Using the RES system, lysosomes within macrophages or monocytes may degrade mAbs following binding between the Fc region and Fcγ receptors, which is a similar process to endogenous IgG elimination.[24] The target-mediated elimination occurs where mAbs target a specific tumor antigen and contact with the Fv portion on the antigen leads to degradation. This process does not require Fab binding to a cell surface receptor and therefore can become saturated due to a limited expression of the target.[25] mAbs may also be degraded within the target cells. Some antibody-target complexes internalize and are degraded in lysosomes.[26] Following an immune reaction due to mAbs, endogenous antibodies against the administered therapy can develop. These human antibodies against mouse (HAMAs), chimeric (HACAs), and human (HAHAs) antibodies can bind to mAbs and often modify the therapeutic effect and elimination processes.[27,28]

Mechanisms of Action

The ideal antigen targets for mAbs are expressed at high density and consistency of expression by malignant cells, do not shed into the circulation, and have a limited tendency to down-regulate and produce antigen-negative variants.[29] mAbs may interact with tumor antigens in various ways to lead to cell death (Fig. 29.2). Certain antibody drugs may use more than one mechanism to cause cell death. For example, rituximab has been shown to exert both CDC and ADCC when binding to CD20 on malignant B-cell lymphoma cells.[30] The effects of rituximab may include cell cycle arrest and induction of apoptosis. Some of the mechanisms are described below.

Complement-Dependent Cytotoxicity

CDC is an immune-mediated process where an antibody can cause cell death by harnessing the effects of the complement pathway. The process of CDC initiation starts with binding of two or more IgG molecules to the cell surface, which then leads to binding between the Fc region on the antibody with the complement component 1 (C1q) region.[31] A study by Racila et al. demonstrated that among patients with follicular lymphoma treated with rituximab, polymorphisms of C1qA affected the clinical response.[32] IgG1 and IgG3, which are subclasses of IgG, are potent activators of the complement pathway as compared with IgG4, which does not have an ability to bind to C1q. CDC can depend on mAb isotype, the antigen concentration, the orientation of the antigen in the membrane, and whether the antigen is present on the surface as a monomer or polymer. This leads to activation of downstream complement proteins, which results in the formation of pores by the membrane attack complex (MAC) on the tumor cell surface and subsequent tumor cell lysis. Two similar mAb isotypes that target the same antigen can vary in the effect. Type I human IgG1 CD20-specific mAbs cross-link

CD20 tetramers and fix complement, which is noted with rituximab. This is in contrast to type II IgG1 CD20-specific mAbs that do not cross-link tetramers or fix complement, for example, obinutuzumab.[33] This typing of anti-CD20 antibodies based on their effector functions and distribution of antigen in the cell after binding has not been widely applied to other antibodies. Four antibodies that recognize CD20 are now FDA approved (Table 29.1).

Antibody-Dependent Cellular Cytotoxicity

ADCC is the process resulting in the lysis of a target cell by an immune effector cell (such as a natural killer cell, monocyte, macrophage, or granulocyte) induced by the recognition of an antibody bound to the surface of the target cell. mAbs can induce binding to FcγRs, which are expressed by natural killer cells, granulocytes, monocytes, and macrophages. FcγRs can differ in their affinity for IgG isotypes and their ability to elicit ADCC.[34] Furthermore, polymorphisms of FcγRs can also affect mAb response. FcγRs can activate or inhibit cellular signaling using immunoreceptor tyrosine-based activation motif (ITAM) and immunoreceptor tyrosine-based inhibitor motif (ITIM). ITAM is a sequence of amino acids in the cytoplasmic domains of various cell surface immunoreceptors.[35] ITAMs function as docking sites for tyrosine kinases using the SRC homology 2 domain, thereby facilitating intracellular signaling cascades. ITIM is similar in structure to ITAM, and this motif is phosphorylated by enzymes of the SRC kinase family that decrease the activation of molecules involved in cell signaling.[36] The main inhibitory FcγR is FcγRIIB or CD32.

Activating signals involve ITAM and FcγRI (CD64) and are expressed on macrophages, neutrophils, and dendritic cells and FcγIIA (CD16A), which are expressed on natural killer cells (NK cells), dendritic cells, and macrophages. These are components required for NK cell ADCC.[37] Tumor cells to which IgG antibodies are bound can be recognized by immune effector populations that

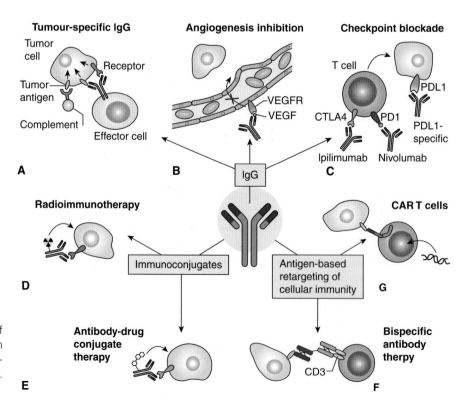

FIGURE **29.2** Mechanisms and applications of monoclonal antibodies. (Reprinted by permission from Nature: Weiner GJ. Building better monoclonal antibody-based therapeutics. *Nat Rev Cancer.* 2015;15(6):361-370. Copyright © 2015 Springer Nature.)

TABLE

29.1   Monoclonal antibodies and their approval statuses in the EU and USA

International Nonproprietary Name (INN)	Trade Name	Target and Type	Therapeutic Indication(s)	Year of First EU EMA Approval	Year of First FDA Approval
Inotuzumab ozogamicin	Besponsa	CD22; humanized IgG4, ADC	Hematological malignancy	2017	2017
Durvalumab	Imfinzi	PD-L1; human IgG1	Bladder cancer	NA	2017
Ocrelizumab	Ocrevus	CD20; humanized IgG1	Multiple sclerosis	Review	2017
Avelumab	Bavencio	PD-L1; human IgG1	Merkel cell carcinoma	Review	2017
Atezolizumab	Tecentriq	PD-L1; humanized IgG1	Bladder cancer	Review	2016
Olaratumab	Lartruvo	PDGFRα; human IgG1	Soft-tissue sarcoma	2016	2016
Daratumumab	Darzalex	CD38; human IgG1	Multiple myeloma	2016	2015
Elotuzumab	Empliciti	SLAMF7; humanized IgG1	Multiple myeloma	2016	2015
Necitumumab	Portrazza	EGFR; human IgG1	Non–small cell lung cancer	2015	2015
Dinutuximab	Unituxin	GD2; chimeric IgG1	Neuroblastoma	2015	2015
Nivolumab	Opdivo	PD-1; human IgG4	Melanoma, non–small cell lung cancer	2015	2014
Blinatumomab	Blincyto	CD19, CD3; murine bispecific tandem scFv	Acute lymphoblastic leukemia	2015	2014
Pembrolizumab	Keytruda	PD-1; humanized IgG4	Melanoma	2015	2014
Ramucirumab	Cyramza	VEGFR-2; human IgG1	Gastric cancer	2014	2014
Siltuximab	Sylvant	IL-6; chimeric IgG1	Castleman disease	2014	2014
Obinutuzumab	Gazyva	CD20; humanized IgG1; glycoengineered	Chronic lymphocytic leukemia	2014	2013
Ado-trastuzumab emtansine	Kadcyla	HER2; humanized IgG1, ADC	Breast cancer	2013	2013
Pertuzumab	Perjeta	HER2; humanized IgG1	Breast cancer	2013	2012
Brentuximab vedotin	Adcetris	CD30; chimeric IgG1, ADC	Hodgkin's lymphoma, systemic anaplastic large cell lymphoma	2012	2011
Ipilimumab	Yervoy	CTLA-4; human IgG1	Metastatic melanoma	2011	2011
Ofatumumab	Arzerra	CD20; human IgG1	Chronic lymphocytic leukemia	2010	2009
Catumaxomab	Removab	EPCAM/CD3; rat/mouse bispecific mAb	Malignant ascites	2009	NA
Panitumumab	Vectibix	EGFR; human IgG2	Colorectal cancer	2007	2006
Bevacizumab	Avastin	VEGF; humanized IgG1	Colorectal cancer	2005	2004
Cetuximab	Erbitux	EGFR; chimeric IgG1	Colorectal cancer	2004	2004
Tositumomab I-131	Bexxar	CD20; murine IgG2a	Non-Hodgkin's lymphoma	NA	2003
Ibritumomab tiuxetan	Zevalin	CD20; murine IgG1	Non-Hodgkin's lymphoma	2004	2002
Alemtuzumab	MabCampath, Campath-1H; Lemtrada	CD52; humanized IgG1	Chronic myeloid leukemia; multiple sclerosis	2013; 2001	2014; 2001
Gemtuzumab ozogamicin	Mylotarg	CD33; humanized IgG4, ADC	Acute myeloid leukemia	In review	In review; 2000
Trastuzumab	Herceptin	HER2; humanized IgG1	Breast cancer	2000	1998
Rituximab	MabThera, Rituxan	CD20; chimeric IgG1	Non-Hodgkin's lymphoma	1998	1997

Several antibody therapeutics are approved for marketing in regions other than the EU or United States. These products include:
Nimotuzumab (TheraCIM®, BIOMAB-EGFR®), humanized anti-EGFR IgG1 approved in numerous countries for various forms of solid tumors starting in the 2000s.
Mogamulizumab (POTELIGEO®), humanized anti-CCR4 IgG1 first approved in Japan on March 30, 2012, for relapsed or refractory CCR4-positive adult T-cell leukemia-lymphoma. NA, not approved.

express Fcγ receptors such as NK cells, neutrophils, dendritic cells, and mononuclear phagocytes.[31,38] The Fc portions of the coating antibodies interact with Fc receptors that are expressed by effector cells, thereby initiating signaling cascades that result in the release of cytotoxic granules (containing perforin and granzyme B) that induce apoptosis of the antibody-coated cell. Following tumor cell lysis, antigen-presenting cells can present tumor-derived peptides on MHC class II molecules and promote CD4+ T-cell activation. Tumor-derived peptides can be presented on MHC class I molecules resulting in inactivation of CD8+ cytotoxic T-cells.

FcRn is related to MHC class I molecules and is known to be involved in passive transfer of maternal humoral immunity to the fetus. FcRn is distinct from Fcγ and is expressed on the vascular endothelium. FcRn can bind to the IgG Fc domain and can return it to the circulation and increase the half-life of the immunoglobulin.[39,40]

Transmembrane Signaling

The process by which an extracellular signal, mediated by a natural ligand or a monoclonal antibody that binds to a membrane receptor, generates an intercellular signal that can affect cellular functions such as apoptosis. In vitro and animal model data have shown that transmembrane signaling may be a mechanism of action for mAbs that leads to apoptosis of tumor cells.[29,41] Examples of antibodies that affect the cancer cell via transmembrane signaling include cetuximab (antibody to epidermal growth factor receptor [EGFR]). In the case of HER2 inhibition, trastuzumab blocks the receptor dimerization.[42,43] Interruption of signaling at the cell surface may also block growth factors downstream that control cell functions such as angiogenesis.[44-46]

Immune Mediation

The control of T-cell immunity and its regulation has been studied extensively over the last decade. The power of T-cells to destroy tissue is clear from diseases like scleroderma and rheumatoid arthritis. The efficacy of T-cells in killing tumors is demonstrated by the graft-versus-leukemia effects seen in allogeneic hematopoietic cell transplantation. So why is the immune system so poorly effective in eliminating cancer cells?

Given that we live in a world of foreign antigens, the immune system must strike a balance between ignoring an antigen that might be dangerous and overreacting to it. We are still learning how the immune system detects danger and discriminates between self and nonself. One set of adaptations tumors make to avoid immune recognition is to mimic self as much as possible. And if a tumor begins to arouse the attention of the immune system, it can hide in plain sight by downregulating expression of MHC class I genes. T-cells do not kill cells that do not express MHC molecules.

A second level of tumor subterfuge is to render T-cells inactive or unresponsive. Several mechanisms limit a normal immune response. The coregulation of ligand-receptor pairs plays a key role in maintaining a balance between activating and inhibiting antigen-specific T-cells. Cytotoxic T-lymphocyte antigen-4 (CTLA4), also known as CD152, is a receptor expressed by activated T-cells that signals the cell that it is time to dampen the response.[47] This and other negative regulators (e.g., TGF-beta) are important for avoiding autoimmunity and a hyperactive immune response. Tumors are able to activate CTLA4 expression and prevent T-cells from exerting an antitumor response. One approach to overcoming this tumor adaptation is to block CTLA4.[48] mAbs to checkpoint inhibitors like CTLA4 (e.g., ipilimumab) interfere with inhibitory signals and enhance T-cell–mediated lysis.[49,50]

The programmed cell death protein (PD-1) receptor-PD-1 ligand (PD-L1) axis is another T-cell regulatory pathway that has led to new forms of cancer therapy. PD-1 is an immune-checkpoint receptor expressed by antigen-stimulated T-cells that inhibits T-cell proliferation, cytokine release, and cytotoxicity. PD-1 and PD-L1 ligands are expressed on the cell surface of tumor cells, stromal cells, or both. Anti–PD-1 and PD-L1 antibodies can reverse T-cell suppression and induce long-lasting antitumor responses in some patients with advanced solid tumors. They may also induce autoimmunity, the effects of which can be long-lasting. Ipilimumab, nivolumab, pembrolizumab, atezolizumab, and others (see Table 29.1) are mAbs developed to activate a robust antitumor T-cell response. They are active in a variety of tumor types that have been unresponsive to conventional cancer treatments. However, we still do not understand the factors that distinguish patients whose tumors respond from patients whose tumors do not respond or why tumors stop responding. One idea for which some evidence exists is that tumor cells defective in DNA repair express a larger number of mutated peptides that may be recognized by the immune system.[51] This has not been shown to be a generalizable marker of responsiveness to checkpoint blockade. Similarly, the evidence is conflicting on the degree to which PD-L1 expression on the tumor cell predicts for response.

Bispecific Antibodies

Bispecific antibodies are engineered to simultaneously target different specific antigens or epitopes. One arm will bind to the tumor-associated antigen, and the other arm can bind to activating receptors on cytotoxic effector cells such as T-cells or NK cells.[52] The resulting effect is retargeting the immune effector cell toward the target cancer cell. They are divided into two classes, those that bear an Fc region and are considered immunoglobulin G (IgG)-like and those that do not have an Fc region, which are non–IgG-like molecules. Those that lack an Fc region are generally smaller than the former class. Where a bispecific antibody lacks an Fc region, the therapeutic effects will rely on the antigen-binding capacity. Smaller bifunctional molecules lacking the Fc components have short half-lives and require a continuous infusion, but these molecules result in less nonspecific immune activation than do intact bifunctional mAbs.[53] Presence of the Fc region in a bispecific antibody can lead to greater solubility and stability and can facilitate ADCC and CDC effects on the target cell. Intact Fc fragments can lead to nonspecific activation of T-cells; therefore, careful manufacturing is needed to avoid serious adverse events and patient harm.

There are several different strategies that may be used to develop both classes of bispecific antibodies. Among the IgG-like class, the quadroma, though to be the first generation of bispecific antibodies, relies on the fusion of two distinct hybridomas. The random pairing of Ig heavy and light chains results in a symmetric bispecific antibody.[53] However, this can result in redundant homodimers or undesirable products that make purification of one desired bispecific antibody difficult. This was improved by development of the "knobs-into-holes" technology where within the CH3 domain (the "knob") a large amino acid is substituted for a small amino acid of one antibody and vice versa (the "hole") for the other antibody.[54] Where heavy chain heterodimerization is forced using mutations in the two CH3 domains, this resulted in asymmetric bispecific antibodies. There are several non–IgG-like variations where bispecific antibodies can also be developed with two different antibody fragments (scFv) that can be fused with albumin or any other nonimmunoglobulin protein. Alternatively, two antigen-binding fragments can be fused.

Trifunctional bispecific antibodies (Triomab) consist of two half antibodies, each with one light and heavy chain that originate from a mouse and rat IgG2 isotypes. These antibodies bind to tumor cell surface antigens, to a T lymphocyte, and to an antigen-presenting cell such as a macrophage and natural killer cell via the heavy chain, which triggers an immune response.

Chimeric Antigen Receptor (CAR) T-cell Therapy (See Chapter 31 on Adoptive Cellular Therapy)

Chimeric antigen receptors are proteins that enable T-cells to recognize an antigen on tumor cells. A patient's polyclonal T-cells are harvested by pheresis and genetically manipulated to express a tumor-specific antibody on the cell surface (e.g., antibody to CD19, a B-cell antigen) connected to T-cell activating signal transducing intracellular elements like the T-cell receptor zeta chain, CD28, OX-40 (CD134), 4-1BB (CD137), or combinations of these proteins. The engineered cells are then administered to the patient.[55]

CAR T-cell therapy has been shown to elicit a response among patients with relapsed acute lymphoblastic leukemia (ALL) where up to 90% of children and adults with ALL who had progressed on standard therapies achieve remission following CAR T-cell therapy.[56,57] These therapies have also demonstrated benefit in small studies of patients with multiple myeloma, diffuse large B-cell lymphoma, and chronic lymphocytic leukemia. Use of CAR T-cell therapy against IL13Rα2 antigen found in glioblastoma has also resulted in regression in a published case report.[58] Among some patients administered this form of treatment, CAR T memory cells have been observed, which may prolong clinical responses. However, this may also be disadvantageous as it may eliminate cells that express the target antigen. As many target antigens may also be expressed on physiological tissue or benign cells, long-term adverse effects could emerge with longer follow-up.

In the case of both bifunctional antibodies and CAR T-cell therapy, a large number of T-cells are exposed to cells expressing the target antigen.[59] This can cause a sudden release of cytokines or cytokine storm characterized by hypotension, capillary leak syndrome, respiratory distress, and CNS toxicity that can be fatal. Management of these toxicities requires close monitoring and specialist input.[60]

Safety and Toxicities

mAbs are generally safe to use in humans. Toxicities may range from those that are immediate and transient to long-term effects that can be life-threatening. These toxicities may depend on the type and intended target of the antibody being used.

Immediate toxicities for patients receiving these infusional therapies include local site injection erythema, pyrexia, and influenza-like syndrome to systemic inflammatory response syndrome. Infusion reactions may occur in over 50% of cases of patients administered with rituximab or alemtuzumab.[61] Nearly all infused antibodies produce infusion reactions of varying degrees of seriousness and may include IgE-mediated anaphylactic reactions. Although the exact mechanism of infusion reactions is unclear, cytokine release from lymphocytes as a result of the antibody-antigen interaction has been proposed as the mechanism. In the case of cetuximab, the anaphylactoid reaction is attributed to the development of galactose-α-1,

3-galactose.[62] Recognizing risk factors such as a history of allergic disorders, reaction to tick bites, or allergic reactions to eating meat, pork, and lamb may help identify those who may be susceptible to cetuximab infusion reactions. In addition, pretreatment with antihistamines and adequate monitoring during the infusion may help ameliorate these reactions. In general, the reactions are most severe with the first infusion and tend to be less severe with subsequent administrations.

Cytokine release syndrome (CRS) is a non–antigen-specific toxicity that occurs as a result of high-level immune activation.[60] It can manifest when large numbers of lymphocytes or myeloid cells become activated and release inflammatory cytokines. Patients present with systemic inflammatory response symptoms of hypotension, pyrexia, and rigors shortly after the infusion, and this may result in multiple organ failure if not managed aggressively. This is a risk for virtually every monoclonal antibody-based therapy.

Infections can occur following treatment with mAbs and can occur due to acquired immune deficiency following the loss of the normal cells expressing the target ligand.[63] For example, alemtuzumab is associated with loss of CD52-bearing cells (nearly all lymphocytes) and immunosuppression, thereby increasing the risk of opportunistic infection. Tuberculosis is less commonly seen among mAbs associated used for cancer treatment compared with the anti-TNF antibodies (e.g., adalimumab) used to treat rheumatoid arthritis. Progressive multifocal leukoencephalopathy (PML) is a rapidly progressive demyelinating disease that can occur due to reactivation of latent infection in the central nervous system with the polyoma virus John Cunningham virus (JCV). Following treatment with rituximab, 57 cases of PML were described.[64] It is hypothesized that B-cell depletion as a result of rituximab may cause reactivation of latent JCV. However, this mechanism may not fully explain the pathophysiological process.[65,66]

mAbs such as rituximab and alemtuzumab may cause drug-induced thrombocytopenia.[67] While alemtuzumab with its cytolytic effect is likely to cause multilineage hematopoietic toxicity, the mechanism of action of drug-induced thrombocytopenia with rituximab is unclear. The anti-VEGF antibody bevacizumab has been associated with venous and arterial thromboembolism. Some studies report an increased risk of 1% to 3% of arterial thromboembolisms among patients treated with bevacizumab.[68,69] However, a meta-analysis and pooled studies have suggested that this risk is not statistically significant.[70,71]

Organ-specific toxicities may also result from mAbs, such as cardiotoxicity and dermatitis. Early clinical trials evaluating trastuzumab in combination with anthracycline-based chemotherapy in patients with metastatic breast cancer found that 27% of trial participants, with no previous cardiac history, experienced symptomatic heart failure or asymptomatic cardiac dysfunction.[72] Following these trials, it was assumed that the combination of an anthracycline chemotherapy with trastuzumab resulted in higher rates of cardiac toxicity. Subsequent trials have shown that the incidence of heart failure was 2% to 4% and cardiac dysfunction is 3% to 19%.[73] Trastuzumab is implicated in impaired contractility and cardiac dysfunction due to on-target effects of ERBB2 and downstream signaling causing mitochondrial membrane, cytochrome c, and caspase activation. Trastuzumab inhibits the activity of neuregulin 1 (NRG-1) in cardiac myocytes, thereby interfering with the structural maintenance and integrity of the heart.[74,75]

Bevacizumab, an anti-VEGF antibody, is also known to cause hypertension due to the effect on vascular endothelial growth factor (VEGF) signaling inhibition. VEGF induces the production of two vasodilators, nitric oxide and prostacyclin, and decreases the production of endothelin-1, a potent vasoconstrictor. VEGF is also expressed on endothelial cells and kidney and has a role in cell proliferation and homeostasis. VEGF signaling can lead to an imbalance between vasodilators and vasoconstrictors, loss of capillary circulation, and alteration in glomerular function that can contribute to hypertension.[76]

Cardiac toxicity and inflammation of other organs such as the thyroid, lungs, and skin can occur when antibodies are directed against programmed death-1 (PD-1). These effects are related to the immune mechanism of checkpoint inhibitors.[77] Dry skin and an acne-like rash can present over the face and torso among patients who are treated with cetuximab and panitumumab, an EGFR-specific mAb. This a target-related effect as EGFR is a transmembrane glycoprotein that is expressed on epithelial cells. There is a correlation between the presence of the skin rash and response to treatment.[78,79]

The general rule of managing mAb-related toxicities involves addressing the symptoms, addressing any organ-specific toxicities and changes in the dose, or cessation of the mAb. Cessation of mAb is dependent on the toxicity and the impact that these adverse events have on quality of life. In the case of PD-1–related toxicity, which are immune mediated, systemic glucocorticoids may improve symptoms.[77] However, there is concern about ameliorating the effect of tumor cells in the process. As with any cancer therapies, clinicians in discussion with their patients need to balance the intent, risks, and benefits when using mAbs.

Monoclonal Antibodies Used in Cancer Treatment

As of August 2017, 31 monoclonal antibodies are FDA approved for use in patients with cancer (Table 29.1). They are directed at 19 different targets, CD20 (rituximab, tositumomab I-131, ibritumomab tiuxetan, ofatumumab, obinutuzumab, ocrelizumab [CD20-directed but approved for multiple sclerosis]), EGFR (cetuximab, panitumumab, necitumumab), HER-2/neu (trastuzumab, pertuzumab, trastuzumab emtansine), PD-L1 (atezolizumab, avelumab, durvalumab), PD-1 (pembrolizumab, nivolumab), CD33 (gemtuzumab ozogamicin), VEGF (bevacizumab), VEGF receptor (ramucirumab), CD52 (alemtuzumab), IL-6 (siltuximab), CD22 (inotuzumab ozogamicin), CD38 (daratumumab), SLAM7 (elotuzumab), CD30 (brentuximab vedotin), the diganglioside GD2 (dinutuximab), CTLA4 (ipilimumab), CD19 (blinatumomab), platelet-derived growth factor receptor alpha (olaratumab), and epithelial cell adhesion molecule (catumaxomab). Five of them are drug conjugates, two are radioconjugates, and two are bispecific antibodies. One monoclonal antibody, nofetumomab (NR-LU10, anti-CD56) labeled with technetium-99m, is approved for use as an imaging agent in the staging of small cell lung cancer. Many more antibodies directed at other targets are in development. Most target tumor cells directly. Bevacizumab (anti-VEGF) and siltuximab (anti-IL-6) are directed at soluble growth factors. Some target receptors (anti-CTLA4, anti–PD-1, anti–PD-L1) aimed at activating the immune system.

CD20 Antibodies

Rituximab (Rituxan)

CD20, the target of rituximab, is expressed mainly on normal and neoplastic B-cells. CD20 is a hydrophobic transmembrane protein of molecular weight 35 kDa. CD20 is not expressed on hematopoietic stem cells, pro-B-cells or plasma cells, or nonlymphoid tissues. The role of CD20 is unclear; some data have suggested that it functions as a calcium channel. It is not shed or internalized upon antibody binding.[80]

Rituximab is a chimeric IgG1, κ antibody with human constant regions and murine variable regions. Its molecular weight is about 145 kDa and it binds CD20 with an affinity of 8 nM. Its antitumor effects are thought to be related to its activation of complement and ADCC. In addition, signaling through CD20 may activate apoptosis mechanisms. Rituximab has been used successfully in combination with chemotherapeutic agents to augment the antitumor effects.

The pharmacokinetics of the agent are influenced by a variety of factors including the tumor burden. Early doses tend to achieve lower serum levels because the tumor and normal B-cells bind a larger fraction of an administered dose. The empirically derived treatment schedule is weekly doses of 375 mg/m^2 IV. After the 4th weekly dose, the half-life averages 205 hours with a maximum serum concentration of 486 µg/mL. Levels continue to increase with additional weekly administrations. Delivery of rituximab with chemotherapy does not alter its pharmacology. A dose of 500 mg/m^2 has been tolerated, but a maximum tolerated dose has not been identified. Rituximab should be infused at an initial rate of 50 mg/h due to toxicity issues related to activation of immune effector mechanisms.

Toxicities from rituximab are mainly related to the initial infusion. Symptoms generally develop within 30 to 120 minutes of starting infusion. In most cases, the symptom complex includes one or more of the following: fever and chills, nausea, pruritis, angioedema, asthenia, headache, bronchospasm, throat irritation, rhinitis, urticaria, myalgia, dizziness, or hypertension. These symptoms are related to complement activation. The reactions resolve entirely with either slowing the infusion or temporarily interrupting it. The infusion-related symptoms generally decrease in incidence with each administration from nearly 80% incidence with the first to around 14% with the eighth. Diphenhydramine, acetaminophen, and intravenous fluids are often required to suppress the symptoms. Once symptoms resolve, the administration of rituximab can be reinitiated at about half the rate of the initial infusion. In some rare and severe cases, patients can develop adult respiratory distress syndrome, myocardial infarction, ventricular fibrillation, or cardiogenic shock.

Other uncommon problems include the development of tumor lysis syndrome from rapid killing of tumor cells and occasional Stevens-Johnson syndrome with severe mucocutaneous inflammation. When rituximab is administered with chemotherapy, some patients have experienced reactivation of hepatitis B. In general, rituximab is very well tolerated. It only rarely elicits a host antibody response (approximately 1% of patients). The suppression of normal B-cells by rituximab is variable in duration depending on the age of the patient and the length of treatment, but most patients recover normal B-cell function within a year of stopping rituximab. No late effects of B-cell suppression have been reported.

Rituximab is effective in nearly all B-cell–derived malignancies that express CD20. It is particularly active when used in combination chemotherapy and has become a component of standard therapy for diffuse large B-cell lymphoma. In addition to its standard use in patients with diffuse large B-cell lymphoma, it is also active in follicular lymphoma, mantle cell lymphoma, chronic lymphoid leukemia, and hairy cell leukemia. It is also being used increasingly to treat autoimmune diseases in which autoreactive antibodies play a pathogenetic role. These include idiopathic thrombocytopenic purpura, thrombotic thrombocytopenic purpura, autoimmune hemolytic anemia, and some cases of pure red cell aplasia.

Ocrelizumab

This is a recombinant humanized monoclonal antibody against CD20 B-cells that has been approved in patients with multiple sclerosis. It is administered intravenously, has a molecular mass of approximately 145 kDa, and has a half-life of 26 days. Ocrelizumab differs from rituximab as it is derived from a different allotype of human Fc than rituximab. In vitro studies have shown that ocrelizumab may have greater ADCC, lower CDC, and greater binding to low-affinity variants of the Fcγ receptor IIIa.[81]

Ofatumumab

Ofatumumab is a human IgG1 κ anti-CD20 mAB that, compared to rituximab, targets the membrane-proximal epitope on CD20 that encompasses two loops. Rituximab's binding site on CD20 is distal to the ofatumumab binding site and involves a large loop only. This intravenous therapy has a half-life of 14 days. It has been approved for treatment of chronic lymphocytic leukemia that is refractory to fludarabine and alemtuzumab.

Preclinical studies have demonstrated that as a result of these differences, ofatumumab has a higher affinity and activates CDC effectively as compared to rituximab. Ofatumumab demonstrated greater activity in rituximab-sensitive or rituximab-resistant cell line models compared with rituximab.[82] However, in a randomized clinical trial of patients with relapsed or refractory diffuse large B-cell lymphoma who were treated with ofatumumab or rituximab, there was difference in efficacy.[83]

Obinutuzumab

Obinutuzumab should not be considered a "biosimilar" to rituximab. It is a humanized IgG1 κ glycoengineered molecule that has been designed to increase affinity to the Fc receptor involved in ADCC and also induces Fv-mediated direct cell effects. It has a molecular mass of 150 kDa and it is administered intravenously. It has an elimination half-life of 28.4 days with a binding affinity to CD20 (using Scatchard analysis) of 4 nM.[84] As compared with rituximab and ofatumumab, which are type I monoclonal antibodies, obinutuzumab is classified as a type II monoclonal antibody. Both these subtypes function using ADCC and demonstrate efficient phagocytosis. Type I monoclonal antibodies are known to activate complement, whereas type II mAbs are ineffective in CDC but can evoke greater homotypic adhesion and direct killing of cells.[85]

To increase ADCC within type II mAbs, the affinity between the Fc portion of the antibody and the FcγRIIIa expressed by effector cells should be improved. Obinutuzumab was engineered to modify the carbohydrate between the two Fc arms. This results in a reduction of fructose on the IgG oligosaccharide, which improved binding to FcγRIII and ADCC.[86]

In 2013, the FDA approved obinutuzumab for use in combination with chlorambucil for patients with previously untreated chronic lymphocytic leukemia.[87] The toxicities related to obinutuzumab are similar to those seen with rituximab. A black box warning has been issued for hepatitis B virus reactivation and PML, which can be fatal.

Ibritumomab Tiuxetan (Zevalin)

Ibritumomab tiuxetan is a murine IgG1 κ antibody chelated to yttrium-90, a beta-emitting isotope. Ibritumomab binds to human CD20 with an affinity of about 14 to 18 nM. Tiuxetan is the chelating agent that attaches yttrium-90 to exposed amino groups in lysines and arginines in the antibody sequence. Ibritumomab tiuxetan is used as a salvage regimen for the treatment of CD20-expressing B-cell malignancies.

Like I-131 tositumomab, the ibritumomab tiuxetan therapeutic regimen consists of two steps: dosimetry followed by therapy. Dosimetry is performed by injecting unlabeled rituximab (250 mg/m²) followed by 5 mCi of indium-111–labeled ibritumomab tiuxetan (containing 1.6 mg of antibody) over 10 minutes to assess biodistribution of the label. If the biodistribution shows too much lung, renal, or bowel uptake, the therapeutic dose is not given. However, if the biodistribution of the In-111 compound is acceptable, 7 to 9 days after dosimetry dose, the patient receives a therapeutic dose of 250 mg/m² rituximab followed by 0.4 mCi/kg of ibritumomab tiuxetan labeled with Y-90 over 10 minutes. The physical half-life of the isotope is just under 3 days and the mean half-life of Y-90 activity in the blood is 30 hours.[88]

The efficacy of ibritumomab tiuxetan appears similar to that of I-131 tositumomab. Patients who have impaired bone marrow reserve (prior hematopoietic stem cell transplantation, radiation to more than 25% of marrow, current low platelet or neutrophil counts) have been treated with ibritumomab tiuxetan at a lower specific activity (0.3 miCi/kg) with response rates of 67% and median response durations of 12 months. The most common toxicity of ibritumomab tiuxetan therapy is myelosuppression. In initial studies, platelet counts less than 50,000/μL were noted in 61% of patients, and neutrophil counts less than 1,000/μL were seen in 57% of patients. The risk of severe thrombocytopenia and neutropenia increased to 75% in patients whose platelet counts were between 100 and 150 K at the start of treatment. Median time to nadir is 7 to 9 weeks and median duration of cytopenias is 3 to 5 weeks. The duration of the myelosuppression complicates subsequent therapeutic decisions. As would be expected, myeloid malignancies and myelodysplasias have been noted in patients surviving more than a year. Gastrointestinal symptoms (nausea, vomiting, abdominal pain, diarrhea) occur in 10% of patients. Human antimouse antibodies or human antichimeric protein antibodies develop in about 4% of cases. Normal B-cells are eliminated but recover after 12 to 16 weeks. Hypogammaglobulinemia is not a clinically significant sequela. A general problem with the radiopharmaceuticals (both I-131 and Y-90) is the long-term compromise of marrow function. Patients who receive these therapies are not easily treated with subsequent courses of myelotoxic drugs because of the long-term loss of physiologic reserve in the hematopoietic system.

CD52 Antibody

Alemtuzumab (Campath)

CD52, the target of alemtuzumab, is a 21- to 28-kDa cell surface glycoprotein expressed on normal and malignant B- and T-cells, NK cells, monocytes, macrophages, a subpopulation of granulocytes, a subpopulation of CD34+ bone marrow cells, and on epididymis, sperm, and seminal vesicle, but not on spermatogonia. Its function is unknown. CD52 does not shed or internalize. Alemtuzumab is an IgG1, κ chimeric antibody with human constant and variable framework regions and rat CDRs. It binds to CD52 with a nanomolar affinity and is thought to act through ADCC.[89]

Alemtuzumab clearance is nonlinear. Its plasma half-life is much shorter for early doses (11 hours) than late doses (6 days) presumably because of the depletion of CD52-bearing cells over time. After 12 weeks of doses, the mean area under the plasma drug concentration-time curve (AUC) is sevenfold higher than the mean AUC after the first dose. No dosage adjustments are required based on age or sex.

Because of infusion-related toxicity, doses are begun at 3 mg/d administered as a 2-hour infusion. When infusion-related toxicities are less than or equal to grade 2, the daily dose is escalated to 10 mg. Once that dose is tolerated, one can advance the dose to 30 mg/d. The usual maintenance dose is 30 mg/d three times a week, usually a Monday-Wednesday-Friday schedule. Weekly doses exceeding 90 mg total are not recommended because of an increased risk of pancytopenia. Dose escalation from 3 to 30 mg doses can generally be accomplished in a week.

Like rituximab, alemtuzumab is associated with significant infusion-related toxicity with the first dose, decreasing with subsequent administration. The symptoms include fever, chills, hypotension, shortness of breath, bronchospasm, and rashes. Rarely, the symptoms may progress to adult respiratory distress syndrome, cardiac arrhythmias, myocardial infarction, and heart failure. Routine premedication with diphenhydramine 50 mg and acetaminophen 650 mg 30 minutes before the infusion is recommended.

The next most common serious toxicity of alemtuzumab is immunosuppression. Because of the widespread expression of CD52 on cells involved in host defenses, patients receiving alemtuzumab become severely immunosuppressed and are susceptible to opportunistic infections such as *Pneumocystis carinii*, aspergillosis, and other fungal infections and intracellular pathogens like *Listeria monocytogenes*. The antibody produces profound lymphopenia. CD4+ T-cell counts do not recover above 200/μL for at least 2 months after stopping treatment and full recovery may take more than 1 year. Opportunistic infection prophylaxis with antiherpetic (acyclovir) and anti-infective (trimethoprim/sulfamethoxazole) therapies is recommended and should be continued until lymphocyte recovery. Because of the immunosuppression, patients on alemtuzumab who receive blood products should have those products irradiated to prevent graft-versus-host disease. Patients on alemtuzumab should not receive any live vaccines.

The third serious toxicity associated with alemtuzumab is myelosuppression. Neutropenia, anemia, and thrombocytopenia are common, and rarely patients have developed prolonged and occasionally fatal pancytopenia. The mechanism of the cytopenia may be either direct cytotoxicity or autoimmune; idiopathic thrombocytopenic purpura and autoimmune hemolytic anemia have both been documented. Grade 3 or 4 myelosuppression is noted in 50% to 70% of patients.

Nearly 2% of patients receiving alemtuzumab generate antibodies to it, but no adverse effects on toxicity or response have been documented.

The main clinical use for alemtuzumab has been as a salvage therapy for chronic lymphocytic leukemia that is unresponsive to alkylating agents and nucleosides. It is being tested as salvage therapy for other lymphomas and is particularly promising in the treatment of T-cell lymphomas. It is being tested as an immunosuppressive agent in graft-versus-host disease and other conditions of immune hyperreactivity. It is effective at depleting marrow and peripheral blood collections of T-cells in vitro before reinfusing the cells in the setting of allogeneic hematopoietic stem cell transplantation.

CD38 Antibody

Daratumumab

Daratumumab is a human IgG1 monoclonal antibody that targets CD38, which is a type II transmembrane glycoprotein highly expressed on myeloma and other hematopoietic cell types. Daratumumab induces apoptosis with ADCC, CDC, and immune-modulatory functions that deplete CD38-positive regulator immune suppressor cells.

In 2016, the FDA approved daratumumab in combination with lenalidomide and dexamethasone or bortezomib and dexamethasone for patients with relapsed multiple myeloma who had received at least one prior therapy.[90,91] It can be administered as monotherapy for patients with multiple myeloma who received at least three prior lines of therapy including a proteasome inhibitor and immunemodulatory agent. In patients with relapsed multiple myeloma who were heavily pretreated, the overall response rate with daratumumab monotherapy was 31%.[92] Adverse reactions noted in clinical trials of daratumumab were infusion reactions, diarrhea, upper respiratory tract infection, and nausea. Daratumumab is administered intravenously at a dose of 16 mg/kg. The molecular weight of daratumumab is approximately 148 kDa. The affinity to human CD38 is 4.36 nM.[93]

Vascular Endothelial Growth Factor Antibodies

Bevacizumab (Avastin)

Bevacizumab is an IgG1 recombinant humanized monoclonal antibody that binds to VEGF. The efficacy of the antibody is surprising. Because VEGF is generally secreted locally and acts locally, it would not be expected that a systemically administered antibody to the growth factor itself would achieve relevant concentrations at the sites of production in tissues. The antibody should circulate and be cleared without ever encountering the physiologically relevant VEGF. In general, growth factor receptors make better targets than growth factors themselves because blocking the effects of the ligand at its binding site should be more efficient than attempting to sop up the ligand like a sponge. The proposed mechanism of action of bevacizumab is to prevent the interaction of VEGF with its receptors, Flt-1 (VEGFR1) and KDR (VEGF2), on the surface of endothelial cells. This should inhibit endothelial cell proliferation and new blood vessel formation and decrease the tumor blood supply. Antiangiogenic drugs also decrease blood vessel permeability, decrease tumor interstitial pressure, and improve delivery of chemotherapy to the tumor.[94]

The half-life of bevacizumab varies according to body weight, sex, and tumor burden; however, the median half-life is around 20 days. The usual dose is 10 mg/kg every 2 weeks. Steady-state serum levels are generally reached by 100 days. It is unknown whether doses need to be adjusted in the setting of renal or hepatic impairment.

Toxicities are overall mild in degree if certain features are monitored and certain clinical situations avoided. Bevacizumab can impair wound healing and has led to wound dehiscences and/or perforations and abscesses in 2% to 4% of patients. If possible, the interval between surgery and initiation of therapy should be 4 weeks. After bevacizumab is administered, elective surgery should be delayed at least 4 weeks, if possible, given the 20-day half-life. A second major side effect is bleeding. Mild bleeding in the form of epistaxis occurs in some patients. However, of greater concern is the risk for major pulmonary or gastrointestinal hemorrhage, which has occurred in up to 20% of patients. Active bleeding from the GI tract and hemoptysis are contraindications to bevacizumab use. It should not be used in lung cancer patients with tumor masses that involve the central bronchial airway because of the risk of fatal bronchial hemorrhage. Severe hypertension may also be seen in 7% to 10% of patients and should be discontinued in cases of uncontrolled or malignant hypertension. Bevacizumab is also associated with proteinuria in up to 20% of patients, but less than 1% develop nephrotic syndrome. Bevacizumab may also worsen congestive heart failure, particularly in patients who have received anthracyclines or radiation therapy involving the heart. Infusion reactions are uncommon and antibodies to bevacizumab have not been documented.

Ramucirumab

Ramucirumab is a IgG1 recombinant humanized monoclonal antibody that binds to vascular endothelial growth factor receptor-2 (VEGFR-2). It is the main receptor that mediates the downstream effects of VEGF-A. Ramucirumab binds with high affinity (approximately 50 pM) to the extracellular VEGF-binding domain of VEGFR-2.[95] It is administered intravenously at a dose of 8 mg/kg every 2 to 3 weeks for gastrointestinal tumors. The half-life of ramucirumab is 14 days. Patients with mild or moderate hepatic or renal impairment did not have any pharmacokinetic differences in comparison to those with normal hepatic or renal function.

In the phase III randomized controlled RAINBOW study, there was a marginal but statistically significant overall survival difference among patients with advanced gastroesophageal junction adenocarcinoma who were treated with ramucirumab and paclitaxel (9.6 months) as compared with those treated with placebo and paclitaxel (7.4 months; HR 0.64 [95% CI 0.54, 0.75] $P < 0.001$).[96] Toxicities are similar to bevacizumab with several clinical trials reporting hypertension and the myelosuppression when administered in combination with cytotoxic chemotherapy.

Human Epidermal Growth Factor Receptor 2 Antibodies

Trastuzumab (Herceptin)

Trastuzumab is a humanized IgG1 κ antibody that binds to the extracellular domain of HER-2/neu, a transmembrane tyrosine kinase growth factor receptor in the EGFR family. The target is a 185-kDa protein expressed on the surface of about 25% of breast cancers. Tumors with amplification of HER-2/neu are generally more refractory to therapy and more aggressive in their rate of progression than HER-2/neu–negative tumors. Trastuzumab binding affinity for its target is about 5 nM; it appears to act both by direct tumor growth inhibition and the activation of ADCC.

The usual method of administration is to give a loading dose of 4 mg/kg intravenously by a 90-minute infusion followed by a maintenance dose of 2 mg/kg weekly by a 30-minute infusion. The mean serum half-life is about 6 days. Steady-state concentrations are achieved between 16 and 32 weeks of therapy with mean trough levels of 79 µg/mL and peak levels of 123 µg/mL. Some patients with HER-2/neu–positive breast cancers have detectable levels of soluble receptor in the serum; the presence of circulating target delays the achievement of steady-state levels by a week or two. The disposition of the antibody is not affected by age or renal function. Coadministration with taxanes results in higher trough levels of the antibody (about 50% higher); other chemotherapeutic agents commonly used in breast cancer do not alter trastuzumab clearance.[97]

Trastuzumab produces a 14% response rate when used as a single agent in metastatic HER-2/neu–positive (at least 2+ by immunohistology) breast cancer. Responses are more common in patients with higher levels of expression. In combination with chemotherapeutic agents, trastuzumab improves response rates and survival in patients with metastatic disease and improves disease-free and overall survival in the adjuvant setting. In early breast cancer, addition of trastuzumab to adjuvant chemotherapy reduces recurrence rate by 50% and reduces mortality by 30%. In the setting of metastatic disease, addition of trastuzumab to chemotherapy increases response rates by 18% to 27%, prolongs disease-free survival by 3 to 5 months, and improves overall survival by 5 to 9 months.

Adverse reactions from trastuzumab are generally rare. The usual initial infusion reaction from human antibodies occurs in 40% of patients receiving trastuzumab for the first time. The incidence of diarrhea in patients taking trastuzumab alone is about 25%. Use of trastuzumab with myelotoxic chemotherapy may result in an increase in myelosuppression. The most significant toxicity from trastuzumab is heart failure. It occurs in about 4% of patients and affects up to 20% of patients in the setting of past or concurrent treatment with anthracyclines. Patients may present with the usual symptoms and signs of heart failure including dyspnea, peripheral edema, and an S3 gallop. Some patients progress to intractable heart failure, but most can be effectively managed by discontinuing the trastuzumab and treating the heart failure. Most of these patients experience gradual improvement in cardiac function with time off therapy. In general, trastuzumab is not withheld in patients with mild decreases in ejection fraction who are asymptomatic. Immunogenicity is low; generally less than 5% of patients make antibodies to trastuzumab.

Small molecular weight inhibitors of HER2/EGFR are in late stages of clinical development and appear to have activity in trastuzumab-resistant patients.

Pertuzumab

Pertuzumab is a humanized IgG1 monoclonal antibody, which binds to the extracellular domain II of HER2. It is involved in inhibiting heterodimerization of HER2 with the other HER family members such as EGFR, HER3, and HER4. This results in interference with two intracellular signaling pathways—mitogen-activated protein (MAP) and phosphatidylinositol 3-kinase (PI3K) resulting in cell growth arrest and apoptosis. The actions of pertuzumab are thought to be complementary to trastuzumab; therefore, both drugs are administered in combination with chemotherapy.

It is administered intravenously at an initial dose of 840 mg as a 60-minute infusion, following by 420 mg over 30 to 60 minutes. The median half-life for pertuzumab was 18 days. Pertuzumab has been studied for treatment of breast cancer in the metastatic, adjuvant, and neoadjuvant settings. The TRYPHAENA and NEOSPHERE studies investigated treatment with pertuzumab, trastuzumab, and chemotherapy (docetaxel and combination chemotherapy) in the neoadjuvant setting.[98] In the TRYPHAENA study, up to 16% of patients receiving an anthracycline-based regimen followed by pertuzumab plus trastuzumab and docetaxel developed left ventricular dysfunction.[99] Patients treated with pertuzumab, trastuzumab, and docetaxel had higher incidence of LVD (8.4%) as compared with trastuzumab and docetaxel alone (1.9%). As with trastuzumab, careful assessment of the patient is required prior to treatment with these agents.

Ado-trastuzumab Emtansine

Ado-trastuzumab emtansine (T-DM1) is an antibody conjugate that is used in the treatment of breast cancer. It consists of two agents—the monoclonal antibody trastuzumab and DM1, a derivative of maytansine, which is a cytotoxic antimicrotubule agent. The DM1 molecule is conjugated to trastuzumab with a nonreducible thioether linker, which renders the drug stable and safe.[100] Ado-trastuzumab contains an average of 3.5 DM1 molecules per antibody. Binding of T-DM1 to HER2 leads to internalization of the HER2-T-DM1 complex via receptor-mediated endocytosis.[101] DM1 is released within target cells upon degradation of the human epidermal growth factor receptor-2 (HER2). This substance specifically inhibits microtubule assembly and leads to cell cycle arrest and apoptosis.[102]

A key study that investigated T-DM1 was the EMILIA trial where 991 patients with locally advanced or metastatic breast cancer were randomized to receive T-DM1 or lapatinib plus capecitabine. The study identified a survival benefit as patients treated with T-DM1 had a median overall survival of 30.9 months as compared with 25.1 months among those treated with lapatinib plus capecitabine (HR 0.68 [95% CI 0.55 to 0.77] $P < 0.001$).[103] Since this trial and other studies, T-DM1 is licensed in patients with HER2-positive metastatic breast cancer who have previous treatment with trastuzumab and a taxane, in combination or as separate agents. The treatment is administered intravenously at a dose of 3.6 mg/kg every 3 weeks. The elimination half-life of T-DM1 is approximately 4 days.

Patients may experience trastuzumab-related toxicities such as cardiotoxicity. Toxicities associated with T-DM1 include thrombocytopenia and increased serum aminotransferases. There are dose modifications that are required in the event patients have T-DM1–related hepatotoxicity.

Epidermal Growth Factor Receptor Antibodies

Cetuximab (Erbitux)

Cetuximab is a chimeric human/mouse monoclonal antibody with constant regions of human IgG1 **κ** origin with murine variable regions that recognize the extracellular domain of the human epidermal growth factor (EGF) receptor. The antibody is thought to work mainly by blocking the EGF receptor and starving the tumor of a needed growth factor. This hypothesis is undermined somewhat by data suggesting that some responding patients have tumors that do not express EGF receptors. EGF receptors are overexpressed in most epithelial malignancies.

The usual method of administration is to give a test dose of 20 mg. Patients then receive a loading dose of 400 mg/m^2 by 2-hour infusion followed by weekly administration of 250 mg/m^2 by 1-hour infusion. Using this regimen, steady-state levels are usually achieved by week 3 with mean peak serum levels being about 200 μg/mL and mean trough serum levels being about 63 μg/mL. Women have about 25% lower clearance rate than men. The half-life is about 5 days (114 hours).

Cetuximab was approved for use based on results obtained in patients with metastatic colorectal cancer. In a randomized trial of patients who had previously progressed on irinotecan, cetuximab plus irinotecan produced a 23% overall response rate compared to about 11% for cetuximab alone. Median response duration was about 6 months for cetuximab plus irinotecan. Other single-arm cetuximab trials showed response rates of 9% to 14% in patients with metastatic colorectal cancer that had progressed following an irinotecan-containing regimen. Although patients were required to have immunohistochemical evidence of EGF receptor expression to be enrolled on these early studies, response did not correlate with either the percentage of positive cells or the intensity of the expression. In a number of other epithelial malignancies, encouraging activity is seen in combination with radiation therapy or chemotherapy in head and neck cancer, non–small cell lung cancer, and pancreatic cancer. Investigations are ongoing to assess the role of antibodies to the EGF receptor versus the small-molecule inhibitors of EGF receptor signaling such as gefitinib and erlotinib and whether various combinations or sequences of agents may boost response rates.[104]

Upon first exposure, cetuximab produces the same syndrome associated with other humanized monoclonal antibodies including hives, bronchospasm, and hypotension. Severe reactions are encountered in about 3% of treated patients. Slowing the administration rate and use of antihistamines controls most such reactions. Patients with pre-existing interstitial lung disease may have a worsening of symptoms with cetuximab. This problem generally emerges between the 4th and 11th doses of antibody. The antibody causes an acneiform rash in nearly 90% of patients, but is severe in grade in about 10%. The lesions can progress to abscesses requiring incision and drainage and sepsis can be a complication. Other mucosal surfaces may also be affected by the antibody including nasal, oral, esophageal, and gastrointestinal. Patients on cetuximab also experience malaise (48%), nausea (29%), fever (27%), constipation or diarrhea (25% each), abdominal pain (26%), and headache (26%). Patients should be followed for the development of hypomagnesemia throughout the course of treatment. Low magnesium levels are detected in about half of treated patients and can progress to dangerous levels with attendant hypocalcemia and hypokalemia if not monitored carefully. Antibodies to cetuximab develop in less than 5% of patients and do not influence response rates.[104]

Panitumumab (Vectibix)

Panitumumab, a second antibody to EGF receptor, is a human IgG2 κ antibody with CDRs of murine origin. Overall, it contains a smaller proportion of murine sequences than does cetuximab. Like cetuximab, it acts to block the binding of EGF to its receptor, and its antitumor effects are thought to be related to loss of EGF receptor signaling.

The recommended regimen is 6 mg/kg given once every 2 weeks by 1-hour infusion. Steady-state levels are usually reached by the third dose and mean peak concentrations are 213 µg/mL and mean trough concentrations are 39 µg/mL. The elimination half-life is about 7.5 days. Age, sex, race, renal dysfunction, hepatic dysfunction, and level of EGF receptor staining on tumor cells make no noticeable impact on the pharmacokinetics of panitumomab.[105]

Panitumumab was approved based on an 8% response rate in patients with metastatic colorectal cancer whose tumors expressed EGF receptor and whose disease had progressed on or following treatment containing 5-fluorouracil, oxaliplatin, and irinotecan. The median duration of responses was about 4 months. No relationship was found between level of expression of EGF receptors and response rate or duration.

The toxicity profile is nearly identical to cetuximab and includes the initial infusion reaction, skin toxicity, diarrhea, hypomagnesemia, and a 1% risk of pulmonary fibrosis. Its use together with irinotecan is not recommended because it may increase the incidence of severe diarrhea (58% grades 3 to 4 in one study). Sunlight exposure may worsen the skin reaction to panitumumab. Antibodies are elicited to panitumumab in less than 4% of patients and are not associated with any alteration in activity or pharmacokinetics. As the most recently approved antibody for a cancer indication, its

activity profile is still actively being defined. There is no reason to suspect that its activity will be substantially different from that of cetuximab.

Necitumumab

Necitumumab is a second-generation recombinant human IgG1 EGFR monoclonal antibody. It binds to EGFR and inhibits EGFR-dependent tumor proliferation and metastasis. In the SQUIRE phase III study, 1,093 patients with squamous non–small lung cancer were randomized to receive necitumumab plus gemcitabine and cisplatin or gemcitabine and cisplatin alone. The overall survival among patients who received necitumumab, gemcitabine, and cisplatin was 11.5 months as compared with 9.9 months in patients who received gemcitabine and cisplatin alone.[106] In 2015, necitumumab was approved in combination with gemcitabine and cisplatin for the first-line treatment of patient with metastatic squamous non–small cell lung cancer.

Necitumumab is administered intravenously at a dose of 800 mg on days 1 and 8 of a 3-week cycle in combination with gemcitabine and cisplatin. Necitumumab binds to EGFR with high affinity ($K_D = 0.32$ nmol/L).[107] The elimination half-life is approximately 14 days. The molecular weight of necitumumab is 147.8 kDa. The common adverse events are similar to other EGFR antagonists and include rash, vomiting, diarrhea, and dermatitis acneiform. Hypomagnesemia, the risk of cardiopulmonary arrest, and sudden death are part of the boxed warnings for necitumumab.

Glycolipid Antigen Disialoganglioside (GD2) Antibody

Dinutuximab

Dinutuximab is a chimeric human-mouse monoclonal antibody that binds to the glycolipid antigen disialoganglioside (GD2). GD2 is expressed on the surface of neuroblastoma cells. Dinutuximab is administered intravenously for 4 days every 4 weeks in combination with granulocyte-macrophage colony–stimulating factor (GM-CSF), interleukin-2 (IL-2), and isotretinoin for patients with high-risk neuroblastoma.[108] The elimination half-life is approximately 10 days.

Adverse reactions include hematological toxicities, infections, hypokalemia, hypotension, and pyrexia. Infusion reactions, anaphylaxis, and peripheral neuropathy are part of the boxed warning for dinutuximab.

Interleukin-6 (IL-6) Antibody

Siltuximab

Siltuximab is a glycosylated chimeric human-mouse monoclonal antibody to IL-6 and was approved for the treatment of patients with multicentric Castleman disease (MCD) who are human immune deficiency virus (HIV) negative and human herpesvirus-8 (HHV8) negative.[109] This is a rare condition associated with lymphadenopathy, fevers, and elevated IL-6 levels, which is an important factor of the acute phase response. Although MCD can occur among patients with HHV8 and HIV, preclinical studies demonstrated that siltuximab does not bind to virally produced IL-6.[110]

Siltuximab is administered as an intravenous infusion at a dose of 11 mg/kg every 3 weeks. It binds to soluble human IL-6 with high selectivity and affinity (K_D = 34 pmol/L). Siltuximab has a molecular weight of 69 kDa and an elimination half-life of 20.6 days. Adverse reactions include anaphylactic reactions, pruritus, hyperuricemia, and upper respiratory tract infection.

Tocilizumab

Tocilizumab is a recombinant humanized monoclonal antibody against the IL-6 receptor that prevents IL-6 from binding to soluble and membrane-bound IL-6 receptor. It is FDA approved for treatment of juvenile idiopathic arthritis (JIA) and adult rheumatoid arthritis. In initial case reports on the use of CAR T-cell therapy in ALL, one patient had severe cytokine-release syndrome.[57] This patient responded to treatment with tocilizumab, which has now been used in association with CAR T-cells to treat CRS.[111] Furthermore, it does not adversely affect the infusion of CD19 CAR T-cells (CTL019).

The dose of treatment is 8 to 12 mg/kg for patients less than 30 kg and 4 to 8 mg/kg for patients greater than or equal to 30 kg. The elimination half-life is concentration-dependent with a half-life of up to 13 days at a dose of 8 mg/kg. Patients should respond and clinical improvement is seen almost immediately. Treatment is administered again in case a response is not seen within 24 to 48 hours.[60] Common adverse events include elevation of liver enzymes and cytopenias, including thrombocytopenia and neutropenia.[112] These side effects improve following cessation of therapy.

Bispecific Monoclonal Antibodies

Catumaxomab

Catumaxomab is a part of the trifunctional monoclonal family and the first bispecific antibody that received market approval. It is produced by coexpression of a rat IgG2b and a mouse IgG2a in a single host cell.[113] Catumaxomab is an antiepithelial cell adhesion molecule (EpCAM)/anti-CD3 bispecific antibody that also activates Fcγ receptor I-, IIa-, and III-positive accessory cells via its functional Fc domain.[114]

Epithelial tumors such as breast, ovarian, and gastric cancer commonly cause ascites and these tumor cells express EpCAM. Therefore, these tumor cells, which circulate and exist within peritoneal cavities, are targeted by catumaxomab. It is administered using an intraperitoneal route in small doses (10 to 150 μg) four to five times over 9 to 13 days. Catumaxomab binds to human epithelial tumor cells with varying levels of EpCAM, and antitumor activity was seen at concentrations of less than 10 ng/mL.[115] Catumaxomab has a half-life of approximately 2.5 days.

Due to the structure of this antibody, side effects are related to CRS and may include fever, chills, nausea, and vomiting. Abdominal pain may be related to the mode of administration but also due to CRS. One study hypothesized that CRS effects may be a predictive marker for catumaxomab efficacy. Patients who had CRS

had a longer interval to repeat paracentesis (48 days) compared to patients who did not have CRS (27 days), but this was not a statistically significant different (log rank P = 0.15).[116]

Blinatumomab

Blinatumomab is a bispecific CD19-directed CD3 T-cell engager (BiTE) approved for the second-line treatment for Philadelphia chromosome–negative relapsed or refractory ALL.[117] This drug allows a patient's T-cells to recognize malignant B-cells. Blinatumomab, which was engineered using the diabody approach, has two binding sites: a CD3 site on T-cell receptors and the CD19 on leukemia B-cells.[118] Following activation, a cytolytic synapse is formed and this also leads to the release of perforin and granzymes in the cytotoxic T-cell that induces apoptosis. T-cells can remain activated and continues to target and attack additional B-cells. Therapy schedule involves a continuous treatment course of blinatumomab for 28 days followed by a 14-day treatment-free interval. Blinatumomab has a molecular weight of 54.1 kDa, which is approximately one third the size of a monoclonal antibody.[119] The half-life of blinatumomab is 2 hours. Renal excretion is minimal; therefore, the manufacturer does not advise dose modifications for renal dysfunction.

Following administration of blinatumomab, IL-10, IL-6, and IFN-γ cytokines are released and peripheral B-cell counts are depleted within 2 days.[120] Compared to chemotherapy, blinatumomab has less myelosuppressive adverse events. However, higher incidences of serious immune-mediated adverse events were noted including neurologic events and effects related to CRS.

Antibody Conjugates

Gemtuzumab Ozogamicin (Mylotarg)

Gemtuzumab ozogamicin has an antibody portion of the molecule that is a humanized IgG4 κ antibody, which binds to CD33, an adhesion glycoprotein expressed on cells of the myelocytic lineage (but not on pluripotent hematopoietic stem cells or nonhematopoietic cells) and on acute myeloid leukemia cells. The antibody is mainly composed of human sequences with murine CDRs. The antibody is conjugated to calicheamicin, a potent antitumor antibiotic isolated from the bacterium, *Micromonospora echinospora calichensis*. Once the conjugate binds to CD33, it is internalized. The calicheamicin is cleaved away from the antibody and released from the lysosomes intracellularly and binds DNA in the minor groove to initiate double-strand breaks and cell death.

Gemtuzumab ozogamicin is usually administered at a dose of 9 mg/m² by 2-hour infusion followed by a second dose of 9 mg/m² 2 weeks later. The elimination half-lives of total and unconjugated calicheamicin are about 45 hours and 4 days, respectively, after the first dose, and the half-life increases about 50% with the second dose. Clearance is not affected by age, sex, weight, or body surface area.

Gemtuzumab ozogamicin is used as a salvage agent in the treatment of acute myeloid leukemia. It was approved for use by the U.S. Food and Drug Administration based on achieving a 26% response rate (13% complete responses) in patients with relapsed acute myeloid leukemia. Response rate and duration of response correlate with the duration of the initial remission. Response rates are 11% for those whose first remission was 6 months or less, 22% for those whose initial remission was 6 to 12 months, and 35% for those whose first remission was a year or longer. Responding patients survive a median of 1 year following treatment. Response is not influenced by patient age or cytogenetic abnormalities. Because of the many options for younger patients, gemtuzumab ozogamicin, used as a single agent, is often used in patients older than 60 years. It is being assessed for its role in postremission therapy as an alternative to bone marrow transplantation in patients who are not candidates or who lack a suitable donor. Data on combination of gemtuzumab ozogamicin with other chemotherapy are limited. The dose is usually reduced to 3 mg/m^2 when it is used together with other chemotherapeutic agents. CD33 is also expressed on the malignant cells of acute promyelocytic leukemia; gemtuzumab ozogamicin has been used with all-trans retinoic acid with promising results in pilot studies.[121]

In addition to infusion reactions, gemtuzumab ozogamicin causes severe myelosuppression. Delayed recovery of platelet counts is often observed in patients who enter complete remission. Patients with peripheral WBC counts above 30,000/μL are susceptible to serious pulmonary dysfunction from cells blocking the pulmonary vessels. Fever, chills, dyspnea, pulmonary infiltrates, pleural effusions, pulmonary edema, and acute respiratory distress syndrome may occur. The WBC count should be reduced below 30,000/μL (with leukapheresis or hydroxyurea) before starting gemtuzumab ozogamicin. The antibody conjugate also increases the risk of developing venoocclusive disease of the liver. Patients undergoing subsequent hematopoietic stem cell transplantation are at higher risk (15%) than patients not undergoing transplantation (1%). Though rare, the syndrome (rapid weight gain, right upper quadrant pain, hepatomegaly, ascites, hyperbilirubinemia, elevated liver enzymes) can progress to death. Another serious complication of gemtuzumab ozogamicin therapy is rapid tumor lysis. Patients with large tumor burdens should receive prophylaxis for tumor lysis syndrome. Like other myelotoxic agents, mucositis, bleeding, and febrile neutropenia may complicate its use. The development of antibodies to gemtuzumab ozogamicin is very rare and does not affect the treatment course.

Brentuximab Vedotin

Brentuximab vedotin is an antibody conjugate in which a chimeric anti-CD30 antibody is combined with a synthetic microtubule-disrupting agent—monomethyl auristatin E, using a protease-cleavable liver.[122] This drug has been used in patients with classical Hodgkin's lymphoma and anaplastic large cell lymphoma. CD30, which is highly expressed on Reed-Sternberg cells, is a member of the tumor necrosis factor (TNF) receptor family and has a range of effects from cell proliferation, cell survival, or cell death. The CD30 ligand increases cytokine production and growth and proliferation of Reed-Sternberg cells.

Brentuximab vedotin has a molecular weight of 153 kDa. It is administered every 3 weeks as an intravenous infusion at a dose of 1.8 mg/kg. It is usually administered as a single agent. It has been combined with ABVD chemotherapy at a dose of 1.2 mg/kg

in trials of patients with Hodgkin's lymphoma.[123] The combination therapy did result in cases of pulmonary toxicity. The half-life of brentuximab vedotin is 4 to 6 days. It is used in patients with Hodgkin's lymphoma following failure of autologous stem cell transplant or treated with two prior lines of multiagent chemotherapy in patients who are not candidates for autologous stem cell therapy. It is also administered for patients with systemic anaplastic lymphoma following failure of at least one prior multiagent chemotherapy treatment.

Adverse events include peripheral neuropathy and are cumulative.[124] In clinical trials, up to 54% of patients experienced peripheral neuropathy. Following completion of treatment, 51% had residual neuropathy. Hematologic toxicities such as neutropenia and thrombocytopenia may also occur. Hepatotoxicity can range from elevations of transaminases or bilirubin to fatal outcomes. Therefore, dose adjustments, delays, or cessation of brentuximab vedotin may be required.

Inotuzumab Ozogamicin

Inotuzumab ozogamicin is an antibody conjugate. It is a humanized anti-CD22 IgG4 monoclonal antibody that is conjugated to calicheamicin, which is a cytotoxic antibiotic agent. CD22 is a sialic acid–binding immunoglobulin-type lectin, or Siglec, that is expressed on the B-cell surface. It inhibits coreceptors of the B-cell antigen receptor–induced signaling.[125] Similar to the mechanism of action of gemtuzumab ozogamicin, when the conjugate of inotuzumab ozogamicin binds to CD22, the complex is internalized and the calicheamicin is released. This drug binds to the minor groove of DNA and can result in double-strand cleavage and apoptosis.

Inotuzumab ozogamicin has a molecular mass of 160 kDa and has been shown to bind to CD22 with a high affinity (KD = 234 pM).[126] Inotuzumab ozogamicin has an elimination half-life of 12.3 days. It is administered intravenously at a dose of 1.8 mg/m^2 per cycle divided in three doses. CD22 is a glycoprotein that is expressed in more than 90% of diffuse large B-cell non-Hodgkin's lymphomas, follicular lymphomas, and from 60% to 100% on B-cell precursor ALL. Dose-limiting toxicities include neutropenia and thrombocytopenia. Hepatic adverse events such as hyperbilirubinemia and venoocclusive disease are also more common among patients who receive inotuzumab ozogamicin. In August 2017, the FDA approved use of inotuzumab ozogamicin treatment of adults with relapsed or refractory B-cell precursor ALL.

Tositumomab and I-131 Tositumomab

Tositumomab is a murine IgG2a λ monoclonal antibody that binds to human CD20 antigen on normal and malignant B-cells (see rituximab above). I-131 tositumomab is the same antibody conjugated to I-131, a beta- and gamma-emitting isotope. The physical half-life of the isotope is 8 days. I-131 tositumomab is targeted to CD20, and it kills cells to which it binds and also kills neighboring cells in the vicinity of the cell to which it binds by delivering radiation.[127]

The use of tositumomab and I-131 tositumomab is divided into two stages; the first step is for dosimetry and the second for therapy. Each step involves the sequential administration of tositumomab followed by I-131 tositumomab. The first injection of unconjugated anti-CD20 antibody was demonstrated to saturate the spleen and improve the tumor specificity of the subsequently delivered radiopharmaceutical. In the dosimetry phase, 450 mg of tositumomab is given intravenously over 1 hour on day 0. Then, a dose of I-131 tositumomab containing 5 mCi of I-131 and 35 mg of tositumomab is infused over 20 minutes. Dosimetry (by external counting of I-131 radioactivity) and biodistribution measurements are then made within 1 hour of infusion, on days 2, 3, or 4 and again on days 6 or 7. Certain criteria are then applied to the biodistribution calculation, and if the biodistribution is acceptable, a therapeutic dose of I-131 tositumomab is calculated. Then, sometime between day 7 and day 14, the therapeutic step is begun with an infusion of 450 mg tositumomab over 1 hour followed by the calculated dose of I-131 tositumomab to deliver 75 cGy of total body radiation. The dosimetry and therapeutic steps together are a course of therapy and patients do not ever receive more than one course.

The activity of labeled and unlabeled tositumomab was defined mainly in patients with follicular lymphoma. Overall response rates in patients with relapsed follicular lymphoma were 63% to 68% with 29% to 33% of the responses defined as complete. Median response duration is about 12 to 18 months. Some complete remissions appear to be durable.

The main toxicity of unlabeled plus labeled tositumomab is myelosuppression, which can be severe. Platelets decrease to less than 50,000/µL in 53% of patients. Neutrophil counts fall below 1,000/µL in 63% of patients. Hemoglobin levels fall below 8 g/dL in 29% of patients. The myelotoxicity is particularly common in the setting of significant marrow involvement with lymphoma; thus, this regimen is not indicated if tumor occupies 25% of more of the marrow space. Febrile neutropenia and other infections were noted in 45% of treated patients. In addition, although patients are pretreated with three doses of supersaturated potassium iodide solution, the uptake of radioactive iodine by the thyroid can produce hypothyroidism early on and increase the risk of thyroid cancer years later. The risk of hypothyroidism is about 15% at 4 years. Second malignancies are a problem with this therapy. About 10% of patients develop secondary acute leukemia or myelodysplastic syndrome by 4 years after treatment. In addition, skin, breast, lung, and head and neck cancers may be increased. Other grade 3 to 4 toxicities are rare. Normal B-cells are depleted, but this does not lead to hypogammaglobulinemia. About 10% of patients develop human antimurine antibodies, but this is of minor consequence in this group of patients who are unlikely to be exposed to other murine antibodies.

Signaling Lymphocytic Activation Molecule F7 Antibody

Elotuzumab

Elotuzumab is a humanized IgG1 immunostimulatory monoclonal antibody that targets signaling lymphocytic activation molecule F7 (SLAMF7, also called the cell surface glycoprotein CD2 subset 1). SLAMF7 is a glycoprotein that is expressed on myeloma and natural killer cells. This mAb is able to bind to natural killer cells and enhance multiple myeloma cell death with this interaction. Furthermore,

elotuzumab may also affect the tumor microenvironment in multiple myeloma due to its inhibitory effects on the bone marrow stromal cells.[128] Elotuzumab has a molecular weight of 148.1 kDa and is administered intravenously at a dose of 10 mg/kg every week for the first two cycles and every 2 weeks thereafter until disease progression.

Preclinical studies have demonstrated that more than 95% of bone marrow myeloma cells express SLAMF7. In the phase 3 ELOQUENT-2 trial, patients with relapsed or refractory multiple myeloma were randomized to receive elotuzumab in combination with lenalidomide and dexamethasone or lenalidomide and dexamethasone alone (control group). The overall response rate among patients treated with elotuzumab was 79% as compared with 66% in the control group.[91] In 2015, the FDA granted approval for elotuzumab in combination with lenalidomide and dexamethasone for patients with relapsed multiple myeloma.

Adverse events related to this drug include infusion reactions, infections, and hepatotoxicity. Invasive secondary malignancies, such as hematological malignancies, solid tumor, or skin cancers, were noted among 9.1% of patients treated with elotuzumab, lenalidomide, and dexamethasone as compared with 5.7% in the control group.

Platelet-Derived Growth Factor Receptor α (PDGFRα) Antibody

Olaratumab

Olaratumab is a recombinant human immunoglobulin G subclass 1 (IgG1) monoclonal antibody that binds to platelet-derived growth factor receptor α (PDGFRα). This is a type III receptor tyrosine kinase that is expressed on many tumor subtypes and is involved in growth, differentiation, and angiogenesis of mesenchymal stem cells. PDGF and the associated receptor are involved in regulating the tumor microenvironment and metastatic capabilities in several tumor subtypes.[129]

Olaratumab has a molecular weight of 154 kDa and has a high affinity for PDGFRα. The elimination half-life is approximately 11 days. It is administered as an intravenous infusion at a dose of 15 mg/kg on days 1 and 8 of a 21-day cycles. Olaratumab is licensed for use in combination with doxorubicin for eight cycles for the treatment of adults with metastatic or locally advanced soft-tissue sarcoma not previously treated with anthracycline therapy.

Common adverse reactions in a phase 2 trial included nausea, mucositis, musculoskeletal pain, and diarrhea.[130] Common biochemical and hematological abnormalities included hypokalemia, hypophosphatemia, neutropenia, and thrombocytopenia.

Cytotoxic T-lymphocyte–Associated Protein 4 (CTLA-4)

Ipilimumab

Ipilimumab is a fully humanized IgG antibody that binds to CTLA4, which blocks an inhibitory signal and affects T-cell regulation. Ipilimumab, a CTLA4 inhibitor, has been approved by the

FDA and has dramatically changed the management of patients with metastatic melanoma.

Ipilimumab was the first immunotherapy to demonstrate a survival benefit among patients with metastatic melanoma in 2011. The half-life for ipilimumab is 15.4 days. It is administered at 10 mg/kg in the adjuvant setting for melanoma and at 3 mg/kg for patients with metastatic melanoma.

In the registration trial reported by Hodi et al., 676 patients with previously treated metastatic melanoma were randomized to receive 3 mg/kg of ipilimumab and placebo, ipilimumab in combination with a peptide vaccine gp100 or gp100 and placebo.[131] The median overall survival was significantly greater with ipilimumab with gp100 as compared with gp100 alone (10 versus 6.4 months; hazard ratio 0.68; $P < 0.001$). Several trials since this study have repeatedly demonstrated a survival benefit for patients with metastatic melanoma. In the adjuvant setting, among patients with stage III resected melanoma, a randomized control trial demonstrated a recurrence-free survival of 40.8% among those treated with ipilimumab as compared with 30.3% in the placebo group.[132] Furthermore, overall survival at 5 years was 54.4% among those treated with ipilimumab as compared with 38.9% for those in the placebo group.

The toxicity of checkpoint blockade mAbs such as ipilimumab is related to the inhibition of T-cell activation and is related to the mechanism of action. Over 90% of patients administered with ipilimumab may experience adverse events. The most common adverse events include gastrointestinal effects (i.e., diarrhea, nausea, abdominal pain) and skin toxicities such as rash and pruritus. These immune-related adverse events may vary in severity and if left untreated can be fatal. Management of these immune-related toxicities requires a multidisciplinary approach.

Programmed Death-1 (PD-1) Antibodies

Pembrolizumab and Nivolumab

Both programmed death-1 (PD-1) and its ligand (PD-L1) are important coinhibitory molecules involved in regulating T-cell–mediated immune responses. PD-1, which is expressed on the surface of activated T-cells in peripheral tissues, is a type I membrane protein with a single extracellular immunoglobulin superfamily V-set domain.[133] PD-L1 and PD-L2 are ligands expressed on dendritic cells and macrophages. Following engagement with its ligands, PD-1 using phosphatase SHP2 inhibits kinases that are involved in T-cell activation.[49] Therefore, in normal conditions, PD-1 signaling maintains immune tolerance to self-antigens. In the context of cancer therapy, PD-L1 is overexpressed on tumors, and it has been noted that the interaction with PD-1 on T-cells permits cancer cells to escape T-cell–mediated immune responses.[134] By blocking PD-1 or PD-L1, it is presumed that tumor cells will be recognized by T-cells and destroyed.

In 2014, pembrolizumab and nivolumab, which are both anti–PD-1 antibodies, were granted breakthrough therapy designation by the FDA in various cancer subtypes such as lung cancer, melanoma, and Hodgkin's lymphoma. These drugs have since been incorporated into clinical management guidelines.[135]

Pembrolizumab is a humanized IgG4***κ*** isotype antibody with an affinity of 29 pmol/L and a half-life between 11 and 22 days.

Randomized controlled trials of pembrolizumab investigated dosing schedules between 2 and 10 mg/kg. A flat-dosing schedule may be instituted as patients can be treated with a 200 mg of pembrolizumab every 3 weeks for a variety of cancer subtypes. Nivolumab is also human IgG4 antibody with an affinity of 3 nM and a half-life between 17 and 27.5 days. The dose of nivolumab is dependent on the indication and cancer subtype. For patients with Hodgkin's lymphoma or metastatic head and neck cancer, nivolumab is dosed at 3 mg/kg every 2 weeks. Flat-dose regimens of 200 mg may be instituted for cases of metastatic melanoma, metastatic non–small cell lung cancer, and advanced renal cell cancer. Both nivolumab and pembrolizumab target epitopes on the PD-1 molecule. These drugs bind on different loops of PD-1, the N-terminal loop of PD-1 for nivolumab interaction, and the C'D loop for pembrolizumab. Furthermore, pembrolizumab has greater overlap with the PD-L1 binding site than the epitope region of nivolumab.[136] However, despite these structural differences, there are many who believe that these drugs could be used interchangeably to target PD-1.

In metastatic melanoma, PD-1–specific mAb has been found to be effective in patients who have been treated with CTLA-4, indicating that this regulatory pathway may be involved with ongoing T-cell immune responses.[137] There have been studies that have shown that the combination of both CTLA4 and PD-1 therapy is efficacious among patients with metastatic melanoma. However, a combination of both agents results in greater toxicity.

In a seminal phase III trials of nivolumab and ipilimumab for patients with metastatic melanoma, PD-L1 status on the tumor was used as a biomarker.[138] Those with PD-L1 positive, nivolumab alone and nivolumab plus ipilimumab resulted in a similar prolongation of progression-free survival as compared with ipilimumab alone. The combination of nivolumab and ipilimumab compared with nivolumab alone had the greatest benefit in the context of negative PD-L1 tumor expression. Use of PD-L1 tumor expression as a biomarker remains an issue that requires further research and assessment.

In a subset of patients who are administered with pembrolizumab or nivolumab, measures of imaging response using standard Response Evaluation Criteria in Solid Tumors, or RECIST, may be misinterpreted. Tumor burden may decrease after an initial increase, which is termed pseudoprogression. Immune-related response criteria (irRC) have attempted to accurately measure response to checkpoint inhibitor antibody therapy. In this criteria, two consecutive scans, performed 4 weeks apart, the inclusion of new lesions in the sum of lesion measurements are meant to delineate progression from pseudoprogression. However, validating the dimensions of measurement and the definition of pseudoprogression itself is difficult.[139] There have been studies that have shown that this phenomenon may occur beyond 12 weeks of therapy.

Programmed Death Ligand-1 (PD-L1) Antibodies

Atezolizumab, Durvalumab, and Avelumab

Agents that target PD-1 and PD-L1 are licensed for use in several cancer subtypes and are also being investigated in clinical trials as monotherapy, or in combination with other agents.

Atezolizumab is a nonglycosylated humanized IgG1κ anti–PD-L1 monoclonal antibody that is Fc-engineered and blocks interaction with PD-1 and B7.1 receptors. It has a molecular mass of 145 kDa and an elimination half-life of 27 days. The affinity for PD-L1 is 1.75 nM. It is administered intravenously at a dose of 1,200 mg over 60 minutes. Atezolizumab was the first humanized IgG1 anti–PD-L1 agent licensed for the treatment of metastatic non–small cell lung cancer and advanced bladder cancer.

Durvalumab is humanized IgG1 anti–PD-L1 monoclonal antibody that blocks the binding to PD-1 and B7.1 receptors, thereby permitting T-cells to recognize and target tumor cells. It has been approved for use in advanced bladder cancer and has shown benefit in a clinical trial of patients with stage III non–small cell lung cancer.[140] It has a molecular weight of 149 kDa and an elimination half-life of 21 days. It has a similar affinity to PD-L1 as atezolizumab (0.67 nM). It is administered as an intravenous infusion at a dose of 10 mg/kg every 2 weeks.

Avelumab is a human IgG1 anti–PD-L1 monoclonal antibody that has been approved for use in Merkel cell carcinoma. It has a molecular weight of 147 kDa and an elimination half-life of 6.1 days, which is shorter as compared with atezolizumab and durvalumab. As compared with the other PD-L1 inhibitors, the binding affinity of avelumab is higher (0.05 nM).[141] It is administered as an intravenous infusion of 10 mg/kg every 2 weeks.

The binding of durvalumab to PD-L1 involves the heavy chain, light chain, and all three CDRs, whereas avelumab interrupts PD-1/PD-L1 interaction with the VH domain.[141] It is not clear whether these molecular differences translate to differences in therapeutic efficacy between these three agents.

Clinicians continue to learn more about checkpoint inhibitor therapies and both the short-term and long-term toxicities. All members of this class (both PD-1 and PD-L1 inhibitors) can cause immune-related adverse events, which are related to the mechanism of action. Adverse events are related to inflammation, or "-itis." Common side effects include dermatitis, hypophysitis, colitis, hepatitis, and pneumonitis. In rare cases, immune-mediated myocarditis can also occur, with nonspecific symptoms, and can be fatal (ref). Immune-checkpoint inhibitors improve outcomes for patients with metastatic melanoma; clinicians need to be vigilant of nonspecific symptoms among those who are administered with combination therapy. Patients are managed with high-dose glucocorticoids, which are slowly tapered till resolution of symptoms or biochemical abnormalities.

Future Directions

Since the initial clinical study over 30 years ago that pioneered the use of monoclonal antibodies in a single patient with non-Hodgkin's lymphoma, millions of patients with a cancer diagnosis have been treated with this class of drug. Components of mAb structure have been introduced into T-cells and used to develop CAR T-cell therapy, a potentially revolutionary way to treat cancer. Owing to the structure and function of mAbs, several applications for this class in cancer management range from diagnosis to treatment both in the adjuvant and metastatic settings. mAbs have been able to target important functional hallmarks of cancer such as angiogenesis, cell growth, and evasion from the immune system. This therapeutic class continues to evolve rapidly as physicians and scientists seek new ways to specifically target tumor components while reducing the risk of adverse events to the patient.

Acknowledgments

David A. Scheinberg, Todd L. Rosenblat, Joseph G. Jurcic, George Sgouros, and Richard P. Junghans contributed this chapter in the last edition, and portions of their chapter have been retained.

References

1. Schwartz RS. Paul Ehrlich's magic bullets. *N Engl J Med.* 2004;350(11):1079-1080.
2. Kohler G, Milstein C. Continuous cultures of fused cells secreting antibody of predefined specificity. *Nature.* 1975;256(5517):495-497.
3. Nadler LM, Stashenko P, Hardy R, et al. Serotherapy of a patient with a monoclonal antibody directed against a human lymphoma-associated antigen. *Cancer Res.* 1980;40(9):3147.
4. Nelson AL, Dhimolea E, Reichert JM. Development trends for human monoclonal antibody therapeutics. *Nat Rev Drug Discov.* 2010;9(10):767-774.
5. Liu JKH. The history of monoclonal antibody development—progress, remaining challenges and future innovations. *Annu Med Surg.* 2014;3(4):113-116.
6. National Comprehensive Cancer Network. *Colon Cancer;* 2017. Available at https://www.nccn.org/professionals/physician_gls/pdf/colon.pdf
7. National Comprehensive Cancer Network. *B-cell Lymphomas;* 2017. Available at https://www.nccn.org/professionals/physician_gls/pdf/b-cell.pdf
8. Scott AM, Wolchok JD, Old LJ. Antibody therapy of cancer. *Nat Rev Cancer.* 2012;12(4):278-287.
9. Roskos LK, Davis CG, Schwab GM. The clinical pharmacology of therapeutic monoclonal antibodies. *Drug Dev Res.* 2004;61(3):108-120.
10. Kuo TT, Aveson VG. Neonatal Fc receptor and IgG-based therapeutics. *MAbs.* 2011;3(5):422-430.
11. Tonegawa S. Somatic generation of antibody diversity. *Nature* 1983;302:575-581.
12. Burrows PD, Cooper MD. B cell development and differentiation. *Curr Opin Immunol.* 1997;9(2):239-244.
13. Villamor N, Montserrat E, Colomer D. Mechanism of action and resistance to monoclonal antibody therapy. *Semin Oncol.* 2003;30(4):424-433.
14. Carter PJ. Potent antibody therapeutics by design. *Nat Rev Immunol.* 2006;6(5):343-357.
15. Keizer RJ, Huitema ADR, Schellens JHM, Beijnen JH. Clinical pharmacokinetics of therapeutic monoclonal antibodies. *Clin Pharmacokinet.* 2010;49(8):493-507.
16. Jackisch C, Kim SB, Semiglazov V, et al. Subcutaneous versus intravenous formulation of trastuzumab for HER2-positive early breast cancer: updated results from the phase III HannaH study. *Ann Oncol.* 2015;26(2):320-325.
17. Ismael G, Hegg R, Muehlbauer S, et al. Subcutaneous versus intravenous administration of (neo)adjuvant trastuzumab in patients with HER2-positive, clinical stage I-III breast cancer (HannaH study): a phase 3, open-label, multicentre, randomised trial. *Lancet Oncol.* 2012;13(9):869-878.
18. Thurber GM, Schmidt MM, Wittrup KD. Factors determining antibody distribution in tumors. *Trends Pharmacol Sci.* 2008;29(2):57.
19. Stohrer M, Boucher Y, Stangassinger M, Jain RK. Oncotic pressure in solid tumors is elevated. *Cancer Res.* 2000;60(15):4251.
20. Graff CP, Wittrup KD. Theoretical analysis of antibody targeting of tumor spheroids. *Cancer Res.* 2003;63(6):1288.
21. Fujimori K, Covell DG, Fletcher JE, Weinstein JN. Modeling analysis of the global and microscopic distribution of immunoglobulin G, F(ab[prime])2, and Fab in tumors. *Cancer Res.* 1989;49:5656-5663.
22. Rudnick SI, Adams GP. Affinity and avidity in antibody-based tumor targeting. *Cancer Biother Radiopharm.* 2009;24(2):155-161.
23. Adams GP, Weiner LM. Monoclonal antibody therapy of cancer. *Nat Biotechnol* 2005;23:1147-1157.
24. Waldmann H, Strober W. Metabolism of immunoglobulins. *Prog Allergy* 1969;13:1-110.
25. Wang W, Wang EQ, Balthasar JP. Monoclonal antibody pharmacokinetics and pharmacodynamics. *Clin Pharmacol Ther.* 2008;84(5):548-558.

26. Press OW, Hansen JA, Farr A, Martin PJ. Endocytosis and degradation of murine anti-human CD3 monoclonal antibodies by normal and malignant T-lymphocytes. *Cancer Res.* 1988;48(8):2249.

27. Nechansky A. HAHA—nothing to laugh about. Measuring the immunogenicity (human anti-human antibody response) induced by humanized monoclonal antibodies applying ELISA and SPR technology. *J Pharm Biomed Anal.* 2009;51:252-254.

28. DeNardo GL, Bradt BM, Mirick GR, DeNardo SJ. Human antiglobulin response to foreign antibodies: therapeutic benefit? *Cancer Immunol Immunother.* 2003;52(5):309-316.

29. Weiner GJ. Building better monoclonal antibody-based therapeutics. *Nat Rev Cancer.* 2015;15(6):361-370.

30. Maloney DG. Mechanism of action of rituximab. *Anticancer Drugs* 2001;12: S1-S4.

31. Weiner LM, Surana R, Wang S. Antibodies and cancer therapy: versatile platforms for cancer immunotherapy. *Nat Rev Immunol.* 2010;10(5):317-327.

32. Racila E, Link BK, Weng W-K, et al. A polymorphism in the complement component C1qA correlates with prolonged response following rituximab therapy of follicular lymphoma. *Clin Cancer Res.* 2008;14(20):6697-6703.

33. Alduaij W, Ivanov A, Honeychurch J, et al. Novel type II anti-CD20 monoclonal antibody (GA101) evokes homotypic adhesion and actin-dependent, lysosome-mediated cell death in B-cell malignancies. *Blood.* 2011;117(17): 4519-4529.

34. Presta LG. Engineering antibodies for therapy. *Curr Pharm Biotechnol.* 2002; 3:237-256.

35. Janeway CA Jr, Travers P, Walport M, et al. *Immunobiology: The Immune System in Health and Disease.* 5th ed. New York: Garland Science; 2001.

36. Getahun A, Cambier JC. Of ITIMs, ITAMs and ITAMis, revisiting immunoglobulin Fc receptor signaling. *Immunol Rev.* 2015;268(1):66-73.

37. Lazar GA, Dang W, Karki S, et al. Engineered antibody Fc variants with enhanced effector function. *Proc Natl Acad Sci U S A.* 2006;103(11):4005-4010.

38. Nimmerjahn F, Ravetch JV. Fcγ receptors: Old friends and new family members. *Immunity.* 2006;24(1):19-28.

39. Rath T, Baker K, Dumont JA, et al. Fc-fusion proteins and FcRn: structural insights for longer-lasting and more effective therapeutics. *Crit Rev Biotechnol.* 2015;35(2):235-254.

40. Pyzik M, Rath T, Lencer WI, Baker K, Blumberg RS. FcRn: the architect behind the immune and non-immune functions of IgG and albumin. *J Immunol (Baltimore, MD: 1950).* 2015;194(10):4595-4603.

41. Tutt AL, French RR, Illidge TM, et al. Monoclonal antibody therapy of B cell lymphoma: signaling activity on tumor cells appears more important than recruitment of effectors. *J Immunol.* 1998;161(6):3176.

42. Gajria D, Chandarlapaty S. HER2-amplified breast cancer: mechanisms of trastuzumab resistance and novel targeted therapies. *Expert Rev Anticancer Ther.* 2011;11(2):263-275.

43. Cuello M, Ettenberg SA, Clark AS, et al. Down-regulation of the erbB-2 receptor by trastuzumab (Herceptin) enhances tumor necrosis factor-related apoptosis-inducing ligand-mediated apoptosis in breast and ovarian cancer cell lines that overexpress erbB-2. *Cancer Res.* 2001;61(12):4892.

44. Ellis LM, Hicklin DJ. VEGF-targeted therapy: mechanisms of anti-tumour activity. *Nat Rev Cancer.* 2008;8:579-591.

45. Carter P, Presta L, Gorman CM, et al. Humanization of an anti-p185HER2 antibody for human cancer therapy. *Proc Natl Acad Sci U S A.* 1992;89(10): 4285-4289.

46. Kim KJ, Li B, Winer J, et al. Inhibition of vascular endothelial growth factor-induced angiogenesis suppresses tumour growth in vivo. *Nature.* 1993; 362(6423):841-844.

47. Brunet JFF, Denizot MF, Luciani M, et al. A new member of the immunoglobulin superfamily—CTLA-4. *Nature.* 1987;328:267-270.

48. Peggs KS, Quezada SA, Korman AJ, Allison JP. Principles and use of anti-CTLA4 antibody in human cancer immunotherapy. *Curr Opin Immunol.* 2006;18(2):206-213.

49. Pardoll DM. The blockade of immune checkpoints in cancer immunotherapy. *Nat Rev Cancer.* 2012;12(4):252-264.

50. Page DB, Postow MA, Callahan MK, et al. Immune modulation in cancer with antibodies. *Annu Rev Med.* 2014;65:185-202.

51. Le DT, Uram JN, Wang H, et al. PD-1 blockade in tumors with mismatch-repair deficiency. *N Engl J Med.* 2015;372(26):2509-2520.

52. Segal DM, Weiner GJ, Weiner LM. Bispecific antibodies in cancer therapy. *Curr Opin Immunol.* 1999;11(5):558-562.

53. Kontermann RE, Brinkmann U. Bispecific antibodies. *Drug Discov Today.* 2015;20(7):838-847.

54. Ridgway JB, Presta LG, Carter P. 'Knobs-into-holes' engineering of antibody CH3 domains for heavy chain heterodimerization. *Protein Eng.* 1996;9(7): 617-621.

55. Barrett DM, Singh N, Porter DL, Grupp SA, June CH. Chimeric antigen receptor therapy for cancer. *Annu Rev Med.* 2014;65:333-347.

56. Maude SL, Frey N, Shaw PA, et al. Chimeric antigen receptor T cells for sustained remissions in leukemia. *N Engl J Med.* 2014;371(16):1507-1517.

57. Grupp SA, Kalos M, Barrett D, et al. Chimeric antigen receptor-modified T cells for acute lymphoid leukemia. *N Engl J Med.* 2013;368(16):1509-1518.

58. Brown CE, Alizadeh D, Starr R, et al. Regression of glioblastoma after chimeric antigen receptor T-cell therapy. *N Engl J Med.* 2016;375(26):2561-2569.

59. Maude SL, Barrett D, Teachey DT, Grupp SA. Managing cytokine release syndrome associated with novel T cell-engaging therapies. *Cancer J (Sudbury, Mass).* 2014;20(2):119-122.

60. Lee DW, Gardner R, Porter DL, et al. Current concepts in the diagnosis and management of cytokine release syndrome. *Blood.* 2014;124(2):188-195.

61. Chung CH. Managing predictions and the risk for reactions to infusional monoclonal antibody therapy. *Oncologist.* 2008;13(6):725-732.

62. Chung CH, Mirakhur B, Chan E, et al. Cetuximab-induced anaphylaxis and IgE specific for galactose-α-1,3-galactose. *N Engl J Med.* 2008;358(11): 1109-1117.

63. Hansel TT, Kropshofer H, Singer T, et al. The safety and side effects of monoclonal antibodies. *Nat Rev Drug Discov.* 2010;9:325-338.

64. Carson KR, Evens AM, Richey EA, et al. Progressive multifocal leukoencephalopathy after rituximab therapy in HIV-negative patients: a report of 57 cases from the Research on Adverse Drug Events and Reports project. *Blood.* 2009;113(20):4834-4840.

65. Aksoy S, Harputluoglu H, Kilickap S, et al. Rituximab-related viral infections in lymphoma patients. *Leuk Lymphoma.* 2007;48(7):1307-1312.

66. Weber F, Goldmann C, Kramer M, et al. Cellular and humoral immune response in progressive multifocal leukoencephalopathy. *Ann Neurol.* 2001;49(5): 636-642.

67. Aster RH, Bougie DW. Drug-induced immune thrombocytopenia. *N Engl J Med.* 2007;357(6):580-587.

68. Scappaticci FA, Skillings JR, Holden SN, et al. Arterial thromboembolic events in patients with metastatic carcinoma treated with chemotherapy and bevacizumab. *J Natl Cancer Inst.* 2007;99(16):1232-1239.

69. Ranpura V, Hapani S, Chuang J, Wu S. Risk of cardiac ischemia and arterial thromboembolic events with the angiogenesis inhibitor bevacizumab in cancer patients: a meta-analysis of randomized controlled trials. *Acta Oncol.* 2010;49(3):287-297.

70. Hurwitz HI, Saltz LB, Van Cutsem E, et al. Venous thromboembolic events with chemotherapy plus bevacizumab: a pooled analysis of patients in randomized phase II and III studies. *J Clin Oncol.* 2011;29(13):1757-1764.

71. Azzi GR, Schutz FA, Je Y, et al. Bevacizumab (BEV) and the risk of arterial thromboembolic events (ATE) in patients with renal cell carcinoma and other cancers: a large comprehensive meta-analysis of more than 13,000 patients. *J Clin Oncol.* 2010;28(369):abstr 4609.

72. Slamon DJ, Leyland-Jones B, Shak S, et al. Use of chemotherapy plus a monoclonal antibody against HER2 for metastatic breast cancer that overexpresses HER2. *N Engl J Med.* 2001;344(11):783-792.

73. Moslehi JJ. Cardiovascular toxic effects of targeted cancer therapies. *N Engl J Med.* 2016;375(15):1457-1467.

74. Keefe DL. Trastuzumab-associated cardiotoxicity. *Cancer.* 2002;95(7): 1592-1600.

75. Yarden Y, Sliwkowski MX. Untagling the ErbB signalling network. *Nat Rev Mol Cell Biol.* 2001;2(2):127-137.

76. Lankhorst S, Saleh L, Danser AHJ, van den Meiracker AH. Etiology of angiogenesis inhibition-related hypertension. *Curr Opin Pharmacol.* 2015;21:7-13.

77. Naidoo J, Page DB, Li BT, et al. Toxicities of the anti-PD-1 and anti-PD-L1 immune checkpoint antibodies. *Ann Oncol.* 2015;26(12):2375-2391.

78. Pinto C, Barone CA, Girolomoni G, et al. Management of skin toxicity associated with cetuximab treatment in combination with chemotherapy or radiotherapy. *Oncologist.* 2011;16(2):228-238.

79. Peeters M, Siena S, Van Cutsem E, et al. Association of progression-free survival, overall survival, and patient-reported outcomes by skin toxicity and KRAS status in patients receiving panitumumab monotherapy. *Cancer.* 2009;115(7):1544-1554.

80. Rastestter W, Molina A, White CA. Rituximab: expanding role in therapy for lymphoma and autoimmune diseases. *Annu Rev Med.* 2004;55: 477-503.

81. Morschhauser F, Marlton P, Vitolo U, et al. Results of a phase I/II study of ocrelizumab, a fully humanized anti-CD20 mAb, in patients with relapsed/refractory follicular lymphoma. *Ann Oncol.* 2010;21(9):1870-1876.

82. Barth MJ, Hernandez-Ilizaliturri FJ, Mavis C, et al. Ofatumumab demonstrates activity against rituximab-sensitive and -resistant cell lines, lymphoma xenografts and primary tumour cells from patients with B-cell lymphoma. *Br J Haematol.* 2012;156(4):490-498.

83. van Imhoff GW, McMillan A, Matasar MJ, et al. Ofatumumab versus rituximab salvage chemoimmunotherapy in relapsed or refractory diffuse large B-cell lymphoma: the ORCHARRD study. *J Clin Oncol.* 2016;35(5):544-551.

84. Mössner E, Brünker P, Moser S, et al. Increasing the efficacy of CD20 antibody therapy through the engineering of a new type II anti-CD20 antibody with enhanced direct and immune effector cell-mediated B-cell cytotoxicity. *Blood.* 2010;115(22):4393-4402.

85. Beers SA, Chan CHT, French RR, Cragg MS, Glennie MJ. CD20 as a target for therapeutic type I and II monoclonal antibodies. *Semin Hematol.* 2010; 47(2):107-114.

86. Gagez A-L, Cartron G. Obinutuzumab: a new class of anti-CD20 monoclonal antibody. *Curr Opin Oncol.* 2014;26(5).

87. Goede V, Fischer K, Busch R, et al. Obinutuzumab plus chlorambucil in patients with CLL and coexisting conditions. *N Engl J Med.* 2014; 370(12):1101-1110.

88. Gordon LI. Practical considerations and radiation safety in radioimmunotherapy with yttrium 90 ibritumomab tiuxetan (zevalin). *Semin Oncol.* 2003; 30:23-28.

89. Ravandi F, O'Brien S. Alemtuzumab. *Expert Rev Anticancer Ther.* 2005;5(1): 39-51.

90. Palumbo A, Chanan-Khan A, Weisel K, et al. Daratumumab, bortezomib, and dexamethasone for multiple myeloma. *N Engl J Med.* 2016;375(8):754-766.

91. Dimopoulos MA, Oriol A, Nahi H, et al. Daratumumab, lenalidomide, and dexamethasone for multiple myeloma. *N Engl J Med.* 2016;375(14):1319-1331.

92. Usmani SZ, Weiss BM, Plesner T, et al. Clinical efficacy of daratumumab monotherapy in patients with heavily pretreated relapsed or refractory multiple myeloma. *Blood.* 2016;128(1):37.

93. van de Donk NWCJ, Janmaat ML, Mutis T, et al. Monoclonal antibodies targeting CD38 in hematological malignancies and beyond. *Immunol Rev.* 2016;270(1): 95-112.

94. Gordon MS, Cunningham D. Managing patients treated with bevacizumab combination therapy. *Oncology.* 2005;69(suppl 3):25-33.

95. Spratlin JL, Cohen RB, Eadens M, et al. Phase I pharmacologic and biologic study of ramucirumab (IMC-1121B), a fully human immunoglobulin G(1) monoclonal antibody targeting the vascular endothelial growth factor receptor-2. *J Clin Oncol.* 2010;28(5):780-787.

96. Wilke H, Van Cutsem E, Oh SC, et al. RAINBOW: a global, phase III, randomized, double-blind study of ramucirumab plus paclitaxel versus placebo plus paclitaxel in the treatment of metastatic gastroesophageal junction (GEJ) and gastric adenocarcinoma following disease progression on first-line platinum- and fluoropyrimidine-containing combination therapy rainbow IMCL CP12-0922 (I4T-IE-JVBE). *J Clin Oncol.* 2014;32(3_suppl):LBA7-LBA.

97. Plosker GL, Keam SJ. Trastuzumab: a review of its use in the management of HER2-positive metastatic and early-stage breast cancer. *Drugs.* 2006; 66(4):449-475.

98. Gianni L, Pienkowski T, Im Y-H, et al. 5-year analysis of neoadjuvant pertuzumab and trastuzumab in patients with locally advanced, inflammatory, or early-stage HER2-positive breast cancer (NeoSphere): a multicentre, open-label, phase 2 randomised trial. *Lancet Oncol.* 2016;17(6):791-800.

99. Schneeweiss A, Chia S, Hickish T, et al. Pertuzumab plus trastuzumab in combination with standard neoadjuvant anthracycline-containing and anthracycline-free chemotherapy regimens in patients with HER2-positive early breast cancer: a randomized phase II cardiac safety study (TRYPHAENA). *Ann Oncol.* 2013;24(9):2278-2284.

100. Erickson HK, Lewis Phillips GD, Leipold DD, et al. The effect of different linkers on target cell catabolism and pharmacokinetics/pharmacodynamics of trastuzumab maytansinoid conjugates. *Mol Cancer Ther.* 2012;11(5):1133.

101. Kovtun YV, Goldmacher VS. Cell killing by antibody-drug conjugates. *Cancer Lett.* 2007;255(2):232-240.

102. Lewis Phillips GD, Li G, Dugger DL, et al. Targeting HER2-positive breast cancer with trastuzumab-DM1, an antibody-cytotoxic drug conjugate. *Cancer Res.* 2008;68(22):9280.

103. Verma S, Miles D, Gianni L, et al. Trastuzumab emtansine for HER2-positive advanced breast cancer. *N Engl J Med.* 2012;367(19):1783-1791.

104. Chong G, Cunningham D. The role of cetuximab in the therapy of previously treated advanced colorectal cancer. *Semin Oncol.* 2006;32(suppl 9): S55-S58.

105. Saif MW, Cohenuram M. Role of panitumumab in the management of metastatic colorectal cancer. *Clin Colorectal Cancer.* 2006;6(2):118-124.

106. Thatcher N, Hirsch FR, Luft AV, et al. Necitumumab plus gemcitabine and cisplatin versus gemcitabine and cisplatin alone as first-line therapy in patients with stage IV squamous non-small-cell lung cancer (SQUIRE): an open-label, randomised, controlled phase 3 trial. *Lancet Oncol.* 2015;16(7): 763-774.

107. Kuenen B, Witteveen PO, Ruijter R, et al. A phase I pharmacologic study of necitumumab (IMC-11F8), a fully human IgG1 monoclonal antibody directed against EGFR in patients with advanced solid malignancies. *Clin Cancer Res.* 2010;16(6):1915.

108. Mueller BM, Romerdahl CA, Gillies SD, Reisfeld RA. Enhancement of antibody-dependent cytotoxicity with a chimeric anti-GD2 antibody. *J Immunol.* 1990;144(4):1382.

109. van Rhee F, Fayad L, Voorhees P, et al. Siltuximab, a novel anti-interleukin-6 monoclonal antibody, for Castleman's disease. *J Clin Oncol.* 2010;28(23):3701-3708.

110. Deisseroth A, Ko C-W, Nie L, et al. FDA approval: siltuximab for the treatment of patients with multicentric Castleman disease. *Clin Cancer Res.* 2015; 21(5):950.

111. Fitzgerald JC, Weiss SL, Maude SL, et al. Cytokine release syndrome after chimeric antigen receptor T cell therapy for acute lymphoblastic leukemia. *Crit Care Med.* 2017;45(2):e124-e131.

112. Barrett DM, Teachey DT, Grupp SA. Toxicity management for patients receiving novel T-cell engaging therapies. *Curr Opin Pediatr.* 2014;26(1): 43-49.

113. Lindhofer H, Mocikat R, Steipe B, Thierfelder S. Preferential species-restricted heavy/light chain pairing in rat/mouse quadromas. Implications for a single-step purification of bispecific antibodies. *J Immunol.* 1995;155(1):219.

114. Heiss MM, Murawa P, Koralewski P, et al. The trifunctional antibody catumaxomab for the treatment of malignant ascites due to epithelial cancer: Results of a prospective randomized phase II/III trial. *Int J Cancer.* 2010; 127(9):2209-2221.

115. Seimetz D, Lindhofer H, Bokemeyer C. Development and approval of the trifunctional antibody catumaxomab (anti-EpCAM×anti-CD3) as a targeted cancer immunotherapy. *Cancer Treat Rev.* 2010;36(6):458-467.

116. Bokemeyer C, Heiss M, Gamperl H, et al. Safety of catumaxomab: cytokine-release-related symptoms as a possible predictive factor for efficacy in a pivotal phase II/III trial in malignant ascites. *J Clin Oncol.* 2009;27(15_suppl):3036.

117. Kantarjian H, Stein A, Gökbuget N, et al. Blinatumomab versus chemotherapy for advanced acute lymphoblastic leukemia. *N Engl J Med.* 2017; 376(9):836-847.

118. Löffler A, Kufer P, Lutterbüse R, et al. A recombinant bispecific single-chain antibody, CD19 × CD3, induces rapid and high lymphoma-directed cytotoxicity by unstimulated T lymphocytes. *Blood.* 2000;95(6):2098.

119. Wu J, Fu J, Zhang M, Liu D. Blinatumomab: a bispecific T cell engager (BiTE) antibody against CD19/CD3 for refractory acute lymphoid leukemia. *J Hematol Oncol.* 2015;8(1):104.

120. Newman MJ, Benani DJ. A review of blinatumomab, a novel immunotherapy. *J Oncol Pharm Pract.* 2015;22(4):639-645.

121. Fenton C, Perry CM. Gemtuzumab ozogamicin: a review of its use in acute myeloid leukaemia. *Drugs.* 2005;65:2405-2427.

122. Francisco JA, Cerveny CG, Meyer DL, et al. cAC10-vcMMAE, an anti-CD30-monomethyl auristatin E conjugate with potent and selective antitumor activity. *Blood.* 2003;102(4):1458.

123. Younes A, Connors JM, Park SI, et al. Brentuximab vedotin combined with ABVD or AVD for patients with newly diagnosed Hodgkin's lymphoma: a phase 1, open-label, dose-escalation study. *Lancet Oncol.* 2013;14(13): 1348-1356.

124. Ansell SM. Brentuximab vedotin. *Blood.* 2014;124(22):3197.

125. Muller J, Nitschke L. The role of CD22 and Siglec-G in B-cell tolerance and autoimmune disease. *Nat Rev Rheumatol.* 2014;10(7):422-428.

126. DiJoseph J, Khandke K, Dougher M, et al., eds. CMC-544 (inotuzumab ozogamicin): a CD22-targeted immunoconjugate of calicheamicin. *Hematol Meeting Rep (formerly Haematologica Reports).* 2009;2:5.

127. Friedberg JW, Fisher RI. Iodine-131 tositumomab (Bexxar®): radioimmunoconjugate therapy for indolent and transformed B-cell non-Hodgkin's lymphoma. *Expert Rev Anticancer Ther.* 2004;4(1):18-26.

128. Tai Y-T, Dillon M, Song W, et al. Anti-CS1 humanized monoclonal antibody HuLuc63 inhibits myeloma cell adhesion and induces antibody-dependent cellular cytotoxicity in the bone marrow milieu. *Blood.* 2008; 112(4):1329.

129. Loizos N, Xu Y, Huber J, et al. Targeting the platelet-derived growth factor receptor α with a neutralizing human monoclonal antibody inhibits the growth of tumor xenografts: Implications as a potential therapeutic target. *Mol Cancer Ther.* 2005;4(3):369.

130. Tap WD, Jones RL, Van Tine BA, et al. Olaratumab and doxorubicin versus doxorubicin alone for treatment of soft-tissue sarcoma: an open-label phase 1b and randomised phase 2 trial. *Lancet.* 2016;388(10043):488-497.

131. Hodi FS, O'Day SJ, McDermott DF, et al. Improved survival with ipilimumab in patients with metastatic melanoma. *N Engl J Med.* 2010;363(8): 711-723.

132. Eggermont AMM, Chiarion-Sileni V, Grob J-J, et al. Prolonged survival in stage III melanoma with ipilimumab adjuvant therapy. *N Engl J Med.* 2016;375(19):1845-1855.

133. Lenschow DJ, Walunas TL, Bluestone JA. CD28/B7 system of T cell costimulation. *Annu Rev Immunol.* 1996;14(1):233-258.

134. Lee HT, Lee JY, Lim H, et al. Molecular mechanism of PD-1/PD-L1 blockade via anti-PD-L1 antibodies atezolizumab and durvalumab. *Sci Rep.* 2017;7(1):5532.

135. National Comprehensive Cancer Network. *Non-Small Cell Lung Cancer* 2017 [Available from: https://www.nccn.org/professionals/physician_gls/pdf/nscl.pdf.]

136. Fessas P, Lee H, Ikemizu S, Janowitz T. A molecular and preclinical comparison of the PD-1-targeted T-cell checkpoint inhibitors nivolumab and pembrolizumab. *Semin Oncol.* 2017;44(2):136-140.

137. McDermott DF, Atkins MB. PD-1 as a potential target in cancer therapy. *Cancer Med.* 2013;2(5):662-673.

138. Larkin J, Chiarion-Sileni V, Gonzalez R, et al. Combined nivolumab and ipilimumab or monotherapy in untreated melanoma. *N Engl J Med.* 2015;373(1):23-34.

139. Nishino M, Ramaiya NH, Hatabu H, et al. Monitoring immune-checkpoint blockade: response evaluation and biomarker development. *Nat Rev Clin Oncol.* 2017;14(11):655-668.

140. Antonia SJ, Villegas A, Daniel D, et al. Durvalumab after chemoradiotherapy in stage III non-small-cell lung cancer. *N Engl J Med* 2017;377: 1919-1929.

141. Tan S, Liu K, Chai Y, et al. Distinct PD-L1 binding characteristics of therapeutic monoclonal antibody durvalumab. *Protein Cell.* 2017;9(1):135-139.

Cytokine Therapy for Cancer

David C. Yao, David F. McDermott, and Henry B. Koon

Cytokines play critical roles in regulating immune responses and maintaining immunologic homeostasis. These molecules are secreted or membrane-bound proteins that act as mediators of intercellular signaling to facilitate diverse biologic activities. Much progress has made in elucidating the roles of cytokines in tumor immunology. This chapter will review clinically tested cytokines in the framework of cancer immunosurveillance. The biological activities and mechanisms of action of these molecules in immunosurveillance and in shaping tumor immunogenicity (immunoediting) will be discussed. This chapter will then describe functions, signaling, and recent clinical applications of these cytokines in cancer immunotherapy.

Cancer Immunity

Ehrlich proposed the concept of immunosurveillance in the early 1900s, and subsequent observations from the field of transplant inferred there was a role for the immune system cancer surveillance. It was not until the early 1990s when genetically engineered animal models became available to elucidate the multistep nature of host immune response to tumor via the regulation of immunity.[1,2] These data did not only validate the cancer immunosurveillance concept but also supported the notion that immune system shapes tumor immunogenicity. These findings prompted Schreiber and his colleagues to develop cancer immunoediting model that describe the complex interaction between host immunity and tumor development.[3,4] Cancer immunoediting has three phases: elimination, equilibrium, and escape.

In the elimination phase of cancer immunosurveillance, both innate immunity, a nonspecific defense mechanism that responds rapidly to stress or environmental insults, and adaptive immunity, a highly restricted immune response that occurs after exposure to antigens derived from tumors, work together to eradicate tumors before they become clinically relevant. If successful, the host will remain tumor-free. The first step of the immune response toward neoplastic development includes the recognition of tumors by innate immune cells via pattern recognition receptors and other cell surface molecules. Tumors often express stress-induced molecules on the surface, which can be recognized by NKG2D receptors on natural killer (NK) cells, macrophages, and cytotoxic T lymphocytes (CTLs).[5] NK cells can further monitor tumor cells that suppress the expression of MHC class I molecules using killer-cell immunoglobulin-like receptors (KIRs).[6] Alternatively, various innate immune effector cells such as NK cells, NKT cells, and γδ T-cells are activated by inflammatory molecules that are

secreted by growing tumor cells and surrounding stromal cells. The activation of these innate effector cells favors an inflammatory condition that facilitates both tumor killing and release of tumor-specific antigens in the microenvironment. This process instigates the adaptive immune responses. Tumor cell turnover activates the local production of type I interferons (IFNs). This cytokine induces the activation of infiltrating dendritic cells (DCs), which takes up tumor-specific antigens. Following which, these cells acquire C-C chemokine receptor (CCR) 7 expression and migrate to the tumor-draining lymph nodes.[7] Once settled in the draining lymph nodes, DCs present tumor-specific antigens to CD4+ T-cells via MHC class II molecules. This engagement facilitates the priming and proliferation of type 1 CD4+ T-helper cells (Th1) in the presence of interleukin (IL)-12 and IL-18.[8] The Th1 cells will then license DCs to cross-present the antigens to CD8+ T-cells, which enable the development of CD8+ CTLs. These cells will undergo clonal expansion in the lymph node and enter the peripheral circulation. They are subsequently recruited to the tumor microenvironment by CXCL9- and CXCL10-mediated chemokine attraction.[9] Once infiltrating the tumors, CTLs are activated upon the recognition of cognate class I tumor-specific molecule on tumor cells. These CTLs will exert tumor-specific killing by secreting specific cytokines, activating death receptors, and releasing granzyme B and perforin. This antigen-specific cytotoxic response is augmented, at least partly, by IL-15 and IL-21.[10,11] Tumor cell death will further the production of additional tumor-specific antigens and thus robust cellular adaptive immune response. Throughout this process, cytokines serve as critical factors that permit the generation of coordinated and robust immune response to tumor antigens. Besides those aforementioned, endogenous type II IFNs, IL-2, and IL-7 have been shown to enhance effector cellular function, while GM-CSF up-regulates the tumor antigen–presenting activity by DCs.[12–14]

Alternatively, the equilibrium phase of immunosurveillance represents the immune-mediated latency of tumor development. In this phase, adaptive immunity appears to play a critical role in maintaining the tumor dormancy. The adaptive effector cells that exert tumor-specific killing function can contain the tumor growth effectively by eliminating a majority of the original tumor cells. Under the chronic immune selection pressure, tumor variants emerge from the remaining live tumor cells due to genetic instability. These variants carry a reduced immunogenicity phenotype by increasing resistance to immune rejection. A less efficacious adaptive immunity in the equilibrium phase leads to the development of a new population of tumor cells. A clinical scenario that characterizes the equilibrium phase is the transmission of cancer from organ transplant donors who have no prior history of cancer or have been in long period of remission prior to transplant.[15,16] These observations have suggested that tumors were kept in the equilibrium phase in organ transplant donors before undergoing rapid expansion in recipients whose immune system was suppressed.

Tumor cells growing out of the equilibrium phase enter the escape period. In this phase, tumor cells acquire the ability to circumvent both innate and adaptive immune-mediated tumor killing. A wide spectrum of effective escape mechanisms has been characterized. Several studies have provided evidence that tumor escape can be attributed to changes occurring in edited tumor targets. These alterations lead to poor immune recognition. For instance, class I molecules are often absent in many human tumor specimens. Other components that are essential for the class I tumor antigen processing and presenting machinery are frequently deficient in human tumors.[17] Alterations to other molecules, such as type II IFN signaling axis, in tumor cells can also indirectly lead to defective antigen processing and presentation. Tumor cells harboring these faulty signaling pathways have shown to fail to up-regulate class I molecules in response to type II IFN stimulation that leads to immune-resistant tumor progression.[18]

Alternatively, tumor cells may develop resistance against immune-mediated cytotoxic effector activities. This escape mechanism occurs when tumors acquire genetic changes that result in either qualitative or quantitative increased of oncogenic and prosurvival factors. Studies have documented that constitutive activation of signal transducer and activator of transcription (STAT) 3 in tumors inhibits mediators necessary for antitumor immune activation. Moreover, STAT3 activity promotes the secretion of immunosuppressive factors, thereby restricting immune-mediated tumor rejection.[19,20] In addition, other prosurvival pathways including mitogen-activated protein kinase (MAPK), epidermal growth factor receptor (EGFR), and tyrosine protein kinase kit (c-KIT) have been implicated in mechanisms of tumor immune evasion.[21–23]

Significant attention has recently focused on the molecular and cellular events that contribute to the establishment of immunosuppressive tumor microenvironment. These events have shown to facilitate tumor escape. Tumor variants surviving the equilibrium secrete immunosuppressive cytokines, such as vascular endothelial growth factor (VEGF) or transforming growth factor beta (TGF-β) that orchestra the immune inhibitory activities.[24,25] Additionally, metabolic products, including adenosine, arginase, indoleamine 2,3-dioxygenase (IDO), inducible nitric oxide synthase (iNOS), and prostaglandin E2 released by the tumor and host cells, contribute to immune inhibition.[26–31] These soluble molecules can curtail the activity of DCs, inhibit innate and adaptive effector cell activation, promote the development of regulatory T cells (Treg), and down-regulate the recruitment of T-cells while encouraging myeloid-derived suppressive cells (MDSCs) to traffic to the tumor microenvironment. These data suggest that a tumor may use a variety of soluble factors to develop a complex local immunosuppressive network.

Besides secretory molecules, cellular populations including CD4+ CD25+ Tregs and MDSCs have garnered considerable interest due to their pathologic roles in the tumor microenvironment. Tregs were first characterized as a subset of CD4+ T-cells that prevent autoimmunity by maintaining self-tolerance.[32] It is now established that Tregs suppress antitumor immune response and

infiltration of Tregs into the tumor bed is associated with poor clinical outcome.[33] Selectively depleting Tregs and blocking their cellular function serve as potentials for unleashing antitumor effector responses. MDSCs represent another major cellular component that negatively regulate the immune response. These cells are a heterogeneous group of cells that are recruited to the tumor site by tumor-derived inflammatory chemokines. They promote immune escape by down-regulating adaptive effector responses and by aiding tumor growth.[34] Analogous to findings in Tregs, accumulation of MDSCs in the microenvironment has been associated with the human tumor progression.[35] Together, these immune inhibitory cells hold clinical significance in human cancer, and active investigations pinpointing the molecular basis of their suppressive functions are ongoing.

Finally, tumor escape can be facilitated through activation of checkpoint receptors and ligands. These immunosuppressive molecules have gained significant interest due to their clinical success in treating cancer recently.[36] Blocking of cytotoxic T-lymphocyte antigen 4 (CTLA-4), the prototypical immune-checkpoint receptor, led to tumor regression in animal models.[37] This finding prompted further clinical development and led to eventual approval of CTLA-4 blockade in advanced melanoma.[38] Recently, blocking agents targeting programmed cell death protein-1 (PD-1) and its ligand have demonstrated clinical efficacy in a variety of human tumors.[39–44] These findings have invigorated further studies that characterize other checkpoint molecules for potential clinical applications. CTLA-4, along with PD-1, T-cell immunoglobulin and mucin-domain containing-3 (TIM-3), lymphocyte-activation gene 3 (LAG-3), T-cell immunoglobulin and ITIM domain (TIGIT) and many others are essential checkpoints that modulate adaptive immune activation.[36] These checkpoint receptors are expressed on the surface of immune cells that recognize one or more surface expressing ligands. There activities are initiated through a cell-cell interaction where receptor molecules on one cell surface bind to specific ligands on neighboring cells. As a consequence, effector T-cells harboring checkpoint receptors are down-regulated. Despite these commonalities, different checkpoint receptors exert immune inhibition differently based on patterns of expression, signaling pathways, and mechanisms of action.[36] For example, CTLA-4–mediated T-cell suppression primarily occurs in the draining lymph node since CTLA-4 ligands are expressed on DCs. In addition, CTLA-4 receptors are found mostly on CD4+ T-cells. Thus, increased adaptive immunity against tumors in response to CTLA-4 blockade is through CD4+ T-cells during priming. Conversely, PD-1 receptors are expressed on CTLs whose ligands are overexpressed in selected tumors and infiltrating inflammatory cells.[45,46] Blocking PD-1 signaling axis preserves TCR-mediated CTL tumor-killing functions. This blockade is thought to work predominantly in the tumor microenvironment. These mechanistic differences between CTLA-4 and PD-1 may reflect the differential toxicity profiles, onset of actions, and spectrum of antitumor activity in the clinical setting. Despite current clinical focus on CTLA-4 and PD-1, preclinical studies have supported that additional checkpoints, including LAG-3, TIGIT, and TIM-3, may contribute to favorable clinical outcomes.[47] These will facilitate innovative strategies to target both immunostimulatory and inhibitory pathways as potential therapeutic targets that could be combined with cytokines.

Cytokine Biology and Cytokine Receptors

Interferon was the first cytokine that was described by Isaacs and Lindenmann in 1957.[48] Subsequently, numerous IFNs and ILs have been identified and characterized. In general, these molecules are mostly secretory whose functions are to maintain proper host immunity. The biological activities of cytokines on the immune system are pleiotropic and redundant, depending on the local cytokine composition and concentration, the differential pattern of cytokine receptor expression on the target cells, and the molecular to epigenetic state of the effected cells. Cytokines induce physiological activities through cognate transmembrane receptors. Based on these receptors, a functional classification of cytokines has been widely accepted.[49] Currently, there are seven receptor families: type I cytokine receptors, type II cytokine receptors, immunoglobulin superfamily receptors, tumor necrosis factor (TNF) receptors, G-protein–coupled receptors, TGF-β, and IL-17 receptors. In the following sections, this chapter will focus on the review of type I receptors, type II receptors, and immunoglobulin superfamily receptors.

Type I Cytokine Receptors

Type I cytokine receptors share a common signaling subunit that dimerizes/multimerizes with a cytokine-specific subunit or subunits to propagate intracellular signals. Three major classes of receptors can be categorized based on a shared common subunit: γ chain (γc), gp130, and β chain (βc). The prototypic type I cytokine receptor is the IL-2 receptor family whose members, including IL-2, IL-4, IL-7, IL-9, IL-15, and IL-21, share a common γc. Upon engagement with corresponding cytokines, these receptors initiate and propagate their signals via Janus kinase (JAK) and signal transducers of activated T (STAT) pathway. GP130 serves as another shared signaling subunit for receptors of IL-6, IL-11, IL-27, leukemia inhibitory factor (LIF), ciliary neurotrophic factor, oncostatin M, cardiotrophin 1, and cardiotrophin-like cytokine. The gp130-mediated biologic activities on immune, hematopoietic, and nervous systems are pleiotropic in nature. They are accomplished through a complex interplay of multiple intracellular signaling pathways. The last group of type I cytokine receptors shares βc as a signaling subunit. IL-3, IL-5, and GM-CSF receptors belong to this family that initiates the intracellular signaling cascade through JAK2 (see Fig. 30.1).

Type II Cytokine Receptors

Type II cytokine receptors are a collection of transmembrane proteins that recognize type I and II interferons, as well as IL-10 and its homologous cytokines, including IL-19, IL-20, IL-22, IL-24, and IL-26. These molecules are stratified based on their structural similarities. There are 12 members of this receptor family with a majority of them are composed of a signaling chain and a ligand binding chain whose extracellular regions share sequence homologies of tandem Ig-like domains. One of these receptor complexes may recognize multiple cytokines, while one particular cytokine can bind to one or two different receptor complexes. For instance, IL-20 receptor complex recognizes soluble IL-19, IL-20, and IL-24 molecules. Conversely, IL-20 can bind to either IL-20 type 1 or type 2 receptor complex.

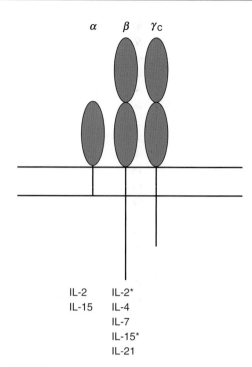

FIGURE **30.1** The IL-2 receptor family is the prototypic type I cytokine receptors. All members of the family share the common gamma chain (γc). IL-2 and IL-15 share a common β signaling subunit (*) but have a distinct subunit that determines their affinity for the receptor.

Signal transduction initiates when cytokine binds to the receptor complex. This engagement activates JAK/STAT pathway and upregulates the transcription of a series of targeted genes. All type II cytokine receptors can activate STAT1 and STAT3, while some can promote STAT2 activity. Besides JAK/STAT, some of these receptors, including type I IFNR, propagate intracellular signals through CRKL-, MAPK-, and PI3K-dependent pathways. Each of these pathways will be described in more detail later in this chapter.

Despite their physical resemblance, the physiological roles of these receptors are vast and different. For instance, type II IFN is a proinflammatory cytokine that activates host defense immunity. In contrast, IL-10 inhibits the expression of costimulatory molecules and macrophage-mediated proinflammatory cytokines. This functional divergence stems from different patterns of receptor expression, complex interaction between cytokine and receptor, and distinct signaling pathway that each cytokine activates.

Immunoglobulin (Ig) Superfamily Receptors

Ig superfamily receptors share a common extracellular homology of immunoglobulin domain. These transmembrane molecules recognize IL-1, IL-18, mast/stem cell factor, and monocyte colony–stimulating factor.

Formulations

The initial availability of cytokines was limited by the need to isolate them from biologically active cultures. The advent of recombinant DNA technology allowed for cytokines to be produced in quantities that would allow them to be used clinically. This technology also allows for the introduction of structural modifications that alter the pharmacokinetic profiles of cytokine. Newer production strategies include structural alterations that change the pharmacodynamic profiles of cytokines. These pharmacodynamic alterations may have clinical utility in cytokines such as interleukin-2 (IL-2) that has pleiotropic effects due to its ability to interact with multiple receptors. Modification of cytokines can be grouped into three categories: (a) structural, (b) fusions, and (c) pegylation.

Structural Modification

One of the earliest structural modifications was to recombinant IL-2, which was altered to improve drug stability. Aldesleukin (Prometheus Therapeutics, San Diego, CA) is the recombinant IL-2 variant that is clinically available in the United States. Aldesleukin differs from natural human IL-2 in that a cysteine residue at amino acid 125 is replaced by serine, and it also lacks the N-terminal alanine.[50] Of historical interest is the Hoffmann-La Roche rIL-2 preparation that lacks the amino acid substitution at position 125 and has an additional N-terminal methionine residue.[51] These initial structural variants had the same biologic activity as native IL-2 and their main effect was on drug stability. Subsequent structural IL-2 variants (muteins) have also been developed with the goal of altering cytokine/receptor interactions to favors specific immune effects.[52,53]

Fusions

Recombinant fusion proteins can be designed to alter the pharmacokinetic/pharmacodynamic properties of the native proteins or to use the binding specificity of the native protein of biologically to facilitate restricted delivery of toxins or radionucleotides. The addition of the Fc region of human immunoglobulin G or covalent binding to albumin to small biologically active proteins that are rapidly cleared by the kidney is used as a strategy to extend their half-life.[54,55] The effect of these modifications can be twofold. By increasing the size of the molecule, the modification reduces clearance by glomerular filtration. The addition of albumin or an Fc modification allows for the molecules to be recycled by the FcRn system within the renal tubules.[54,55] Etanercept, a Fc moiety linked to soluble tumor necrosis factor receptor (TNFR2), was the first fusion approved by the FDA for the treatment of rheumatoid arthritis in 1998.[56] Subsequently, this paradigm has been not only used for receptor fusions but has also been used for soluble factors with short-lived half-life such as factor VIII and factor IX.[57,58]

The use of fusion proteins for cytokine therapy has been limited. Denileukin diftitox (Ontak—no longer available in the United States) is a fusion of IL-2 and diphtheria toxin that was approved by the FDA in 1999 to treat cutaneous T-cell lymphoma (CTCL).[59] ALKS–4230, is a fusion of IL-2 and CD25 (IL-2 and alpha chain receptor) that has differential effects on T-cells that are dependent on whether they express the high-affinity or intermediate-affinity IL-2 receptors is currently in clinical investigation.[60]

Pegylation

The covalent addition of polyethylene glycol (PEG) has been used to alter their pharmacokinetic profiles. IFN-α conjugated to polymer polyethylene glycol (PEG-IFN) has an increased half-life allowing for longer dosing intervals and long exposure times (see below).[61] However, new site-directed pegylation strategies are being used to alter receptor affinity of cytokines such as IL-2. NKTR-214 is a pegylated version of IL-2 that is engineered to preferentially interact with the IL-2 intermediate-affinity receptor as opposed to the high-affinity IL-2 receptor.[62,63] This modification appears to alter the T-cell response in a way that is potentially favorable to tumor immunity and at the same time appears to reduce the toxicity profile of IL-2 (discussed in IL-2 section). NKTR-214 is currently being studied in combination with the PD-1 antibody nivolumab in multiple solid tumors.

Interferons

IFNs are characterized based on their ability to bind to specific receptors. There are currently three distinct types of IFNs.[64–66]

Type I Interferons

Type I IFN family is a gene family that encodes 13 IFN-α subtypes, one IFN-β, and various individual gene products of IFN-ε, IFN-τ, IFN-κ, IFN-ω, IFN-δ, and IFN-ζ. Among these molecules, IFN-α and IFN-β are the most well defined and characterized.[67] The production of these molecules is mediated by the activation of pattern recognition receptors (PRRs) in response to microbial products, and they signal via either homodimeric or heterodimeric receptors.[67] The activation of these receptors can enhance IFN-stimulated genes (ISGs), which will lead to a variety of immunostimulatory activities.[67]

Type I IFNs have been shown to possess strong antitumor activities. It was first thought that these molecules exert antineoplastic effects by direct stimulation of IFNAR signaling on tumor cells to inhibit mitotic division, promote terminal lineage differentiation, and induce cell apoptosis.[68] It is now evident that type I IFN-mediated tumor rejection is, at least in part, dependent on immunosurveillance and response. To elucidate the roles of type I IFNs in immunological function, mice carrying a targeted deficiency in the IFNAR1 locus, which encodes a transmembrane receptor subunit for IFN-α and IFN-β, were studied.[69] These mice exhibit an increasing rate of carcinogen-induced tumor formation. Similarly, mice carrying homozygous STAT1-null allele, which encodes a nonredundant intracellular messenger downstream of type I IFN receptor, yield a complete deficiency in type I IFN activity with phenotypes that include, but not limited to, de novo tumor development.[69] These findings support the hypothesis that type I IFNs are essential in immunosurveillance of oncogenesis.

Type I IFNs are able to activate both innate and adaptive immunities due to the ubiquitous expression of their binding receptors.[69] Previous studies have demonstrated that these molecules mobilize innate immunity against tumor by various mechanisms: First, they down-regulate NK cell–mediated CTL elimination[70,71]; second, they induce expression of proinflammatory cytokines by macrophages[72]; and lastly, they inhibit the suppressive function of Tregs.[73] Type I IFNs can further facilitate the tumor-specific adaptive immune response. They promote cross-priming of DCs to CD8$^+$ T-cells by stimulating the maturation of DCs and the migration of DC to the draining lymph nodes.[74,75] These molecules can further up-regulate the expression of effector molecules in CTLs when encountering cognate tumor antigens.[76] Finally, they promote the survival of memory CTLs.[77] Taken together, type I IFNs exhibit a broad range of cellular activities of the immune systems that coordinate innate and adaptive immune responses. Further understanding toward the regulations of type I IFNs may lead to new strategies of therapeutic potentials while minimizing side effects.

Type I Interferon Production

Type I IFNs are highly pleiotropic. They are produced in almost all cells in the body after PRRs that are stimulated by viral and bacterial nucleic acids and bacterial cell wall. On exposure to these microbial products, PRRs on the cell surface, in the endosomal compartment, and in the cytosol activate diverse intracellular signaling pathways. These signals converge at key proteins that lead to the upregulation of IFNA or IFNB transcripts via IFN regulatory factors (IRFs) and nuclear factor-*κ*B (NF-*κ*B).

Type I Interferon Signal Transduction

JAK-STAT Pathway

Type I IFNs bind to a heterodimeric transmembrane receptor comprising IFNAR1 and IFNAR2. This intracellular signaling is mediated through numerous pathways that regulate various biological responses. The JAK-STAT pathway was the first signaling pathway shown to be activated by IFNs. Since its discovery in the 1990s, the JAK-STAT signaling cascade is proven to be critical to regulate IFN-mediated functions. The canonical pathway is initiated by the binding of type I IFN to its receptor that results in the rapid activation of JAK1 and TYK2, members of JAK family.[78,79] The intracellular tail of the receptors is then phosphorylated, which endorses the docking of STAT1 and STAT2.[80] Other STAT heterodimers and homodimers including STAT3 and STAT5 may be activated on binding to type I IFN, while STAT4 and STAT6 can also be activated by IFN-*α* in restricted cell types.[80] The close proximity of JAK and STAT aids the phosphorylation of STATs, which leads to the dimerization of STATs. Type I IFN-mediated signal transduction continues when dimerized STAT1/STAT2 translocates to the nucleus where this complex binds to IFN regulatory factor 9 (IRF9) to form the IFN-stimulated gene factor 3 (ISGF3) transcriptional machinery.[81,82] This complex binds to its cognate sequences, IFN-stimulated response elements (ISREs), that drives the expression of type I IFN-specific transcripts. Other STAT complexes recognize IFN-*γ*-activated site (GAS) element.[81,82] Given IFN-stimulated genes (ISGs) are regulated by promoter sites containing either ISREs, GAS, or both elements, combinations of various STAT complexes are to optimize the activation of genes and thus biological responses.

CRKL-Mediated Pathway

It is now evident that JAK-STAT activity alone is not adequate to account for all the biological activities generated by type I IFNs. Other pathways including the CRK-like (CRKL) family, mitogen-activated protein kinase (MAPK), and phosphatidylinositol 3-kinase (PI3K) operate either independently or in concert with STATs to coordinate proper downstream transcriptional activities.[80]

CRKL is a family of adaptor proteins comprising SRC homology (SH) 2 and SH3 domains.[83] Upon type I IFN (IFN-*α*, IFN-*β*, and IFN-*ω*)-mediated activation of JAK, the SH2 domain of CRKL interacts with TYK2 and undergoes tyrosine phosphorylation.[84] The phosphorylated CRKL forms a complex with STAT5.[85] This complex then translocates to the nucleus where it recognizes GAS element and promotes the expression of ISGs. Alternatively, type I IFN can exert a broad range of functions through CRKL in STAT5-independent manner. In response to type I IFN stimulation, CRKL binds to C3G, a guanine nucleotide exchange factor, to activate a

small G-protein RAP1.[86] Similar to other RAS family proteins, activated RAP1 can further interact with multiple downstream effectors that control cellular proliferation, differentiation, and other biological activities.

p38-Regulated Pathway

MAPKs are a group of serine and threonine kinases that mediate signals for the regulation of cellular behaviors. p38, a family of four MAP kinase homologs, is a key player for the generation of a plethora of type I IFN-initiated signals. P38*α*, the first member of the family identified, was shown to undergo tyrosine phosphorylation, which led to the activity of other catalytic enzymes in response to cellular stress. Subsequently, three additional members, p38*β*, p38*γ*, and p38*δ*, were cloned.[87–89] These proteins are encoded by different genes. They share structural homology and have different differential tissue expression. To date, the precise pathway of p38 in response to type I IFN stimulation is little known. The current working model starts with the phosphorylation of VAV, an SH2- and SH3-domain–containing adaptor protein, by IFN-activated JAKs. The activation of VAV leads to RAC1-mediated MAPKK3/6 activity that directly phosphorylates p38 and its activation.[80] Interestingly, cells maintaining targeted deficiency in MAPKK have preserved IFN-mediated p38 activity, which suggests that these kinases are redundant in this signaling cascade. Numerous downstream targets for p38, including MAPK-activated protein kinase (MAPKAPK) 2, MAPKAPK3, heat shock protein 27, lymphocyte-specific protein 1, cAMP response element-binding protein, transcription factor ATF1, tyrosine hydroxylase, mitogen- and stress-activated kinase 1 (MSK1), and MAPK-interacting protein kinase 1 (MNK1), drive the modulation of mRNA stability, maintain the stability of translational machinery, stabilize the integrity of transcriptional complexes, regulate the remodeling of chromatin, and up-regulate the activity of transcription function.[90] It is now clear that p38 signaling cascade is necessary and is independent of the canonical JAK-STAT pathway in the induction of type I IFN-dependent gene transcription and thus response.

PI3K-Mediated Pathway

Another well-documented regulatory molecule that is immediately downstream of the type I IFN receptor is PI3K. The first report implicating PI3K signaling pathway in IFN-mediated signaling was published in 1995.[91] In which, IFN-*α*–, IFN-*β*–, and IFN-*ω*–mediated JAK activity is shown to induce tyrosine phosphorylation of insulin receptor substrate 1 (IRS1), which supports the docking of PI3K. PI3K activation results in the production of phosphatidylinositol-4,5-bisphosphate (PIP2) and phosphatidylinositol-3,4,5-triphosphate (PIP3). These messengers bring phosphoinositide-dependent kinase 1 (PDK1) and protein kinase B (AKT) in close physical proximity that triggers sequential phosphorylation of AKT. PDK1 first phosphorylates AKT on threonine 308. Full AKT activity is optimized when serine 473 is phosphorylated, a reaction catalyzed by enzymes such as mammalian target of rapamycin (mTOR) complex 2. Activated AKT exerts biological effects through downstream regulatory partners, including mTOR and nuclear factor kappa-light-chain-enhancer of activated B-cells (NF-*κ*B).[92,93]

mTOR is a well-conserved serine/threonine protein kinase that has two distinct protein complexes, mTORC1 and mTORC2. They differ in their subunit composition and rapamycin sensitivity.

mTORC1 is a rapamycin-sensitive complex of mTOR kinase, mLST8 (mTOR-associated protein, LST8 homolog Saccharomyces cerevisiae), DEPTOR, the Tti/Tel2 complex, PRAS40 (proline-rich AKT1 substrate), and RAPTOR (regulatory-associated protein of mTOR, complex 1).[94] Activation of mTORC1 in response to type I IFN enhances mRNA translation of ISGs by phosphorylating ribosomal S6 kinases (S6K) and eukaryotic initiation factor 4E (eIF4E), leading to synthesis of proteins that play a role in autophagy and cell survival.[95] mTORC2 is the rapamycin-insensitive complex of mTOR kinase, mLST8, DEPTOR, the Tti/Tel2 complex, Sin1 and Rictor (rapamycin-insensitive companion of mTOR).[94] This protein complex is less sensitive to the rapamycin treatment. Studies using mouse embryonic fibroblast cells maintaining targeted deficiency in either the Rictor or the Sin1 locus have demonstrated that defective IFN-mediated AKT engagement, ISG transcription, and mTORC1 activation can be attributed to faulty mTORC2 activity.[96] Thus, it is evident that mTORC2 is indispensible in the generation of proper IFN response.

NF-κB, a ubiquitously expressed transcription factor, is a homo- or heterodimeric complex containing subunits from a family of five DNA-binding proteins, including c-Rel, NF-κB1 p50, NF-κB2 p52, RelA (p65), and RelB.[97,98] These proteins share a Rel homology domain, which holds sites for dimerization, DNA binding, and interaction with regulatory partners. The most abundant NF-κB is the p50/p65 heterodimer, which expresses in nearly all cell types.[97] At baseline, the inactive form of NF-κB p50/p65 dimer is bound to IκB inhibitory unit in the cytoplasm. Upon type I IFN-mediated stimulation, AKT induces NF-κB activity via IKKβ and PKCθ.[75] These intermediate messengers phosphorylate IκB, which results in its proteolytic degradation. NF-κB is then liberated for nuclear translocation, DNA binding, and transcriptional activity. Alternatively, type I IFN can activate NF-κB through TNF receptor-associated factors (TRAFs), NF-κB–inducing kinase (NIK), and

IKKα signaling cascade without the involvement of AKT.[75] In this setting, activation of IKKα leads to the processing and the nuclear translocation of RelB/p52 NF-κB heterodimeric complex. Both canonical and noncanonical activation of NF-κB by type I IFN regulate cell survival and molecular events leading to antigen processing and presentation (see Fig. 30.2).

Pharmaceutical Preparations

IFN-α, initially referred to as leukocyte IFN because of how it was originally isolated, is comprised of a group of at least twelve distinct proteins.[64] Recombinant IFN-α2a, IFN-α2b, and IFN-α2c differ by one to two amino acids and are the forms of IFN-α that have been tested clinically.[64] In the United States, IFN-α2a is sold under the trade name Roferon (Hoffmann-La Roche; Nutley, NJ), and IFN-α2b is available as Intron A (Schering; Kenilworth, NJ). IFN-α2c is available in Europe as Berofor (Bender; Vienna, Austria). These three compounds have never been compared in a randomized trial; however, their spectrum of activity is likely similar. The approved indications for these agents include treatment of viral diseases such as hepatitis C and Kaposi's sarcoma as well as treatment of cancers such as melanoma and chronic myeloid leukemia (CML).[99–101] IFN-α conjugated to polymer polyethylene glycol (PEG-IFN) has an increased half-life allowing for longer dosing intervals and long exposure times (see below).[61] Pegylated IFN-α2a (Pegasys, Hoffmann-La Roche; Nutley, NJ) and pegylated IFN-α2b (PEG-Intron, Schering; Kenilworth, NJ) are the two forms of PEG-IFN available in the United States.[102,103] These agents are widely used in combination with ribavirin in the treatment of hepatitis C. The role of the PEG-IFNs as monotherapies for cancer is still under study.[104,105]

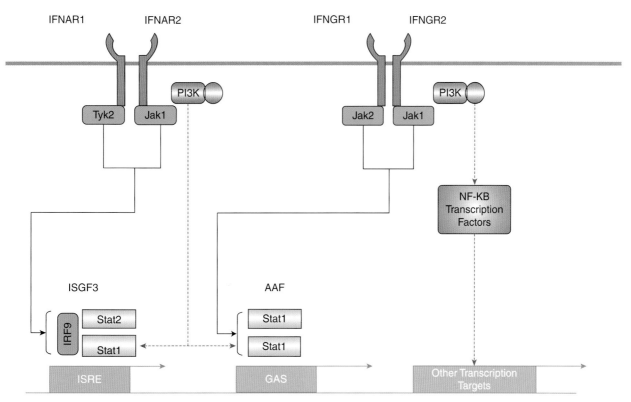

FIGURE 30.2 Interferon signaling.

Clinical Pharmacology of Type I Interferons

IFN-α

The pharmacokinetics of the IFNs were initially measured in serum using bioassays, which measure protection from viral cytopathic effect, prior to the development of direct immunological tests such as enzyme-linked immunosorbent assays. When given subcutaneously or intramuscularly to humans, approximately 80% of IFN-α is absorbed.[106] These routes of administration lengthen its distribution phase, with peak serum levels occurring at 1 to 8 hours. Clearance varies between 4.8 and 48 L/hour, and the terminal elimination half-life is 4 to 16 hours.[106] The high-dose IFN-α2b regimen used for adjuvant therapy of melanoma may yield peak serum levels of 2,500 IU/mL at the end of the intravenous phase and 150 IU/mL after subcutaneous administration[106–108] (Table 30.1).

In order to improve the pharmacokinetic profile of IFN-α, these agents have chemically modified by linkage to a PEG molecule.[61] The PEG modification increases the serum half-life resulting in a less frequent dosing interval. A monopegylated IFN-α2b was developed by Schering-Plough/Merck (Kenilworth, New Jersey). This species has a 70-fold increase in serum half-life compared with native IFN-α2a.[109] Linkage of a 40-kd branched PEG molecule to IFN-α2a or a 12-kd linear PEG moiety to IFN-α2b markedly altered the pharmacokinetic profile and increased activity against hepatitis C in a direct clinical comparison of subcutaneous PEG-IFN with the parent compound.[110,111] The larger PEG moiety of PEG–IFN-α2a leads to the slowest absorption half-life and a longer elimination half-life[110,111] (Table 30.2).

PEG–IFN-α2b at 1 μg/kg/week induced a biological response similar to that of IFN-α2b at 3 million IU administered subcutaneously three times a week.[112] Anticancer activity against solid tumors was demonstrated in a phase I/II trial of PEG–IFN-α2b, which determined 6 μg/kg/week as the maximal tolerated dose (MTD) and showed evidence of drug accumulation with an area under the curve (AUC) of 374 pg/hour/mL for week 1, compared with 480 pg/hour/mL at week 4 for patients treated with the MTD.[113] PEG–IFN-α2b has been directly compared with the parent drug as initial treatment for chronic phase CML in a phase III study, where it showed efficacy and toxicity at 6 μg/kg/week similar to those of IFN-α2b at 5 million IU/m^2 per day.[114] The toxicity of

TABLE 30.1 Pharmacokinetics of interferons

Route of Administration	Dose (mU)	Serum Concentration (U/mL)	Peak Time	Duration (from–to)	IFN Type	Reference
IFN-α						
IM	50	2,000 pg/mL	6 h	<0.5 to >24 h	α2a	106
	36	1,000 pg/mL	6 h	<0.5 to 24 h		
	18	500 pg/mL	6 h	<0.5 to 24 h		
Continuous SC infusion	2 to 5/day	20 to 60	Steady state	24 to 72 h	α2b	391
IV	4 to 10	10 to 300	30 min		Fibroblast β	392
	40 to 80	200 to 10,000	30 min			
	160 to 320	2,000 to 20,000	30 min			
IFN-β						
SC	90	10^2		1 to 8 h	β1b	393
IV	90	10^3	5 min	5 min–12 h		
IV 4-h infusion	0.01 to 1.00	<10			β1b	394
	10	25–30	6 h	0.5 to 24 h		
	30	140	4 h	0.05 to 24 h		
IV	18	1,386	<0.5 h	n.a	β1a	395
I.M.	18	7.5	10 h	n.a		
SC	18	10.4	3 h	n.a		
IFN-γ						
IV 10-min infusion	0.01 MU/m^2	150	n.a.	n.a.	γ	396
	1.0 MU/m^2	250	n.a.	n.a.		
	30.0 MU/m^2	1,000-2,000	n.a.	60 to 90 min		
	75.0 MU/m^2	n.a.	n.a.	30 to 60 min		
IV	100 mcg/m^2	n.a.	n.a.	38 min	γ-1b	397
IM	100 mcg/m^2	1.5 ng/mL	4 h	2.9 h	γ-1b	
SC	100 mcg/m^2	0.6 ng/mL	7 h	5.9 h	γ-1b	

TABLE
30.2 *Pharmacokinetics of pegylated parental IFN-alphas*

	IFN-α2a	PEG–IFN-α2a	IFN-α2b	PEG–IFN-α2b
Volume of distribution	31 to 73 L	8 to 12 L	1.4 L/kg	0.99 L/kg
Absorption t½	2.3 h	50 h	2.3 h	4.6 h
Elimination t½	3 to 8 h	65 h	4 h	~40 h
Time to max. conc.	7.3 to 12 h	80 h	7.3 to 12 h	15 to 44 h
Peak/trough		1.5		>10

t½, half-life; max. conc., maximal concentration; ∞, infinitesimal.

both agents appears comparable to historical controls treated with the parental compound.[104] Whether the alteration of IFN-α pharmacokinetics will increase antitumor activity must be addressed in future studies.

IFN-β

A single species in humans, IFN-β exists as a 23-kd glycoprotein containing 166 amino acids, and IFN-β appears to be metabolized primarily in the liver.[106] After intravenous injection, the terminal elimination half-life is about 1 to 2 hours, and IFN-β remains measurable for up to 4 hours (Table 30.1).[106] In contrast, after a single subcutaneous or intramuscular injection, serum IFN-β is barely detectable.[106] However, intravenous and subcutaneous administration of the same dose elicited similar pharmacodynamic responses, including 2 to 5 A synthetase induction—a known interferon response gene that has been correlated to dose and serum level in some studies.[106,115]

Three modifications of IFN-β to improve the pharmacokinetic profile have been developed. Albuferon is a recombinant protein resulting from fusion of the IFN-β peptide with albumin. In monkeys, the bioavailability of subcutaneous Albuferon was 87%, plasma clearance was reduced by 140-fold, and the terminal half-life increased 5-fold, while in vitro and in vivo activity was preserved.[116] Fusion of IFN-β to soluble recombinant type I IFN receptor subunit (sIFNAR-2) prolonged the half-life and increased antitumor activity in mice.[117] Finally, pegylation of IFN-β1a with a linear 20-kd molecule increased the maximum serum concentration, which is achieved 4-fold, while the AUC increased 10-fold and the half-life increased 3-fold.[118]

Since IFN-α and IFN-β signal through the same receptor, they would be expected to have similar biologic effects and have overlapping indications. However, this is not always the case. Although both IFN-α and IFN-β have activity against gliomas, one small study suggests that IFN-β has a higher response rate compared to IFN-α.[119] In contrast to IFN-α, IFN-β has been reported to have no clinical activity against CML, and no responses were seen in a phase I trial of 35 patients with metastatic solid tumors.[120,121] Two forms of IFN-β, originally named fibroblast IFN, have been approved for use in patients with relapsing multiple sclerosis—IFN-β1a (Avonex, Biogen Idec; Cambridge, MA) and IFN-β1b (Betaseron, Berlex; Montville, NJ). Their use in treatment of malignancy is currently limited to clinical trials.

IFN-γ-Type II Interferon

In contrast to type I IFN, there is only one type II IFN, IFN-γ. This molecule, a soluble homodimeric protein, is produced by DCs, lymphocyte subsets, NK cells, and natural killer T (NKT) cells.[122] IFN-γ signals through type II cytokine receptor consisting of two subunits, IFNGR1 and IFNGR2, which are associated with JAK1 and JAK2, respectively. Ligation of IFN-γ to its receptor leads to autophosphorylation and activation of JAKs that endorses the formation of STAT1 homodimerization.[123] Subsequent nuclear translocation of this homodimer complex leads to the transcription of IFN-γ–targeted genes. Through the activation of downstream molecules, IFN-γ plays diverse biological roles that orchestrate host defense immunity. IFN-γ up-regulates the expression of MHC class I, costimulatory molecules, and proteasome subunits.[124] All of which support the priming and presentation of DCs. IFN-γ can also facilitate Th1-mediated immune response while inhibiting Th2 development.[124] IFN-γ production can further recruit effector cells to the site of inflammation by up-regulating the inducible chemokines, including MIG, IP10, and I-TAC.[125–127] Recently, IFN-γ expression in the tumor microenvironment has been shown to drive "fragility" of Tregs, which plays a role in tumor immune response mediated by PD-1 blockade.[128] These positive immune-modulatory functions may suggest a role of IFN-γ in tumor surveillance, which is supported by the increased risk of spontaneous and chemically induced tumors in mice maintaining targeted disruption of IFN-γ or its receptor.

Unfortunately, IFN-γ–mediated antitumor immunity is dampened by the expression of PD-L1 checkpoint molecules in the tumor microenvironment.[129] Using shRNA hairpin screening and CRISPR technologies, studies have demonstrated that IFN-γ–mediated JAK/STAT/IRF1 signaling axis plays essential roles in PD-L1 and PD-L2 promotion. The presence of an IFN-γ gene signature has been correlated with response to PD-1 blockade across multiple tumor types.[130,131] Conversely, IFN-γ induces the expression of IDO potentially contributing to an immunosuppressive tumor microenvironment.[132,133] These findings offer the rationale for the development of PD-1 blockade therapies in combination with IFN-γ or IDO inhibitors in clinical studies.[134,135]

Clinical Pharmacology of Type II Interferon (IFN-γ)

After subcutaneous or intramuscular administration, 30% to 70% of IFN-γ is absorbed, and the terminal elimination half-life is 25 to

35 minutes; after intravenous injection, IFN-γ remains detectable in serum up to 4 hours (Table 30.1). Like IFN-β, IFN-γ appears to be metabolized primarily by the liver.[106] A phase I trial in colon cancer patients achieved IFN-γ concentrations greater than 5 U/mL for more than 6.5 hours following subcutaneous administration of 100 $\mu g/m^{2.106}$ Preclinical studies of PEG-IFN-γ show an increased elimination half-life activity with preserved activity, but this molecule has not yet been evaluated in patients.[106]

The antitumor effects of IFN-γ suggested it would be effective against a wide spectrum of malignancies. Although IFN-γ has demonstrated limited clinical utility in cancer, it likely plays a critical role in the in vivo effects of other cytokines.[136–138] Actimmune (InterMune; Brisbane, CA) is an IFN-γ preparation that has been approved for the treatment of chronic granulomatous disease.[139] Clinically significant benefit in treatment of malignancies has been largely restricted to type I interferons.

Type III Interferons

In contrast to type I IFNs, the family of type III interferons (IFN-λ) was discovered more recently in 2003. The biologic activity of IFN-λ is somewhat similar to type I IFNs. The production of these cytokines is first induced when viral infection is recognized by various PRRs. Upon binding to a cell surface expressing heterodimeric receptor consisting of IL10Rβ and IL28Rα (or IFNLR1), IFN-λ transmits signals via JAK1/TYK2-STAT1/STAT2 pathway. As a consequence, IFN-stimulated regulatory element is upregulated to orchestrate host immune responses against virus. IFN-λ exhibits antiviral activity in the epithelial lining of the respiratory, gastrointestinal, and urogenital tracts, as well as the liver. The tissue specificity is secondary to the differential expression of IL28Rα. Given IFN-λ shares similar downstream activities with type I IFNs, its therapeutic utility in malignancy is undergoing active investigation.

Clinical Indications

Hematologic Malignancies: Hairy Cell Leukemia

In clinical usage, the type I IFNs have had their most success against two hematologic malignancies, hairy cell leukemia (HCL) and CML. A regimen of IFN-α2b 2 million units/m^2 subcutaneously 3 times a week for 52 weeks produced an overall response rate of 77% with a complete response rate of 5% in patients with HCL.[140] The vast majority of these patients (61 out of 64) had undergone splenectomy, but were otherwise untreated. Subsequent studies demonstrated complete responses in 25% to 35% of patients who had not had splenectomies leading to regulatory approval for IFN in this patient population.[141] Although IFN has a significant response rate and improves survival in HCL, the majority of patients relapse after discontinuation of therapy.[142] Subsequent studies demonstrated that 80% of patients who relapsed would respond to another course of IFN.[142] It remains unclear whether IFNs effect in HCL is mediated by immune mechanisms or direct effects on the leukemic cells.[143–145] Although IFN was once considered first-line therapy, the introduction of the nucleoside analogues, which have a greater than 90% CR rate, has limited the use of IFN therapy to patients who have disease that is refractory to nucleosides or with contraindications to these agents.[146,147]

Hematologic Malignancies: Chronic Myelogenous Leukemia

Initial trials of IFN-α in CML suggested that as a single agent, IFN produced complete hematologic responses in over 50% of patients and a complete cytogenic response in up to 25% of patients.[101,148] Follow-up randomized studies demonstrated that IFN was superior to hydroxyurea or busulfan or both.[149–153] Four of these studies demonstrated an improved overall survival (OS) for the IFN-treated patients.[149,150,152–155] A meta-analysis of the randomized trials demonstrated an improvement in the 5-year survival in the IFN-treated group of 12 % over hydroxyurea and 20% over busulfan-treated patients, respectively.[156] Additionally, the meta-analysis showed the benefit extended to all risk groups. All three commercially available IFN-α were used in the CML trials, and although not formally compared, their activity in CML appeared similar.

The mechanism of response of CML to IFN has been extensively investigated. Reports that human leukocyte antigen (HLA) type and development of an immune response to BCR-Abl correlate with a complete response suggest that IFN works through an immune mechanism in patients with CML.[157] Further evidence supporting an immune mechanism of response in CML is the observation that patients who obtain a complete response correct abnormalities in the secretion of Th1 cytokines.[158] However, IFN also exerts a direct antiproliferative effect in CML through inhibition of DNA polymerase.[159] These data suggest the mechanism of action of IFN in CML is multifactorial.

In an effort to enhance the efficacy of IFN in CML, a number of trials were conducted with IFN combined with chemotherapy.[160] The combination of IFN and low-dose Ara-C was shown to improve the number of cytogenetic remissions compared to IFN alone. However, the beneficial impact of the combination on OS is small and was achieved with a substantial increase in toxicity.[161–163]

Cases of prolonged cytogenetic remission after discontinuing IFN treatment in CML have been reported.[164] Furthermore, clinical efficacy of kinase inhibitors is limited by drug resistance and intolerance. Together, these factors have reinvigorated recent interest in IFN in CML. A large multicenter and randomized trial combining weekly 90 μg of PEG-IFN with the first generation of kinase inhibitor has demonstrated significantly faster and better molecular response rates, including 12-, 18-, and 24-month rates and cumulative incidences of major molecular responses, when compared with kinase inhibitor alone.[165] Studies assessing safety and clinical efficacy of combining IFN and second generation of kinase inhibitors are actively undergoing investigation. Although largely supplanted as first-line therapy by kinase inhibitors,[166] IFN and IFN-containing regimens remain a valid second-line therapeutic option for patients with CML.[166–169]

Hematologic Malignancies: Non-Hodgkin's Lymphoma

Early studies of IFN-α monotherapy in follicular lymphomas demonstrated a response rate of over 50%.[170–172] Subsequently, a number of trials combined IFN with chemotherapy in an induction regimen or as maintenance therapy after induction were performed. The results of these trials were mixed in terms of OS benefit. The Groupe d'Etude des Lymphoma Folliculaires (GELF) study demonstrated an advantage in response rate (85% versus 69%, $P < 0.001$) and OS (34 months versus 19 months, $P = 0.02$) for chemotherapy plus IFN-**α** 5 MIU thrice weekly for 18 months compared to chemotherapy alone using an anthracycline-based regimen.[173,174] These results were a major impetus for the approval of IFN-**α** for the treatment of follicular lymphoma. A meta-analysis of the IFN trials supports a survival advantage for intensive chemotherapy regimens containing IFN.[175] Interestingly, a large SWOG trial did not show any survival advantage for IFN-**α** at 2 MIU thrice weekly for 24 months versus observation.[176] These data suggest that the dose of IFN-**α** used may be critical to the beneficial effect in patients with follicular lymphomas. IFN is approved for treatment of follicular lymphoma, but its use is limited due to associated toxicities and the activity of a variety of other agents.

Melanoma

The natural history of melanoma suggests that it is an immune-responsive tumor. Up to 25% of primary cutaneous melanomas show histologic regression at the time of biopsy.[177] All three IFN-**α**s have been investigated in patients with metastatic (stage IV) melanoma. Multiple dose levels and schedules have been tested, and the overall response rate for single-agent IFN in patients with metastatic melanoma is approximately 15%.[178–186] There is no clear best regimen in terms of response rate; however, IFN administered on thrice-weekly schedule is the most widely used schedule because it has a significantly better toxicity profile than a daily administration schedule with no diminution in response rates.[187,188] It is unknown if IFN provides a survival advantage because there are no randomized

trials in metastatic melanoma comparing IFN to either cytotoxic chemotherapy or best supportive care.[189] IFN works best in patients with low metastatic tumor burden, perhaps presaging its clinical activity in the adjuvant setting.[190]

IFN has proved most useful in the management of melanoma in the adjuvant setting. Multiple IFN regimens have been used in the adjuvant setting for patients with intermediate- and high-risk melanoma (Tables 30.3 and 30.4).[191–202] IFN was approved in Europe based on studies that used lower dose of regimens. Two trials of low-dose IFN-**α**2a given for 12 to 18 months demonstrated a benefit in relapse-free survival (RFS) in patients with melanomas greater that 1.5 mm or locoregional disease, but neither trial showed an OS benefit.[192,196] Subsequent trials using low-dose IFN-**α**2a and IFN-**α**2b have failed to demonstrate a durable RFS or an OS benefit (Table 30.3).[191,194,195,197,198,203]

In the United States, IFN was approved for adjuvant therapy in patients with high-risk melanoma based on the ECOG 1684 trial (Table 30.4).[107] In this trial, patients with high-risk melanoma defined as primary tumors greater than 4 mm or pathologic or clinical regional lymph node involvement who had undergone lymphadenectomy were treated with 1 year of high-dose IFN-**α**2b (HDI).[107] The high-dose IFN regimen consists of 20 million units/m²/d 5 days/wk for 4 weeks followed by 10 million units/m²/d thrice weekly for 48 weeks.[107] This initial trial demonstrated an overall improvement in median RFS from 1 to 1.7 years and median OS from 2.8 to 3.8 years.[107] In addition, there was a significant (42%)

TABLE

30.3   *Adjuvant trials of low- to intermediate-dose IFN for melanoma*

Trial	Number of Patients	Dose	Population	RFS	OS
WHO-16[398]	218	3 MIU SC 3×/wk × 3 y	>1.5 mm		
	208	Observation	Clinically node negative	NS	NS
NCCTG 83-7052[194]	131	20 MIU/m² IM 3×/wk × 3 mo	>1.5 mm and/or		
	131	Observation	Resected regional disease	NS	NS
French Cooperative Group[192]	244	3 MIU SC 3×/wk × 18 mo	>1.5 mm		
	245	Observation	Clinically node negative	P = 0.04	NS
Austrian Melanoma Cooperative Group[196]	154	3 MIU/d × 3 wk and then 3 MIU SQ/wk × 1 y	>1.5 mm		
	157	Observation	Clinically node negative	P = 0.02	NS
EORTC 18871[195]	244	1 MIU q od SQ × 1 y	>3.0 mm and/or		
	240	IFNg × 1 y	Resected regional disease	NS	NS
	244	observation			
Scottish Melanoma Group[197]	46	3 MIU SC 3×/wk × 6 mo	>3.0 mm and/or		
	49	Observation	Resected regional disease	NS	NS
EORTC 18952[191]	553	10 MIU/d × 4 wk then 10 MIU SQ 3×/wk × 1 y	>4.0 mm and/or		
	556	5 MIU SQ 3×/wk × 2 y	Resected regional disease	NS	NS
	279	Observation			
AIM HIGH[198]	338	3 MIU SQ 3×/wk × 2 y	>4.0 mm and/or		
	336	Observation	Resected regional disease	NS	NS

MIU, million international units; NS, not statistically significant.

TABLE

30.4 *Adjuvant trials of high-dose IFN for melanoma*

Trial	Number of Patients	Dose	Population	RFS	OS
ECOG 1684[107]	143	IFN-α2b 20 MIU/m² 5×/wk × 1 mo then 10 MIU/m² 3×/wk × 48 wk	>4.0 mm and/or Resected regional disease	$P = 0.004$	$P = 0.046$
	137	Observation			
ECOG 1690[204]	215	IFN-α2b 20 MIU/m² 5×/wk × 1 mo then 10 MIU/m² 3×/wk × 48 wk	>4.0 mm and/or Resected regional disease	$P = 0.05$	NS
	215	3 MIU SC 3×/wk × 3 y		$P = 0.17$	NS
	212	Observation			
ECOG 1694[199]	385	IFN-α2b 20 MIU/m² 5×/wk × 1 mo then 10 MIU/m² 3×/wk × 48 wk	>4.0 mm and/or Resected regional disease	$P = 0.0027$	$P = 0.0147$
	389	GM2-KLH/QS-21 vaccine			
EORTC 18991[207]	627	PEG-IFN 6 μg/kg weekly × 8 wk then 3 μg/kg weekly to 5 y	Resected regional disease	$P = 0.01$	NS
	629	Observation			
Sunbelt[202]	112	20 MIU/m² 5×/wk × 1 month then 10 MIU/m² 3×/wk × 48 wk	Single tumor-positive lymph node after SLN followed by completion lymph node dissection	NS	NS
	106	Observation			
ECOG 1697[399]	385	IFN-α2b 20 MIU/m² 5×/wk × 1 mo	>1.5 mm and/or up to three lymph nodes with microscopic disease followed by completion lymph node dissection	NS	NS
	389	Observation			
DeCOG[400]	451	PEG-IFN 180 μg subcutaneously 1×/ wk for 24 mo	stage IIa (T3a)–stage IIIb	NS	NS
	458	IFN-α2a 3 MIU subcutaneously 3×/wk; 24 mo			

MIU, million international units; NS, not statistically significant.

reduction in the risk of relapse. In a subsequent intergroup trial, ECOG 1690, an improvement in median and overall RFS was seen in the HDI arm compared to observation, but there was no difference in OS (Table 30.4).[204] The reason for the lack of an OS advantage for the HDI in this trial appeared to be related to improved survival in patients on the observation arm following relapse (6 years versus 2.8 years in ECOG 1984).[204] Multiple explanations have been postulated for this observation. In contrast to E1684, patients on E1690 were not required to undergo elective node dissection prior to enrollment on study.[107,204] Consequently, many patients were enrolled with greater than 4-mm-thick primary tumors who had no evaluation of their regional nodal basin.[204] Additionally, IFN-α received FDA approval in 1996, while E1690 was ongoing.

Consequently, many patients on the observation arm who relapsed in previously unsampled regional nodes received off protocol adjuvant IFN following therapeutic node dissection, perhaps contributing to their better than anticipated survival, while obscuring the survival benefit related to upfront IFN administration.[204]

As ECOG 1684 and1690 completed accrual, the surgical approach for melanoma was evolving, and sentinel lymph node biopsy (SLN) was being adopted as the standard of care for melanoma staging. SLN biopsy allows for accurate mapping of the draining nodal basin. SLN biopsy allows for detailed examination of the lymph node that includes standardized evaluation of more tumor sections and by immunohistochemical staining. Multiple studies have demonstrated that SLN status is the most important predictor of prognosis. Subsequent studies investigated SLN tumor burden (intranodal location, tumor penetrative depth, and maximum size of tumor deposits) as prognostic factors.[205,206] Maximum tumor size greater than 1 mm in the sentinel lymph node was the most reliable and consistent parameter independently associated with higher rates of nonsentinel lymph node involvement, poorer disease-free survival (DFS), and poorer MSS[205] and has been used to define the SLN positivity in recent EORTC adjuvant trials.

EORTC 18991 was the first large study of pegylated interferon for the treatment of melanoma in the adjuvant setting. This study randomized 1,256 patients with stage III melanoma (with the exclusion in-transit metastases) to observation or 5 years of pegylated IFN-α2b for patients.[207] During the first 8 weeks, pegylated IFN-α2b was administered at 6 μg/kg/wk for 8 weeks followed by 3 μg/kg/wk maintenance therapy for up to 5 years. Overall survival was not significantly different in the two groups; however, the IFN-treated patients showed a significant improvement in recurrence-free survival (HR 0.84, $P = 0.02$) with a median follow-up of 3.8 years. Subgroup analysis shows the greatest improvement in relapse-free survival was in the patients with microscopic nodal disease (HR 0.73 $P = 0.02$) as opposed to those with macroscopic disease (HR 0.86 $P = 0.12$)[207] supporting a role for pegylated interferon in the adjuvant treatment of melanoma. A combined subset analysis of EORTC18952 and EORTC18991 showed improvement in DFS and OS in patients with ulcerated primaries. The prognostic value of ulceration in the adjuvant setting will be investigated prospectively in EORTC 18081.[208]

The Sunbelt Melanoma Trial investigated the role of HDI in a population who underwent SLN biopsy. In this study, stage IIIA melanoma with only 1 positive LN was randomized to HDI ($n = 112$) or observation ($n = 106$) after SLN/CLND, while patients with greater than 1 LN were assigned HDI.[202] No difference in RFS or overall was seen between the arms with a median of 71 months follow-up suggesting there was no benefit associated with HDI in patients with minimal nodal disease. When the effect of ulceration was assessed, HDI was associated with improved RFS but no change in OS in contrast with the observations of the EORTC studies.[202]

ECOG 1694, a trial that compared HDI to the GM2 ganglioside conjugated to keyhole limpet hemocyanin (GM2-KLH) vaccine, showed an improvement in both RFS and OS for patients receiving HDI (Table 30.4).[199] However, the utility of GM2-KLH vaccine as a comparator was called into question after the EORTC 18961, which compared GM2-KLH vaccine to observation in patients with stage II melanoma, was stopped for futility. There was a trend toward decreased RFS rate of 1.2% (HR, 1.03; 95% CI, 0.84 to 1.25) and OS rate of 2.1% (HR, 1.16; 95% CI, 0.90 to 1.51) in the vaccine arm with 4 years of follow-up.

The ECOG adjuvant trials were stratified based on stage to ensure balance between the arms. Although not powered for subset analysis, these data were reviewed to determine if any populations disproportionately benefited from adjuvant interferon.[107,204] In ECOG 1684, the patients with microscopic involvement of their lymph nodes (stage IIIaT4pN1) had the greatest improvement in their hazard ratio when treated with IFN.[107,204] Since patients were not required to have lymphadenectomies, the group of patients who had microscopic disease was mixed in with the T4N0 subgroup in the E1690 trial.[107,204] In both studies, there was an improvement in node-positive disease that

proportionate to the patient's risk. The Sunbelt and EORTC studies in which patients had undergone SLN staging suggest the benefit in there may be limited benefit in patients with stage II and IIIA disease in the absence of ulceration. Meta-analyses of the adjuvant melanoma that have reported no RFS or OS benefit or confirmed the RFS and OS benefit have done little to clarify the utility of interferon.[209–211] An individual patient data meta-analysis of the only trials using observation as a control arm demonstrated improved RFS HR 0.86 (0.81 to 0.91) and OS HR 0.90 (0.85 to 0.97).[212] This meta-analysis demonstrated a correlation with ulceration but did not demonstrate any effect of dose on outcome.[212]

The results from adjuvant studies of newer agents including BRAF inhibitors and immune-checkpoint inhibitors report are becoming available. Ipilimumab, a fully human anti–CTLA-4 antibody, given 10 mg/kg every 3 weeks for four doses followed by dosing every 12 weeks up to 3 years was compared to placebo in stage III melanoma patients who had undergone a completion lymph node dissection. The relapse-free survival (HR = 0.76; 95% CI, 0.64 to 0.89) and overall survival (HR = 0.72; 95% CI, 0.58 to 0.88) were significantly better for the ipilimumab arm and resulted in the approval of adjuvant ipilimumab in the United States.[213] Stage III patients with mutant BRAF melanoma (V600E or V600K) who had undergone a completion lymph node dissection were randomized to the combination of dabrafenib and trametinib or placebo.[214] The 3-year relapse-free survival (HR 0.47; 95% CI 0.39 to 0.58) and overall survival (HR = 0.57; 95% CI, 0.42 to 0.79) were significantly better for the combination arm. An early report of nivolumab 3 mg/kg compared to ipilimumab 10 mg/kg both given for 1 year demonstrated an improvement in relapse-free survival for nivolumab (HR = 0.65; 97.56% CI, 0.51 to 0.83).[215] Other studies using these newer agents compared to placebo and IFN have completed accrual, but the results are not mature. Given the data from the recent IFN trials and the emergence of newer agents, the role of IFN in the adjuvant setting may become limited to patients with stage II disease with ulceration.

As with CML and NHL, combinations of IFN with chemotherapies and other cytokines have been studied in the metastatic melanoma setting in hopes of improving clinical benefit. One early single institution randomized phase II trial reported that combined IFN and dacarbazine demonstrated an improved response rate (53% versus 20%) and improved OS (18 versus 10 months) relative to dacarbazine alone.[216] Unfortunately, this benefit could not be confirmed in a larger randomized phase III trial (E3690).[189,217,218] In addition to chemotherapy, IFN has been combined with other cytokines. A trial testing the combination of a type I IFN combined with IFN-γ did not demonstrate any substantial benefit over type I IFN alone.[219] IFN-α retains a diminishing role care for adjuvant treatment of patients with high-risk melanoma, while its role in metastatic melanoma has been limited to its use in combination with other drugs in various clinical trials.

Renal Cell Carcinoma

In advanced RCC, both recombinant IFN-α2a (Roferon, Hoffmann-La Roche, Basel, Switzerland) and IFN-α2b (Intron A, Schering-Plough International, Kenilworth, NJ) have undergone extensive clinical evaluation.[220–223] There is no clinically meaningful difference between these two interferons and thus the generic

IFN-α will be used to describe these data. Despite the use of a variety of preparations, doses, and schedules, most studies have shown modest antitumor activity, with the overall response rate being approximately 10% to 15%. Responses are often delayed in onset, with median time to response being approximately 4 months. Most responses are partial and short-lived (median response duration, 6 to 7 months). Only a small number of patients have had complete responses, with only an occasional patient having a response persist in excess of 1 year after therapy. Although no clear dose-response relationship exists, daily doses in the 5- to 10-MU range appear to have the highest therapeutic index.[160,221–228]

In order to investigate a possible survival benefit to IFN-α in RCC, several randomized trials have been performed. Table 30.5 is a summary of randomized trials that have investigated the effect of IFN-α on OS in metastatic RCC patients. More recent studies have suggested the antitumor effects of IFN-α are quite limited. For example, a French Immunotherapy Group Phase III trial comparing IFN-α to both IL-2 and IL-2 plus IFN-α reported a response rate of only 7.5% for the interferon arm with a 1-year event-free survival rate of only 12%.[229] In addition, a Southwestern Oncology Group (SWOG) study comparing IFN-α alone to debulking nephrectomy followed by IFN-α reported tumor responses in less than 5% of patients receiving either treatment approach.[230]

While the role of low-dose single-agent cytokines is limited, combinations of cytokines with targeted therapy may have merit. Sorafenib and interferon have been combined in two separate single-arm phase II trials.[231,232] These trials demonstrated objective response rates of 18% and 35%. Toxicity observed was typical of that observed with each single agent with a notable reduction in hand-foot syndrome compared to sorafenib monotherapy data. Given limited efficacy and increased toxicity, a full exploration of this combination regimen was not explored in randomized trials. Two large phase III trials of interferon plus bevacizumab versus interferon alone have demonstrated superior efficacy with the combination regimen compared to cytokine monotherapy and suggested the potential of an additive effect.[233,234] However, while this combination has received FDA approval, its application has been limited by the superior therapeutic index of VEGF tyrosine kinase inhibitors.[235] Given the modest survival impact of IFN-α seen in phase III studies and its widespread application worldwide, regulatory agencies have supported the use of IFN as control arm for randomized trials with targeted therapies (e.g., sunitinib, temsirolimus) that are

described elsewhere in this book (Chapter 26). The results of these investigations have essentially eliminated the use of IFN as a single agent in advanced RCC.

Kaposi's Sarcoma

AIDS-related Kaposi's sarcoma (KS) is a multifocal vascular proliferative disease associated with HIV and Kaposi's sarcoma herpesvirus (KSHV)/human herpes virus-8 (HHV-8) coinfection.[236] Histologically, these lesions are composed of clusters of spindle-shaped cells (KS spindle cells) with prominent microvasculature. This angiogenic lesion is driven by autocrine and paracrine cytokine loops.[110,237,238] Because of the antiangiogenic activity of IFN in hemangiomas, it was tested in patients with KS.[239–241]

As a single agent for the treatment of KS, IFN has a response rate of 30% to 40% that appears to be dose-dependent.[100,242–244] When combined with antiretroviral therapy, the response rate appears to be over 40%.[245,246] Although IFN is useful in KS, initiation of effective antiretroviral therapy, cytotoxic chemotherapy, and local therapy are currently the first-line treatments.[247]

Management of Treatment-Related Adverse Events (See Table 30.6)

The enthusiasm for IFN use is tempered by its side effects. Nonetheless, the side effects are typically dose related and mostly are resolved quickly with discontinuation of treatment. The toxicities can be broken down into five major categories—constitutional, neuropsychiatric, gastrointestinal, hematologic, and autoimmune.

Constitutional symptoms are the most common with more than 80% of the patients in the high-dose IFN trials reporting fever and fatigue.[248] Additionally, more than half of patients report headache and myalgias.[248] The majority of these symptoms can be controlled with acetaminophen or NSAIDs; however, severe fatigue often requires a break from therapy with a subsequent dose reduction for amelioration.

Neuropsychiatric issues are not as common, but are potentially life-threatening. As many as 10% of patients complain of confusion and rarely (<1%) patients develop mania.[248,249] In some studies, up to 45% of patients reported depression and suicides were occasionally reported.[250,251] In one small double-blind placebo-controlled trial in patients receiving HD IFN for high-risk melanoma, prophylactic use of antidepressants significantly reduced the risk of depression from 45% to 11% after 12 weeks.[250] These data suggest that at a minimum, patients with a history of depression should be

TABLE 30.5	Interferon alpha in metastatic renal cell carcinoma			
Trial Design	No. of Patients	Response Rate Advantage for IFN-α	Overall Survival Impact	
IFN-α versus medroxyprogesterone[160]	335	10%	2.5 mo advantage for IFN-α ($P = 0.017$)	
IFN-α plus vinblastine versus vinblastine[228]	160	14%	7.0 mo advantage for IFN-α ($P = 0.0049$)	
Meta-analysis of randomized, controlled trials of IFN-α[224]	4,216 (42 trials)	11%	3.8 mo advantage for IFN-α ($P = 0.0005$)	

TABLE 30.6 Interferon-associated toxicities

Acute effects

Fever
Chills and rigors
Myalgia
Fatigue
Headache
Nausea/vomiting

Chronic effects

Constitutional
Anorexia
Fatigue
Weight loss
Headache
Nausea

Laboratory abnormalities

Transaminase elevations
Leukopenia/neutropenia
Thrombocytopenia
Anemia

Neuropsychiatric

Depression
Confusion
Dizziness/ataxia

Autoimmunity

Thyroiditis
Vitiligo

thrombocytopenia purpura (TTP) has been reported in association with IFN.[252–255] Hemolytic anemia and TTP require permanent drug discontinuation.[256–259]

In addition to autoimmune hemolytic anemia and thrombocytopenia, other manifestations of immune dysfunction can also be observed. Thyroid dysfunction in the form of hyperthyroidism or hypothyroidism occurs in about 15% of patients, and, therefore, thyroid function test should be routinely monitored in patients receiving IFN therapy.[260] The hyperthyroidism often presents as fatigue, restlessness, and/or significant weight loss and may be attributed to other causes if thyroid function tests are not checked. Sarcoidosis can occur in patients receiving IFN and can also present a diagnostic dilemma. It can present as skin lesions masquerading as subcutaneous metastases or as FDG-avid lymph nodes on PET scan.[261,262] Vitiligo, lupus, rheumatoid arthritis, polymyalgia rheumatica, and psoriasis are among the other autoimmune disorders that have been observed.[263,264] Of interest, patients who develop vitiligo or autoantibodies such as antithyroid and antinuclear antibodies during adjuvant interferon therapy for high-risk melanoma appear to have an improved relapse-free and OS relative to the total IFN-treated population, perhaps suggesting that at least in patients with melanoma, IFN mediates its antitumor effect through an autoimmune mechanism.[265] The clinician using IFN should be aware that a change in symptomatology of a patient on long-term IFN might herald the development of an autoimmune disease.

Interleukins

Interleukins have pleiotropic effects on innate and cellular immunity as well as hematopoiesis. Studies of cytokines in animal tumor models suggested that they would have broad antitumor activity. Unfortunately, only IL-2 has shown sufficient activity to obtain regulatory approval.

Interleukin-2

Biology

Interleukin-2 is one of the first immunotherapy that demonstrates clinical efficacy in cancer treatment. With careful selection criteria and appropriate supportive care, 10% of patients with metastatic melanoma and renal cell carcinoma (RCC) who received high doses of IL-2 have achieved complete response. This clinical response is durable with approximately 70% of patients maintaining complete remission for more than 25 years. The clinical application of IL-2 in cancer, however, has been limited by short in vivo half-life due to rapid clearance, significant toxicity profiles, including vascular leak syndrome, and regulatory T-cell expansion. Over the last 10 years, a better understanding of IL-2 biology has led to the development of strategies that address some of these challenges. The generation of more stable IL-2 formulations with improved selective immunostimulatory capacity has supported the further development of IL-2 immunotherapy for cancer treatment.

IL-2 was first described in 1976 as a T-cell growth factor. It is a four–alpha-helix bundle cytokine that transduces signals through IL-2 receptors. These receptors can express as monomers (IL-2Rα), dimers (IL-2Rβ and IL-2Rγ, or IL-2Rβγ), or trimers (IL-2Rα,

treated with antidepressants if they are not currently taking them at the time of IFN initiation. All other patients should be monitored closely and antidepressant therapy should be instituted at the earliest sign of depression.

Gastrointestinal side effects are common with up to one third of patients having diarrhea, which is usually well controlled with over-the-counter antidiarrheal medications.[248] Two thirds of patients have problems with nausea and anorexia. Antiemetics often alleviate the nausea; however, the combination of nausea and anorexia can lead to significant weight loss.[248] Additionally, IFN can produce significant hepatic toxicity, which requires serial monitoring of liver function tests. In the early trials, some patients had fatal hepatic failure. Usually, a drug holiday until the liver function improves followed by dose reduction allows the majority of patients with liver toxicity to continue treatment.

IFN can affect all of the hematopoietic lineages. Thrombocytopenia, leukopenia, and neutropenia are common and are typically managed with dose reductions.[248] Anemia, if not hemolytic, can be treated with transfusions or dose reductions. Rarely thrombotic

IL-2Rβ, and IL-2Rγ, or IL-2R$\alpha\beta\gamma$). IL-2 binds to these receptors at different affinities. Monomeric IL-2 receptors are either membrane bound or soluble. They recognize IL-2 with low affinity and this binding does not yield a signal. Conversely, dimeric and trimeric IL-2 receptors bind to IL-2 that lead to the stimulation of signaling cascade through multiple pathways including JAK1/3-STAT5, MAPK, and PI3K-AKT. Dimeric IL-2 receptors interact with IL-2 directly with intermediate affinity; thus, stimulation requires higher concentrations of cytokine. In the presence of all three receptor subunits, IL-2Rα sensitizes cells to low levels of IL-2 by capturing the cytokine and presenting it to IL-2R$\beta\gamma$. This reaction allows the trimeric IL-2Rs bind to IL-2 with high affinity.

IL-2 elicits a wide range of biological activities that are pleiotropic and contextual. It is both immunostimulatory and immunosuppressive. While IL-2 activates and amplifies the effector response following antigen stimulation, it promotes the survival of Tregs, which in turn maintains peripheral immune tolerance by down-regulating effector functions. These different biological effects can be attributed, at least partly, to the different expression patterns of IL-2 receptor complex on the target cells. Recent studies have established that IL-2R$\beta\gamma$ is highly expressed on effector T and NK cells, while high levels of IL-2Rα and intermediate levels of IL-2R$\beta\gamma$ are detected on Tregs. At low doses, IL-2 preferentially binds to trimeric IL-2 receptors, which expands immunosuppressive Tregs. At higher doses, once high-affinity IL-2 receptors on Tregs are saturated, IL-2 binds to dimeric IL-2 receptors leading to expansion of tumor-killing effector cells. Unfortunately, high doses of IL-2 can also trigger vascular leak syndrome and pulmonary edema in an IL-2Rα–dependent fashion.

IL-2 Signaling (See Figure 30.3)

There are several modified IL-2 formulations that are actively undergoing evaluation for the treatment of cancer. These strategies are designed with a goal to favor IL-2 to IL-2Rβ binding, biasing activity toward the expansion of effector T and NK cells. The first such preclinical data were that S4B6, a murine anti–IL-2-specific monoclonal antibody, could preferentially expand effector T-cells. It was thought that S4B6 treatment increased half-lives of IL-2 resulting in differential binding and stimulation of effector lymphocytes.[266] Alternatively, S4B6 engagement could mask the IL-2Rα binding domain on IL-2, which led to stimulation of effector cells expressing high levels of IL-2R$\beta\gamma$. Subsequently, a human IL-2 harboring structural modifying mutation that provided higher binding affinity for IL-2R$\beta\gamma$ was developed. This molecule was able to preferentially induce the activation of effector cells lacking IL-2Rα receptor.[53] Unfortunately, much like high-dose IL-2 therapy, this IL-2 formulation yielded significant toxicity when assessed in the clinical setting. Most recently, NKTR-214, a molecule comprising IL-2 bound by six releasable PEG chains with biased IL-2Rβ engagement, has demonstrated clinical efficacy as monotherapy or combined with CTLA-4 blockade in mouse melanoma.[63] Furthermore, NKTR-214 did not produce extensive toxicity from vascular leak syndrome in nonhuman primates.[63] Early-phase trials evaluating NKTR-214 as a single agent demonstrated an increase in NK cells as well as PD-1+ CD4+ and PD-1+CD8+T-cells in the peripheral blood and tumor of patients. Grade 3 hypotension that was controllable with fluids was seen in 3 of 25 patients. The toxicity profile at the doses tested appeared to be manageable in the outpatient setting which would potentially allow NKTR-214 to be combined with other immunotherapeutics in ambulatory regimens.[267]

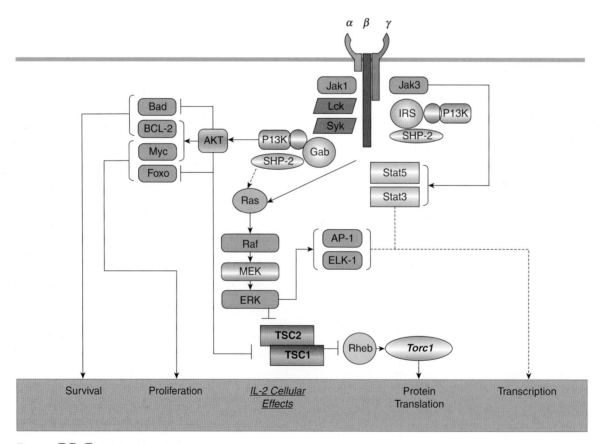

FIGURE **30.3** IL-2 signal transduction.

Pharmacologic Preparations

Several recombinant preparations of IL-2 (rIL-2) have been used clinically; however, the only preparation currently available for clinical use in the United States is aldesleukin (Prometheus Therapeutics, San Diego, CA). Aldesleukin is a recombinant IL-2 that differs from natural human IL-2 in that a cysteine residue at amino acid 125 is replaced by serine, and it also lacks the N-terminal alanine.[50] Of historical interest is the Hoffmann-La Roche rIL-2 preparation that lacks the amino acid substitution at position 125 and has an additional N-terminal methionine residue.[51] The measure of activity of IL-2 evolved during the development of these agents and understanding the differences is critical in reviewing the literature.

The international unit (IU) is the accepted standard for calculating dose of IL-2. One IU of IL-2 is defined as the reciprocal of the dilution that produces 50% of the maximal proliferation of murine HT2 cells in a short-term tritium-labeled thymidine incorporation assay described by the World Health Organization.[268] 1.1 milligram of aldesleukin contains 18 million IU of drug.[269] The Cetus unit was commonly used in the past to express doses of this cytokine, with 3×10^6 Cetus units equaling 1.1 mg of aldesleukin.[269] Hoffmann-La Roche rIL-2 contained 15.0×10^6 Cetus U/mg of protein.[269] Hank et al. found that 3 to 6 IU of Chiron rIL-2 is required for induction of the same biologic effects as 1 IU of Hoffmann-La Roche rIL-2 and a dosage of 4.5×10^6 IU/m^2/d of aldesleukin were equivalent in toxicity to a dose of 1.5×10^6 IU/m^2/d of Roche rIL-2.[269] Given these differences, care must be used in extrapolating date from the initial IL-2 literature.

Aldesleukin has a short half-life when administered as an intravenous (IV) bolus with a $t_{1/2}\alpha$ of 12.9 minutes, followed by a slower phase with a $t_{1/2}\beta$ of 85 minutes.[270] Injection of 6×10^6 IU/m^2 produces serum levels of 1,950 IU/mL, and reported clearance rate of 117 mL/min is consistent with renal filtration being the major route of elimination.[271] In an effort to simplify the dosing of IL-2, alternative routes of administration have been investigated.

Il-2 has been widely used by subcutaneous (SC) injection, and in this setting, peak serum concentrations occur at 120 to 360 minutes, the median peak serum levels of 32.1 IU/mL to 42 IU/mL with SC doses of 6×10^6 IU/m^2, which are over 50-fold lower than the levels achieved with IV dosing.[270] The serum bioavailability of IL-2 administered by the SC route can be improved by split dosing. Kirchner et al. demonstrated that the same dose of IL-2 given as two doses (10 MIU/m^2 twice daily) versus a single dose (20 MIU/m^2 daily) resulted in an almost twofold increase in the AUC with the twice-daily regimen.[272] IL-2 has also been administered by continuous infusion (c.i.) and steady-state levels are generally achieved within 2 hours.[270] Median steady-state levels of 123 IU/mL are produced by infusion of 6×10^6 IU/m^2 over 6 hours, and the levels then fall rapidly after termination of rIL-2 infusion. The clearance rate with c.i. administration is similar to that seen with bolus administration.[270] Although c.i. provides prolonged IL-2 levels, the high rate of catheter infections seen in studies has limited enthusiasm for this route of administration.[273,274]

Clinical Investigations Involving High-Dose IL-2

Investigators at the NCI Surgery Branch developed a regimen that involved the administration of high-dose intravenous bolus IL-2.[275]

In this regimen, IL-2 was administered at 600,000 to 720,000 IU/kg intravenously every 8 hours days 1 to 5 and 15 to 19 of a treatment course. A maximum of 28 to 30 doses per course was administered; however, doses were frequently withheld for excessive toxicity. Treatment courses were repeated at 8- to 12-week intervals in responding patients. During initial studies, patients underwent daily leukapheresis on days 8 to 12 during which large numbers of lymphocytes were obtained to be cultured in IL-2 for 3 to 4 days to generate lymphokine-activated killer (LAK) cells. These LAK cells were then reinfused into the patient during the second 5 day period of IL-2 administration. This high-dose IL-2 regimen with or without LAK cells produced overall tumor responses in 15% to 20% of patients with metastatic melanoma or renal cell cancer in clinical trials conducted at either the NCI Surgery Branch or within the Cytokine Working Group (formerly the Extramural IL-2 and LAK Working Group).[276] Complete responses were noted in 4% to 6% of patients with each disease and were frequently durable. Rare responses, usually partial and of shorter duration, were also noted in patients with either Hodgkin's or non-Hodgkin's lymphoma, or non–small cell lung, colorectal, or ovarian carcinoma.[277] Randomized and sequential clinical trials comparing IL-2 plus LAK cells with high-dose IL-2 alone failed to show sufficient benefit for the addition of LAK cells to justify their continued use.[278] Long-term follow-up data on patients with melanoma and renal cell cancer who were treated on the initial trials of high-dose bolus IL-2 have confirmed the durability of responses with median duration for complete responses yet to be reached. Few, if any, relapses being observed in patients in ongoing response for more than 30 months.[279,280] A substantial proportion of responding patients remain free of disease in excess of 10 years since initiating treatment. These data suggest that high-dose IL-2 treatment may actually have led to the cure of some patients with these previously incurable advanced malignancies.

Renal Cell Carcinoma

High-dose bolus interleukin 2 (IL-2) was granted Food and Drug Administration approval in 1992 based on its ability to produce durable complete responses in a small number of patients with metastatic RCC. However, the substantial toxicity and limited efficacy of IL-2 narrowed its application to highly selected patients treated at specialized centers.[279,281-284] In an attempt to reduce toxicity, several investigators evaluated alternative schedules of high-dose IL-2 and lower doses of IL-2.[285-287] Attempts were also made to improve treatment efficacy by adding IFN-α and then fluorouracil to lower-dose IL-2 regimens.[285-293] These lower-dose IL-2 regimens were reported to produce response rates and survival comparable to those reported for high-dose IL-2 with much less toxicity but possibly less durable responses. The relative merits of these low- and high-dose IL-2 regimens were clarified by four randomized trials.[229,294-296]

Taken together, these studies suggest that high-dose IV bolus IL-2 is superior in response rate and possibly response quality to regimens that involve either low-dose IL-2 and IFN-α, intermediate- or low-dose IL-2 alone, or low-dose IFN-α alone (Table 30.7). The superiority of high-dose IL-2 is particularly apparent in patients with tumor metastases in the liver or bone or who have their primary tumor in place. As a result of these trials, and the advent of molecularly targeted therapy, the application of low-dose IL-2

30.7   *Select Randomized Trials of Cytokine Therapy in Metastatic RCC*

Trial	Treatment Regimens	N	Response Rate	Durable CR (%)	Overall Survival (months)	OS Difference
FIG[229]	CIV IL-2 18 MIU/m² CIV d 1–5, 12–16	138	6.5	1	12	NS
	LD SC IFN-α 18 MIU SC TIW	147	7.5	2	13	
	CIV IL-2 + IFN-α 18 MIU/m² CIV. d 1–5, 12–16 6 × MIU SC TIW	140	18.6	5	17	
FIG[401]	MPA 200 mg PO QD	123	2.5	1	14.9	
	LD SC IFN-α 9 × MIU SC TIW	122	4.4	3	15.2	NS
	LD SC IL-2 9 MIU SC QD	125	4.1	0	15.3	
	SC IFN + SC IL-2 IFN 9 MIU SC TIW, IL-2 9 MIU SC QD	122	10.9	0	16.8	
NCI SB[296]	HD IV IL-2 720,000 IU/kg q8h D 1–5, 15–19 (max 28 doses)	156	21%	8	NR	
	LD IV IL-2 72,000 IU/kg q8h D 1–5, 15–19 (max 28 doses)	150	13%	3	NR	NS
	LD SC IL-2 250,000 IU/kg/QD × 5d wk 1, then 125,000 IU/kg/QD × 5d wk 2-6	94	10%	1	NR	
CWG[294]	LD SC IL-2/ IFN-α IL-2 5 MIU/m² sc Q8 h × 3 on day 1, then 5 d/wk for 4 wk, IFN 5 MIU/m² sc Q8 h × 3 on day 1, then TIW for 4 wk	91	10%	2	13	NS
	HD IV IL-2 600,000 IU/kg q8h D 1–5, 15–19 (max 28 doses)	95	23%	9	17.5	

HD, high dose; LD, low dose; IV, intravenous; SC, subcutaneous; PO, orally; QD, once per day; IU, international units; MIU, million IU; CIV, continuous IV infusion; NS, not statistically significant; TIW, three times per week; MPA, medroxyprogesterone acetate; NCI SB, National Cancer Institute Surgery Branch; CWG, Cytokine Working Group; FIG, French Immunotherapy Group; RR, response rate; CR, complete response.

therapy has largely ended in metastatic RCC, and high-dose IV IL-2 remains an option for appropriately selected patients with access to such therapy. However, given the toxicity and limited efficacy of high-dose IV IL-2 therapy, additional efforts should be directed at better defining the patient population for whom this therapy is appropriate.

Melanoma

HD IL-2 received regulatory approval for patients with advanced melanoma in 1998. This approval was also largely based on its demonstrated ability to produce durable complete responses in a minority of patients.[280] Data collected from multiple phase II studies showed a response rate of 16% with 6% of patients achieving a CR and 10% a PR.[280] The median response duration was 11.2 months for all responders and exceeded 59 months for patients with a CR (Fig. 30.4).[280,297] At the time of this report, no patient achieving a response lasting in excess of 30 months had relapsed. Given that follow-up on many of these patients exceeds 15 years, this durability suggests that some, if not all, of these patients may actually be cured of their disease (Fig. 30.4).

A variety of IL-2–containing regimens have been tested in patients with melanoma in an effort to improve the effectiveness of general applicability of IL-2. A study from the NCI Surgery Branch suggested the addition of a gp100 peptide vaccine to HD IL-2 might increase the response rate to 40%.[298,299] A randomized phase III trial comparing high-dose IL-2 + gp-100 vaccine to high-dose IL-2

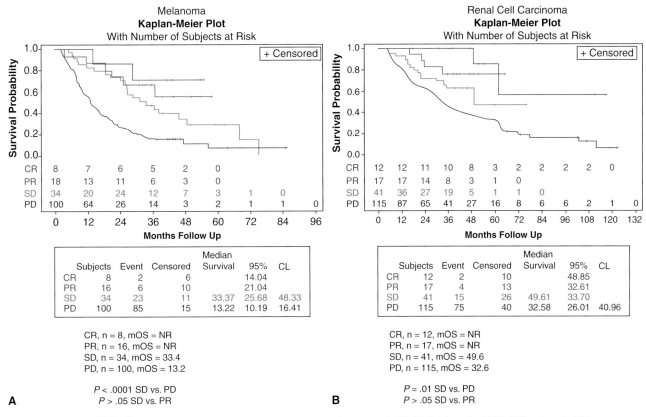

FIGURE **30.4** Kaplan-Meier estimates of overall survival in patients treated with HD IL-2 from the PROCLAIM registry **A.** OS by response (melanoma). **B.** OS by response (renal cell carcinoma). *Vertical bars* represent censored subjects. NR, not reached; F/U, follow-up.

alone revealed significant improvements in both response rate and progression-free survival in patients receiving the combination.[300] This trial offered the first evidence of a clinical benefit with vaccination in patients with melanoma, although it has not become a new standard of care.

In the 1990s, biochemotherapy regimens were developed under the hypothesis that the combination of chemotherapy and cytokines would increase response rates and lead to an increase in the number of durable responses. The phase II data suggested these regimens had response rates in excess of 40% with up to 10% of patients achieving a durable benefit.[301–305] Unfortunately, randomized trials showed no survival advantage to biochemotherapy compared to chemotherapy alone.[306–311]

Investigators have also continued to pursue IL-2 together with cellular therapy approaches. IL-2 and tumor-infiltrating lymphocyte (TIL) combinations were extremely promising in animal tumor models.[312] Interest in adoptive immunotherapy has been revived by an NCI Surgery Branch study involving the administration of clonally expanded, tumor antigen–specific CD8$^+$ lymphocytes and IL-2 following chemotherapy and radiation-induced lymphodepletion that showed encouraging antitumor activity in patients with refractory melanoma.[313–315] Clinical studies are underway to determine if this approach can be streamlined and exported outside the NIH.[316]

Toxicity

The utility of high-dose IL-2 has been limited by toxicity, many features of which resemble bacterial sepsis. Side effects are dose-dependent and, fortunately, largely predictable and rapidly reversible. Common side effects include fever, chills, lethargy, diarrhea, nausea, anemia, thrombocytopenia, eosinophilia, diffuse erythroderma, hepatic dysfunction, and confusion.[317] Myocarditis also occurs in approximately 5% of patients. IL-2 therapy also commonly produces a "capillary leak syndrome," leading to fluid retention, hypotension, early adult respiratory distress syndrome, prerenal azotemia, and occasionally myocardial infarction. As a consequence of these side effects, few patients are able to receive all of the scheduled therapy. IL-2 has also been shown to produce a neutrophil chemotactic defect that predisposes patients to infection with gram-positive and occasionally gram-negative bacteria.[318] Early high-dose IL-2 studies were associated with 2% to 4% mortality, largely related to infection or cardiac toxicity.[280,317] The routine use of antibiotic prophylaxis, more extensive cardiac screening, and the more judicious IL-2 administration have greatly enhanced the safety of this therapy; since 1990, the mortality rates at experienced treatment centers have been less than 1% (Table 30.8).[319,320] Nonetheless, the considerable toxicity of the high-dose IL-2 regimen has continued to limit its application to highly selected patients with excellent performance status and adequate organ function treated at medical centers with considerable experience with this approach.

Laboratory studies have suggested that the toxicity of IL-2 appears to be in part mediated by the release of secondary cytokines such as TNF-α, IL-1, and IL-6.[321] Nonetheless, attempts to block the toxicity of IL-2 by the coadministration of soluble receptors of IL-1 or TNF; CNI-1493, an inhibitor of IL-1 and TNF signaling; or M40403, a nonpeptidyl mimic of superoxide dismutase, have yielded only a modest reduction in the hypotension, vascular leak, and other serious side effects routinely observed in patients receiving high-dose IL-2.[322–326]

30.8 *Safety of High-Dose IV Bolus rIL-2 Therapy (720,000 IU/kg q8h): The NCI Experience*

- Incidence of grade 3 to 4 adverse events has been greatly reduced*

Adverse Event	1985 Incidence	1997 Incidence
Hypotension	81%	31%
Diarrhea	92%	12%
Neuropsychiatric toxicity	19%	8%
Line sepsis	18%	4%
Pulmonary complications	12%	3%

- With patient selection and experience managing side effects, high-dose rIL-2 is safe
- No treatment-related deaths in 809 consecutive patients treated at the NCI[319]
- No treatment-related deaths in 362 patients 2005 to 2012 in PROCLAIM registry[320]

Management of Patients Receiving High-Dose Interleukin-2

The safe administration of high-dose IL-2 requires a careful selection of patients capable of tolerating the fever, hypotension, and edema that often develops during treatment. As such, high-dose IL-2 should be considered a reasonable treatment option only in patients without significant cardiac disease (i.e., angina, congestive heart failure, arrhythmia, or prior myocardial infarction). Patients over 40 years of age should undergo stress testing and those found to have exercise-induced ischemia should be excluded. Patients should be specifically screened for CNS metastases, and those with a positive head CT scan or MRI should not be given high-dose IL-2. Patients should also have adequate renal, hepatic, and pulmonary function with a serum creatinine less than 1.6 mg/dL, bilirubin less than 1.5 mg/dL, and a forced expiratory volume (FEV1) of greater than 2 L. They should also have an ECOG performance status of less than 2.

Once a decision is made to offer high-dose IL-2 to a patient, the various treatment-associated side effects can be ameliorated by the concomitant administration of acetaminophen and indomethacin to reduce fever and chills, H2 blockers to prevent gastritis, and prophylactic antibiotics to prevent central line–associated infections.[317] Patients should receive antiemetics and antidiarrheals as needed. IL-2–induced pruritus and dermatitis can be minimized with diphenhydramine, gabapentin, and various skin creams. Glucocorticoids should be avoided since they antagonize the immunostimulatory properties of IL-2. Hypotension is best managed initially with fluid replacement, but many patients require intravenous dopamine and, in some instances, both dopamine and phenylephrine. Most patients require supplemental IV sodium bicarbonate to prevent acidosis. In the event of life-threatening toxicity (e.g., hypotension refractory to pressors), the IL-2 is discontinued but may be resumed after the resolution of the problem. Generally, doses of IL-2 withheld because of toxicity are not made up at the end of a treatment cycle. With careful patient selection and the appropriate use of concurrent medications, most patients can safely receive high-dose IL-2; however, the unusual array and severity of treatment side effects mandate that this form of immunotherapy be administered by a team of physicians and nurses experienced in the use of this agent.

Summary

While the clinical application of IL-2 has benefited only a small portion of patients with either melanoma or renal cancer to date, it can produce durable benefit in a small but reproducible portion of patient with these diseases. Unfortunately, efforts to build on the successes seen with high-dose IL-2 alone have been disappointing. The hurdles of the inpatient high-dose IL-2 regimen in the era of immune-checkpoint inhibitors has helped accelerate the development of new IL-2 formulations. These newer formulations appear to have a reduced toxicity profile while still maintaining efficacy and thus may be more amenable to combination with newer agents. Correlative biomarker investigations associated with clinical trials suggest that the potential exists for identifying predictors of response (or resistance) and limiting IL-2 therapy to those most likely to benefit. This will be discussed in more detail below.

Interleukin-7

Interleukin-7 (IL-7) was first described in the 1980s as a member of IL-2 superfamily. It is mostly secreted from the inflammatory cells and the stromal structure in the bone marrow and the thymus. This molecule binds to a γc receptor subunit. Productive signaling through this complex results in activation of JAK1 or JAK3. This reaction transduces molecular signals through STAT5, PI3 kinase, and SRC kinases that ultimately drive the IL-7–specific gene expression. Preclinical studies in animal models have demonstrated the fundamental role of IL-7 in the remodeling, development, proliferation, and homeostasis of T-cells.[327] This critical role is underscored in patients with severe combined immune deficiency (SCID) whose IL-7 pathway is functional deficient due to loss-of-function mutations in IL-7R.[328,329]

Given its role in T-cell proliferation, IL-7 has been an attractive therapeutic target in immunotherapy. It has been shown that IL-7 induces tumoricidal activity against human melanoma line through the promotion of IL-1α, IL-1β, and TNFα production.[330] When compared to IL-2, IL-7 appears to differentially expand CTL population more effectively.[331] IL-7 can further augment antigen-specific CTL activity. Two early-phase clinical studies have shown that the administration of recombinant IL-7 led to the improvement of CD4$^+$ and CD8$^+$ T-cell counts in a dose-dependent manner without significant systemic toxicity observed.[332] This increase did not change the number of other cell lineages significantly, including B-cell, NK cell, or Treg. In view of these observations, clinical applications of IL-7 may stem from improving immune function without significant undesirable outcomes.

Interleukin-10

Interleukin-10 (IL-10), a secretory homodimeric protein, was first discovered as a major modulator for the induction of tolerance by impeding the activity of effector T-cells and type II IFN-mediated immunity. IL-10 is produced by a wide variety of hematopoietic cells, notably DCs, macrophages, Tregs, and among others. Productive binding between IL-10 and its receptor instigates a cascade of molecular events that activate JAK/STAT3 pathway. IL-10–mediated signal transduction subsequently upregulates anti-inflammatory signature that leads to lower expression of MHC class II and costimulatory molecules B7-1/B7-2 on macrophages, as well as limited production of proinflammatory cytokines.[333] Furthermore, IL-10–expressing DCs receive autocrine IL-10 signaling that can lead to restricted draining lymph node trafficking. Together, the suppressive effects of IL-10 on DCs and macrophages indirectly inhibit T-cell effector function and Th1 response. While IL-10 functions as an efficient suppressive cytokine, it has the ability to activate T-cells against tumor.

Exogenous IL-10 has been shown to reduce growth of syngeneic melanoma and TSA mammary adenocarcinoma.[334] Interestingly, the mechanisms by which IL-10 controls cancer stem from its stimulation on NK and effector T-cells: increasing the intratumoral CTLs infiltration, enhancing the production of IFN-γ, and intratumoral tumor antigen presentation.[335] There have been several early-phase efforts that assessed the safety of pegylated recombinant IL-10. One report has demonstrated that the pegylated formulation of IL-10 is immunologically active in patients with advanced solid tumors.[336] Although grade 3 or 4 treatment-related rash, transaminitis, anemia, or thrombocytopenia was observed, all treatment-related adverse effects seemed to be manageable. Further assessment of pegylated IL-10 as monotherapy or in combination with chemotherapy or checkpoint inhibitor targeting PD-1 is actively pursued.

Interleukin-12

Interleukin-12 (IL-12) was first recognized in the late 1980s as a cytotoxic lymphocyte maturation factor and a natural killer-cell stimulatory factor. It possesses a broad spectrum of physiologic functions, encompassing both immune and nonimmune activities. This perhaps stems from the ability of IL-12 to potently induce the production of IFN-γ. IL-12, a cytokine family of four heterodimeric members comprising a 35-kD and a 40-kD subunit, acts through JAK/STAT-associated type I cytokine receptor. This molecule is primarily produced by DCs and phagocytes in response to toll-like receptor engagement. IL-12 production can further be intricately regulated by proinflammatory and immunosuppressive molecules. To date, the most well-documented biological activity of IL-12 involves the differentiation of naïve CD4+ T-cells into Th1 lineage. Other essential roles of IL-12 in immune modulation include the potentiation of the effector function of NK, CTLs, and CD4+ T-cells, the augmentation of antibody-dependent cellular cytotoxicity (ADCC), and the manipulation of immunoglobulin production from B-cells.

Despite the proinflammatory immune activities that make IL-12 an ideal candidate for immunotherapy, its potent antiangiogenic property ignited a flurry of research activity in antitumor analysis.[337] This antiangiogenic property is IFN-γ dependent. In experimental models, IL-12 has proven to be an effective agent against glioma, hepatocellular carcinoma, leukemia, mammary carcinoma, melanoma, and sarcoma.[338] Although its application against tumor was promising in mice, the application of IL-12 was

challenged by both life-threatening toxicities and insufficient clinical efficacy in clinical trials. In one of the original early-phase trials, the administration of recombinant IL-12 led to 2 deaths and 12 hospitalizations in 17 renal cell cancer patients who received the experimental regimen. This resulted in a thorough investigation with a conclusion that the systemic administration of IL-12 carries a significant schedule-dependent adverse toxicity, which can be reduced with a single test dose of IL-12 2 weeks prior to the initiation of the treatment dose.[339] In other clinical studies, IL-12, used as monotherapy or combined with other agents, has produced marginal clinical efficacy.[338] It was found that repeated administration of recombinant IL-12 led to a progressive decline of IFN-γ concentration in the serum and a steadily increase of IL-10 production that may limit the overall durable therapeutic effect.[340] Strategies to overcome this negative feedback mechanism are actively under investigation in local delivery and in tumor vaccine therapy, especially in the context of a therapeutic combination, such as checkpoint blockade.

Interleukin-15

Interleukin-15 (IL-15), a member of the four–alpha-helix bundle family of cytokines, was first reported in 1994 as a T-cell growth factor. The main sources of this cytokine are monocytes, macrophages, and DCs. The expression of IL-15 protein is strictly regulated by posttranscriptional machinery despite the abundant expression of IL-15 transcripts. These regulatory mechanisms maintain a pool of IL-15 transcripts and limit its protein production at homeostasis. When cells are stimulated by soluble molecules, such as GM-CSF, double-strand mRNA, or lipopolysaccharide (LPS) in the presence of surrounding insults, IL-15 transcripts are translated into final protein product for secretion. Once secreted, IL-15 facilitats the establishment of of a proinflammatory environment through regulation of transcription, translation, and protein trafficking. IL-15 molecules signal through a heterotrimeric receptor that is composed of a unique IL-15α subunit, a shared β subunit with IL-2R, and a common γc receptor subunit. IL-15 activity is initiated through a cell-cell interaction where IL-15Rα subunits on one cell surface present bound IL-15 molecules to β-γc on neighboring effector NK or T-cells. Presentation of membrane-bound IL-15 to γc complex activates the JAK/STAT pathways, Syk kinase and PLCγ, Lck kinase, and Shc resulting in the expression of prosurvival and antiapoptotic signals. As a consequence, IL-15 induces T-cell proliferation that resembles IL-2 activity. Based on the functional characterization, IL-15 can further facilitate the generation of CTLs and NK cells, as well as the long-term maintenance of effector memory T-cells. Unlike IL-2, IL-15 maintains effector cell population and function without affecting the Treg cohort.[10] This may offer a potential immunotherapeutic advantage that optimizes immunostimulation. To date, several clinical trials using recombinant IL-15 as monotherapy or in combination with patient-derived tumor-infiltrating CTLs or NK cells as immunotherapeutic strategy in patients with advanced solid malignancies are ongoing.[341,342] However, recent studies have suggested that the clinical utility of recombinant IL-15 may be limited by a short half-life in vivo. Moreover, soluble IL-15Rα has been shown to stabilize IL-15 with a heightened pharmacokinetic property; therapeutic strategies using soluble IL-15Rα-IL-15 complex in various clinical scenarios are under active investigation.[343]

Interleukin-18

Structurally related to IL-1, IL-18 was first identified as a cytokine that stimulates the production of type II IFNs. In addition, IL-18 has been shown to stimulate immune effector response that activates macrophages, promotes lineage differentiation of Th1 CD4[+] T-cells, and enhances cytotoxicity activity of CTLs by upregulating FasL expression. Preclinical data suggest that administration of IL-18 results in tumor rejection through activation of NK and effector T lymphocytes. Early-phase clinical trial of recombinant IL-18 has demonstrated safety without reaching dose-limiting toxicity although clinical efficacy has been modest.[344] Thus, its application in immunotherapy requires further clinical investigation.

Interleukin-21

Analogous to other members of IL-2 superfamily, IL-21, a four–alpha-helix bundle cytokine, signals through a heterodimeric receptor consisting of a IL-21 receptor subunit and a shared common γc receptor subunit. IL-21 transduces signals via JAK/STAT1 or STAT3, PI3K, and MAPK pathways that ultimately translates into cellular behavior, proliferation, survival, lineage commitment, and other biological activities.[11] Given its pleiotropism, IL-21 can orchestrate innate and adaptive immune response by modulating behaviors of almost all lymphocyte subsets, DCs, and to a lesser degree monocyte. IL-21 is first secreted by activated CD4[+] T-cells and NKT cells. IL-21 can work in concert with other activating cytokines or molecules to enhance NK cell cytotoxicity and to promote CD4+ T cell and CTL proliferation. IL-21 can further facilitate the molecular machinery that supports the production of antigen-specific antibody in B-cells without promoting non–specific B-cell activation.

The broad spectrum of proinflammatory immune-modulatory activities of IL-21 has made it a promising immunotherapeutic target in cancer care. In orthotopic transplantation models, administration of exogenous IL-21 alone or in combination that targets multiple pathways results in syngeneic tumor regression.[345] In the experience of first two phase I clinical studies, recombinant IL-21 in melanoma or RCC patient cohort was generally well tolerated with manageable toxicity.[346,347] The clinical responses have been modest. More recent efforts have been focused on combination regimens targeting immunostimulation, specifically checkpoint blockade targeting CTLA-4 and PD-1.

GM-CSF

Granulocyte-macrophage colony–stimulating factor (GM-CSF) was first described as a hematopoietic growth factor. GM-CSF has now been assigned a role in regulating mature myeloid compartment in steady state and inflammation. GM-CSF is secreted as a monomeric glycoprotein. The cognate receptor for GM-CSF, a heterodimer comprising a GM-CSF–specific α subunit and a common β subunit (shared with IL-3 and IL-5 receptors), transduces inflammatory and prosurvival signatures via JAK2/STAT5 and PI3K pathways, respectively.[348,349]

GM-CSF maintains a low basal level under homeostatic conditions, but it is inducible at sites of infection or inflammation. Many cells have been identified as significant sources of GM-CSF, including endothelial cells, fibroblasts, hematopoietic cells, stromal cells, and tumors.[348,349] Proinflammatory molecules and microbial particles are potent positive modulators of GM-CSF. Once expressed, GM-CSF favors an inflammatory milieu by inducing proinflammatory cytokine production, promoting M1 macrophage development, and enhancing the recruitment of inflammatory monocytes. Furthermore, GM-CSF may facilitate the development of monocyte-derived DCs and the activation of conventional DCs in the skin and the gut lining. Its clinical utility in cancer treatment has been suggested in a report that forced expression of GM-CSF in a murine melanoma vaccine led to robust and specific antitumor immunity.[350] In this setting, it was thought that exogenous GM-CSF would recruit and activate inflammatory DCs to enhance tumor-specific antigen presentation. This concept laid the foundation for the development of clinical trials that utilize GM-CSF as a part of tumor vaccines.

Although early-phase clinical trials using GM-CSF in solid tumors demonstrated safety and activity, a phase III study in which patients with high-risk resected melanoma was given adjuvant GM-CSF yielded a negative result.[351] Recent success of immunotherapy with a favorable toxicity profile in a wide spectrum of cancers has revitalized the application of GM-CSF. Thus, the combination of checkpoint blockade and GM-CSF is actively undergoing investigation. In another notable approach, local administration of oncolytic virus talimogene laherparepvec/T-VEC (Amgen, Thousand Oaks, CA), an attenuated strain of herpes simplex virus type 1 encoding GM-CSF, has provided durable disease control in patients with unresectable recurrent melanoma leading to its approval in the use.[352] How best to integrate oncolytic viral-based therapies with cytokines or newer immunotherapies is an area of active investigation.[353]

Predictors of Response to Cytokine Therapy

Cytokine therapy has produced durable responses in melanoma and RCC. The majority of patients, however, are exposed to substantial toxicity with only a small percentage obtaining clinical benefit. Potential predictive markers have been studied in an effort to prospectively identify the subset of patients most likely to benefit from cytokines.

In melanoma patients receiving high-dose IL-2, tumor responses were more likely in patients who exhibited a good performance status (ECOG performance status 0) and who had not received prior systemic therapy.[354] Patients with cutaneous metastases and HLA Cw7 have been reported to be more likely to respond IL-2–containing therapy.[190,355,356] Response to HD IL-2 for melanoma also has been reported to be higher in patients with autoimmunity phenomenon such as thyroid dysfunction or vitiligo, low pretreatment IL-6 levels, and low pretreatment CRP levels.[356–359] More recently, response to IL-2 therapy has been correlated with pretreatment serum levels of VEGFs and fibronectin and tumor RNA expression of immunoregulatory genes as well as normal baseline LDH.[360–362] The mutational status of melanomas predicts for higher responses in patients treated with high-dose IL-2 tumors with NRAS-mutant melanomas having a response rate of 47% in contrast to BRAF mutant (23%) and WT (12%).[362] Unfortunately, the presence of specific mutations did not correlate with relapse-free or OS. While these investigations have enhanced the understanding of the mechanisms underlying the antitumor effects of IL-2 activity, for the most part, they do not aid in the selection of patients with melanoma for IL-2–based therapy as they lack prospective validation.

The development of autoimmunity during adjuvant IFN treatment for melanoma is associated with a dramatic improvement in survival.[265] These data combined with the observation that patients with ulcerated primaries have an improved outcome with adjuvant interferon therapy supports the hypothesis that only a subgroup of patients benefit from interferon therapy.[208] Whether patients who present with ulcerated primaries and those who develop autoimmunity while receiving IFN represent groups of patients who have IFN-responsive disease remains to be determined in prospective trials.

The correlation of autoimmunity with response has led to the investigation of polymorphisms of immune pathways as predictors of response. Single nucleotide polymorphisms (SNPs) may serve as prognostic or predictive markers due to their linkage to variable expression of critical genes. For example, SNPs that reportedly alter IL-10 and IFN-γ expression are associated with response to biochemotherapy.[363] Perhaps paradoxically, SNPs related to increased IL-10 and decreased IFN-γ expression have been associated with good prognosis calling into question the mechanism of this linkage or the validity of these results.[363-366] Clearly more research is needed to sort out the influence of genotype variations on the antitumor effects of various cytokine-based immunotherapies.

For patients with kidney cancer, tumor response has been associated with ECOG performance status, number of metastatic sites, the degree of treatment-related thrombocytopenia, thyroid dysfunction, rebound lymphocytosis erythropoietin production, low pretreatment IL-6 levels, and posttreatment elevations of blood TNFα and IL-1 levels.[367] Additional retrospective studies suggested that the histologic pattern of the renal cancer also correlates with the probability of response to IL-2.[368] Response rates as high as 40% have been seen in patients whose primary tumors possessed favorable histologic features, such as clear cell histology with alveolar, but no papillary or granular, cell components, while patients whose tumors displayed papillary or greater than 50% granular features were unlikely to respond. While this correlation was independently confirmed in an examination of metastatic lesions, prospective validation is lacking. Additional immunohistochemical studies suggested that the expression of the G250 antigen (carbonic anhydrase IX) on a large percentage of renal cancer cells is also associated with an increased likelihood of benefit from IL-2 treatment.[369,370] Unfortunately, a prospective trial designed to validate these biomarkers in RCC did not meet its primary endpoint. It is possible that additional molecular studies (e.g., RNA expression signatures) on tumor tissue obtained before therapy may ultimately lead to more definitive predictors of responsiveness to cytokine-based therapy and thereby limit this intensive and toxic therapy to those most likely to benefit.

Strategies for Overcoming Resistance to Immunotherapy

The immunosurveillance hypothesis suggests that tumors are constantly under attack from the immune system. The natural extension of this hypothesis, "immunoediting," suggests tumors are constantly under selective pressure that favors clones that can escape the onslaught of the immune system.[4] Thus, even when immune responses are seen in patients, they often do not correlate with clinical benefit since the tumors may have already undergone "immune escape."

Tumors utilize two broad strategies to escape immunosurveillance—altered antigen presentation/T-cell response and immunosuppression. Tumor cells have down-regulated MHC class I molecules, CD80 (B7-1), CD86 (B7-2), and ICAM-1, which are important for antigen presentation and activation of CD8$^+$ CTLs.[371] In addition to tumor-specific defects, down-regulation of the T-cell signaling components, zeta chain and Lck, is seen in a number of malignancies.[372,373] The IFNs upregulate MHC I and MHC II and IL-2 has been shown to restore zeta chain and Lck expression on T-cells.[372,373]

Malignancies induce an immunosuppressive microenvironment by multiple mechanisms. Tumors secrete a number of cytokines that are potentially immunosuppressive such as IL-10, TGF-β, and IL-6.[374-378] Also, nutrient-catabolizing enzymes such as IDO and arginase contribute to an immunosuppressive environment and are attractive therapeutic targets.[379,380] Multiple arginase and IDO inhibitors are undergoing clinical investigation, and early studies suggest these agents may improve efficacy when combined with immune-checkpoint inhibitors with little change in the toxicity profile.[134,381-383] The utility of these agents when combined with cytokines has yet to be tested.

Tumor cells are protected by mechanisms designed to prevent autoimmune disease. Expression of CLTA-4 on activated T-cells and PD-L1 expression on tumors limits the immune response. Invariant NKT (iNKT) cells, CD4$^+$CD25$^+$ T-regulatory cells (Tregs), Th3 cells, and type I regulatory cells are all immunoregulatory T-cells that are part of the natural course of an immune response. The fact that the induction of a tumor-focused immune response does not correlate with clinical benefit suggests that some of these of immune escape mechanisms are operating in vivo.

Treg numbers increase with HD IL-2 in most patients.[384,385] In one study, objective response in melanoma and RCC patients correlated with a subsequent decrease in Tregs four weeks after HD IL-2 therapy.[384] These data support the hypothesis that regulatory cells may inhibit responses to immunotherapy.

Efforts to deplete Tregs, Th3 cells, and type I regulatory T-cells have included the use of the anti-CD25 agent, denileukin diftitox (Ontak), and lymphodepletion. A single dose of Ontak has been shown to deplete circulating regulatory T-cell populations and enhances the antitumor response to DC-based vaccines.[386,387] Ontak as a single agent induced responses in 5 out of 16 melanoma patients that were associated with transient depletion of Tregs with the development of MART-1–specific CD8$^+$ T cells in one patient.[388] In contrast, investigators at the NCI using a different dosing schedule did not observe reductions of Tregs based on Foxp3 expression.[389] Whether these differences are due to patient selection or methodology remains to be determined. The NCI Surgery Branch piloted a strategy of lymphodepletion using fludarabine and cyclophosphamide to deplete immunoregulatory cells followed by adoptive transfer of T-cells and IL-2 therapy. This regimen produced a response rate of 50% in patients who were previously resistant to IL-2–based immunotherapy.[313,314] Ipilimumab that blocks the activation CTLA-4 has resulted in a survival benefit in melanoma patients leading to FDA approval in 2011.[38] The addition of this agent to HD IL-2 therapy in a phase Ib/II study resulted in a higher response than would have been expected with either agent alone but did not appear to be synergistic.[390] The early reports of enhanced clinical activity with NKTR-214 combined with PD-1 blockade are promising but need to be confirmed with Phase III studies.[402] These early results suggest that strategies to disrupt the immunosuppressive microenvironment of the tumor may significantly enhance the efficacy of cytokines in the treatment of cancer.

Conclusion

Preclinical data suggested cytokine-based therapies would have efficacy against a broad spectrum of malignancies. Unfortunately, only IFN and IL-2 have found a place in the therapeutic armamentarium against cancer. IL-2 can reproducibly produce long-term remissions in patients with metastatic melanoma or RCC; however, the use of high-dose IL-2 is waning since the introduction of immune-checkpoint inhibitors. Efforts focused on improved patient selection for IFN and IL-2 therapy have not as of yet allowed for the selection patients with low likelihood of response to pursue other treatment options and avoid significant toxicity. The development of novel formulations such as those being pursued for IL-2 that result lower toxicity while maintaining efficacy holds the promise of extending the clinical benefits of cytokines to larger populations of patients as monotherapy and combined with newer agents. While the success of cytokines has been modest to date, the development of novel immune response modulators offers multiple avenues to expand the use of cytokines as a critical component of a curative strategy in the treatment of metastatic solid tumors.

References

1. Dunn GP, et al. A critical function for type I interferons in cancer immunoediting. *Nat Immunol.* 2005;6(7):722-729.
2. Kaplan DH, et al. Demonstration of an interferon gamma-dependent tumor surveillance system in immunocompetent mice. *Proc Natl Acad Sci U S A.* 1998;95(13):7556-7561.
3. Dunn GP, et al. Cancer immunoediting: from immunosurveillance to tumor escape. *Nat Immunol.* 2002;3(11):991-998.
4. Dunn GP, Old LJ, Schreiber RD. The immunobiology of cancer immunosurveillance and immunoediting. *Immunity.* 2004;21(2):137-148.
5. Spear P, et al. NKG2D ligands as therapeutic targets. *Cancer Immun.* 2013;13:8.
6. Guillerey C, Huntington ND, Smyth MJ. Targeting natural killer cells in cancer immunotherapy. *Nat Immunol.* 2016;17(9):1025-1036.
7. Martín-Fontecha A, et al. Regulation of dendritic cell migration to the draining lymph node: impact on T lymphocyte traffic and priming. *J Exp Med.* 2003;198(4):615-621.
8. Dranoff G. Cytokines in cancer pathogenesis and cancer therapy. *Nat Rev Cancer.* 2004;4(1):11-22.
9. Chow MT, Luster AD. Chemokines in cancer. *Cancer Immunol Res.* 2014;2(12):1125-1131.
10. Steel JC, Waldmann TA, Morris JC. Interleukin-15 biology and its therapeutic implications in cancer. *Trends Pharmacol Sci.* 2012;33(1):35-41.
11. Spolski R, Leonard WJ. Interleukin-21: basic biology and implications for cancer and autoimmunity. *Annu Rev Immunol.* 2008;26:57-79.
12. Gardner A, Ruffell B. Dendritic cells and cancer immunity. *Trends Immunol.* 2016;37(12):855-865.
13. Dunn GP, Koebel CM, Schreiber RD. Interferons, immunity and cancer immunoediting. *Nat Rev Immunol.* 2006;6(11):836-848.

14. Ma, A., Koka R, Burkett P. Diverse functions of IL-2, IL-15, and IL-7 in lymphoid homeostasis. *Annu Rev Immunol.* 2006;24:657-679.
15. Morris-Stiff G, et al. Transmission of donor melanoma to multiple organ transplant recipients. *Am J Transplant.* 2004;4(3):444-446.
16. Kauffman HM, McBride MA, Delmonico FL. First report of the United Network for Organ Sharing Transplant Tumor Registry: donors with a history of cancer. *Transplantation.* 2000;70(12):1747-1751.
17. Stewart TJ, Abrams SI. How tumours escape mass destruction. *Oncogene.* 2008;27(45):5894-5903.
18. Sucker A, et al. Acquired IFNgamma resistance impairs anti-tumor immunity and gives rise to T-cell-resistant melanoma lesions. *Nat Commun.* 2017;8:15440.
19. Yu H, Pardoll D, Jove R. STATs in cancer inflammation and immunity: a leading role for STAT3. *Nat Rev Cancer.* 2009;9(11):798-809.
20. Yu H, Kortylewski M, Pardoll D. Crosstalk between cancer and immune cells: role of STAT3 in the tumour microenvironment. *Nat Rev Immunol.* 2007;7(1):41-51.
21. Sharma P, et al. Primary, adaptive, and acquired resistance to cancer immunotherapy. *Cell.* 2017;168(4):707-723.
22. Rabinovich GA, Gabrilovich D, Sotomayor EM. Immunosuppressive strategies that are mediated by tumor cells. *Annu Rev Immunol.* 2007;25:267-296.
23. Sumimoto H, et al. The BRAF-MAPK signaling pathway is essential for cancer-immune evasion in human melanoma cells. *J Exp Med.* 2006;203(7):1651-1656.
24. Mellman I, Coukos G, Dranoff G. Cancer immunotherapy comes of age. *Nature.* 2011;480(7378):480-489.
25. Bierie B, Moses HL. Transforming growth factor beta (TGF-beta) and inflammation in cancer. *Cytokine Growth Factor Rev.* 2010;21(1):49-59.
26. Munn DH, Mellor AL. IDO in the tumor microenvironment: inflammation, counter-regulation, and tolerance. *Trends Immunol.* 2016;37(3):193-207.
27. Deaglio S, et al. Adenosine generation catalyzed by CD39 and CD73 expressed on regulatory T cells mediates immune suppression. *J Exp Med.* 2007;204(6):1257-1265.
28. Zou W. Immunosuppressive networks in the tumour environment and their therapeutic relevance. *Nat Rev Cancer.* 2005;5(4):263-274.
29. Bogdan C. Nitric oxide and the immune response. *Nat Immunol.* 2001;2(10):907-916.
30. Rodriguez PC, et al. Arginase I in myeloid suppressor cells is induced by COX-2 in lung carcinoma. *J Exp Med.* 2005;202(7):931-939.
31. Talmadge JE. Pathways mediating the expansion and immunosuppressive activity of myeloid-derived suppressor cells and their relevance to cancer therapy. *Clin Cancer Res.* 2007;13(18 Pt 1):5243-5248.
32. Vignali DA, Collison LW, Workman CJ. How regulatory T cells work. *Nat Rev Immunol.* 2008;8(7):523-532.
33. Tanaka A, Sakaguchi S. Regulatory T cells in cancer immunotherapy. *Cell Res.* 2017;27(1):109-118.
34. Khaled YS, Ammori BJ, Elkord E. Myeloid-derived suppressor cells in cancer: recent progress and prospects. *Immunol Cell Biol.* 2013;91(8):493-502.
35. Bronte V, et al. Recommendations for myeloid-derived suppressor cell nomenclature and characterization standards. *Nat Commun.* 2016;7:12150.
36. Topalian SL, Drake CG, Pardoll DM. Immune checkpoint blockade: a common denominator approach to cancer therapy. *Cancer Cell.* 2015;27(4):450-461.
37. Leach DR, Krummel MF, Allison JP. Enhancement of antitumor immunity by CTLA-4 blockade. *Science.* 1996;271(5256):1734-1736.
38. Hodi FS, et al. Improved survival with ipilimumab in patients with metastatic melanoma. *N Engl J Med.* 2010;363(8):711-723.
39. Antonia SJ, et al. Durvalumab after chemoradiotherapy in stage III non-small-cell lung cancer. *N Engl J Med.* 2017;377:1919-1929.
40. Melani C, et al. PD-1 blockade in mediastinal gray-zone lymphoma. *N Engl J Med.* 2017;377(1):89-91.
41. Choueiri TK, Motzer RJ. Systemic therapy for metastatic renal-cell carcinoma. *N Engl J Med.* 2017;376(4):354-366.
42. Ferris RL, et al. Nivolumab for recurrent squamous-cell carcinoma of the head and neck. *N Engl J Med.* 2016;375(19):1856-1867.
43. Nghiem PT, et al. PD-1 blockade with Pembrolizumab in advanced Merkel-cell carcinoma. *N Engl J Med.* 2016;374(26):2542-2552.
44. Ansell SM, et al. PD-1 blockade with nivolumab in relapsed or refractory Hodgkin's lymphoma. *N Engl J Med.* 2015;372(4):311-319.

45. Herbst RS, et al. Predictive correlates of response to the anti-PD-L1 antibody MPDL3280A in cancer patients. *Nature.* 2014;515(7528):563-567.

46. Okazaki T, Honjo T. PD-1 and PD-1 ligands: from discovery to clinical application. *Int Immunol.* 2007;19(7):813-824.

47. Anderson AC, Joller N, Kuchroo VK. Lag-3, Tim-3, and TIGIT: co-inhibitory receptors with specialized functions in immune regulation. *Immunity.* 2016;44(5):989-1004.

48. Isaacs A, Lindenmann J. Virus interference. I. The interferon. *Proc R Soc Lond B Biol Sci.* 1957;147(927):258-267.

49. Abbas AK, Lichtman AH, Pober JS. *Cellular and Moleuclar Immunology*, 4th ed. Philadelphia, PA: W.B. Saunders Company; 2000.

50. Lotze MT, et al. Clinical effects and toxicity of interleukin-2 in patients with cancer. *Cancer.* 1986;58(12):2764-2772.

51. Sosman JA, et al. Repetitive weekly cycles of recombinant human interleukin-2: responses of renal carcinoma with acceptable toxicity. *J Natl Cancer Inst.* 1988;80(1):60-63.

52. Carmenate T, et al., Human IL-2 mutein with higher antitumor efficacy than wild type IL-2. *J Immunol.* 2013;190(12):6230-6238.

53. Levin AM, et al. Exploiting a natural conformational switch to engineer an interleukin-2 'superkine'. *Nature.* 2012;484(7395):529-533.

54. Roopenian DC, Akilesh S. FcRn: the neonatal Fc receptor comes of age. *Nat Rev Immunol.* 2007;7(9):715-725.

55. Anderson CL, et al. Perspective—FcRn transports albumin: relevance to immunology and medicine. *Trends Immunol.* 2006;27(7):343-348.

56. Moreland LW, et al. Treatment of rheumatoid arthritis with a recombinant human tumor necrosis factor receptor (p75)-Fc fusion protein. *N Engl J Med.* 1997;337(3):141-147.

57. Powell JS, et al. Phase 3 study of recombinant factor IX Fc fusion protein in hemophilia B. *N Engl J Med.* 2013;369(24):2313-2323.

58. Powell JS, et al. Safety and prolonged activity of recombinant factor VIII Fc fusion protein in hemophilia A patients. *Blood.* 2012;119(13):3031-3037.

59. Olsen E., et al. Pivotal phase III trial of two dose levels of denileukin diftitox for the treatment of cutaneous T-cell lymphoma. *J Clin Oncol.* 2001;19(2):376-388.

60. Vaishampayan UN, et al. A phase I trial of ALKS 4230, an engineered cytokine activator of NK and effector T cells, in patients with advanced solid tumors. *J Clin Oncol.* 2017;35(15 suppl):TPS3111-TPS3111.

61. Harris, J.M., N.E. Martin, and M. Modi, Pegylation: a novel process for modifying pharmacokinetics. *Clin Pharmacokinet.* 2001;40(7):539-551.

62. Charych D, et al. Modeling the receptor pharmacology, pharmacokinetics, and pharmacodynamics of NKTR-214, a kinetically-controlled interleukin-2 (IL2) receptor agonist for cancer immunotherapy. *PLoS One.* 2017;12(7):e0179431.

63. Charych DH, et al. NKTR-214, an engineered cytokine with biased IL2 receptor binding, increased tumor exposure, and marked efficacy in mouse tumor models. *Clin Cancer Res.* 2016;22(3):680-690.

64. Pestka S, Krause CD, Walter MR. Interferons, interferon-like cytokines, and their receptors. *Immunol Rev.* 2004;202:8-32.

65. Pestka S, et al. Interferons and their actions. *Annu Rev Biochem.* 1987;56:727-777.

66. Stewart WE II. Interferon nomenclature recommendations. *J Infect Dis.* 1980;142(4):643.

67. McNab F, et al., Type I interferons in infectious disease. *Nat Rev Immunol.* 2015;15(2):87-103.

68. Borden EC, et al. Interferons at age 50: past, current and future impact on biomedicine. *Nat Rev Drug Discov.* 2007;6(12):975-990.

69. Zitvogel L, et al., Type I interferons in anticancer immunity. *Nat Rev Immunol.* 2015;15(7):405-414.

70. Crouse J, et al. Type I interferons protect T cells against NK cell attack mediated by the activating receptor NCR1. *Immunity.* 2014;40(6):961-973.

71. Xu HC, et al. Type I interferon protects antiviral CD8+ T cells from NK cell cytotoxicity. *Immunity.* 2014;40(6):949-960.

72. Park SH, et al. Type I interferons and the cytokine TNF cooperatively reprogram the macrophage epigenome to promote inflammatory activation. *Nat Immunol.* 2017;18(10):1104-1116.

73. Bacher N, et al. Interferon-alpha suppresses cAMP to disarm human regulatory T cells. *Cancer Res.* 2013;73(18):5647-5656.

74. Diamond MS, et al. Type I interferon is selectively required by dendritic cells for immune rejection of tumors. *J Exp Med.* 2011;208(10):1989-2003.

75. Hervas-Stubbs S, et al. Direct effects of type I interferons on cells of the immune system. *Clin Cancer Res.* 2011;17(9):2619-2627.

76. Curtsinger JM, et al. Type I IFNs provide a third signal to CD8 T cells to stimulate clonal expansion and differentiation. *J Immunol.* 2005;174(8):4465-4469.

77. Ilander M, et al. Enlarged memory T-cell pool and enhanced Th1-type responses in chronic myeloid leukemia patients who have successfully discontinued IFN-alpha monotherapy. *PLoS One.* 2014;9(1):e87794.

78. Colamonici OR, Domanski P. Identification of a novel subunit of the type I interferon receptor localized to human chromosome 21. *J Biol Chem.* 1993;268(15):10895-10899.

79. Lutfalla G, et al. The structure of the human interferon alpha/beta receptor gene. *J Biol Chem* 1992;267(4):2802-2809.

80. Platanias LC. Mechanisms of type-I- and type-II-interferon-mediated signalling. *Nat Rev Immunol.* 2005;5(5):375-386.

81. Aaronson DS, Horvath CM. A road map for those who don't know JAK-STAT. *Science.* 2002;296(5573):1653-1655.

82. Darnell JE Jr. STATs and gene regulation. *Science.* 1997;277(5332):1630-1635.

83. Feller SM. Crk family adaptors-signalling complex formation and biological roles. *Oncogene.* 2001;20(44):6348-6371.

84. Ahmad S, et al. The type I interferon receptor mediates tyrosine phosphorylation of the CrkL adaptor protein. *J Biol Chem.* 1997;272(48):29991-29994.

85. Fish EN, et al. Activation of a CrkL-stat5 signaling complex by type I interferons. *J Biol Chem.* 1999;274(2):571-573.

86. Braiman A, Isakov N. The role of Crk adaptor proteins in T-cell adhesion and migration. *Front Immunol.* 2015;6:509.

87. Lisnock J, et al. Molecular basis for p38 protein kinase inhibitor specificity. *Biochemistry.* 1998;37(47):16573-16581.

88. Jiang Y, et al. Characterization of the structure and function of a new mitogen-activated protein kinase (p38beta). *J Biol Chem.* 1996;271(30):17920-17926.

89. Lechner C, et al. ERK6, a mitogen-activated protein kinase involved in C2C12 myoblast differentiation. *Proc Natl Acad Sci U S A.* 1996;93(9):4355-4359.

90. Zarubin T, Han J. Activation and signaling of the p38 MAP kinase pathway. *Cell Res.* 2005;15(1):11-18.

91. Uddin S, et al. Interferon-alpha engages the insulin receptor substrate-1 to associate with the phosphatidylinositol 3′-kinase. *J Biol Chem.* 1995;270(27):15938-15941.

92. Ivashkiv LB, Donlin LT. Regulation of type I interferon responses. *Nat Rev Immunol.* 2014;14(1):36-49.

93. Luo J, Manning BD, Cantley LC. Targeting the PI3K-Akt pathway in human cancer: rationale and promise. *Cancer Cell.* 2003;4(4):257-262.

94. Kim LC, Cook RS, Chen J. mTORC1 and mTORC2 in cancer and the tumor microenvironment. *Oncogene.* 2017;36(16):2191-2201.

95. Kroczynska B, et al. Regulatory effects of SKAR in interferon alpha signaling and its role in the generation of type I IFN responses. *Proc Natl Acad Sci U S A.* 2014;111(31):11377-11382.

96. Kaur S, et al. Regulatory effects of mTORC2 complexes in type I IFN signaling and in the generation of IFN responses. *Proc Natl Acad Sci U S A.* 2012;109(20):p. 7723-7728.

97. Hoesel B, Schmid JA. The complexity of NF-kappaB signaling in inflammation and cancer. *Mol Cancer.* 2013;12:86.

98. Oeckinghaus A, Ghosh S. The NF-kappaB family of transcription factors and its regulation. *Cold Spring Harb Perspect Biol.* 2009;1(4):a000034.

99. Greenberg HB, et al. Effect of human leukocyte interferon on hepatitis B virus infection in patients with chronic active hepatitis. *N Engl J Med.* 1976;295(10):517-522.

100. Krown SE, et al. Preliminary observations on the effect of recombinant leukocyte A interferon in homosexual men with Kaposi's sarcoma. *N Engl J Med.* 1983;308(18):1071-1076.

101. Talpaz M, et al. Hematologic remission and cytogenetic improvement induced by recombinant human interferon alpha A in chronic myelogenous leukemia. *N Engl J Med.* 1986;314(17):1065-1069.

102. Reddy KR. Development and pharmacokinetics and pharmacodynamics of pegylated interferon alfa-2a (40 kD). *Semin Liver Dis.* 2004;24(Suppl 2):33-38.

103. Youngster S, et al. Structure, biology, and therapeutic implications of pegylated interferon alpha-2b. *Curr Pharm Des.* 2002;8(24):2139-2157.

104. Motzer RJ, et al. Phase II trial of branched peginterferon-alpha 2a (40 kDa) for patients with advanced renal cell carcinoma. *Ann Oncol.* 2002;13(11):1799-1805.

105. Talpaz M, et al., Phase 1 study of polyethylene glycol formulation of interferon alpha-2B (Schering 54031) in Philadelphia chromosome-positive chronic myelogenous leukemia. *Blood.* 2001;98(6):1708-1713.

106. Wills RJ. Clinical pharmacokinetics of interferons. *Clin Pharmacokinet.* 1990;19(5):390-399.

107. Kirkwood JM, et al. Interferon alfa-2b adjuvant therapy of high-risk resected cutaneous melanoma: the Eastern Cooperative Oncology Group Trial EST 1684. *J Clin Oncol.* 1996. 14(1): p. 7-17.

108. Tagliaferri P, et al. New pharmacokinetic and pharmacodynamic tools for interferon-alpha (IFN-alpha) treatment of human cancer. *Cancer Immunol Immunother.* 2005;54(1):1-10.

109. Bailon P, et al. Rational design of a potent, long-lasting form of interferon: a 40 kDa branched polyethylene glycol-conjugated interferon alpha-2a for the treatment of hepatitis C. *Bioconjug Chem.* 2001;12(2):195-202.

110. Karnam US, Reddy KR. Pegylated interferons. *Clin Liver Dis.* 2003;7(1):139-148.

111. Zeuzem S, Welsch C, Herrmann E. Pharmacokinetics of peginterferons. *Semin Liver Dis.* 2003;23(Suppl 1):23-28.

112. Glue P, et al. Pegylated interferon-alpha2b: pharmacokinetics, pharmacodynamics, safety, and preliminary efficacy data. Hepatitis C Intervention Therapy Group. *Clin Pharmacol Ther.* 2000;68(5):556-567.

113. Bukowski R, et al. Pegylated interferon alfa-2b treatment for patients with solid tumors: a phase I/II study. *J Clin Oncol.* 2002;20(18):3841-3849.

114. Michallet M, et al. Pegylated recombinant interferon alpha-2b vs recombinant interferon alpha-2b for the initial treatment of chronic-phase chronic myelogenous leukemia: a phase III study. *Leukemia.* 2004;18(2):309-315.

115. Goldstein D, et al., Human biologic response modification by interferon in the absence of measurable serum concentrations: a comparative trial of subcutaneous and intravenous interferon-beta serine. *J Natl Cancer Inst.* 1989;81(14):1061-1068.

116. Sung C, et al. An IFN-beta-albumin fusion protein that displays improved pharmacokinetic and pharmacodynamic properties in nonhuman primates. *J Interferon Cytokine Res.* 2003;23(1):25-36.

117. McKenna SD, et al. Formation of human IFN-beta complex with the soluble type I interferon receptor IFNAR-2 leads to enhanced IFN stability, pharmacokinetics, and antitumor activity in xenografted SCID mice. *J Interferon Cytokine Res.* 2004;24(2):119-129.

118. Pepinsky RB, et al. Improved pharmacokinetic properties of a polyethylene glycol-modified form of interferon-beta-1a with preserved in vitro bioactivity. *J Pharmacol Exp Ther.* 2001;297(3):1059-1066.

119. Nagai M, Arai T. Clinical effect of interferon in malignant brain tumours. *Neurosurg Rev.* 1984;7(1):55-64.

120. Bukowski RM, et al. Phase I trial of natural human interferon beta in metastatic malignancy. *Cancer Res.* 1991;51(3):836-840.

121. Aulitzky WE, et al. Divergent in vivo and in vitro antileukemic activity of recombinant interferon beta in patients with chronic-phase chronic myelogenous leukemia. *Ann Hematol.* 1993;67(5):205-211.

122. Green DS, Young HA, Valencia JC. Current prospects of type II interferon gamma signaling and autoimmunity. *J Biol Chem.* 2017;292(34):13925-13933.

123. Zaidi MR, Merlino G. The two faces of interferon-gamma in cancer. *Clin Cancer Res.* 2011;17(19):6118-6124.

124. Schroder K, et al. Interferon-gamma: an overview of signals, mechanisms and functions. *J Leukoc Biol.* 2004;75(2):163-189.

125. Cole KE, et al. Interferon-inducible T cell alpha chemoattractant (I-TAC): a novel non-ELR CXC chemokine with potent activity on activated T cells through selective high affinity binding to CXCR3. *J Exp Med.* 1998;187(12):2009-2021.

126. Farber JM. A macrophage mRNA selectively induced by gamma-interferon encodes a member of the platelet factor 4 family of cytokines. *Proc Natl Acad Sci U S A.* 1990;87(14):5238-5242.

127. Luster AD, Ravetch JV. Biochemical characterization of a gamma interferon-inducible cytokine (IP-10). *J Exp Med.* 1987;166(4):1084-1097.

128. Overacre-Delgoffe AE, et al. Interferon-gamma drives Treg fragility to promote anti-tumor immunity. *Cell.* 2017;169(6):1130.e11-1141.e11.

129. Mandai M, et al. Dual faces of IFNgamma in cancer progression: a role of PD-L1 induction in the determination of pro- and antitumor immunity. *Clin Cancer Res.* 2016;22(10):2329-2334.

130. Ayers M, et al. IFN-gamma-related mRNA profile predicts clinical response to PD-1 blockade. *J Clin Invest.* 2017;127(8):2930-2940.

131. Sharma P, et al. Nivolumab in metastatic urothelial carcinoma after platinum therapy (CheckMate 275): a multicentre, single-arm, phase 2 trial. *Lancet Oncol.* 2017;18(3):312-322.

132. Takikawa O, et al. Interferon-gamma-dependent/independent expression of indoleamine 2,3-dioxygenase. Studies with interferon-gamma-knockout mice. *Adv Exp Med Biol.* 1999;467:553-557.

133. Taylor MW, Feng GS. Relationship between interferon-gamma, indoleamine 2,3-dioxygenase, and tryptophan catabolism. *FASEB J.* 1991;5(11):2516-2522.

134. Zakharia Y, et al. Interim analysis of the Phase 2 clinical trial of the IDO pathway inhibitor indoximod in combination with pembrolizumab for patients with advanced melanoma. *Cancer Res.* 2017;77(13 Suppl):CT117.

135. Dorand RD, et al. Cdk5 disruption attenuates tumor PD-L1 expression and promotes antitumor immunity. *Science* 2016;353(6297):399-403.

136. Elhilali MM, et al. Placebo-associated remissions in a multicentre, randomized, double-blind trial of interferon gamma-1b for the treatment of metastatic renal cell carcinoma. The Canadian Urologic Oncology Group. *BJU Int.* 2000;86(6):613-618.

137. Koziner B, et al. Double-blind prospective randomized comparison of interferon gamma-1b versus placebo after autologous stem cell transplantation. *Acta Haematol.* 2002;108(2):66-73.

138. Small EJ, et al. The treatment of metastatic renal cell carcinoma patients with recombinant human gamma interferon. *Cancer J Sci Am.* 1998;4(3):162-167.

139. Todd PA, Goa KL. Interferon gamma-1b. A review of its pharmacology and therapeutic potential in chronic granulomatous disease. *Drugs.* 1992;43(1):111-122.

140. Golomb HM, et al. Alpha-2 interferon therapy of hairy-cell leukemia: a multicenter study of 64 patients. *J Clin Oncol.* 1986;4(6):900-905.

141. Quesada JR, et al. Treatment of hairy cell leukemia with recombinant alpha-interferon. *Blood.* 1986;68(2):493-497.

142. Golomb HM, et al. Interferon treatment for hairy cell leukemia: an update on a cohort of 69 patients treated from 1983-1986. *Leukemia.* 1992;6(11):1177-1180.

143. Dadmarz R, et al. The mechanism of action of interferon-alpha (IFN-alpha) in hairy-cell leukaemia; Hu-IFN-alpha 2 receptor expression by hairy cells and other normal and leukaemic cell types. *Leuk Res.* 1986;10(11):1279-1285.

144. Paganelli KA, et al. B cell growth factor-induced proliferation of hairy cell lymphocytes and inhibition by type I interferon in vitro. *Blood.* 1986;67(4):937-942.

145. Huber C, et al. Studies on the optimal dose and the mode of action of alpha-interferon in the treatment of hairy cell leukemia. *Leukemia.* 1987;1(4):355-357.

146. Goodman GR, Bethel KJ, Saven A. Hairy cell leukemia: an update. *Curr Opin Hematol.* 2003;10(4):258-266.

147. Seymour JF, et al. Response to interferon-alpha in patients with hairy cell leukemia relapsing after treatment with 2-chlorodeoxyadenosine. *Leukemia.* 1995;9(5):929-932.

148. Talpaz M, et al. Leukocyte interferon-induced myeloid cytoreduction in chronic myelogenous leukemia. *Blood.* 1983;62(3):689-692.

149. The Italian Cooperative Study Group on Chronic Myeloid Leukemia; Tura S, Baccarani M, Zuffa E, Russo D, Fanin R, Zaccaria A, Fiacchini M. Interferon alfa-2a as compared with conventional chemotherapy for the treatment of chronic myeloid leukemia. *N Engl J Med.* 1994;330(12):820-825.

150. Allan NC, Richards SM, Shepherd PC. UK Medical Research Council randomised, multicentre trial of interferon-alpha n1 for chronic myeloid leukaemia: improved survival irrespective of cytogenetic response. The UK Medical Research Council's Working Parties for Therapeutic Trials in Adult Leukaemia. *Lancet.* 1995;345(8962):1392-1397.

151. Broustet A, et al. Hydroxyurea versus interferon alfa-2b in chronic myelogenous leukaemia: preliminary results of an open French multicentre randomized study. *Eur J Cancer.* 1991;27(suppl 4):S18-S21.

152. Hehlmann R, et al. Randomized comparison of interferon-alpha with busulfan and hydroxyurea in chronic myelogenous leukemia. The German CML Study Group. *Blood*. 1994;84(12):4064-4077.

153. Ohnishi K, et al. A randomized trial comparing interferon-alpha with busulfan for newly diagnosed chronic myelogenous leukemia in chronic phase. *Blood*. 1995;86(3):906-916.

154. Long-term follow-Up of the Italian trial of interferon-alpha versus conventional chemotherapy in chronic myeloid leukemia. The Italian Cooperative Study Group on Chronic Myeloid Leukemia. *Blood*. 1998;92(5):1541-1548.

155. Hehlmann R, et al. Randomized comparison of interferon alpha and hydroxyurea with hydroxyurea monotherapy in chronic myeloid leukemia (CML-study II): prolongation of survival by the combination of interferon alpha and hydroxyurea. *Leukemia*. 2003;17(8):1529-1537.

156. Interferon alfa versus chemotherapy for chronic myeloid leukemia: a meta-analysis of seven randomized trials: Chronic Myeloid Leukemia Trialists' Collaborative Group. *J Natl Cancer Inst*. 1997;89(21):1616-20.

157. Yasukawa M, et al. CD4(+) cytotoxic T-cell clones specific for bcr-abl b3a2 fusion peptide augment colony formation by chronic myelogenous leukemia cells in a b3a2-specific and HLA-DR-restricted manner. *Blood*. 1998;92(9):3355-3361.

158. Aswald JM, Lipton JH, Messner HA. Intracellular cytokine analysis of interferon-gamma in T cells of patients with chronic myeloid leukemia. *Cytokines Cell Mol Ther*. 2002;7(2):75-82.

159. Nicolson NL, Talpaz M, Nicolson GL. Interferon-alpha directly inhibits DNA polymerase activity in isolated chromatin nucleoprotein complexes: correlation with IFN-alpha treatment outcome in patients with chronic myelogenous leukemia. *Gene*. 1995;159(1):105-111.

160. Interferon-alpha and survival in metastatic renal carcinoma: early results of a randomised controlled trial. Medical Research Council Renal Cancer Collaborators. Lancet, 1999. 353(9146): p. 14-7.

161. Kuhr T, et al. A randomized study comparing interferon (IFN alpha) plus low-dose cytarabine and interferon plus hydroxyurea (HU) in early chronic-phase chronic myeloid leukemia (CML). *Leuk Res*. 2003;27(5):405-411.

162. Giles FJ, et al. A prospective randomized study of alpha-2b interferon plus hydroxyurea or cytarabine for patients with early chronic phase chronic myelogenous leukemia: the International Oncology Study Group CML1 study. *Leuk Lymphoma*. 2000;37(3-4):367-377.

163. Guilhot F, et al. Interferon alfa-2b combined with cytarabine versus interferon alone in chronic myelogenous leukemia. French Chronic Myeloid Leukemia Study Group. *N Engl J Med*. 1997;337(4):223-229.

164. Talpaz M, et al. Re-emergence of interferon-alpha in the treatment of chronic myeloid leukemia. *Leukemia*. 2013;27(4):803-812.

165. Preudhomme C, et al. Imatinib plus peginterferon alfa-2a in chronic myeloid leukemia. *N Engl J Med*. 2010;363(26):2511-2521.

166. O'Brien SG, Deininger MW. Imatinib in patients with newly diagnosed chronic-phase chronic myeloid leukemia. *Semin Hematol*. 2003;40(2 suppl 2):26-30.

167. Anstrom KJ, et al. Long-term survival estimates for imatinib versus interferon-alpha plus low-dose cytarabine for patients with newly diagnosed chronic-phase chronic myeloid leukemia. *Cancer*. 2004;101(11):2584-2592.

168. Kantarjian HM, et al. Imatinib mesylate therapy improves survival in patients with newly diagnosed Philadelphia chromosome-positive chronic myelogenous leukemia in the chronic phase: comparison with historic data. *Cancer*. 2003;98(12):2636-2642.

169. Branford S, et al. Imatinib produces significantly superior molecular responses compared to interferon alfa plus cytarabine in patients with newly diagnosed chronic myeloid leukemia in chronic phase. *Leukemia*. 2003;17(12):2401-2409.

170. Foon KA, et al. Treatment of advanced non-Hodgkin's lymphoma with recombinant leukocyte A interferon. *N Engl J Med*. 1984;311(18):1148-1152.

171. Siegert W, et al. Treatment of non-Hodgkin's lymphoma of low-grade malignancy with human fibroblast interferon. *Anticancer Res*. 1982;2(4):193-198.

172. Louie AC, et al. Follow-up observations on the effect of human leukocyte interferon in non-Hodgkin's lymphoma. *Blood*. 1981;58(4):712-718.

173. Solal-Celigny P, et al. Doxorubicin-containing regimen with or without interferon alfa-2b for advanced follicular lymphomas: final analysis of survival and toxicity in the Groupe d'Etude des Lymphomes Folliculaires 86 Trial. *J Clin Oncol*. 1998;16(7):2332-2338.

174. Solal-Celigny P, et al. Recombinant interferon alfa-2b combined with a regimen containing doxorubicin in patients with advanced follicular lymphoma. Groupe d'Etude des Lymphomes de l'Adulte. *N Engl J Med*. 1993;329(22):1608-1614.

175. Rohatiner AZ, et al. Meta-analysis to evaluate the role of interferon in follicular lymphoma. *J Clin Oncol*. 2005;23(10):2215-2223.

176. Fisher RI, et al. Interferon alpha consolidation after intensive chemotherapy does not prolong the progression-free survival of patients with low-grade non-Hodgkin's lymphoma: results of the Southwest Oncology Group randomized phase III study 8809. *J Clin Oncol*. 2000;18(10):2010-2016.

177. Barnetson RS, Halliday GM. Regression in skin tumours: a common phenomenon. *Australas J Dermatol*. 1997;38(Suppl 1):S63-S65.

178. Coates A, et al. Phase-II study of recombinant alpha 2-interferon in advanced malignant melanoma. *J Interferon Res*. 1986;6(1):1-4.

179. Creagan ET, et al. Phase II study of low-dose recombinant leukocyte A interferon in disseminated malignant melanoma. *J Clin Oncol*. 1984;2(9):1002-1005.

180. Dorval T, et al. Clinical phase II trial of recombinant DNA interferon (interferon alpha 2b) in patients with metastatic malignant melanoma. *Cancer*. 1986;58(2):215-218.

181. Hersey P, et al. Effects of recombinant leukocyte interferon (rIFN-alpha A) on tumour growth and immune responses in patients with metastatic melanoma. *Br J Cancer*. 1985;51(6):815-826.

182. Mughal TI, et al. Role of recombinant interferon alpha 2 and cimetidine in patients with advanced malignant melanoma. *J Cancer Res Clin Oncol*. 1988;114(1):108-109.

183. Neefe JR, et al. Phase II study of recombinant alpha-interferon in malignant melanoma. *Am J Clin Oncol*. 1990;13(6):472-476.

184. Robinson WA, et al. Treatment of metastatic malignant melanoma with recombinant interferon alpha 2. *Immunobiology*. 1986;172(3-5):275-282.

185. Sertoli MR, et al. Phase II trial of recombinant alpha-2b interferon in the treatment of metastatic skin melanoma. *Oncology*. 1989;46(2):96-98.

186. Steiner A, Wolf C, Pehamberger H. Comparison of the effects of three different treatment regimens of recombinant interferons (r-IFN alpha, r-IFN gamma, and r-IFN alpha + cimetidine) in disseminated malignant melanoma. *J Cancer Res Clin Oncol*. 1987;113(5):459-465.

187. Decatris M, Santhanam S, O'Byrne K. Potential of interferon-alpha in solid tumours: part 1. *BioDrugs*. 2002;16(4):261-281.

188. Legha SS, et al. Clinical evaluation of recombinant interferon alfa-2a (Roferon-A) in metastatic melanoma using two different schedules. *J Clin Oncol*. 1987;5(8):1240-1246.

189. Falkson CI, et al. Phase III trial of dacarbazine versus dacarbazine with interferon alpha-2b versus dacarbazine with tamoxifen versus dacarbazine with interferon alpha-2b and tamoxifen in patients with metastatic malignant melanoma: an Eastern Cooperative Oncology Group study. *J Clin Oncol*. 1998;16(5):1743-1751.

190. Creagan ET, et al. Recombinant leukocyte A interferon (rIFN-alpha A) in the treatment of disseminated malignant melanoma. Analysis of complete and long-term responding patients. *Cancer*. 1986;58(12):2576-2578.

191. Eggermont AM, et al. Post-surgery adjuvant therapy with intermediate doses of interferon alfa 2b versus observation in patients with stage IIb/III melanoma (EORTC 18952): randomised controlled trial. *Lancet*. 2005;366(9492):1189-1196.

192. Grob JJ, et al. Randomised trial of interferon alpha-2a as adjuvant therapy in resected primary melanoma thicker than 1.5 mm without clinically detectable node metastases. French Cooperative Group on Melanoma. *Lancet*. 1998;351(9120):1905-1910.

193. Ascierto PA, et al. 3-year treatment with recombinant interferon-alpha as adjuvant therapy of cutaneous malignant melanoma. *Int J Mol Med*. 1999;3(3):303-306.

194. Creagan ET, et al. Randomized, surgical adjuvant clinical trial of recombinant interferon alfa-2a in selected patients with malignant melanoma. *J Clin Oncol*. 1995;13(11):2776-2783.

195. Kleeberg UR, et al. Final results of the EORTC 18871/DKG 80-1 randomised phase III trial. rIFN-alpha2b versus rIFN-gamma versus ISCADOR M versus observation after surgery in melanoma patients with either high-risk primary (thickness >3 mm) or regional lymph node metastasis. *Eur J Cancer*. 2004;40(3):390-402.

196. Pehamberger H, et al. Adjuvant interferon alfa-2a treatment in resected primary stage II cutaneous melanoma. Austrian Malignant Melanoma Cooperative Group. *J Clin Oncol.* 1998;16(4):1425-1429.

197. Cameron DA, et al. Adjuvant interferon alpha 2b in high risk melanoma—the Scottish study. *Br J Cancer.* 2001;84(9):1146-1149.

198. Hancock BW, et al. Adjuvant interferon in high-risk melanoma: the AIM HIGH Study—United Kingdom Coordinating Committee on Cancer Research randomized study of adjuvant low-dose extended-duration interferon Alfa-2a in high-risk resected malignant melanoma. *J Clin Oncol.* 2004;22(1):53-61.

199. Kirkwood JM, et al. High-dose interferon alfa-2b significantly prolongs relapse-free and overall survival compared with the GM2-KLH/QS-21 vaccine in patients with resected stage IIB-III melanoma: results of intergroup trial E1694/S9512/C509801. *J Clin Oncol.* 2001;19(9):2370-2380.

200. Kirkwood JM, et al. A pooled analysis of eastern cooperative oncology group and intergroup trials of adjuvant high-dose interferon for melanoma. *Clin Cancer Res.* 2004;10(5):1670-1677.

201. Hillner BE, et al. Economic analysis of adjuvant interferon alfa-2b in high-risk melanoma based on projections from Eastern Cooperative Oncology Group 1684. *J Clin Oncol.* 1997;15(6):2351-2358.

202. McMasters KM, et al., Final results of the Sunbelt Melanoma Trial: a Multi-Institutional Prospective Randomized Phase III Study Evaluating the Role of Adjuvant High-Dose Interferon Alfa-2b and Completion Lymph Node Dissection for Patients Staged by Sentinel Lymph Node Biopsy. *J Clin Oncol.* 2016;34(10):1079-1086.

203. Castello G, et al. Immunological and clinical effects of intramuscular rIFN alpha-2a and low dose subcutaneous rIL-2 in patients with advanced malignant melanoma. *Melanoma Res.* 1993;3(1):43-49.

204. Kirkwood JM, et al. High- and low-dose interferon alfa-2b in high-risk melanoma: first analysis of intergroup trial E1690/S9111/C9190. *J Clin Oncol.* 2000;18(12):2444-2458.

205. van der Ploeg AP, et al. The prognostic significance of sentinel node tumour burden in melanoma patients: an international, multicenter study of 1539 sentinel node-positive melanoma patients. *Eur J Cancer.* 2014;50(1):111-120.

206. van Akkooi AC, et al. Sentinel node tumor burden according to the Rotterdam criteria is the most important prognostic factor for survival in melanoma patients: a multicenter study in 388 patients with positive sentinel nodes. *Ann Surg.* 2008;248(6):949-955.

207. Eggermont AM, et al. Adjuvant therapy with pegylated interferon alfa-2b versus observation alone in resected stage III melanoma: final results of EORTC 18991, a randomised phase III trial. *Lancet.* 2008;372(9633):117-126.

208. Eggermont AM, et al. Ulceration of primary melanoma and responsiveness to adjuvant interferon therapy: analysis of the adjuvant trials EORTC18952 and EORTC18991 in 2,644 patients. *J Clin Oncol.* 2009;27(15s):9007.

209. Wheatley K, et al. Does adjuvant interferon-alpha for high-risk melanoma provide a worthwhile benefit? A meta-analysis of the randomised trials. *Cancer Treat Rev.* 2003;29(4):241-252.

210. Lens MB, Dawes M. Interferon alfa therapy for malignant melanoma: a systematic review of randomized controlled trials. *J Clin Oncol.* 2002;20(7):1818-1825.

211. Mocellin S, et al. Interferon alpha adjuvant therapy in patients with high-risk melanoma: a systematic review and meta-analysis. *J Natl Cancer Inst.* 2010;102(7):493-501.

212. Ives NJ, et al. Adjuvant interferon-alpha for the treatment of high-risk melanoma: an individual patient data meta-analysis. *Eur J Cancer.* 2017;82:171-183.

213. Eggermont AM, et al. Prolonged survival in stage III melanoma with ipilimumab adjuvant therapy. *N Engl J Med.* 2016;375(19):1845-1855.

214. Long GV, et al. Adjuvant dabrafenib plus trametinib in stage III BRAF-mutated melanoma. *N Engl J Med.* 2017;377(19):1813-1823.

215. Weber J, et al. Adjuvant nivolumab versus ipilimumab in resected stage III or IV melanoma. *N Engl J Med.* 2017;377(19):1824-1835.

216. Falkson CI, Falkson G, Falkson HC. Improved results with the addition of interferon alfa-2b to dacarbazine in the treatment of patients with metastatic malignant melanoma. *J Clin Oncol.* 1991;9(8):1403-1408.

217. Thomson DB, et al. Interferon-alpha 2a does not improve response or survival when combined with dacarbazine in metastatic malignant melanoma:

218. Bajetta E, et al. Multicenter randomized trial of dacarbazine alone or in combination with two different doses and schedules of interferon alfa-2a in the treatment of advanced melanoma. *J Clin Oncol.* 1994;12(4):806-811.

219. Creagan ET, et al. A phase I-II trial of the combination of recombinant leukocyte A interferon and recombinant human interferon-gamma in patients with metastatic malignant melanoma. *Cancer.* 1988;62(12):2472-2474.

220. Rinehart J, et al. Phase I/II trial of human recombinant beta-interferon serine in patients with renal cell carcinoma. *Cancer Res.* 1986;46(10):5364-5367.

221. McDermott DF, Rini BI. Immunotherapy for metastatic renal cell carcinoma. *BJU Int.* 2007;99(5 Pt B):1282-1288.

222. Muss HB, et al. Recombinant alfa interferon in renal cell carcinoma: a randomized trial of two routes of administration. *J Clin Oncol.* 1987;5(2):286-291.

223. Parton M, Gore M, Eisen T. Role of cytokine therapy in 2006 and beyond for metastatic renal cell cancer. *J Clin Oncol.* 2006;24(35):5584-5592.

224. Coppin C, et al. Immunotherapy for advanced renal cell cancer. *Cochrane Database Syst Rev.* 2005;(1):CD001425.

225. Muss HB. Interferon therapy for renal cell carcinoma. *Semin Oncol.* 1987;14(2 suppl 2):36-42.

226. Negrier S, et al. Treatment of patients with metastatic renal carcinoma with a combination of subcutaneous interleukin-2 and interferon alfa with or without fluorouracil. Groupe Francais d'Immunotherapie, Federation Nationale des Centres de Lutte Contre le Cancer. *J Clin Oncol.* 2000;18(24):4009-4015.

227. Neidhart JA. Interferon therapy for the treatment of renal cancer. *Cancer.* 1986;57(8 suppl):1696-1699.

228. Pyrhonen S, et al. Prospective randomized trial of interferon alfa-2a plus vinblastine versus vinblastine alone in patients with advanced renal cell cancer. *J Clin Oncol.* 1999. 17(9): p. 2859-2867.

229. Negrier S, et al. Recombinant human interleukin-2, recombinant human interferon alfa-2a, or both in metastatic renal-cell carcinoma. Groupe Francais d'Immunotherapie. *N Engl J Med.* 1998;338(18):1272-1278.

230. Flanigan RC, et al. Nephrectomy followed by interferon alfa-2b compared with interferon alfa-2b alone for metastatic renal-cell cancer. *N Engl J Med.* 2001;345(23):1655-1659.

231. Gollob JA, et al., Phase II trial of sorafenib plus interferon alfa-2b as first- or second-line therapy in patients with metastatic renal cell cancer. *J Clin Oncol.* 2007;25(22):3288-3295.

232. Ryan CW, et al. Sorafenib with interferon alfa-2b as first-line treatment of advanced renal carcinoma: a phase II study of the Southwest Oncology Group. *J Clin Oncol.* 2007;25(22):3296-3301.

233. Escudier B, et al. Bevacizumab plus interferon alfa-2a for treatment of metastatic renal cell carcinoma: a randomised, double-blind phase III trial. *Lancet.* 2007;370(9605):2103-2111.

234. Rini BI, et al., Bevacizumab plus interferon alfa compared with interferon alfa monotherapy in patients with metastatic renal cell carcinoma: CALGB 90206. *J Clin Oncol.* 2008;26(33):5422-5428.

235. Motzer RJ, et al. Sunitinib versus interferon alfa in metastatic renal-cell carcinoma. *N Engl J Med.* 2007;356(2):115-124.

236. Schalling M, et al. A role for a new herpes virus (KSHV) in different forms of Kaposi's sarcoma. *Nat Med.* 1995;1(7):707-708.

237. Ensoli B, et al. AIDS-Kaposi's sarcoma-derived cells express cytokines with autocrine and paracrine growth effects. *Science.* 1989;243(4888):223-226.

238. Sinkovics JG. Kaposi's sarcoma: its 'oncogenes' and growth factors. *Crit Rev Oncol Hematol.* 1991;11(2):87-107.

239. Folkman J. Successful treatment of an angiogenic disease. *N Engl J Med.* 1989;320(18):1211-1212.

240. White CW, et al. Treatment of pulmonary hemangiomatosis with recombinant interferon alfa-2a. *N Engl J Med.* 1989;320(18):1197-1200.

241. Ezekowitz A, Mulliken J, Folkman J. Interferon alpha therapy of haemangiomas in newborns and infants. *Br J Haematol.* 1991;79(suppl 1):67-68.

242. Real FX, Oettgen HF, Krown SE. Kaposi's sarcoma and the acquired immunodeficiency syndrome: treatment with high and low doses of recombinant leukocyte A interferon. *J Clin Oncol.* 1986;4(4):544-551.

243. Gelmann EP, et al. Human lymphoblastoid interferon treatment of Kaposi's sarcoma in the acquired immune deficiency syndrome. Clinical response and prognostic parameters. *Am J Med.* 1985;78(5):737-741.

244. Groopman JE, et al. Recombinant alpha-2 interferon therapy for Kaposi's sarcoma associated with the acquired immunodeficiency syndrome. *Ann Intern Med.* 1984;100(5):671-676.

245. Mauss S, Jablonowski H. Efficacy, safety, and tolerance of low-dose, long-term interferon-alpha 2b and zidovudine in early-stage AIDS-associated Kaposi's sarcoma. *J Acquir Immune Deific Syndr Hum Retrovirol.* 1995;10(2):157-162.

246. Krown SE, et al. Interferon-alpha with zidovudine: safety, tolerance, and clinical and virologic effects in patients with Kaposi sarcoma associated with the acquired immunodeficiency syndrome (AIDS). *Ann Intern Med.* 1990;112(11):812-821.

247. Dezube BJ, Pantanowitz L, Aboulafia DM. Management of AIDS-related Kaposi sarcoma: advances in target discovery and treatment. *AIDS Read.* 2004;14(5):236-238; 243-244, 251-253.

248. Jonasch E, Haluska FG. Interferon in oncological practice: review of interferon biology, clinical applications, and toxicities. *Oncologist.* 2001;6(1):34-55.

249. Greenberg DB, et al. Adjuvant therapy of melanoma with interferon-alpha-2b is associated with mania and bipolar syndromes. *Cancer.* 2000;89(2):356-362.

250. Musselman DL, et al. Paroxetine for the prevention of depression induced by high-dose interferon alfa. *N Engl J Med.* 2001;344(13):961-966.

251. Jonasch E, et al. Adjuvant high-dose interferon alfa-2b in patients with high-risk melanoma. *Cancer J.* 2000;6(3):139-145.

252. Lacotte L, et al. Thrombotic thrombocytopenic purpura during interferon alpha treatment for chronic myelogenous leukemia. *Acta Haematol.* 2000;102(3):160-162.

253. Ravandi-Kashani F, et al. Thrombotic microangiopathy associated with interferon therapy for patients with chronic myelogenous leukemia: coincidence or true side effect? *Cancer.* 1999;85(12):2583-2588.

254. Rachmani R, et al. Thrombotic thrombocytopenic purpura complicating chronic myelogenous leukemia treated with interferon-alpha. A report of two successfully treated patients. *Acta Haematol.* 1998;100(4):204-206.

255. Iyoda K, et al. Thrombotic thrombocytopenic purpura developed suddenly during interferon treatment for chronic hepatitis C. *J Gastroenterol.* 1998;33(4):588-592.

256. Gentile I, et al. Hemolytic anemia during pegylated IFN-alpha2b plus ribavirin treatment for chronic hepatitis C: ribavirin is not always the culprit. *J Interferon Cytokine Res.* 2005;25(5):283-285.

257. Braathen LR, Stavem P. Autoimmune haemolytic anaemia associated with interferon alfa-2a in a patient with mycosis fungoides. *BMJ.* 1989;298(6689):1713.

258. Pangalis GA, Griva E. Recombinant alfa-2b-interferon therapy in untreated, stages A and B chronic lymphocytic leukemia. A preliminary report. *Cancer.* 1988;61(5):869-872.

259. Akard LP, et al. Alpha-interferon and immune hemolytic anemia. *Ann Intern Med.* 1986;105(2):306.

260. Jones TH, Wadler S, Hupart KH. Endocrine-mediated mechanisms of fatigue during treatment with interferon-alpha. *Semin Oncol.* 1998;25(1 suppl 1):54-63.

261. Brudin LH, et al. Fluorine-18 deoxyglucose uptake in sarcoidosis measured with positron emission tomography. *Eur J Nucl Med.* 1994;21(4):297-305.

262. Lewis PJ, Salama A. Uptake of fluorine-18-fluorodeoxyglucose in sarcoidosis. *J Nucl Med.* 1994;35(10):1647-1649.

263. Brenard R. Practical management of patients treated with alpha interferon. *Acta Gastroenterol Belg.* 1997;60(3):211-213.

264. Dalekos GN, et al. A prospective evaluation of dermatological side-effects during alpha-interferon therapy for chronic viral hepatitis. *Eur J Gastroenterol Hepatol.* 1998;10(11):933-939.

265. Gogas H, et al. Prognostic significance of autoimmunity during treatment of melanoma with interferon. *N Engl J Med.* 2006;354(7):709-718.

266. Kamimura D, et al. IL-2 in vivo activities and antitumor efficacy enhanced by an anti-IL-2 mAb. *J Immunol.* 2006;177(1):306-314.

267. Bernatchez C, Haymaker C, Tannir N, et al. A CD122-biased agonist increases CD8+T Cells and natural killer cells in the tumor microenvironment; making cold tumors hot with NKTR-214. In Society for Immunotherapy of Cancer (SITC) Annual Meeting. National Harbor, Maryland, 2016, pp Abs 387.

268. Gearing AJ, Thorpe R. The international standard for human interleukin-2. Calibration by international collaborative study. *J Immunol Methods.* 1988;114(1-2):3-9.

269. Hank JA, et al. Distinct clinical and laboratory activity of two recombinant interleukin-2 preparations. *Clin Cancer Res.* 1999;5(2):281-289.

270. Konrad MW, et al. Pharmacokinetics of recombinant interleukin 2 in humans. *Cancer Res.* 1990;50(7):2009-2017.

271. Hersh EM, et al. Phase I study of cancer therapy with recombinant interleukin-2 administered by intravenous bolus injection. *Biotherapy.* 1989;1(3):215-226.

272. Kirchner GI, et al. Pharmacokinetics of recombinant human interleukin-2 in advanced renal cell carcinoma patients following subcutaneous application. *Br J Clin Pharmacol.* 1998;46(1):5-10.

273. Vlasveld LT, et al. Catheter-related complications in 52 patients treated with continuous infusion of low dose recombinant interleukin-2 via an implanted central venous catheter. *Eur J Surg Oncol.* 1994;20(2):122-129.

274. Eastman ME, et al. Central venous device-related infection and thrombosis in patients treated with moderate dose continuous-infusion interleukin-2. *Cancer.* 2001;91(4):806-814.

275. Rosenberg SA, et al. Observations on the systemic administration of autologous lymphokine-activated killer cells and recombinant interleukin-2 to patients with metastatic cancer. *N Engl J Med.* 1985;313(23):1485-1492.

276. Rosenberg SA, et al. Treatment of 283 consecutive patients with metastatic melanoma or renal cell cancer using high-dose bolus interleukin 2. *JAMA.* 1994;271(12):907-913.

277. Sznol M, Hawkins MJ. Interleukin-2 in Malignancies Other than Melanoma and Renal Cell Carcinoma. In: M.B. Atkins and J.W. Mier. Therapeutic Applications of Interleukin-2. ed. . 1993, Marcel Dekker Inc.: New York, NY. 177-188.

278. Rosenberg SA, et al. Prospective randomized trial of high-dose interleukin-2 alone or in conjunction with lymphokine-activated killer cells for the treatment of patients with advanced cancer. *J Natl Cancer Inst.* 1993;85(8):622-632.

279. Fisher RI, Rosenberg SA, Fyfe G. Long-term survival update for high-dose recombinant interleukin-2 in patients with renal cell carcinoma. *Cancer J Sci Am.* 2000;6(suppl 1):S55-S57.

280. Atkins MB, et al. High-dose recombinant interleukin-2 therapy in patients with metastatic melanoma: long-term survival update. *Cancer J Sci Am.* 2000;6(suppl 1):S11-S14.

281. Belldegrun A, et al. Renal toxicity of interleukin-2 administration in patients with metastatic renal cell cancer: effect of pre-therapy nephrectomy. *J Urol.* 1989;141(3):499-503.

282. Fyfe G, et al. Results of treatment of 255 patients with metastatic renal cell carcinoma who received high-dose recombinant interleukin-2 therapy. *J Clin Oncol.* 1995;13(3):688-696.

283. Margolin KA, et al. Interleukin-2 and lymphokine-activated killer cell therapy of solid tumors: analysis of toxicity and management guidelines. *J Clin Oncol.* 1989;7(4):486-498.

284. Rosenberg SA, et al. Durability of complete responses in patients with metastatic cancer treated with high-dose interleukin-2: identification of the antigens mediating response. *Ann Surg.* 1998;228(3):307-319.

285. Lopez Hanninen E, Kirchner H, Atzpodien J. Interleukin-2 based home therapy of metastatic renal cell carcinoma: risks and benefits in 215 consecutive single institution patients. *J Urol.* 1996;155(1):19-25.

286. Sleijfer DT, et al. Phase II study of subcutaneous interleukin-2 in unselected patients with advanced renal cell cancer on an outpatient basis. *J Clin Oncol.* 1992;10(7):1119-1123.

287. Yang JC, et al. Randomized comparison of high-dose and low-dose intravenous interleukin-2 for the therapy of metastatic renal cell carcinoma: an interim report. *J Clin Oncol.* 1994;12(8):1572-1576.

288. Atzpodien J, et al. Subcutaneous recombinant interleukin-2 and alpha-interferon in patients with advanced renal cell carcinoma: results of a multicenter phase II study. *Cancer Biother.* 1993;8(4):289-300.

289. Atzpodien J, et al. Multiinstitutional home-therapy trial of recombinant human interleukin-2 and interferon alfa-2 in progressive metastatic renal cell carcinoma. *J Clin Oncol.* 1995;13(2):497-501.

290. Figlin RA, et al. Concomitant administration of recombinant human interleukin-2 and recombinant interferon alfa-2A: an active outpatient regimen in metastatic renal cell carcinoma. *J Clin Oncol.* 1992;10(3):414-421.

291. Vogelzang NJ, Lipton A, Figlin RA. Subcutaneous interleukin-2 plus interferon alfa-2a in metastatic renal cancer: an outpatient multicenter trial. *J Clin Oncol.* 1993;11(9):1809-1816.

292. Acquavella N, et al. Toxicity and activity of a twice daily high-dose bolus interleukin 2 regimen in patients with metastatic melanoma and metastatic renal cell cancer. *J Immunother.* 2008;31(6):569-576.

293. Finkelstein SE, et al. Changes in dendritic cell phenotype after a new high-dose weekly schedule of interleukin-2 therapy for kidney cancer and melanoma. *J Immunother.* 2010;33(8):817-827.

294. McDermott DF, et al. Randomized phase III trial of high-dose interleukin-2 versus subcutaneous interleukin-2 and interferon in patients with metastatic renal cell carcinoma. *J Clin Oncol.* 2005;23(1):133-141.

295. Negrier S, et al. Medroxyprogesterone, interferon alfa-2a, interleukin 2, or combination of both cytokines in patients with metastatic renal carcinoma of intermediate prognosis: results of a randomized controlled trial. *Cancer.* 2007;110(11):2468-2477.

296. Yang JC, et al. Randomized study of high-dose and low-dose interleukin-2 in patients with metastatic renal cancer. *J Clin Oncol.* 2003;21(16):3127-3132.

297. Atkins MB. Cytokine-based and biochemo-therapy for advanced melanoma. *Clin Cancer Res.* 2006;12:2353s-2358s.

298. Rosenberg SA, et al. Immunizing patients with metastatic melanoma using recombinant adenoviruses encoding MART-1 or gp100 melanoma antigens. *J Natl Cancer Inst.* 1998;90(24):1894-1900.

299. Rosenberg SA, et al. Impact of cytokine administration on the generation of antitumor reactivity in patients with metastatic melanoma receiving a peptide vaccine. *J Immunol.* 1999;163(3):1690-1695.

300. Schwartzentruber DJ, Richards J. A phase III multi-institutional randomized study of immunization with the gp100:209-217(210M) peptide followed by high-dose IL-2 compared with high-dose IL-2 alone in patients with metastatic melanoma. *J Clin Oncol.* 2009;27(18 suppl):Abstr CRA9011.

301. Feun L, et al. Cyclosporine A, alpha-interferon and interleukin-2 following chemotherapy with BCNU, DTIC, cisplatin, and tamoxifen: a phase II study in advanced melanoma. *Cancer Invest.* 2005;23(1):3-8.

302. Atkins MB, et al. A phase II pilot trial of concurrent biochemotherapy with cisplatin, vinblastine, temozolomide, interleukin 2, and IFN-alpha 2B in patients with metastatic melanoma. *Clin Cancer Res.* 2002;8(10):3075-3081.

303. McDermott DF, et al. A phase II pilot trial of concurrent biochemotherapy with cisplatin, vinblastine, dacarbazine, interleukin 2, and interferon alpha-2B in patients with metastatic melanoma. *Clin Cancer Res.* 2000;6(6):2201-2208.

304. Gibbs P, et al. A phase II study of biochemotherapy for the treatment of metastatic malignant melanoma. *Melanoma Res.* 2000;10(2):171-179.

305. Johnston SR, et al. Randomized phase II trial of BCDT [carmustine (BCNU), cisplatin, dacarbazine (DTIC) and tamoxifen] with or without interferon alpha (IFN-alpha) and interleukin (IL-2) in patients with metastatic melanoma. *Br J Cancer.* 1998;77(8):1280-1286.

306. Atkins MB, et al. Phase III trial comparing concurrent biochemotherapy with cisplatin, vinblastine, dacarbazine, interleukin-2, and interferon alfa-2b with cisplatin, vinblastine, and dacarbazine alone in patients with metastatic malignant melanoma (E3695): a trial coordinated by the Eastern Cooperative Oncology Group. *J Clin Oncol.* 2008;26(35):5748-5754.

307. Bajetta E, et al. Multicenter phase III randomized trial of polychemotherapy (CVD regimen) versus the same chemotherapy (CT) plus subcutaneous interleukin-2 and interferon-alpha2b in metastatic melanoma. *Ann Oncol.* 2006;17(4):571-577.

308. Eton O, et al. Sequential biochemotherapy versus chemotherapy for metastatic melanoma: results from a phase III randomized trial. *J Clin Oncol.* 2002;20(8):2045-2052.

309. Hauschild A, et al. Dacarbazine and interferon alpha with or without interleukin 2 in metastatic melanoma: a randomized phase III multicentre trial of the Dermatologic Cooperative Oncology Group (DeCOG). *Br J Cancer.* 2001;84(8):1036-1042.

310. Ridolfi R, et al. Cisplatin, dacarbazine with or without subcutaneous interleukin-2, and interferon alpha-2b in advanced melanoma outpatients: results from an Italian multicenter phase III randomized clinical trial. *J Clin Oncol.* 2002;20(6):1600-1607.

311. Rosenberg SA, et al. Prospective randomized trial of the treatment of patients with metastatic melanoma using chemotherapy with cisplatin, dacarbazine, and tamoxifen alone or in combination with interleukin-2 and interferon alfa-2b. *J Clin Oncol.* 1999;17(3):968-975.

312. Rosenberg SA. A new era of cancer immunotherapy: converting theory to performance. *CA Cancer J Clin,* 1999. 49(2): p. 70-73, 65.

313. Dudley, M.E., et al., Cancer regression and autoimmunity in patients after clonal repopulation with antitumor lymphocytes. *Science.* 2002;298(5594):850-854.

314. Dudley ME, et al. A phase I study of nonmyeloablative chemotherapy and adoptive transfer of autologous tumor antigen-specific T lymphocytes in patients with metastatic melanoma. *J Immunother.* 2002;25(3):243-251.

315. Dudley ME, et al. Adoptive cell therapy for patients with metastatic melanoma: evaluation of intensive myeloablative chemoradiation preparative regimens. *J Clin Oncol.* 2008;26(32):5233-5239.

316. Sarnaik A, et al. *J Clin Oncol.* 2017;35(suppl):Abstr 3045.

317. Margolin, K., *The clinical toxicities of high-dose interleukin-2., in Therapeutic Applications of Interleukin-2, A.* MB, Editor. Marcel Dekker Inc: New York. 1993;331-362.

318. Klempner MS, et al. An acquired chemotactic defect in neutrophils from patients receiving interleukin-2 immunotherapy. *N Engl J Med.* 1990;322(14):959-965.

319. Kammula US, White DE, Rosenberg SA. Trends in the safety of high dose bolus interleukin-2 administration in patients with metastatic cancer. *Cancer.* 1998;83(4):797-805.

320. Alva A, et al. Contemporary experience with high-dose interleukin-2 therapy and impact on survival in patients with metastatic melanoma and metastatic renal cell carcinoma. *Cancer Immunol Immunother.* 2016;65(12):1533-1544.

321. Gemlo BT, et al. Circulating cytokines in patients with metastatic cancer treated with recombinant interleukin 2 and lymphokine-activated killer cells. *Cancer Res.* 1988;48(20):5864-5867.

322. Atkins MB, et al. A phase I study of CNI-1493, an inhibitor of cytokine release, in combination with high-dose interleukin-2 in patients with renal cancer and melanoma. *Clin Cancer Res.* 2001;7(3):486-492.

323. Du Bois JS, et al. Randomized placebo-controlled clinical trial of high-dose interleukin-2 in combination with a soluble p75 tumor necrosis factor receptor immunoglobulin G chimera in patients with advanced melanoma and renal cell carcinoma. *J Clin Oncol.* 1997;15(3):1052-1062.

324. Kilbourn RG, et al. Strategies to reduce side effects of interleukin-2: evaluation of the antihypotensive agent NG-monomethyl-L-arginine. *Cancer J Sci Am.* 2000;6(Suppl 1):S21-S30.

325. McDermott DF, et al. A two-part phase I trial of high-dose interleukin 2 in combination with soluble (Chinese hamster ovary) interleukin 1 receptor. *Clin Cancer Res.* 1998;4(5):1203-1213.

326. Samlowski WE, et al. A nonpeptidyl mimic of superoxide dismutase, M40403, inhibits dose-limiting hypotension associated with interleukin-2 and increases its antitumor effects. *Nat Med.* 2003;9(6):750-755.

327. Fry TJ, Mackall CL. The many faces of IL-7: from lymphopoiesis to peripheral T cell maintenance. *J Immunol.* 2005;174(11):6571-6576.

328. Roifman CM, et al. A partial deficiency of interleukin-7R alpha is sufficient to abrogate T-cell development and cause severe combined immunodeficiency. *Blood.* 2000;96(8):2803-2807.

329. Puel A, et al. Defective IL7R expression in T(-)B(+)NK(+) severe combined immunodeficiency. *Nat Genet.* 1998;20(4):394-397.

330. Alderson MR, et al. Interleukin 7 induces cytokine secretion and tumoricidal activity by human peripheral blood monocytes. *J Exp Med.* 1991;173(4):923-930.

331. Rosenberg SA, et al. IL-7 administration to humans leads to expansion of CD8+ and CD4+ cells but a relative decrease of CD4+ T-regulatory cells. *J Immunother.* 2006;29(3):313-319.

332. Mackall CL, Fry TJ, Gress RE. Harnessing the biology of IL-7 for therapeutic application. *Nat Rev Immunol.* 2011;11(5):330-342.

333. Dennis KL, et al. Current status of interleukin-10 and regulatory T-cells in cancer. *Curr Opin Oncol.* 2013;25(6):637-645.

334. Zheng LM, et al. Interleukin-10 inhibits tumor metastasis through an NK cell-dependent mechanism. *J Exp Med.* 1996;184(2):579-584.

335. Mumm JB, et al. IL-10 elicits IFNgamma-dependent tumor immune surveillance. *Cancer Cell.* 2011;20(6):781-796.

336. Naing A, et al. Safety, antitumor activity, and immune activation of pegylated recombinant human interleukin-10 (AM0010) in patients with advanced solid tumors. *J Clin Oncol.* 2016;34(29):3562-3569.

337. Voest EE, et al. Inhibition of angiogenesis in vivo by interleukin 12. *J Natl Cancer Inst.* 1995;87(8):581-586.

338. Lasek W, Zagozdzon R, Jakobisiak M. Interleukin 12: still a promising candidate for tumor immunotherapy? *Cancer Immunol Immunother.* 2014;63(5):419-435.

339. Leonard JP, et al. Effects of single-dose interleukin-12 exposure on interleukin-12-associated toxicity and interferon-gamma production. *Blood.* 1997;90(7):2541-2548.

340. Portielje JE, et al. Repeated administrations of interleukin (IL)-12 are associated with persistently elevated plasma levels of IL-10 and declining IFN-gamma, tumor necrosis factor-alpha, IL-6, and IL-8 responses. *Clin Cancer Res.* 2003;9(1):76-83.

341. Pilipow K, et al. IL15 and T-cell stemness in T-cell-based cancer immunotherapy. *Cancer Res.* 2015;75(24):5187-5193.

342. Conlon KC, et al. Redistribution, hyperproliferation, activation of natural killer cells and CD8 T cells, and cytokine production during first-in-human clinical trial of recombinant human interleukin-15 in patients with cancer. *J Clin Oncol.* 2015;33(1):74-82.

343. Waldmann TA, The shared and contrasting roles of IL2 and IL15 in the life and death of normal and neoplastic lymphocytes: implications for cancer therapy. *Cancer Immunol Res.* 2015;3(3):219-227.

344. Tarhini AA, et al. A phase 2, randomized study of SB-485232, rhIL-18, in patients with previously untreated metastatic melanoma. *Cancer.* 2009;115(4):859-868.

345. Davis MR, et al. The role of IL-21 in immunity and cancer. *Cancer Lett.* 2015;358(2):107-114.

346. Bhatia S, et al. Recombinant interleukin-21 plus sorafenib for metastatic renal cell carcinoma: a phase 1/2 study. *J Immunother Cancer.* 2014;2:2.

347. Petrella TM, et al. Interleukin-21 has activity in patients with metastatic melanoma: a phase II study. *J Clin Oncol.* 2012;30(27):3396-3401.

348. Becher B, Tugues S, Greter M. GM-CSF: from growth factor to central mediator of tissue inflammation. *Immunity.* 2016;45(5):963-973.

349. Wicks IP, Roberts AW, Targeting GM-CSF in inflammatory diseases. *Nat Rev Rheumatol.* 2016;12(1):37-48.

350. Dranoff G, et al. Vaccination with irradiated tumor cells engineered to secrete murine granulocyte-macrophage colony-stimulating factor stimulates potent, specific, and long-lasting anti-tumor immunity. *Proc Natl Acad Sci U S A.* 1993;90(8):3539-3543.

351. Lawson DH, et al. Randomized, placebo-controlled, phase III trial of yeast-derived granulocyte-macrophage colony-stimulating factor (GM-CSF) versus peptide vaccination versus GM-CSF plus peptide vaccination versus placebo in patients with no evidence of disease after complete surgical resection of locally advanced and/or stage IV melanoma: a trial of the Eastern Cooperative Oncology Group-American College of Radiology Imaging Network Cancer Research Group (E4697). *J Clin Oncol.* 2015;33(34):4066-4076.

352. Wall LM, Baldwin-Medsker A. Safe and effective standards of care: supporting the administration of T-VEC for patients with advanced melanoma in the outpatient oncology setting. *Clin J Oncol Nurs.* 2017;21(5):E260-E266.

353. Long GV, et al. Efficacy analysis of MASTERKEY-265 phase 1b study of talimogene laherparepvec (T-VEC) and pembrolizumab (pembro) for unresectable stage IIIB-IV melanoma. *J Clin Oncol.* 2016;34(15 suppl):9568-9568.

354. Atkins MB, et al. High-dose recombinant interleukin 2 therapy for patients with metastatic melanoma: analysis of 270 patients treated between 1985 and 1993. *J Clin Oncol.* 1999;17(7):2105-2116.

355. Scheibenbogen C, et al. HLA class I alleles and responsiveness of melanoma to immunotherapy with interferon-alpha (IFN-alpha) and interleukin-2 (IL-2). *Melanoma Res.* 1994;4(3):191-194.

356. Tartour E, et al. Predictors of clinical response to interleukin-2–based immunotherapy in melanoma patients: a French multiinstitutional study. *J Clin Oncol.* 1996;14(5):1697-1703.

357. Atkins MB, et al. Hypothyroidism after treatment with interleukin-2 and lymphokine-activated killer cells. *N Engl J Med.* 1988;318(24):1557-1563.

358. Phan GQ, et al. Immunization of patients with metastatic melanoma using both class I- and class II-restricted peptides from melanoma-associated antigens. *J Immunother.* 2003;26(4):349-356.

359. Rosenberg SA, White DE. Vitiligo in patients with melanoma: normal tissue antigens can be targets for cancer immunotherapy. *J Immunother Emphasis Tumor Immunol.* 1996;19(1):81-84.

360. Wang E, et al. Prospective molecular profiling of melanoma metastases suggests classifiers of immune responsiveness. *Cancer Res.* 2002;62(13):3581-3586.

361. Sabatino, M., et al., Serum vascular endothelial growth factor and fibronectin predict clinical response to high-dose interleukin-2 therapy. *J Clin Oncol.* 2009;27(16):2645-2652.

362. Joseph RW, et al. Correlation of NRAS mutations with clinical response to high-dose IL-2 in patients with advanced melanoma. *J Immunother.* 2012;35(1):66-72.

363. Liu D, et al. Impact of gene polymorphisms on clinical outcome for stage IV melanoma patients treated with biochemotherapy: an exploratory study. *Clin Cancer Res.* 2005;11(3):1237-1246.

364. Garcia-Hernandez ML, et al. Interleukin-10 promotes B16-melanoma growth by inhibition of macrophage functions and induction of tumour and vascular cell proliferation. *Immunology.* 2002;105(2):231-243.

365. Huang S, et al. Interleukin 10 suppresses tumor growth and metastasis of human melanoma cells: potential inhibition of angiogenesis. *Clin Cancer Res.* 1996;2(12):1969-1979.

366. Howell WM, et al. IL-10 promoter polymorphisms influence tumour development in cutaneous malignant melanoma. *Genes Immun.* 2001;2(1):25-31.

367. Atkins M, Garnick M, Renal Neoplasia, in The Kidney, B. Brenner, Editor. 2000, WB Saunders Co p 1844-1868.

368. Upton, M.P., et al., Histologic predictors of renal cell carcinoma response to interleukin-2-based therapy. *J Immunother.* 2005;28(5):488-495.

369. Atkins M, et al. Carbonic anhydrase IX expression predicts outcome of interleukin 2 therapy for renal cancer. *Clin Cancer Res.* 2005;11(10):3714-3721.

370. Bui MH, et al. Carbonic anhydrase IX is an independent predictor of survival in advanced renal clear cell carcinoma: implications for prognosis and therapy. *Clin Cancer Res.* 2003;9(2):802-811.

371. Rivoltini L, et al. Immunity to cancer: attack and escape in T lymphocyte-tumor cell interaction. *Immunol Rev.* 2002;188:97-113.

372. De Paola F, et al. Restored T-cell activation mechanisms in human tumour-infiltrating lymphocytes from melanomas and colorectal carcinomas after exposure to interleukin-2. *Br J Cancer.* 2003;88(2):320-326.

373. Bukowski RM, et al. Signal transduction abnormalities in T lymphocytes from patients with advanced renal carcinoma: clinical relevance and effects of cytokine therapy. *Clin Cancer Res.* 1998;4(10):2337-2347.

374. Piancatelli D, et al. Local expression of cytokines in human colorectal carcinoma: evidence of specific interleukin-6 gene expression. *J Immunother.* 1999;22(1):25-32.

375. Lissoni P, et al. Correlation between pretreatment serum levels of neopterin and response to interleukin-2 immunotherapy in cancer patients. *J Biol Regul Homeost Agents.* 1995;9(1):21-23.

376. Chen CK, et al. T lymphocytes and cytokine production in ascitic fluid of ovarian malignancies. *J Formos Med Assoc.* 1999;98(1):24-30.

377. Nemunaitis J, et al. Comparison of serum interleukin-10 (IL-10) levels between normal volunteers and patients with advanced melanoma. *Cancer Invest.* 2001;19(3):239-247.

378. Chen Q, et al. Production of IL-10 by melanoma cells: examination of its role in immunosuppression mediated by melanoma. *Int J Cancer.* 1994;56(5):755-760.

379. Kim R, et al. Tumor-driven evolution of immunosuppressive networks during malignant progression. *Cancer Res.* 2006;66(11):5527-5536.

380. Prendergast GC, Metz R, Muller AJ. IDO recruits Tregs in melanoma. *Cell Cycle.* 2009;8(12):1818-1819.

381. Witkiewicz AK, et al. Genotyping and expression analysis of IDO2 in human pancreatic cancer: a novel, active target. *J Am Coll Surg.* 2009;208(5):781-787; discussion 787-789.

382. Agnello G, et al. Depleting blood arginine with AEB1102 (Pegzilarginase) exerts additive anti-tumor and synergistic survival benefits when combined with immunomodulators of the PD-1 pathway. *J ImmunTher Cancer.* 2017;5(suppl 2):255.

383. Luke JJ, et al. Preliminary antitumor and immunomodulatory activity of BMS-986205, an optimized indoleamine 2,3-dioxygenase 1 (IDO1) inhibitor, in combination with nivolumab in patients with advanced cancers. In Society for Immunotherapy of Cancer (SITC) Annual Meeting. National Harbor, Maryland; 2017.

384. Cesana GC, et al. Characterization of CD4+CD25+ regulatory T cells in patients treated with high-dose interleukin-2 for metastatic melanoma or renal cell carcinoma. *J Clin Oncol.* 2006;24(7):1169-1177.

385. van der Vliet HJ, et al. Effects of the administration of high-dose interleukin-2 on immunoregulatory cell subsets in patients with advanced melanoma and renal cell cancer. *Clin Cancer Res.* 2007;13(7):2100-2108.

386. Barnett B, et al. Depleting CD4+ CD25+ regulatory T-cells improves immunity in cancer-bearing patients. In: Proceedings of AACR; 2004.

387. Vieweg J, Su Z, Dannuli J. Enhancement of antitumor immunity following depletion of CD+CD25+ regulatory T-cells. In: Proceedings of ASCO; 2004.

388. Rasku MA, et al. Transient T cell depletion causes regression of melanoma metastases. *J Transl Med.* 2008;6:12.

389. Attia P, et al. Inability of a fusion protein of IL-2 and diphtheria toxin (denileukin diftitox, DAB389IL-2, ONTAK) to eliminate regulatory T lymphocytes in patients with melanoma. *J Immunother.* 2005;28(6):582-592.

390. Maker AV, et al. Tumor regression and autoimmunity in patients treated with cytotoxic T lymphocyte-associated antigen 4 blockade and interleukin 2: a phase I/II study. *Ann Surg Oncol.* 2005;12(12):1005-1016.

391. Dorr RT, et al. Phase I-II trial of interferon-alpha 2b by continuous subcutaneous infusion over 28 days. *J Interferon Res.* 1988;8(6):717-725.

392. Kirkwood JM, et al. Comparison of intramuscular and intravenous recombinant alpha-2 interferon in melanoma and other cancers. *Ann Intern Med.* 1985;103(1):32-36.

393. Chiang J, et al. Pharmacokinetics of recombinant human interferon-beta ser in healthy volunteers and its effect on serum neopterin. *Pharm Res.* 1993;10(4):567-572.

394. Grunberg SM, et al. Phase I study of recombinant beta-interferon given by four-hour infusion. *Cancer Res.* 1987;47(4):1174-1178.

395. Buchwalder PA, et al. Pharmacokinetics and pharmacodynamics of IFN-beta 1a in healthy volunteers. *J Interferon Cytokine Res.* 2000;20(10):857-866.

396. Rinehart JJ, et al. Phase I/II trial of human recombinant interferon gamma in renal cell carcinoma. *J Biol Response Mod.* 1986;5(4):300-308.

397. ACTIMMUNE® (Interferon Gamma-1b); Horizon Pharma Ireland Ltd. Dublin, Ireland; August 2015.

398. Cascinelli N, et al. Results of adjuvant interferon study in WHO melanoma programme. *Lancet.* 1994;343(8902):913-914.

399. Agarwala SS, et al. Phase III randomized study of 4 weeks of high-dose interferon-alpha-2b in stage T2bNO, T3a-bNO, T4a-bNO, and T1-4N1a-2a (microscopic) Melanoma: a trial of the Eastern Cooperative Oncology Group-American College of Radiology Imaging Network Cancer Research Group (E1697). *J Clin Oncol.* 2017;35(8):885-892.

400. Eigentler TK, et al. Adjuvant treatment with pegylated interferon alpha-2a versus low-dose interferon alpha-2a in patients with high-risk melanoma: a randomized phase III DeCOG trial. *Ann Oncol.* 2016;27(8):1625-1632.

401. Negrier S, et al. Medroxyprogesterone, interferon alfa-2a, interleukin 2, or combination of both cytokines in patients with metastatic renal carcinoma of intermediate prognosis: results of a randomized controlled trial. *Cancer.* 2007;110(11):2468-2477.

402. Diab A, Tannir N, Cho D, et al. Preliminary safety, efficacy and biomarker results from the Phase 1/2 study of CD-122-biased agonist NKTR-214 plus nivolumab in patients with locally advanced/metastatic solid tumors. In Society for Immunotherapy of Cancer (SITC) Annual Meeting. National Harbor, Maryland, 2017, pp Abs 020.

Adoptive Cellular Therapy

Marco Ruella, Antonella Rotolo, Katherine D. Cummins, and Carl H. June

Introduction and Definition

Adoptive cellular therapy (ACT) is the transfer of immune cells into a patient with the goal of obtaining a therapeutic benefit. In the last few years, ACT has gained renewed attention largely, thanks to the impressive clinical results obtained with anti-CD19 chimeric antigen receptor (CAR) T cells in B-cell leukemias and lymphomas. Indeed, the Food and Drug Administration (FDA) achieved an historical milestone in 2017 when tisagenlecleucel, the CAR developed at the University of Pennsylvania and by Novartis, became the first ACT therapy to be approved, closely followed by the approval of axicabtagene ciloleucel by Kite of the CD19 CAR developed at the National Cancer Institute (NCI). ACT is indeed revolutionizing the treatment of B-cell leukemia and lymphoma, and it is poised to become a routine therapeutic option for cancer types.[1]

In most cases, ACT has been developed for cancer patients; however, ACT could also be employed to treat infectious diseases and autoimmune disorders. The most common immune cells used in ACT are lymphocytes but also other immune cells like natural killer cells, monocytes, and dendritic cells can be modified ex vivo and reinfused. Commonly, lymphocytes are isolated, ex vivo activated, genetically engineered, and infused into the patient. This chapter describes the background, rationale, and current clinical use and experimental approaches of adoptive cellular therapies using lymphocytes for the treatment of cancer.

History

The sentinel observations made by William B. Coley in the 1890s that patients with certain malignancies responded to the intratumoral inoculation of live bacteria or toxins provided the impetus for the development of immunotherapy for cancers. However, it is only several decades later that Bellingham and coworkers first coined the term adoptive immunity to describe the transfer of lymphocytes to mediate an effector function in a series of experiments addressing mechanisms of skin allograft rejection.[2] In the 1950s, the concept of ACT for tumor allografts was first reported in rodents by Mitchison.[3] For the early development of ACT, see Ref.[4]

The cloning of T-cell growth factors made possible the first ex vivo expansion of tumor-specific T cells for ACT in mouse syngeneic tumor models. In the following years, significant additional improvements to T-cell growth and expansion allowed the clinical transition of ACT besides the transplant setting. The first clinical experience of ACT in humans was reported by the Seattle group in 1991 in the context of cytomegalovirus (CMV) prophylaxis during immune reconstitution post transplantation, where CMV-specific T-cell clones were expanded ex vivo and infused into patients at high risk of CMV infection, resulting in the establishment of a protective immune response.[5] This important report demonstrated that the fundamental requirements for successful ACT, namely, ex vivo manipulation, expansion, and reinfusion, into patients were technically feasible and precipitated concerted efforts to apply ACT to target malignancy.

Early efforts to target malignancy focused on the use of bulk populations of expanded lymphocytes, tumor-infiltrating lymphocytes (TILs) pioneered by the Rosenberg group at the NCI.[6] Significant progress has been achieved over the past 30 years, but it is only in the last 6 to 8 years that, thanks to the orthogonal technologies of gene engineering and synthetic biology, ACT has become progressively more successful, culminating with the FDA approvals. Table 31.1 summarizes the main characteristics of the most commonly used ACT approaches.

Scientific Rationale for Adoptive Cellular Therapy

Allogeneic Cell Transplantation

Allogeneic hematopoietic stem cell transplant (allo-HSCT) can be considered the first successful form of ACT as the infused donor CD34$^+$ stem cells will regenerate the full immune system of the host, including lymphocytes with potential antitumor activity. Indeed, in a seminal study published in 1979, it was observed that stem cell transplantation from syngeneic donors was less effective than sibling donors in preventing relapse of leukemia,[7] suggesting a "graft-versus-leukemia" (GVL) effect contributed to the efficacy of allogeneic transplantation. Subsequently, it was demonstrated that relapse rates were higher when T cells were removed from the allograft and that relapse could successfully be treated by infusion of donor lymphocytes (DLI) or withdrawal of T-cell–directed immunosuppression, all pointing to the importance of T cells in the anticancer response after allogeneic transplant. For these reasons, allo-HSCT can be considered the first form of successful ACT.

Two key factors can negatively impact on the outcome of allo-HSCT. First, immune reconstitution can be slow and incomplete, potentially resulting in disease relapse. Furthermore, in the case of post–allo-HSCT relapse, patients are generally unfit for chemotherapy and therapeutic options remain limited.[8] Second, donor lymphocytes often recognize as nonself and kill recipient

TABLE

31.1   *Characteristics of the main strategies for ACT*

Parameter	DLI	TIL	TCR T	CAR T
Tissue of origin	Donor PB	Tumor	PB	PB
Ease of generation	High	Low	Moderate	Moderate
Efficiency of generation	High	Moderate	High	High
Time of ex vivo manipulation	0 (unmanipulated) up to 5 weeks (NK DLI)	20 to 60 d	Generally 8 to 12 d	Generally 6 to 10 d
Genetic modification	Not necessary	Not necessary	Required	Required
Antigens targeted	All	All	All	Surface only
Antigen specificity	Undefined	Undefined	Defined	Defined
Need for antigen processing and HLA presentation	Yes	Yes	Yes	No
Effector functionality	Undefined	Undefined	High	High
Proven clinical efficacy	1. CML, relapsed chronic phase 2. Indolent B-NHL, PTLD, MM, AML: only if low burden and in combination with cytoreductive chemotherapy 3. AML—NK DLI	1. Melanoma 2. HCC 3. Colorectal carcinoma	1. Melanoma 2. Synovial cell sarcoma 3. Multiple myeloma 4. NAML	1. CD19⁺ B-cell neoplasms: ALL, DLBCL, CLL 2. Multiple myeloma 3. Glioblastoma
Potential for on-target, off-tumor toxicity	High	Low	High	High
Potential for off-target toxicity	High (GVHD)	Low	Moderate	Low
Feasibility of commercialization	Low	Low	Moderate	Two FDA-approved products: 1. Kymriah™ (tisagenlecleucel, UPENN/ Novartis) for difficult-to-treat or relapsed ALL, up to 25-year-old patients 2. Yescarta™ (axicabtagene ciloleucel, NCI/Kite) for DLBCL

DLI, donor lymphocyte infusions; TIL, tumor-infiltrating lymphocytes; TCRT, T-cell receptor–engineered T cells; CART, chimeric antigen receptor–modified T cells; PB, peripheral blood; CML, chronic myeloid leukemia; B-NHL, B-lineage non-Hodgkin lymphoma; PTLD, posttransplant lymphoproliferative disorder; MM, multiple myeloma; AML, acute myeloid leukemia; NK DLI, donor natural killer cell infusion; HCC, hepatocellular carcinoma; ALL, B-lineage acute lymphoblastic leukemia; DLBCL, diffuse large B-cell lymphoma; CLL, chronic lymphocytic leukemia; GBM, glioblastoma multiforme; GVHD, graft-versus-host disease; UPENN, University of Pennsylvania; NCI, National Cancer Institute.

healthy tissues causing graft-versus-host disease (GVHD). In an effort to solve the first issue, donor lymphocyte infusions (DLIs) were developed, that is, a form of ACT consisting of infusions of mature donor effector cells aimed to exert prompt antitumor activity in individuals with florid relapse (therapeutic DLI) and boost immune surveillance in patients at high risk of relapse (prophylactic DLI). Although successful in chronic myeloid leukemia (CML), the therapeutic effect of DLI remained limited in other malignancies. The relative inefficacy in acute disorders such as acute myeloid leukemia (AML) and acute lymphoblastic leukemia (ALL) might be explained by the contrast between the rapid kinetics of highly proliferative blasts and the delayed onset of the DLI-induced antileukemic effect, usually peaking 6 to 8 months after infusion. Similarly,

loss of expression of HLA molecules by a process termed uniparental disomy,[9] impaired antigen presentation, lack of costimulation, and immunosuppressive microenvironment may be responsible for the poorer results in other malignancies with slower kinetics, for example, myelodysplastic syndromes (MDS) and multiple myeloma (MM). Lymphodepleting chemotherapy regimens given prior to DLI have been associated with greater responses, possibly due to the effect on the immunosuppressive microenvironment, including depletion of regulatory T cells (Treg cells) and on the cytokine milieu. In addition, ex vivo activation of donor lymphocytes by IL-2 and/or anti–CD3-and anti–CD28-coated beads[10] resulted in significant improvement of T-cell reactivity even in patients who were previously resistant to unmanipulated DLI.

However, clinical responses to conventional DLI correlate with the occurrence of GVHD, with a proportional relationship between the magnitude of the therapeutic response and the severity of the adverse event. Hence, there has been a growing interest in the manipulation of the graft cellular components to modulate allogeneic T-cell reactivity. Pioneer work demonstrated that durable remissions with tolerable GVHD could be attained by using either CD8[+]-depleted (or CD4[+]-enriched) grafts[11] or donor PBMCs endowed with a suicide gene to allow fast elimination of alloreactive CD3[+] cells in the event of severe GVHD.[12] Alternatively, the composition of the donor graft could be manipulated to enrich for specific T-cell subsets according to their differentiation state.[13] Specifically, more mature CD8[+] effector T cells (CD8[+] T_E) have been associated with swift and potent reactivity in vitro and high potential for robust GVT/GVL effect, while the less differentiated central memory T subset (T_{CM}) showed greater engraftment, expansion, and proliferation in vivo, features that are crucial to achieve sustained immune surveillance, although at the cost of increased risk of GVHD. Therefore, it can be envisioned that better outcomes may stem from the infusion of more balanced allograft products carrying equal proportions of more mature (cytotoxic) and less differentiated (long-term persistent) cells. Finally, there is evidence that regulatory T cells (Tregs), a heterogeneous population of immunosuppressive lymphocytes identified by the natural (nTreg) or acquired (iTreg) expression of the master transcription factor Foxp3,[14] could help prevent/abrogate GVHD while preserving GVL/GVT effect. Preclinical and clinical observations demonstrated an inverse correlation between the number of donor Treg and the risk of GVHD. In agreement with this, administration of ex vivo activated and expanded Treg cells prevents GVHD in animal models[15] and appears safe and may prevent GVHD in umbilical cord blood transplants.[16] DLIs with cells depleted for Treg cells have been successfully used in AML patients, with no increased risk of GVHD-enhanced antileukemic activity.[17]

ACT with Natural Killer (NK) Lymphocytes

First hypothesized by Kiessling and Wigzell in the 1970s as naturally occurring lymphoid cells with innate reactivity against a variety of tumor cells,[18] NK cells were conclusively demonstrated by Ljunggren and Karre (reviewed in Ref. [19]). NK cells can discriminate between normal (self) and aberrant (nonself) cells on the basis of the expression of MCH class I molecules, constitutively expressed by most healthy cells. When aberrant cells lacking MHC class I molecules do not engage NK inhibitory receptors, the activating pathways prevail; NK cells achieve full activation and kill the target cell.[20] On this basis, NK cells can potentially exert potent antitumor activity.

In the setting of auto-HSCT, early recovery of NK cells is associated with improved survival in a variety of hematologic malignancies.[21] In allo-HSCT, early recovery of donor-derived NK cells, which are the first population to repopulate the lymphoid compartment upon stem cell engraftment, was associated with improved relapse-free survival.[22] Since NK cell recovery and maturation may be delayed or impaired by a number of factors, including the use of nonlymphodepleting chemotherapy regimens pretransplant and immunosuppression posttransplant,[23] NK-DLIs have been tested in the management of allotransplanted patients.

Initial studies of ACT with NK cells have been hampered by their short-term survival. Several strategies have been tested to improve survival and to enhance the activity of NK cells in vivo. The presence of contaminating monocytes as well as the incorporation of monocyte-derived DC within the NK preparations correlated with better clinical outcomes. Likewise, the addition of IL-15 significantly improved NK cell life span and has become a key component of most Good Manufacturing Practices (GMP)-compliant protocols.[24]

The most recent advance has been the transduction of NK cells to express CARs to enhance cytotoxicity. Substantial preclinical data have been amassed with respect to the transduction of CAR molecules targeting a range of different tumor antigens using NK-92, an immortalized NK cell line, for the treatment of a range of solid organ and hematological cancers.[25] The results from clinical trials evaluating CAR+ NK cells are currently awaited. As numerous different approaches with NK cells are being evaluated, the anticipated benefits and drawbacks are as follows: (a) autologous NK cells are safe; however, they have low efficacy; (b) allogeneic NK cells are effective against some malignancies especially if KIR mismatched, though needing substantial T-cell depletion to avoid risk of GVHD; (c) NK cell lines are readily expanded and are safe for ACT after irradiation; however, efficacy remains unknown; and (d) CAR+ NK cells have the capacity to direct NK cell activity against specific tumor antigens; however, they are difficult to manufacture in large numbers.[26]

Cytokine-Induced Killer T Cells

Cytokine-induced killer (CIK) cells are a heterogeneous population of activated polyclonal CD3[+]CD56[+] effector cells, with a coexisting CD3[+]CD56[−] subset, expressing variable levels of CD16. CIK cells are generated from CD3[+] T cell by exposure to IFN-γ, OKT3 (anti-CD3 activating antibody), and IL-2, added in a rigorous time-sensitive manner. They promptly react and proliferate in response to cytokine stimulation by 3-log fold change within 2 weeks and exert potent antitumor activity against a wide range of hematological and solid cancers.[27] However, to date, clinical trials have shown modest clinical activity of CIK. Preclinical models of various cancers suggest that CIK cell antitumor activity could be even enhanced in combination with immune checkpoint inhibitors.[28] There is an emerging interest in the opportunity of redirecting unmanipulated CIK cells by exploiting the expression of CD16 in combination with infusions of monoclonal Ab to selectively induce potent antibody-dependent cell-mediated cytotoxicity (ADCC) against cancer cells.

Tumor-Infiltrating Lymphocytes

TILs have been evaluated as a source for tumor-reactive lymphocytes for ACT.[6] In most cancers, the degree and pattern of T-cell infiltration at diagnosis correlate with good prognosis and response to treatment, although the actual prognostic value also depends on the nature of the infiltrating lymphocytes and the surrounding microenvironment. In the late 1980s, Steven Rosenberg and colleagues at the NCI established a method to ex vivo generate a large amount of TIL starting from tumor specimens (Fig. 31.1A). The final TIL product is generally composed by CD8[+] and CD4[+] T cells, with no or little contamination from other cells, and is eventually reinfused into the patient after lymphodepleting chemotherapy.

Such approach has been successful in melanoma patients, with reports of unprecedented complete and durable regression of metastatic lesions (as further detailed in the "Clinical Outcomes of ACT—Solid Tumors" section).

To further select and expand truly tumor-specific TILs, the NCI group developed a strategy to detect T cells that are reactive to tumor-associated genetic mutations (Fig. 31.1B). Whole-exome sequencing of tumor-normal pair samples revealed somatic nonsynonymous mutations occurring in malignant cells, some of them encoding for peptides with immunogenic potential.[29] Several groups have developed manufacturing approaches to expand TILs specific for these neoantigens, and infusion of these TILs has led to remission in melanoma patients, leading to complete remissions in some patients with no off-tumor toxicity.[30] The same approach can be applied to other solid tumors such as cholangiocarcinoma.[31] In addition, in a patient with metastatic colorectal cancer, autologous

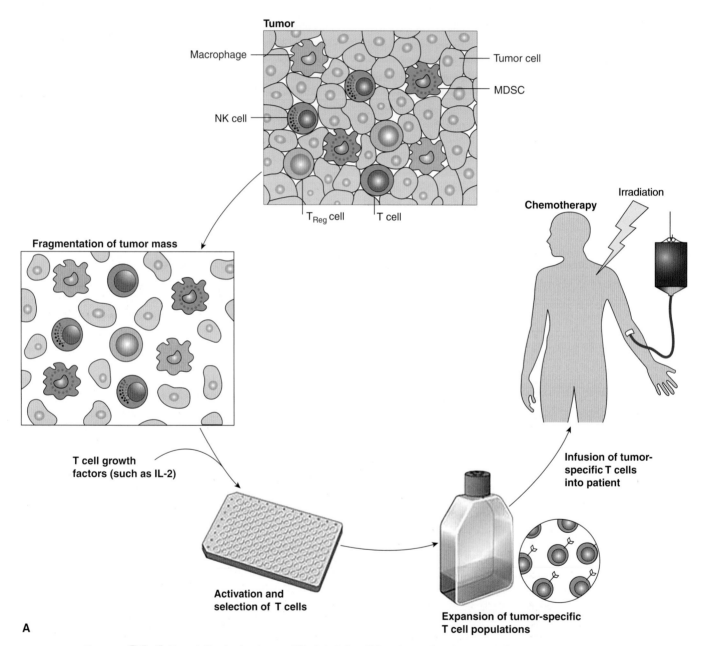

A

FIGURE **31.1** Tumor-infiltrating lymphocytes (TIL). **A.** Isolation of TIL and expansion of tumor-specific populations. Tumor masses are surgically resected and fragmented and the cells cultured with a T-cell growth factor, such as interleukin-2. Antitumor T cells can be selected, expanded, and then adoptively transferred into patients with cancer. Typically, before TIL infusion, patients undergo lymphodepletion by either chemotherapy alone or chemotherapy in combination with total body irradiation. MDSC, myeloid-derived suppressor cell; NK, natural killer; T_{Reg}, regulatory T cell. (Reprinted by permission from Nature: Restifo NP, Dudley ME, Rosenberg SA. Adoptive immunotherapy for cancer: harnessing the T cell response. *Nat Rev Immunol.* 2012;12(4):269-281. Copyright © 2012 Springer Nature.)

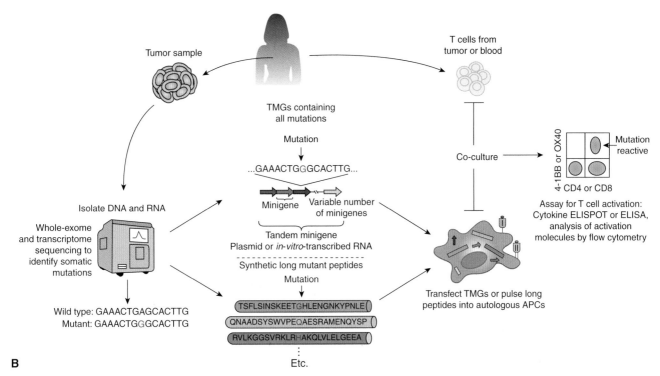

B

FIGURE 31.1 (*Continued*) **B.** Expansion of T cells specifically recognizing mutated proteins in cancer cells. Next-generation sequencing (whole exome and whole transcriptome) is performed on tumor and matched normal cells to identify nonsynonymous somatic mutations expressed by the cancer **(left)**. Next, minigenes encoding the mutation flanked by nucleotides from the wild-type gene can be synthesized in tandem to create TMG constructs, which are then cloned into an appropriate viral vector **(top)** or long peptides **(bottom)** and introduced into the appropriate antigen-presenting cells (APCs), such as autologous dendritic cells or B cells, through techniques such as electroporation or lipid-based transfection, to allow processing and presentation of the neoantigens in the context of the patient's own HLA class I and II molecules. T cells derived from tumor (TILs) or from the blood **(right)** are then cocultured with the antigen-presenting cells expressing the TMGs, and T-cell reactivity is evaluated by immunological methods. (Reprinted by permission from Nature: Tran E, Robbins PF, Rosenberg SA. 'Final common pathway' of human cancer immunotherapy: targeting random somatic mutations. *Nat Immunol.* 2017;18(3):255-262. Copyright © 2017 Springer Nature.)

CD8[+] TILs reactive to a KRAS G12D mutated variant were expanded ex vivo and reinfused into the patient, leading to regression of all metastases.[32]

Although targeting individual mutated immunogenic epitopes may appear impractical at present, in the future, this may provide an acceptable option particularly for poor prognosis cancers that would not normally be considered immunogenic.[33] Further implementation may require refinement of the T-cell expansion protocols. To this end, exposure to IL-21 or AKT inhibitors during the ex vivo manipulation may help preserve a less differentiated state and improve in vivo persistence.

T-Cell Receptor–Engineered T Cells (TCR T)

T cell can identify cancer cells mainly by recognizing mutated peptides or peptides that are overexpressed in tumor cells as compared to normal cells. This recognition is mediated by the interaction between the T-cell receptor (TCR) and the MHC-peptide complex in target cells (Fig. 31.2). The TCR affinity and T-cell avidity are key determinants of antitumor reactivity. Comparative analyses have demonstrated that TCRs against tumor have substantially lower antigen affinity (approximately 0.5 logs) compared to TCRs directed against virus-derived antigens.[34]

Therefore, increasing the affinity of antitumor TCR has been a strategy to improve antitumor killing of redirected T cells. Affinity-tuned TCRs have been generated against an array of candidate targets in several malignancies, including MDM-2, p53, CEA, gp100, MAGE-A3, and NY-ESO-1. High-affinity TCR-engineered T-cell clones exhibited a greater reactivity in patients with advanced, chemotherapy refractory blood cancers and metastatic solid tumors that were associated with more robust and durable clinical responses.[35,36] However, caution is warranted because cases of severe toxicity, including lethal events, have also been reported due to off-target reactivity with epitopes shared by peptide expressed in normal tissues.[37,38]

Most recently, neoantigens generated from somatic point mutations, as well as epigenetic, transcriptional, translational, and posttranslational alterations in tumor but not normal tissues,[39] have become attractive targets for TCR ACT.[40] For example, TCR-engineered CD4[+] T cells recognizing an ERBB2 neoantigen induced sustained remission in a patient with cholangiocarcinoma.[31] A similar approach is used for TIL therapy where T-cell clones reactive to mutated peptides are expanded and reinfused back to the patient (please refer to the previous section "Tumor-infiltrating Lymphocytes" of this chapter).

Several aspects of redirected TCR ACT are under active investigation with the goal of increasing clinical responses and safety. First, the variable and heterogeneous expression of the targeted peptide-MHC within the tumor mass can reduce the efficacy of redirected TCR T cell; therefore, infusions of pools of TCR-engineered T-cell lines recognizing different neoantigens may represent a valid option

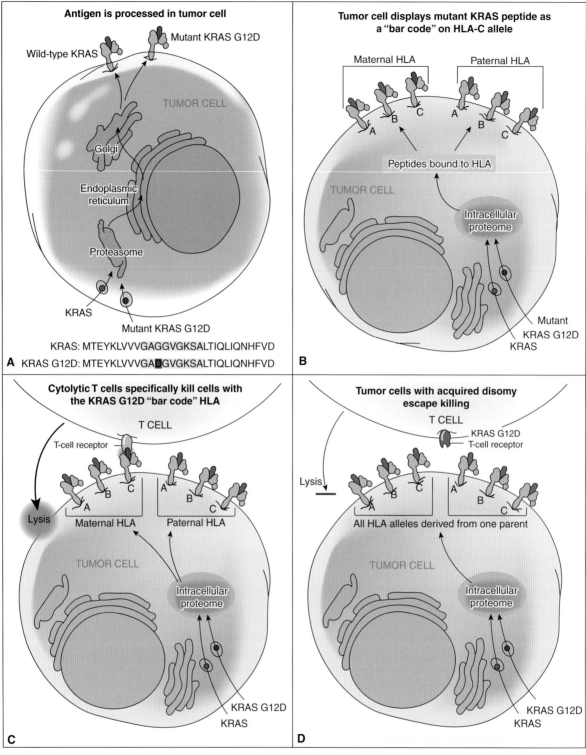

FIGURE **31.2** Presentation of neoantigen peptides by tumor to T cells. **Panel A** shows tumor cells that have a heterozygous nonsense point mutation in KRAS. Wild-type and mutant KRAS peptides are degraded into a series of peptides in the proteasome and are then bound to HLA molecules in the endoplasmic reticulum and Golgi apparatus before being displayed on the surface of tumor cells. The HLA molecules are "bar-coded" by displaying unique wild-type or mutant peptides derived from KRAS for recognition on their surface. The sequence of the first 20 amino acids of wild-type KRAS and mutant KRAS G12D is depicted; the nonamer peptide is shown in *yellow*, and the mutant amino acid residue is shown in *red*. **Panel B** shows tumor cells that display mutant KRAS peptides as a "bar code" on the HLA allele. The intracellular proteome is displayed on HLA genes A, B, and C. The HLA genes are codominant and are inherited from both maternal and paternal DNA. **Panel C** shows T cells that specifically kill tumor cells with a T-cell receptor specific for HLA molecules expressing mutant KRAS G12D while ignoring HLA molecules that have wild-type KRAS peptides. **Panel D** shows the development of tumor resistance to the T cells through down-regulation of the MHC allele capable of presenting the antigen to the T cell. In this instance, the tumor has stopped expressing the maternal MHC alleles; therefore, the T cell cannot recognize the peptide antigen. (Redrawn from June CH. Drugging the Undruggable Ras — Immunotherapy to the Rescue? *N Engl J Med.* 2016;375(23):2286-2289.)

to prevent immune evasion.[41] Second, cotransfer of CD3 molecule, which is part of the TCR complex and is required for TCR surface expression but is generally produced in limiting amounts, has been associated with increased membrane levels of the exogenous TCR and improved antitumor activity in preclinical in vivo models.[42] Third, expression of heterodimeric TCR $\alpha\beta$ transgenes must be highly regulated, ensuring a balanced production and preventing mispairing with the endogenous counterparts. Mispairing with endogenous $\alpha\beta$ TCR chains not only can reduce transduction efficiency but also confer new specificities against autoantigens, thus resulting in off-target toxicity.[43] To circumvent this, three main approaches have been used: (a) usage of improved clinical vectors employing modified promoters, codon optimization, and bicistronic elements to promote higher levels and coordinated expression of TCR$\alpha\beta$ transgenes,[44] (b) editing of the constant region and additional disulfide bonds to maximize correct pairing of the exogenous chains, and (c) gene editing to reduce or eliminate expression of the endogenous TCR.[45]

Further refinement of TCR-engineered T cells includes measures to prevent T-cell tolerance in vivo. The use of anti–PD-1 antibody in combination with NY-ESO-1-TCR–specific T cells has been proven to effectively restore T-cell function.[46] Evidence generated from CAR T-cell studies suggests that TCR-modified T cells may benefit from transgenic chemokine receptors to improve homing at the tumor site.[47] The main advantage of TCR T cells is the ability to detect low levels of mutated target antigenic peptides, while the requirement for HLA restriction represents the main limitation for clinical translation of TCR-based adoptive therapy.

Chimeric Antigen Receptor-Engineered T Cells

CARs are synthetic proteins consisting of an antibody-derived antigen-binding moiety coupled with the TCR complex signaling domains (Fig. 31.3). Such a protein can redirect an otherwise non–tumor-specific T cell against a specific tumor surface protein. The idea of endowing T cells with an antibody specificity dates back to the late 1980s, when Gross and Eshhar described an innovative "T-body," that is, a protein consisting of two chains joining the immunoglobulin recognition function with TCR constant regions.[48] A similar concept, that is, the expression of chimeric receptor composed of immunoglobulin-derived V regions and T-cell receptor-derived C regions, was developed by Kuwana and colleagues.[49] Since then, new designs have been proposed to refine and implement such technology, although the basic tetramodular structure has remained substantially the same and is characterized by the following: (a) a binding moiety, mostly derived from monoclonal antibodies (mAbs) and less frequently from ligand analogues, peptides, receptors, and nanobodies; (b) an extracellular spacer/hinge borrowed from Ig, CD4, CD8, or CD28 molecules, crucial in determining the optimal distance between T-and target cells at the immunological synapse as well as the outcome of nonspecific interactions with bystander cells, that is, off-target activation and macrophage-mediated clearance; (c) a transmembrane domain,

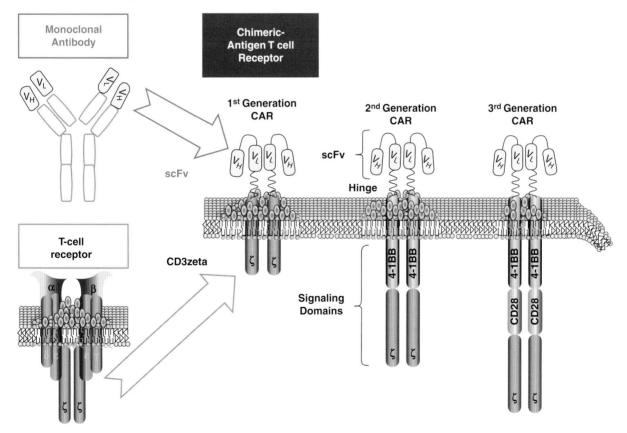

FIGURE **31.3** The structure of a chimeric antigen receptor compared to antibody and T-cell receptor. A chimeric antigen receptor (CAR) is a synthetic protein derived from the fusion of the antigen-recognizing domains of a monoclonal antibody (in the form of a single-chain variable fragment) and the intracellular signaling domain of the T-cell receptor CD3ζ chain. Second-and third-generation CARs also include costimulatory domains (typically 4-1BB or CD28). (Modified from Garfall AL, Fraietta JA, Maus MV. Immunotherapy with Chimeric Antigen Receptors for Multiple Myeloma. *Discov Med.* 2014;17(91):37-46. Reprinted with permission from Discovery Medicine.)

with variable impact on the final CAR T activation and effector functions; and (d) an activating CD3ζ/FcRγ chain endodomain. Further second-and third-generation CARs incorporate one or two costimulatory components, respectively, to compensate for the lack of costimulatory signals on malignant cells. Different costimulatory domains have been associated with distinct T-cell functional profiles and can be accordingly chosen to modulate the outcome of the desired AR cell response. Of the various costimulatory domains, it has been observed that CD28 induces higher levels of IL-2 and TNF-α, ICOS promotes greater cytotoxicity, and 4-1BB enhances survival.[50]

The first clinical experiences with CART were reported in the late 1990s. First-generation CAR T immunotherapy was initially investigated in patients with colorectal carcinoma (TAG72 and carcinoembryonic antigen, CEA), breast cancer (CEA), ovarian cancer (folate receptor-α), renal cell carcinoma (carbonic anhydrase IX, CAIX), and neuroblastoma (L1 cell adhesion molecule and GD2 ganglioside). Grade 3 and 4 adverse events were observed, including unexpected on-target off-tumor toxicity, that is, cholangitis in a renal cell carcinoma patient treated with CAIX-specific CART cells due to unanticipated CAIX expression on the bile duct epithelial cells,[51] thus providing important insights into the potential danger inherent in the choice of CAR targets. Importantly, CAR cells were proved to traffic to tumor sites and react against malignant cells, although with minimal or no clinical benefit due to poor in vivo activation and rapid immune-mediated clearance of CART cells.[52] Subsequently, CD20-and CD19-specific CAR T cells were used in a cohort of hematological patients with relapsed/refractory B-cell lymphoma. All patients received lymphodepleting chemotherapy and some of them concomitant low-dose IL-2. In contrast with solid tumor trials, there were no severe toxicity, no adverse events attributable to T-cell infusions, and no immune responses against CAR-engineered cells. Although clinical responses remained disappointing, these proof-of-principle studies (a) confirmed feasibility of viral-based gene engineering of immune cells for the purposes of ACT, (b) supported the relevance of chemotherapy regimens to improve engraftment and contain immune-mediated rejection of CAR T cells, and (c) suggested a link between in vivo CAR T-cell persistence and sustained clinical responses. Hence, to improve CAR T-cell survival, second-generation CARs were developed, which in combination with CD19-scFV led to unprecedented results including sustained complete molecular remissions in advanced relapsed or refractory chronic lymphocytic leukemia (CLL), ALL, B-cell non-Hodgkin lymphoma (B-NHL), and MM.[53]

Optimization of the clinical protocols, that is, preparatory chemotherapy, CAR T-cell dose, schedule, and timing of administration, allowed further implementation with significant reduction of potentially lethal toxicity related to overwhelming T-cell activation, referred to as cytokine release syndrome (CRS) (*discussed in "Toxicity of Modern Adoptive Cellular Therapies"*).

Figure 31.4 summarizes the main steps for CAR T-cell manufacturing. Briefly, patients undergo leukapheresis, followed by T-cell activation with anti–CD3-/anti–CD28-coated beads or other technologies. Next, activated T cells are incubated with lentiviral particles carrying the vector encoding for the CAR and expanded up to clinical scale numbers (typically over 10 days). At the end of the expansion, the beads are removed, and the cell culture can be either concentrated or cryopreserved until usage. Modifications to the above procedure may include different starting material (peripheral blood); the method to deliver the CAR transgene, for example,

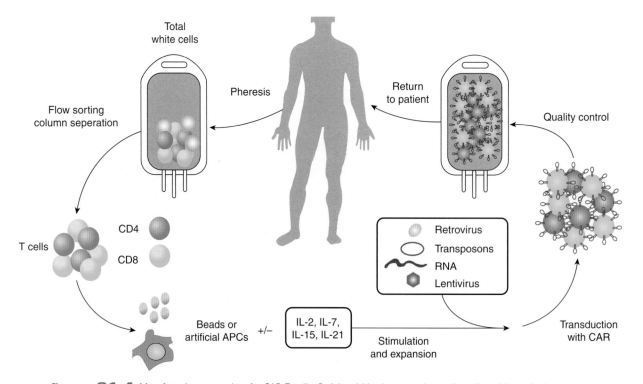

FIGURE 31.4 Manufacturing approaches for CAR T cells. Peripheral blood mononuclear cells collected by leukapheresis are expanded ex vivo and transduced with a lentiviral vector to express the CAR molecule before infusion into the patient. In this example, paramagnetic beads coated with antibodies to CD3 and CD28 are used for ex vivo expansion. (Modified with permission from Barrett DM, Singh N, Porter DL, et al. Chimeric antigen receptor therapy for cancer. *Annu Rev Med.* 2014;65:333-347. Copyright © 2014 by Annual Reviews, http://www.annualreviews.org.)

Sleeping Beauty transposon system or mRNA transfection versus retro-/lentivirus transduction; the usage of artificial APC for CAR T-cell expansion or anti-CD3 MoAb plus IL-2 instead of anti–CD3-/anti–CD28-coated beads; and the choice of specific devices for CAR T-cell culture, for example, G-Rex static systems in case of initial low seeding densities versus bioreactors with rocking platform. Development of fully automated procedures for CAR T manufacturing could potentially be critical to sustain the increase in the demand for CAR immunotherapy.

Despite the impressive results in CD19 malignancies, the outcome of CAR T immunotherapy in CD19-negative disorders remains poor mainly due to lack of potency and specificity. Because of its high and homogeneous expression on virtually all malignant cells and the relative tumor restriction, CD19 is an excellent yet unique molecule to elicit robust immune responses with acceptable off-tumor toxicity. Conversely, the relative dearth of suitable antigens represents one of the main challenges of CAR T immunotherapy in CD19-negative hematologic neoplasm and solid tumors.

Several candidates have been under investigation. CD22 is an attractive target in CD19-negative ALL relapses, frequently occurring after CD19-directed immunotherapies (e.g., NCT02315612, NCT02650414, NCT02650414). Targeting B-cell maturation antigen (BCMA), expressed on normal and malignant plasma cells, with CART cells can elicit potent antitumor activity in myeloma patients (e.g., NCT02215967, NCT02658929, NCT02546167), whereas CD33 and CD123 have been evaluated in AML trials (e.g., NCT03126864, NCT02623582, NCT02159495, NCT03190278). More recently, CD123-specific CART cells have been also proposed to treat Hodgkin lymphoma (HL), given the addiction of the malignant clone to the tumor microenvironment (TME) and the expression of CD123 on tumor-associated macrophages (TAM).[54] In solid tumors, HER2 is under evaluation in several malignancies, including melanoma, breast cancer, and glioblastoma (e.g., NCT02547961, NCT02442297, NCT02713984). Clinical activity has been reported in a glioblastoma patient treated with anti-IL13Ra2 CART,[55] and a new construct directed against a mutant variant of the epidermal growth factor receptor (EGFRvIII) has shown promising preclinical activity in the same disease.[56] Other potential candidates include the receptor tyrosine kinase c-Met, which is also overexpressed in malignant pleural mesothelioma, breast cancer, and melanoma (e.g., NCT01837602, NCT03060356), mesothelin in mesothelioma and pancreatic and ovarian cancers (NCT01355965), and the orphan tyrosine kinase receptor ROR1, which has been involved in survival of several hematological and solid tumors, thus representing an attractive target for a broad range of malignancies (NCT02706392). An overview of the clinical results is provided below in *Clinical outcomes of adoptive cell therapies*.

While the quest for the adequate candidates continues, several strategies have been attempted to improve safety and efficacy. Active elimination of CART cells represents the most obvious way to address toxicity issues. Beyond the administration of nonspecific pharmacological immunosuppression, selective termination of CAR T-cell activity has been achieved by introducing suicide and/or elimination switches. Suicide genes include HSV-TK or proteins with caspase-like activity (iCasp9), in frame with a drug dimerizer domain, that trigger apoptosis upon induction with ganciclovir or specific dimerizer (rimiducid), respectively. Elimination

genes are surface antigens, for example, CD20 and EGFR-derived extracellular epitopes, that can mediate in vivo depletion by clinical grade mAbs. Other approaches rely on transient expression of the CAR construct by means of RNA electroporation.[57] Although powerful, the flip side of in vivo CAR cell ablation would be the concomitant loss of immunosurveillance. Hence, another line of research is focused on the implementation of the CAR design and the generation of affinity-optimized CAR variants that can discriminate between aberrant and healthy cells based on different levels of expression of the target antigen.[36] Specifically, low-affinity CARs have been proven to mediate strong cytotoxicity against transformed cells expressing high levels of the relevant antigen with minimal or no reactivity against antigen-low normal cells. The introduction of microcircuits and transcriptional loops to modulate CAR expression,[50] the use of *trans* 2nd-generation CARs with split costimulatory configuration or multi-CAR platforms, and combining conventional activating constructs with inhibitory CARs (iCAR), carrying CTLA-4- or PD-1–derived inhibitory domains, could potentially add further precision and ensure that the effector cells reach full activation only against targets expressing a defined array of tumor-associated antigens.[58]

Another hurdle, particularly in solid tumors, is the inhibitory influence of the microenvironment that blunts the immune response.[59] To overcome this, new strategies have been conceived to increase CAR cell trafficking to the tumor site, for example, by inducing exogenous coexpression of chemokines and homing receptors, or to target simultaneously both malignant and neighboring immunosuppressive cells. Alternatively, CAR cells could be equipped with novel functions and become "armored CAR cells" or "TRUCKs." These CAR T cells have the ability to express costimulatory ligands, release homeostatic cytokines, and secrete checkpoint-blocking scFv. Constitutive coexpression of CD40L or 4-1BBL by tumor-specific CAR T cells can potentially shape the tumor microenvironment and reactivate endogenous anergized immune cells. Similarly, cytokine-secreting CAR T cells would offer the opportunity to harness the adjuvant effect of recombinant cytokines as living pharmacies, with the advantages of dispensing the drug locally at the tumor site, that is, maximal activity in situ and no systemic toxicity. IL-12, a pleiotropic cytokine produced by APC cells, has been extensively investigated owing to its key role in modulating the hostile tumor microenvironment and rescuing endogenous unresponsive immune cells. IL-12 secreting CAR T cells resulted superior to their unarmored counterpart in a number of preclinical studies in vitro and in vivo, thus providing the foundation for further clinical investigation, for example, in patients with recurrent ovarian cancer. Given the toxicity observed in melanoma patients receiving TILs engineered with NFAT-inducible IL-12, IL-18 expressing CAR T cells have been proposed as a safer format of armored cells. Another way to curb environmental immunosuppression may be to shield CAR T cells from checkpoint proteins. Indeed, CAR T cells are susceptible to immune-checkpoint inhibitory signals, and combinatorial therapy with anti-PD1 mAb has shown the ability to relieve immunosuppression and restore CAR T-cell function. Accordingly, CRISPR-mediated PD1-KO, dominant negative receptors, PD1-CAR, and anti–PD-L1 Ab-secreting CART cells exhibited enhanced anticancer activity, with promising evidence of efficacy in solid tumors. Whether the abrogation of negative immune regulators would lead to increased challenges with control needs to be addressed in clinical trials.

Building upon the paradigm of combination chemotherapy regimens, CAR immunotherapy directed against more than one tumor-associated antigen simultaneously has been proven to be more potent while mitigating against the risk of immune evasion.[60] Pools of CAR T cells, that is, mixtures of CAR T cells with different specificities, or multiplex CAR T cells where a single cell can engage several antigens with distinct CAR constructs or one single CAR with two binding domains in frame, can serve to this scope. More recently, switchable CARs, such as biotin-binding immune receptors (BBIR) and UniCAR, have been developed by creating an array of soluble, modular, tagged scFv domains, equally fitting a constant CAR stalk and supplied as required, thus allowing extra flexibility and multispecificity in a timely controlled manner.

Lastly, there is great interest in developing universal CAR T or TCR-engineered T cells that could be used in any patient without the need of HLA matching. To this goal, universal T-cell rejection by the recipient immune system and GVHD caused by donor T cells need to be overcome. Zinc finger nucleases (ZFN), TAL effector nuclease (TALEN), or CRISPR/Cas9 gene-editing techniques have been used to disrupt the cell surface expression of TCR (prevent GHVD) and HLA I molecules (prevent rejection), with preliminary evidence supporting effective separation of GVL and GVH effects in pediatric patients.[61] Clinical trials to test these products are underway.

ACT with γδ T Lymphocytes and Invariant Natural Killer T Cells

γδ T and invariant natural killer T cells (iNKT) are cytotoxic and immunoregulatory "multitasker" cells, bridging the natural and adaptive arms of the immune system. While γδ T represent up to 10% of circulating T lymphocytes, iNKT cell is less than 0.1%, but with enormous expandability and proliferative potential in vitro and vivo.[62] γδ T lymphocytes are defined by an alternative TCR heterodimer, comprising γ and δ chains, which, unlike conventional αβ, recognize phosphoantigens, including aberrant metabolites such as isopentenyl pyrophosphate (IPP) produced by transformed cells. Conversely, iNKT cells are characterized by an invariant TCRαβ (iTCR) restricted to CD1d; a nonpolymorphic HLA class I–like molecule presenting phospho-/glycol-lipid antigens, which is mainly expressed on antigen-presenting cells (APC), including normal mature B cells as well as their malignant counterpart and tumor-associated macrophages (TAM); and some epithelial tissues.

Owing to their hybrid function between NK and T cells, γδ T cell and iNKT cell are poised for TCR-dependent and TCR-independent responses, characterized by rapid target cell cytolysis and robust cytokine release, features that are highly relevant to tumor immunity and provide the impetus for use in adoptive cell immunotherapy. Their GVL activity could be further enhanced in combination with other technologies, such as CAR, which is currently under investigation in neuroblastoma[63] and CD19+ malignancies (NCT02656147).

Notably, there is growing evidence supporting that donor γδ T cells do not cause GVHD while mediating potent GVL. On this basis, it has been predicted that third-party, "off-the-shelf" γδ T cells could be used for the purposes of adoptive immunotherapy with

minimal or no GVHD, reduced risk of graft rejection, and significantly lower relapse rates. Likewise, owing to CD1d expression on a number of malignant cells and its nonpolymorphic nature, iNKT cells could be used from third-party donors, thus fully exploiting their antitumor potential without inducing GVHD.

Early-phase trials have demonstrated the feasibility of expanding γδ T-and iNKT cells up to clinical scale in vitro without impairing their regulatory and effector functions. Indeed, ex vivo expanded autologous γδ T-and iNKT cells have been safely reinfused into cancer patients suffering from advanced/refractory disease, with reports of metastasis regressions.[64]

T-Cell Dysfunction in Cancer Patients

Impairments of T-cell function have been shown in mature T cells isolated from hosts with chronic antigen exposure, including cancer, autoimmunity, and chronic infection.[65] CD3ζ down-regulation in TILs may be one of the many mechanisms employed by tumor cells to evade immune surveillance. The first report showing CD3ζ down-regulation in the context of cancer came from an experimental model of colon carcinoma, in which cytotoxic T cells showed impaired effector function.[66] In a fully functional T cell following TCR engagement, the lymphocyte-specific protein tyrosine kinase (Lck) phosphorylates residues in the CD3ζ chain ITAMs, allowing the ζ-chain–associated protein kinase of 70 kDa (ZAP70) to bind and the signal to be transmitted downstream. Total or partial loss of CD3ζ expression thus prevents activation of the T cell.

Many enzymes with immune regulatory activity are up-regulated in cancer patients, either in tumor environment or draining lymph nodes, such as arginase 1, inducible nitric oxide synthase, and IDO, along with an increased production of nitric oxide and reactive oxygen and nitrogen species.[67,68] Under certain conditions, ACT can achieve tumor eradication without detectable changes in the composition or phenotype of intratumoral myeloid cells.[69] Conventional radiotherapy and chemotherapy can facilitate antitumor T-cell function by increasing T-cell homing tumors and/or alleviating immunosuppression. T-cell exhaustion as well as immune senescence and tumor mass can impact the response to checkpoint blockade in patients with melanoma,[70] and it is likely that these factors will be important factors determining the success of ACT.

Clinical Outcomes of Adoptive Cellular Therapies

The Evolving Clinical Role of Allogeneic Transplant and DLI

The underlying principles and biological rationale for allo-HSCT and DLI have been discussed in detail in *Scientific Rational for ACT: Allogeneic Cell Transplantation and DLI* earlier in this chapter. The successful treatment in some cases of otherwise incurable diseases with allo-HSCT is the proof of concept of the potency of T-cell–mediated cytotoxicity and is the underlying principle driving development of ACT.

Allogeneic stem cell transplantation remains a highly specialized area of medicine, and the decision to take a patient to allo-HSCT is often a complicated one and includes consideration of patient age, comorbid health problems, physical fitness or frailty, disease status at the time of transplant, availability of a suitable HLA-matched donor, presence of contraindications to long-term immune suppression such as recent malignancy, available social supports to adhere to treatment and attend regular follow-up, and, of course, the wishes of the patient. In addition to all these variables, it can be somewhat difficult to evaluate allo-HSCT in randomized trials, due to the enormity of the proposed intervention being undertaken and also significant regional variation with respect to both conditioning regimen and perceived role of allo-HSCT for a given disease entity. Performing randomized clinical trials to evaluate the efficacy of allo-HSCT is challenging, and in many cases, there exists a paucity of evidence to definitively support or refute the benefit of allo-HSCT. Summary papers are published every few years outlining recommendations with respect to the best practice guidelines for indications for allograft, though these remain controversial for many conditions, and continue to evolve over time as new data from clinical trials emerge. The recently published European guidelines outline the current evidence for the role of allo-HSCT in the treatment of a range of malignant and nonmalignant conditions,[71] and such papers are a good reference to keep up with the constantly evolving recommendations with respect to allo-HSCT. In many cases, the decision to go to transplant is a highly individualized decision, combining the physician's expert opinion, the best available evidence, and the wishes of the patient.

Hematologic Malignancies

B-lineage Acute Lymphoblastic Leukemia

One of the greatest successes of CART therapy has been achieved in the treatment of B-lineage acute lymphoblastic lymphoma (B-ALL), using CART cells directed against the B-lineage antigen CD19. The initial phase 1 clinical trials conducted in pediatric/young adult B-ALL patients achieved exceptional complete remission (CR) rates ranging from 70% to 90%[53]; these results are particularly impressive given the patients were heavily pretreated, with many having already relapsed after allo-HSCT, a point after which few (if any) further therapeutic options remain for most patients. These CR results were replicated in multicenter studies with 25 enrollment centers worldwide,[72] confirming the proof of feasibility of an international chain of supply of the CAR T cells. The CART19 product developed at the University of Pennsylvania and by Novartis was the first ACT to be approved by the FDA in late 2017. While there are some instances where manufacturing failures occur, these are rare, and the process of CAR T cell manufacturing and production is likely to improve with ongoing research and development (Fig. 31.4).

In addition to the successes of CART19 therapy, there have also been significant toxicities related to this treatment, which will be discussed later in this chapter (see "*Toxicity of Modern Adoptive Cellular Therapies*"). Another key advance with CAR T cells is the ability to eradicate leukemic blasts from the central nervous system (CNS), given the ability of T cells to permeate the blood-brain barrier.[73,74] While this also may be a contributing factor to the neurological toxicity of CART therapy (*discussed in more detail later in the chapter*), it has access to and can clear a sanctuary site of CNS leukemia,

addressing a key limitation of monoclonal antibody-based therapy, many of which have only very poor penetration of the blood-brain barrier. The success of CART19 has spurred an explosion of interest in CAR T-cell therapy and led to its evaluation for the potential treatment of numerous other disease entities, some of which are discussed in more detail below. Lastly, additional targets are under clinical investigation for B-ALL in particular to address the issue of CD19-negative relapses. Anti-CD22 CARTs have shown excellent activity in pediatric/young adult patients with B-ALL[75]; however, some patients show low expression of CD22 in leukemic blasts and have limited response to CART22.

While CAR T therapy will likely influence the role of allo-HSCT in the treatment of this disease in years to come as treatments improve and move closer to the frontline of therapy, allo-HSCT currently remains a key therapeutic treatment for many patients with poor-risk or relapsed disease. Of note, however, is Philadelphia chromosome-positive B-lineage acute lymphoblastic leukemia (Ph+ B-ALL), in which the role of allo-HSCT is subject to re-evaluation and debate as increasingly potent tyrosine kinase inhibitors (TKI) enter the therapeutic milieu.[76] For patients who achieve molecular residual disease (MRD)-negative status following chemotherapy and TKI therapy, there are data from several phase 2 trials to suggest that a transplant may not be indicated in first remission, yet the standard of care at this time for transplant-eligible patients remains allo-HSCT in first remission.

Acute Myeloid Leukemia

Conversely to B-ALL, the role of allo-HSCT in the treatment of AML has remained relatively unchanged in recent years. AML remains a disease with a poor prognosis for most patients and as yet has not been successfully treated using CART therapy due primarily to the lack of a suitably "expendable" antigen, such as CD19 in B-ALL. There is increasing interest, however, in the use of modified natural killer (NK) cells in the treatment of AML, which was outlined earlier in *ACT with natural killer lymphocytes* as NK cells have demonstrated antileukemic activity following allo-HSCT but with significantly lower risk of GvHD,[77] with antileukemic activity being enhanced when killer immunoglobulin-like receptor human leukocyte antigen (KIR-HLA) genes are mismatched between donor and recipient. A range of early-phase clinical trials are now under way evaluating the adoptive transfer of NK cells, including both autologous and allogeneic NK cells, and there is an accumulating body of data supporting the modest clinical activity of adoptively transferred NK cells against AML.[78] While there is some evidence of clinical response, the overall response rates are somewhat disappointing when compared with CAR T therapy for B-ALL.

As mentioned, the development of effective ACT for AML is hampered mostly by the lack of suitable targets. In fact, most targets expressed by AML are also expressed by normal hemopoietic cells. One strategy is targeting the Wilms' tumor 1 (WT1) protein that is overexpressed in a subset of AML. T cells engineered with a WT1/HLA-A2–specific TCR have generated promising preliminary results in phase I studies (NCT01640301, NCT01621724).[79] Lastly, several targets (CD33, CD123, and others) are being evaluated for CAR T–based therapy of AML in both the preclinical and clinical settings. Key data will be obtained from early trials and will help in understanding the potential toxicity on the myeloid compartment with CD33 and CD123 CAR T cells.

B-Cell Lymphomas and Chronic Lymphocytic Leukemia

B-cell non-Hodgkin lymphomas (B-NHL) and chronic lymphocytic leukemia (CLL) also express CD19; therefore, CART19 therapy has been tested in these diseases in multiple clinical trials. A phase 1 multicenter study in 111 patients with r/r B-cell lymphoma, primary mediastinal B-cell lymphoma, or transformed follicular lymphoma treated with the CART19 axicabtagene ciloleucel (KTE-19) reported an overall response rate (ORR) of 82%, and the complete response rate was 54%. With a median follow-up of 15.4 months, 42% of the patients continued to have a response, with 40% continuing to have a complete response.[80] Similar response rates were obtained using the University of Pennsylvania construct with 4-1BB costimulation. Out of 28 patients treated with CTL019, 64% of patients showed response, with 43% CR rate in DLBCL and 71% in FL. Sustained remissions were achieved, and at a median follow-up of 28.6 months, 86% of patients with diffuse large B-cell lymphoma who had a response (95% CI, 33 to 98) and 89% of patients with follicular lymphoma who had a response (95% CI, 43 to 98) had maintained the response.[81] A similar response pattern was seen following the treatment of 14 patients with relapsed/refractory chronic lymphocytic leukemia (CLL)—this small cohort of patients was heavily pretreated (median of 5 previous therapies, range 1 to 11) with a deletion of 17p identified in 57% of patients. Following treatment with CART19, the CR rate was relatively low at 29% (4/14 patients); however, in those who achieved a CR, this response was durable, with all 4 of these patients maintaining CR at a median follow-up of 38.5 months (range 21 to 53 months).[82] The 2 patients with the longest durations of remission remain MRD negative at more than 7 years, presenting the tantalizing possibility of long-term disease eradication, even in patients with treatment refractory and poor-risk disease as represented by this cohort.

It has also been observed that the treatment appears to be well tolerated among the generally older cohorts of patients with B-NHL—the median age of patients in the NCI DLBCL trial was 58 years old and 66 years old in the CLL trial. While CRS and/or neurotoxicity did occur in these patients, the treatment was generally well tolerated and certainly deliverable, which is encouraging with respect to the feasibility of CAR T therapy in older patients on a larger scale in the future.

The explanation of the vastly different response rates between B-ALL versus B-NHL and CLL, despite targeting the same antigen, is most likely due to differences in disease biology; for example, the access by the CAR T cells to the malignant cells and the immunosuppressive role of the tumor microenvironment. It is also noted that the traditional chemotherapeutic agents for the treatment of B-NHL are by design lymphocytotoxic and may cause potential differences in T-cell composition (i.e., CD4 subsets, CD8 memory and effector cells, and CD4/CD8 ratios) that comprises the final CAR T product, which in turn may affect its efficacy. The optimal composition of the CAR T product is currently unknown and is another area of ongoing research and development.

Despite its B-cell origin, Hodgkin lymphoma (HL) does not express CD19. However, about 40% of HL is associated with Epstein-Barr virus. As a consequence, adoptive transfer of ex vivo expanded autologous EBV-specific CTLs, recognizing the EBV-derived latent membrane proteins 1 and 2 (LMP1 and LMP2), induces objective responses in patients with r/r EBV+ HL.[83] More recently, T cells specific for intracellular tumor-associated antigens, that is, PRAME, SSX2, MAGEA4, NY-ESO-1, and survivin, were shown to induce complete responses in patients with HL in the absence of conditioning chemotherapy. Lastly, CAR T cells against CD30 have been developed and showed some anti-HL activity in early clinical trials.[84]

A logical way of increasing the potency of CAR T therapy is in combination with other novel therapies that have proved efficacious in lymphomas, such as small molecular inhibitors like ibrutinib that block Bruton's tyrosine kinase, a key component of B-cell signaling and growth. Preclinical data have shown enhanced killing of mantle cell lymphoma (MCL) samples by CART19 when combined with ibrutinib.[85] In addition, data from a preclinical model suggest that the addition of ibrutinib to CART19 therapy is protective against CRS. A clinical trial evaluating this combination is currently recruiting patients at the University of Pennsylvania (NCT02640209).

Another rational combination with CAR T cells is the checkpoint inhibitors, a class of drugs that enhance the ability of endogenous T cells to eradicate tumor cells. Malignant cells often up-regulate expression of proteins that cause T-cell suppression, effectively rendering cancer cells invisible to the patient's T cells. Checkpoint inhibitors are a class of drug that interrupt this interaction between the cancer cell and the T cell and allow the T cell to "see" the malignant cell and thus destroy it. In preclinical studies, anti–PD-1 enhances the efficacy of CAR T cells.[86] This treatment approach proved successful in the treatment of a man with relapsed/refractory (RR) DLBCL that had proved nonresponsive to CART19 therapy at the University of Pennsylvania. He was treated with a checkpoint inhibitor (pembrolizumab), achieved a partial response, and was clinically well at 1 year since the commencement of pembrolizumab. The success of this strategy has led to the opening of a phase I/II clinical trial evaluating the effect of pembrolizumab in other patients with CD19+ B-NHL who have failed treatment with CART19 (NCT02650999).

Looking at the broader history of cancer therapy, where it is rare for a single agent to achieve a long-term remission—with the noted exception of tyrosine kinase inhibitors for a subset of patients with CML—it is likely that CAR T therapy and indeed ACT may ultimately be of utmost clinical utility in combination with novel therapies. The combination of CAR T therapy, in particular with immune-based therapies, is eagerly awaited.

Plasma Cell Myeloma

The treatment of plasma cell myeloma (MM), a disease due to malignant transformation of antibody producing plasma cells, is perhaps one of the most difficult conditions to treat in hematology, with disease progression being the inevitable outcome. Antimyeloma therapy has made incredible progress over the last decade, with the development of proteasome inhibitors such as bortezomib and carfilzomib; immunomodulatory drugs such as thalidomide, lenalidomide, and pomalidomide; and monoclonal antibodies targeting plasma cell antigens, such as daratumumab and elotuzumab. Even with these new therapies, however, disease progression remains a foregone conclusion for most, with only a very small subset of patients achieving long-term disease control following allo-HSCT. It is hoped that by harnessing CAR T-cell therapy, this paradigm may change.

There are several antigens being evaluated for targeting with CART therapy, including CD19, CD38, CD138, and B-cell maturation antigen (BCMA). At present, the largest body of evidence exists with respect to efficacy and safety is with CART19; however, many malignant plasma cells are CD19 negative. There is some early clinical data suggesting efficacy of CART19 in the treatment of myeloma; a patient with early disease progression after high-dose melphalan autologous transplantation (auto-HSCT) was treated with CART19 and, despite the majority (99.95%) of the bone marrow plasma cells lacking CD19 expression, obtained a durable response after a second auto-HSCT and CART19.[87] A phase 1 study at the University of Pennsylvania evaluating this treatment strategy has completed recruitment at the time of writing, and results are awaited (NCT02135406).

BCMA has good credentials as a suitable target for CAR T therapy as it is highly expressed in MM, and the only off-tumor expression is in a B-cell subset.[88] At the 2017 American Society of Clinical Oncology Annual Meeting, high rates of responses after BCMA-CART were reported in 2 clinical trials (NCT03090659, NCT02658929). Fan et al. (#LBA3001) treated 19 MM patients with their LCAR-B38M anti-BCMA CAR T (Nanjing Legend Biotech Inc.) and obtained 100% ORR (1 PR, 4 VGPR, 14 CR). Berdeja et al. (#3010) had 100% ORR in 6 evaluable patients treated with bb2121 anti-BCMA CART (bluebird bio), including 2 stringent complete remissions (sCRs) and 2 MRD-negative responses. While CD38 and CD138 are also being evaluated for myeloma, the expression of these antigens on a wide range of normal tissue, particularly of CD38 on immature erythroid cells, increasing the potential of on-target off-tumor toxicity, a concept which will be discussed in more detail later in the chapter, and cautious evaluation of CAR T-cell therapy against these antigens are being pursued.

Lastly, engineered TCR T cells are also under development for MM. As spontaneous as well as postvaccination humoral and cellular immunity against the NY-ESO157-165/HLAA*02:01 complex has been also observed in myeloma patients, this target was evaluated in phase I/II studies. Promising results in MM (NCT01892293) were observed in patients receiving T cells transduced with NY-ESO-1–specific TCRs.[89]

Solid Organ Tumors

Although the most celebrated successes of ACT to date have been in the treatment of B-ALL leukemia and lymphoma with CD19 CAR T cells, it was in the treatment of solid organ malignancies that ACT had its first successes, specifically in the treatment of melanoma using both TILs and TCR T cells, the theory of which has been covered earlier in this chapter.

Tumor-Infiltrating Lymphocytes

The efficacy of TILs was first demonstrated in 1988; of the 12 patients with metastatic solid organ malignancies (melanoma, breast, colon, and renal cell carcinoma), 2 patients had a partial response (PR) after receiving cyclophosphamide followed by infusion of tumor-derived TILs and interleukin-2, with no treatment-related mortality. While there has been improvement with respect to response rates over the years as changes have been made to conditioning regimen and other variables relating to the TIL manufacture, the application of TILs remains largely in the domain of metastatic melanoma, with overall response rates across a range of trials ranging from 21 to 72%. In the data presented by Rosenberg et al.[90] in 2011, some of these responses were both deep and durable, with 22% (20/93) of heavily pretreated patients achieving completed tumor regression and 19 of these 20 patients maintained complete remissions beyond 3 years. A randomized controlled phase III study is evaluating TIL infusions compared to ipilimumab in stage IV melanoma (NCT02278887).

A recent phase 1 clinical trial showed promising results for the treatment of adoptive transfer of expanded TILs for the treatment of 15 patients with hepatocellular carcinoma, reporting 100% of patients were alive after a median follow-up of 14 months, with no evidence of disease in 12 patients (NCT01462903). Recently, the adoptive transfer of ex vivo expanded TILs directed against driver oncogenes, such as KRAS, was demonstrated by the Rosenberg group to induce regression of multiple pulmonary metastasis of colorectal cancer in a patient being treated on a phase 2 clinical trial (NCT01174121)[91]; a population of CD8+ TILs targeting a common KRAS mutation (KRAS G12D) was isolated from biopsied tissue from 3 metastatic deposits and following ex vivo expansion was reinfused after lymphodepleting chemotherapy (Fig. 31.2). The patient was unable to tolerate ongoing IL-2 therapy beyond 5 doses, yet all 7 metastatic deposits regressed after 40 days of therapy and achieved a partial response for 9 months until progression of 1 lung lesion that had lost presentation of the KRAS G12D peptide. This lesion was resected, and the patient remains clinically disease-free. While these results are promising, there are also many patients who fail to respond to TILs, and ongoing research continues in this field.

TCR-Modified T Cells (TCR T)

The initial clinical results were disappointing when TCR T with low-affinity TCRs were used. Subsequent trials employing modified T cells with higher-affinity binding achieved higher response rates (25%) but also demonstrated on-target off-tumor toxicity in many patients.[92] This phenomenon was also demonstrated in a trial evaluating TCRs targeting the melanoma-melanocyte antigen gp100; 29 of the 36 patients treated demonstrated a widespread erythematous rash, which resolved in some patients, while others experienced ongoing vertigo.[92] A smaller number of patients in this cohort experienced off-tumor toxicity affecting ocular and ototoxicity, where melanocytic cells are also located. A major limitation in the use of ACT for the treatment of solid organ malignancies has been the relative paucity of tumor-specific antigens, with many antigens being common to the malignant and healthy tissue. There have also been some unexpected toxicities, some of them fatal, which have slowed the pace of progression. Progress is being made, with promising results observed with TCR T cells, especially those targeting the cancer-testis antigen NY-ESO-1, with this target being the first to enable responses of 45% to 65% in patients with both melanoma and nonmelanoma cancers (synovial cell sarcoma), using a high-avidity NY-ESO-1 HLA-A2–restricted TCR.[93]

CAR T Cells (CAR T)

Unfortunately, the successes of CAR T therapy have not been achieved yet to date in the treatment of solid organ cancers, with the majority of previously published trials showing negative results.[36,53,58] A third-generation CAR directed against ERBB2 (HER2) was tested in the treatment of metastatic melanoma and had severe toxicity with the first patient treated succumbing to pulmonary toxicity due to on-target, off-tumor toxicity. Given the successes of CAR T cells in the treatment of hematological malignancies, however, there is renewed interest in CAR therapy for solid organ disease, though with very cautious selection of potential target epitopes given this history of off-target toxicity. Examples of key targets that are under clinical evaluation are mesothelin (basket trial at the University of Pennsylvania, NCT02159716), ROR-1 (basket trial at the Fred Hutchinson Cancer Research Center, NCT02706392), HER2 (basket trials targeting breast cancer, glioblastoma, and other HER2-expressing malignancies; NCT02547961, NCT02442297, NCT02713984), cMET (targeting breast cancer and melanoma at the University of Pennsylvania, NCT01837602 and NCT03060356), and others.

One tumor showing potential for suitability for treatment with CAR T cells is glioblastoma multiforme (GBM, an aggressive brain tumor with dismal prognosis) having at least 2 potential targets for CAR T therapy: IL13Rα2 (a glioma-associated antigen associated with poor overall survival) and a particular mutant variant of the epidermal growth factor receptor (EGFRvIII), which is observed in approximately 30% of GBM and is a neoepitope (i.e., is not expressed on nonmalignant tissues). Following evidence of anti-glioma effect with a first-generation CAR T targeting IL13Rα2, the City of Hope reported a 50-year-old man with aggressive GBM whose disease recurred only 6 months after standard-of-care treatment with surgical resection, adjuvant radiotherapy, and temozolomide chemotherapy with rapid progression and multiple intracranial parenchymal and leptomeningeal deposits. The patient received treatment with resection of the largest tumors, followed by IL13Rα2 CAR T cells given both intravenously and via a catheter into the tumor resection bed from the site of the largest lesion in the right temporal-occipital region. While other tumor sites continued to grow, there was disease control at the site of the catheter, so a second catheter was placed in the right lateral ventricle with the rationale that localized delivery to the CSF would enhance CAR T-cell delivery to GBM cells. Remarkably, the patient's cancer regressed and was not visible by MRI or PET scan after the 5th intraventricular CAR T infusion, and the dexamethasone dose was gradually eliminated with an associated improvement in the patient's function and even his return to work. This response was sustained for 7.5 months from the initiation of CAR treatment, although the tumor recurred after cycle 16, notably at different

sites from the original disease and with evidence of decreased IL13Ra2 expression, suggesting antigen loss as the potential mechanism of relapse.

As another approach for CAR T therapy of GBM, Johnson et al. designed a CAR T targeting EGFRvIII, which produced favorable preclinical data,[56] and the subsequent phase 1 trial at the University of Pennsylvania and the University of California reported on-target effects autologous CART-EGFRvIII in the treatment of GBM at recurrence or following resection with residual disease.[94] A study at Duke is currently enrolling patients for a trial evaluating CAR T cells against EGFRvIII in a newly diagnosed cohort (NCT02664363) in combination with standard-of-care therapy.

Clinical Limitations of Adoptive Cellular Therapy

Like all cancer therapies, ACT has limitations of toxicity and treatment failure. The toxicity of allo-HSCT is considerable, and it is well established that following relapsed disease, the main causes of morbidity and mortality are GVHD, infection, organ failure, interstitial pneumonitis, and primary graft failure.[8] While allo-HSCT has for many years been the only potentially curative option for some patients with malignant disease, the development of ACT now provides an avenue by which the potency of T cells may be harnessed more effectively, with greater specificity and with less toxicity.

When considering newer forms of ACT, their unique mechanisms of action create a unique constellation of possible toxicities, which may be grouped conceptually into the following five main categories,[95] some being associated with specific forms of ACT more than others: (a) toxicity due to the immunosuppressive medications given to the patient prior to the infusion of the cellular therapy, for example, cytopenias and other adverse events following the administration of chemotherapy such as fludarabine and cyclophosphamide; (b) toxicity due to the rapid in vivo proliferation of the T cells, typically associated with CAR T therapy and termed CRS; (c) "on-target off-tumor" toxicity occurring when healthy tissues bearing the same antigen being targeted by the cellular therapy are also damaged; (d) aberrant reactivity describes unexpected targeting of healthy tissues by T cells that had not been anticipated (off-target toxicity); and (e) neurotoxicity of uncertain etiology, seen commonly following CAR T therapy.

Toxicity of Modern Adoptive Cellular Therapies

Lymphodepleting Chemotherapy

The primary aim of lymphodepleting chemotherapy is to deplete the recipient's endogenous T cells, creating a cytokine environment that enhances in vivo proliferation and function of the transfused T-cell product. Lymphodepleting regimens commonly contain classic chemotherapeutic agents such as fludarabine, cyclophosphamide, pentostatin, or bendamustine. These drugs are often associated with nausea, fatigue, and other common side effects of chemotherapy and may cause cytopenias, which can predispose the patient to infection or bleeding. Fludarabine is particularly potent in achieving lymphodepletion, but it has also been postulated that there may be increased rates of neurological toxicity following its use as conditioning prior to ACT infusion.

A group of investigators at the Fred Hutchinson Cancer Research Center evaluated the choice of lymphodepleting chemotherapy in a small cohort of patients with B-NHL receiving treatment with CART19.[96] They identified an association between improved T-cell expansion and CAR T-cell persistence in vivo, with lymphodepleting chemotherapy with cyclophosphamide and fludarabine (Cy/Flu) in comparison with cyclophosphamide alone or in combination with etoposide. Improved T-cell expansion and persistence also correlated with superior clinical outcomes and lower rates of CAR T failure. They also found that toxicity, in particular neurotoxicity and CRS, was higher in patients who had received Cy/Flu. Thus, it seems that toxicity and efficacy with respect to lymphodepletion, in particular the inclusion of fludarabine, may be two sides of the same coin, and research into identifying the improved regimens for lymphodepletion is ongoing.

Cytokine Release Syndrome

CRS is a potentially life-threatening inflammatory state induced by cytokines released as the CAR T cells encounter their target antigen and begin rapid in vivo proliferation. The production of cytokine is thought to be driven by CAR T but also macrophages and stromal cells that react to CAR T activation.[97] There is a marked rise in cytokines, including interleukin 6 (IL-6), interleukin gamma, and interleukin 10, resulting in fever, malaise, tachycardia, and capillary leak, with varying degrees of hypotension, organ dysfunction, and disseminated intravascular coagulation (DIC). Given the prevalence of CRS following CAR T therapy, there is now a considerable body of experience guiding its management. While the grading scores and management recommendations vary slightly between institutions, the key aspects are the following: (a) close monitoring and prompt hospitalization of any patient with a fever following CAR T therapy, (b) rapid escalation to critical care if there is evidence of fluid refractory hypotension, (c) inotropic support to preserve organ function, and (d) judicious use of the IL-6–blocking antibody (tocilizumab) +/− systemic corticosteroids in severe CRS.[98] Another important observation in B-ALL has been that the inflammatory response is proportional to the burden of disease (and, thus, antigen burden) present at the time of infusion; many centers have now adopted fractionated split dosing of CAR T cells, in some cases in accordance with blast percentage in the bone marrow, to ameliorate the risk of severe CRS. Fractionated dosing also offers the added benefit of reduced morbidity in the event of an infusion-related adverse event.

On-Target Off-Tumor Toxicity

Antigens targeted by ACT are often common to both malignant and healthy tissues. Despite this, ACT can be highly tolerable if the healthy tissue expressing the antigen can be considered physiologically "expendable." For example, CD19 is expressed both by malignant B-ALL cells and by healthy antibody-producing B-cells; such persistence of the CART19 population is associated with B-cell depletion and subsequent hypogammaglobulinemia. Despite this, patients remain clinically well, and the risk of opportunistic infection due to reduced humeral immunity is low

and may be ameliorated by gamma globulin replacement. The clinical relevance of the observed hypogammaglobulinemia has also been further evaluated, with evidence that while total serum levels of serum immunoglobulin G and A are reduced following CART19, functional humoral immunity appears largely intact, manifested by preservation of vaccine responses.[99] These authors identified polyclonal CD138+ plasma cells by immunohistochemistry and flow cytometry in the bone marrow of patients following CART19 therapy and hypothesized that the preserved humoral vaccine responses may be attributable to long-lived CD19-negative plasma cells. Importantly, B-cell aplasia is a biomarker of persistence of functional CD19 CAR T cells, and current recommendations are to continue gamma globulin replacement in pediatric patients who have serum hypogammaglobulinemia following CAR therapy.

On-target off-tumor toxicity was severe following infusion of CAR T cells expressing scFv derived from Herceptin, probably due to low-level expression of ERBB2 on lung epithelium.[100] TCRs targeting melanoma differentiation antigens (MART-1 and gp100) destroyed normal melanocytes in the skin, ears, and eyes and CAR T cells targeting carbonic anhydrase-IX (CAIX)-mediated on-target destruction of biliary duct epithelial tissue.[51] On-target toxicity has been reported in cases with T cells engineered with a TCR specific for the CEA resulting in severe dose-limiting inflammatory colitis resulting from expression of target antigen in a normal colon.[100] It is possible that CAR T cells directed against CEA may have less toxicity as CEA is expressed in a polarized fashion, with healthy colonic mucosa expressing CEA predominantly on the luminal side and malignant cells expressing the antigen over the entire cell, with the hypothesis that CAR T cells in the vascular compartment would have no access to luminal surfaces and would therefore preferentially target malignant cells. Three recent clinical trials supported this hypothesis, with no evidence of colitis (even at high CART-CEA doses) in small cohorts; however, the associated disease responses were somewhat disappointing with the best treatment responses achieved being stable disease in patients treated (NCT02349724, NCT01212887, NCT01373047).

In conclusion, when developing new targets for ACT, the expression of the target antigen on healthy tissues is a crucial consideration, and the lack of tumor-specific antigens has limited the utility of ACT in the treatment of solid tumors though numerous avenues of investigation are being explored to negotiate this obstacle.

Aberrant/Unexpected Cross-Reactivity

In rare cases, toxicity has occurred due to unexpected binding of modified T cells to an antigen expressed by a physiological tissue in vivo. This phenomenon is demonstrated by the deaths from cardiogenic shock of the first two patients treated with affinity-enhanced T cells directed against HLA-A*01–restricted MAGE-A3, for the treatment of melanoma and plasma cell myeloma, respectively. No myocardial MAGE-A3 protein expression was identifiable at autopsy, yet there was extensive myocardiocyte death and T-cell infiltration. After extensive investigation, it was found that the cardiac toxicity was due to cross-reactivity against a striated muscle peptide titin expressed in cardiac tissue.[38] In another trial using anti–MAGE-A3 T-cell receptor–modified T cells, 2 of the 9 patients who received treatment died from irreversible neurotoxicity, likely attributable to cross-reactivity with a different member of the MAGE protein family (MAGE-A12), which was found to be expressed on neuronal tissue and was established after necrotizing leukomalacia was identified at autopsy.[37] These unexpected cross-reactivities, which have been postulated as attributable to "supraphysiological affinity tuning of the TCR," are perhaps the most difficult adverse event to manage due to their fulminant toxicity and idiosyncratic nature and highlight the need for better methods to improve the specificity of ACT.[38]

Neurotoxicity from CART Therapy

There is a classic form of neurological toxicity that is seen following CAR T therapy, which does not fit neatly into any of the preceding classifications, as its etiology is not completely understood. The manifestations of this toxicity vary from altered conscious state, encephalopathy, aphasia, seizures, and obtundation. While it is likely that the high fevers seen during CRS likely contribute to delirium, as is also seen in many critically ill patients, there is a distinct encephalopathy syndrome that is particular to CAR T therapy. It is generally "brief and self-limited, resolving over several days without intervention or apparent long-term sequelae",[101] and can include atypical features such as word-finding difficulties in the absence of an identifiable cerebral vascular or inflammatory pathology. While this syndrome is generally self-limiting, there have been a small number of patient deaths due to cerebral edema following CART therapy, which led to the discontinuation of the clinical trial evaluating JCAR015 (a CART19 product featuring a CD28 costimulatory domain manufactured by Juno Therapeutics, NCT02535364). The mechanism of the neurotoxicity remains poorly understood; however, there is evidence of endothelial cell activation and disruption of the blood-brain barrier in 2 autopsy cases.[102]

Not all patients receiving CART19 experience neurotoxicity, leading others to hypothesize that an idiosyncratic pattern of CD19 expression in the neurons of some patients renders them more susceptible to a neuroinflammatory response from blinatumomab, a bispecific antibody binding CD19 and CD3.[103] It is noted, however, that a similar pattern of neurotoxicity following CAR T therapy targeting other antigens has been observed in phase 1 clinical trials investigating CART-22 and CART-BCMA (for the treatment of B-ALL and plasma cell myeloma, respectively). The common manifestation of similar neurological toxicities despite the targeting of different antigens suggests that the toxicity is unlikely to be antigen-specific. A recent analysis at the Fred Hutchinson Cancer Research Center identified an elevated serum interleukin-6 (IL-6) above 30 pg/mL the day following CAR T therapy to be a sensitive and independent predictor for the subsequent development of severe neurotoxicity, suggesting that early measurement of serum IL-6 may be used to identify patients at high risk of neurotoxicity and to evaluate early intervention strategies,[104,105] which are necessary to reduce the risk of this potentially lethal adverse event.

Strategies to Reduce Toxicity of ACT

Many strategies are being pursued to reduce the toxicity associated with ACT, not only to reduce patient morbidity and mortality but also to extend the range of patients for whom ACT may have a therapeutic role. As outlined previously, protocols to identify and manage CRS are now well established, and centers that frequently administer CAR T therapy have strict protocols with respect to the escalation to critical care units. Research is ongoing to improve specificity of the targets being recognized by the transfused T cells to reduce on-and off-target toxicity. Many ACT products are now being developed that have also been transduced with a "suicide gene" into the T cells such that they can be eradicated in vivo if desired[12] in the event of unacceptable toxicity or relating the clinical paradigm in which the therapy is being used. Transduction of a CAR molecule into cells may also be achieved by RNA electroporation, with the result being a "biodegradable" short-acting ACT product that can be given as a series of multiple infusions, again to offset potential toxicity.[106]

Treatment Failure and Relapse

Some diseases cannot be currently treated with ACT due to the lack of a suitable antigen that is expressed by the tumor but not shared by healthy tissues. In some patients, there are technical failures in the manufacture of the ACT product, or their disease progresses too rapidly such that treatment cannot be initiated in a timely fashion. Some patients fail ACT despite their tumor's expression of the target antigen against which the T cell is expressed, and treatment failure by this mechanism may be due to a range of factors including antigen expression and density, tumor heterogeneity, vascular access to the tissue, and the immunosuppressive role of the tumor microenvironment.[107] Despite the use of lymphodepleting chemotherapy, in some patients, there is inadequate in vivo expansion or persistence of the CAR T population. The optimal duration of CART19 persistence remains unknown; however, data from the CART19-treated B-ALL patients at the University of Pennsylvania suggest that at least 2 to 3 months are required for long-term remission.[73] The requirement for CAR T persistence will need to be established for all other CAR T-cell subtypes going forward.

The other route of relapse identified to date is via emergence of antigen-negative cells—that is, the emergence of a population of malignant cells that lack the antigen against which the modified T cells are targeted and are therefore immune to its surveillance and cytotoxic effect. It is unclear if these cells are present in the initial cancer and gain a selective advantage under pressure from the T-cell therapy or if they develop mutations to facilitate their survival. This has been studied extensively in B-ALL, where CD19-negative relapse is becoming increasingly common with increased duration of follow-up. It has been demonstrated in some patients with B-ALL that CD19-negative blasts were indeed present prior to CART19 therapy and may have undergone clonal expansion, while CD19-positive blasts were removed by the CART19 therapy.[108] Another research group identified the presence of an alternative exon splicing of CD19, such that the CD19 epitope recognized by CART19 was lost, while retaining a truncated version of the protein with preserved receptor functionality.[109] An additional strategy being evaluated to mitigate the problem of antigen-negative relapse is to target more than one antigen with T-cell therapy simultaneously, thus reducing the chance of clonal evolution.[110]

Commercialization of ACT

In the absence of changes in health care reimbursement policies, the advent of numerous but often noncurative targeted therapies will increase the life span and the prevalence of patients living with cancer.[111] The financial toxicities imposed by effective but noncurative therapies currently encountered by patients with hematologic malignancies, particularly CLL and MM, are challenging. CLL is the most common form of leukemia in the United States with approximately 100,000 patients living with the disease in 2000, and because of improved but noncurative targeted therapies such as ibrutinib and idelalisib, an increase in prevalence to approximately 200,000 cases in the United States is projected.[112] However, targeted therapies for CLL present a significant economic burden for both patients and the economy, currently estimated at $604,000 lifetime costs per patient, and the total cost of CLL management in the United States alone is estimated to exceed $5 billion per year by 2025.[112] A cost-effectiveness analysis of targeted therapies versus CAR T-cell therapies has not yet been completed.

ACT is a powerful approach that provides durable responses and the potential for cure in patients with previous refractory cancer such as CLL, ALL, and myeloma. While autologous cell therapies offer great clinical promise, the only previous FDA-approved cell therapy for cancer (Sipuleucel-T) has not achieved commercial success, in part due to the complicated manufacturing logistics and high cost of manufacturing.[113] Due to their personalized nature, the bespoke manufacturing processes of TIL, CAR T-, and TCR T cells are associated with high development and manufacturing costs, stringent regulatory requirements pertaining to gene transfer, and reimbursement challenges. The current high cost of CAR T manufacturing might be mitigated by an approach such as annuity payments with risk sharing, also known as pay for performance.[114] Novartis has implemented this approach in the United States and charges for tisagenlecleucel CAR T cells only upon clinical benefit. A detailed analysis of the public health considerations on the pricing of gene-modified cells is beyond the scope of this chapter, but some aspects have been summarized.[115]

Conclusions and Perspectives

In this chapter, we have highlighted and discussed a number of topics of direct relevance for the application of ACT, within space and scope constraints. The field of ACT is exponentially growing, and new strategies and ideas are being developed at a rapid pace. The scientific community is intensively studying strategies to increase T-cell efficacy, to optimize T-cell production, to develop off-the-shelf T cells, to reduce clinical toxicity, to reduce T-cell exhaustion, to avoid tumor-microenvironment immunosuppression, and finally to test commercialization approaches.

With the FDA approval of tisagenlecleucel (Kymriah™) in 2017, the ACT field has capitalized on the multitude of lessons learned as a result of combining the commitment, insights, and innovations of a multitude of scientists with the profound bravery and generosity of

patients. In the last few years, ACT has progressively demonstrated dramatic potency in clinical trials of TIL, redirected TCR T and CAR T, leading to complete and durable responses in patients with late stage and treatment refractory disease (Table 31.2). However, subsets of patients are still not responding, are relapsing, or do not have an adequate ACT strategy for their disease. There is therefore much to be done in the field to ensure that most cancer patients respond in the long term.

Immunotherapy is now a pillar of cancer treatment and will likely represent the backbone of future treatment algorithms. ACT has led to excellent results in some cancers, and the ongoing research efforts will hopefully broaden its application to most cancers (Fig. 31.5). For cancer with high-mutational burden, checkpoint inhibitors and TIL represent a viable option. When the mutational burden is low, redirected high-affinity TCR T could represent a possible strategy, together with CAR T cells when an appropriate surface marker is available. Indeed, after tisagenlecleucel (CART19), other ACT are close to FDA approval, including CART-BCMA, CART-22, and likely NY-ESO-1 TCR-engineered T cells. Combination treatments and off-the-shelf cellular products will hopefully also be available to patients in the next few years. Delivering these treatments to patients in a fair and sustainable way will be the next challenge.

T-cell production has achieved high levels of efficiency; however, there is still a significant difference in efficiency between products, and studies are evaluating the expansion of T cells in the presence of small molecules potentially able to improve their effect in vivo. Other groups are selecting specific T-cell subsets that are potentially endowed with higher antitumor activity (naive, memory-stem cell subsets). Lastly, given that for some patients ACT product cannot be manufactured in a timely fashion, shortened (less than a week) manufacturing protocols are under investigation.

An appealing perspective for the field of ACT is developing a universal, off-the-shelf product. Several groups are pursuing this goal using the amazing new technologies of gene editing such as CRISPR-Cas9, TALEN, and zinc finger nucleases. Using these tools, their T-cell–naive TCR can be knocked out to reduce GVHD, and beta-2-microglobulin can also be knocked out to avoid recognition by recipient T cells. Universal CART19 that lack TCR are currently being tested in clinical trials.[61]

T-cell exhaustion[116] is a known mechanism of reduced antitumor T-cell function. Combining checkpoint inhibitors with ACT is under evaluation in several trials; however, other interesting approaches include specific knockout of exhaustion markers (e.g., PD-1 and CTLA-4) in effector T cells using gene-editing technologies such as CRISPR-Cas9. In solid tumors and lymphomas, the immunosuppression of the TME can potentially lead to ACT failure. T-cell products armed with cytokines, directly targeting the TME or able to revert immunosuppression, are currently under clinical evaluation.

Finally issues of scale-up, automation, commercialization, and intellectual property[117] and addressing regulatory hurdles unique to cell therapy[118] need to be addressed as more ACT products are being approved for clinical use and patients treated at large scale.

TABLE
31.2 *Key targets for ACT and established clinical results*

Disease	Target	Effector	Efficacy	Toxicity	Citation
Acute leukemia					
AML (pediatric and young adult)	MHC class 1 self versus non–self-recognition	Ex vivo expanded KIR-HLA mismatched allogeneic NK cells	MRD(−) 100% at 4 mo EFS 100% at 2 y	Injection (IL2) site reaction 10% [1/10] Other toxicity likely 2° febrile neutropenia	Rubnitz et al. 2010[119]
B-ALL (pediatric)	CD19	CART19 (CTL019, TCRζ/4-1BB)	CR 90% [27/30]	CRS 100% [37/37] sCRS 27% [9/37] Neurotoxicity 43% [13/30]	Maude et al. 2014[73]
B-ALL (adult)	CD19	CART19 (19-28z)	CR/CRi 88% [14/16]	sCRS 44% [7/16] Neurotoxicity 44% [7/16]	Davila et al. 2014[120]
B-NHL					
DLBCL/PMBCL/SMZL/B-NHL	CD19	CART19 (CD3ζ/CD28)	ORR 80% [12/15] CR 53% [8/15] PR 27% [4/15] SD 7% [1/15] NE 13% [2/15]	Hypotension 27% [4/15] Neurotoxicity 40% [6/15] Death of unknown cause [1/15]	Kochenderfer et al. 2015[121]
CLL	CD19	CART19 (CTL019, TCRζ/4-1BB)	ORR 57% [8/14] CR 29% [4/14] PR 29% [4/14]	CRS 64% [9/14] sCRS 29% [4/14] Neurotoxicity 36% [5/14]	Porter et al. 2015[82]
DLBCL	CD19	KTE-C19 (CD3ζ/CD28)	ORR 71% [5/7] CR 57% [4/7]	Grade ≥3 CRS and neurotoxicity 57% [4/7]	Locke et al. 2016[122]
Plasma cell neoplasms					
MM	NY-ESO-1/LAGE-1	TCR-engineered T cells	CR/nCR 70% [14/20] VGPR 10% [2/20] PR 5% [1/20] SD 5% [1/20] PD [1/20]	Skin rash with lymphocytosis 15% [3/20] Auto-GVHD 15% [3/20]	Rapoport et al. 2015[89]
MM	BCMA	LCAR-B38M CAR T	ORR 100% [19/19] CR 32% [6/19] nCR [32% 12/19]	CRS 74% [14/19] sCRS	Fan et al. 2017[123]
MM	BCMA	BCMA-CART (4-1BB/CD3ζ)	ORR 100% [11/11] sCR 18% [2/11]	CRS 73% [8/11]	Bergdeja et al. 2017[124]

Disease	Target	Effector	Efficacy	Toxicity	Citation
Skin malignancies					
Metastatic melanoma	MART1	Low-affinity TCR-modified T cells (MART-1:27-35/ DMF4)	ORR 12% [2/17]	None reported	Morgan et al. 2006[125]
Metastatic melanoma	MART1 (melan-A) and gp100	Higher-affinity TCR-modified T cells (MART-1:27-35/ DMF5 & gp100:154)	ORR (DMF5): 30% [6/20] ORR: (gp100:154) 19% [3/16]	Widespread rash 81% [29/36] Uveitis (DMF5) 55% [11/20] Uveitis (Gp100:154) 25% [4/16] Ototoxicity (DMF5) 50% [10/20] Ototoxicity 31% (Gp100:154) [5/16]	Johnson et al. 2009[92]
Metastatic melanoma	n/a	TIL	ORR 22% [20/93] CR 20% [19/93]	TRM (sepsis) 1% [1/93] PHT 1% [1/93] Nephropathy 1% [1/93]	Rosenberg et al. 2011[90]
Solid organ malignancies					
Melanoma, renal cell ca, breast ca, colorectal ca	n/a	TIL	PR 17% [2/12] (responses in 1 pt with melanoma, 1 pt with renal cell cancer)	No treatment-related mortality	Topalian et al. 1988[26]
Synovial cell sarcoma/ metastatic melanoma	NY-ESO-1	TCR-modified T cells (1G4-α95:LY)	ORR (sarcoma) 65% [4/6] ORR (melanoma) 45% [5/11]	No toxicity attributed to the transferred cells, though transient chemotherapy and IL2 toxicities occurred	Robbins et al. 2011[93]
Hepatocellular ca	n/a	TIL	ORR 100% [15/15] CR	Gr 1 malaise/flu-like symptoms 20% [3/15]	Jiang et al. 2015[127]
GBM	IL13rα2	IL13rα2-CART	Case report from phase 2 study; CR on MRI after IV and CSF administration of CART, clinical response lasting 7.5 mo	None reported	Brown et al. 2016[128]
Colorectal ca	KRAS G12D	CD8+ TIL	Case report from phase 2 study; PR for 9 mo until progression (lung metastasis), then ongoing remission after resection of lesion	Intolerant of IL2 therapy	Rosenberg et al. 2017[91]

B-ALL, B-lineage acute lymphoblastic leukemia; KIR-HLA, killer immunoglobulin-like receptor human leukocyte antigen genes; B-NHL, B-lineage non-Hodgkin lymphoma; PMBCL, primary mediastinal B-cell lymphoma; SMZL, splenic marginal zone lymphoma; CLL, chronic lymphocytic leukemia; MM, plasma cell myeloma; ORR, overall response rate; CR, complete remission; CRi, complete remission with incomplete count recovery; PR, partial response; SD, stable disease; NE, not evaluable; MRD(−), minimal residual disease negative; sCR, stringent CR; nCR, near CR; VGRP, very good partial response; CRS, cytokine release syndrome; sCRS, severe cytokine release syndrome; auto-GVHD, autologous graft-versus-host disease; n/a, not applicable; TIL, tumor-infiltrating lymphocytes; TRM, treatment-related mortality; PHT, pulmonary hypertension; ca, cancer; GBM, glioblastoma multiforme.

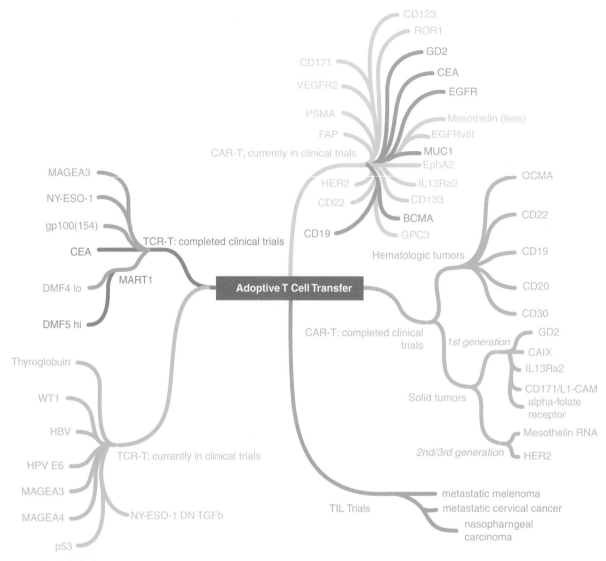

FIGURE **31.5** Examples of completed and ongoing TIL, TCR T-, and CAR T-cell immunotherapy clinical trials identified on ClinicalTrials.gov.

References

1. Tran E, Longo DL, Urba WJ. A milestone for CAR T cells. *N Engl J Med.* 2017;377:2593-2596.

2. Billingham RE, Brent L, Medawar PB. Quantitative studies on tissue transplantation immunity. II. The origin, strength and duration of actively and adoptively acquired immunity. *Proc R Soc Lond B Biol Sci.* 1954;143:58-80.

3. Mitchison NA. Studies on the immunological response to foreign tumor transplants in the mouse. I. The role of lymph node cells in conferring immunity by adoptive transfer. *J Exp Med.* 1955;102:157-177.

4. Rosenberg SA, Terry WD. Passive immunotherapy of cancer in animals and man. *Adv Cancer Res.* 1977;25:323-388.

5. Greenberg PD, Reusser P, Goodrich JM, et al. Development of a treatment regimen for human cytomegalovirus (CMV) infection in bone marrow transplantation recipients by adoptive transfer of donor-derived CMV-specific T cell clones expanded in vitro. *Ann NY Acad Sci.* 1991;636:184-195.

6. Rosenberg SA, Restifo NP. Adoptive cell transfer as personalized immunotherapy for human cancer. *Science.* 2015;348:62-68.

7. Weiden PL, Flournoy N, Thomas ED, et al. Antileukemic effect of graft-versus-host disease in human recipients of allogeneic-marrow grafts. *N Engl J Med.* 1979;300:1068-1073.

8. Barrett AJ, Battiwalla M. Relapse after allogeneic stem cell transplantation. *Expert Rev Hematol.* 2010;3:429-441.

9. Vago L, Perna S, Zanussi M, et al. Loss of mismatched HLA in leukemia after stem-cell transplantation. *N Engl J Med.* 2009;361:478.

10. Porter DL. Allogeneic immunotherapy to optimize the graft-versus-tumor effect: concepts and controversies. *Hematology.* 2011;2011:292-298.

11. Giralt S, Hester J, Huh Y, et al. CD8-depleted donor lymphocyte infusion as treatment for relapsed chronic myelogenous leukemia after allogeneic bone marrow transplantation. *Blood.* 1995;86:4337-4343.

12. Di Stasi A, Tey S-K, Dotti G, et al. Inducible apoptosis as a safety switch for adoptive cell therapy. *N Engl J Med.* 2011;365:1673-1683.

13. Klebanoff CA, Gattinoni L, Restifo NP. Sorting through subsets: which T-cell populations mediate highly effective adoptive immunotherapy? *J Immunother.* 2012;35:651-660.

14. Hori S, Nomura T, Sakaguchi S. Control of regulatory T cell development by the transcription factor Foxp3. *Science.* 2003;299:1057-1061.

15. Godfrey WR, Spoden DJ, Ge Y, et al. In vitro expanded human CD4+CD25+ T regulatory cells markedly inhibit allogeneic dendritic cell stimulated MLR cultures. *Blood.* 2004;104:453-461.

16. Brunstein CG, Miller JS, McKenna DH, et al. Umbilical cord blood-derived T regulatory cells to prevent GVHD: kinetics, toxicity profile, and clinical effect. *Blood.* 2016;127:1044-1051.

17. Maury S, Lemoine FM, Hicheri Y, et al. CD4+CD25+ regulatory T cell depletion improves the graft-versus-tumor effect of donor lymphocytes after allogeneic hematopoietic stem cell transplantation. *Sci Transl Med.* 2010;2:41ra52.

18. Kiessling R, Wigzell H. An analysis of the murine NK cell as to structure, function and biological relevance. *Immunol Rev.* 1979;44:165-208.

19. Ljunggren HG, Karre K. In search of the 'missing self': MHC molecules and NK cell recognition. *Immunol Today.* 1990;11:238-244.

20. Vivier E, Ugolini S, Blaise D, et al. Targeting natural killer cells and natural killer T cells in cancer. *Nat Rev Immunol.* 2012;12:239-252.

21. Porrata LF, Gertz MA, Inwards DJ, et al. Early lymphocyte recovery predicts superior survival after autologous hematopoietic stem cell transplantation in multiple myeloma or non-Hodgkin lymphoma. *Blood.* 2001;98:579-585.

22. Kumar S, Chen MG, Gastineau DA, et al. Lymphocyte recovery after alloge-neic bone marrow transplantation predicts risk of relapse in acute lympho-blastic leukemia. *Leukemia.* 2003;17:1865-1870.

23. Zhao XY, Chang YJ, Huang XJ. Conflicting impact of alloreactive NK cells on transplantation outcomes after haploidentical transplantation: do the reconstitution kinetics of natural killer cells create these differences? *Biol Blood Marrow Transplant.* 2011;17:1436-1442.

24. Benjamin JE, Gill S, Negrin RS. Biology and clinical effects of natural killer cells in allogeneic transplantation. *Curr Opin Oncol.* 2010;22:130-137.

25. Zhang C, Oberoi P, Oelsner S, et al. Chimeric antigen receptor-engineered NK-92 cells: an off-the-shelf cellular therapeutic for targeted elimination of cancer cells and induction of protective antitumor immunity. *Front Immunol.* 2017;8:533.

26. Guillerey C, Huntington ND, Smyth MJ. Targeting natural killer cells in can-cer immunotherapy. *Nat Immunol.* 2016;17:1025-1036.

27. Schmidt TL, Negrin RS, Contag CH. A killer choice for cancer immuno-therapy. *Immunol Res.* 2014;58:300-306.

28. Poh SL, Linn YC. Immune checkpoint inhibitors enhance cytotoxicity of cytokine-induced killer cells against human myeloid leukaemic blasts. *Cancer Immunol Immunother.* 2016;65:525-536.

29. Wolfel T, Hauer M, Schneider J, et al. A p16INK4a-insensitive CDK4 mutant targeted by cytolytic T lymphocytes in a human melanoma. *Science.* 1995;269:1281-1284.

30. Robbins PF, Lu YC, El-Gamil M, et al. Mining exomic sequencing data to identify mutated antigens recognized by adoptively transferred tumor-reac-tive T cells. *Nat Med.* 2013;19:747-752.

31. Tran E, Turcotte S, Gros A, et al. Cancer immunotherapy based on muta-tion-specific CD4+ T cells in a patient with epithelial cancer. *Science.* 2014;344:641-645.

32. Tran E, Robbins PF, Lu Y-C, et al. T-cell transfer therapy targeting mutant KRAS in cancer. *N Engl J Med.* 2016;375:2255-2262.

33. Schumacher TN, Schreiber RD. Neoantigens in cancer immunotherapy. *Science.* 2015;348:69-74.

34. Aleksic M, Liddy N, Molloy PE, et al. Different affinity windows for virus and cancer-specific T-cell receptors: implications for therapeutic strategies. *Eur J Immunol.* 2012;42:3174-3179.

35. Barrett DM, Singh N, Porter DL, et al. Chimeric antigen receptor therapy for cancer. *Annu Rev Med.* 2014;65:333-347.

36. Johnson LA, June CH. Driving gene-engineered T cell immunotherapy of cancer. *Cell Res.* 2017;27:38-58.

37. Morgan RA, Chinnasamy N, Abate-Daga D, et al. Cancer regression and neu-rological toxicity following anti-MAGE-A3 TCR gene therapy. *J Immunother.* 2013;36:133-151.

38. Linette GP, Stadtmauer EA, Maus MV, et al. Cardiovascular toxicity and titin cross-reactivity of affinity enhanced T cells in myeloma and melanoma. *Blood.* 2013;122:863-871.

39. Coulie PG, Van den Eynde BJ, van der Bruggen P, et al. Tumour antigens recognized by T lymphocytes: at the core of cancer immunotherapy. *Nat Rev Cancer.* 2014;14:135-146.

40. Bobisse S, Foukas PG, Coukos G, et al. Neoantigen-based cancer immuno-therapy. *Ann Transl Med.* 2016;4:262.

41. Verdegaal EM, de Miranda NF, Visser M, et al. Neoantigen landscape dynam-ics during human melanoma-T cell interactions. *Nature.* 2016;536:91-95.

42. Morris EC, Stauss HJ. Optimizing T-cell receptor gene therapy for hemato-logic malignancies. *Blood.* 2016;127:3305-3311.

43. Bendle GM, Linnemann C, Hooijkaas AI, et al. Lethal graft-versus-host disease in mouse models of T cell receptor gene therapy. *Nat Med.* 2010;16:565-570.

44. Schmitt TM, Stromnes IM, Chapuis AG, et al. New strategies in engineering T-cell receptor gene-modified T cells to more effectively target malignan-cies. *Clin Cancer Res.* 2015;21:5191.

45. Provasi E, Genovese P, Lombardo A, et al. Editing T cell specificity towards leukemia by zinc finger nucleases and lentiviral gene transfer. *Nat Med.* 2012;18:807-815.

46. Moon EK, Ranganathan R, Eruslanov E, et al. Blockade of programmed death 1 augments the ability of human T cells engineered to target NY-ESO-1 to control tumor growth after adoptive transfer. *Clin Cancer Res.* 2016;22:436-447.

47. Di Stasi A, De Angelis B, Rooney CM, et al. T lymphocytes coexpressing CCR4 and a chimeric antigen receptor targeting CD30 have improved homing and antitumor activity in a Hodgkin tumor model. *Blood.* 2009;113:6392-6402.

48. Gross G, Waks T, Eshhar Z. Expression of immunoglobulin-T-cell receptor chimeric molecules as functional receptors with antibody-type specificity. *Proc Natl Acad Sci U S A.* 1989;86:10024-10028.

49. Kuwana Y, Asakura Y, Utsunomiya N, et al. Expression of chimeric receptor composed of immunoglobulin-derived V regions and T-cell receptor-derived C regions. *Biochem Biophys Res Commun.* 1987;149:960-968.

50. Lim WA, June CH. The principles of engineering immune cells to treat can-cer. *Cell.* 2017;168:724-740.

51. Lamers CHJ, Sleijfer S, Vulto AG, et al. Treatment of metastatic renal cell carcinoma with autologous T-lymphocytes genetically retargeted against car-bonic anhydrase IX: first clinical experience. *J Clin Oncol.* 2006;24:e20-e22.

52. Hege KM, Bergsland EK, Fisher GA, et al. Safety, tumor trafficking and immunogenicity of chimeric antigen receptor (CAR)-T cells specific for TAG-72 in colorectal cancer. *J Immunother Cancer.* 2017;5:22.

53. June CH, Sadelain M. Chimeric antigen receptor T cells. *N Engl J Med.* 2018;in press.

54. Ruella M, Klichinsky M, Kenderian SS, et al. Overcoming the immunosup-pressive tumor microenvironment of Hodgkin lymphoma using chimeric antigen receptor T cells. *Cancer Discov.* 2017;7:1154–1167.

55. Brown CE, Badie B, Barish ME. Bioactivity and safety of IL13Ralpha2-redirected chimeric antigen receptor CD8+ T cells in patients with recur-rent glioblastoma. *Clin Cancer Res.* 2015;21:4062-4072.

56. Johnson LA, Scholler J, Ohkuri T. Rational development and characteriza-tion of humanized anti-EGFR variant III chimeric antigen receptor T cells for glioblastoma. *Sci Transl Med.* 2015;7:275ra22.

57. Kenderian SS, Ruella M, Shestova O, et al. CD33-specific chimeric anti-gen receptor T cells exhibit potent preclinical activity against human acute myeloid leukemia. *Leukemia.* 2015;29:1637-1647.

58. Sadelain M, Rivière I, Riddell S. Therapeutic T cell engineering. *Nature.* 2017;545:423-431.

59. Joyce JA, Fearon DT. T cell exclusion, immune privilege, and the tumor microenvironment. *Science.* 2015;348:74-80.

60. Navai Shoba A, Ahmed N. Targeting the tumour profile using broad spec-trum chimaeric antigen receptor T-cells. *Biochem Soc Trans.* 2016;44:391.

61. Qasim W, Zhan H, Samarasinghe S, et al. Molecular remission of infant B-ALL after infusion of universal TALEN gene-edited CAR T cells. *Sci Transl Med.* 2017;9: pii: eaaj2013.

62. Bendelac A, Savage PB, Teyton L. The biology of NKT cells. *Annu Rev Immunol.* 2007;25:297-336.

63. Tian G, Courtney AN, Jena B, et al. CD62L+ NKT cells have prolonged per-sistence and antitumor activity in vivo. *J Clin Investig.* 2016;126:2341-2355.

64. Kobayashi H, Tanaka Y, Shimmura H, et al. Complete remission of lung metastasis following adoptive immunotherapy using activated autologous gammadelta T-cells in a patient with renal cell carcinoma. *Anticancer Res.* 2010;30:575-579.

65. Staveley-O'Carroll K, Sotomayor E, Montgomery J, et al. Induction of anti-gen-specific T cell anergy: an early event in the course of tumor progression. *Proc Natl Acad Sci U S A.* 1998;95:1178-1183.

66. Mizoguchi H, O'Shea JJ, Longo DL, et al. Alterations in signal trans-duction molecules in T lymphocytes from tumor-bearing mice. *Science.* 1992;258:1795-1798.

67. Rabinovich GA, Gabrilovich D, Sotomayor EM. Immunosuppressive strate-gies that are mediated by tumor cells. *Annu Rev Immunol.* 2007;25:267-296.

68. Arina A, Bronte V. Myeloid-derived suppressor cell impact on endogenous and adoptively transferred T cells. *Curr Opin Immunol.* 2015;33:120-125.

69. Arina A, Schreiber K, Binder DC, et al. Adoptively transferred immune T cells eradicate established tumors despite cancer-induced immune suppres-sion. *J Immunol.* 2014;192:1286-1293.

70. Huang AC, Postow MA, Orlowski RJ, et al. T-cell invigoration to tumour burden ratio associated with anti-PD-1 response. *Nature.* 2017;545:60-65.

71. Sureda A, Bader P, Cesaro S, et al. Indications for allo-and auto-SCT for haematological diseases, solid tumours and immune disorders: current practice in Europe, 2015. *Bone Marrow Transplant.* 2015;50:1037-1056.

72. Maude S, Laetsch TW, Buechner J, et al. Tisagenlecleucel in children and young adults with acute lymphoblastic leukemia. *N Engl J Med.* 2018;378:439-448.

73. Maude SL, Frey N, Shaw PA, et al. Chimeric antigen receptor T cells for sustained remissions in leukemia. *N Engl J Med.* 2014;371:1507-1517.

74. Sampson JH, Maus MV, June CH. Immunotherapy for brain tumors. *J Clin Oncol.* 2017;35:2450-2456.

75. Fry TJ, Shah NN, Orentas RJ, et al. CD22-targeted CAR T cells induce remission in B-ALL that is naive or resistant to CD19-targeted CAR immunotherapy. *Nat Med.* 2018;24:20-28.

76. Khaled SK, Thomas SH, Forman SJ. Allogeneic hematopoietic cell transplantation for acute lymphoblastic leukemia (ALL) in adults. *Curr Opin Oncol.* 2012;24:182-190.

77. Ruggeri L, Capanni M, Urbani E, et al. Effectiveness of donor natural killer cell alloreactivity in mismatched hematopoietic transplants. *Science.* 2002;295:2097-2100.

78. Rezvani K, Rouce RH. The application of natural killer cell immunotherapy for the treatment of cancer. *Front Immunol.* 2015;6:578.

79. Chapuis AG, Ragnarsson GB, Nguyen HN, et al. Transferred WT1-reactive CD8+ T cells can mediate antileukemic activity and persist in post-transplant patients. *Sci Transl Med.* 2013;5:174ra27.

80. Neelapu SS, Locke FL, Bartlett NL, et al. Axicabtagene ciloleucel CAR T-cell therapy in refractory large B-cell lymphoma. *N Engl J Med.* 2017;377:2531-2544.

81. Schuster SJ, Svoboda J, Chong EA, et al. Chimeric antigen receptor T cells in refractory B-cell lymphomas. *N Engl J Med.* 2017;377:2545-2554.

82. Porter DL, Hwang W-T, Frey NV, et al. Chimeric antigen receptor T cells persist and induce sustained remissions in relapsed refractory chronic lymphocytic leukemia. *Sci Transl Med.* 2015;7:303ra139.

83. Bollard CM, Aguilar L, Straathof KC, et al. Cytotoxic T lymphocyte therapy for Epstein-Barr virus+ Hodgkin's disease. *J Exp Med.* 2004;200:1623-1633.

84. Ramos CA, Ballard B, Zhang H, et al. Clinical and immunological responses after CD30-specific chimeric antigen receptor-redirected lymphocytes. *J Clin Investig.* 2017;127:3462-3471.

85. Ruella M, Kenderian SS, Shestova O, et al. The addition of the BTK inhibitor ibrutinib to anti-CD19 chimeric antigen receptor T cells (CART19) improves responses against mantle cell lymphoma. *Clin Cancer Res.* 2016;22:2684-2696.

86. John LB, Devaud C, Duong CP, et al. Anti-PD-1 antibody therapy potently enhances the eradication of established tumors by gene-modified T cells. *Clin Cancer Res.* 2013;19:5636–5646.

87. Garfall AL, Maus MV, Hwang WT, et al. Chimeric antigen receptor T cells against CD19 for multiple myeloma. *N Engl J Med.* 2015;373:1040-1047.

88. Carpenter RO, Evbuomwan MO, Pittaluga S, et al. B-cell maturation antigen is a promising target for adoptive T-cell therapy of multiple myeloma. *Clin Cancer Res.* 2013;19:2040-2060.

89. Rapoport AP, Stadtmauer EA, Binder-Scholl GK, et al. NY-ESO-1-specific TCR-engineered T cells mediate sustained antigen-specific antitumor effects in myeloma. *Nat Med.* 2015;21:914-921.

90. Rosenberg SA, Yang JC, Sherry RM, et al. Durable complete responses in heavily pretreated patients with metastatic melanoma using T-cell transfer immunotherapy. *Clin Cancer Res.* 2011;17:4550-4557.

91. Rosenberg SA, Tran E, Robbins PF. T-cell transfer therapy targeting mutant KRAS. *N Engl J Med.* 2017;376:e11.

92. Johnson LA, Morgan RA, Dudley ME, et al. Gene therapy with human and mouse T-cell receptors mediates cancer regression and targets normal tissues expressing cognate antigen. *Blood.* 2009;114:535-546.

93. Robbins PF, Morgan RA, Feldman SA, et al. Tumor regression in patients with metastatic synovial cell sarcoma and melanoma using genetically engineered lymphocytes reactive with NY-ESO-1. *J Clin Oncol.* 2011;29:917-924.

94. O'Rourke DM, Nasrallah MP, Desai A, et al. A single dose of peripherally infused EGFRvIII-directed CAR T cells mediates antigen loss and induces adaptive resistance in patients with recurrent glioblastoma. *Sci Transl Med.* 2017;9(399): pii: eaaa0984.

95. Yang JC. Toxicities associated with adoptive T-cell transfer for cancer. *Cancer J.* 2015;21:506-509.

96. Turtle CJ, Hanafi L-A, Berger C, et al. Immunotherapy of non-Hodgkin's lymphoma with a defined ratio of CD8+/CD4+ CD19-specific chimeric antigen receptor–modified T cells. *Sci Transl Med.* 2016;8:355ra116.

97. Obstfeld AE, Frey NV, Mansfield K, et al. Cytokine release syndrome associated with chimeric-antigen receptor T-cell therapy; clinicopathological insights. *Blood.* 2017;130:2569-2572.

98. Lee DW, Gardner R, Porter DL, et al. Current concepts in the diagnosis and management of cytokine release syndrome. *Blood.* 2014;124:188-195.

99. Bhoj VG, Arhontoulis D, Wertheim G, et al. Persistence of long-lived plasma cells and humoral immunity in individuals responding to CD19-directed CAR T-cell therapy. *Blood.* 2016;128:360-370.

100. Hinrichs CS, Restifo NP. Reassessing target antigens for adoptive T cell therapy. *Nat Biotechnol.* 2013;31:999-1008.

101. Maude SL, Teachey DT, Porter DL, et al. CD19-targeted chimeric antigen receptor T-cell therapy for acute lymphoblastic leukemia. *Blood.* 2015;125:4017-4023.

102. Gust J, Hay KA, Hanafi LA, et al. Endothelial activation and blood-brain barrier disruption in neurotoxicity after adoptive immunotherapy with CD19 CAR-T cells. *Cancer Discov.* 2017;7:1404-1419.

103. Benjamin JE, Stein AS. The role of blinatumomab in patients with relapsed:refractory acute lymphoblastic leukemia. *Ther Adv Hematol.* 2016;7:142-156.

104. Turtle CJ, Hanafi L-A, Berger C, et al. CD19 CAR–T cells of defined CD4+:CD8+ composition in adult B cell ALL patients. *J Clin Investig.* 2016;126:2123-2138.

105. Hay KA, Hanafi LA, Li D, et al. Kinetics and biomarkers of severe cytokine release syndrome after CD19 chimeric antigen receptor-modified T cell therapy. *Blood.* 2017;130:2295-2306.

106. Schutsky K, Song DG, Lynn R, et al. Rigorous optimization and validation of potent RNA CAR T cell therapy for the treatment of common epithelial cancers expressing folate receptor. *Oncotarget.* 2015;6:28911-28928.

107. Almåsbak H, Aarvak T, Vemuri MC. CAR T cell therapy: a game changer in cancer treatment. *J Immunol Res.* 2016;2016:5474602.

108. Ruella M, Barrett DM, Kenderian SS, et al. Dual CD19 and CD123 targeting prevents antigen-loss relapses after CD19-directed immunotherapies. *J Clin Investig.* 2016;126:3814-3826.

109. Sotillo E, Barrett DM, Black KL, et al. Convergence of acquired mutations and alternative splicing of CD19 enables resistance to CART-19 immunotherapy. *Cancer Discov.* 2015;5:1282-1295.

110. Ruella M, Maus MV. Catch me if you can: leukemia escape after CD19-directed T cell immunotherapies. *Comput Struct Biotechnol J.* 2016;14:357-362.

111. Neumann PJ, Cohen JT. Measuring the value of prescription drugs. *N Engl J Med.* 2015;373:2965-2967.

112. Chen Q, Jain N, Ayer T, et al. Economic burden of chronic lymphocytic leukemia in the era of oral targeted therapies in the United States. *J Clin Oncol.* 2017;35:166-174.

113. Jaroslawski S, Toumi M. Sipuleucel-T (Provenge®)-autopsy of an innovative paradigm change in cancer treatment: why a single-product biotech company failed to capitalize on its breakthrough invention. *BioDrugs.* 2015;29:301.

114. Carr DR, Bradshaw SE. Gene therapies: the challenge of super-high-cost treatments and how to pay for them. *Regen Med.* 2016;11:381-393.

115. Hettle R, Corbett M, Hinde S, et al. The assessment and appraisal of regenerative medicines and cell therapy products: an exploration of methods for review, economic evaluation and appraisal. *Health Technol Assess.* 2017;21:1-204.

116. Wherry EJ, Kurachi M. Molecular and cellular insights into T cell exhaustion. *Nat Rev Immunol.* 2015;15:486-499.

117. Levine BL, June CH. Perspective: assembly line immunotherapy. *Nature.* 2013;498:S17.

118. McGarrity GJ, Hoyah G, Winemiller A, et al. Patient monitoring and follow-up in lentiviral clinical trials. *J Gene Med.* 2013;15:78-82.

119. Rubnitz JE, Inaba H, Ribeiro RC, et al. NKAML: a pilot study to determine the safety and feasibility of haploidentical natural killer cell transplantation in childhood acute myeloid leukemia. *J Clin Oncol.* 2010;28:955-959.

120. Davila ML, Riviere I, Wang X, et al. Efficacy and toxicity management of 19-28z CAR T cell therapy in B cell acute lymphoblastic leukemia. *Sci Transl Med.* 2014;6:224ra25.

121. Kochenderfer JN, Dudley ME, Kassim SH, et al. Chemotherapy-refractory diffuse large B-cell lymphoma and indolent B-cell malignancies can be effectively treated with autologous T cells expressing an anti-CD19 chimeric antigen receptor. *J Clin Oncol.* 2015;33:540-549.

122. Locke FL, Neelapu SS, Bartlett NL, et al. Phase 1 clinical results of the ZUMA-1 (KTE-C19-101) study: a phase 1-2 multi-center study evaluating the safety and efficacy of anti-CD19 CAR T cells (KTE-C19) in subjects with refractory aggressive non-Hodgkin lymphoma (NHL). *Blood.* 2015;126:3991.

123. Fan F, Zhao W, Liu J, et al. Durable remissions with BCMA-specific chimeric antigen receptor (CAR)-modified T cells in patients with refractory/relapsed multiple myeloma. *J Clin Oncol.* 2017;35:LBA3001.

124. Berdeja JG, Lin Y, Raje NS, et al. First-in-human multicenter study of bb2121 anti-BCMA CAR T-cell therapy for relapsed/refractory multiple myeloma: updated results. *J Clin Oncol.* 2017;35:3010.

125. Morgan RA, Dudley ME, Wunderlich JR, et al. Cancer regression in patients after transfer of genetically engineered lymphocytes. *Science.* 2006;314:126-129.

126. Topalian SL, Solomon D, Avis FP, et al. Immunotherapy of patients with advanced cancer using tumor-infiltrating lymphocytes and recombinant interleukin-2: a pilot study. *J Clin Oncol.* 1988;6:839-853.

127. Jiang SS, Tang Y, Zhang YJ, et al. A phase I clinical trial utilizing autologous tumor-infiltrating lymphocytes in patients with primary hepatocellular carcinoma. *Oncotarget.* 2015;6:41339-41349.

128. Brown CE, Alizadeh D, Starr R, et al. Regression of glioblastoma after chimeric antigen receptor T-cell therapy. *N Engl J Med.* 2016;375:2561-2569.

Section V

Supportive Care

Antiemetics

Rudolph M. Navari

Introduction

Chemotherapy-induced nausea and vomiting (CINV) is associated with a significant deterioration in quality of life and is perceived by patients as a major adverse effect of the treatment.[1-3] Increased risk of CINV is associated with the type of chemotherapy administered (Table 32.1) and specific patient characteristics (Table 32.2).[3] CINV can result in serious complications, such as weakness, weight loss, electrolyte imbalance, dehydration, or anorexia and is associated with a variety of complications, including fractures, esophageal tears, decline in functional and mental status, and wound dehiscence.[1-3] Patients who are dehydrated, debilitated, or malnourished, as well as those who have an electrolyte imbalance or those who have recently undergone surgery or radiation therapy, are at greater risk of experiencing serious complications from CINV.[1-3]

The type of chemotherapy to be given defines the degree of emetogenicity (Table 32.3) and the risk of CINV for patients. Tables 32.4 to 32.6 lists the emetogenicity of the various intravenous chemotherapy agents, and Table 32.7 lists the emetogenicity of some of the oral chemotherapy agents. The type and number of antiemetics to be used for the control of CINV are dictated by whether the chemotherapy is of high, moderate, or low emetogenic potential.

Physicians and nursing staff may underestimate the CINV experienced by patients[4] and significant increases in cost of health care expenditures may ensue when CINV is not well controlled.[5]

The use of first-generation 5-hydroxytryptamine-3 (5-HT$_3$) receptor antagonists plus dexamethasone has improved the control of CINV.[3,6] Further improvement in the control of CINV has been achieved with the use of a second-generation 5-HT$_3$ receptor antagonist (palonosetron),[7] neurokinin-1 receptor antagonists (aprepitant, netupitant, and rolapitant)[8-10] and olanzapine, an antipsychotic that blocks multiple neurotransmitters in the central nervous system.[11-15]

The primary endpoint used for studies evaluating various agents for the control of CINV has been complete response (no emesis, no use of rescue medication) over the acute (24 hours postchemotherapy), delayed (24 to 120 hours), and overall (0 to 120 hours) periods.[3] The combination of a 5-HT$_3$ receptor antagonist, dexamethasone, and an NK-1 receptor antagonist has improved the control of emesis in patients receiving either highly emetogenic chemotherapy (HEC) or moderately emetogenic chemotherapy (MEC) over a 120-hours period following chemotherapy administration.[3,7-13] When nausea is measured as a secondary endpoint, it often has not been well controlled.[16,17]

Emesis is a well-defined event that is easily measured, but nausea may be more subjective and more difficult to measure. However, two well-defined measures of nausea are the visual analogue scale (VAS) and the Likert scale.[18] The VAS is a scale from 0 to 10 or 0 to 100, with 0 representing no nausea and 10 or 100 representing maximal nausea. The Likert scale asks patients to rate nausea as "None, Mild, Moderate, or Severe."

Many studies have reported the secondary end point of "no significant nausea" or "only mild nausea".[3,8,17] Studies that have reported "no nausea" may be more useful in identifying the most effective available antinausea agents.[14,16]

Despite the introduction of more effective antiemetic agents, emesis and nausea remain important complications of

32.1 *Emetic potential of chemotherapy agents*

Emetogenic Potential	Typical Agents	Definition (no CINV Prevention)
High	Cisplatin, dacarbazine, melphalan (high dose), nitrogen mustard, cyclophosphamide plus an anthracycline	Emesis in nearly all patients
Moderate	Anthracyclines, carboplatin, carmustine (high dose), cyclophosphamide, ifosfamide, irinotecan, methotrexate (high dose), oxaliplatin, topotecan	Emesis in >70% of patients
Low	Etoposide, 5-fluorouracil, gemcitabine, mitoxantrone, taxanes, vinblastine, vinorelbine	Emesis in 10% to 70% of patients
Minimal	Bortezomib, hormones, vinca alkaloids, bleomycin	Emesis in <10% of patients

CINV, chemotherapy-induced nausea and vomiting.

TABLE

32.2 *Patient-related risk factors for emesis following chemotherapy*

Major Factors	Minor Factors
Female	History of motion sickness
Age <50 y	Emesis during past
History of low prior chronic alcohol intake (<1 ounce of alcohol/d)	pregnancy
History of previous chemotherapy-induced emesis	
Emetogenicity of chemotherapy regimen	

TABLE

32.4 *Highly emetogenic chemotherapy*

* >90% emetic risk:
  ○ Anthracycline + cyclophosphamide combination (defined as either doxorubicin or epirubicin with cyclophosphamide)
  ○ Carboplatin AUC $\geq$4
  ○ Carmustine >250 mg/m^2
  ○ Cisplatin
  ○ Cyclophosphamide >1,500 mg/m^2
  ○ Dacarbazine
  ○ Doxorubicin $\geq$60 mg/m^2
  ○ Epirubicin >90 mg/m^2
  ○ Ifosfamide $\geq$2 g/m^2 per dose
  ○ Streptozocin

chemotherapy. The purpose of this chapter is to evaluate the clinical agents available for the prevention and treatment of CINV. The use of these agents in various clinical settings is described using the recently established guidelines from the Multinational Association of Supportive Care in Cancer (MASCC) and the European Society of Medical Oncology (ESMO)[19], the American Society of Clinical Oncology (ASCO)[20] and the National Comprehensive Cancer Network (NCCN) guidelines.[21] The literature cited consists of the primary clinical trials used for the U.S. FDA approval of the various agents as well as comprehensive reviews.

Pathophysiology of Nausea and Vomiting

The sensation of nausea and the act of vomiting are protective reflexes that rid the intestine and stomach of toxic substances. The experience of nausea is subjective, and nausea may be considered a prodromal phase to the act of vomiting[18] although significant nausea may occur without vomiting. Vomiting consists of a pre-ejection phase, retching, and ejection and is accompanied by shivering and salivation. Vomiting is triggered when afferent impulses from the cerebral cortex, chemoreceptor trigger zone (CTZ), and pharynx and vagal afferent fibers of the gastrointestinal (GI) tract travel to the vomiting center, located in the medulla (Fig. 32.1). Efferent impulses then travel from the VC to the abdominal muscles, salivation center, cranial nerves, and respiratory center, causing vomiting. It is thought that chemotherapeutic agents cause vomiting by activating neurotransmitter receptors located in the CTZ, GI tract, and vomiting center. The mechanisms of emesis are not well defined, but emesis may be primarily mediated through neurotransmitters

(serotonin, dopamine, substance P) in the GI tract and the central nervous system.[18] Figure 32.1 shows that chemotherapy agents may directly affect areas in the cerebral cortex and the medulla oblongata or may stimulate the small intestine of the GI tract via the vagus nerve. A vomiting center, termed the "central pattern generator" by some authors[22] appears to be located in the lateral reticular formation of the medulla, which coordinates the mechanism of nausea and vomiting. An additional important area, also located in the medulla, is the CTZ in the area postrema near the fourth ventricle.[22] The nucleus tractus solitarius (NTS) neurons lying ventrally to the area postrema initiate emesis.[23] This medullary area is a convergence point for projections arising from the area postrema and the vestibular and vagal afferents.[23] The NTS is a good candidate for the site of action of centrally acting antiemetics.

The main approach to the control of emesis has been to identify the active neurotransmitters and their receptors in the central nervous system and the GI tract that mediate the afferent inputs to the vomiting center (Fig. 32.2). Agents that may block these neurotransmitter receptors in the CTZ, the vomiting center, or the GI tract may be useful in preventing or controlling emesis (Table 32.8).

TABLE

32.3 *Chemotherapy emetogenicity risk classification*

Risk Classification	Definition
High emetic risk	>90% frequency of emesis
Moderate emetic risk	30% to 90% frequency of emesis
Low emetic risk	10% to 30% frequency of emesis
Minimal emetic risk	<10% frequency of emesis

TABLE

32.5 *Moderately emetogenic chemotherapy*

* 30% to 90% emetic risk:
  ○ Bendamustine
  ○ Oxaliplatin
  ○ Carboplatin AUC <4
  ○ Carmustine $\leq$250 mg/m^2
  ○ Cyclophosphamide $\leq$1,500 mg/m^2
  ○ Ifosfamide <2 g/m^2 per dose
  ○ Irinotecan
  ○ Cytarabine >200 mg/m^2
  ○ Doxorubicin <60 mg/m^2, daunorubicin, idarubicin
  ○ Temozolomide
  ○ Methotrexate $\geq$250 mg/m^2

TABLE **32.6**	*Low emetogenic chemotherapy*

- 10% to 30% emetic risk:
  - 5-Fluorouracil
  - Ado-trastuzumab emtansine
  - Cytarabine (low dose) 100 to 200 mg/m^2
  - Docetaxel
  - Eribulin
  - Gemcitabine
  - Topotecan
  - Paclitaxel
  - Pemetrexed
  - Ziv-aflibercept
  - Vismodegib

TABLE **32.7**	*Oral chemotherapy agents with moderate to high emetogenic potential*

- Altretamine
- Busulfan (≥4 mg/d)
- Ceritinib
- Crizotinib
- Cyclophosphamide (≥100 mg/m^2/d)
- Estramustine
- Etoposide
- Lenvatinib
- Lomustine (single day)
- Mitotane
- Olaparib
- Panobinostat
- Procarbazine
- Temozolomide (>75 mg/m^2/d)

Nausea is a difficult-to-describe, sick, or queasy sensation, usually perceived as being in the stomach that is sometimes followed by emesis.[18] The experience of nausea is difficult to describe in another person. Nausea and emesis are not necessarily on a continuum. One can experience nausea without emesis, and one can have sudden emesis without nausea. Nausea has been assumed to be the conscious awareness of unusual sensations in the "vomiting center" of the brainstem (Fig. 32.1), but the existence of such a center and its relationship to nausea remain controversial.[18]

The study of the receptors that are illustrated in Figure 32.2 has guided the development of antagonists to the serotonin and the

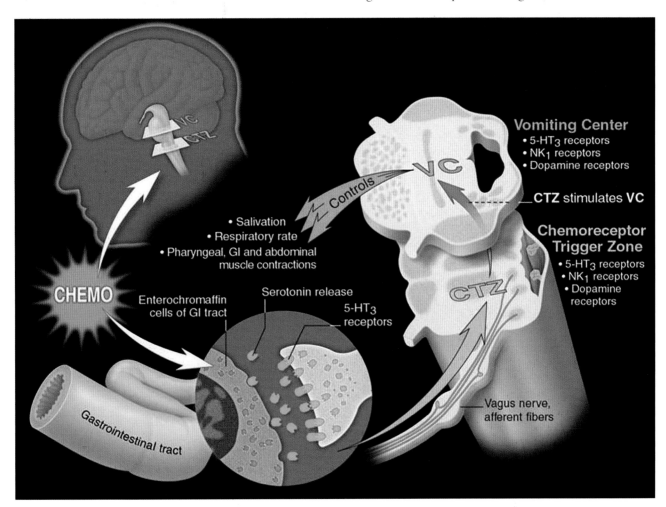

FIGURE **32.1** Physiology of chemotherapy-induced emesis.

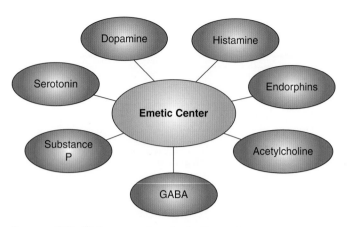

FIGURE **32.2** Neurotransmitters involved in emesis.

substance P receptors with improved success in controlling emesis. It is not clear whether the serotonin and/or the substance P receptors are important in the control of nausea. Other receptors, such as dopaminergic, histaminic, and muscarinic, may be the dominant receptors in the control of nausea.[3,16,17]

Types of Chemotherapy-Induced Nausea and Vomiting

Five categories are used to classify CINV: acute, delayed, anticipatory, breakthrough, and refractory. Nausea and vomiting may occur any time after the administration of chemotherapy, but the mechanisms appear different for CINV occurring in the first 24 hours after chemotherapy in contrast to that which occurs in the period of 1 to 5 days after chemotherapy.

Acute CINV

The term acute-onset CINV refers to nausea and/or vomiting occurring within 24 hours of chemotherapy administration[3] and usually peaks within the first 5 to 6 hours after the initiation of chemotherapy. The incidence of acute emesis and/or nausea reflects several treatment-related factors, including the environment in which chemotherapy is administered, the emetogenicity of the chemotherapy, the dosage of the emetogenic agents, and patient-related factors.[21]

Delayed CINV

Nausea and/or vomiting that develop more than 24 hours after chemotherapy administration is known as delayed emesis and/or nausea. Typically occurring with administration of cisplatin, carboplatin, doxorubicin, or cyclophosphamide, delayed emesis/nausea is more common in those who experience acute emesis/nausea. Other predictive factors include the dose and the emetogenicity of the chemotherapeutic agent, patient sex and age, and protection against nausea and vomiting in previous cycles of chemotherapy.[3,21] For cisplatin, which has been most extensively studied, delayed emesis reaches peak intensity 2 to 3 days subsequent to chemotherapy administration and can last up to a week.[3,19–21]

Breakthrough CINV

Vomiting and/or nausea that occurs within 5 days after chemotherapy despite prophylactic use of antiemetic agents and/or requires additional antiemetics ("rescue") is called breakthrough emesis.

Refractory CINV

Vomiting and/or nausea occurring after chemotherapy in subsequent chemotherapy cycles when antiemetic prophylaxis and/or rescue have failed in earlier cycles is known as refractory emesis.[3,21]

Anticipatory CINV

If patients experience CINV, they may develop a conditioned response known as anticipatory nausea and/or vomiting, which occurs before the administration of chemotherapy in future chemotherapy cycles and is attributed to the memory of prior CINV. Incidence rates for this type of nausea and vomiting range from 10% to 45%, with nausea occurring more frequently.[3,21]

Antiemetic Agents

Dopamine Receptor Antagonists

Dopamine receptors are known to exist in the CTZ, the main area of activity of the dopamine antagonists, such as the phenothiazines and the butyrophenones (droperidol, haloperidol). However, a high

TABLE **32.8**	*Antiemetic receptor antagonists*		
Dopamine Receptor Antagonists	**5-HT₃ Receptor Antagonists**	**Dopa–5-HT₃ Receptor Antagonists**	**NK-1 Receptor Antagonists**
Butyrophenones, olanzapine, phenothiazines	Azasetron, dolasetron (not recommended for use per U.S. FDA), granisetron, olanzapine, ondansetron (IV dose restriction per FDA), palonosetron, ramosetron, tropisetron	Metoclopramide	Aprepitant (MK-869), fosaprepitant, netupitant, rolapitant

IV, intravenous; NK, neurokinin; 5-HT₃, serotonin.

level of blockade of the dopamine receptors results in extrapyramidal reactions, as well as disorientation and sedation, limiting the clinical use of these agents. Their current use is primarily to treat established nausea and emesis and not for CINV prophylaxis.[21]

Serotonin (5-HT₃) Receptor Antagonists

Serotonin receptors, specifically the 5-HT_3 receptors, exist in the central nervous system and in the GI tract. The 5-HT_3 receptor antagonists appear to act through both the central nervous system and the GI tract via the vagus and splanchnic nerves.

The introduction of 5-HT_3 receptor antagonists for the prevention of CINV, as well as postoperative and radiotherapy-induced nausea and vomiting, has resulted in an improvement in supportive care.[3] Treatment guidelines for the prevention of CINV recommended by a number of international groups[19–21] suggest the use of a 5-HT_3 receptor antagonist and dexamethasone alone or in combination with other antiemetics prechemotherapy for the prevention of acute CINV and the use of dexamethasone alone or in combination with other antiemetics following chemotherapy for the prevention of delayed nausea and vomiting in patients receiving either moderately or HEC.

First-Generation 5-HT₃ Receptor Antagonists

Table 32.9 shows the 5-HT_3 receptor antagonists currently in use. The first-generation 5-HT_3 receptor antagonists (dolasetron, granisetron, ondansetron, tropisetron[24] azasetron[25] and ramosetron[26]) are equivalent in efficacy and toxicities when used in the recommended doses and compete only on an economic basis.[27] They have not been associated with major toxicities; the most commonly reported adverse events are mild headache, constipation, and, occasionally, mild diarrhea.[3] Azasetron and ramosetron are not available in North America and Europe and have not been compared extensively with the other 5-HT_3 receptor antagonists. They are marketed primarily in Southeast Asia.

TABLE 32.9	Serotonin antagonists and dosage before chemotherapy [a]	
Antiemetic	**Route**	**Dosage**
Azasetron	IV	10 mg
Dolasetron[b]	IV	100 mg or 1.8 mg/kg
	PO	100 mg
Granisetron	IV	10 µg/kg or 1 mg
	PO	2 mg (or 1 mg twice daily)
Ondansetron	IV	8 mg (restricted to <16 mg)
	PO	24 mg
Palonosetron	IV	0.25 mg
Ramosetron	IV	0.30 mg
Tropisetron	IV or PO	5 mg

[a]The same doses are used for highly and moderately emetogenic chemotherapy.
[b]Not recommended for use per U.S. FDA.
IV, intravenous; PO, oral.

Differences in metabolism of the 5-HT_3 receptor antagonists may occur due to genetic variability in individuals that may lead to a difference in response to these agents, but no documented clinical reports of this phenomenon have been noted.[3,19–21,24–27]

In 2006, Canada issued a drug alert for dolasetron due to potential serious cardiovascular adverse events (cardiac arrhythmias)[28] stating that dolasetron was not indicated for use in children but only for prevention of CINV in adults.[28] Subsequently, in 2010, the U.S. FDA announced that the intravenous form of dolasetron should no longer be used to prevent CINV in any patient. New data suggested that dolasetron injection can increase the risk of developing a prolongation of the QT interval, which may potentially precipitate life-threatening ventricular arrhythmias.[29]

In 2012, the FDA placed a restriction on the doses of intravenous ondansetron due to the risk of prolongation of the QT interval.[30] Patients who may be at particular risk for QT prolongation with the use of ondansetron are those with congenital long QT syndrome, congestive heart failure, bradyarrhythmias, or taking concomitant medications that prolong the QT interval. The use of a single 32-mg intravenous dose of ondansetron should be avoided. QT prolongation occurs in a dose-dependent manner and specifically at a single intravenous dose of 32 mg. The lower-dose intravenous regimen of 0.15 mg/kg every 4 hours for three doses may be used in adults with CINV. However, no single intravenous dose of ondansetron should exceed 16 mg due to the risk of QT prolongation. None of the recommended oral dosing regimens for ondansetron, including the single oral dose of 24 mg for CINV, are altered.[30] Mason et al.[31] recently reported that intravenous granisetron had no clinically significant effect on the QTc interval at supratherapeutic concentrations.

The first-generation 5-HT_3 receptor antagonists have not been as effective against delayed emesis as they are against acute CINV.[32–34] The first-generation 5-HT_3 receptor antagonists alone do not add significant efficacy to that obtained by dexamethasone in the control of delayed emesis.[33] Hickok et al.[34] reported that the first-generation 5-HT_3 receptor antagonists used in the delayed period were no more effective than prochlorperazine in controlling nausea. The antiemetic effects of prochlorperazine can be attributed to postsynaptic dopamine receptor blockade in the CTZ. A meta-analysis[33] showed that there was neither clinical evidence nor cost-effectiveness advantages to justify the use of the first-generation 5-HT_3 receptor antagonists beyond 24 hours after chemotherapy for the prevention of delayed emesis. Delayed nausea is poorly controlled by the first-generation 5-HT_3 receptor antagonists in patients receiving HEC or MEC.[12,35,36]

Extended-Release Granisetron

A randomized, double-blind, phase III clinical trial evaluated the antiemetic efficacy of transdermal granisetron compared to oral granisetron in patients receiving MEC and HEC.[37] No significant difference in the control of acute or delayed emesis was noted between transdermal and oral granisetron. Transdermal granisetron was effective and safe in the control of acute emesis induced by MEC and HEC.[37]

APF530 is a new, subcutaneously (SC) administered polymeric formulation of granisetron that was developed to provide slow, controlled, and sustained release of granisetron to prevent both acute and delayed CINV associated with MEC and HEC.[38] APF530 consists of 2% granisetron and a polymer vehicle of tri(ethylene glycol) poly(orthoester) (TEG-POE) that undergoes controlled hydrolysis, resulting in slow, controlled, and sustained drug release. The novel biodegradable polymeric excipient is hydrolyzed in vivo, generating nontoxic biodegradable metabolites. This Biochronomer™ drug delivery system (Heron Therapeutics, Inc., Redwood City, CA) allows therapeutic levels of granisetron to be maintained for greater than 5 days with a single subcutaneous injection. In a clinical study[38] of patients undergoing chemotherapy, single-dose APF530 (5 to 15 mg granisetron) administered SC in the abdomen provided circulating levels of granisetron within 30 minutes, a maximum plasma concentration at approximately 24 hours, and sustained therapeutic levels for greater than 120 hours. In a phase 3 noninferiority trial, the clinical efficacy of APF530 250 and 500 mg SC (containing granisetron 5 and 10 mg, respectively) was compared with that of the approved dose of palonosetron (0.25 mg intravenously) in combination with dexamethasone for prevention of acute and delayed CINV following single-day administration of MEC or HEC in patients with cancer. APF530 was noninferior to palonosetron with injection site reactions and constipation as the most commonly reported adverse events.[30] In a QTc study, the APF530 formulation had no clinically significant effect on the QTc interval at supratherapeutic concentrations.[31]

Second-Generation 5-HT₃ Receptor Antagonists: Palonosetron

Palonosetron is a second-generation 5-HT₃ receptor antagonist that has antiemetic activity at both central and GI sites.[3,6,7] In comparison with the first-generation 5-HT₃ receptor antagonists, it has a higher potency, a significantly longer half-life, and a different molecular interaction with 5-HT₃ receptors[3,6,7,39] (Table 32.10). Palonosetron may have efficacy in controlling delayed CINV compared with the first-generation 5-HT₃ receptor antagonists.[3,6,7,39]

Palonosetron demonstrated a 5-HT₃ receptor binding affinity at least 30-fold higher than other 5-HT₃ receptor antagonists.[34] Rojas et al.[40] reported that palonosetron exhibited allosteric binding and positive cooperativity when binding to the 5-HT₃ receptor compared with simple bimolecular binding for both granisetron and ondansetron. Additional studies by Rojas et al.[40] suggested that palonosetron triggers 5-HT₃ receptor internalization and causes prolonged inhibition of receptor function. Differences in binding

and effects on receptor function may explain some differences between palonosetron and the first-generation 5-HT₃ receptor antagonists.[7,40] These differences may explain palonosetron's efficacy in delayed CINV compared with the first-generation receptor antagonists.[3,7,39]

In a systematic review and meta-analysis of all randomized controlled trials comparing a single dose of palonosetron with other 5-HT₃ receptor antagonists, Botrel et al.[41] concluded that palonosetron was more effective than the first-generation receptor antagonists in preventing acute and delayed CINV in patients receiving MEC or HEC, regardless of the use of concomitant glucocorticoids. Schwartzberg et al.[42] concluded that palonosetron is more effective than the first-generation 5-HT₃ receptor antagonists in controlling CINV in the delayed and overall postchemotherapy periods based on a pooled analysis of phase III clinical studies of palonosetron versus ondansetron, dolasetron, and granisetron. In an additional review, Popovic et al.[43] concluded that palonosetron is safer and more efficacious than the other 5-HT₃ receptor antagonists. The international antiemetic guidelines[19–21] recommend palonosetron as the preferred 5-HT₃ receptor antagonist.

The safety and tolerability of palonosetron have been well documented in multiple, large phase III trials. No clinically relevant differences were seen among palonosetron, ondansetron, or dolasetron in laboratory, electrocardiographic, or vital sign changes over multiple cycles of chemotherapy.[7,39,43–45] The adverse reactions reported were the most common reactions reported for the 5-HT₃ receptor antagonist drug class. No reports document any adverse cardiac events with palonosetron, specifically no prolongation of the QT interval in healthy volunteers or patients receiving repeated cycles of emetogenic chemotherapy.[7,39,43–45] Table 32.11 summarizes the reported adverse events of the antiemetic guideline-directed serotonin antagonists.

No other second-generation 5-HT₃ receptor antagonists are on the market, and no information is available on other second-generation agents in development.

Dopamine-Serotonin Receptor Antagonists

Metoclopramide has antiemetic properties both in low doses as a dopamine antagonist and in high doses as a serotonin antagonist. The use of metoclopramide may be somewhat efficacious in relatively high doses (20 mg orally, three times daily) in the delayed period[46] but may result in sedation and extrapyramidal side effects.[3,21,47]

TABLE 32.10 *5-HT₃ receptor antagonists' binding affinity and plasma half-life*

Drug	pKi [-log(Ki)]	Half-life (hours)
Palonosetron	10.45	40
Ondansetron	8.39	4
Granisetron	8.91	9
Dolasetron[a]	7.60	7.3

[a]Half-life reported for hydrodolasetron, the active metabolite of dolasetron.

TABLE 32.11 *Safety and tolerability of the antiemetic guideline-directed serotonin antagonists[19–21,30,31]*

Antiemetic	Route	Adverse Events
Granisetron	IV, PO	Constipation, headache, diarrhea, mild dizziness
Ondansetron	IV, PO	Constipation, headache, diarrhea, mild dizziness, QTc prolongation with IV doses >16 mg
Palonosetron	IV, PO	Constipation, headache, diarrhea

Metoclopramide has been used both as a preventative agent for CINV[46] and a treatment for breakthrough CINV.[21,47] In 2013, the European Medicines Agency issued use restrictions for metoclopramide due to the risk of:

- Extrapyramidal disorders
- Involuntary movement disorders that may include muscle spasms
- Tardive dyskinesia

The risk of side effects is increased at high doses or with long-term treatment. The review recommended that treatment duration be restricted to short-term use (up to 5 days) and that the maximum dose be limited in adults to 10 mg three times daily. It was also recommended that metoclopramide not be used in children under 1 year old.[48] The reduced dose of 10 mg three times daily may be less efficacious as a preventative agent for CINV and as a treatment for breakthrough CINV.[3,21,46,47]

Neurokinin (NK-1) Receptor Antagonists

Substance P is a mammalian tachykinin that is found in vagal afferent neurons innervating the brainstem NTS, which sends impulses to the vomiting center.[49] Substance P induces vomiting and binds to NK-1 receptors in the abdominal vagus, the NTS, and the area postrema.[49] Compounds that block NK-1 receptors lessen emesis after cisplatin, ipecac, apomorphine, and radiation therapy.[49] These observations have led to the development of NK_1 receptor antagonists and the study of the role they may play in controlling CINV.

Aprepitant

Aprepitant is an NK_1 receptor antagonist that blocks the emetic effects of substance P.[3,8,50] When combined with a standard regimen of the glucocorticoid, dexamethasone, and a 5-HT$_3$ receptor antagonist, aprepitant is effective in the prevention of CINV in patients receiving cisplatin-based HEC.[3,50] This regimen is recommended in the guidelines of multiple international groups for the control of CINV in patients receiving HEC.[19–21]

Combined data from two large phase III trials of aprepitant plus a first-generation 5-HT$_3$ receptor antagonist and dexamethasone for the prevention of CINV in patients receiving HEC demonstrated an improvement in complete response when aprepitant was added to ondansetron and dexamethasone, but no improvement was noted in nausea when the pooled data were analyzed for sex (no nausea, overall period: 46% for women, aprepitant group; 38% for women, control group; 50% for men, aprepitant group; 44% for men, control group).[51] Using the same pooled data, a separate analysis[52] showed a statistical but small improvement in no nausea with the use of aprepitant (no nausea, overall period: 48%, aprepitant group; 42%, control group).

In a similar study involving breast cancer patients receiving cyclophosphamide and doxorubicin or epirubicin, aprepitant was added to ondansetron and dexamethasone for the prevention of CINV. The addition of aprepitant to the 5-HT$_3$ receptor antagonist plus dexamethasone improved the complete response, but no improvement in nausea was noted (no nausea, overall period: 33% aprepitant group; 33% control group).[36]

Palonosetron and aprepitant have been combined with dexamethasone for the prevention of CINV in a phase II study of 58 patients who received doxorubicin and cyclophosphamide.[53] This three-drug antiemetic regimen was found to be safe and highly effective in preventing emesis and rescue in the acute, delayed, and overall periods, but control of nausea was poor (no nausea, overall period: 30%).

Fosaprepitant

Fosaprepitant (also known as MK-0517 and L-758,298) is a water-soluble phosphoryl prodrug for aprepitant that, when administered intravenously, is converted to aprepitant within 30 minutes via the action of ubiquitous phosphatases. The pharmacological effect of fosaprepitant is attributed to aprepitant. Due to the rapid conversion of fosaprepitant to the active form (aprepitant) by phosphatase enzymes, it is expected to provide the same aprepitant exposure in terms of area under the curve (AUC) and a correspondingly similar antiemetic effect.[54,55] A single dose of intravenous fosaprepitant, 150 mg on day 1 of cisplatin chemotherapy, was noninferior to a 3-day oral regimen of aprepitant in the prevention of CINV in the 120 hours postchemotherapy.[55]

Both standard 3-day dosing of aprepitant and single-dose fosaprepitant are well tolerated after ondansetron and dexamethasone in patients receiving cisplatin.[55] The tolerability profiles of the two regimens were similar, except for a higher incidence of infusion site adverse events and significantly more thrombophlebitis with intravenous fosaprepitant. Higher incidence of infusion site adverse events was observed in a retrospective review of 98 patients treated with fosaprepitant.[56]

Aprepitant is metabolized extensively by liver enzymes, primarily CYP3A4. CYP3A4 inhibitors can increase aprepitant exposure, and CYP3A4 inducers can reduce aprepitant exposure.[57] Aprepitant is also both an inducer and a moderate inhibitor of CYP3A4.[58] Consequently, the potential for drug-drug interactions exists when aprepitant is coadministered with other drugs that are metabolized by CYP enzymes, including chemotherapeutic agents.[59] Results from several clinical efficacy trials and pharmacokinetic studies showed that most drug-drug interactions with aprepitant had little or no clinical consequence and that no differences in severe adverse events were noted between treatment arms with or without aprepitant.[52,59] Aprepitant had minimal effect on the AUC of several chemotherapeutic agents tested, including cyclophosphamide, docetaxel, and vinorelbine.[59] Coadministration of aprepitant causes a significant increase in the AUC of some glucocorticoids, including a 2.2-fold increase in dexamethasone and a 2.5-fold increase in oral methylprednisolone, necessitating up to 50% dose reduction of these drugs.[59] Aprepitant causes reduced AUC of oral contraceptives, and this has prompted the recommendation of a secondary barrier contraceptive for patients receiving aprepitant.[59] Ifosfamide and aprepitant are both substrates of CYP3A4, and theoretical questions have been raised as to whether aprepitant could be involved in rare cases of ifosfamide encephalopathy, but no clinical data exist demonstrating an association.[8,57,59]

The success of NK-1 receptor antagonists with 5-HT$_3$ receptor antagonists and dexamethasone in preventing emesis in patients receiving single-day HEC[3,6] prompted the use of the NK-1 receptor antagonist aprepitant combined with a 5-HT$_3$ receptor antagonist and dexamethasone in patients receiving multiday, high-dose chemotherapy prior to hematopoietic stem cell transplant. A number of phase III studies have been reported with the use of the NK-1 aprepitant added to a 5-HT₃ receptor antagonists and dexamethasone[60–63] in patients receiving multiday, high-dose chemotherapy before autologous or allogeneic stem cell transplant. In a randomized, placebo-controlled, phase III clinical trial, Stiff et al.[62] randomized 179 patients receiving multiday, high-dose chemotherapy before autologous or allogeneic transplants to aprepitant or placebo in combination with ondansetron and dexamethasone before chemotherapy. Significant improvement in emesis was observed with the use of aprepitant, but no difference in the use of rescue medications or nausea. No adverse events were noted with the use of aprepitant.

Schmitt et al.[60] randomized 362 patients receiving 2 days of high-dose melphalan chemotherapy before autologous transplant to aprepitant or placebo in combination with granisetron and dexamethasone before and after chemotherapy. A significant improvement in complete response of vomiting was seen with the use of aprepitant, but no difference in the use of rescue medications or nausea. No adverse events were noted with the use of aprepitant. Svanberg and Birgegard[10] randomized 96 patients receiving multiday, high-dose chemotherapy before autologous transplant to aprepitant or placebo in combination with tropisetron and a glucocorticoid before and after chemotherapy. Emesis was significantly improved with the use of aprepitant, but no difference in the use of rescue medications or nausea was seen. No adverse events were noted with the use of aprepitant.

Pielichowski et al.[61] used aprepitant, palonosetron, and dexamethasone to prevent nausea and vomiting following BEAM chemotherapy before autologous transplant in patients with non-Hodgkin's or Hodgkin's lymphoma. Emesis was improved in the acute and delayed phases postchemotherapy compared to historical controls who received ondansetron or palonosetron plus dexamethasone alone.

One retrospective study and two prospective (phase II, III) studies, each with a small number of patients (25-40 patients), also demonstrated improvement in emesis with the addition of aprepitant to a 5-HT₃ receptor antagonist with or without a glucocorticoid in patients receiving autologous or allogeneic stem cell transplant.[64–66]

As a result of the studies cited above, the 2017 ASCO and the 2017 MASCC/ESMO Antiemetic Guidelines have recommended the use of a NK-1 receptor antagonist, a 5-HT₃ receptor antagonist, and dexamethasone as the preferred prophylaxis for patients receiving high-dose, multiday chemotherapy before autologous or allogeneic stem cell transplantation.[67,68] The studies discussed above have demonstrated that the addition of aprepitant to a 5-HT₃ receptor antagonist and dexamethasone results in improved control of emesis postchemotherapy, but not nausea. The control of nausea remains a significant problem, not only in multiday, high-dose chemotherapy but also in single-day HEC. Neither 5-HT₃ receptor antagonists nor aprepitant appear to be effective antinausea agents in the postchemotherapy period.[3,6,16]

Netupitant/NEPA

Netupitant is a NK-1 receptor antagonist approved by the FDA in 2014 as the second NK-1 for the prevention of CINV. In vitro and in vivo pharmacologic characterization demonstrated that netupitant inhibits substance P in NK-1 receptors but was inactive for NK-2

and NK-3 receptors. This was demonstrated with intrathecal injections in mice and intraperitoneally in both mice and gerbils. In all assays, aprepitant exhibited similar effects.[69]

Netupitant behaves as a brain penetrant, is orally active, and is a potent and selective NK-1 antagonist.[69,70] Rossi et al.[69] and Spinelli et al.[70] reported that positive emission tomography demonstrates that netupitant is a potent agent targeting NK-1 receptors. It has a high degree of occupancy (90%) for a long duration (96 hours) when given as a single oral dose and appears to be safe.[69–71] Netupitant has a high binding affinity and a long half-life of 90 hours compared to a 9- to 13-hour half-life of aprepitant.[8,9,69–71] It is metabolized by CYP3A4 and is a moderate inhibitor of CYP3A4.[9,69–71] Due to netupitant's interaction with CYP3A4, it potentially could increase the concentration of docetaxel when administered simultaneously. However, netupitant would be expected to have similar interactions as aprepitant, which has been shown not to cause any clinically significant alterations in the pharmacokinetics of docetaxel or of its toxicity (adverse events and neutropenia) compared with administration of docetaxel alone in cancer patients.[59]

NEPA is an oral fixed-dose combination of netupitant and palonosetron that has been employed in phase II and phase III clinical trials for the prevention of CINV in patients receiving the chemotherapy combination of an anthracycline and cyclophosphamide and HEC.[9,72–74] Clinical trials demonstrated that NEPA (300 mg of netupitant plus 0.50 mg of palonosetron) plus dexamethasone significantly improved the prevention of CINV compared to the use of palonosetron and dexamethasone alone in patients receiving either HEC[72] or a combination of an anthracycline and cyclophosphamide.[73] The significant improvement in the delayed period (24 to 120 hours) and the overall period (0 to 120 hours) postchemotherapy was maintained over multiple cycles of chemotherapy.[74] Adverse events (hiccups, headache, constipation) were few in number (<3.5%) and were mild to moderate in severity.[9,72–74] No cardiac adverse events were noted. On October 10, 2014, NEPA (Akynzeo) was approved by the U.S. FDA to treat nausea and vomiting in patients undergoing cancer chemotherapy.[75]

Rolapitant

Rolapitant is a high-affinity, highly selective NK-1 receptor antagonist.[63] It penetrates the central nervous system following oral administration and has a high affinity for the human NK-1 receptor. It is highly selective for the NK-1 receptor over the human NK-2 and NK-3 receptor subtypes. It is a competitive antagonist and reversed NK-1 agonist-induced foot tapping in a gerbil animal model following both intravenous and oral administration.[76] Rolapitant reverses both apomorphine- and cisplatin-induced emesis in ferrets.[76]

The pharmacokinetics of rolapitant demonstrates that it has a long half-life (approximately 180 hours) with high affinity ($K_i = 0.66$ nM) for the NK-1 receptor,[76,77] and it does not induce or inhibit CYP3A4. Poma et al.[77] reported that rolapitant and its major metabolite SCH720 881 do not affect the pharmacokinetics of midazolam, a sensitive CYP3A4 substrate. Administration of rolapitant, unlike other NK-1 receptor antagonists such as aprepitant and netupitant, does not require dose adjustment of concomitantly administered drugs metabolized by CYP34A. Rolapitant is a moderate CYP2D6 inhibitor suggesting potential interactions with metoprolol or venlafaxine.

A phase I clinical trial in 14 healthy volunteers demonstrated that a 180-mg rolapitant dose provided ≥90% NK-1 receptor occupancy in the brain for up to 5 days following a single dose.[10,78] A phase II randomized, double-blind, active-controlled dose-finding study showed that a 180-mg dose of rolapitant plus granisetron and dexamethasone was safe and effective in the prevention of CINV in patients receiving HEC.[10,79] Complete response was significantly improved with rolapitant compared to placebo with all patients receiving ondansetron and dexamethasone.

The 180-mg dose of rolapitant was used in three large phase III clinical trials demonstrating that rolapitant, granisetron, and dexamethasone significantly improved complete response compared to granisetron and dexamethasone alone in patients receiving MEC and HEC.[10,80,81] Approximately 80% of the patients in the MEC study[80] received a combination of an anthracycline and cyclophosphamide chemotherapy or carboplatin chemotherapy. No serious adverse events were noted in the clinical trials, and no differences in the number of adverse events were seen in the rolapitant or control arms. On September 2, 2015, the U.S. FDA approved rolapitant (Varubi) for the prevention of nausea and vomiting associated with cancer chemotherapy.

Safety and Tolerability of Neurokinin-1 Receptor Antagonists

A 10-year review of the safety and efficacy of aprepitant and fosaprepitant[8] demonstrated that these agents are safe and no specific adverse events are associated with their use. In comparison studies, aprepitant-treated patients have had patterns and incidences of adverse events similar to those associated with standard control antiemetic therapy[8] (Table 32.12).

Rolapitant and netupitant have also demonstrated a low level of adverse events, not different from comparison control antiemetic therapy, in patients receiving either MEC or HEC[72,73,80,81] (Table 32.12). Headache, constipation, hiccups, and fatigue appear to be the most commonly reported events. Dos Santos et al.[82] reported a retrospective review of sixteen studies of the NK-1 receptor antagonists; the incidence of severe infection increased from 2% to 6% in the NK-1 receptor antagonist group in three RCTs with a total of 1,480 patients. The increased infection rate was not seen in the other thirteen studies and was not reported in a 10-year review of aprepitant[8] or in phase III clinical trials of netupitant[72,73] or rolapitant.[80,81] A meta-analysis by Zhang et al.[83] reported

that NK-1 receptor antagonist-based triple regimens were effective in the prevention of CINV with few significant toxicities.

Dexamethasone

Dexamethasone has been an effective antiemetic in controlling both acute and delayed CINV when combined with 5-HT$_3$ receptor antagonists and NK-1 receptor antagonists and is the main glucocorticoid used as an antiemetic.[19–21] Dexamethasone added to a 5-HT$_3$ receptor antagonist improves the control of acute CINV, and it has been used as a single agent or in combination with NK-1 receptor antagonists in an attempt to control delayed CINV.[19–21]

Concern has been expressed with the potential toxicity of the use of multiple-day dexamethasone to control CINV.[84] Patients receiving dexamethasone as prophylaxis for CINV reported moderate to severe problems with insomnia, hyperglycemia, indigestion, epigastric discomfort, agitation, increased appetite, weight gain, and acne.[84] Some studies have demonstrated that dexamethasone use might be decreased from multiple days to 1 day in an antiemetic regimen when used with other agents that are effective in controlling CINV in both the acute and the delayed periods.[13,21,85,86]

Celio et al.[85] used palonosetron in combination with 1 day versus 3 days of dexamethasone to prevent CINV in patients receiving MEC. No improvement in complete response or no nausea over the 5-day overall period was obtained with the use of 3 days of dexamethasone versus 1 day of dexamethasone. A similar study[86] using palonosetron plus dexamethasone for 1 day versus 3 days for breast cancer patients receiving an anthracycline and cyclophosphamide chemotherapy showed similar results: no improvement in complete response or in no nausea over the 5-day period with the use of 3 days versus 1 day of dexamethasone. Navari et al.[13,21] reported that 4 days of olanzapine with 1 day of a 5-HT$_3$ receptor antagonist and 1 day of dexamethasone was effective in the prevention of CINV in patients receiving HEC.

Olanzapine

Olanzapine is an atypical antipsychotic agent of the thienobenzodiazepine class and was approved by the FDA for the treatment of the manifestations of psychotic disorders in 1996[87,88] with a generic formulation becoming available in 2011. This drug blocks multiple neurotransmitter receptors including dopaminergic (D$_1$, D$_2$, D$_3$, D$_4$ brain receptors), serotonergic (5-HT$_{2a}$, 5-HT$_{2c}$, 5-HT$_3$, 5-HT$_6$ receptors), catecholaminergic (alpha$_1$-adrenergic receptors), cholinergic

TABLE

32.12   *Safety and tolerability of NK-1 receptor antagonists*

Agent	Chemotherapy	No. of Patients	Adverse Events	Reference
Rolapitant	HEC	1070	Dyspepsia, headache Constipation, hiccups (not different from control)	83
	MEC	1344	Constipation, fatigue Headache, fatigue (not different from control)	82
Netupitant	HEC	694	Hiccups, headache (not different from control)	74
	MEC	1455	Headache, constipation (not different from control)	75
Aprepitant	HEC	521	Asthenia, fatigue (not different from control)	8

(muscarinic receptors), and histaminergic (H_1 receptors).[89] Olanzapine has five times the affinity for 5-HT_2 receptors than for D_2 receptors.[90] The effect of olanzapine on the serotonin-mediated 5-HT_{2C} receptor as well as other dopamine and serotonin receptors may explain, in part, its efficacy in alleviating nausea and vomiting.

A benefit of olanzapine is that it is not a cytochrome P-450 inhibitor and thus appears to have fewer drug interactions than many other drugs.[89,90] Common side effects are sedation and weight gain.[90] The sedation is short term and may be dose-dependent.[91] The weight gain can occur after higher doses given over a period of months and can lead to diabetes mellitus when given for a period of greater than 6 months.[92]

Phase III clinical trials have demonstrated the effectiveness of olanzapine in the prevention of CINV.[12–14,93] Olanzapine improved the control of nausea and emesis when added to azasetron and dexamethasone compared to azasetron and dexamethasone alone in patients receiving MEC and HEC.[12] Olanzapine, palonosetron, and dexamethasone improved the control of nausea compared to aprepitant, palonosetron, and dexamethasone in patients receiving HEC.[13] This antiemetic regimen has been recommended by the NCCN guidelines as an option for the prevention of CINV in patients receiving HEC.[21]

The National Cancer Institute recently approved a multi-institutional phase III clinical trial (Alliance A221301) for the prevention of CINV in patients receiving HEC using olanzapine plus standard antiemetics compared to placebo plus standard antiemetics.[14] This randomized, double-blind, phase III trial was performed in chemotherapy-naïve patients receiving cisplatin, greater than 70 mg/m^2, or cyclophosphamide-anthracycline-based chemotherapy, comparing olanzapine to placebo in combination with aprepitant, a 5-HT_3 receptor antagonist (5-HT_3), and dexamethasone. The olanzapine regimen was 10 mg of oral olanzapine, 125 mg of oral aprepitant, a 5-HT_3, and oral dexamethasone of 12 mg prechemotherapy on day 1, 10 mg/d of oral olanzapine on days 2 to 4 postchemotherapy, 80 mg of oral aprepitant on days 2 to 3 postchemotherapy, and 8 mg of oral dexamethasone on days 2 to 4 postchemotherapy. The placebo regimen was oral placebo, on day 1, and oral placebo on days 2 to 4 postchemotherapy, with the aprepitant, 5-HT_3, and dexamethasone pre and postchemotherapy being the same as in the olanzapine regimen. Fosaprepitant (150 mg IV), on day 1, could be substituted for the oral aprepitant. Palonosetron, ondansetron, and granisetron were the permitted 5-HT_3 options. Nausea was measured on a 0 to 10 VAS, with 0 being no nausea at all and 10 being nausea as bad as it can be. Four hundred one patients were enrolled with 380 patients evaluable (192 patients receiving the olanzapine regimen and 188 patients receiving the placebo regimen). The proportion of patients with no nausea was significantly improved for the olanzapine regimen compared to the placebo regimen for the acute period (24 hours postchemotherapy) (74% versus 45%, $P = 0.002$), for the delayed period (25 to 120 hours postchemotherapy) (42% versus 25%, $P = 0.002$), and for the overall period (0 to 120 hours) (37% versus 22%, $P = 0.002$). Complete response (no emesis, no rescue medications) was significantly improved on olanzapine compared to placebo patients for the acute (86% versus 65%, $P < 0.001$), the delayed (67% versus 52%, $P = 0.007$), and the overall periods (64% versus 41%, $P < 0.001$). No grade 3 or 4 toxicities were encountered. No nausea, the primary endpoint,

and complete response, a secondary endpoint, were significantly improved with olanzapine compared to placebo.[14]

Olanzapine has been compared to metoclopramide for the treatment of breakthrough emesis and nausea in patients receiving HEC and guideline-directed antiemetic prophylaxis. Olanzapine was significantly better than metoclopramide for the treatment of breakthrough emesis and nausea.[47]

Based on the studies discussed, olanzapine has been recommended for use for the prevention of CINV and for the treatment of breakthrough CINV by both the NCCN Antiemetic Guidelines[21] and the new ASCO Antiemetic Guidelines.[68]

Gabapentin

Gabapentin is a gamma-aminobutyric acid (GABA) analogue that has been used for the treatment of seizures, chronic neuropathic pain, and postherpetic neuralgia.[94] The mechanism of action of gabapentin is unknown. Gabapentin does not interact with GABA receptors, is not converted metabolically into GABA or a GABA agonist, and is not an inhibitor of GABA uptake or degradation.[94]

Guttuso et al[95] reported an improvement in CINV in six of nine breast cancer patients when gabapentin was used to prevent nausea. Cruz et al.[96] added gabapentin to ondansetron, dexamethasone, and ranitidine to prevent CINV in patients receiving HEC. The complete response was significantly improved in the patients receiving gabapentin, but nausea was not significantly improved (no nausea, overall: 62% versus 45%). A phase III double-blind, placebo-controlled study of gabapentin for the prevention of CINV in patients receiving HEC has been reported. All patients received a 5-HT_3 receptor antagonist and dexamethasone before chemotherapy and dexamethasone postchemotherapy. Patients were randomized to 5 days of gabapentin or placebo starting with the day of chemotherapy. Gabapentin did not significantly improve delayed CINV.[97]

Cannabinoids

Studies in animal models have suggested that delta-9-tetrahydrocannabinoid (dronabinol) selectively acts on CB1 receptors in specific regions of the dorsal vagal complex to inhibit emesis.[98,99] A few reported studies have explored this mechanism in patients.[100,101] Meiri et al.[100] looked at the efficacy of dronabinol versus ondansetron in patients receiving chemotherapy for a wide variety of neoplasms. Dronabinol and ondansetron were similarly effective antiemetic treatments in 61 patients receiving MEC and HEC.

Nabilone is a synthetic cannabinoid, a racemic mixture of isomers, that mimics the main ingredient of cannabis (dronabinol). A review of the published English literature on the use of oral nabilone in the treatment of CINV concluded that cannabinoids do not add to the benefits of the 5-HT_3 receptor antagonists.[101]

At this time, insufficient data support the routine use of dronabinol or nabilone[101,102] as preventative antiemetics in all chemotherapeutic regimens. Limited data suggest that dronabinol may be effective for some patients in the breakthrough CINV setting.[102]

Ginger

Ginger is an herbal supplement that has been used for reducing the severity of motion sickness, pregnancy-induced nausea, and postoperative nausea and vomiting.[103] The mechanism of action by which ginger might exert antiemetic effects is unclear. Animal studies have described enhanced GI transport, anti–5-HT activity, and possible central nervous system antiemetic effects. Human experiments to determine the mechanism of action show varying results regarding gastric motility and corpus motor response.[103]

Pillai et al.[104] added ginger to ondansetron and dexamethasone in children and young adults receiving HEC and reported a reduction in the severity of acute and delayed CINV, but all patients had some nausea in days 1 to 4 postchemotherapy. Zick et al.[105] reported that ginger provided no additional benefit for reduction of the prevalence or severity of acute or delayed CINV when given with 5-HT$_3$ receptor antagonists and/or aprepitant in 162 cancer patients receiving chemotherapy. Ryan et al.[106] gave ginger before and after chemotherapy to 644 patients receiving a wide variety of chemotherapy regimens and found a reduction in nausea during the first day of chemotherapy.

At present, the available studies do not support recommending ginger as an agent for CINV prevention; ongoing studies aim to determine if there is a role for ginger.[107]

Clinical Management of CINV

Principles in the Management of CINV

International antiemetic guidelines[19–21,68] form the basis for the recommendations for the management of CINV. As new information emerges, these guidelines will evolve to provide the highest-quality evidence-based clinical practice.

Single-Day Chemotherapy (Table 32.13)

For patients receiving HEC, current evidence suggests the following[19–21,68]:

■ Prechemotherapy—olanzapine with any of the 5-HT$_3$ receptor antagonists, plus an NK-1 plus dexamethasone. The guidelines suggest that the combination of cyclophosphamide and doxorubicin should be considered as HEC and the appropriate preventative agents should be used.
■ Postchemotherapy—olanzapine with or without dexamethasone or dexamethasone alone.

For patients receiving MEC, current evidence suggests the following.[19–21,68]

■ Prechemotherapy—the 5-HT$_3$ receptor antagonist palonosetron plus dexamethasone. If palonosetron is not available, ondansetron or granisetron may be employed.
■ Postchemotherapy—dexamethasone on days 2 to 4.

Antiemetic guidelines of the past have included the available oral first-generation 5-HT$_3$ receptor antagonists as optional therapy for the prevention of delayed emesis, but the level of evidence supporting this practice is low.[33,34] The first-generation 5-HT$_3$ receptor antagonists are no longer recommended for use postchemotherapy.[19–21,68]

For patients receiving low emetogenic chemotherapy, a single agent in the form of a 5-HT$_3$ receptor antagonist, dexamethasone, or a phenothiazine, depending on the clinical situation, should be used prechemotherapy, and an antiemetic following chemotherapy should be given only as needed.

Treatment of Breakthrough CINV

Phenothiazine, metoclopramide, dexamethasone, or olanzapine may be effective in the treatment of breakthrough nausea and vomiting.[21] A 5-HT$_3$ receptor antagonist may also be effective unless a patient presents with nausea and vomiting that developed following the use of a 5-HT$_3$ receptor antagonist as prophylaxis for chemotherapy or radiotherapy-induced emesis. It is very unlikely that breakthrough nausea and vomiting will respond to an agent in the same drug class after unsuccessful prophylaxis with an agent of that same class.

Patients who develop nausea or vomiting postchemotherapy (days 1 to 5) despite adequate prophylaxis should be considered for treatment with a regimen of 3 days of oral or sublingual olanzapine or oral metoclopramide. A phase III study demonstrated that oral olanzapine (10 mg/d for 3 days) was significantly better than oral metoclopramide (10 mg three times daily for 3 days) in controlling both emesis and nausea in patients receiving HEC who developed breakthrough CINV despite guideline-directed prophylactic antiemetics.[47] Aprepitant has been approved as an additive agent to a 5-HT$_3$ receptor antagonist and dexamethasone for the prevention of CINV. It has not been studied and should not be used to treat breakthrough nausea and vomiting.

Refractory CINV

Patients who develop CINV during subsequent cycles of chemotherapy when antiemetic prophylaxis has not been successful in controlling CINV in earlier cycles should be considered for a change in the prophylactic antiemetic regimen. If anxiety is considered to be a major patient factor in the CINV, a benzodiazepine such as lorazepam or alprazolam can be added to the prophylactic regimen. If the patient is receiving HEC, olanzapine (days 1 to 4) can be substituted for aprepitant or fosaprepitant in the prophylactic antiemetic regimen.[13,21] If the patient is receiving MEC, an NK-1 receptor antagonist can be added to the palonosetron and dexamethasone antiemetic regimen.[21]

Anticipatory CINV

In order to prevent the occurrence of anticipatory CINV, patients should be counseled before the initial course of treatment concerning their "expectations" of CINV. Patients should be informed that very effective prophylactic antiemetic regimens will be used and that 70% to 75% of patients will have a complete response (no emesis, no use of rescue medications). The most effective prophylactic antiemetic regimen for the patient's specific type of chemotherapy should be used before the first course of chemotherapy in order to obtain the optimum control of CINV during the first course of chemotherapy. If CINV is effectively controlled during the first cycle, it is likely that the patient will have effective control during subsequent cycles of the same chemotherapy. If the patient has a poor experience with CINV in the first cycle, it may be more difficult to control CINV in subsequent cycles, and refractory and/or anticipatory CINV may occur. The use of antianxiety medications such as lorazepam or another benzodiazepine may be considered for excess anxiety before the first course of chemotherapy in order to obtain an optimal outcome and prevent anticipatory CINV. If anticipatory CINV occurs despite the use of prophylactic antiemetics, behavioral therapy might be considered.[108,109]

TABLE

32.13 | *Summary of International Antiemetic Guidelines*

Guidelines for High Emetic Risk[a]

	Acute CINV	Delayed CINV (D 2-4)
NCCN	5-HT$_3$ RA + Dex + NK-1 RA[b]	Dex ± Aprepitant
	Netupitant/Palonosetron (300 /0.5 mg)+ Dex	Dex
	Olanzapine + Palonosetron + Dex	Olanzapine
	5-HT$_3$ PA + Aprepitant + Dex + Olanzapine	Olanzapine + Dex ± Aprepitant
ASCO	Olanzapine + 5-HT$_3$ RA + Dex + NK-1 RA	Olanzapine + Dex ± Aprepitant
MASCC	5-HT$_3$ RA + Dex + NK-1 RA	Dex ± Aprepitant

Guidelines for Moderate Emetic Risk[c]

	Acute CINV	Delayed CINV (D 2-3)
NCCN	5-HT$_3$ RA (Palonosetron or granisetron SQ preferred) + Dex (category 1) ± NK-1 RA	Dex ± Aprepitant
	Netupitant/Palonosetron (300 /0.5 mg) + Dex	Dex
	Olanzapine + Palonosetron + Dex	Olanzapine
ASCO	5-HT$_3$ RA (palonosetron preferred) + Dex	Dex
MASCC	Palonosetron + Dex	Dex

Guidelines for Low and Minimal Emetic Risk[d]

	Low Emetic Risk	Minimal Emetic Risk
NCCN	5-HT$_3$ RA OR Dex OR Metoclopramide OR Prochlorperazine	No routine prophylaxis
ASCO	Dex	No routine prophylaxis
MASCC	5-HT$_3$ RA OR Dex OR Dopamine RA	No routine prophylaxis

Dex, dexamethasone; SQ, subcutaneous.

[a]Examples include cisplatin in combination with cyclophosphamide for the treatment of metastatic ovarian cancer and the combination of doxorubicin and cyclophosphamide for the treatment of metastatic breast cancer. Recommendations for HEC are similar across guidelines.[19,21,68]

[b]Aprepitant or fosaprepitant.

[c]Examples include irinotecan in combination with 5-fluorouracil/leucovorin for the treatment of metastatic colorectal cancer and oxaliplatin in combination with 5-fluorouracil/leucovorin for the treatment of advanced colorectal cancer. For acute CINV, the base recommendation is 2-drug regimens. Final treatment decisions are based on patient factors and physician's choice. For delayed CINV, there is slightly more variation (NCCN, 2017; Basch et al, 2011; Roila et al, 2016).

[d]Examples include docetaxel for the treatment of non-small cell lung cancer after platinum therapy failure and gemcitabine for the treatment of pancreatic cancer. References.[19–21,68]

Multiday Chemotherapy and High-Dose Chemotherapy with Stem Cell or Bone Marrow Transplantation

The success of the use of NK-1 receptor antagonists with 5-HT₃ receptor antagonists and dexamethasone in preventing emesis in patients receiving single-day HEC[3,6] prompted the use of the NK-1 receptor antagonist aprepitant combined with a 5-HT₃ receptor antagonist and dexamethasone in patients receiving multiday, high-dose chemotherapy before hematopoietic stem cell transplant. A number of phase II and III studies has been reported with the use of the NK-1 aprepitant added to a 5-HT₃ receptor antagonists and dexamethasone[60–66] in patients receiving multiday, high-dose chemotherapy before transplant. The 2017 ASCO and the 2017 MASCC/ESMO Antiemetic Guidelines have recommended the use of a NK-1 receptor antagonist, a 5-HT3 receptor antagonist, and dexamethasone as the preferred prophylaxis for patients receiving high-dose, multiday chemotherapy before transplant.[67,68] The addition of aprepitant to a 5-HT₃ receptor antagonist and dexamethasone resulted in improved control of emesis postchemotherapy, but not nausea. The control of nausea remains a significant problem, not only in multiday, high-dose chemotherapy but also in single-day HEC. Neither 5-HT₃ receptor antagonists nor aprepitant appear to be effective antinausea agents in the postchemotherapy period.[3,6,16]

Prevention and Treatment of Nausea

Multiple large studies suggest that the first- or second-generation 5-HT₃ receptor antagonists and the NK-1 receptor antagonists have not been effective in the control of nausea in patients receiving either MEC or HEC, despite the marked improvement in the control of emesis with these agents.[16–18] Neither the serotonin nor the substance P receptors may be important in mediating nausea. Phase III studies with olanzapine have demonstrated very good control of both emesis and nausea in patients receiving either MEC or HEC.[12–14] Preliminary small studies with gabapentin, cannabinoids, and ginger are inconclusive in defining their role, if any, in the prevention of CINV. At this time, olanzapine appears to have high potential for the prevention of both emesis and nausea in patients receiving MEC or HEC.[12–14] If patients are having difficulty with significant nausea, consideration should be given in including olanzapine in their prophylactic antiemetic regimen.[12–14] Olanzapine may also be efficacious in the treatment of breakthrough nausea.[47]

References

1. Bloechl-Daum B, Deuson RR, Mavros P, et al. Delayed nausea and vomiting continue to reduce patients' quality of life after highly and moderately emetogenic chemotherapy despite antiemetic treatment. *J Clin Oncol.* 2006;24:4472-4478.
2. Cohen L, de Moor CA, Eisenberg P, et al. Chemotherapy-induced nausea and vomiting: incidence and impact on patient quality of life at community oncology settings. *Support Care Cancer.* 2007;15:497-503.
3. Navari RM, Aapro M. Antiemetic prophylaxis for chemotherapy-induced nausea and vomiting. *N Engl J Med.* 2016;374:1356-1367.
4. Grunberg SM. Chemotherapy-induced nausea and vomiting: prevention, detection, and treatment—how are we doing? *J Support Oncol.* 2004;2(1 Suppl 1):1-10.
5. Broder MS, Faria C, Powers A, et al. The impact of 5HT3RA use on cost and utilization in patients with chemotherapy-induced nausea and vomiting: systematic review of the literature. *Am Health Drug Benefits.* 2014;7:171-182.
6. Navari RM. Management of chemotherapy-induced nausea and vomiting: focus on newer agents and new uses for older agents. *Drugs.* 2013;73:249-262.
7. Navari RM. Palonosetron for the treatment of chemotherapy-induced nausea and vomiting. *Expert Opin Pharmacother.* 2014;15:2599-2608.
8. Aapro M, Carides A, Rapoport BL. Aprepitant and fosaprepitant: a ten-year review of efficacy and safety. *Oncologist.* 2015;20:450-458.
9. Navari RM. Profile of netupitant/palonosetron fixed-dose combination (NEPA) and its potential in the treatment of chemotherapy-induced nausea and vomiting (CINV). *Drug Des Devel Ther.* 2015;9:155-161.
10. Navari RM. Rolapitant for the treatment of chemotherapy induced nausea and vomiting. *Expert Rev Anticancer Ther.* 2015;15:1127-1133.
11. Navari RM, Einhorn LH, Loehrer PJ, et al. A phase II trial of olanzapine, dexamethasone, and palonosetron for the prevention of chemotherapy-induced nausea and vomiting. *Support Care Cancer.* 2007;15:1285-1291.
12. Tan L, Liu J, Piu X, et al. Clinical research of olanzapine for the prevention of chemotherapy-induced nausea and vomiting. *J Exp Clin Cancer Res.* 2009;28:1-7.
13. Navari RM, Gray SE, Kerr AC. Olanzapine versus aprepitant for the prevention of chemotherapy-induced nausea and vomiting: a randomized phase III trial. *J Support Oncol.* 2011;9:188-195.
14. Navari RM, Qin R, Ruddy KJ, et al. Olanzapine for the prevention of chemotherapy-induced nausea and vomiting. *N Engl J Med.* 2016;375:134-142.
15. Mukhopadhyay S, Kwatra G, Alice KP, et al. Role of olanzapine in chemotherapy-induced nausea and vomiting on platinum-based chemotherapy patients: a randomized controlled study. *Support Care Cancer.* 2017;25:145-154.
16. Navari RM. Treatment of chemotherapy-induced nausea. *Community Oncol.* 2012;9:20-26.
17. Ng TL, Hutton B, Clemons M. Chemotherapy-induced nausea and vomiting: time for more emphasis on nausea? *Oncologist.* 2015;20:576-583.
18. Stern RM, Koch KL, Andrews PLR, eds. *Nausea: Mechanisms and Management.* New York: Oxford University Press; 2011.
19. Molassiotis A, Aapro M, Herrstedt J, et al. MASCC/ESMO Antiemetic Guidelines: Introduction to the 2016 guideline update. *Support Care Cancer.* 2017;25:267-269.
20. Hesketh PJ, Bohlke K, Lyman GH, et al. Antiemetics: American society of clinical oncology focused guideline update. *J Clin Oncol.* 2016;34:381-386.
21. NCCN Clinical Practice Guidelines in Oncology version 1 2017. *Antiemesis. National Comprehensive Cancer Network (NCCN)* [online]. Available at http://www.nccn.org/professionals/physician_gls/PDF/antiemesis.pdf. Accessed June, 2017.
22. Koga T, Fukuda H. Neurons in the nucleus of the solitary tract mediating inputs from vagal afferents and the area postrema in the pattern generator in the emetic act in dogs. *Neurosci Res.* 1992;14:366-379.
23. Yates BJ, Grelot L, Kerman IA, et al. Organization of the vestibular inputs to nucleus tractus solitarius and adjacent structures in cat brain stem. *Am J Physiol.* 1994;267:R974-R983.
24. Simpson K, Spencer CM, McClellan KJ. Tropisetron: an update of its use in the prevention of chemotherapy-induced nausea and vomiting. *Drugs.* 2000;59:1297-1315.
25. Kimura E, Niimi E, Watanabe A, et al. Study on clinical effect of a continuous intravenous infusion of azasetron against nausea and vomiting induced by anticancer drugs including CDDP. *Gan To Kagaku Ryoho.* 1996;23:477-481.
26. Taguchi T, Tsukamoto F, Watanabe T, et al. Usefulness of ramosetron hydrochloride on nausea and vomiting in CMF or CEF therapy for breast cancer. *Gan To Kagaku Ryoho.* 1999;26:1163-1170.
27. Hesketh PJ. Comparative review of 5-HT₃ receptor antagonists in the treatment of acute chemotherapy-induced nausea and vomiting. *Cancer Invest.* 2000;18:163-173.
28. World Health Organization. Dolasetron mesylate and serious cardiovascular reactions. *WHO Drug Informat.* 2006;20:185.
29. U.S. Food and Drug Information. FDA drug safety communication: abnormal heart rhythms associated with use of anzemet (dolasetron mesylate) [online]. Available at http://www.fda.gov/Drugs.DrugSafety/usm237081.htm. Accessed June 15, 2017.
30. Ondansetron [online]. Available at www.drugs.com/fda/ondansetron. Accessed 15 June July 2017.
31. Mason JW, Moon TE, O'Boyle E, et al. A randomized, placebo-controlled, four-period cross-over definitive QT study of the effects of APF530 exposure, high-dose intravenous granisetron, and moxifloxacin on QT_C prolongation. *Cancer Manage Res.* 2014;6:183-189.

32. Roila F, Warr D, Clark-Snow R, et al. Delayed emesis: moderately emetogenic chemotherapy. *Support Care Cancer.* 2005;13:104-108.

33. Geling O, Eichler H. Should 5-Hydroxytryptamine-3 receptor antagonists be administered beyond 24 hours after chemotherapy to prevent delayed emesis? Systematic re-evaluation of clinical evidence and drug cost implications. *J Clin Oncol.* 2005;23:1289-1294.

34. Hickok JT, Roscoe JA, Morrow GR, et al. 5-HT₃ receptor antagonists versus prochlorperazine for control of delayed nausea caused by doxorubicin: a URCC CCOP randomized controlled trial. *Lancet Oncol.* 2005;6:765-772.

35. Saito M, Aogi K, Sekine I, et al. Palonosetron plus dexamethasone versus granisetron plus dexamethasone for the prevention of nausea and vomiting during chemotherapy: a double-blind, double dummy, randomized, comparative phase III trial. *Lancet Oncol.* 2009;10:115-124.

36. Warr DG, Hesketh PJ, Gralla RJ, et al. Efficacy and tolerability of aprepitant for the prevention of chemotherapy-induced nausea and vomiting in patients with breast cancer after moderately emetogenic chemotherapy. *J Clin Oncol.* 2005;23:2822-2830.

37. Boccia RV, Gordan LN, Clark G, et al. Efficacy and tolerability of transdermal granisetron for the control of chemotherapy-induced nausea and vomiting associated with moderately and highly emetogenic multi-day chemotherapy: a randomized, double-blind, phase III study. *Support Care Cancer.* 2011;19:1609-1617.

38. Raftopoulos H, Cooper C, O'Boyle E, et al. Comparison of an extended-release formulation of granisetron (APF530) versus palonosetron for the prevention of chemotherapy-induced nausea and vomiting associated with moderately or highly emetogenic chemotherapy: results of a prospective, randomized, double-blind, noninferiority phase III trial. *Support Care Cancer.* 2015;23:723-732.

39. Eisenberg P, MacKintosh FR, Ritch P, et al. Efficacy, safety, and pharmacokinetics of palonosetron in patients receiving highly emetogenic, cisplatin-based chemotherapy: a dose-ranging, clinical study. *Ann Oncol.* 2004;15:330-337.

40. Rojas C, Thomas AG, Alt J, et al. Palonosetron triggers 5-HT₃ receptor internalization and causes prolonged inhibition of receptor function. *J Pharmacol.* 2010;626:193-199; 41.

41. Botrel T, Clark O, Clark L, et al. Efficacy of palonosetron compared to other serotonin inhibitors (5-HT₃R) in preventing chemotherapy-induced nausea and vomiting (CINV) in patients receiving moderately or highly emetogenic treatment: systematic review and meta-analysis. *Support Care Cancer.* 2011;19:823-832.

42. Schwartzberg L, Barbour SY, Morrow GR, et al. Pooled analysis of phase III studies of palonosetron versus ondansetron, dolasetron, and granisetron in the prevention of chemotherapy-induced nausea and vomiting. *Support Care Cancer.* 2014;22:469-477.

43. Popovic M, Warr DG, DeAngelis C, et al. Efficacy and safety of palonosetron for the prophylaxis of chemotherapy-induced nausea and vomiting (CINV): a systematic review and meta-analysis of randomized controlled trials. *Support Care Cancer.* 2014;22:1485-1497.

44. Yavas C, Dogan U, Yavas G, et al. Acute effect of palonosetron electrocardiographic parameters in cancer patients; a prospective study. *Support Care Cancer.* 2012;20:2343-2347.

45. Aogi K, Sakai H, Yoshizawa H, et al. A phase III open-label study to assess safety and efficacy of palonosetron for preventing chemotherapy-induced nausea and vomiting (CINV) in repeated cycles of emetogenic chemotherapy. *Support Care Cancer.* 2012;20:1507-1514.

46. Roila F, Ballatori E, Ruggeri B, et al. Aprepitant versus metoclopramide, both combined with dexamethasone, for the preventing cisplatin-induced delayed emesis: a randomized, double- blind study. *J Clin Oncol.* 2014;32:5s (suppl; abstr 9503).

47. Navari RM, Nagy CK, Gray SE. Olanzapine versus metoclopramide for the treatment of breakthrough chemotherapy-induced nausea and vomiting in patients receiving highly emetogenic chemotherapy. *Support Care Cancer.* 2013;21:1655-1663.

48. European Medicine Agency Metoclopramide use recommendations. 26 July 2013. Available at www.ema.europa.eu. Accessed June 15, 2017.

49. Diemunsch P, Grelot L. Potential of substance P antagonists as antiemetics. *Drugs.* 2000;60:533-546.

50. Sankhala KK, Pandya DM, Sarantopoulos J, et al. Prevention of chemotherapy induced nausea and vomiting: a focus on aprepitant. *Expert Opin Drug Metab Toxicol.* 2009;12:1607-1614.

51. Hesketh PJ, Grunberg SM, Herrstedt J, et al. Combined data from two phase III trials of the NK-1 antagonist aprepitant plus a 5HT₃ antagonist and a corticosteroid for prevention of chemotherapy-induced nausea and vomiting: effect of gender on treatment response. *Support Care Cancer.* 2006;14:354-360.

52. Warr DG, Grunberg SM, Gralla RJ, et al. The oral NK1 antagonist aprepitant for the prevention of acute and delayed chemotherapy-induced nausea and vomiting: pooled data from two randomized, double-blind, placebo controlled trials. *Eur J Cancer.* 2005;41:1278-1285.

53. Grote T, Hajdenberg J, Cartnell A, et al. Combination therapy for chemotherapy-induced nausea and vomiting in patients receiving moderately emetogenic chemotherapy: palonosetron, dexamethasone, and aprepitant. *J Support Oncol.* 2006;4:403-408.

54. Navari RM. Fosaprepitant (MK-0517): a neurokinin-1 receptor antagonist for the prevention of chemotherapy-induced nausea and vomiting. *Expert Opin Investig Drugs.* 2007;16:1977-1985.

55. Grunberg S, Chua D, Maru A, et al. Single-dose fosaprepitant for the prevention of chemotherapy-induced nausea and vomiting associated with cisplatin therapy: randomized, double-blind study protocol—EASE. *J Clin Oncol.* 2011;29:1495-1501.

56. Leal AD, Kadakia KC, Looker S, et al. Fosaprepitant-induced phlebitis: a focus on patients receiving doxorubicin/cyclophosphamide therapy. *Support Care Cancer.* 2014;22:1313–1317.

57. Drug interactions of aprepitant [slide presentation]. Available at http://www.fda.gov/ohrms/dockets/ac/03/slides/3928s1_03_fda-jarugula.ppt. Accessed June 9, 2017.

58. Scientific discussion: This module reflects the initial scientific discussion for the approval of Emend. Available at http://www.ema.europa.eu/docs/en_GB/document_library/EPAR_Scientific_Discussion/human/000527/WC500026534.pdf. Accessed June 9, 2017.

59. Aapro MS, Walko CM. Aprepitant: drug-drug interactions in perspective. *Ann Oncol.* 2010;21:2316-2323.

60. Schmitt T, Goldschmitt H, Nieben K, et al. Aprepitant, granisetron, and dexamethasone for prevention of chemotherapy-induced nausea and vomiting after high-dose melphalan in autologous transplantation for multiple myeloma: results of a randomized, placebo-controlled phase III trial. *J Clin Oncol.* 2014;32:3413-3420.

61. Pielichowski W, Barzal J, Gawronski B et al. A triple-drug combination to prevent nausea and vomiting following BEAM chemotherapy before autologous hematopoietic stem cell transplantation. *Transplant Proc.* 2011;43:3107-3110.

62. Stiff PJ, Fox-Geiman MP, Kiley K, et al. Prevention of nausea and vomiting associated with stem cell transplant: Results of a prospective, randomized trial of aprepitant used with highly emetogenic preparative regimens. *Biol Blood Marrow Transplant.* 2013;19:49-55.

63. Svanberg A, Bergegard C. Addition of aprepitant to standard antiemetic regimen continued for seven days after chemotherapy for stem cell transplantation provide significant reduction of vomiting. *Oncology.* 2015;89:31-36.

64. Uchida M, Ikesue H, Miyamoto T, et al. Effectiveness and safety of antiemetic aprepitant in Japanese patients receiving high-dose chemotherapy prior to autologous hematopoietic stem cell transplantation. *Biol Pharm Bull.* 2013;36:819-824.

65. Sakuri M, Mori T, Kato J, et al. Efficacy of aprepitant in preventing nausea and vomiting due to high-dose melphalan–based conditioning for allogeneic hematopoietic stem cell transplantation. *Int J Hematol.* 2014;99:457-462.

66. Bechtel T, McBride A, Crawford B, et al. Aprepitant for the control of delayed nausea and vomiting associated with the use of high-dose melphalan for autologous peripheral blood stem cell transplants in patients with multiple myeloma: a phase II study. *Support Care Cancer.* 2014;22:2911-2916.

67. Einhorn LH, Rapoport B, Navari RM, et al. 2016 updated MASCC/ESMO consensus recommendations: prevention of nausea and vomiting following multiple-day chemotherapy, high dose chemotherapy, and breakthrough nausea and vomiting. *Support Care Cancer.* 2017;25:303-308.

68. Hesketh PJ, Kris MG, Basch E, et al. Antiemetics: American Society of Clinical Oncology Clinical Practice guideline update. *J Clin Oncol.* 2017;35:3240-3261.

69. Rizzi A, Campi B, Camarda V, et al. In vitro and in vivo pharmacological characterization of the novel NK-1 receptor selective antagonist Netupitant. *Peptides.* 2012;37:86-97.

70. Spinelli T, Calcagneli S, Giuliano C. Netupitant PET imaging and ADME studies in humans. *J Clin Pharmacol.* 2014;54:97-108.

71. National Cancer Institute Drug Dictionary. Available at https://www.cancer.gov/publications/dictionaries/cancer-drug. Accessed June 15, 2017.

72. Hesketh PJ, Rossi G, Rizzi G, et al. Efficacy and safety of NEPA, an oral combination of netupitant and palonosetron, for prevention of chemotherapy-induced nausea and vomiting following highly emetogenic chemotherapy: a randomized dose-ranging pivotal study. *Ann Oncol.* 2014;25:1340-1346.

73. Aapro M, Rugo H, Rossi G, et al. A randomized phase III study evaluating the efficacy and safety of NEPA, a fixed-dose combination of netupitant and palonosetron, for prevention of chemotherapy-induced nausea and vomiting following moderately emetogenic chemotherapy. *Ann Oncol.* 2014;25:1328-1333.

74. Gralla RJ, Bosnjak SM, Hontsa A, et al. A phase III study evaluating the safety and efficacy of NEPA, a fixed-dose combination of netupitant and palonosetron, for prevention of chemotherapy-induced nausea and vomiting over repeated cycles of chemotherapy. *Ann Oncol.* 2014;25:1333-1339.

75. FDA News Release, FDA approves Akynzeo for nausea and vomiting associated with cancer chemotherapy. Available at http://www.fda.gov/NewsEvents/Newsroom/PressAnnouncements. Accessed June 9, 2017.

76. Duffy RA, Morgan C, Naylor R, et al. Rolapitant (SCH 619734): a potent, selective and orally active neurokinin NK-1 receptor antagonist with centrally-mediated antiemetic effects in ferrets. *Pharmacol Biochem Behav.* 2012;102:95-100.

77. Poma A, Christensen J, Pertikis H, et al. Rolapitant and its major metabolite do not affect the pharmacokinetics of midazolam, a sensitive cytochrome P450 3A4 substrate. *Support Care Cancer.* 2013;21:S154. Abstract 441.

78. Poma A, Christensen J, Davis J, et al. Phase 1 positron emission tomography (PET) study of the receptor occupancy of rolapitant, a novel NK-1 receptor antagonist. *J Clin Oncol.* 2014;32, abstr e20690.

79. Rapoport B, Chua D, Poma A, et al. Study of rolapitant, a novel, long acting, NK-1 receptor antagonist, for the prevention of chemotherapy-induced nausea and vomiting (CINV) due to highly emetogenic chemotherapy (HEC). *Support Care Cancer.* 2015;23:3281-3288. doi:10.1007/s00520-015-2738-1.

80. Schwartzberg L, Modiano M, Rapoport B, et al. Safety and efficacy assessment of rolapitant for the prevention of chemotherapy-induced nausea and vomiting following administration of moderately emetogenic chemotherapy in cancer patients in a randomized phase 3 trial. *Lancet Oncol.* 2015;16:1071-1078.

81. Rapoport B, Chasen M, Gridelli C, et al. Safety and efficacy assessment of rolapitant for the prevention of chemotherapy-induced nausea and vomiting following administration of cisplatin-based highly emetogenic chemotherapy in cancer patients in two randomized phase 3 trials. *Lancet Oncol.* 2015;16:1079-1089.

82. dos Santos LV, Souza FH, Brunetto AT, et al. Neurokinin-1 receptor antagonists for chemotherapy-induced nausea and vomiting: a systematic review. *J Natl Cancer Inst.* 2012;104:1280-1292.

83. Zhang Y, Yang Y, Zhang Z, et al. Neurokinin-1 receptor antagonist-based triple regimens in preventing chemotherapy-induced nausea and vomiting: a network meta-analysis. *J Natl Cancer Inst.* 2017;109:1-11. doi:10.1093/jnci/djw217.

84. Vardy J, Chiew KS, Gallica J, et al. Side effects associated with the use of dexamethasone for prophylaxis of delayed emesis after moderately emetogenic chemotherapy. *Br J Cancer.* 1999;94:1011-1015.

85. Celio L, Frustaci S, Denaro A, et al. Palonosetron in combination with 1-day versus 3-day dexamethasone for prevention of nausea and vomiting following moderately emetogenic chemotherapy: a randomized, multi-center, phase III trial. *Support Care Cancer.* 2011;19:1217-1225.

86. Aapro M, Fabi A, Nole F, et al. Double-blind, randomized, controlled study of the efficacy and tolerability of palonosetron plus dexamethasone for 1 day with or without dexamethasone on days 2 and 3 in the prevention of nausea and vomiting induced by moderately emetogenic chemotherapy. *Ann Oncol.* 2010;21:1083-1088.

87. Fulton, B, Goa KL. Olanzapine: a review of its pharmacological properties and therapeutic efficacy in the management of schizophrenia and related psychoses. *Drugs.* 1999;53:281-298.

88. Kando, JC, Shepski JC, Satterlee W, et al. Olanzapine: a new antipsychotic agent with efficacy in the management of schizophrenia. *Ann Pharmacother.* 1997;31:1325-1334.

89. Bymaster FP, Calligaro D, Falcone J, et al. Radioreceptor binding profile of the atypical antipsychotic olanzapine. *Neuropsychopharmacology.* 1996;14:87-96.

90. Stephenson CM, Pilowsky LS. Psychopharmacology of olanzapine: a review. *Br J Psychiatry Suppl.* 1999;174:52-58.

91. Passik S, Navari RM, Loehrer PJ, et al. A phase I trial of olanzapine (Zyprexa) for the prevention of delayed emesis in cancer patients receiving chemotherapy. *Cancer Invest.* 2004;22:383-388.

92. Goldstein LE, Sporn J, Brown S, et al. New-onset diabetes mellitus and diabetic ketoacidosis associated with olanzapine treatment. *Psychosomatics.* 1999;40:438-443.

93. Mizukami N, Yamanchi M, Koike K, et al. Olanzapine for the prevention of chemotherapy-induced nausea and vomiting in patients receiving highly or moderately emetogenic chemotherapy: a randomized, double-blind placebo-controlled study. *J Pain Symptom Manage.* 2014;47:542-550.

94. Irving G, Jensen M, Cramer M, et al. Efficacy and tolerability of gastric-retentive gabapentin for the treatment of post-herpetic neuralgia: results of a double-blind, randomized, placebo-controlled clinical trial. *Clin J Pain.* 2009;25:185-192.

95. Guttuso T, Roscoe J, Griggs J. Effect of gabapentin on nausea induced by chemotherapy in patients with breast cancer. *Lancet.* 2003;361:1703-1705.

96. Cruz FM, de Iracema Gomes Cubero D, Taranto P. Gabapentin for the prevention of chemotherapy-induced nausea and vomiting: a pilot study. *Support Care Cancer.* 2011;20:601-606.

97. Barton DL, Thanarajasingam G, Sloan JA, et al. Phase III double-blind, placebo-controlled study of gabapentin for the prevention of delayed chemotherapy-induced nausea and vomiting in patients receiving highly emetogenic chemotherapy, NCCTG N08C3 (Alliance). *Cancer.* 2014;120:3575-3583.

98. Van Sickle MD, Duncan M, Kingsley PJ, et al. Identification and functional characterization of brainstem cannabinoid CB2 receptors. *Science.* 2005;310:329-332.

99. Darmani NA. Delta-9-tetrahydrocannabinol differentially suppresses cisplatin-induced emesis and indices of motor function via cannabinoid CB1 receptors in the least shrew. *Pharmacol Biochem Behav.* 2001;69:239-249.

100. Meiri E, Jhangiani H, Vredenburgh JJ, et al. Efficacy of dronabinol alone and in combination with ondansetron versus ondansetron alone for delayed chemotherapy-induced nausea and vomiting. *Curr Med Res Opin.* 2007;23:533-543.

101. Davis MP. Oral nabilone capsules in the treatment of chemotherapy-induced nausea and vomiting and pain. *Expert Opin Investig Drugs.* 2008;17:85-95.

102. May MB, Grode AE. Dronabinol for chemotherapy-induced nausea and vomiting unresponsive to antiemetics. *Cancer Manag Res.* 2016;8:49-55.

103. Mills S, Bone K, eds. *Principles and Practice of Phytotherapy*. Oxford: Churchill Livingstone; 2000.

104. Pillai AK, Sharma KK, Gupta YK, et al. Anti-emetic effect of ginger powder versus placebo as an add-on therapy in children and young adults receiving highly emetogenic chemotherapy. *Pediatr Blood Cancer.* 2011;56:234-238.

105. Zick SM, Ruffin MT, Normolle DP, et al. Phase II trial of encapsulated ginger as a treatment for chemotherapy-induced nausea and vomiting. *Support Care Cancer.* 2009;17:563-572.

106. Ryan JL, Heckler C, Roscoe JA, et al. Ginger reduces acute chemotherapy-induced nausea: a URCC CCOP study of 576 patients. *Support Care Cancer.* 2012;20:1479-1489.

107. Bossi P, Cortinovis D, Cossu MR, et al. Searching for evidence to support the use of ginger in the prevention of chemotherapy-induced nausea and vomiting. *J Altern Complement Med.* 2016;22:486-488.

108. Navari RM. Should behavioral therapy be used as the primary treatment to control Anticipatory vomiting? *HemeOnc Today.* 2016;17:13.

109. Navari RM. Cancer patients at high risk for chemotherapy-induced nausea and vomiting—prediction assessments/tools. *Expert Rev Quality Cancer Care.* 2017;2:103-108.

Hematopoietic Growth Factors

Gary H. Lyman and Nicole M. Kuderer

Introduction

The hematopoietic growth factors (HGFs) are an important class of biologic agents for the support of cancer patients receiving myelosuppressive chemotherapy by augmenting the production and functional maturation of hematopoietic cells for the purpose of reducing hematologic complications while enabling the safe delivery of effective treatment. Myelosuppression represents the most common dose-limiting complications of cancer chemotherapy and is associated with considerable morbidity, mortality, and costs. In addition to direct chemotherapy-associated complications such as neutropenia, anemia, and thrombocytopenia, myelosuppression often prompts chemotherapy dose reductions and delays, reducing delivered chemotherapy dose intensity potentially compromising disease control and long-term survival in patients with responsive and potentially curable malignancies.

Biology and Pharmacology of the Hematopoietic Growth Factors

Endogenous production of HGFs occurs in a wide variety of both hematopoietic and nonhematopoietic cells (Table 33.1). Figure 33.1 depicts the hematopoietic lineages derived from the myeloid stem cell and stimulated by the various HGFs. The hematopoietic stem cell gives rise to the early common myeloid progenitor which then leads to the megakaryocyte-erythroid (MK) progenitor which can then lead to either erythroid or megakaryocyte progenitors.

The Myeloid Growth Factors

The term colony-stimulating factor (CSF) reflects that certain glycoproteins support the formation of colonies of hematopoietic elements when bone marrow cells are cultured.[1,2] The genes encoding for G-CSF, GM-CSF, and interleukin-3 (IL-3) were cloned leading to the production of CSF using recombinant DNA technology.[3] The currently approved myeloid growth factors are recombinant human rhu G-CSF (filgrastim, lenograstim), rhu GM-CSF (sargramostim, molgramostim, regramostim), and pegylated rhu G-CSF (pegylated filgrastim). Table 33.2 summarizes some of the pharmacokinetic characteristics of the CSFs.

Granulocyte Colony-Stimulating Factor (G-CSF)

G-CSF is an 18.8-kDa glycoprotein with 174 amino acids encoded by a single gene on chromosome 17 (q21-22). G-CSF is produced endogenously by monocytes, macrophages, endothelial cells, fibroblasts, mesenchymal cells, and bone marrow stromal cells. G-CSF is usually absent or present in low concentration but is highly stimulated by inflammatory cytokines and bacterial cell wall products.[4,5] The G-CSF receptor is composed of 813 amino acids and is encoded by gene located on chromosome 1 (p32-34) and is expressed on mature neutrophils and their precursors. The receptor consists of both a cytokine-specific binding subunit and signal-transducing subunit. Cytokine binding of G-CSF to its receptor leads to dimerization bringing together signaling proteins associated with the cytoplasmic domains. The biologic action of the cytokine is orchestrated by the Janus kinase-signal transducers and activators of transcription (JAK-STAT) signaling pathway. Activated phosphorylated STAT proteins dissociate from the receptor and translocate to the nucleus where they activate transcription. Other important signaling pathways include ras-mitogen activated protein (MAP) kinases which are necessary for G-CSF–directed cellular proliferation.

G-CSF is necessary to sustain normal neutrophil production and to increase neutrophil numbers in response to stress. Endogenous G-CSF levels rise in neutropenic states and most dramatically with febrile neutropenia (FN). G-CSF acts on late myeloid progenitors leading to increase cell division and reduced transit time through the bone marrow to the peripheral blood and tissues. G-CSF also induces the differentiation and functional maturation of neutrophils increasing chemotaxis, phagocytosis, and antibody dependent cellular toxicity.[4,5] The CSFs are metabolized by binding to the receptor with subsequent internalization and by hepatic enzymes. Unpegylated CSFs are cleared by glomerular filtration and excreted in urine.

Pegylated G-CSF (Pegfilgrastim)

Pegfilgrastim is a recombinant G-CSF bioengineered by covalently binding a 20-kDa polyethylene glycol molecule to the N-terminus of filgrastim, increasing the total molecular weight from 18,800 daltons to 39,000 daltons.[6] The pegfilgrastim molecule is too large for renal clearance prolonging the half-life to approximately 33 hours while retaining the biological activity of filgrastim. Pegfilgrastim has saturable and self-regulating neutrophil-mediated elimination with neutrophil production stimulated when neutrophil counts are low and rapid clearance as neutrophil counts recover providing fresh receptors for binding (Figure 33.2). Similar concentration-time profiles of pegfilgrastim are observed in bilateral nephrectomised rats while filgrastim clearance is decreased by 60% to 70%.[7,8] The apparent neutrophil-dependent clearance of pegfilgrastim results in prolonged circulation and action during recovery from neutropenia. Like filgrastim, pegfilgrastim acts on hematopoietic cells by

TABLE

33.1 *Pharmaceutical characteristics of hematopoietic growth factors*

Cytokine	Other Names	Generic Names	Expression Vector	Brand Names	No. of Amino Acids	Human Chromosome Location	Normal Endogenous Sources
G-CSF	Granulocyte colony-stimulating factor	Filgrastim Lenograstim Tbo-filgrastim Filgrastim-sndz	*E. coli* *CHO* *E. coli* *E. coli*	Neupogen (Amgen) Granulocyte (Chugai) Granix Zarxio	174	17	Monocytes/macrophages, fibroblasts, endothelial cells, keratinocytes
GM-CSF	Granulocyte-macrophage colony-stimulating factor	Sargramostim Molgramostim Regramostim	Yeast *E. coli* CHO	Leukine (Immunex) Leucomax (Schering)	127	5	T-lymphocytes, monocytes/macrophages, fibroblasts, endothelial cells, osteoblasts, epithelial cells
EPO	Erythropoietin	Epoetin-α Epoetin-α Epoetin-β Darbepoetin-α	CHO CHO CHO CHO	Epogen (Amgen) Procrit/Eprex (Ortho) NeoRecormon (Roche) Aranesp (Amgen)	165	7	Renal cells, hepatocytes
IL-11	Interleukin-11	Oprelvekin	*E. coli*	Neumega (Genetics Institute)	178	19	Stromal fibroblasts, trophoblasts
TPO	Thrombopoietin, megakaryocyte growth and development factor	Romiplostim Eltrombopag		Nplate Promacta	332	3	Liver, kidney

CHO, Chinese hamster ovary cells; CSF, colony-stimulating factor.

binding to cell surface G-CSF receptors resulting in an increase in cell division, shorter marrow transit, increased differentiation, and end-cell functional activation of neutrophils.[9]

Granulocyte-Macrophage Colony-Stimulating Factor (GM-CSF)

Human GM-CSF, purified in 1984,[10] is a 14- to 35-kDa glycoprotein encoded by a gene located on chromosome 5 (q23-31) close to a cluster of hematopoietic regulatory genes.[10] GM-CSF is produced by monocytes, macrophages, fibroblasts, endothelial cells, and conditioned lymphocytes.[5] The GM-CSF receptor is expressed on neutrophils, monocytes, eosinophils, myeloid progenitors, myeloid leukemia cells, T lymphocytes, and dendritic cells. The GM-CSF receptor is composed of two subunits: an α subunit that is GM-CSF–specific encoded on chromosome X/Y and a β-subunit shared by other cytokines encoded on chromosome 22q31. Binding of GM-CSF to its receptor leads to downstream signaling mainly through the JAK and STAT pathways stimulating functional activity of neutrophils, macrophages, monocytes, and eosinophils.[5]

Recombinant GM-CSF is available as sargramostim (yeast-derived), and molgramostim (*Escherichia coli*–derived) is approved by the U.S. FDA for use in acute myeloid leukemia (AML), autologous and allogeneic stem cell transplantation (SCT), and for stem cell mobilization. GM-CSF augments the survival and proliferation of cells in the granulocytic and macrophage lineages as well as maintains megakaryocyte progenitors at high concentrations.[11] GM-CSF is a potent stimulator of dendritic cells, which are important initiators of primary immune responses.[12]

The Erythropoiesis-Stimulating Agents

The glycoprotein erythropoietin is the primary regulator of red cell production. The erythropoiesis-stimulating agents (ESAs) available in the United States include epoetin alfa and the hyperglycosylated recombinant erythropoietin, darbepoetin alfa.[13] Darbepoetin results from mutagenesis of the gene encoding ESA adding two N-glycosylation sites yielding a 23% increase in molecular weight and a three-fold increase in circulation time through protection from metabolic degradation.[13,14] The therapeutic effects of the ESAs

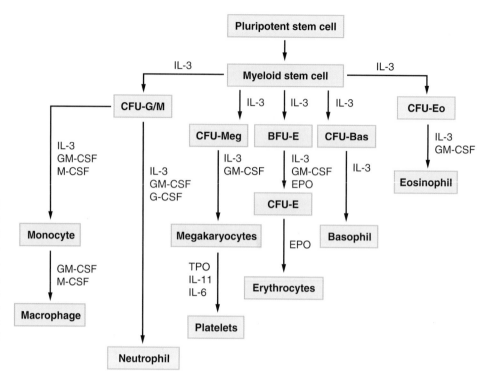

FIGURE **33.1** Representation of myeloid hematopoietic differentiation. Cytokines capable of stimulating specific cells are listed below such cells. BFU-E, burst-forming unit, erythroid; CFU-GEMM, colony-forming unit–granulocyte-erythrocyte-megakaryocyte macrophage; CFU-GM, colony-forming unit–granulocyte-macrophage; EPO, erythropoietin; G-CSF, granulocyte colony-stimulating factor; GM-CSF, granulocyte-macrophage colony-stimulating factor; IL, interleukin; M-CSF, macrophage colony-stimulating factor; SCF, stem cell factor; TPO, thrombopoietin.

include induction, proliferation, and differentiation of erythroid progenitors and may also play a role in the stimulation of early multipotent progenitors.

Erythropoietin (EPO) is primarily produced in the peritubular interstitial cells and regulated by an oxygen sensor. Inappropriately low as well as high EPO concentrations have been reported following chemotherapy due in part to paradoxical elevations of endogenous EPO concentrations immediately following chemotherapy.[15,16] Since the efficacy of EPO is dependent on adequate iron stores, treatment with intravenous iron may further improve the hemoglobin response in cancer patients treated with recombinant EPO.[17]

TABLE
33.2 *Pharmacokinetic studies of hematopoietic growth factors*

CSF	Route	N	Half-life (h)	T_{max} (h)	CI (mL/min/kg)
G-CSF	SQ	37	2.5 to 5.8	4 to 8	19 to 56
Peg G-CSF	SQ	10	27 to 47	72 to 120	0.04 to 0.68
G-CSF	IV	58	(α 8[a], β 1.8) 1.3 to 5.1	NA	4 to 21
GM-CSF	SQ	55	1.6 to 5.8	2.7 to 20	249 to 312
GM-CSF	IV	63	(α 5 to 20[a], β 1.1 to 2.5) 1.1 to 2.4	NA	9.9 to 178
EPO	SQ	125	9 to 38	12 to 28	N/A
EPO	IV	135	4 to 11.2	NA	2.8 to 6.7
DARBO	SQ	14	33 to 49	54 to 86	0.062
DARBO	IV	28	18 to 25	NA	0.027 to 0.033
ELTROMOPAG	PO	73	9 to 12	NA	NA
ROMIPLASTIM	SQ	4	56	24	N/A
IL-11	SQ	18	6.9	3.2	NA[b]

[a]Values are in minutes.
[b]Clearance of IL-11 in infants and children is 1.2-fold to 1.6-fold higher than in adults or adolescents.
CI, systemic clearance (values are "apparent" for SQ route); CSF, colony-stimulating factor; DARBO, darbepoetin alpha; EPO, erythropoietin; G-CSF, granulocyte colony-stimulating factor; GM-CSF, granulocyte macrophage colony-stimulating factor; IL, interleukin; N, number of patients; NA, not applicable; Peg, pegylated; T_{max}, time of maximal concentration after SQ injection.
Data presented are ranges of mean values in the reviewed studies.

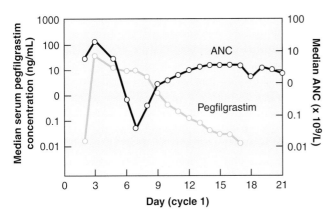

FIGURE **33.2** Pegfilgrastim serum concentrations and absolute neutrophil count (ANC) in patients with breast cancer who received pegfilgrastim as an adjunct to chemotherapy. (Adapted from Green MD, Koelbl H, Baselga J, et al. A randomized double-blind multicenter phase III study of fixed-dose single-administration pegfilgrastim versus daily filgrastim in patients receiving myelosuppressive chemotherapy. *Ann Oncol.* 2003;14(1):29-35. Reproduced by permission of Oxford University Press.)

The Thrombopoietic Agents

As noted above, the megakaryocyte-erythroid (MK) progenitor can lead to either erythroid or megakaryocyte progenitors. Stem cell factor (SCF) or c-Kit ligand and IL-3 act at early stages and stimulate proliferation and differentiation of progenitor cells into the MK lineage. Thrombopoietin (TPO) has broad activity, stimulating growth and maturation of MK progenitor cells into mature megakaryocytes. In a normal state, 10^{11} platelets are produced daily, with platelets lasting about 8 to 9 days in the circulation.[18,19]

TPO was initially identified in 1994 as the primary regulator of thrombopoiesis while also stimulating platelet adhesion and aggregation.[20] TPO is a 332 amino acid glycoprotein with an amino domain essential for thrombopoietic activity and a carboxy domain which increases the half-life. TPO is produced primarily in the liver, and its effects are mediated through the TPO receptor (c-Mpl) on megakaryocytes and platelets. TPO levels are regulated by the number of receptors available for binding[21] with unbound TPO primarily regulating megakaryocytopoiesis. TPO levels are increased in cases of thrombocytopenia due to decreased production while levels are not sufficiently elevated with increased destruction such as in immune thrombocytopenic purpura (ITP) likely due to high turnover of TPO with the platelets and their c-Mpl receptors.[21,22] Recombinant human TPO is identical to endogenous TPO and increases platelet counts in a dose-dependent fashion.[23] No neutralizing antibodies have been found, and serial bone marrow biopsies from patients treated with TPO demonstrated hypercellularity, megakaryocytic hyperplasia, and reticulin fibrosis which resolved within three months after rhTPO was stopped.[20] Pegylated recombinant human megakaryocyte growth and development factor (PEG-rHuMGDF) consists of the receptor binding domain of TPO bound to a polyethylene glycol moiety. Although early trials demonstrated improvement in the time to platelet recovery and need for platelet transfusions in patients undergoing cancer chemotherapy, thrombocytopenia associated with cross-reacting antibody formation were observed in patients receiving PEG-rHuMGDF.[24] Therefore, alternative TPO agonists have been sought lacking any sequence homology with endogenous TPO.

The peptide mimetic, romiplostim, is a recombinant fusion protein with two identical subunits consisting of a peptide with two TPO-binding domains covalently bound to the Fc domain of a human IgG molecule.[25] It was the first TPO receptor agonist to receive FDA approval for treatment of thrombocytopenia in patients with chronic immune thrombocytopenic purpura (ITP) poorly responsive to corticosteroids, immunoglobulins, or splenectomy. The rationale for TPO agonists in ITP relates to the inappropriately normal or low TPO levels in most patients with immune destruction of platelet precursors.[26] Eltrombopag is a small molecule selective nonpeptide agonist of the TPO receptor that stimulates receptor phosphorylation and activation of cytoplasmic tyrosine kinases and signal transducers of transcription (STAT transcription factors). Eltrombopag promotes proliferation and differentiation of marrow stem cells into committed megakaryocyte precursors in a dose-dependent fashion. Preclinical data demonstrated that this agent has good oral bioavailability with consistent increases in platelet counts following daily oral administration.[27]

IL-11 acts synergistically with early- and later-acting cytokines in various stages of hematopoiesis including megakaryopoiesis. Preclinical and in vitro studies indicate that IL-11 directly stimulates megakaryocytes. Recombinant IL-11 (Oprelvekin) was the first cytokine to reach the market for the prevention of chemotherapy-induced thrombocytopenia.

Clinical Application of the Hematopoietic Growth Factors in Oncology

Granulocyte Colony-Stimulating Factor

Solid Tumor and Lymphoma

The colony-stimulating factors (CSFs) are used in clinical practice to reduce the risk of neutropenic complications and to maintain chemotherapy dose intensity.[28-30] Primary prophylaxis with G-CSF starting within 3 to 5 days of the initial cycle of chemotherapy is based on evidence that the risk of neutropenic complications including febrile neutropenia (FN) is greatest during the first cycle of chemotherapy.[31] Multiple randomized controlled trials (RCTs) of primary prophylaxis with G-CSF have been reported in a variety of malignancies and treatment regimens.[32] Filgrastim is approved by the U.S. Food and Drug Administration (FDA) to decrease the incidence of infection, as manifested by FN, in patients with nonmyeloid malignancies receiving myelosuppressive anticancer drugs associated with a significant incidence of severe neutropenia with fever. It is also approved for several other indications including mobilization of hematopoietic progenitors cells in the autologous setting as well as of allogeneic donors and for acute radiation syndrome.[29,30] The efficacy of G-CSF for reducing the risk of FN has been confirmed in real-world studies of unselected patients receiving chemotherapy in clinical practice.[33]

Pegfilgrastim

FDA approval of pegfilgrastim was based on two phase III RCTs using filgrastim as an active control. The pegfilgrastim dose was 100 μg/kg in one trial[34] and fixed dose at 6 mg in the other.[35] (Figure 33.3) Patients received either a single injection of pegfilgrastim starting

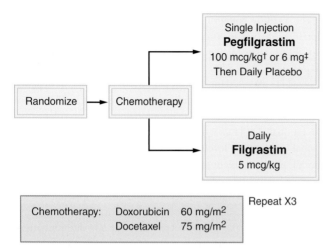

Chemotherapy: Doxorubicin 60 mg/m^2 Repeat X3
Docetaxel 75 mg/m^2

FIGURE **33.3** Design of pegfilgrastim phase III randomized trials in patients receiving chemotherapy for stage II to IV breast cancer. [†]Holmes FA, Jones SE, O'Shaughnessy J, et al. Comparable efficacy and safety profiles of once-per-cycle pegfilgrastim and daily injection filgrastim in chemotherapy-induced neutropenia: a multicenter dose-finding study in women with breast cancer. *Ann Oncol.* 2002;13:903-909; [‡]Green MD, Koelbl H, Baselga J, et al. A randomized double-blind multicenter phase III study of fixed-dose single-administration pegfilgrastim versus daily filgrastim in patients receiving myelosuppressive chemotherapy. *Ann Oncol.* 2003;14:29-35.

24 hours after chemotherapy followed by daily placebo or daily filgrastim 5 μg/kg until neutrophil recovery or a maximum of 14 days. The combined treatment effect from both studies demonstrated further relative risk (RR) reduction of FN with pegfilgrastim

of 44% ($P = 0.015$).[6] Studies of the efficacy of same-day dosing of Pegfilgrastim have been inconclusive.[36] The largest RCT of G-CSF reported to date compared pegfilgrastim to placebo in 928 women with breast cancer receiving docetaxel 100 mg/m^2 every three weeks for four cycles.[37] Patients receiving pegfilgrastim experienced a lower incidence of FN (1% versus 17%; $P < 0.001$), FN-related hospitalization (1% versus 14%, $P < 0.001$), and IV antibiotics (2% versus 10%; $P < 0.001$) compared to placebo control. Pegfilgrastim is approved by the U.S. FDA to decrease the incidence of infection, as manifested by FN, in patients with nonmyeloid malignancies receiving myelosuppressive anticancer drugs associated with an incidence of FN of 17% or greater risk. The recommended dose is 6 mg single subcutaneous injection 24 hours after administration of chemotherapy and not less than 14 days before the next scheduled chemotherapy cycle. Pegfilgrastim is now also available for administration of an on-body injector (OnPro) generally placed on the skin on the day of chemotherapy treatment and set to inject the scheduled dose of pegfilgrastim approximately 24 hours later.

Pooled Analysis of Randomized Controlled Trials

A systematic review of RCTs of primary prophylaxis with G-CSF in patients with solid tumors and lymphoma reported a relative risk for FN with G-CSF prophylaxis 0.54 ($P < 0.0001$).[32] The relative risk for infection-related mortality and early all-cause mortality with G-CSF was 0.55 ($P = 0.018$) and 0.60 ($P = 0.002$), respectively (Figure 33.4). Of note, the median relative dose intensity (RDI) among control subjects was 89% compared to 96% in patients receiving G-CSF in these trials potentially influencing

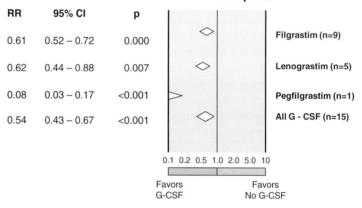

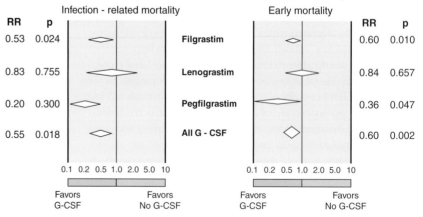

FIGURE **33.4** Forest plots of summary results from a meta-analysis of RCTs of G-CSF prophylaxis in solid tumor and lymphoma patients receiving systemic chemotherapy with or without prophylactic G-CSF including filgrastim, lenograstim, or pegfilgrastim. **Top** figure displays reported rates of FN. (From Kuderer NM, Dale DC, Crawford J, et al. Impact of primary prophylaxis with G-CSF on febrile neutropenia and mortality in adult cancer patients receiving chemotherapy: a systematic review. *J Clin Oncol.* 2007;25(21):3158-3167. Reprinted with permission. Copyright © 2007 American Society of Clinical Oncology. All rights reserved.) **Bottom** graphs reflect results for infection-related mortality and all-cause early mortality reported across trials.

on long-term disease control and mortality. Several studies have reported improved clinical outcomes by increasing the relative dose intensity of chemotherapy utilizing abbreviated treatment schedules (dose dense) with G-CSF support.[38] In a recent systematic review, 61 randomized comparisons in 59 RCTs of patients with solid tumors or lymphoma receiving chemotherapy with or without initial G-CSF were identified.[39,40] The relative risk (RR) for all-cause mortality with G-CSF were 0.93 ($P < 0.001$). Greater RR reduction for mortality was observed among studies with longer follow-up ($P = 0.02$), where treatment was for curative intent [RR = 0.91; $P < 0.001$], with dose-dense regimens [RR = 0.89; $P < 0.001$] and when survival was the primary outcome [RR = 0.91; $P < 0.001$].

Administration of filgrastim prophylaxis only after the development of afebrile neutropenia does not reduce the risk or duration of infection compared to placebo.[41] RCTs permitting a cross-over of control patients after experiencing FN have demonstrated a decrease in the risk and duration of febrile neutropenia in subsequent cycles.[32] A systematic review of 14 RCTs addressing the role of CSF plus antibiotics in the treatment of FN demonstrated that overall and infection-related mortality were not improved compared to antibiotics alone. Patients receiving CSF plus antibiotics were less likely to be hospitalized greater than 10 days, had faster neutrophil recovery, and experienced shorter duration of neutropenia, faster recovery from fever, and shorter duration of antibiotic use, while reporting a higher incidence of bone or joint pain or flu-like symptoms than participants receiving antibiotics alone.[42]

Biosimilar G-CSF

A biosimilar is a biologic product produced in living systems that is highly similar to an approved reference biologic with no meaningful differences in efficacy, safety, and purity.[43] Minor modifications in manufacturing, processing, and packaging may result in differences in both biosimilars as well as originator biologic, potentially leading to small differences in immunogenicity and adverse event profiles appearing over time. Several biosimilar filgrastims have been approved and marketed for the past decade in Europe. Although filgrastim came off patent in the United States in 2012, regulatory guidelines for biosimilar approval in the United States were not yet available. Therefore, although approved as a biosimilar in Europe, tbo-filgrastim was submitted to the FDA as a new agent with supporting clinical studies including three randomized trials comparing tbo-filgrastim to filgrastim in patients with lymphoma, breast cancer, or lung cancer.[44] In 2015, the first biosimilar was approved in the United States, represented by the myeloid growth factor filgrastim-sndz, after demonstrating bioequivalence to the reference originator filgrastim through chemical evaluation and clinical testing including a randomized, double-blind, two-way crossover single dose pharmacokinetic and safety study in healthy volunteers,[45] and a phase III randomized, double-blind, four-arm comparative trial in breast cancer patients receiving neoadjuvant chemotherapy demonstrating clinical equivalence in the primary end point of duration of severe neutropenia.[46] Based on U.S. FDA regulations, the indications for filgrastim-sndz were extrapolated to other approved indications for Neupogen. Additional biosimilar forms of filgrastim and pegfilgrastim have been developed and are currently under review by the U.S. FDA and will likely be approved in the coming year.

Clinical Practice Guidelines

Clinical practice guidelines for the use of myeloid growth factors in patients receiving cancer chemotherapy have been developed by several major professional organizations[29,30] (Table 33.3). Consistent recommendations across these guidelines include primary prophylaxis with the CSFs when the risk of FN is 20% or greater, consideration of prophylactic CSF use with regimens reporting lower risk of FN in cancer patients with additional individual risk factors including older age, poor performance status, and major comorbidities.[31,47] The effectiveness of G-CSF in reducing the risk of neutropenic complications in older patients is well established.

Acute Leukemia and Myelodysplastic Syndrome

The CSFs have been used after induction chemotherapy, priming before induction chemotherapy, and after consolidation chemotherapy in patients with acute myeloid leukemia (AML). The use of CSFs before chemotherapy as priming therapy to increasing the proportion of blasts in growth phase has provided mixed results.[48,49] Most studies of CSF use after induction therapy have demonstrated a shortening of neutropenia and hospitalization but only a single study demonstrated a survival benefit in older patients receiving GM-CSF.[50] CSF use after AML consolidation therapy has been shown to ameliorate the severity and duration of neutropenia.[51,52] In patients with acute lymphocytic leukemia (ALL), the CSFs shorten the duration of neutropenia and are recommended after initial induction and postremission chemotherapy.[53] In patients with neutropenia in the setting of myelodysplastic syndrome (MDS), G-CSF occasionally can increase the granulocyte count.

Stem Cell Transplantation

The CSFs are commonly used in stem cell transplantation (SCT) either for mobilization of peripheral blood progenitor cells (PBPCs) to allow enhanced stem cell collection or after autologous SCT to decrease the duration of neutropenia.[54,55] G-CSF alone or following myelosuppressive chemotherapy is commonly utilized to enhance in vivo production of PBPCs for SCT. Pegfilgrastim is capable of enhancing efficient mobilization of PBPCs when given after salvage therapy inducing rapid multilineage hematopoietic recovery when reinfused. While mobilization kinetics are similar to that of filgrastim, pegfilgrastim is associated with earlier leukocyte recovery and peak levels of CD34$^+$ cells. The feasibility of pegfilgrastim mobilization regimens has been demonstrated in several malignancies.[56]

G-CSF administered after autologous PBPC reinfusion appears to aid engraftment.[57] G-CSF administered following high-dose chemotherapy and autologous SCT accelerates neutrophil recovery.[58] Pegfilgrastim appears to be at least as effective as filgrastim when administered post-SCT resulting in a lower incidence and shorter duration of FN. The use of the CSFs following allogeneic SCT remains controversial. In a retrospective study of patients with AML undergoing allogeneic SCT, CSF support was associated with higher rate of graft versus host disease (GVHD), transplantation-related mortality, and lower disease free and overall survival.[59] Alternatively, a meta-analysis of RCTs of CSFs following allogeneic SCT demonstrated more rapid neutrophil engraftment, shorter durations of hospitalization and intravenous antibiotic use, and lower 100-day transplant-related mortality in patients treated with CSF [$P = 0.046$].[60]

TABLE 33.3	*Summary of primary prophylaxis recommendations*[30]

ASCO White Blood Cell Growth Factor Guidelines Update Summary

Setting/Indication	✓ Recommended	✗ Not Recommended
General circumstances	FN risk in the range of 20% or higher	
Special circumstances	Clinical factors dictate use	
Secondary prophylaxis	Based on chemotherapy reaction among other factors	
Therapy of afebrile neutropenia		Not to be used routinely
Therapy of febrile neutropenia	If high-risk for complications or poor clinical outcomes	Not to be used routinely as adjunctive treatment with antibiotic therapy
Acute myeloid leukemia	Following induction therapy, patients greater than 55 years old most likely to benefit	Not to be used for priming effects
	After the completion of consolidation chemotherapy	
Myelodysplastic syndrome		Intermittent administration for a subset of patients with severe neutropenia and recurrent infection
Acute lymphocytic leukemia	After the completion of initial chemotherapy or first post remission course	
Radiotherapy	Consider if receiving radiation therapy alone and prolonged delays are expected	Avoid in patients receiving concomitant chemotherapy and radiation therapy
Older patients	If ≥65 years old with diffuse aggressive lymphoma and treated with curative chemotherapy	
Pediatric population	For the primary prophylaxis of pediatric patients with a likelihood of FN and the secondary prophylaxis or therapy for high-risk pts.	G-CSF use in children with ALL should be considered carefully

Toxicity and Safety

The CSFs are generally well tolerated with mild to moderate bone pain in approximately 20% to 30% of patients representing the most common side effect.[32] Splenomegaly, splenic rupture, and thrombocytopenia have been rarely reported with CSF use in the setting of stem cell mobilization. Reversible laboratory abnormalities include leukocytosis and elevation of uric acid, alkaline phosphatase, and lactate dehydrogenase. The safety experience with pegfilgrastim is similar to that with filgrastim with the most common adverse event being bone pain. Retrospective analyses of the two randomized phase III studies of pegfilgrastim versus filgrastim have shown no statistically significant differences in incidence, severity, or duration of bone pain.[8,35] Despite label restrictions, studies suggest that pegfilgrastim may also be safely used to support dose-dense regimens.[34]

The presence of G-CSF receptors on the surface of myeloid leukemic cells has led to concern about any risk of acute myeloid leukemia (AML) or myelodysplastic syndrome (MDS) in patients receiving G-CSF. Using SEER-Medicare data, Hershman et al reported an increased risk of AML in elderly women with early-stage breast cancer who received adjuvant chemotherapy supported by G-CSF or GM-CSF.[61] The ability of G-CSF to sustain or increase either chemotherapy dose intensity or cumulative dose confounds any influence of G-CSF on the risk of AML or MDS due to the known leukemogenic potential of ionizing radiation and

many chemotherapeutic agents. In a meta-analysis of 25 RCTs of G-CSF-supported chemotherapy with at least two years of follow-up, AML/MDS was reported in 22 control and 43 G-CSF–treated patients with estimated relative risk of 1.92 [$P = 0.007$] with an absolute risk increase of four per 1,000.[39] At the same time, the relative risk for all-cause mortality across all trials was 0.897 [$P < 0.0001$] with an absolute reduction of 34 deaths per 1,000 patients.

Granulocyte-Macrophage Colony-Stimulating Factor

GM-CSF is indicated in clinical practice to reduce the time to neutrophil recovery and reduce the incidence of severe infections following induction chemotherapy in adults with AML, for mobilization of hematopoietic progenitor cells and acceleration of myeloid reconstitution following autologous or allogeneic transplantation. Like G-CSF, GM-CSF is now approved for increasing survival in the setting of acute radiation syndrome. While sargramostim was shown to improve survival and reduce toxicity when combined with ipilimumab in patients with stage III or IV melanoma, the results need to be confirmed.[62]

Acute Myeloid Leukemia

In a phase III placebo-controlled study in elderly patients with AML, sargramostim enhanced neutrophil recovery, reduced infections, and led to longer survival.[50] In a randomized, placebo-controlled study, 240 older patients with AML received molgramostim during and after induction chemotherapy resulting in shorter time to neutrophil recovery and improved disease-free survival than controls.[63]

High-Dose Therapy with Stem Cell Support

Randomized, placebo-controlled clinical trials of GM-CSF in the setting of high-dose chemotherapy with SCT have demonstrated accelerated neutrophil recovery when bone marrow alone is used.[64,65] GM-CSF therapy has shown no significant effect on the incidence or severity of graft versus host disease in patients receiving allogeneic transplants.

Priming of Peripheral Blood Progenitor Cells

GM-CSF alone or following chemotherapy has been effective in priming PBPCs for subsequent leukapheresis.[66] GM-CSF–primed PBPCs following cytotoxic chemotherapy with autologous marrow rescue are associated with significantly improved myeloid and platelet recovery.[67]

Toxicity and Safety

Fever, dyspnea, fluid retention, myalgias, and bone pain are seen in *E. coli*–derived GM-CSF. Dose-related adverse effects with GM-CSF include capillary leak syndrome, central vein thrombosis, and hypotension while effects seen over a range of doses include fever, pleuritis, myalgia, bone pain, pulmonary infiltrates, rash, and thrombophlebitis. Some patients have experienced a syndrome of transient hypoxia and hypotension following the first dose but not subsequent doses of GM-CSF. GM-CSF is a known inducer of other endogenous cytokines, which are thought to account for at least some of the adverse effects. The simultaneous administration of GM-CSF and cycle-specific chemotherapy or radiation therapy has worsened myelosuppression.[68]

Erythropoiesis-Stimulating Agents (ESAs)

In randomized, placebo-controlled trials in cancer patients receiving chemotherapy with anemia, both epoetin alfa[69] and darbepoetin alfa[70] increase hemoglobin levels and reduce red cell transfusion rates. Pooled analysis of trials comparing early intervention to delayed treatment with ESAs suggest that the former resulted in less

severe anemia and greater reductions in transfusion requirements.[71] While several biosimilar epoetins have been approved in Europe for patients with chronic kidney disease, none are available in the United States.

Toxicity and Safety

While these agents are generally well tolerated, safety concerns have emerged that should be considered by the patient and clinician including early mortality, increased thrombosis, hypertension, and worsening anemia, and rarely pure red cell aplasia and due to ESA-neutralizing antibodies. Placebo-controlled RCTs of the ESAs have suggested that some cancer patients receiving these agents outside of recommended schedules experience worse outcomes.[72,73] While meta-analyses of RCTs of epoetin and darbepoetin alfa have demonstrated a significantly reduction in the need for red blood cell transfusions and improved hematologic response, an increased risk of thromboembolic events has been seen.[74] At the same time, a small increase in overall mortality in cancer patients has been observed notably in trials administering the ESAs outside of guideline-recommended starting and target hemoglobin levels (RR = 1.06; 95% CI: 1.00 to 1.12), while in most randomized trials of ESAs in patients with cancer, no difference in survival has been observed.[74,75] (Figure 33.5) Safety issues concerning the ESAs primarily emerged from the Breast Cancer Erythropoietin Survival Trial [BEST] and the Erythropoietin in Head and Neck Cancer Study [ENHANCE]) trials which targeted high hemoglobin levels or enrolled patients outside the approved utilization. Subsequent clinical trials and meta-analyses continue to provide conflicting results suggesting small but concerning safety signals including increased mortality in some studies with no such indication in other trials.[76–78] The ESAs should be used with caution in patients with advanced cancer receiving systemic chemotherapy with appropriate consideration of potential benefits and harms. However, in 2017, the FDA determined that the ESA Risk Evaluation and Mitigation Strategy (REMS) program was no longer needed to ensure that the benefits of ESA therapy outweigh the harms. The FDA black box warning states that the ESAs should only be used to treat chemotherapy-induced anemia, should be discontinued once

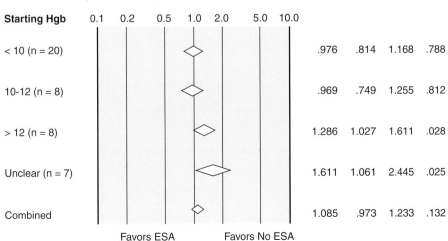

FIGURE **33.5** Forest plot of summary results of overall mortality among RCTs of epoetin alfa and darbepoetin alfa in cancer patients receiving systemic chemotherapy stratified by reported starting hemoglobin. (Derived from Bohlius J, Wilson J, Seidenfeld J, et al. Recombinant human erythropoietins and cancer patients: updated meta-analysis of 57 studies including 9353 patients. *J Natl Cancer Inst.* 2006;98:708-714.)

chemotherapy is complete, and should not be used when the treatment intent is curative. Further studies are needed of the ESAs used for the treatment of chemotherapy-induced anemia according to the common practice and clinical guidelines. There are known risks of transfusions, and it is essential that clinical studies and practice be aimed toward balancing risks against the known benefits in order to achieve optimal outcomes in cancer patients.

Clinical Practice Guidelines

Current clinical practice guidelines from the American Society of Clinical Oncology and the American Society of Hematology for the use of ESA's in patients undergoing myelosuppressive therapy with a hemoglobin less than 10 g/dL, recommend that clinicians discuss potential harms (for example thrombosis, early early mortality) and benefits (for example, decreased transfusions), and compare these with the potential harms and benefits of RBC transfusions. Individual preferences for assumed risk should contribute to shared decisions on managing chemotherapy-induced anemia while cautioning against ESA use under other circumstances. Alternatively, guidelines for the use of ESAs for the management of chemotherapy-induced anemia from the National Comprehensive Cancer Network limit their use to symptomatic patients being treated for noncurative intent.

Thrombopoietic Agents

Interleukin (IL) 11

Early clinical trials of IL-11 in patients with cancer demonstrated an ability to increase steady-state platelet counts and to reduce the risk of chemotherapy-induced thrombocytopenia. A small randomized, placebo-controlled evaluation of IL-11 for secondary prophylaxis of thrombocytopenia in previously transfused patients with chemotherapy-induced thrombocytopenia reported platelet transfusion requirements in 90% and 72% in placebo and IL-11–treated patients, respectively.[79] Administration of IL-11 did not appear to alter platelet recovery or transfusion requirements in patients with breast cancer enrolled in a randomized, placebo-controlled study following high-dose chemotherapy and infusion with G-CSF–primed PBPCs. Constitutional symptoms including myalgia, arthralgia, and fatigue, were the dose-limiting toxicities and approximately 60% of patients treated with IL-11 experience edema secondary to sodium retention. Atrial arrhythmias, tachycardia, conjunctival injection, and worsening of effusions can also occur.

Romiplostim

Romiplostim is approved for use in patients with chronic ITP based on a durable platelet response in two phase III multicenter, double-blind, randomized placebo-controlled trials in splenectomized and nonsplenectomized patients receiving at least one prior treatment for ITP. Romiplostim was associated with significant improvement in quality of life with no significant increase in serious adverse events.[80] No neutralizing antibodies to TPO were observed, and while reticulin formation was observed in 10 patients, no progression to marrow fibrosis was observed in the phase 3 studies. Severe thrombocytopenia following discontinuation of romiplostim in four patients resolving within two weeks prompted implementation of a REMS program. There has only been limited study of TPO utilized for chemotherapy-associated thrombocytopenia.

In a phase II, open label trial, romiplostim was found to reverse chemotherapy-induced thrombocytopenia in solid tumor patients allowing resumption and maintenance of cancer-directed therapy in the large majority of patients.[81]

Eltrombopag

As the first orally absorbed, small molecule thrombopoietin receptor agonist, Eltrombopag was approved by the U.S. FDA for the treatment of thrombocytopenia in patients with chronic ITP with insufficient response to corticosteroids, immunoglobulins, or splenectomy based on data from two double-blind, placebo-controlled clinical studies.[82,83] Major safety findings pertained to a risk for hepatic toxicity, worsening thrombocytopenia with hemorrhage following discontinuation, and reticulin formation in the bone marrow. A global, randomized, placebo-controlled trial demonstrated a significantly better platelet response for eltrombopag and a reduction in bleeding dependent on the platelet response. While liver toxicity was generally mild and reversible, routine monitoring of liver function is encouraged. Approval was accompanied by a REMS program to monitor for further safety signals. A recent Cochrane review of thrombopoietin receptor agonists for prevention and treatment of chemotherapy-induced thrombocytopenia in patients with solid tumors concluded that no conclusions could be drawn to support the use of these agents for the treatment or prevention of chemotherapy-induced thrombocytopenia inpatients with solid tumors.[84]

References

1. Metcalf D. Studies on colony formation in vitro by mouse bone marrow cells. I. Continuous cluster formation and relation of clusters to colonies. *J Cell Physiol.* 1969;74(3):323-332. doi: 10.1002/jcp.1040740313.

2. Metcalf D, Foster R. Bone marrow colony-stimulating activity of serum from mice with viral-induced leukemia. *J Natl Cancer Inst.* 1967;39(6):1235-1245.

3. Clark SC, Kamen R. The human hematopoietic colony-stimulating factors. *Science.* 1987;236(4806):1229-1237.

4. Bagby G, Heinrich M. Growth factors, cytokines, and the control of hematopoiesis. In: Hoffman R, Shattil SJ, eds. *Heamotology Basic Principles and Practice.* Philadelphia: Churchill Livingstone; 2000:154-202.

5. Moore M. Colony stimulating factors: basic principles and preclinical studies. In: Rosenberg S, ed. *Principles and Practice of the Biologic Therapy of Cancer.* Philadelphia: Lippincott Williams & Wilkins; 2000:113-140.

6. Lyman GH. Pegfilgrastim: a granulocyte colony-stimulating factor with sustained duration of action. *Expert Opin Biol Ther.* 2005;5(12):1635-1646.

7. Yang BB, Lum PK, Hayashi MM, Roskos LK. Polyethylene glycol modification of filgrastim results in decreased renal clearance of the protein in rats. *J Pharm Sci.* 2004;93(5):1367-1373. doi: 10.1002/jps.20024.

8. Holmes FA, Jones SE, O'Shaughnessy J, et al. Comparable efficacy and safety profiles of once-per-cycle pegfilgrastim and daily injection filgrastim in chemotherapy-induced neutropenia: a multicenter dose-finding study in women with breast cancer. *Ann Oncol.* 2002;13(6):903-909.

9. Molineux G. The design and development of pegfilgrastim (PEG-rmetHuG-CSF, Neulasta). *Curr Pharm Des.* 2004;10(11):1235-1244.

10. Gough NM, Gough J, Metcalf D, et al. Molecular cloning of cDNA encoding a murine haematopoietic growth regulator, granulocyte-macrophage colony stimulating factor. *Nature.* 1984;309(5971):763-767

11. Peters WP, Stuart A, Affronti ML, Kim CS, Coleman RE. Neutrophil migration is defective during recombinant human granulocyte-macrophage colony-stimulating factor infusion after autologous bone marrow transplantation in humans. *Blood.* 1988;72(4):1310-1315.

12. Demir G, Klein HO, Tuzuner N. Low dose daily rhGM-CSF application activates monocytes and dendritic cells in vivo. *Leuk Res.* 2003;27(12):1105-1108.

13. O'Dwyer PJ, LaCreta FP, Schilder R, et al. Phase I trial of thiotepa in combination with recombinant human granulocyte-macrophage colony-stimulating factor. *J Clin Oncol.* 1992;10(8):1352-1358.

14. Elliott S, Lorenzini T, Asher S, et al. Enhancement of therapeutic protein in vivo activities through glycoengineering. *Nat Biotechnol.* 2003;21(4):414-421. doi: 10.1038/nbt799

15. Birgegard G, Wide L, Simonsson B. Marked erythropoietin increase before fall in Hb after treatment with cytostatic drugs suggests mechanism other than anaemia for stimulation. *Br J Haematol.* 1989;72(3):462-466.

16. Schapira L, Antin JH, Ransil BJ, et al. Serum erythropoietin levels in patients receiving intensive chemotherapy and radiotherapy. *Blood.* 1990;76(11):2354-2359.

17. Auerbach M, Ballard H, Trout JR, et al. Intravenous iron optimizes the response to recombinant human erythropoietin in cancer patients with chemotherapy-related anemia: a multicenter, open-label, randomized trial. *J Clin Oncol.* 2004;22(7):1301-1307. doi: 10.1200/JCO.2004.08.119

18. Gordon MS, McCaskill-Stevens WJ, Battiato LA, et al. A phase I trial of recombinant human interleukin-11 (neumega rhIL-11 growth factor) in women with breast cancer receiving chemotherapy. *Blood.* 1996;87(9):3615-3624.

19. Isaacs C, Robert NJ, Bailey FA, et al. Randomized placebo-controlled study of recombinant human interleukin-11 to prevent chemotherapy-induced thrombocytopenia in patients with breast cancer receiving dose-intensive cyclophosphamide and doxorubicin. *J Clin Oncol.* 1997;15(11):3368-3377.

20. Douglas VK, Tallman MS, Cripe LD, Peterson LC. Thrombopoietin administered during induction chemotherapy to patients with acute myeloid leukemia induces transient morphologic changes that may resemble chronic myeloproliferative disorders. *Am J Clin Pathol.* 2002;117(6):844-850. doi: 10.1309/09NP-3DFG-BLM9-E5LE.

21. Nurden AT, Viallard JF, Nurden P. New-generation drugs that stimulate platelet production in chronic immune thrombocytopenic purpura. *Lancet.* 2009;373(9674):1562-1569.

22. Deutsch VR, Tomer A. Megakaryocyte development and platelet production. *Br J Haematol.* 2006;134(5):453-466. doi: 10.1111/j.1365-2141.2006.06215.x.

23. Kuter DJ, Begley CG. Recombinant human thrombopoietin: basic biology and evaluation of clinical studies. *Blood.* 2002;100(10):3457-3469. doi: 10.1182/blood.V100.10.3457

24. Li J, Yang C, Xia Y, et al. Thrombocytopenia caused by the development of antibodies to thrombopoietin. *Blood.* 2001;98(12):3241-3248

25. Wang B, Nichol JL, Sullivan JT. Pharmacodynamics and pharmacokinetics of AMG 531, a novel thrombopoietin receptor ligand. *Clin Pharmacol Ther.* 2004;76(6):628-638

26. Bussel JB, Kuter DJ, George JN, et al. AMG 531, a thrombopoiesis-stimulating protein, for chronic ITP. *N Engl J Med.* 2006;355(16):1672-1681. doi: 10.1056/NEJMoa054626

27. Jenkins JM, Williams D, Deng Y, et al. Phase 1 clinical study of eltrombopag, an oral, nonpeptide thrombopoietin receptor agonist. *Blood.* 2007;109(11):4739-4741. Epub 2007/03/01. doi: blood-2006-11-057968.

28. Aapro MS, Cameron DA, Pettengell R, et al. EORTC guidelines for the use of granulocyte-colony stimulating factor to reduce the incidence of chemotherapy-induced febrile neutropenia in adult patients with lymphomas and solid tumours. *Eur J Cancer.* 2006;42(15):2433-2453.

29. Crawford J, Becker PS, Armitage JO, et al. Myeloid growth factors, Version 2.2017, NCCN Clinical Practice Guidelines in Oncology. *J Natl Compr Canc Netw.* 2017;15(12):1520-1541. doi: 10.6004/jnccn.2017.0175.

30. Smith TJ, Bohlke K, Lyman GH, et al. Recommendations for the use of WBC growth factors: American Society of Clinical Oncology Clinical Practice Guideline Update. *J Clin Oncol.* 2015;33(28):3199-3212. doi: 10.1200/JCO.2015.62.3488.

31. Lyman GH, Delgado DJ. Risk and timing of hospitalization for febrile neutropenia in patients receiving CHOP, CHOP-R, or CNOP chemotherapy for intermediate-grade non-Hodgkin lymphoma. *Cancer.* 2003;98(11):2402-2409. Epub 2003/11/25. doi: 10.1002/cncr.11827.

32. Kuderer NM, Dale DC, Crawford J, Lyman GH. Impact of primary prophylaxis with granulocyte colony-stimulating factor on febrile neutropenia and mortality in adult cancer patients receiving chemotherapy: a systematic review. *J Clin Oncol.* 2007;25(21):3158-3167.

33. Agiro A, Ma Q, Acheson AK, et al. Risk of neutropenia-related hospitalization in patients who received colony-stimulating factors with chemotherapy for breast cancer. *J Clin Oncol.* 2016;34(32):3872-3879. doi: 10.1200/JCO.2016.67.2899.

34. Holmes FA, O'Shaughnessy JA, Vukelja S, et al. Blinded, randomized, multicenter study to evaluate single administration pegfilgrastim once per cycle versus daily filgrastim as an adjunct to chemotherapy in patients with high-risk stage II or stage III/IV breast cancer. *J Clin Oncol.* 2002;20(3):727-731. Epub 2002/02/01.

35. Green MD, Koelbl H, Baselga J, et al. A randomized double-blind multicenter phase III study of fixed-dose single-administration pegfilgrastim versus daily filgrastim in patients receiving myelosuppressive chemotherapy. *Ann Oncol.* 2003;14(1):29-35. Epub 2002/12/19.

36. Lyman GH, Allcott K, Garcia J, et al. The effectiveness and safety of same-day versus next-day administration of long-acting granulocyte colony-stimulating factors for the prophylaxis of chemotherapy-induced neutropenia: a systematic review. *Support Care Cancer.* 2017;25(8):2619-2629. doi: 10.1007/s00520-017-3703-y.

37. Vogel CL, Wojtukiewicz MZ, Carroll RR, et al. First and subsequent cycle use of pegfilgrastim prevents febrile neutropenia in patients with breast cancer: a multicenter, double-blind, placebo-controlled phase III study. *J Clin Oncol.* 2005;23(6):1178-1184. Epub 2005/02/19. doi: 10.1200/JCO.2005.09.102.

38. Lyman GH, Reiner M, Morrow PK, Crawford J. The effect of filgrastim or pegfilgrastim on survival outcomes of patients with cancer receiving myelosuppressive chemotherapy. *Ann Oncol.* 2015;26(7):1452-1458. doi: 10.1093/annonc/mdv174.

39. Lyman GH, Dale DC, Wolff DA, et al. Acute myeloid leukemia or myelodysplastic syndrome in randomized controlled clinical trials of cancer chemotherapy with granulocyte colony-stimulating factor: a systematic review. *J Clin Oncol.* 2010;28(17):2914-2924. doi: 10.1200/JCO.2009.25.8723.

40. Lyman GH, Dale DC, Culakova E, et al. The impact of the granulocyte colony-stimulating factor on chemotherapy dose intensity and cancer survival: a systematic review and meta-analysis of randomized controlled trials. *Ann Oncol.* 2013;24(10):2475-2484. doi: 10.1093/annonc/mdt226

41. Hartmann LC, Tschetter LK, Habermann TM, et al. Granulocyte colony-stimulating factor in severe chemotherapy-induced afebrile neutropenia. *N Engl J Med.* 1997;336(25):1776-1780. Epub 1997/06/19.

42. Mhaskar R, Clark OA, Lyman G, et al. Colony-stimulating factors for chemotherapy-induced febrile neutropenia, *Cochrane Database Syst Rev.* 2014;(10):CD003039. doi: 10.1002/14651858.CD003039.pub2.

43. Lyman GH, Balaban E, Diaz M, et al. American Society of Clinical Oncology Statement: Biosimilars in Oncology. *J Clin Oncol.* 2018:JCO2017774893. doi: 10.1200/JCO.2017.77.4893.

44. Hirsch BR, Lyman GH. Biosimilars: a cure to the U.S. health care cost conundrum? *Blood Rev.* 2014;28(6):263-268. doi: 10.1016/j.blre.2014.08.003.

45. Sorgel F, Schwebig A, Holzmann J, Prasch S, Singh P, Kinzig M. Comparability of biosimilar filgrastim with originator filgrastim: protein characterization, pharmacodynamics, and pharmacokinetics. *BioDrugs.* 2015;29(2):123-131. doi: 10.1007/s40259-015-0124-7.

46. Blackwell K, Semiglazov V, Krasnozhon D, et al. Comparison of EP2006, a filgrastim biosimilar, to the reference: a phase III, randomized, double-blind clinical study in the prevention of severe neutropenia in patients with breast cancer receiving myelosuppressive chemotherapy. *Ann Oncol.* 2015;26(9):1948-1953. doi: 10.1093/annonc/mdv281

47. Lyman GH, Morrison VA, Dale DC, Crawford J, Delgado DJ, Fridman M. Risk of febrile neutropenia among patients with intermediate-grade non-Hodgkin's lymphoma receiving CHOP chemotherapy. *Leuk Lymphoma.* 2003;44(12):2069-2076. Epub 2004/02/13.

48. Lowenberg B, van Putten W, Theobald M, et al. Effect of priming with granulocyte colony-stimulating factor on the outcome of chemotherapy for acute myeloid leukemia. *N Engl J Med.* 2003;349(8):743-752. Epub 2003/08/22. doi: 10.1056/NEJMoa025406.

49. Pabst T, Vellenga E, van Putten W, et al. Favorable effect of priming with granulocyte colony-stimulating factor in remission induction of acute myeloid leukemia restricted to dose escalation of cytarabine. *Blood.* 2012;119(23):5367-5373. doi: 10.1182/blood-2011-11-389841.

50. Rowe JM, Andersen JW, Mazza JJ, et al. A randomized placebo-controlled phase III study of granulocyte-macrophage colony-stimulating factor in adult patients (>55 to 70 years of age) with acute myelogenous leukemia: a study of the Eastern Cooperative Oncology Group (E1490). *Blood.* 1995;86(2):457-462. Epub 1995/07/15.

51. Harousseau JL, Witz B, Lioure B, et al. Granulocyte colony-stimulating factor after intensive consolidation chemotherapy in acute myeloid leukemia: results of a randomized trial of the Groupe Ouest-Est Leucemies Aigues Myeloblastiques. *J Clin Oncol.* 2000;18(4):780-787. Epub 2000/02/16.

52. Heil G, Hoelzer D, Sanz MA, et al. A randomized, double-blind, placebo-controlled, phase III study of filgrastim in remission induction and consolidation therapy for adults with de novo acute myeloid leukemia. The International Acute Myeloid Leukemia Study Group. *Blood.* 1997;90(12):4710-4718. Epub 1998/01/07.

53. Pui CH, Boyett JM, Hughes WT, et al. Human granulocyte colony-stimulating factor after induction chemotherapy in children with acute lymphoblastic leukemia. *N Engl J Med.* 1997;336(25):1781-1787. Epub 1997/06/19.

54. Klumpp TR, Mangan KF, Goldberg SL, Pearlman ES, Macdonald JS. Granulocyte colony-stimulating factor accelerates neutrophil engraftment following peripheral-blood stem-cell transplantation: a prospective, randomized trial. *J Clin Oncol.* 1995;13(6):1323-1327. Epub 1995/06/01.

55. Nemunaitis J, Appelbaum F, Singer J. Effect of GM-CSF on circulating granulocyte-monocyte progenitors in autologous bone marrow transplantation. *Lancet.* 1989;2(8676):1405-1406. Epub 1989/12/09. doi: S0140-6736(89)92027-8.

56. Noga S, Oroszlan M, Hetherington J. Use of pegfilgrastim for autologous peripheral blood stem cell mobilization: comparison to a daily filgrastim regimen. *Bone Marrow Transplant.* 2003;31:S18

57. Kawano Y, Takaue Y, Mimaya J, et al. Marginal benefit/disadvantage of granulocyte colony-stimulating factor therapy after autologous blood stem cell transplantation in children: results of a prospective randomized trial. The Japanese Cooperative Study Group of PBSCT. *Blood.* 1998;92(11):4040-4046. Epub 1998/12/03.

58. Bishop MR, Tarantolo SR, Geller RB, et al. A randomized, double-blind trial of filgrastim (granulocyte colony-stimulating factor) versus placebo following allogeneic blood stem cell transplantation. *Blood.* 2000;96(1):80-85. Epub 2000/07/13.

59. Ringden O, Labopin M, Gorin NC, et al. Treatment with granulocyte colony-stimulating factor after allogeneic bone marrow transplantation for acute leukemia increases the risk of graft-versus-host disease and death: a study from the Acute Leukemia Working Party of the European Group for Blood and Marrow Transplantation. *J Clin Oncol.* 2004;22(3):416-423. Epub 2003/12/24. doi: 10.1200/JCO.2004.06.102.

60. Komrokji RS, Lyman GH. The colony-stimulating factors: use to prevent and treat neutropenia and its complications. *Expert Opin Biol Ther.* 2004;4(12):1897-1910. Epub 2004/12/02. doi: 10.1517/14712598.4.12.1897.

61. Hershman D, Neugut AI, Jacobson JS, et al. Acute myeloid leukemia or myelodysplastic syndrome following use of granulocyte colony-stimulating factors during breast cancer adjuvant chemotherapy. *J Natl Cancer Inst.* 2007;99(3):196-205.

62. Hodi FS, Lee S, McDermott DF, et al. Ipilimumab plus sargramostim vs ipilimumab alone for treatment of metastatic melanoma: a randomized clinical trial. *JAMA.* 2014;312(17):1744-1753. doi: 10.1001/jama.2014.13943.

63. Witz F, Sadoun A, Perrin MC, et al. A placebo-controlled study of recombinant human granulocyte-macrophage colony-stimulating factor administered during and after induction treatment for de novo acute myelogenous leukemia in elderly patients. Groupe Ouest Est Leucemies Aigues Myeloblastiques (GOELAM). *Blood.* 1998;91(8):2722-2730. Epub 1998/05/16.

64. Advani R, Chao NJ, Horning SJ, et al. Granulocyte-macrophage colony-stimulating factor (GM-CSF) as an adjunct to autologous hemopoietic stem cell transplantation for lymphoma. *Ann Intern Med.* 1992;116(3):183-189. Epub 1992/02/01.

65. De Witte T, Gratwohl A, Van Der Lely N, et al. Recombinant human granulocyte-macrophage colony-stimulating factor accelerates neutrophil and monocyte recovery after allogeneic T-cell-depleted bone marrow transplantation. *Blood.* 1992;79(5):1359-1365. Epub 1992/03/01.

66. Elias AD, Ayash L, Anderson KC, et al. Mobilization of peripheral blood progenitor cells by chemotherapy and granulocyte-macrophage colony-stimulating factor for hematologic support after high-dose intensification for breast cancer. *Blood.* 1992;79(11):3036-3044. Epub 1992/06/01.

67. Ballestrero A, Ferrando F, Garuti A, et al. Comparative effects of three cytokine regimens after high-dose cyclophosphamide: granulocyte colony-stimulating factor, granulocyte-macrophage colony-stimulating factor (GM-CSF), and sequential interleukin-3 and GM-CSF. *J Clin Oncol.* 1999;17(4):1296. Epub 1999/11/24.

68. Shaffer DW, Smith LS, Burris HA, et al. A randomized phase I trial of chronic oral etoposide with or without granulocyte-macrophage colony-stimulating factor in patients with advanced malignancies. *Cancer Res.* 1993;53(24):5929-5933. Epub 1993/12/15.

69. Case DC, Jr., Bukowski RM, Carey RW, et al. Recombinant human erythropoietin therapy for anemic cancer patients on combination chemotherapy. *J Natl Cancer Inst.* 1993;85(10):801-806. Epub 1993/05/19.

70. Vansteenkiste J, Pirker R, Massuti B, et al. Double-blind, placebo-controlled, randomized phase III trial of darbepoetin alfa in lung cancer patients receiving chemotherapy. *J Natl Cancer Inst.* 2002;94(16):1211-1220. Epub 2002/08/22.

71. Lyman GH, Glaspy J. Are there clinical benefits with early erythropoietic intervention for chemotherapy-induced anemia? A systematic review. *Cancer.* 2006;106(1):223-233.

72. Henke M, Laszig R, Rube C, et al. Erythropoietin to treat head and neck cancer patients with anaemia undergoing radiotherapy: randomised, double-blind, placebo-controlled trial. *Lancet.* 2003;362(9392):1255-1260. Epub 2003/10/25. doi: S0140-6736(03)14567-9

73. Leyland-Jones B. Breast cancer trial with erythropoietin terminated unexpectedly. *Lancet Oncol.* 2003;4(8):459-460. Epub 2003/08/07. doi: S147020450301163X.

74. Bohlius J, Wilson J, Seidenfeld J, et al. Recombinant human erythropoietins and cancer patients: updated meta-analysis of 57 studies including 9353 patients. *J Natl Cancer Inst.* 2006;98(10):708-714.

75. Bohlius J, Schmidlin K, Brillant C, et al. Recombinant human erythropoiesis-stimulating agents and mortality in patients with cancer: a meta-analysis of randomised trials. *Lancet.* 2009;373(9674):1532-1542.

76. Aapro M, Moebus V, Nitz U, et al. Safety and efficacy outcomes with erythropoiesis-stimulating agents in patients with breast cancer: a meta-analysis. *Ann Oncol.* 2015;26(4):688-695. doi: 10.1093/annonc/mdu579.

77. Leyland-Jones B, Bondarenko I, Nemsadze G, et al. A randomized, open-label, multicenter, phase III study of epoetin alfa versus best standard of care in anemic patients with metastatic breast cancer receiving standard chemotherapy. *J Clin Oncol.* 2016;34(11):1197-1207. doi: 10.1200/JCO.2015.63.5649.

78. Marchetti C, De Felice F, Palaia I, et al. Erythropoiesis-stimulating agents in gynecological malignancies: A study-level meta-analysis. *Crit Rev Oncol Hematol.* 2016;99:123-128. doi: 10.1016/j.critrevonc.2015.12.013.

79. Tepler I, Elias L, Smith JW, 2nd, et al. A randomized placebo-controlled trial of recombinant human interleukin-11 in cancer patients with severe thrombocytopenia due to chemotherapy. *Blood.* 1996;87(9):3607-3614. Epub 1996/05/01.

80. Kuter DJ, Bussel JB, Lyons RM, et al. Efficacy of romiplostim in patients with chronic immune thrombocytopenic purpura: a double-blind randomised controlled trial. *Lancet.* 2008;371(9610):395-403.

81. Parameswaran R, Lunning M, Mantha S, et al. Romiplostim for management of chemotherapy-induced thrombocytopenia. *Support Care Cancer.* 2014;22(5):1217-1222. doi: 10.1007/s00520-013-2074-2.

82. Bussel JB, Cheng G, Saleh MN, et al. Eltrombopag for the treatment of chronic idiopathic thrombocytopenic purpura. *N Engl J Med.* 2007;357(22):2237-2247. Epub 2007/11/30. doi: 357/22/2237.

83. Bussel JB, Provan D, Shamsi T, et al. Effect of eltrombopag on platelet counts and bleeding during treatment of chronic idiopathic thrombocytopenic purpura: a randomised, double-blind, placebo-controlled trial. *Lancet.* 2009;373(9664):641-648. Epub 2009/02/24. doi: S0140-6736(09)60402-5.

84. Zhang X, Chuai Y, Nie W, Wang A, Dai G. Thrombopoietin receptor agonists for prevention and treatment of chemotherapy-induced thrombocytopenia in patients with solid tumours. *Cochrane Database Syst Rev.* 2017;11:CD012035. doi: 10.1002/14651858.CD012035.pub2.

Cancer and Coagulopathy

Rachel P.G. Rosovsky

Introduction

The association between cancer and thrombosis was first proposed by Armand Trousseau (Fig. 34.1) when he recognized the condition of *thrombophlebitis migrans*, as a forewarning of occult malignancy.[1] In 1865, he remarked, "when in doubt as to the nature of an affection of the stomach, should you when hesitating between chronic gastritis, simple ulcer, and cancer, observe a vein become infected in the arm or leg, you may dispel your doubt, and pronounce in a positive manner that there is a cancer …".[1] Although the association of hemostatic disorders and cancer has been studied extensively over the past 150 years, venous thromboembolism (VTE), defined herein as pulmonary embolus (PE) or deep vein thrombosis (DVT), remains a major cause of morbidity and mortality in cancer patients as well as a high economic burden.

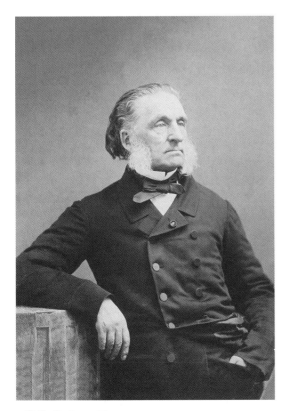

FIGURE **34.1** Armand Trousseau.

This chapter will explore the pathogenesis of thrombosis in cancer as well as the epidemiology and risk factors. This review will also focus on novel risk assessment models and the emergence of biomarkers to classify patients at high risk of developing VTE. Current diagnostic and management strategies for VTE in cancer patients and the challenges of antithrombotic therapy in this population will be examined including the emerging role of direct oral anticoagulants (DOACs). This update will also review the results of several randomized controlled trials aimed at assessing the clinical benefit of antithrombotic prophylaxis in cancer outpatients. Finally, new therapeutic developments in this area will be addressed.

Pathogenesis

The pathophysiological mechanisms of thrombosis in cancer patients are complex and involve multiple clinical and biological factors including tumor cells, the hemostatic system, inherited and acquired thrombophilia, and exogenous contributors such as chemotherapy and radiotherapy.[2-4] Tumors contribute to thrombosis through the expression of procoagulant factors including tissue factor, cancer procoagulant, and adhesion molecules. Numerous experimental models of human cancers have shown that an integral feature of neoplastic transformation from cancer cells is through activation of clotting proteins.[5-8] Tumor-related release of various cytokines, growth factors, and proteases including tumor necrosis factor-α (TNF-α), interleukin-1β, and vascular endothelial growth factor (VEGF) contribute not only to angiogenesis and inflammation but also to the activation of the hemostatic system. A growing body of evidence demonstrates that the same mechanisms that promote tumor growth and metastases also appear to activate the hemostatic system.

The role of tissue factor–bearing microparticles (MP) contributing to thrombin generation has also been explored in in vitro and in vivo studies. Zwicker et al. found that VTE developed in 34.8% of cancer patients with elevated levels of MP compared to 0% in those without detectable levels.[9] Tumor cells can also induce platelet activation and aggregation through secretion of proteases. Furthermore, tumor cells interact directly with the host blood vessels, endothelial cells, leukocytes, and monocytes leading to host cell inflammatory responses.[2] These many and varied interactions lead to both a direct and indirect activation of the clotting system, an increase in thrombin generation, and ultimately a hypercoagulable state.

Epidemiology

Venous thrombosis is a common complication in patients with cancer. Presently, it is the second leading cause of death in cancer patients, with cancer progression being number one.[10] Although the exact incidence of VTE in cancer patients is unknown, reports range from 4% to 30% depending on tumor type.[11,12] These numbers likely underestimate the problem as VTE often causes no symptoms. In a recent study, clinically unsuspected PE was present in up to 4.4% of oncology patients undergoing CT scans for other indications.[13] If symptoms are present, they are often nonspecific or attributed to a patient's underlying malignancy.

Certain malignancies exhibit high rates of VTE such as hematological malignancies and neoplasms, especially if high grade, of the pancreas, gastrointestinal tract, ovary, brain, colon, kidney, lung, and prostate.[14–19] However, it is unclear if the high rates are due to the underlying properties of particular cancers or merely reflect the high prevalence of certain cancers. Nevertheless, it is well documented that cancers diagnosed at the same time as an episode of VTE are more likely to have distant metastases and lower survival rates.[20,21] One study showed that cancer patients with VTE had a 1-year survival of 12% as compared to 36% in cancer patients without VTE.[21] Similarly, patients who develop VTE within a year after a cancer diagnosis are more likely to have advanced stage and poorer prognosis when compared to analogous cancer patients without VTE.[21] It also appears that cancer patients with VTE are two to three times more likely to have recurrent VTE and two to six times more likely to experience hemorrhagic complications from anticoagulant therapy than noncancer patients with VTE.[22,23] These findings clearly indicate that VTE may be more aggressive and difficult to treat in cancer patients than in noncancer patients.

The association between cancer and thrombosis is further supported by the many studies, suggesting that an idiopathic VTE is often associated with occult cancer. Approximately 5% to 10% of patients who present with an idiopathic or unprovoked VTE are diagnosed with cancer within the subsequent 1 to 2 years.[24–29] These provocative findings raise the unanswered question as to whether all patients with idiopathic VTE should undergo extensive cancer screening. Recently, several prospective studies, meta-analyses, and Cochrane reviews attempted to address this issue.[25–30]

In the Screening for Occult Malignancy in Unprovoked Venous Thromboembolism study, patients with a first unprovoked VTE were randomized to either limited occult-cancer screening (basic blood tests, chest radiograph, and screening for breast, cervical, and prostate cancer as per age-specific cancer screening guidelines) or limited occult-cancer screening plus an abdominal and pelvic CT. At 1-year follow-up, there was no difference in the number of new cancers identified (3.2% in limited and 4.5% in limited + CT group) or in the number of cancers missed by each strategy. Furthermore, there was no difference in time to cancer diagnosis or in cancer-related mortality demonstrating that routine screening with the abdominal and pelvic CT provided no clinically significant benefit.[25] In a subsequent cost-effective analysis, the addition of a comprehensive CT scan was associated with higher costs ($551 Canadian dollar) but with no improvement in detecting occult cancer.[31] A similar trial demonstrated that a CT-based diagnostic strategy, which included thoracic, abdominal, and pelvic CT in combination with fecal occult blood test did not provide a clinically significant benefit over more limited cancer screening for detecting occult cancer in patients with unprovoked VTE.[26]

The use of PET-CT was also recently investigated to screen for occult malignancy. Patients with an unprovoked VTE were randomized to a limited screening strategy (physical examination, usual laboratory tests, and basic radiographs) or a limited screening strategy plus an (18)F-FDG PET/CT scan. The rate of cancer diagnosis was similar in both groups during the initial screening assessment; however, the rate of subsequent cancer diagnosis was lower in the patients who had a negative initial screening in the (18)F-FDG PET/CT group compared to the limited screening group (absolute risk difference 4.1%, 95% CI 0.8 to 8.4, P = 0.01). This raises the possibility that (18)F-FDG PET/CT might be useful in high-risk patients.[27]

Recent systematic reviews found that testing for occult malignancy in patients who presented with an unprovoked VTE may lead to an earlier diagnosis of cancer at an earlier stage, but there was insufficient evidence to know if this practice reduces cancer or VTE-related morbidity or mortality.[29,30] However, in one review, the probability of cancer diagnosis was strongly associated with age; cancer prevalence was sevenfold higher in patients ≥50 years than in younger patients.[29] This finding may help guide future screening strategies. Indeed, to better stratify patients, the REITE (Registro Informatizado Enfermedad TromboEmbólica) investigators developed a risk scoring system to help detect occult cancers in patients with VTE. Selected variables included male sex, age greater than 70 years, chronic lung disease, anemia, elevated platelet count, prior VTE, and recent surgery. The proportion of patients with cancer who scored ≤2 points was 5.8%, whereas that proportion in those who scored ≥3 points was 12%. This clinical prediction rule needs to be externally validated.[32]

None of the published literature to date has shown that extensive screening over limited screening has led to a decrease in morbidity or mortality in this patient population. Current recommendations are to provide age-appropriate cancer screening for patients who present with idiopathic VTE, and any additional testing should be driven by what is discovered in a thorough medical history, physical examination, and basic laboratory tests (complete blood count, calcium, urinalysis, and liver function tests).[33,34] Future studies evaluating extensive cancer screening for patients with idiopathic VTE may be warranted, especially in high-risk patients.

Risk Factors

Many inherited and acquired risk factors are associated with the development of VTE, and they are often divided into patient-, cancer-, and treatment-related factors (Table 34.1). The patient-related factors include advanced age, obesity, prior history of VTE, comorbid conditions, obesity, inherited thrombophilia, elevated platelet count, and certain ethnicities such as African Americans.[15,16,35,36] In addition to high-risk tumors, additional cancer-related factors include advanced stage, liver metastases, and time of VTE occurrence from cancer diagnosis.[37] Patients are at the highest risk of developing VTE within the first 6 months of their diagnosis.[15,38]

Cancer patients may have additional risk factors related to their treatment including surgery, immobilization, chemotherapy, some

TABLE

34.1 *Risk factors for venous thromboembolism*

- Patient-Related Factors
  - Inherited
    - Antithrombin deficiency
    - Protein C deficiency
    - Protein S deficiency
    - Factor V Leiden
    - Prothrombin G20210A mutation
    - Dysfibrinogenemias
  - Comorbid states and disease
    - Advanced age
    - Prior thrombotic event
    - Smoking
    - Obesity
    - Prolonged air travel
    - Prolonged immobilization, paresis
    - Pregnancy and the postpartum period
    - Major trauma
    - Congestive heart failure
    - Antiphospholipid syndrome
    - Myeloproliferative disorders (e.g., essential thrombocytopenia, polycythemia vera)
    - Inflammatory bowel disease
    - Paroxysmal nocturnal hemoglobinuria
    - Nephrotic syndrome
    - High platelet count
- Cancer-Related Factors
  - High-risk tumors (e.g., high-grade tumors of the pancreas, gastrointestinal tract, ovary, brain, colon, kidney, lung, and prostate)
  - Hematological malignancies and neoplasms
  - Advanced stage
  - Liver metastases
  - Time of VTE occurrence from cancer diagnosis
- Treatment-Related Factors
  - Hormones (e.g., estrogen, tamoxifen)
  - Chemotherapy (lenalidomide, L-asparaginase, cisplatin)
  - Vascular endothelial growth factor (VEGF; e.g., bevacizumab)
  - Central venous catheterization
  - Surgery
  - Heparin-induced thrombocytopenia
  - Immobilization
  - Erythropoiesis-stimulating agents

forms of hormone therapy, and the presence of indwelling central venous catheters (CVCs). Without appropriate prophylaxis, cancer patients have twice the risk of developing postoperative DVT and three times the risk of developing a fatal PE than patients without cancer.[39] Long-term immobilization, often due to lengthy hospital stays, also increases the risk of developing VTE.

Other treatment-related risks include cancer medications such as tamoxifen, estrogen, thalidomide, L-asparaginase, cisplatin, and VEGF inhibitors; these are especially prothrombotic when used in combination with other chemotherapeutic agents. In a trial involving women with advanced-stage breast cancer, the incidence of VTE was 2.6% with tamoxifen alone versus 13.6% with tamoxifen plus chemotherapy.[40] Similarly, in studies involving multiple myeloma, treatment with thalidomide alone had a risk of 2%. The risk increased to 33% with the addition of chemotherapy.[41] Cancer patients who receive either cytotoxic or immunosuppressive therapy have a 6.5-fold increased risk of developing a VTE when compared to noncancer patients and a twofold increased risk compared to cancer patients not receiving chemotherapy.[42] In a recent systematic review of 8,216 cancer patients, those receiving cisplatin-based chemotherapy had a significantly increased rate of VTE compared to patients who did not (RR, 1.67l 95% CI, 1.25 to 2.23; $P = 0.01$).[43] Furthermore, venous thrombosis, and in particular, cortical sinus thrombosis, is a frequent complication of L-asparaginase treatment, and it may be related to inhibition of the synthesis of anticoagulant factors, protein C, and protein S.[44,45]

Many of the new antiangiogenic agents used in practice to treat a variety of cancers appear to increase the risk of both venous events and arterial events. In a recent systematic review of 15 RCT, patients receiving bevacizumab, the recombinant humanized monoclonal antibody to VEGF, had an increased risk of VTE compared to controls (RR 1.3; 95% CI, 1.13 to 1.56; $P < 0.001$).[46] Similar findings were seen with patients on anti–epidermal growth factor receptors (EGFR) especially with the use of cetuximab and panitumumab.[16,47]

Other agents may also contribute to creating a prothrombotic state. Erythropoiesis-stimulating agents (ESAs) are often given to patients with chemotherapy-induced anemia. However, studies show that ESAs administered to patients with cancer not only increase the risk of VTE but also mortality.[16,48,49] As such, the Food and Drug Administration (FDA) label limits the use of ESA to patients receiving chemotherapy for palliative intent. ESAs are no longer indicated for patients receiving chemotherapy for curative intent. Other supportive therapies such as red blood cell and platelet transfusions may also add to the risk of VTE in cancer patients.

CVCs are another common treatment-related risk factor for VTE. These devices are commonplace among cancer patients who require long-term chemotherapy. The reported incidence of catheter-related thrombosis ranges from 5% to 75%, and this wide range likely reflects the distinct types of malignancy, the kind of catheter used, and the duration of its implantion.[50] In addition, the complications associated with CVC-related thrombosis can result in loss of catheter function, postphlebitic syndrome of the upper extremity, PE, and even mortality. There have been major efforts to identify disease management approaches to decrease the risk of VTE with CVC, and these mechanisms are discussed in Prevention section of this chapter.

Risk Predictive Models

Trying to predict the risk of VTE in cancer patients is a major clinical challenge. Patients at high risk of developing VTE may benefit from prophylactic anticoagulation, whereas patients at low risk may have unnecessary and unfavourable consequences from this practice such as bleeding. Therefore, the development of risk assessment tools and predictive biomarkers to identify high-risk patients is clinically relevant and important (Table 34.2).

TABLE

34.2   *Risk scoring systems to predict venous thromboembolism risk in ambulatory cancer patients*

Name of Risk Scoring System Characteristic	Khorana[51]	Vienna-CATS[52]	Protecht[53]
Site of cancer			
Very high risk (pancreas, stomach)	+2	+2	+2
High risk (lung, lymphoma, gynecological, genitourinary)	+1	+1	+1
Platelet count ≥ 350,000/mm³	+1	+1	+1
Leukocyte count ≥ 11,000/mm³	+1	+1	+1
Hemoglobin < 10 g/dL or use of ESA	+1	+1	+1
Body mass index ≥ 35 kg/m²	+1	+1	+1
D-dimer >1.44 g/L		+1	
Soluble P-selectin > 53.1		+1	
Chemotherapy			
Gemcitabine			+1
Platinum based			+1
Score (percentage [%] of patients who developed VTE with that score)	High risk ≥ 3 (6.7%) Inter risk 1-2 (2%) Low risk 0 (0.3%)	High risk ≥ 5 (35%) Inter risk 3 (10.3%) Low risk 0 (1.0%)	On placebo: High risk ≥ 3 (8.1%) Low/inter risk 0-2 (2%) On nadroparin: High risk ≥ 3 (2.2%) Low/inter risk 0-2 (1.9%)

Inter, Intermediate; VTE, venous thromboembolism.
The Khorana and Vienna-CATS score identified ambulatory cancer patients who developed VTE while on no prophylactic medication. The VTE rates in the Khorana score are from the validation study. The Protecht study assessed the effect of nadroparin for VTE prophylaxis in ambulatory cancer patients receiving chemotherapy according to the Khorana and Protecht scores, but only the Protecht score are reported.
Adapted from Maraveyas A, Muazzam I, Noble S, Bozas G. Advances in managing and preventing thromboembolic disease in cancer patients. *Curr Opin Support Palliat Care.* 2017;11:347-354, Ref.[54]

A well-cited tool is the Khorana score (KS), which uses baseline clinical and laboratory variables to predict the risk of chemotherapy-associated VTE.[51] The score assigns points to cancer site (2 points for very high-risk sites such as pancreatic or gastric and 1 point for high-risk sites such as the lung, ovarian, or bladder), platelet count ≥350 × 10⁹/L (1 point), hemoglobin ≤10 g/dL or the use of erythropoietin-stimulating agents (1 point), leukocyte count ≥11 × 10⁹/L (1 point), and body mass index ≥35 kg/m² (1 point). A score of ≥3 is considered high risk and correlates with a rate of symptomatic VTE in 6.7% of patients undergoing chemotherapy. This model was recently expanded to include biomarkers in the Vienna Cancer and Thrombosis Study (CATS) score[52] (see Biomarker section below) and modified to include platinum or Gemcitabine-based chemotherapies in the Protecht score.[53]

The Ottawa score is another clinical prediction rule aimed at identifying recurrent VTE risk in patients with cancer-associated VTE.[55] The independent variables include sex, primary tumor site, tumor-node-metastasis (TNM) stage, and prior VTE. High-risk predictors include female, lung cancer, and history of VTE and are given 1 point each. Low-risk predictors include breast cancer and stage 1 cancer of any origins and are given -1 and -2 points, respectively. A score of ≤0 correlates with a low clinical probability of recurrent VTE (≤4.5%), whereas a score of ≥1 correlates with a high clinical probability of recurrent VTE (≥19%).

Implementing these scoring systems may be challenging, and a recent innovative approach, a computerized Care Process Management System (CPMS), was developed to automatically assess electronic medical records to calculate the risk of VTE in active cancer patients in real time. This approach may be used to readily risk stratify patients and ultimately help customize management decisions regarding the use of VTE prophylaxis.[56]

Future prospective trials are warranted to demonstrate the reproducibility, generalizability, and safety of the KS, Vienna (CATS), Protecht, and Ottawa scores as well as to determine their effectiveness and ease of implementation tools for treating cancer patients at risk of VTE.

Biomarkers

Identifying biomarkers to help predict the risk of VTE in cancer patients is one of the largest growing areas of research. Data from the prospective Vienna CATS demonstrated that elevated levels P-selectin were predictive of VTE in cancer patients.[57] The probability of developing VTE at 6 months was 11.9% in patients with high levels of P-selectin compared to 3.7% in patients with low levels. This group also found that patients with elevated D-dimer and high prothrombin fragment 1+2 (F 1+2) compared to patients with nonelevated levels were associated with an increased risk of VTE (15.5% versus 5%).[58] Thrombin generation is another potential biomarker studied by the Vienna CATS group.[59] Elevated peak thrombin levels conferred an 11% risk of developing VTE compared to 4% in patients with lower levels. An expansion of the original KS to include D-dimer and P-selectin appears to improve the VTE risk prediction tool.[52] There was a 26-fold higher probability of developing VTE in the patients with a high score compared to patients with a low score. However, this expanded risk score requires further validation studies and may be limited by the lack of widely available P-selectin assays.

In the last few years, the role of tissue factor–bearing MP in connection with cancer progression and thrombosis has been investigated. In an immunohistochemical study, high levels versus low levels of MP in pancreatic cancer patients correlated with the development of VTE (26.3% versus 4.5%).[60] Similarly, Zwicker et al. found that VTE developed in 34.8% cancer patients with detectable levels of MP compared to 0% in patients with undetectable levels.[9]

Biomarkers may improve the stratification of cancer patients in regard to their risk of VTE. The efficacy and safety of prophylactic anticoagulation in patients with these elevated biomarkers are currently being addressed in well-designed RCTs. Indeed, Zwicker et al. reported on the first RCT evaluating a novel biomarker-based anticoagulation strategy for thromboprophylaxis.[61] Patients with metastatic or locally advanced pancreatic, lung or colorectal cancers were evaluated based on levels of tissue factor MP. Patients with low levels of MP were observed, and patients with elevated levels of MP were randomized to prophylactic enoxaparin versus observation. The incidence of VTE at 2 months was 7.2% in the patients with low levels of MP, 5.6% in the patient with high levels of MP in the enoxaparin arm, and 27.3% in patients with high levels of MP in the observation arm. Future studies are underway to confirm these encouraging findings.

Clinical Manifestations

Cancer patients can present with a wide range of thromboembolic events. The two most commonly recognized are DVT (Fig. 34.2) and pulmonary embolism (PE; Fig. 34.3). However, symptoms and signs

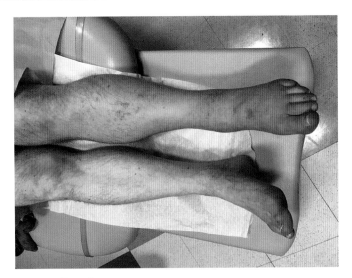

FIGURE **34.2** Deep vein thrombosis.

may result from migratory thrombophlebitis, nonbacterial thrombotic endocarditis, disseminated intravascular coagulopathy (DIC), thrombotic microangiography, and arterial thrombosis. Cancer patients may also present with multiple clinical sequelae as was originally reported in 1977 by Sack et al. in a review of 182 cases of neoplasia associated with alterations in blood coagulation.[62] Figure 34.4 is an expansion of the original Venn diagram created by Sack et al., which represents the interrelations between the various clinical phenomena. Discussion of all these clinical presentations is beyond the scope of this chapter and, therefore, only DVT and PE will be presented in detail.

Patients with DVT may experience complaints of leg pain, swelling, tenderness, discoloration, venous distension, or a palpable cord. Nonspecific symptoms of PE include dyspnea, tachypnea, tachycardia, pleuritic chest pain, cough, and wheeze. Signs may include hemoptysis, hypotension, syncope, coma, pleural effusion, or pulmonary infiltrates. Each of these clinical features can be a manifestation of other cardiac or pulmonary processes, such as pneumonia or heart failure, making the diagnosis of PE difficult.

Data from the MASTER registry in Italy demonstrated that the clinical presentation of acute VTE in cancer patients is different and more extensive than in patients without cancer.[63] The incidence of

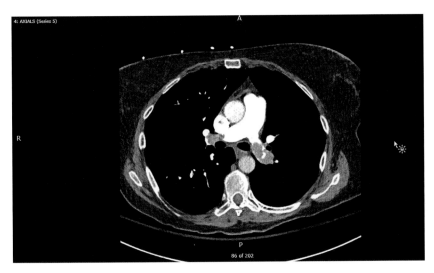

FIGURE **34.3** Pulmonary embolism.

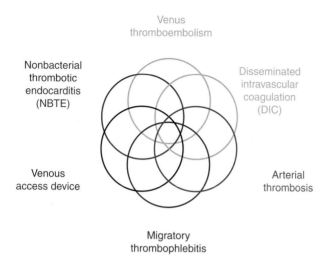

FIGURE **34.4** Venn diagram of relationships between clinical signs.

bilateral DVT and rates of iliocaval thrombosis were higher in the cancer patients. The management of VTE in the cancer patients was also more problematic with a higher incidence of hemorrhage and need for inferior vena cava (IVC) filters.

Other consequences of DVT and PE include acute morbidity or even death. Some of the short- and long-term complications due to thrombotic events consist of extension of the clot, embolization, post-thrombotic syndrome, pulmonary hypertension, and recurrent VTE. Furthermore, there may be significant morbidity associated with long-term anticoagulation or with placement of an IVC filter. The psychological stress and fear that patients face when suffering from a thromboembolic event must also be appreciated. Moreover, the presence of VTE or its complications may cause delays in chemotherapy or other treatments, which may have considerable consequences for the patient. In one of the largest outcome studies of DVT in cancer patients, the most common complication was bleeding, which occurred in 13% of patients.[64] PE, death from DVT, and death from anticoagulation were also observed. In this study, over 99% of patients were hospitalized and the mean length of stay was 11 days with a mean cost of hospitalization of $20,065. VTE as the cause of death was also shown in an autopsy-based study where one out of every seven cancer deaths in the hospital was due to PE.[65] Over 60% of those who died of a PE had either limited metastatic or local disease indicating a reasonable chance of prolonged survival if not for the fatal PE.[65]

Diagnosis of VTE

Diagnosing VTE in cancer patients, as in other patients, may be difficult. The signs and symptoms of VTE are often variable and non-specific, and available diagnostic tests have varying sensitivities and specificities. Moreover, commonly employed models for predicting the probability of VTE have limited value in cancer patients because of the significant additional risk factors at play. Ultimately, a diagnosis requires a combination of modalities.

If VTE is clinically suspected, a common first test is the D-dimer, which reflects the degradation product of cross-linked fibrin. This test is highly sensitive but not specific.[66] Because it is elevated in a variety of situations including malignancy, acute VTE, underlying lung abnormalities, recent surgery, hospitalization, and aging, the

primary value of the D-dimer test is a negative result, which constitutes strong evidence against significant thrombosis.[66] Two recent studies demonstrated that the combination of a normal D-dimer and a low clinical pretest probability was useful in excluding the diagnosis of DVT in cancer patients.[67,68] If the D-dimer test is positive, however, additional diagnostic tests should be performed.

Duplex venous ultrasound (US) imaging, the most widely available modality for diagnosing DVT, is highly sensitive for detecting proximal vein thrombosis but less so for detecting calf vein clots. Therefore, if a patient presents with symptoms suggestive of a calf vein thrombosis, but has a negative US test, a repeat test at 3 to 5 days may be warranted, especially if symptoms persist and no alternative diagnosis has been established. If the US is inconclusive, magnetic resonance imaging (MRI) of the lower extremities is usually definitive.

If PE is suspected, a variety of imaging tests may aid in making the diagnosis, including lung radionuclide scans (VQ), spiral computed tomography (CT), pulmonary angiography, MRI, and magnetic resonance angiography (MRA). Although pulmonary angiography has been the gold standard, it is invasive and often unavailable or impractical and, therefore, has been replaced by CT angiography.

VQ scans, formerly a frequently used diagnostic tool, are now employed only when there is a contraindication to CT scans with contrast, such as renal failure or iodine allergy. VQ scans are helpful when they are either positive or negative, but their results are often inconclusive or confounded by underlying lung abnormalities.

The spiral CT or computerized tomographic angiography (CTA) is highly sensitive for large emboli. Multidetector scanners can visualize the subsegmental arteries effectively. Simultaneous imaging of the lower extremities, which is helpful in identifying an associated DVT, can further increase the diagnostic sensitivity of CTA. Moreover, the spiral CT may help identify alternative etiologies for a patient's symptoms if a PE is not identified.

One of the newest diagnostic tools to diagnose PE, MRI/MRA of the chest, has been incompletely evaluated and standardized. Currently studies are underway to assess its accuracy and safety.

Treatment

The management of VTE in cancer patients is a challenge due to the frequent presence of a hypercoagulable state, physical obstructions to blood flow, patient immobility, and the general impression that these patients may be resistant to anticoagulant therapy. The goals of treatment are to prevent fatal PE, recurrent VTE, and long-term VTE complications. This section will outline current treatment recommendations for both the acute and long-term treatment of VTE in cancer patients based on several studies and guidelines (American College of Chest Physicians [ACCP], National Comprehensive Cancer Network [NCCN], American Society of Clinical Oncology [ASCO]).[34,69–72]

Acute Treatment

The initial treatment for DVT and PE is similar. Historically, there have been three options for anticoagulation: low molecular weight heparin (LMWH), unfractionated heparin (UFH), and fondaparinux sodium. The use of the DOACs to treat VTE in cancer patients is discussed under the section of New Developments. Table 34.3 outlines the major properties of these medications.

TABLE

34.3 *Anticoagulants for prevention and treatment of venous thrombosis*

Class	PK (T1/2) (h)	Clearance Mechanism	Assay	Toxicity	Antidote	Adjust Dose	Drug Interactions
Warfarin (oral)	35 h	CYP2C9	INR	Bleeding, cutaneous necrosis	Vitamin K	Hepatic dysfunction	Numerous, CYP inducers, and inhibitors
Fondaparinux	17 h	Renal excretion	Anti-Xa	Bleeding	None	Renal dysfunction	—
Apixaban (oral)	12 h	CYP3A4, 25% renal	Anti-Xa	Bleeding	None	Renal or hepatic dysfunction	CYP3A4 inducers or inhibitors, PGP inhibitors
Rivaroxaban (oral)	5–9 h	Renal excretion	Anti-Xa	Bleeding	None	Renal dysfunction	CYP3A4 inducers or inhibitors, PGP inhibitors
Edoxaban (oral)	8 h	Renal excretion	Anti-Xa	Bleeding	None	Renal dysfunction	PGP inhibitors
Dabigatran (oral)	12 h	Renal excretion	Dilute thrombin time	Dyspepsia, bleeding	Idarucizumab	Renal dysfunction	Proton pump inhibitors, PGP inhibitors
Heparin, unfractionated (intravenous or subcutaneous)	1–5 h	Reticuloendothelial degradation	PTT	Bleeding, HIT, osteoporosis	Protamine	—	—
Heparin, fractionated (subcutaneous)	4–17 h	Renal excretion	Anti-Xa	Bleeding, HIT <1%	Protamine	Renal dysfunction	—

PGP, P-glycoprotein.

For almost 2 decades, LMWH has been the preferred treatment of choice for cancer-associated VTE. A recent Cochrane review of 15 RCT enrolling 1,615 patients compared the efficacy and safety of three types of parenteral anticoagulants (LMWH, UFH, and fondaparinux) for the initial treatment of VTE in people with cancer and found that LMWH is possibly superior to UFH in the initial treatment of VTE in people with cancer.[73]

LMWH is a fragment of UFH and exerts its anticoagulant effect through antifactor Xa and antithrombin activities. It is cleared from plasma by metabolism in the liver, and a small portion is excreted in the urine. LMWH has largely replaced the use of UFH as the initial treatment for VTE because of its similar efficacy, superior safety profile, and pharmacokinetic advantages that allow for once or twice daily subcutaneous administration without laboratory monitoring, lower risk of complications such as heparin-induced thrombocytopenia (HIT) or heparin-induced osteoporosis and potential for outpatient treatment. LMWH, a weight-based therapy, may need to be episodically monitored in two particular situations: in patients who are at the extremes of body weight or in those suffering from renal failure, the latter situation because of LMWH clearance by renal excretion. This monitoring involves measuring the antifactor Xa activity 3 to 4 hours after subcutaneous injection with a therapeutic goal generally of 0.5 to 1.3 U/mL, depending on the assay used.

If a patient requires a short-acting initial anticoagulant or one that needs to be carefully monitored, is anticipating an invasive procedure, or has a contraindication to LMWH such as severe renal failure, UFH is the favored treatment. UFH, a glycosaminoglycan, exerts its anticoagulant effect at several steps in the formation of fibrin clots. Specifically, when combined with antithrombin III, it inactivates activated factor X and inhibits the conversion of prothrombin to thrombin. UFH is metabolized in the liver and can be reversed with the antidote, protamine sulfate, if necessary. However, unlike LMWH, UFH is usually given intravenously and needs to be monitored frequently, and the dose must be adjusted with the use of nomograms to maintain an activated partial thromboplastin time (aPPT) of 1.5 to 2.5 times the normal.

A third anticoagulant option is the synthetic pentasaccharide, fondaparinux sodium, which works by indirectly inhibiting factor Xa. It has similar efficacy and safety for the initial treatment of PE and DVT as UFH or LMWH. It is an attractive medication because of its once-daily subcutaneous administration and linear pharmacokinetic profile. In addition, it does not cause a syndrome akin to HIT to date. However, it cannot be reversed, and its 17-hour half-life makes it an unreasonable option in patients who require a short-acting therapy. In addition, because fondaparinux is excreted unchanged in the urine, monitoring is essential in patients with mild or moderate renal insufficiency, and the medication is contraindicated in patients with severe renal failure. The efficacy of fondaparinux for the initial VTE treatment in cancer patients is limited. Results from a post hoc analysis of the MATISSE trials suggest that fondaparinux may be more efficacious than UFH but less efficacious than LMWH.[74]

Other options for the initial treatment of DVT and PE that are not anticoagulants include thrombolytic therapy, thromboendarterectomy, and IVC filters. The data investigating the use of thrombolytics in cancer patients specifically are lacking, and therefore, the risks and benefits of this therapy are extrapolated from the general population. Thrombolytic therapy is controversial in DVT and currently should be considered only for patients with massive iliofemoral thrombosis and at risk for limb gangrene.[34,75,76] A meta-analysis has helped clarify the use of thrombolytics for the initial treatment of PE.[77] While there was no overall benefit of thrombolytics in terms of recurrent PE or death, patients who were hemodynamically unstable (systolic blood pressure <90 to 100 mm Hg) had a significantly lower rate of recurrent PE and death and a significantly higher rate of major bleeding.[77] The use of thrombolytics has also been considered in patients who are hemodynamically stable but exhibit evidence of severe right ventricular dysfunction. In a meta-analysis of 16 trials comprising 2,115 patients with PE who were hemodynamically stable with right ventricular (RV) dysfunction, thrombolytic therapy was associated with lower rates of all-cause mortality but increased risks of major bleeding and intracranial hemorrhage (ICH).[78] In this same population, a study investigating the long-term prognosis of patients who underwent thrombolytic therapy found that thrombolysis did not affect long-term mortality rates or did it appear to reduce residual dyspnea or RV dysfunction in these patients.[79]

Thrombolytic drugs in current use include tissue-type plasminogen activator (t-PA), urokinase, and streptokinase. t-PA, the most commonly used of the group, is given as a 100-mg infusion over 2 hours, followed by heparin. In patients refractory to t-PA, one should consider the presence of a saddle embolus, which might require thromboendarterectomy.

Inferior vena cava filters (IVCF) are another option for the initial treatment of VTE. They are primarily used in patients with recurrent DVT or PE on anticoagulation or in patients in whom anticoagulation is contraindicated. There is little published evidence to document an improvement in outcomes after their use, and the few studies available are conflicting. One recent retrospective review found that stable patients with PE and greater than 60 years of age had a lower in-hospital all-cause mortality with an IVCF than in those who did not receive a filter.[80] Conversely, a larger retrospective review found that cancer patients with IVCF had poorer overall survival but also greater contraindication to anticoagulation possibly reflecting poorer cancer prognosis.[81] A prospective study would be helpful to clarify if IVCF are beneficial in cancer patients. Importantly, if necessary, removable filters are preferred.

Long-Term Treatment

Similar to the initial treatment for VTE, the long-term treatment for VTE in cancer patients can be complicated by the concomitant need for chemotherapy, hormone therapy, invasive procedures, CVCs, and more recently, immunotherapy. In addition, cancer patients have higher rates of recurrent VTE and bleeding with traditional anticoagulant therapy than noncancer patients, which adds a further challenge to their management. For many years, the long-term treatment recommendation for VTE in cancer patients was similar to that of the general population, the vitamin K antagonist (VKA), warfarin (Coumadin). After the initiation of UFH, LMWH, or fondaparinux, warfarin is started on day 1 and adjusted to maintain an INR of 2 to 3. Given the slow onset of action, there needs to be a 5- to 7-day overlap between the two medications. Although warfarin has the advantage of being an oral medication, it has significant disadvantages. It requires regular laboratory monitoring, has significant drug interactions because of its CYP3A4-dependent metabolism, and is influenced by nutritional status. Fortunately, several trials have shown that LMWH and, more recently, DOACs (see section on New Developments) are attractive alternatives.

The RCT, CLOT (Randomized Comparison of LMWH versus Oral Anticoagulant Therapy for the Prevention of Recurrent VTE in Cancer Patients), demonstrated a clear benefit to LMWH compared with warfarin in cancer patients for long-term treatment or secondary prophylaxis after VTE.[82] After 6 months of therapy, cancer patients who received LMWH had a significantly lower rate of recurrent VTE (9%) than those who received warfarin (17%), with no difference in the rates of bleeding (Fig. 34.5). In addition, a post hoc analysis of the patients with nonmetastatic solid tumors revealed a survival advantage in the LMWH group. Twelve-month cumulative mortality in this population was 20% in the LMWH group versus 36% in the warfarin group.[83] In a similar design, the 900 patient CATCH (Comparison of Acute Treatment in Cancer Haemostasis) study demonstrated a 30% lower rate of recurrent VTE in the LMWH arm (6.9%) compared to warfarin arm (10%).[84] Although these findings did not reach statistical significance ($P = 0.07$), the overall rates of VTE identified were lower in CATCH versus CLOT, and recent meta-analyses, prior to the DOAC versus LMWH trials, continue to show that LMWH is superior to warfarin.[85]

The mechanism by which anticoagulants may decrease cancer mortality is not clear. However, in the past decade, multiple trials have suggested a survival advantage in cancer patients receiving LMWH as compared to UFH or warfarin for treatment or prevention of VTE.[82] Interestingly, the survival advantages were not solely attributable to decreases in the rate of fatal pulmonary emboli. Three trials studying the value of LMWH in patients without VTE found a significant survival advantage in patients who received LMWH versus placebo.[86–88] A systematic review and meta-analysis of four studies enrolling 898 patients randomized to LMWH versus

placebo suggested that LMWH may improve overall survival in cancer patients.[89] However, two more recent studies did not find a survival benefit with the use of LMWH.[28,90] Furthermore, a number of trials investigating the use of LMWH for thromboprophylaxis in cancer patients receiving chemotherapy have failed to show any survival benefit.[91–94] Several ongoing and compelling in vivo and in vitro studies are underway to further evaluate this question and to possibly define the tumor types, disease stages, and dosing schedules most likely to have a survival benefit.[95–97]

LMWHs, up until December 2017, were the most attractive antithrombotic choice for the long-term treatment or secondary prophylaxis in cancer patients. Indeed, the ACCP, ASCO, NCCN guidelines have recommended LMWH for the first 3 to 6 months of long-term anticoagulant therapy for cancer patients with VTE.[71,72,76] Osteoporosis is a potential complication of LMWH, and if no contraindications, these patients should be placed on calcium and vitamin D.

The duration of long-term treatment of acute VTE in cancer patients has not been clearly established. For noncancer patients, in whom the inciting factor has been removed, the recommendation is to treat for 3 to 6 months. However, in patients with idiopathic VTE, where the inciting factor is unknown and may still exist or in patients with a provoked VTE who have ongoing risk factors, several trials have demonstrated decreased recurrence with prolonged anticoagulation beyond 3 months.[87,98–100] Patients with active cancer are similar to these patients.

There were two recent RCT, ALICAT and LONGEVA, designed to address the question of extending anticoagulation in cancer patients beyond 6 months but both failed to recruit.[101] The only other available data in this area is from two single cohort, prospective studies. DALTECAN aimed to determine the safety of dalteparin between 6 and 12 months in patients with cancer-associated VTE (CAT) and demonstrated that the risk of developing major bleeding or recurrent VTE was greatest in the first month of therapy

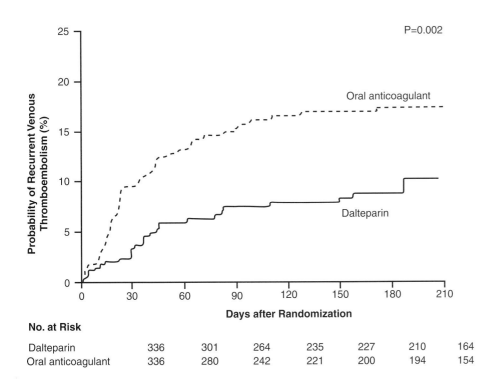

FIGURE **34.5** Recurrent VTE. Kaplan-Meier estimates of the probability of symptomatic recurrent VTE among cancer patients who were randomized to secondary prophylaxis with dalteparin versus warfarin treatment for acute VTE (22).

P=0.002

No. at Risk

Dalteparin	336	301	264	235	227	210	164
Oral anticoagulant	336	280	242	221	200	194	154

and lower in the subsequent 11 months.[102] The TiCAT (Tinzaparin in CAT) evaluated the safety of LMWH beyond 6 months of therapy and found that it was safe in patients with CAT, although male gender showed greater risk for clinically relevant bleeding.[103]

Thus, current ACCP, ASCO NCCN guidelines recommend continuing anticoagulant therapy for as long as there is evidence of active cancer or ongoing cancer therapy, whichever is longer.[71,72,76] Indefinite therapy is recommended for patients with known metastases because their risk of recurrent VTE remains high. However, in the current age of targeted and immunotherapies that may enable metastatic cancer patients to live for years, the need for ongoing anticoagulation is unknown. Therefore, it is prudent to reevaluate patients frequently to reassess the risk-benefit ratio of continuing anticoagulation. Despite the present recommendations, a recent study found that one in five cancer patients stopped their LMWH injections after a median of 90 days due to side effects.[104] Ongoing studies, especially those with the DOACs are investigating this issue.

Recurrent VTE

Recurrent thrombosis is not uncommon in cancer patients with a reported incidence of up to 17%.[22,23,82] Cancer patients who develop recurrent VTE also have decreased survival.[82] In a population-based study, risks associated with recurrence included certain solid tumors (brain, lung, and ovarian), myeloproliferative or myelodysplastic disorders, stage IV cancers, progressive cancers, and leg paresis.[105] A more recent multicenter, prospective cohort study aimed at evaluating whether serial measurements of procoagulant markers can identify cancer patients at high risk of recurrent VTE demonstrated that baseline P-selectin but not D-dimer levels predicted recurrent VTE.[106] In addition, in a prespecified analysis of the CATCH trial, patients in the highest quartile of tissue factor experienced the greatest rate of VTE recurrence.[107] These predictors and biomarkers could be used to develop a prediction rule to identify high-risk patients who may benefit from more intensive therapy or closer observation especially since cancer patients who develop recurrent VTE have decreased survival.[82,105]

In patients who develop a recurrent VTE, one should first determine medication compliance, and if on heparin, rule out HIT. If the patient is on VKA, the recommendation is to switch to LMWH. In patients who develop recurrent VTE while on LMWH, there is evidence to support dose escalation.[108] In a small retrospective cohort study of cancer patients who developed a recurrent VTE while on LMWH, increasing the dose by 20% to 25% was effective in preventing additional recurrences. In these patients, it may also be useful to check an anti-Xa level at 3 to 4 hours after injection to determine peak plasma concentrations. If the patient is on daily LMWH dosing and develops a recurrent VTE, switching to twice-daily dosing is also reasonable. Changing to another anticoagulant such as fondaparinux is an attractive alternative option. There are not enough data on the DOACs to make a recommendation regarding their use in this setting.

The use of IVC filters in cancer patients with recurrent VTE is controversial. There is no definitive evidence to support this practice, and in retrospective series, the risk of recurrent DVT after IVC insertion is as high as 32%.[64] Furthermore, these recurrences are associated with significant morbidity and decreased quality of life. These findings are not surprising as filters have no ability to dampen the activated coagulation system in these patients.

Complications of Treatment

The treatment of VTE in cancer patients is not without morbidity. Potential complications include bleeding, HIT, heparin-induced osteoporosis, or warfarin- or heparin-induced skin necrosis. In two trials involving the use of warfarin, patients with cancer had a clinically and statistically significant increase in the overall incidence of major bleeding compared with noncancer patients: 12.4% and 13.3 per 100 patient-years in patients with cancer versus 4.9% and 2.1 per 100 patient-years in patients without cancer.[22,23] Importantly, the use of LMWH has not been associated with an increased risk of bleeding when compared to warfarin, and some evidence even suggests a decreased risk.[82] Similarly, treatment doses of fondaparinux have the same bleeding episodes as compared to LMWH or UFH.[74,109]

In addition to bleeding, there is a 3% risk of HIT with UFH and 1% risk with LMWH.[110] Skin necrosis due to heparins or warfarin is another infrequent but serious complication. Skin necrosis presents first with erythema then purpura and hemorrhage and eventually necrosis. Specific complications are associated with therapeutic devices, including an increased risk of DVT with IVC filters, and an increased risk of infection with CVCs.

Prevention

Because of the high rate of VTE in cancer patients, primary prophylaxis has become a major area of interest. This section will briefly discuss preventive strategies associated with surgery, hospitalization, chemotherapy, and CVC. Table 34.4 outlines the current guidelines from ASCO, NCCN, ACCP, Anticoagulation Forum (AC Forum), and International Society of Thrombosis and Hemostasis (ISTH).[34,70,71,76,111,112]

Surgery

Cancer patients have a twofold higher risk of developing a postoperative DVT and threefold higher risk of fatal PE than noncancer patients undergoing similar procedures.[39,113,114] Advanced stage of disease, increased duration of anesthesia, prolonged postoperative immobilization, and prior VTE all increase the risk of VTE in the postoperative setting. Trials have led to the conclusion that antithrombotic therapy can reduce the rate of postoperative PE and clinical DVT when comparing LMWH or UFH with no treatment.

Additional studies have shown a significant reduction in postoperative VTE in cancer patients who receive prophylaxis beyond their hospitalization. The ENOXACAN II trial found a 60% reduction in the rate of VTE in cancer patients who received extended LMWH prophylaxis (up to 30 days) after their abdominal or pelvic surgery versus those who received prophylaxis only during their hospital stay (approximately 6 to 10 days).[115] A meta-analysis comparing the safety and efficacy of extended use of LMWH (for 3 to 4 weeks after surgery) to conventional in-hospital prophylaxis found that the administration of extended LMWH prophylaxis significantly reduced the incidence of VTE (5.93% versus 13.6%, RR 0.44 [CI 95% 0.28 to 0.7]), with no significant difference in major or minor bleeding.[116]

Other anticoagulants have also been investigated in this setting. The PEGASUS trial compared fondaparinux to LMWH and found no difference in the rates of postoperative VTE or bleeding in the

TABLE

34.4 Consensus guidelines for the use of primary prophylactic anticoagulation in cancer patients

Organization Situation[g]	ASCO	NCCN	ACCP	AC Forum	ISTH
Major surgery	Yes for major cancer surgery	Yes	Yes	Suggest	Yes
Abdominal/pelvic surgery plus high-risk features (ASCO, NCCN, ISTH)	Consider extending to 4 weeks[a]	Extend up to 4 weeks[b]	Consider extending	Suggest extending up to 4 weeks	Consider extending to 4 weeks
Hospitalized with active cancer, acute medical illness, reduced mobility, or high risk	Yes	Yes	Yes	Suggest	Yes
Hospitalized with minor procedures/chemo	Inadequate data	No comment	No comment	No comment	No comment
Ambulatory, low risk	Not routine	No	No	Suggest against	No
Ambulatory, high risk[h]	Consider	Consider	Suggest	Consider	Suggest
Multiple myeloma	Yes[c]	Yes[d]	Suggest	Suggest[e]	Yes[f]
To extend overall survival	No	No	No	No comment	No comment

[a]High-risk features may include restricted mobility, obesity, history of VTE. Additional risk factors can be found in guideline update.[71]

[b]High-risk features may include surgery for gastrointestinal malignancies, patients with previous VTE, anesthesia time greater than 2 hours, bed rest greater than 4 days, advanced-stage disease, patient age greater than 60 years. Additional risk factors can be found in guidelines.[111]

[c]Patients receiving thalidomide or lenalidomide-based regimens with chemotherapy and/or dexamethasone.[71]

[d]Patients receiving thalidomide/lenalidomide/pomalidomide: in combination with high-dose dexamethasone or doxorubicin or multi-agent chemotherapy or for patients with two or more individual or myeloma risk factors (Refer to guidelines for specific risks).[111]

[e]Patients receiving IMiDs-based regimens.[70]

[f]Patients receiving IMiDs combined with steroids and/or chemotherapy (doxorubicin).[112]

[g]Consensus guidelines are based on expert opinions, which often come from extrapolated data involving other patient populations. Providers are encouraged to discuss VTE risk factors and the risks and benefits of VTE prevention with their patients prior to initiating any therapy. Recommendations are made assuming no existing contraindications to pharmacological prophylaxis.

[h]High risk is defined by each professional society differently, and they can be located in each specific guidelines. In general, risk factors for cancer-associated VTE often include but are not limited to Khorana score (KS) $\geq$ 3, advanced-stage disease, use of hormonal therapy or erythropoiesis-stimulating agents, older age, obesity, and prior VTE.

general population[117]. However, in a post hoc analysis of cancer patients, there was a statistically significant reduction in VTE in the fondaparinux group (4.7%) but not in the LMWH group (7.7%).[117] Further studies are needed to confirm this finding. However, it is likely that anticoagulant therapy reduces the postoperative risk of VTE in cancer.

Occasionally, cancer patients may have a contraindication to anticoagulant therapy. In these situations, mechanical forms of prevention can be employed such as intermittent pneumatic compression devices or compression stockings. However, the efficacy of these measures has not been established by rigorous trials.

Detailed and specific recommendations for prophylactic anticoagulation in cancer patients undergoing surgical procedures can be found in the ASCO, ACCP, NCCN, AC Forum, and ISTH guidelines.[39,71,111,112,118]

Hospitalizations

Cancer patients who are immobile or bedridden with an acute medical illness or because of cancer-related morbidity are at increased risk of developing VTE. Although there are no cancer-specific RCT evaluating thromboprophylaxis in hospitalized cancer patients,[119] in one study where the vast majority of patients had cancer, the risk of VTE was reduced by 41% in the patients whose physicians received a computer-generated alert reminding them to provide VTE prophylaxis.[120] A more recent prospective study found that pharmacologic thromboprophylaxis was frequently administered to hospitalized patients with cancer but that nearly one third of these patients were considered to have relative contraindications for prophylactic anticoagulation, the most common being thrombocytopenia followed by active hemorrhage.[121] Thus, perhaps the most effective strategy is to establish a risk assessment tool to predict VTE in hospitalized cancer patients. Such an approach was recently investigated and found that a KS of greater than 3, male gender, older age, and use of anticoagulation were significantly associated with VTE occurrence in this population.[122] Future studies are needed to further validate this prediction tool. For now, the ACCP and JNCCN currently recommend that in the absence of contraindications, "high-risk" immobilized and hospitalized cancer patients receive VTE prophylaxis, a LMWH such as dalteparin (5,000 U subcutaneously [sc] everyday [qd]), enoxaparin (40 mg sc qd), or tinzaparin (4,500 U sc qd); UFH (5,000 U sc three times daily); or fondaparinux (2.5 mg sc qd).[39,72,123,124] For patients with a contraindication to anticoagulant prophylactic therapy, graduated compression stockings or pneumatic compression devices can be used as alternatives.

Chemotherapy

High rates of VTE are associated with the use of chemotherapy. Therefore, the value of thromboprophylaxis has emerged as important research topic. In one of the earliest studies, over 300 women with metastatic breast cancer were randomized to chemotherapy plus or minus warfarin. There was an 85% relative risk reduction of VTE (4.4% versus 0.66%) in the warfarin group with no difference in bleeding rates.[125] Despite these significant findings, thromboprophylaxis was not adopted as standard practice at that time.

In the last several years, there has been a surge of trials focusing on the potential benefit of primary thrombosis prophylaxis in ambulatory cancer patients. TOPIC I and TOPIC II investigated the use of the LMWH, certoparin, versus placebo in patients with breast and lung cancer, respectively. In the breast cancer patients, there was no difference in the rates of VTE (4% in both groups); however, there was an increase in major bleeding complications in the LMWH arm (1.7% versus 0%).[126] In the lung cancer patients, there was a nonsignificant trend toward decrease VTE in the LMWH arm compared to placebo (4.5% versus 8.3%, P = 0.07).[126] Another thromboprophylaxis study, PROTECHT (Prophylaxis of Thromboembolism During Chemotherapy), randomized ambulatory patients receiving chemotherapy for advanced cancers to nadroparin or placebo and showed a noteworthy 50% reduction in the rates of symptomatic VTE (2.0% versus 3.9%; P = 0.02) with no difference in bleeding.[92] A combined analysis of data from PROTECHT and TOPIC II in metastatic or locally advanced lung cancer patients found that LMWHs compared to placebo significantly decreased the rate of VTE (3.2% versus 6.4%) with no difference in major bleeding.[127]

Another approach in evaluating the role of prophylactic anticoagulation is to focus on a single site of cancer known to be at high risk of VTE. Two prospective studies concentrated on MM. In one study, newly diagnosed MM patients receiving a thalidomide-containing regimen were randomized to aspirin (ASA), VKA, or enoxaparin. The incidence of VTE revealed 7.3% in the ASA group, 9.5% in the VKA group, and 4.6% in the LMWH. Historical rates of VTE in this population are reported to be as high as 35%.[41] A comparable study randomized newly diagnosed MM patients receiving lenalidomide plus dexamethasone to ASA or enoxaparin and found similar rates of VTE (2.27% ASA and 1.20% enoxaparin).[128] Based on these and other trials, current guidelines recommend outpatient VTE prophylaxis in the form of LMWH or VKA for cancer patients receiving highly thrombogenic thalidomide or lenalidomide-based combination chemotherapy regimens.[72,129,130] Trials investigating the DOACs in this population are underway.

Given the increased risk of VTE in glioma patients, the PRODIGE study evaluated the use of dalteparin versus placebo in patients with malignant gliomas. Although the trial was closed early due to expiration of study medication, the investigators noted a trend toward reduced rates of VTE and an increased rate of ICH in the LMWH group (5.1% versus 1.2%).[94] High rates of VTE are also associated with pancreatic cancers, and two trials evaluated the use of LMWH exclusively in this population. In CONKO-04, advanced pancreatic cancer patients randomized to enoxaparin had a major reduction in VTE rates compared to patients randomized to placebo (6.4% versus 15.1%; P = < 0.01), but no difference in survival.[131,132] Similarly, the FRAGEM study demonstrated that pancreatic patients receiving gemcitabine plus nadroparin compared to gemcitabine alone had a

58% risk reduction in VTE (12% versus 28%; P = 0.002) with no difference in bleeding.[93] Of note, lethal VTE occurred in 8.3% of the control arm and 0% in the LMWH arm.

The largest study of thromboprophylaxis in ambulatory patients receiving chemotherapy, SAVE-ONCO, randomized 3212 patients with metastatic or locally advanced solid tumors to semuloparin or placebo.[91] With a median treatment duration of 3.5 months, semuloparin proved superior to placebo in reducing the risk of VTE (1.2% versus 3.4%; P = <0.001) with no apparent increase in major bleeding. The most recent study examining the role of thromboprophylaxis in ambulatory cancer patients employed the KS. A prophylactic dose of dalteparin given to patients with a KS ≥3 starting a new systemic therapy was associated with a nonsignificant reduced risk of VTE but a significantly increased risk of clinically relevant bleeding.[133]

Several recent meta-analyses were performed to assess the efficacy and safety of LMWH in cancer patients without VTE. A Cochrane review of 9 trials (none after 2009) enrolling 2,857 patients found that the effect of heparin therapy on mortality was not statistically significant at 12 months (risk ratio [RR] 0.93; 95% CI 0.85 to 1.02); however, heparin therapy was associated with a statistically and clinically important reduction in VTE (RR 0.55; 95% CI 0.37 to 0.82) with no significant effect on bleeding.[134] A second analysis including over 7,000 patients from 11 studies showed a significant increase in bleeding (RR: 1.32; 95% CI, 1.08 to 1.62) but a decrease in VTE (RR: 0.53; 95% CI, 0.42 to 0.64) in cancer patients who received LMWH compared to placebo or no anticoagulation.[135] There was no difference in 1-year mortality rate or major bleeding. The most recent Cochrane systematic review of 7 RCT (6 with warfarin and 1 with apixaban) involving 1,498 patients found that the existing evidence showed no mortality benefit to oral anticoagulation in patients with cancer but suggested an increased risk of bleeding.[73] A similar review of parenteral anticoagulation found that heparin reduced symptomatic VTE but likely increased major and minor bleeding and appeared to have no effect on mortality in 9,575 patients from 18 RCT.[136]

The numerous thromboprophylaxis studies, to date, demonstrate that outpatient prophylactic anticoagulation is feasible, safe, and effective. However, it is important to note that these studies do not show a statistically significant reduction in fatal VTE or improvement in overall survival. Consequently, current guidelines (ACCP, ASCO, NCCN, ESMO, AC Forum, and ISTH) recommend against primary thromboprophylaxis for most ambulatory cancer patients.[72,111,112,123,129,130] Multiple myeloma is the exception and the only malignancy in which thromboprophylaxis is recommended for patients receiving immunomodulatory agents in combination with chemotherapy and/or corticosteroids.[34,71,76,111] Given the available data, the FDA has voted against approving LMWHs for primary prophylaxis in cancer patients and emphasized the need to create clinically useful tools to better risk stratify patients for thromboprophylaxis.

In an effort to create risk stratification models, a new scoring system, the COMPASS-CAT score, was used on 1,023 ambulatory patients with breast, colorectal, lung, and ovarian cancers. Based on several variables including cancer-related risk factors, predisposing risk factors, and biomarkers, patients were identified as low/intermediate risk or high risk.[137] At 6 months, the patients in the low/intermediate-risk group had a 1.7% rate of VTE compared to 13.3% patients in the high-risk group. This model appears promising and is currently undergoing external validation.

Presently, there are little data on the utilization of the DOACs as thromboprophylaxis in ambulatory cancer patients. A small pilot study examining the role of apixaban for primary thromboprophylaxis in patients receiving chemotherapy found that patients randomized to apixaban (5, 10, or 20 mg daily) had lower rates of VTE compared to placebo (0% versus 10.3%) with no significant difference in bleeding.[138] The safety and efficacy of DOACs in ambulatory cancer patients is currently being studied in two large RCT. The AVERT study is enrolling 574 cancer patients at high risk of VTE to receive apixaban (2.5 mg bid) or placebo and similarly, the CASSININ trial is enrolling 700 cancer patients at high risk of VTE to receive rivaroxaban (10 mg daily) or placebo. Results from these trials are expected in 2018.

Central Venous Catheters

There have been major efforts to decrease catheter-related clotting and its complications with prophylactic anticoagulation. Although the initial studies of CVC thromboprophylaxis demonstrated effectiveness in preventing CVC-related thrombosis, subsequent RCTs showed no benefit.[50] Moreover, a recent Cochrane review of 12 RCTs examined the safety and efficacy of VTE prophylaxis in cancer patients with CVC and found no statistically significant effect of UFH, LMWH, or VKA on death, DVT, bleeding, infection, or thrombocytopenia.[139] Current guidelines state that low-dose warfarin or LMWH to prevent thrombosis related to long-term indwelling CVCs in cancer patients is not warranted.[72,123,130] Studies aimed at identifying high-risk patients who may benefit from thromboprophylaxis are needed. Indeed, a recent prospective study confirmed a high incidence of CVP-associated VTE in cancer patients (5.9% at 3 months and 11.3% at 12 months) and found that a high KS and lung cancer were the most significant predictors for the development of CVP-associated VTE.[140] Further validation studies as well as studies to assess the safety and efficacy of DOACs in this setting are warranted.

New Developments

Direct Oral Anticoagulants

In view of the limitations and side effects associated with the current antithrombotic therapies, better treatments are needed for cancer patients who have unique risks and comorbidities. There is a particular need for longer acting, oral agents that have few drug interactions, do not depend on nutritional status, and do not require monitoring. Thus, there is great interest in the DOACs that target the active site of factor Xa or thrombin and their potential role in cancer patients.

The DOACs have a highly predictable pharmacological profile, which allows them to be taken in fixed doses without laboratory monitoring. Although they have few drug and food interactions, there is little information in how they interact with chemotherapeutic agents. Another limitation is the lack of a reversible agent or an assay to measure their anticoagulant effect. There is also a dearth of experience in how to adjust these medications

in patients with thrombocytopenia, which can be common in cancer patients undergoing chemotherapy. The use of these new agents needs to be rigorously investigated in cancer patients, and many studies are underway, some of which have been recently published.

DOACs in Medically Ill Patients

Three factor Xa inhibitors, rivaroxaban, apixaban, and betrixaban, have been recently tested in large phase III trials for VTE prophylaxis in acutely ill medical patients. The ADOPT trial that compared extended duration prophylaxis of apixaban to a shorter course of enoxaparin in medically ill patients found that apixaban was not superior to a shorter course with enoxaparin but was associated with significantly more major bleeding than enoxaparin[141]. This trial included only 10% cancer patients, and the authors mentioned no significant difference in these patients with respect to the primary safety end point. In a similar design, the MAGELLAN trial, an extended duration of rivaroxaban, was compared to a standard course of enoxaparin[142]. There were 7.3% active cancer patients in this trial, and in a post hoc analysis, rivaroxaban showed a nonsignificant trend to less efficacy than enoxaparin in this population (RR 1.34; 95% CI 0.71 to 2.54).[143] A more recent trial evaluating betrixaban as extended thromboprophylaxis in acutely medical ill patients with an elevated D-dimer level found that there was no significant difference between extended-duration betrixaban and standard regimen of enoxaparin in the rate of proximal DVT or symptomatic VTE.[144] This study enrolled 11% to 13% patients with a history of cancer and makes no mention of any difference in outcomes or safety in this group or if the patients had active cancer.

DOACs Versus Warfarin in VTE Patients

There are currently three factor Xa inhibitors (rivaroxaban, apixaban, and edoxaban) and one direct thrombin inhibitor (dabigatran) that have gained FDA approval for the treatment of acute VTE in the general population. Each trial compared a DOAC to warfarin.

In the EINSTEIN-acute DVT and the EINSTEIN-PE trial, rivaroxaban was noninferior when compared to enoxaparin followed by VKA in terms of VTE and bleeding rates.[145,146] Cancer patients accounted for 9% to 12% patients in these trials, and the primary efficacy and safety outcomes were no different in this group as compared to the total group of patients. In the RECOVER trials, dabigatran, a direct thrombin inhibitor, was compared to VKA, and the rates of VTE and bleeding were similar in both groups.[147] Cancer patients made up 10% of the population, and there was no mention of any difference in outcomes or safety in this group. In the AMPLIFY trial, apixaban was noninferior to conventional therapy (subcutaneous enoxaparin, followed by warfarin) for the treatment of acute VTE and was associated with significantly less bleeding.[148] In a subgroup analysis of 9% cancer patients (3% active cancer and 7% with history of cancer), there was no difference in the safety and efficacy of the two approaches.[149]

DOACs Versus LMWH in VTE Patients

A major limitation to the aforementioned studies is that the DOACs were compared to warfarin, and it is well established that warfarin is inferior to LMWH in cancer patients. Furthermore, in the trials comparing warfarin to DOACs for the treatment of VTE, cancer patients represented only a small percentage of the patients. Recently, two trials were presented comparing a DOAC to LMWH for long-term VTE treatment in cancer patients.[150,151]

In Select-D, an open-label study comparing rivaroxaban to dalteparin in 406 cancer patients, recurrent VTE occurred in 4% (95% CI, 2% to 9%) in the rivaroxaban group and 11% (95% CI, 7% to 17%) in the dalteparin group.[151] Major bleeding was similar across both arms, but overall, there was more bleeding (categorized as either major or clinically relevant nonmajor) in the rivaroxaban arm (17%; 95% CI, 12% to 22%) compared to the dalteparin arm (5%; 95% CI, 3% to 8%). The majority of patients (59% in each arm) had metastatic cancer, and over 50% in each arm had incidental PEs. The original trial sample size was reduced when the second randomization designed to evaluate duration of anticoagulation was closed due to a high attrition rate. Furthermore, patients with esophageal and gastroesophageal cancers were excluded due to an apparent imbalance in major bleeding rates compared to other tumor types.

A similar finding in regard to bleeding was seen in the Hokusai VTE Cancer trial. This open-label, noninferiority study compared edoxaban to dalteparin in 1,046 patients and found no difference in the primary composite end point of recurrent VTE or major bleeding between the groups: 12.8% in the edoxaban arm and 13.5% in the dalteparin arm (hazard ratio [HR], 0.97; 95% CI, 0.70 to 1.36; $P = 0.006$ for noninferiority; $P = 0.87$ for superiority).[150] There was a nonsignificant reduction in the rate recurrent VTE in the edoxaban arm compared to the dalteparin arm (7.9% versus 11.3%, respectively; HR, 0.71; 95% CI, 0.48 to 1.06; $P = 0.09$). However, the rate of major bleeding over the 12 months of therapy was significantly higher in the edoxaban arm compared to the dalteparin arm (6.9% and 4.0%, respectively; HR, 1.77; 95% CI, 1.03 to 3.04; $P = 0.04$). Patients with gastrointestinal cancers were more likely to have an increase in the risk of bleeding with edoxaban than with dalteparin. This finding is consistent with results from SELECT-D as well as previous studies of DOACs. Importantly, the increase in upper gastrointestinal bleeding occurred mainly in patients with gastrointestinal cancers.

Current studies are underway to assess the efficacy and safety of apixaban as compared to dalteparin in cancer patients with VTE as it is unknown even within the same class of agents, whether there are differences among the DOACs.

Overall, the role of DOACs in the treatment of CAT is evolving, and the evidence appears favorable in select patients. However, there are still many unanswered questions, and further investigations are necessary to address patients with thrombocytopenia, brain metastases, catheter-related thrombosis, or those who are on immunotherapies or at increased risk of bleeding. For now, clinicians must balance the risk of recurrent thrombosis with the risk of bleeding when thinking about whether to treat cancer patients with a DOAC and engage in shared decision-making with their patients. Ultimately, more research and a greater understanding of the safety and efficacy of these novel therapies will enable clinicians to develop individualized treatment plans with the goal of decreasing the morbidity and mortality associated with CAT.

Future Directions

Many questions regarding the prevention and treatment of VTE in cancer patients remain unanswered. The evidence linking the use of LMWH to increases in cancer survival in both patients with and without VTE is compelling and is presently being explored. Future investigations will need to address the ideal type and duration of treatment in cancer patients with VTE. Due to the unique challenges in cancer patients, the antithrombotic impact of the DOACs is being evaluated specifically in this population. The role of thromboprophylaxis should be investigated with the use of risk stratification approaches combining biomarkers with risk assessment tools. The decision to initiate anticoagulation therapy must not only balance the benefits and risks but also integrate the patient's values and preferences. Lastly, quality of life measures and cost analyses should be included in future studies.

Conclusion

VTE in cancer patients is a challenging clinical problem. The pathogenesis is complex and multifactorial, and the additional risk factors for cancer patients are often unavoidable. Identifying biomarkers to help predict which patients are at risk of developing VTE are underway and preliminary results are promising. Diagnosing VTE has become more successful and easier with newer noninvasive modalities. The practice of providing extensive screening to identify occult malignancies in patients who present with an idiopathic VTE is intriguing and needs to be explored further. The treatment for VTE can often be difficult and risky, especially given the unique risk factors such as chemotherapy, hormonal therapy and CVCs, and the comorbidities that are often associated with cancer patients. Moreover, the complications that are related to both VTE and their therapy can cause significant morbidity and even mortality in cancer patients.

LMWH has become a valuable tool for preventing and treating VTE and may have independent beneficial effects on the progression of cancer. The DOACs are an attractive alternative and their efficacy and safety in cancer patients in recently published trials is encouraging. Thromboprophylaxis in patients undergoing surgery or hospitalization appears safe and effective in lowering the risk of VTE. Additional studies employing risk stratification models and measurement of biomarkers are needed to determine the benefit of targeted thromboprophylaxis for primary prevention of VTE in cancer patients.

Given all the limitations and challenges associated with cancer patients and the current available therapies, it is clear that better, safer, and easier treatments are urgently needed. In order to discover these much needed novel treatments, well-designed prospective RCTs specifically for cancer patients are required.

References

1. Trousseau A. Phlegmasia alba dolens. *Clinique Medicale de l'Hotel-Dieu de Paris.* 1865;3:654-712.
2. Falanga A, Marchetti M, Vignoli A. Coagulation and cancer: biological and clinical aspects. *J Thromb Haemost.* 2013;11:223-233.
3. Falanga A, Russo L, Milesi V, Vignoli A. Mechanisms and risk factors of thrombosis in cancer. *Crit Rev Oncol Hematol.* 2017;118:79-83.

4. Magnus N, D'Asti E, Meehan B, Garnier D, Rak J. Oncogenes and the coagulation system--forces that modulate dormant and aggressive states in cancer. *Thromb Res.* 2014;133(Suppl 2):S1-S9.

5. Boccaccio C, Comoglio PM. Genetic link between cancer and thrombosis. *J Clin Oncol.* 2009;27:4827-4833.

6. Boccaccio C, Sabatino G, Medico E, et al. The MET oncogene drives a genetic programme linking cancer to haemostasis. *Nature.* 2005;434:396-400.

7. Garnier D, Magnus N, D'Asti E, et al. Genetic pathways linking hemostasis and cancer. *Thromb Res.* 2012;129(Suppl 1):S22-S29.

8. Rong Y, Post DE, Pieper RO, Durden DL, Van Meir EG, Brat DJ. PTEN and hypoxia regulate tissue factor expression and plasma coagulation by glioblastoma. *Cancer Res.* 2005;65:1406-1413.

9. Zwicker JI, Liebman HA, Neuberg D, et al. Tumor-derived tissue factor-bearing microparticles are associated with venous thromboembolic events in malignancy. *Clin Cancer Res.* 2009;15:6830-6840.

10. Khorana AA. Venous thromboembolism and prognosis in cancer. *Thromb Res.* 2010;125:490-493.

11. Deitcher SR. Cancer-related deep venous thrombosis: clinical importance, treatment challenges, and management strategies. *Semin Thromb Hemost.* 2003;29:247-258.

12. Falanga A, Rickles FR. Pathophysiology of the thrombophilic state in the cancer patient. *Semin Thromb Hemost.* 1999;25:173-182.

13. Browne AM, Cronin CG, English C, NiMhuircheartaigh J, Murphy JM, Bruzzi JF. Unsuspected pulmonary emboli in oncology patients undergoing routine computed tomography imaging. *J Thorac Oncol.* 2010;5:798-803.

14. Ahlbrecht J, Dickmann B, Ay C, et al. Tumor grade is associated with venous thromboembolism in patients with cancer: results from the Vienna Cancer and Thrombosis Study. *J Clin Oncol.* 2012;30:3870-3875.

15. Blom JW, Doggen CJ, Osanto S, Rosendaal FR. Malignancies, prothrombotic mutations, and the risk of venous thrombosis. *JAMA.* 2005;293:715-722.

16. Khorana AA, Dalal M, Lin J, Connolly GC. Incidence and predictors of venous thromboembolism (VTE) among ambulatory high-risk cancer patients undergoing chemotherapy in the United States. *Cancer.* 2012;119:648-655.

17. Khorana AA, Francis CW, Culakova E, Kuderer NM, Lyman GH. Frequency, risk factors, and trends for venous thromboembolism among hospitalized cancer patients. *Cancer.* 2007;110:2339-2346.

18. Paneesha S, McManus A, Arya R, et al. Frequency, demographics and risk (according to tumour type or site) of cancer-associated thrombosis among patients seen at outpatient DVT clinics. *Thromb Haemost.* 2008;103:338-343.

19. Petterson TM, Marks RS, Ashrani AA, Bailey KR, Heit JA. Risk of site-specific cancer in incident venous thromboembolism: a population-based study. *Thromb Res.* 2015;135:472-478.

20. Chew HK, Wun T, Harvey D, Zhou H, White RH. Incidence of venous thromboembolism and its effect on survival among patients with common cancers. *Arch Intern Med.* 2006;166:458-464.

21. Sorensen HT, Mellemkjaer L, Olsen JH, Baron JA. Prognosis of cancers associated with venous thromboembolism. *N Engl J Med.* 2000;343:1846-1850.

22. Hutten BA, Prins MH, Gent M, Ginsberg J, Tijssen JG, Buller HR. Incidence of recurrent thromboembolic and bleeding complications among patients with venous thromboembolism in relation to both malignancy and achieved international normalized ratio: a retrospective analysis. *J Clin Oncol.* 2000;18:3078-3083.

23. Prandoni P, Lensing AW, Piccioli A, et al. Recurrent venous thromboembolism and bleeding complications during anticoagulant treatment in patients with cancer and venous thrombosis. *Blood.* 2002;100:3484-3488.

24. Prandoni P, Lensing AW, Buller HR, et al. Deep-vein thrombosis and the incidence of subsequent symptomatic cancer. *N Engl J Med.* 1992;327:1128-1133.

25. Carrier M, Lazo-Langner A, Shivakumar S, et al. Screening for occult cancer in unprovoked venous thromboembolism. *N Engl J Med.* 2015;373:697-704.

26. Prandoni P, Bernardi E, Valle FD, et al. Extensive computed tomography versus limited screening for detection of occult cancer in unprovoked venous thromboembolism: a multicenter, controlled, randomized clinical trial. *Semin Thromb Hemost.* 2016;42:884-890.

27. Robin P, Le Roux PY, Planquette B, et al. Limited screening with versus without (18)F-fluorodeoxyglucose PET/CT for occult malignancy in unprovoked venous thromboembolism: an open-label randomised controlled trial. *Lancet Oncol.* 2016;17:193-199.

28. Van Doormaal FF, Terpstra W, Van Der Griend R, et al. Is extensive screening for cancer in idiopathic venous thromboembolism warranted? *J Thromb Haemost.* 2011;9:79-84.

29. van Es N, Le Gal G, Otten HM, et al. Screening for occult cancer in patients with unprovoked venous thromboembolism: a systematic review and meta-analysis of individual patient data. *Ann Intern Med.* 2017;167:410-417.

30. Robertson L, Yeoh SE, Stansby G, Agarwal R. Effect of testing for cancer on cancer-and venous thromboembolism (VTE)-related mortality and morbidity in people with unprovoked VTE. *Cochrane Database Syst Rev.* 2017;8:CD010837.

31. Coyle K, Carrier M, Lazo-Langner A, et al. Cost effectiveness of the addition of a comprehensive CT scan to the abdomen and pelvis for the detection of cancer after unprovoked venous thromboembolism. *Thromb Res.* 2017;151:67-71.

32. Jara-Palomares L, Otero R, Jimenez D, et al. Development of a risk prediction score for occult cancer in patients with VTE. *Chest.* 2017;151:564-571.

33. Delluc A, Antic D, Lecumberri R, Ay C, Meyer G, Carrier M. Occult cancer screening in patients with venous thromboembolism: guidance from the SSC of the ISTH. *J Thromb Haemost.* 2017;15:2076-2079.

34. Kearon C, Akl EA, Ornelas J, et al. Antithrombotic therapy for VTE disease: CHEST guideline and expert panel report. *Chest.* 2016;149:315-352.

35. Khorana AA, Francis CW, Culakova E, Fisher RI, Kuderer NM, Lyman GH. Thromboembolism in hospitalized neutropenic cancer patients. *J Clin Oncol.* 2006;24:484-490.

36. Khorana AA, Francis CW, Culakova E, Lyman GH. Risk factors for chemotherapy-associated venous thromboembolism in a prospective observational study. *Cancer.* 2005;104:2822-2829.

37. Ashrani AA, Gullerud RE, Petterson TM, Marks RS, Bailey KR, Heit JA. Risk factors for incident venous thromboembolism in active cancer patients: a population based case-control study. *Thromb Res.* 2016;139:29-37.

38. Walker AJ, Card TR, West J, Crooks C, Grainge MJ. Incidence of venous thromboembolism in patients with cancer—a cohort study using linked United Kingdom databases. *Eur J Cancer.* 2013;49:1404-1413.

39. Geerts WH, Pineo GF, Heit JA, et al. Prevention of venous thromboembolism: the Seventh ACCP Conference on Antithrombotic and Thrombolytic Therapy. *Chest.* 2004;126:338S-400S.

40. Pritchard KI, Paterson AH, Paul NA, Zee B, Fine S, Pater J. Increased thromboembolic complications with concurrent tamoxifen and chemotherapy in a randomized trial of adjuvant therapy for women with breast cancer. National Cancer Institute of Canada Clinical Trials Group Breast Cancer Site Group. *J Clin Oncol.* 1996;14:2731-2737.

41. Zangari M, Barlogie B, Anaissie E, et al. Deep vein thrombosis in patients with multiple myeloma treated with thalidomide and chemotherapy: effects of prophylactic and therapeutic anticoagulation. *Br J Haematol.* 2004;126:715-721.

42. Heit JA, Silverstein MD, Mohr DN, Petterson TM, O'Fallon WM, Melton LJ III. Risk factors for deep vein thrombosis and pulmonary embolism: a population-based case-control study. *Arch Intern Med.* 2000;160:809-815.

43. Seng S, Liu Z, Chiu SK, et al. Risk of venous thromboembolism in patients with cancer treated with Cisplatin: a systematic review and meta-analysis. *J Clin Oncol.* 2012;30:4416-4426.

44. Duarte X, Esteves S, Neto AM, Pereira F. Incidence and risk factors for Central Nervous System thrombosis in paediatric acute lymphoblastic leukaemia during intensive asparaginase treatment: a single-centre cohort study. *Br J Haematol.* 2016;174:280-291.

45. Grace RF, Dahlberg SE, Neuberg D, et al. The frequency and management of asparaginase-related thrombosis in paediatric and adult patients with acute lymphoblastic leukaemia treated on Dana-Farber Cancer Institute consortium protocols. *Br J Haematol.* 2011;152:452-459.

46. Nalluri SR, Chu D, Keresztes R, Zhu X, Wu S. Risk of venous thromboembolism with the angiogenesis inhibitor bevacizumab in cancer patients: a meta-analysis. *JAMA.* 2008;300:2277-2285.

47. Petrelli F, Cabiddu M, Borgonovo K, Barni S. Risk of venous and arterial thromboembolic events associated with anti-EGFR agents: a meta-analysis of randomized clinical trials. *Ann Oncol.* 2012;23:1672-1679.

48. Bennett CL, Silver SM, Djulbegovic B, et al. Venous thromboembolism and mortality associated with recombinant erythropoietin and darbepoetin administration for the treatment of cancer-associated anemia. *JAMA.* 2008;299:914-924.

49. Bohlius J, Wilson J, Seidenfeld J, et al. Recombinant human erythropoietins and cancer patients: updated meta-analysis of 57 studies including 9353 patients. *J Natl Cancer Inst.* 2006;98:708-714.

50. Rosovsky RP, Kuter DJ. Catheter-related thrombosis in cancer patients: pathophysiology, diagnosis, and management. *Hematol Oncol Clin North Am.* 2005;19:183-202, vii.

51. Khorana AA, Kuderer NM, Culakova E, Lyman GH, Francis CW. Development and validation of a predictive model for chemotherapy-associated thrombosis. *Blood.* 2008;111:4902-4907.

52. Ay C, Dunkler D, Marosi C, et al. Prediction of venous thromboembolism in cancer patients. *Blood.* 2010;116:5377-5382.

53. Verso M, Agnelli G, Barni S, Gasparini G, LaBianca R. A modified Khorana risk assessment score for venous thromboembolism in cancer patients receiving chemotherapy: the Protecht score. *Intern Emerg Med.* 2012;7:291-292.

54. Maraveyas A, Muazzam I, Noble S, Bozas G. Advances in managing and preventing thromboembolic disease in cancer patients. *Curr Opin Support Palliat Care.* 2017;11:347-354.

55. Louzada ML, Carrier M, Lazo-Langner A, et al. Development of a clinical prediction rule for risk stratification of recurrent venous thromboembolism in patients with cancer-associated venous thromboembolism. *Circulation.* 2012;126:448-454.

56. Lustig DB, Rodriguez R, Wells PS. Implementation and validation of a risk stratification method at The Ottawa Hospital to guide thromboprophylaxis in ambulatory cancer patients at intermediate-high risk for venous thrombosis. *Thromb Res.* 2015;136:1099-1102.

57. Ay C, Simanek R, Vormittag R, et al. High plasma levels of soluble P-selectin are predictive of venous thromboembolism in cancer patients: results from the Vienna Cancer and Thrombosis Study (CATS). *Blood.* 2008;112:2703-2708.

58. Ay C, Vormittag R, Dunkler D, et al. D-dimer and prothrombin fragment 1 + 2 predict venous thromboembolism in patients with cancer: results from the Vienna Cancer and Thrombosis Study. *J Clin Oncol.* 2009;27:4124-4129.

59. Ay C, Dunkler D, Simanek R, et al. Prediction of venous thromboembolism in patients with cancer by measuring thrombin generation: results from the Vienna Cancer and Thrombosis Study. *J Clin Oncol.* 2011;29:2099-2103.

60. Khorana AA, Ahrendt SA, Ryan CK, et al. Tissue factor expression, angiogenesis, and thrombosis in pancreatic cancer. *Clin Cancer Res.* 2007; 13:2870-2875.

61. Zwicker JI, Liebman HA, Bauer KA, et al. Prediction and prevention of thromboembolic events with enoxaparin in cancer patients with elevated tissue factor-bearing microparticles: a randomized-controlled phase II trial (the Microtec study). *Br J Haematol.* 2012;160:530-537.

62. Sack GH Jr, Levin J, Bell WR. Trousseau's syndrome and other manifestations of chronic disseminated coagulopathy in patients with neoplasms: clinical, pathophysiologic, and therapeutic features. *Medicine (Baltimore).* 1977; 56:1-37.

63. Imberti D, Agnelli G, Ageno W, et al. Clinical characteristics and management of cancer-associated acute venous thromboembolism: findings from the MASTER Registry. *Haematologica.* 2008;93:273-278.

64. Elting LS, Escalante CP, Cooksley C, et al. Outcomes and cost of deep venous thrombosis among patients with cancer. *Arch Intern Med.* 2004; 164:1653-1661.

65. Shen VS, Pollak EW. Fatal pulmonary embolism in cancer patients: is heparin prophylaxis justified? *South Med J.* 1980;73:841-843.

66. Stein PD, Hull RD, Patel KC, et al. D-dimer for the exclusion of acute venous thrombosis and pulmonary embolism: a systematic review. *Ann Intern Med.* 2004;140:589-602.

67. Carrier M, Le Gal G, Bates SM, Anderson DR, Wells PS. D-dimer testing is useful to exclude deep vein thrombosis in elderly outpatients. *J Thromb Haemost.* 2008;6:1072-1076.

68. Di Nisio M, Rutjes AW, Buller HR. Combined use of clinical pretest probability and D-dimer test in cancer patients with clinically suspected deep venous thrombosis. *J Thromb Haemost.* 2006;4:52-57.

69. Di Nisio M, Baudo F, Cosmi B, et al. Diagnosis and treatment of disseminated intravascular coagulation: guidelines of the Italian Society for Haemostasis and Thrombosis (SISET). *Thromb Res.* 2012;129:e177-e184.

70. Khorana AA, Carrier M, Garcia DA, Lee AY. Guidance for the prevention and treatment of cancer-associated venous thromboembolism. *J Thromb Thrombolysis.* 2016;41:81-91.

71. Lyman GH, Khorana AA, Kuderer NM, et al. Venous thromboembolism prophylaxis and treatment in patients with cancer: American Society of Clinical Oncology clinical practice guideline update. *J Clin Oncol.* 2013; 31:2189-2204.

72. Streiff MB. The National Comprehensive Cancer Center Network (NCCN) guidelines on the management of venous thromboembolism in cancer patients. *Thromb Res.* 2010;125(Suppl 2):S128-S133.

73. Hakoum MB, Kahale LA, Tsolakian IG, et al. Anticoagulation for the initial treatment of venous thromboembolism in people with cancer. *Cochrane Database Syst Rev.* 2018;1:CD006649.

74. van Doormaal FF, Raskob GE, Davidson BL, et al. Treatment of venous thromboembolism in patients with cancer: subgroup analysis of the Matisse clinical trials. *Thromb Haemost.* 2009;101:762-769.

75. Buller HR, Agnelli G, Hull RD, Hyers TM, Prins MH, Raskob GE. Antithrombotic therapy for venous thromboembolic disease: the Seventh ACCP Conference on Antithrombotic and Thrombolytic Therapy. *Chest.* 2004;126:401S-428S.

76. Kearon C, Akl EA, Comerota AJ, et al. Antithrombotic therapy for VTE disease: Antithrombotic Therapy and Prevention of Thrombosis, 9th ed: American College of Chest Physicians Evidence-Based Clinical Practice Guidelines. *Chest.* 2012;141:e419S-e494S.

77. Wan S, Quinlan DJ, Agnelli G, Eikelboom JW. Thrombolysis compared with heparin for the initial treatment of pulmonary embolism: a meta-analysis of the randomized controlled trials. *Circulation.* 2004;110:744-749.

78. Chatterjee S, Chakraborty A, Weinberg I, et al. Thrombolysis for pulmonary embolism and risk of all-cause mortality, major bleeding, and intracranial hemorrhage: a meta-analysis. *JAMA.* 2014;311:2414-2421.

79. Konstantinides SV, Vicaut E, Danays T, et al. Impact of thrombolytic therapy on the long-term outcome of intermediate-risk pulmonary embolism. *J Am Coll Cardiol.* 2017;69:1536-1544.

80. Stein PD, Matta F, Hughes MJ. Inferior vena cava filters in stable patients with acute pulmonary embolism who receive thrombolytic therapy. *Am J Med.* 2018;131:97-99.

81. Coombs C, Kuk D, Devlin S, et al. Outcomes after inferior vena cava filter placement in cancer patients diagnosed with pulmonary embolism: risk for recurrent venous thromboembolism. *J Thromb Thrombolysis.* 2017;44:489-493.

82. Lee AY, Levine MN, Baker RI, et al. Low-molecular-weight heparin versus a coumarin for the prevention of recurrent venous thromboembolism in patients with cancer. *N Engl J Med.* 2003;349:146-153.

83. Lee AY, Rickles FR, Julian JA, et al. Randomized comparison of low molecular weight heparin and coumarin derivatives on the survival of patients with cancer and venous thromboembolism. *J Clin Oncol.* 2005;23:2123-2129.

84. Lee AYY, Kamphuisen PW, Meyer G, et al. Tinzaparin versus warfarin for treatment of acute venous thromboembolism in patients with active cancer: a randomized clinical trial. *JAMA.* 2015;314:677-686.

85. Carrier M, Cameron C, Delluc A, Castellucci L, Khorana AA, Lee AY. Efficacy and safety of anticoagulant therapy for the treatment of acute cancer-associated thrombosis: a systematic review and meta-analysis. *Thromb Res.* 2014;134:1214-1219.

86. Altinbas M, Coskun HS, Er O, et al. A randomized clinical trial of combination chemotherapy with and without low-molecular-weight heparin in small cell lung cancer. *J Thromb Haemost.* 2004;2:1266-1271.

87. Kearon C, Ginsberg JS, Kovacs MJ, et al. Comparison of low-intensity warfarin therapy with conventional-intensity warfarin therapy for long-term prevention of recurrent venous thromboembolism. *N Engl J Med.* 2003;349:631-639.

88. Klerk CP, Smorenburg SM, Otten HM, et al. The effect of low molecular weight heparin on survival in patients with advanced malignancy. *J Clin Oncol.* 2005;23:2130-2135.

89. Lazo-Langner A, Goss GD, Spaans JN, Rodger MA. The effect of low-molecular-weight heparin on cancer survival. A systematic review and meta-analysis of randomized trials. *J Thromb Haemost.* 2007;5:729-737.

90. Sideras K, Schaefer PL, Okuno SH, et al. Low-molecular-weight heparin in patients with advanced cancer: a phase 3 clinical trial. *Mayo Clin Proc.* 2006;81:758-767.

91. Agnelli G, George DJ, Kakkar AK, et al. Semuloparin for thromboprophylaxis in patients receiving chemotherapy for cancer. *N Engl J Med.* 2012;366:601-609.

92. Agnelli G, Gussoni G, Bianchini C, et al. Nadroparin for the prevention of thromboembolic events in ambulatory patients with metastatic or locally advanced solid cancer receiving chemotherapy: a randomised, placebo-controlled, double-blind study. *Lancet Oncol.* 2009;10:943-949.

93. Maraveyas A, Waters J, Roy R, et al. Gemcitabine versus gemcitabine plus dalteparin thromboprophylaxis in pancreatic cancer. *Eur J Cancer.* 2012;48:1283-1292.

94. Perry JR, Julian JA, Laperriere NJ, et al. PRODIGE: a randomized placebo-controlled trial of dalteparin low-molecular-weight heparin thromboprophylaxis in patients with newly diagnosed malignant glioma. *J Thromb Haemost.* 2010;8:1959-1965.

95. Kevane B, Egan K, Allen S, et al. Endothelial barrier protective properties of low molecular weight heparin: a novel potential tool in the prevention of cancer metastasis? *Res Pract Thromb Haemost.* 2017;1:23-32.

96. Vianello F, Sambado L, Goss A, Fabris F, Prandoni P. Dabigatran antagonizes growth, cell-cycle progression, migration, and endothelial tube formation induced by thrombin in breast and glioblastoma cell lines. *Cancer Med.* 2016;5:2886-2898.

97. Guasti L, Squizzato A, Moretto P, et al. In vitro effects of Apixaban on 5 different cancer cell lines. *PLoS One.* 2017;12:e0185035.

98. Ridker PM, Goldhaber SZ, Danielson E, et al. Long-term, low-intensity warfarin therapy for the prevention of recurrent venous thromboembolism. *N Engl J Med.* 2003;348:1425-1434.

99. Agnelli G, Buller HR, Cohen A, et al. Apixaban for extended treatment of venous thromboembolism. *N Engl J Med.* 2013;368:699-708.

100. Weitz JI, Lensing AWA, Prins MH, et al. Rivaroxaban or aspirin for extended treatment of venous thromboembolism. *N Engl J Med.* 2017;376:1211-1222.

101. Noble SI, Nelson A, Fitzmaurice D, et al. A feasibility study to inform the design of a randomised controlled trial to identify the most clinically effective and cost-effective length of Anticoagulation with Low-molecular-weight heparin In the treatment of Cancer-Associated Thrombosis (ALICAT). *Health Technol Assess.* 2015;19:vii-xxiii, 1-93.

102. Francis CW, Kessler CM, Goldhaber SZ, et al. Treatment of venous thromboembolism in cancer patients with dalteparin for up to 12 months: the DALTECAN Study. *J Thromb Haemost.* 2015;13:1028-1035.

103. Jara-Palomares L, Solier-Lopez A, Elias-Hernandez T, et al. Tinzaparin in cancer associated thrombosis beyond 6 months: TiCAT study. *Thromb Res.* 2017;157:90-96.

104. van der Wall SJ, Klok FA, den Exter PL, et al. Continuation of low-molecular-weight heparin treatment for cancer-related venous thromboembolism: a prospective cohort study in daily clinical practice. *J Thromb Haemost.* 2017;15:74-79.

105. Chee CE, Ashrani AA, Marks RS, et al. Predictors of venous thromboembolism recurrence and bleeding among active cancer patients: a population-based cohort study. *Blood.* 2014;123:3972-3978.

106. van Es N, Louzada M, Carrier M, et al. Predicting the risk of recurrent venous thromboembolism in patients with cancer: a prospective cohort study. *Thromb Res.* 2018;163:41-46.

107. Khorana AA, Kamphuisen PW, Meyer G, et al. Tissue factor as a predictor of recurrent venous thromboembolism in malignancy: biomarker analyses of the CATCH trial. *J Clin Oncol.* 2017;35:1078-1085.

108. Carrier M, Le Gal G, Cho R, Tierney S, Rodger M, Lee AY. Dose escalation of low molecular weight heparin to manage recurrent venous thromboembolic events despite systemic anticoagulation in cancer patients. *J Thromb Haemost.* 2009;7:760-765.

109. Buller HR, Davidson BL, Decousus H, et al. Fondaparinux or enoxaparin for the initial treatment of symptomatic deep venous thrombosis: a randomized trial. *Ann Intern Med.* 2004;140:867-873.

110. Warkentin TE. Heparin-induced thrombocytopenia: pathogenesis and management. *Br J Haematol.* 2003;121:535-555.

111. Streiff MB, Holmstrom B, AShrani A. Cancer-Associated Venous Thromboembolic Disease. *J Natl Compr Canc Netw.* 2018. Available at: https://www.nccn.org/professional/physician_gls/pdf/vte.pdf.

112. Farge D, Debourdeau P, Beckers M, et al. International clinical practice guidelines for the treatment and prophylaxis of venous thromboembolism in patients with cancer. *J Thromb Haemost.* 2013;11:56-70.

113. Huber O, Bounameaux H, Borst F, Rohner A. Postoperative pulmonary embolism after hospital discharge. An underestimated risk. *Arch Surg.* 1992;127:310-313.

114. White RH, Zhou H, Romano PS. Incidence of symptomatic venous thromboembolism after different elective or urgent surgical procedures. *Thromb Haemost.* 2003;90:446-455.

115. Bergqvist D, Agnelli G, Cohen AT, et al. Duration of prophylaxis against venous thromboembolism with enoxaparin after surgery for cancer. *N Engl J Med.* 2002;346:975-980.

116. Bottaro FJ, Elizondo MC, Doti C, et al. Efficacy of extended thromboprophylaxis in major abdominal surgery: what does the evidence show? A meta-analysis. *Thromb Haemost.* 2008;99:1104-1111.

117. Agnelli G, Bergqvist D, Cohen AT, Gallus AS, Gent M. Randomized clinical trial of postoperative fondaparinux versus perioperative dalteparin for prevention of venous thromboembolism in high-risk abdominal surgery. *Br J Surg.* 2005;92:1212-1220.

118. Gould MK, Garcia DA, Wren SM, et al. Prevention of VTE in nonorthopedic surgical patients: Antithrombotic Therapy and Prevention of Thrombosis, 9th ed: American College of Chest Physicians Evidence-Based Clinical Practice Guidelines. *Chest.* 2012;141:e227S-e277S.

119. Carrier M, Khorana AA, Moretto P, Le Gal G, Karp R, Zwicker JI. Lack of evidence to support thromboprophylaxis in hospitalized medical patients with cancer. *Am J Med.* 2014;127:82.e1-86.e1.

120. Kucher N, Koo S, Quiroz R, et al. Electronic alerts to prevent venous thromboembolism among hospitalized patients. *N Engl J Med.* 2005;352:969-977.

121. Zwicker JI, Rojan A, Campigotto F, et al. Pattern of frequent but nontargeted pharmacologic thromboprophylaxis for hospitalized patients with cancer at academic medical centers: a prospective, cross-sectional, multicenter study. *J Clin Oncol.* 2014;32:1792-1796.

122. Patell R, Rybicki L, McCrae KR, Khorana AA. Predicting risk of venous thromboembolism in hospitalized cancer patients: utility of a risk assessment tool. *Am J Hematol.* 2017;92:501-507.

123. Kahn SR, Lim W, Dunn AS, et al. Prevention of VTE in nonsurgical patients: Antithrombotic Therapy and Prevention of Thrombosis, 9th ed: American College of Chest Physicians Evidence-Based Clinical Practice Guidelines. *Chest.* 2012;141:e195S-e226S.

124. Wagman LD, Baird MF, Bennett CL, et al. Venous thromboembolic disease. Clinical practice guidelines in oncology. *J Natl Compr Canc Netw.* 2006;4:838-869.

125. Levine M, Hirsh J, Gent M, et al. Double-blind randomised trial of a very-low-dose warfarin for prevention of thromboembolism in stage IV breast cancer. *Lancet.* 1994;343:886-889.

126. Haas SK, Freund M, Heigener D, et al. Low-molecular-weight heparin versus placebo for the prevention of venous thromboembolism in metastatic breast cancer or stage III/IV lung cancer. *Clin Appl Thromb Hemost.* 2012;18:159-165.

127. Verso M, Gussoni G, Agnelli G. Prevention of venous thromboembolism in patients with advanced lung cancer receiving chemotherapy: a combined analysis of the PROTECHT and TOPIC-2 studies. *J Thromb Haemost.* 2010;8:1649-1651.

128. Larocca A, Cavallo F, Bringhen S, et al. Aspirin or enoxaparin thromboprophylaxis for patients with newly diagnosed multiple myeloma treated with lenalidomide. *Blood.* 2012;119:933-939; quiz 1093.

129. Lyman GH, Kuderer NM. Prevention and treatment of venous thromboembolism among patients with cancer: the American Society of Clinical Oncology Guidelines. *Thromb Res.* 2010;125(Suppl 2):S120-S127.

130. Mandala M, Falanga A, Roila F. Management of venous thromboembolism (VTE) in cancer patients: ESMO Clinical Practice Guidelines. *Ann Oncol* 2011;22(Suppl 6):vi85-vi92.

131. Riess H, Pelzer U, Opitz B, et al. A prospective, randomized trial of simultaneous pancreatic cancer treatment with enoxaparin and chemotherapy: final results of the CONKO-004 trial. *J Clin Oncol.* 2010;28:4033.

132. Pelzer U, Opitz B, Deutschinoff G, et al. Efficacy of prophylactic low-molecular weight heparin for ambulatory patients with advanced pancreatic cancer: outcomes from the CONKO-004 trial. *J Clin Oncol.* 2015;33:2028-2034.

133. Khorana AA, Francis CW, Kuderer NM, et al. Dalteparin thromboprophylaxis in cancer patients at high risk for venous thromboembolism: a randomized trial. *Thromb Res.* 2017;151:89-95.

134. Akl EA, Kahale LA, Hakoum MB, et al. Parenteral anticoagulation in ambulatory patients with cancer. *Cochrane Database Syst Rev* 2011;4:CD006652..

135. Che DH, Cao JY, Shang LH, Man YC, Yu Y. The efficacy and safety of low-molecular-weight heparin use for cancer treatment: a meta-analysis. *Eur J Intern Med.* 2013;24:433-439.

136. Akl EA, Kahale LA, Hakoum MB, et al. Parenteral anticoagulation in ambulatory patients with cancer. *Cochrane Database Syst Rev.* 2017;9:CD006652.

137. Abdel-Razeq H, Mansour A. Venous thromboembolism prophylaxis for ambulatory cancer patients, can we do better? *J Thromb Thrombolysis.* 2017; 44:399-405.

138. Levine MN, Gu C, Liebman HA, et al. A randomized phase II trial of apixaban for the prevention of thromboembolism in patients with metastatic cancer. *J Thromb Haemost.* 2012;10:807-814.

139. Akl EA VS, Gunukula S, Yosuico VED, Barba M, Sperati F, Cook D, Schünemann H. Anticoagulation for patients with cancer and central venous catheters (Review). *Cochrane Database Syst Rev.* 2011;2:CD006468.

140. Hohl Moinat C, Periard D, Grueber A, et al. Predictors of venous thromboembolic events associated with central venous port insertion in cancer patients. *J Oncol.* 2014;2014:743181.

141. Goldhaber SZ, Leizorovicz A, Kakkar AK, et al. Apixaban versus enoxaparin for thromboprophylaxis in medically ill patients. *N Engl J Med.* 2011; 365:2167-2177.

142. Cohen AT, Spiro TE, Buller HR, et al. Rivaroxaban for thromboprophylaxis in acutely ill medical patients. *N Engl J Med.* 2013;368:513-523.

143. Cohen AT, Spiro T, Buller HR, et al. Rivaroxaban versus enoxaparin for the prevention of venous thromboembolism in acutely ill medical patients: Magellan subgroup analyses. *J Thromb Haemost.* 2011;9:20 (O-MO-034).

144. Cohen AT, Harrington RA, Goldhaber SZ, et al. Extended thromboprophylaxis with betrixaban in acutely ill medical patients. *N Engl J Med.* 2016;375:534-544.

145. Bauersachs R, Berkowitz SD, Brenner B, et al. Oral rivaroxaban for symptomatic venous thromboembolism. *N Engl J Med.* 2010;363:2499-2510.

146. Buller HR, Prins MH, Lensin AW, et al. Oral rivaroxaban for the treatment of symptomatic pulmonary embolism. *N Engl J Med.* 2012;366:1287-1297.

147. Schulman S, Kearon C, Kakkar AK, et al. Dabigatran versus warfarin in the treatment of acute venous thromboembolism. *N Engl J Med.* 2009;361:2342-2352.

148. Agnelli G, Buller HR, Cohen A, et al. Oral apixaban for the treatment of acute venous thromboembolism. *N Engl J Med.* 2013;369:799-808.

149. Agnelli G, Buller HR, Cohen A, et al. Oral apixaban for the treatment of venous thromboembolism in cancer patients: results from the AMPLIFY trial. *J Thromb Haemost.* 2015;13:2187-2191.

150. Raskob GE, van Es N, Verhamme P, et al. Edoxaban for the treatment of cancer-associated venous thromboembolism. *N Engl J Med.* 2018;378:615-624.

151. Young A, Marshall A, Thirwall J, et al. Anticoagulation therapy in selected cancer patients at risk of recurrence of venous thromboembolism: results of the Select-D pilot trial. *Blood.* 2017;130.

Note: Page numbers followed by "f" indicate figures; those followed by "t" indicate tables.